Oxford Medical Publications
Coronary Heart Disease
Epidemiology

Coronary Heart Disease Epidemiology

from aetiology to public health

SECOND EDITION

Edited by

MICHAEL MARMOT
Department of Epidemiology and
Public Health, University College London

and

PAUL ELLIOTT
Department of Epidemiology and
Public Health, Imperial College London

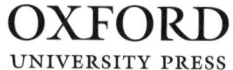

OXFORD
UNIVERSITY PRESS

OXFORD

UNIVERSITY PRESS

Great Clarendon Street, Oxford OX2 6DP

Oxford University Press is a department of the University of Oxford.
It furthers the University's objective of excellence in research, scholarship,
and education by publishing worldwide in

Oxford New York

Auckland Cape Town Dar es Salaam Hong Kong Karachi
Kuala Lumpur Madrid Melbourne Mexico City Nairobi
New Delhi Shanghai Taipei Toronto

With offices in

Argentina Austria Brazil Chile Czech Republic France Greece
Guatemala Hungary Italy Japan Poland Portugal Singapore
South Korea Switzerland Thailand Turkey Ukraine Vietnam

Oxford is a registered trade mark of Oxford University Press
in the UK and in certain other countries

Published in the United States
by Oxford University Press Inc., New York

British Library Cataloguing in Publication Data
Data available

Library of Congress Cataloging in Publication Data
Coronary heart disease epidemiology: from aetiology to public health / edited
by Michael Marmot and Paul Elliott.–2nd ed.
Includes bibliographical references and index.
1. Coronary heart disease–Epidemiology. [DNLM: 1. Coronary Disease–epidemiology.
2. Community Health Services.   3. Risk Factors.   WG 300 C8233 2005]
I. Marmot, M. G.   II. Elliott, P. (Paul)
RA645.C68C67 2005   614.5'912—dc22   2005006679

Typeset by Newgen Imaging Systems (P) Ltd., Chennai, India
Printed in Great Britain
on acid-free paper by
Biddles Ltd., King's Lynn

ISBN 0–19–852573–7 (pbk.: alk. paper)   978–0–19–852573–8
ISBN 0–19–856806–1 (hbk.: alk. paper)   978–0–19–856806–3

10 9 8 7 6 5 4 3 2 1

Preface to the second edition

Just over a decade has passed since the publication of the first edition of this book, which was originally intended as a Festschrift to Geoffrey Rose, but took on an independent existence as a reference book on coronary heart disease epidemiology and prevention. The aim of the book was to capture Geoffrey Rose's approach of establishing the scientific basis for prevention of coronary heart disease (CHD) and then evaluating efforts to translate these findings into public health and individual actions to prevent CHD.

We were delighted when Oxford University Press approached us to commission a second edition and have had the pleasure of making contact and welcoming contributions from a number of the previous authors. Sadly, we have lost a few contributors over the years, but are happy to welcome new ones, all acknowledged experts in their respective fields.

The basic scientific framework of CHD epidemiology has not changed greatly in the last ten years, but a huge amount of new information has accumulated and so the book has grown from 36 to 51 chapters. It is not possible to cover the entire field as adequately as we would wish in one volume, but we have attempted to represent the main areas of interest in this text. We have maintained the basic structure of the book, and include reprints of three chapters: that by Epstein, which provides insightful historical context; that by Morris, a pioneer in recognizing the importance of exercise as a protective factor against CHD (accompanied by a commentary by Bill Haskell); and that by Rose on his hypothesis for preventive strategies relating to sick populations and for sick individuals, which has had such a major effect on epidemiological thinking and is still of fundamental relevance today.

The introduction leads to Section II, which looks at the global picture of patterns and trends in CHD in various areas of the world. There are three chapters which cover some of the extensive work done under the auspices of World Health Organization on the global burden of disease in relation to smoking, lipids, and blood pressure. Section III contains a series of chapters on specific risk factors and a subsection devoted to risk factors from a life course perspective. New chapters are included on homocysteine, alcohol, metabolic syndrome, chronic infection, air pollution, temperature and gene–environment interactions, and expanded themes that include three chapters on psychological and social factors. Section IV, on aetiology as related to public health, again concentrates on strategies relating to clinical and risk factor assessment, primary and secondary prevention, methods of intervention, and ways of effecting behavioural change at individual, community, and national levels, with specific examples from around the world.

We asked the authors to contribute a lively and up-to-date discourse on their particular topic and are pleased to offer some quite personal accounts within the text. Inevitably there is a wide range of views, and in editing the text we have had some interesting exchanges that reflect the continuing debate about many aspects of CHD epidemiology. We hope that this new edition will appeal to those who are both learning and practising in the field of epidemiology and public health as applied to CHD, and will prove as interesting in its final content as we have found it to be in preparation of the text.

Finally, we wish to convey our sincere thanks and appreciation to Jennifer Wells for her tireless efforts behind the scenes to help bring this volume to fruition, and to Helen Liepman at Oxford University Press for her understanding and patience.

London   M. M.
May 2004   P. E.

Preface to first edition

The idea for this book took shape in the editors' minds as a tribute to the work of Geoffrey Rose. We considered whether the book might be a collection of pieces by former students, friends, and colleagues – a good deal of overlap in these categories – and whether it might cover the topics to which Geoffrey Rose contributed. It quickly became apparent that such an effort would be a textbook of coronary heart disease epidemiology and prevention.

The aim of the book is not simply to review knowledge of well-established factors. A book on coronary heart disease must include them, but there are any number of reviews by expert committees and government bodies. Rather, our aim is to look forward, equipped with lessons learnt from the past. Thus we included major areas of new work that hold great promise for future knowledge. The authors, each at the forefront of his/her field, took seriously the charge to be topical or fresh, and reflect current thinking. The results are up-to-date personal accounts, rather than simply comprehensive reviews. The aim was to cover the frontiers of work on aetiology, on appropriate methodology, and on application of scientific knowledge to the development of policy.

A book that started life as a Festschrift and ended as a textbook might have posed a conflict of interest: should the invited contributors be Geoffrey Rose's friends and colleagues or should they be acknowledged experts in the field? In the event, there was no conflict. These two categories overlapped to a high degree. Our considerable dilemma was in having an embarrassment of riches from which to choose. We offer our profound apologies to those whom the pressures of space excluded.

Geoffrey Rose's work reflects, and often led, the progress of a whole field of scientific endeavour. His work covered the epidemiology of coronary heart disease, including studies within a single population and international studies, important areas of methodological development, trials to test preventive strategies, and the application of epidemiological and other knowledge to the development of public health policy for the prevention of this widespread disease. The sub-title of this book, *From aetiology to public health*, and its contents cover this spectrum. They exemplify the use and application of epidemiological research: to go from studies of aetiology to implementing public health policies and evaluating their effects.

For many of us, a significant development of recent years has been Geoffrey Rose's transition from epidemiology to public health. His initial position was 'pure': the epidemiologist should assemble the facts and leave them to others to act on. The danger in becoming an activist was seen to be loss of scientific 'objectivity'. There was also no particular reason to believe that people who were good at research were also good at effecting and implementing policy change. A natural transition, however, was to move to using epidemiological insights to plan public health strategies. The promotion by the World Health Organization (WHO) of the population approach to heart disease prevention began with Geoffrey Rose's chairmanship of the 1982 WHO Expert Committee on the Prevention of Coronary Heart Disease.

This provides an instructive model. It does not suggest that epidemiologists must become public health activists – they may if they are so inclined – but that they should use their knowledge to inform and analyse public health policy decisions.

This informs the structure of the book. A brief introduction sets the scene by (a) charting changes that have occurred in coronary heart disease mortality, following its emergence in countries undergoing economic development and other changes, and (b) giving an overview of the contribution of epidemiology to development of knowledge on aetiology and occurrence of coronary heart disease. The next part, on aetiology, starts with a chapter by Stamler summarizing evidence on the established risk factors and providing the knowledge base on which the newer developments, covered in this part, are built. Up-to-date accounts of the main areas of current research in coronary heart disease epidemiology are then given. The final part of the book is, appropriately, on public health – appropriate not only because an important purpose of epidemiological research is to improve the public health, but because this is an exciting and developing field of which we shall see much more in the future. This field has progressed to the point where scientific debate takes place alongside debates about the translation of research findings into health policy. It is to be expected, therefore, that there would not be complete accord. Some disagreement is to be found among authors, which reflects cogently argued current policy positions.

The book is aimed at two groups of readers: those interested in an up-to-date view of coronary heart disease epidemiology, and those who will appreciate that coronary heart disease serves as an instructive example of the application of research to the formation and evaluation of public health policy. We anticipate that this would serve as a reference work for medical students and as a text for postgraduate students and practitioners of epidemiology and public health, but would also be read by those actively concerned with prevention of cardiovascular disease.

We wish to acknowledge the special contribution of Gaye Woolven who, in effect, served as an executive editor for the book. It has been a pleasure to work with Oxford University Press in producing this volume.

June 1991   M. M.
                                                                                                      P. E.

Contents

Section III **Aetiology**

III.I **Risk factors**

Contributors

K. George M. M. Alberti (Sir)
Professor of Metabolic Medicine, Faculty of
Medicine, Imperial College London,
St Mary's Campus, Norfolk Place, London
W2 1PG and Professor of Medicine at School
of Clinical Medical Sciences, Faculty of
Medical Sciences, University of Newcastle
upon Tyne, NE1 7RU, UK.

Sonia Anand
Associate Professor of Medicine,
Department of Medicine, Division of
Cardiology, Population Health Research
Institute, McMaster University, 1200 Main
Street West, Hamilton, Ontario ON L8L 3Z5,
Canada.

Lawrence J. Appel
Associate Professor of Medicine,
Epidemiology and International Health,
Welch Center for Prevention, Epidemiology
and Clinical Research, Johns Hopkins
Medical University, 2024 East Monument
Street (Suite 2-645), Baltimore,
MD 21205-2223, USA.

David J. P. Barker
Professor of Clinical Epidemiology,
University of Southampton, Southampton,
SO 16 6YD, UK, and Professor in the
Department of Medicine, Oregon Health and
Science University, 3181 S W Sam Jackson
Park Road, L-464 Portland, Oregon OR
97201-3098, USA.

Robert Beaglehole
Director, Department of Chronic Diseases
and Health Promotion, World Health
Organization, Avenue Appia, CH 1211
Geneva 27, Switzerland.

Martin Bobak
Reader in Epidemiology,
International Centre for Health and Society,
Department of Epidemiology and Public
Health, University College London, Gower
Street Campus, 1–19 Torrington Place,
London WC1E 6BT, UK.

Richard S. Cooper
Department of Preventive Medicine and
Epidemiology, Loyola University Medical
Center, Stritch School of Medicine, 2160
South First Avenue, Maywood, Illinois,
IL 60153, USA.

Lucy J. Cooke
Research Psychologist, Cancer Research UK
Health Behaviour Unit, University College
London, Gower Street Campus, 2–16
Torrington Place, London WC1E 6BT, UK.

John Danesh
Professor of Epidemiology and Medicine,
Department of Public Health and Primary
Care, University of Cambridge, Strangeways
Site, Cambridge CB1 8RN, UK.

George Davey Smith
Professor of Clinical Epidemiology,
Department of Social Medicine, Canynge
Hall, University of Bristol, Whiteladies Road,
Bristol BS8 2PR, UK.

Martha L. Daviglus
Department of Preventive Medicine,
Feinberg School of Medicine, Northwestern
University, 680 North Lake Shore Drive
(Suite 1102), Chicago, Illinois, IL
60611-4402, USA.

Annette Dobson
Professor of Biostatistics, School of
Population Health, Faculty of Health
Sciences, University of Queensland, Herston
Road, Herston, Qld 4006, Australia.

Alan R. Dyer
Professor of Preventive Medicine,
Department of Preventive Medicine,
Feinberg School of Medicine, Northwestern
University, 680 North Lake Shore Drive
(Suite 1102), Chicago, Illinois, IL
60611-4402, USA.

Paul Elliott
Professor of Epidemiology and Public Health
Medicine, and Head of Department of
Epidemiology and Public Health, Faculty
of Medicine, Imperial College London,
St Mary's Campus, Norfolk Place, London
W2 1PG, UK.

Thomas P. Erlinger
Assistant Professor of Medicine, Johns
Hopkins Medical University, Welch Center
for Prevention, Epidemiology and Clinical
Research, Suite 2-624, 2024 E. Monument
Street, Baltimore, MD 21205-2223, USA.

Majid Ezzati
Department of Population and International
Health, Harvard School of Public Health,
Harvard University, 665 Huntington Avenue,
Boston, MA 02115, USA.

Caroline M. Fichtenberg
Research Fellow, Division of Cardiology,
Department of Medicine, Center for
Tobacco Control Research and Education,
and Institute for Health Policy Studies and
Cardiovascular Research Institute,
University of California, Box 1390,
San Francisco, CA 94143-1390, USA.

Daniel B. Garside
Department of Preventive Medicine,
Feinberg School of Medicine, Northwestern
University, 680 North Lake Shore Drive
(Suite 1102), Chicago, Illinois IL
60611-4402, USA.

Stanton A. Glantz
Professor of Medicine, Division of
Cardiology, Department of Medicine,
Director, Center for Tobacco Control
Research and Education and Institute for

Health Policy Studies and Cardiovascular
Research Institute, University of California,
Box 1390, San Francisco, CA 94143-1390,
USA.

Ian F. Godsland
Wynn Reader in Human Metabolism,
Department of Endocrinology and
Metabolic Medicine, Imperial College
London, St Mary's Campus, Norfolk Place,
London W2 1PG, UK.

Philip Greenland
Harry W. Dingman Professor and Chairman,
Department of Preventive Medicine,
Feinberg School of Medicine, Northwestern
University, 680 North Lake Shore Drive
(Suite 1102), Chicago, Illinois, IL
60611-4402, USA.

Diederick E. Grobbee
Professor of Clinical Epidemiology and
Chairman, Julius Center for Health Sciences
and Primary Care, Utrecht University
Medical School, Box 85500, 3508 GA
Utrecht, The Netherlands.

William L. Haskell
Stanford Prevention Research Center, School
of Medicine, Stanford University, Hoover
Pavilion, Room N229, 211 Quarry Road,
Stanford, CA 94305-5705, USA.

Harry Hemingway
Reader in Clinical Epidemiology,
Department of Epidemiology and Public
Health, University College London Medical
School, 1–19 Torrington Place, London
WC1E 6BT, UK.

Frank B. Hu
Associate Professor of Nutrition and
Epidemiology, Departments of Nutrition
and Epidemiology, Brigham and Women's
Hospital and Harvard School of Public
Health, 665 Huntingdon Avenue, Boston,
MA 02115, USA.

Gang Hu
Senior Researcher, Diabetes and Genetic
Epidemiology Unit, Department of
Epidemiology and Health Promotion,
National Public Health Institute,
Mannerheimintie 166 FIN-00300, Helsinki,
Finland, and Department of Public Health,
University of Helsinki, Finland.

Steve E. Humphries
Professor of Cardiovascular Genetics, Centre
for Cardiovascular Genetics, The Rayne
Building, Royal Free and University College
School of Medicine, British Heart
Foundation Laboratories, 5 University
Street, London WC1E 6JJ, UK.

W. Philip T. James
Honorary Professor, London School of
Hygiene and Tropical Medicine. Chairman,
International Obesity Task Force, 231 North
Gower Street, London NW1 2NS, UK.

Martin J. Jarvis
Professor of Health Psychology, Cancer
Research UK Health Behaviour Unit,
Department of Epidemiology and Public
Health, University College London, Gower
Street Campus, 1–19 Torrington Place,
London WC1E 6BT, UK.

Desmond G. Johnston
Professor of Endocrinology and Metabolic
Medicine, Department of Endocrinology
and Metabolic Medicine, Imperial College
London, Faculty of Medicine, St Mary's
Campus, Norfolk Place, London
W2 1PG, UK.

Jozef V. Joossens
Emeritus Professor, Department of
Epidemiology, School of Public Health,
Katholieke Universiteit Leuven,
Kapucijnenvoer 35, Leuven B-3000,
Belgium.

Hugo Kesteloot
Emeritus Professor, Department of
Epidemiology, School of Public Health,
Katholieke Universiteit Leuven,
Kapucijnenvoer 35, Leuven B-3000,
Belgium.

Kornelia Kotseva
Senior Clinical Research Fellow,
Cardiovascular Medicine, National Heart
and Lung Institute, Imperial College
London, Charing Cross Campus, Charing
Cross Hospital, Fulham Palace Road, London
W6 8RF, UK.

Daan Kromhout
Director of Division of Public Health
Research, National Institute for Public
Health and The Environment (RIVM),
PO Box 1, 3720 BA Bilthoven, The
Netherlands.

Lewis H. Kuller
Professor of Epidemiology, Department of
Epidemiology, Bellefield Professional
Building, Room 550, University of
Pittsburgh, 130 North Bellefield Avenue,
Pittsburgh, PA 15213, USA.

Hannah E. Kuper
Clinical Research Unit, London School of
Hygiene and Tropical Medicine, Keppel
Street, London WC1E 7HT, UK.

Darwin R. Labarthe
Associate Director for Cardiovascular Health
Policy and Research and Acting Chief,
Cardiovascular Health Branch, Division of
Adult and Community Health, National
Center for Chronic Disease Prevention and
Health Promotion, Centers for Disease
Control and Prevention, 4770 Buford
Highway, NE, Mailstop K-47, Atlanta,
Georgia 30341-3717, USA.

Malcolm R. Law
Professor of Preventive Medicine, Wolfson
Institute of Preventive Medicine, Bart's and
The London Queen Mary's School of
Medicine and Dentistry, Charterhouse
Square, London EC1M 6BQ, UK.

Carlene M. M. Lawes
Research Fellow, Clinical Trials Research Unit, Department of Medicine, Faculty of Medicine and Health Science, University of Auckland, Private Bag 92019, Auckland, New Zealand.

Eva Lonn
Associate Professor of Medicine, Department of Medicine, Division of Cardiology, Population Health Research Institute, McMaster University, 1200 Main Street West, Hamilton, Ontario ON L8L 3Z5, Canada.

Alan D. Lopez
Professor of Medical Statistics and Head of School of Population Health, University of Queensland, Herston Road, Herston Qld 4006, Australia.

Russell V. Luepker
Mayo Professor and Head of Division, Division of Epidemiology, School of Public Health, University of Minnesota, 1300 South Second Street (Suite 300), Minneapolis, MN 55454-1015, USA.

John W. Lynch
Department of Epidemiology, School of Public Health, University of Michigan, 109 Observatory Street, Ann Arbor, MI 48109-2029, USA.

Peter K. MacCallum
Senior Lecturer in Haematology, Cardiovascular Research Group, Department of Environmental and Preventive Medicine, Wolfson Institute of Preventive Medicine, Bart's and The London Queen Mary's School of Medicine and Dentistry, Charterhouse Square, London EC1M 6BQ, and Honorary Consultant Haematologist, Bart's and The London NHS Trust.

Stephen MacMahon
Principal Director, The George Institute for International Health, University of Sydney, PO Box M201, Missenden Road, Sydney NSW 2050, Australia.

Michael Marmot (Sir)
Professor of Epidemiology and Public Health, Director of International Centre for Health and Society, Department of Epidemiology and Public Health, University College London, Gower Street Campus, 1–19 Torrington Place, London WC1E 6BT, UK.

Thomas W. Meade
Emeritus Professor of Epidemiology, Department of Epidemiology and Population Health, London School of Hygiene and Tropical Medicine, Keppel Street, London WC1E 7HT and Queen Mary, University of London.

Edgar R. Miller III
Associate Professor of Medicine and Epidemiology, Welch Center for Prevention, Epidemiology and International Health, Johns Hopkins Medical University, 2024 East Monument Street (Suite 2-624), Baltimore, MD 21205-2223, USA.

Joan K. Morris
Reader, Wolfson Institute of Preventive Medicine, Bart's and The London Queen Mary's School of Medicine and Dentistry, Charterhouse Square, London EC1M 6BQ, UK.

James D. Neaton
Professor of Biostatistics, Division of Biostatistics, School of Public Health, University of Minnesota, 2221 University Avenue SE, Suite 200, Minneapolis MN 55414-3080, USA.

Mary Pierce
Clinical Senior Lecturer, School of Health and Social Studies, University of Warwick, Coventry, Warwickshire CV4 7AL, UK.

C. Arden Pope III
Department of Economics, Brigham Young University, 142 Faculty Office Building, Provo, Utah, UT 84602-2363, USA.

Neil R. Poulter
Professor of Preventive Cardiovascular
Medicine, International Centre for
Circulatory Health, National Heart and Lung
Institute, Imperial College London, Faculty
of Medicine, St Mary's Campus,
International Centre for Circulatory Health
Building, 59 North Wharf Road, London
W2 1NY, UK.

Pekka Puska
Director-General, National Public Health
Institute, Mannerheimintie 166 FIN-00300,
Helsinki, Finland.

Qing Qiao
Senior Researcher, Diabetes and Genetic
Epidemiology Unit, Department of
Epidemiology and Health Promotion,
National Public Health Institute,
Mannerheimintie 166 FIN-00300, Helsinki,
Finland, and Department of Public Health,
University of Helsinki, Finland.

Farhat Rasul
Research Fellow, Department of Psychiatry,
Bart's and The Royal London School of
Medicine and Dentistry, Queen Mary
University of London, Basic Medical
Sciences Building, Mile End Road, London
E1 4NS, UK.

K. Srinath Reddy
Professor and Head of Cardiology, All India
Institute of Medical Sciences, Ansari Nagar,
New Delhi 110 029, India, and Coordinator,
Initiative for Cardiovascular Health Research
in Developing Countries.

Neville J. Rigby
Director of Policy and Public Affairs, the
International Obesity Task Force of the
International Association for the Study of
Obesity, 231 North Gower Street, London
NW1 2NS, UK.

Anthony Rodgers
Director, Clinical Trials Research Unit,
Department of Medicine, Faculty of
Medicine and Health Science, University of
Auckland, Private Bag 92019, Auckland,
New Zealand.

Peter S. Sever
Professor of Clinical Pharmacology,
International Centre for Circulatory Health,
National Heart and Lung Institute, Imperial
College London, International Centre for
Circulatory Health Building, 59 North Wharf
Road, London W2 1NY, UK.

Gavin Shaddick
Lecturer in Statistics, Department of
Mathematical Sciences, University of
Bath, Claverton Down, Bath
BA2 7AY, UK.

Sasha Shepperd
Department of Public Health, University
of Oxford, Rosemary Rue Building,
Old Road Campus Headington,
Oxford OX3 7LF, UK.

Jeremiah Stamler
Emeritus Professor, Department of
Preventive Medicine, Feinberg School of
Medicine, Northwestern University, 680
North Lake Shore Drive (Suite 1102),
Chicago, Illinois IL 60611-4402, USA.

Stephen Stansfeld
Professor of Psychiatry, Head of Department,
Department of Psychiatry, Bart's and The
Royal London School of Medicine and
Dentistry, Queen Mary University of
London, Basic Medical Sciences Building,
Mile End Road, London E1 4NS, UK.

Andrew Steptoe
British Heart Foundation Professor of
Psychology, Department of Epidemiology
and Public Health, University College
London, Gower Street Campus, 1–19
Torrington Place, London
WC1E 6BT, UK.

Mireille B. Toledano
Lecturer in Epidemiology, Department of
Epidemiology and Public Health, Faculty of
Medicine, Imperial College London, St
Mary's Campus, Norfolk Place, London
W2 1PG, UK.

Jaako Tuomilehto
Professor, Diabetes and Genetic
Epidemiology Unit, Department of
Epidemiology and Health Promotion,
National Public Health Institute,
Mannerheimintie 166 FIN-00300, Helsinki,
Finland, and Department of Public Health,
Helsinki, Finland.

Hugh Tunstall-Pedoe
Cardiovascular Epidemiology Unit,
University of Dundee, Ninewells Hospital
and Medical School, Dundee
DD1 9SY, UK.

Hirotsugu Ueshima
Professor and Head of Department,
Department of Health Science, Faculty of
Medicine, Shiga University of Medical
Science, Tsukinowa-cho Seta, Otsu, Shiga
520-2192, Japan.

Johanna G. van der Bom
Associate Professor of Clinical Epidemiology,
Department of Clinical Epidemiology,
Leiden University Medical Center, PO Box
9600, 2300 R C Leiden, The Netherlands.

Stephen Vander Hoorn
Biostatistics Manager, Clinical Trials
Research Unit, Department of Medicine,
Faculty of Medicine and Health Science,
University of Auckland, Private Bag 92019,
Auckland, New Zealand.

David S. Wald
Wolfson Institute of Preventive Medicine,
Bart's and The London Queen Mary's School
of Medicine and Dentistry, Charterhouse
Square, London, EC1M 6BQ, UK.

Nicholas J Wald
Director, Wolfson Institute of Preventive
Medicine, Bart's and The London Queen
Mary's School of Medicine and Dentistry,
Charterhouse Square, London EC1M
6BQ, UK.

Jane Wardle
Professor of Clinical Psychology, and Director
of Cancer Research UK Health Behaviour
Unit, Department of Epidemiology and
Public Health, University College London,
Gower Street Campus, 2–16 Torrington
Place, London WC1E 6BT, UK.

Peter Whincup
Professor of Cardiovascular Epidemiology,
Department of Community Health Sciences,
St George's Hospital Medical School,
Cranmer Terrace, London
SW17 0RE, UK.

Margaret Whitehead
W. H. Duncan Professor of Public Health,
Department of Public Health, University of
Liverpool, Whelan Building, The
Quadrangle, Liverpool L69 3GB, UK.

Walter C. Willett
Fredrick John Stare Professor of
Epidemiology and Nutrition, Chair,
Department of Nutrition, Harvard School of
Public Health, 665 Huntingdon Avenue,
Boston, MA 2115, USA.

David A. Wood
Garfield Weston Professor of Cardiovascular
Medicine, Cardiovascular Medicine, National
Heart and Lung Institute, Imperial College
London, Charing Cross Campus, Charing
Cross Hospital, Fulham Palace Road, London
W6 8RF, UK.

Salim Yusuf
Professor of Medicine, Director of Division
of Cardiology, Director, Population Health
Research Institute, McMaster University,
Ontario, L8L 2X2, Canada.

Abbreviations

ABI	ankle–brachial (blood pressure) index	DM	diabetes mellitus
AC	all-cause (mortality)	DR	detection rate
ACE	angiotensin-converting enzyme	DVT	deep vein thrombosis
ACS	American Cancer Society	EB	ectopic beat
ADA	American Diabetes Association	EB(C)T	electron beam (computed) tomography
ADP	adenosine disphosphate	ECG	electrocardiogram
AGE	advanced glycosylation end product	EME	established market economies
AHA	American Heart Association	EPA	Environmental Protection Agency,
ALA	alpha-linolenic acid		eicosapentaenoic acid
AMI	acute myocardial infarction	ESRD	end-stage renal disease
ARB	angiotensin receptor blocker	ETS	environmental tobacco smoke
BDI	Beck Depression Inventory	FA	fatty acid
BMI	body mass index	FAO	Food and Agriculture Organization
BP	blood pressure	FDA	Federal Development Agency
BSE	bovine spongiform encephalopathy	FIBB	beta fibrinogen gene
CABG	coronary artery bypass graft	FFA	free fatty acid
CAD	coronary artery disease	FFQ	food frequency questionnaire
CAGS	coronary artery graft surgery	FPG	fasting plasma glucose
CAP	Common Agricultural Policy	FSE	former socialist economies
CC	coronary calcium	FSU	former Soviet Union
CCB	calcium channel blocker	GBD	Global Burden of Disease Study
CDC	Center for Disease Control (USA)	GDM	gestational diabetes mellitus
CEE	Central and Eastern Europe	GFR	glomerular filtration rate
CETP	cholesterol ester transfer protein	GHQ	general health questionnaire
CHD	coronary heart disease	GI	glycaemic index
CHF	congestive heart failure	GITS	gastro-intestinal transport system
CI	confidence interval	GL	glycaemic load
CIMT	carotid intima–media thickness	HBP	high blood pressure
CK	creatinine kinase	HDL-C	high-density lipoprotein cholesterol
CMV	cytomegalovirus		
COPD	chronic obstructive pulmonary disease	HPLC	high-performance liquid chromatography
CPB	cardiopulmonary bypass		
CRP	C-reactive protein	HR	hazard ratio / heart rate
CT	computed tomography	HRT	hormone replacement therapy
CV	coefficients of variation, cardiovascular	HRV	heart-rate variability
CVA	cerebrovascular accident	HT	hormone therapy
CVD	cardiovascular disease	IARC	International Agency of Research into Cancer
DALYs	disability-adjusted life years		
DBP	diastolic blood pressure	ICD	International Classification of Diseases/implanted cardioverter defibrillator
DHA	docosahexaenoic acid		
DHEA	dehydroepiandrosterone		
DIS	diagnostic interview schedule	IDL	intermediate-density lipoprotein
		IDL-C	intermediate-density lipoprotein cholesterol

IFG	impaired fasting glucose/glycaemia
IGR	impaired glucose regulation
IGT	impaired glucose tolerance
IHD	ischaemic heart disease
IL-1, IL-6	interleukin-1, interleukin-6
ILSI	International Life Sciences Institute
IMT	intima–media thickness
IPCC	Intergovernmental Panel on Climate Change
ISH	isolated systolic hypertension
IVUS	intravascular ultrasound
JAS	Jenkins activity survey
LDL-C	low-density lipoprotein cholesterol
LF	low frequency
Lp(a)	lipoprotein a
LR	low risk
LVEF	left ventricular ejection fraction
LVH	left ventricular hypertrophy
MCS	mental component summary
MET (score)	metabolic equivalents score
MFA	monounsaturated fatty acids
MI	myocardial infarction
MMP	matrix metaloprotease
MMPI	Minnesota Multiphasic Personality Inventory
MMSE	mini mental state examination
MSIMI	mental stress-induced myocardial ischaemia
MTHFR	methylenetetrahydrofolate reductase
NBW	normal birth weight
NCD	non-communicable disease
NCEP	National Cholesterol Education Program
NEFA	non-esterified fatty acid
NGO	non-governmental organization
NHANES	National Health and Nutrition Examination Survey
NHLBI	National Heart, Lung, and Blood Institute
NIDDM	non-insulin dependent diabetes mellitus
NMR	nuclear magnetic resonance imaging
NO	nitric oxide
OC	oral contraceptive
OGTT	oral glucose tolerance test
OR	odds ratio
PAD	peripheral arterial disease
PAI-1	plasminogen activator inhibitor type 1
PCO(S)	polycystic ovary syndrome
PCS	physical component summary

PE	pulmonary embolism
PET	positron emission tomography
PFA	polyunsaturated fatty acids
PMN	polymorphonuclear leukocytes
P/S ratio	polyunsaturated/saturated fat ratio
PTCA	percutaneous transluminal coronary angioplasty
PUFA	polyunsaturated fatty acid
PVC	premature cardiovascular constriction
PVP	predictive value positive
QALYs	quality-adjusted life years
RAS	renin–angiotensin system
RCT	randomized controlled trial
RDA	recommended daily allowance
RH	relative hazard
RO	relative odds
ROC	receiver operating characteristic
RR	relative risk
RRR	Relative risk reduction
SBP	systolic blood pressure
SCD	sudden cardiac death
SCM	Stages of Change Model
SD	standard deviation
SEP	socio-economic position
SERMS	selective oestrogen receptor modulators
SES	socio-economic status/strata
SFA	saturated fatty acid
SI	special risk intervention
SIDS	sudden infant death syndrome
SIR	smoking impact ratio
SMR	standardized mortality ratio
SSA	sub-Saharan Africa
TABP	type A behaviour pattern
TC	total cholesterol
TCV	total cardiovascular (mortality)
TFA	trans fatty acid
TH2	T helper
TIA	transient ischaemic attack
TNF-α	tumour necrosis factor-α
TSP	total suspended particulates
TTM	Transtheoretical Model of Behaviour Change
vCJD	variant Creutzfeldt–Jakob disease
VLDL	very low-density lipoprotein
VLDL-C	very low-density lipoprotein cholesterol
VTE	venous thromboembolic disease
vWF	von Willebrand factor
WHO	World Health Organization

Section I

Introduction

Chapter 1

Coronary heart disease epidemiology: from aetiology to public health

M. Marmot and P. Elliott

1.1 Introduction

Some years ago a colleague told us that he had been active in coronary heart disease epidemiology in the 1960s and then moved on to other areas. After twenty years he again attended a scientific meeting on CHD epidemiology and felt like he had not been away. Little had changed. We suggest that were he able now to return, a further twenty years on, he would find much that is new and of interest. This can be summarized in four trends.

First, the decline in CHD rates in the rich countries of the world, which he would have seen a little of in the early 1980s, has been a dominant feature of the epidemiological landscape. But these trends have been uneven. In Europe, as heart disease declined in frequency in the west it increased in the east, opening up an east–west gap. Within countries there has been the emergence of big socio-economic differences in CHD. In general, the decline in rates has been steeper in subgroups of the population in more favoured socio-economic positions. As a result, socio-economic differences in CHD have increased.

A second major trend has been the increasing importance of cardiovascular disease, including CHD, in developing countries.

Third, there has been intense research on 'newer' risk factors. Our colleague may complain that some of these risk factors are not so new – he had heard of all of them twenty years ago. Perhaps, but there has been a good deal more research on early life effects, antioxidants, fish intake, plasma homocysteine, the metabolic syndrome and diabetes, psychosocial factors, air pollution, temperature, oral contraceptives, and gene–environment interactions than when he last tuned out in the 1980s.

Fourth, the established risk factors are even more established. Research since the 1980s has confirmed their importance, together with the concept of low risk based on the *absence* of risk factors. There has been much activity in converting yesterday's risk factor research into today's public health.

All four of these trends are well represented in this book. We wish to draw attention to these themes in a little more detail.

1.2 Trends in the developed countries

1.2.1 Rethink 'premature'

Several chapters in this book pick up the theme of the decline in CHD mortality rates in many rich countries. Despite this decline, it is still the major cause of death. In particular, as the population ages, and the proportion of people over 65 increases, the fact that more than 80%

of coronary deaths occur in people over age 65 becomes increasingly salient. The very label, 'premature' disease, implies an acceptance that CHD may be a frequent mode of exit when an old person eventually dies, and that it is premature disease that claims attention. With an ageing population, however, our definition of 'premature' may need to change. WHO calculates healthy life expectancy at age 60 (WHO 2003). In Japan and Sweden, the usual benchmarks for good health, healthy life expectancy at age 60 is 17 years for men and 19.6 (Sweden) and 21.7 (Japan) for women. With an expectation of living healthily to at least 80 if you are a woman, or 77 if a man, we may start to think of a CHD death before age 75 as 'premature'. Certainly the evidence reviewed in this book gives grounds for believing that CHD is preventable up to at least this age.

1.2.2 Social inequalities

The welcome decline in CHD rates has not been uniform within countries. Figure 1.1 shows trends in CHD death rates within England and Wales (Acheson 1998; Drever and Whitehead 1997; White *et al.* 2003). The gap in CHD rates between people in more and those in less favoured socio-economic positions had been growing and has now started to diminish. This is not simply a problem of British social classes, but is seen elsewhere (Kunst *et al.* 1998, 1999; Pappas *et al.* 1993; Valkonen *et al.* 1993).

There has been much discussion about the reasons for the trends in CHD. Explanations are likely to include some or all of changes in society, action on specific risk factors and health behaviours, and trends in treatment. Whichever of these proves to be the dominant explanation,

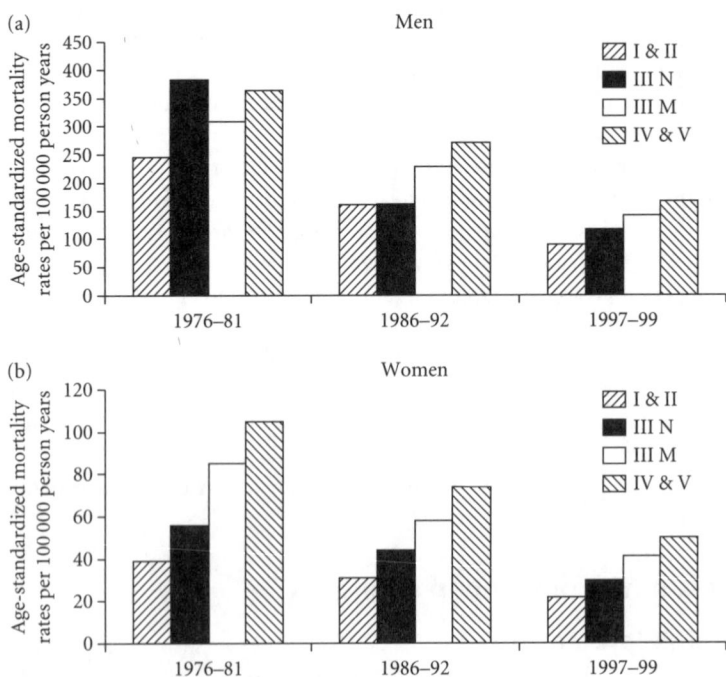

Fig. 1.1 Trends in coronary heart disease death rates within England and Wales. (From Drever and Whitehead 1997, and White *et al.* 2003.)

it would appear that the benefits are not being spread equally to all social classes. This will continue to be a major challenge for the future.

1.2.3 Heterogeneity among developed countries

To be middle-aged man in Russia in 2002 was to face a higher risk of death than in Nigeria or Senegal, India or Indonesia, Guatemala or El Salvador, Brazil or Ecuador. The evidence to support this statement comes from WHO's calculation of probability of dying between ages 15 and 60 per 1000 in 2002 (WHO 2003). The figures for men are: Russia, 464; Nigeria, 453; Senegal, 349; India, 291; Indonesia, 244; Guatemala, 283; El Salvador, 257; Brazil, 246; Ecuador, 216. By contrast, in the USA it is 140, UK, 107; Japan, 95; and in Sweden, 83. The fact that the probability of a 15-year-old dying by age 50 is more than four times higher in Russia than in Sweden suggests how far we have to go in understanding and applying this knowledge to improving public health.

The health disadvantage of being Russian was the most extreme among the former Communist countries of Central and Eastern Europe, but all suffered badly in life expectancy compared with Western Europe. The major contributor to this health disadvantage has been CHD (Bobak *et al.* 1996).

All the usual subjects have been rounded up to explain the trends in Central and Eastern Europe: smoking, diet, obesity, poor standards of treatment, alcohol, psychosocial factors. There are no grounds for complacency. It remains a major public health problem.

1.3 A major problem in developing countries

The fact that CHD has rightly claimed attention in developed countries should not blind us to its emerging importance in the developing world. Figure 1.2, from the *World health report 2003*, shows that cardiovascular diseases are the major cause of death in many developing countries (WHO 2003). Twice as many deaths from cardiovascular diseases now occur in developing countries as in developed. Increasingly, CHD is playing a major part.

An important question arises as to the approach to be taken to this new epidemic. To what extent do the research findings from the last half century in developed countries have to be

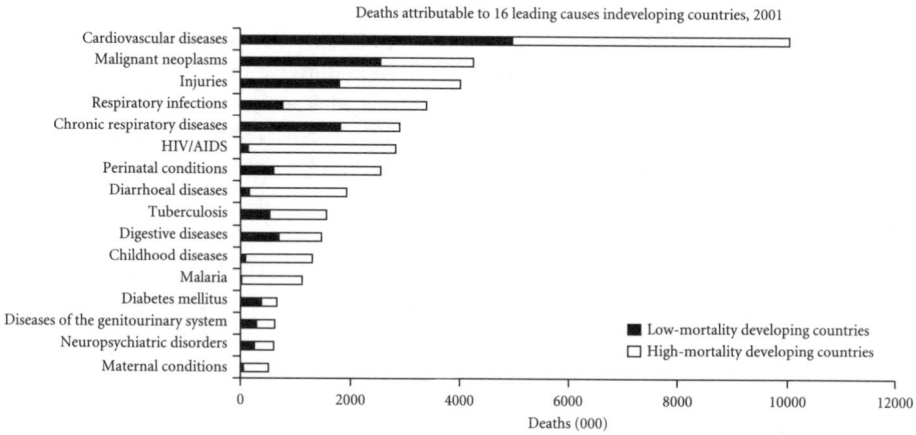

Fig. 1.2 Deaths attributable to 16 leading causes in developing countries, 2001. (From WHO 2003.)

reproduced in the developing? WHO is in no doubt that the knowledge needed for action is now in place. Indeed, none would doubt that smoking is a major cause of morbidity and mortality in developing, as in developed countries. It hardly needs new large-scale epidemiological studies to be confident of that conclusion. The same applies to high blood pressure

On the other hand, new epidemiological studies in developing countries, such as those of David Barker and colleagues in India and of Salim Yusuf internationally, are likely to yield important new information on aetiology.

1.4 New risk factors or applying what we know?

This question brings together themes three and four. There is a view that we now know enough to take action to prevent CHD and that further research for new risk factors is 'occupational therapy for epidemiologists' (Beaglehole and Magnus 2002). We do not hold to the view that we know so much already that the only research that is needed is about how to apply what we know. Nor do we take the view that we know so little that no action is warranted until more research is in. We see no contradiction between further research on newer risk factors and taking action on those that are well established. Chapter 4 and Section III in this book reflect that dual approach.

To illustrate, one of us has been much exercised in trying to understand the reasons for the social gradient in coronary heart and other diseases (Marmot 2004a). In the Whitehall studies of British civil servants, a combination of plasma cholesterol, blood pressure level, obesity, smoking, sedentary life style, and height explain less than a third of the social gradient in CHD mortality: higher rates as the occupational hierarchy is descended (Marmot et al. 1984, 1997; van Rossum et al. 2000). This has stimulated us to look for 'new' risk factors, among them psychosocial factors. This in no way contradicts the importance of the established risk factors. We calculated that if everyone in the population had plasma cholesterol levels in the bottom quintile, blood pressure in the bottom quintile, and were never smokers, CHD mortality rates would be predicted to be two-thirds lower (Marmot 2004b). This could indeed be taken as saying that we know all we need to know to reduce CHD mortality rates by two-thirds. But, the low-risk group constituted about 5% of the population. It is a worthwhile goal to try and reduce the whole population's level of risk factors to that of the healthiest 5%. It will be major challenge.

There is, however, a different question: why, among people with fairly uniform exposure to levels of blood pressure and cholesterol (smoking shows an inverse social gradient), is there a social gradient in CHD. These two approaches – applying what we know and discovering what we don't – should therefore go on at the same time. As the chapters in this book reveal, that is indeed the case, and the activities in both areas are vibrant and healthy.

References

Acheson, D. (1998). *Inequalities in health: report of an independent inquiry*. HMSO, London.

Beaglehole, R. and Magnus, P. (2002). The search for new risk factors for coronary heart disease: occupational therapy for epidemiologists? *International Journal of Epidemiology*, **31**, 1117–22.

Bobak, M. and Marmot, M. G. (1996). East-West mortality divide and its potential explanations: proposed research agenda. *British Medical Journal*, **312**, 421–5.

Drever, F. and Whitehead, M. (1997). *Health inequalities: decennial supplement. Series DS No.15*, pp. 125–7. The Stationery Office, Office for National Statistics, London.

Kunst, A. E., Groenhof, F., and Mackenbach, J. P. (1998). The EU Working Group on Socioeconomic Inequalities in Health. Occupational class and cause specific mortality in middle aged men in 11 European countries: comparison of population based studies. *British Medical Journal*, 316, 1636–8.

Kunst, A. E., Groenhof, F., Andersen, O., Borgan, J-K., Costa, G., Desplanques, G. *et al.* (1999). Occupational class and ischemic heart disease mortality in the United States and 11 European countries. *American Journal of Public Health*, 89, 47–53.

Marmot, M. (2004*a*). *Status syndrome*. London, Bloomsbury.

Marmot, M. (2004*b*). Commentary. Risk factors or social causes? *International Journal of Epidemiology*, 33, 297–8.

Marmot, M. G., Shipley, M. J., and Rose, G. (1984). Inequalities in death: specific explanations of a general pattern. *Lancet*, 323, 1003–6.

Marmot, M. G., Bosma, H., Hemingway, H., Brunner, E., and Stansfeld, S. (1997). Contribution of job control and other risk factors to social variations in coronary heart disease. *Lancet*, 350, 235–40.

Pappas, G., Queen, S., Hadden, W., and Fisher, G. (1993). The increasing disparity in mortality between socio-economic groups in the United States, 1960 and 1986. *New England Journal of Medicine*, 329, 103–9.

Valkonen, T., Martelin, T., Rimpela, A., Notkola, V., and Savela, S. (1993). *Socio-economic mortality differences in Finland 1981–90*. Statistics Finland, Helsinki.

van Rossum, C. T. M., Shipley, M. J., Van de Mheen, H., Grobbee, D. E., and Marmot, M. G. (2000). Employment grade differences in cause specific mortality: a 25 year follow up of civil servants from the first Whitehall study. *Journal of Epidemiology and Community Health*, 54, 178–84.

White, C., Van Galen, F., and Chow, Y. H. (2003). Trends in social class differences in mortality by cause, 1986 to 2000. *Health Statistics Quarterly*, 20, 25–37.

WHO (World Health Organization) (2003). *World health report 2003: shaping the future*. WHO, Geneva.

Chapter 2

Contribution of epidemiology to understanding coronary heart disease

(reprinted from first edition)*

F. H. Epstein

2.1 Introduction

Understanding a disease means being able to explain its clinical and preclinical manifestations in terms of the responsible pathobiological mechanisms and to account for its occurrence in different populations and social groups within the community. In this context, epidemiology has played a crucial role in understanding CHD and has provided a model, only beginning to be applied, for the potential contributions of epidemiology towards the prevention of other non-communicable disorders. Epidemiology is both a science and a method. It has contributed to the study of CHD on both levels. Surgeon Rear-Admiral Sheldon Dudley, in his presidential address to the Section of Epidemiology and State Medicine of the Royal Society of Medicine, has spoken of ecology as an 'attitude of mind' (Dudley 1936–37). Epidemiology, being in one of its metamorphoses human or medical ecology, is also an attitude of mind. As such, it has extended the clinical horizon to include the picture of health and disease in the community and it has influenced clinical scientists in their study designs. Epidemiology has become an integral part of the interdisciplinary approaches towards understanding CHD.

2.2 Historical background

It might almost seem as if CHD epidemiology started with a 'big bang' around 1948, shortly after the end of the Second World War. This is certainly true for epidemiological research in this field as a deliberate effort under the term 'epidemiology'. The beginnings reach back into the nineteenth century, particularly under the description 'geographical pathology'. It is a sobering experience to read the contributions of Aschoff and, especially, Anitschkow in the Proceedings of the Conference on Geographical Pathology held in the Netherlands in 1934 in which a good many of the currently accepted causes of atherosclerosis and its main clinical consequence, CHD, are foreshadowed (*Deuxième Conférence Internationale de Pathologie Géographique* 1934). The question of why CHD epidemiology came over the horizon so suddenly and so forcefully in the brief period between 1947 and 1949 is part of the mystery of creative ideas and falls outside the present task of describing the impact of the studies conducted over the past 45 years which led to present knowledge and understanding.

Two great currents can be distinguished: the era of prospective studies which started in the late 1940s, and the era of intervention studies, with explorations in the 1960s, which started

---

* Copyright rests with the estate holders of Professor F. H. Epstein.

with full force in the early 1970s. The first era culminated in the discovery of CHD risk factors. These had become so firmly established, within a remarkably short period of time, by the early 1960s that preventive trials to test their cause and effect relationship to the disease were called for as an imperative need. The two eras overlap. The first era rose to a peak in the late 1960s and declined in the 1970s as the emphasis shifted to the second era of intervention studies, but has emerged from this partial eclipse during the last decade. This resurgence related to the deepening of knowledge concerning established, and the search for new, risk factors. The second era reached its peak around 1980 and has maintained its level, with a shift from large-scale to more clinical types of trials. Alongside these randomized trials involving individuals, intervention projects concerned with entire communities have gained in prominence.

In parallel with the developments just outlined, geographical differences in the frequency of CHD have continued to be in the centre of interest. They revolve around the question of why the disease is more common in some parts of the world and why secular mortality trends are steeper in some countries than others. In more recent years, there have been intensive efforts to explain the unexpected downward trends in CHD mortality in a number of countries.

During the past decade, the problem of how preventive cardiovascular care can be organized most effectively for individuals and on the community level – the matter of the high-risk and population strategies of prevention – has moved more and more into the foreground. The issue is not strictly concerned with understanding CHD and will therefore not be further discussed here, being covered elsewhere in this book. However, those strategies are at the core of the question of why understanding CHD is essential for the practice of preventive cardiology.

So far this brief historical review has dealt with the interrelationships between CHD and its precursors within their epidemiological context. Investigations into the epidemiology of the precursors themselves have been of equal importance. The basic studies into the determinants of serum lipid levels within the broader field of lipid metabolism rank first and foremost, not only in number, but also because of their direct relationship to the development of atherosclerosis from youth into older ages. The presence of cholesterol in atherosclerotic lesions has been known since 1843, and there were numerous studies on the role of cholesterol in atherogenesis prior to the Second World War (Epstein 1990). However, it is beyond question that Ancel Keys, whose pioneering research started in the late 1940s, was chiefly responsible for the wide interest in the 'cholesterol hypothesis' as it developed into the 'cholesterol theory'. Keys himself traced back some of this history (Keys 1953, 1975, 1983), but a full account of his contributions remains to be written, not only in terms of his own work but also of the wave of research by others which he stimulated. Keys' contributions range from nutritional experiments under controlled metabolic conditions to extensive international epidemiological field studies. During the intervening years, an enormous amount of data have been accumulated to identify the nutritional determinants of serum lipids, including cholesterol, and their interaction with genetic dispositions is beginning to be understood. This knowledge, based to a considerable extent on epidemiological studies, had an important impact on nutritional science in general and forms the basis of nutritional counselling as one cornerstone of CHD prevention programmes in the community and of nutritional advice in medical practice.

Epidemiology has also played an important part in understanding the determinants of blood pressure. It is of interest that the pioneers in epidemiological research were not always professional epidemiologists. Keys' original training was in human biology, and the first epidemiological study of blood pressure was promoted by Sir George Pickering, the renowned clinical scientist. It would be fair to say that a large part of current knowledge on the distribution of blood pressure levels and its determinants in different populations comes from epidemiological observations, opening the way for the control of hypertension by non-pharmacological means. Epidemiological investigations have also contributed substantially to the identification of the factors influencing glucose intolerance and diabetes. Similar advances in the emerging field of thrombogenesis and haemostasis as precursors of heart attacks are being made.

The strength of the epidemiological approach lies partly in its ability not only to identify risk factors for CHD, but also to determine their relative importance singly and in combination in the population at large. It also permits a quantitative estimate of how much of the disease can be accounted for in terms of known risk factors and what proportion may remain to be explained. This knowledge is important for the practice of preventive cardiology, public health planning of preventive services, and for the design of research still needed.

The achievements of cardiovascular disease epidemiology during recent decades give reason for much satisfaction and provide hope that these approaches will continue to be useful. As new methods are being developed, it will be possible to identify persons at increased risk with greater precision and to focus the need for preventive measures more sharply for the purposes of the high-risk strategy. Further knowledge is going to be gained as to how preventive services can be established most effectively in the community. Community programmes for the prevention of cardiovascular diseases will be linked with programmes for the prevention of other chronic diseases, moving toward comprehensive approaches for the preservation of health (Epstein and Holland 1983).

2.3 Lessons from changes over time

Around 1950, the view was still widely held that atherosclerosis, as often as not called arteriosclerosis, is a degenerative condition and an inevitable concomitant of ageing. It was recognized from autopsy studies that the extent of lesions may vary greatly from one individual to another, but this was attributed to constitutional rather than environmental differences. With the advent of epidemiology around this time, there was an intensified attempt to show that the increasing mortality from 'arteriosclerotic heart disease' in the preceding years could not be explained solely by changing fashions of death certification but reflected a true change, with the implication that environmental factors were responsible. Alongside the information from international mortality statistics, Morris's report (Morris 1951), based on autopsy records at the London Hospital, that ischaemic heart disease but not atherosclerotic lesions had become more common over time, received much attention.

International mortality statistics since 1950, despite the changes in the World Health Organization (WHO) nomenclature of causes of death certification, left no reasonable doubt that death from CHD was increasing in most Western countries. It came as a totally unexpected surprise in the 1970s that the trend had reversed in the USA and some other countries. This constitutes an important epidemiological contribution to understanding CHD because upward or downward secular changes in mortality are amongst the most persuasive pieces of evidence that disease occurrence is strongly influenced by environmental changes.

2.4 Lessons from cross-cultural variations

Geographical variations in disease frequency constitute further convincing evidence for the relationship between lifestyles and the disorders largely due to atherosclerosis. They were discussed at the Conference on Geographic Pathology in 1934, mentioned earlier. At the same conference, reference was also made to variations related to social class and occupation, investigated intensively since, which can also be attributed to environmental conditions. The term 'lifestyle', which came to be extraordinarily useful, was first used by Keys in the early 1950s. The suggestion that geographical differences in mortality are correlated with differences in dietary fat consumption and therefore with serum cholesterol levels was made by Keys (1953), opening up a field of research which has remained prominent. The Seven Countries Study, started by Keys in 1958, is the single most convincing piece of evidence that not only CHD mortality but also its incidence are associated with differences in fat consumption and serum cholesterol levels (Keys 1980). On the basis of a large number of studies around the world, it can no longer be questioned that marked differences in lifestyles, particularly in regard to diet, run parallel with corresponding differences in CHD frequency. The fact that differences in CHD mortality, particularly within Europe, can exist in the absence of marked dietary differences does not in any way run counter to the view just expressed; it merely means that there are regional differences which must be due to other influences. Nor do these findings indicate that dietary changes in a favourable direction could not further reduce CHD frequency in countries with already relatively low risk.

Migrant studies constitute another approach to understanding geographical variations. The first of three prominent examples is the British–Norwegian–United States Migrant Study, initiated primarily by the late Professor D. D. Reid, who preceded Professor Rose in the position from which he has now retired. It is one of Reid's many contributions towards creating foundations of chronic disease epidemiology and was published posthumously (Feinleib *et al.* 1982). The second example, the Japan–Honolulu–San Francisco Study, provided strong evidence that lifestyle is a key determinant of CHD risk (Robertson *et al.* 1977). Thirdly, in the Tokelau Island Study, a pioneering effort was made by Dr I. A. M. Prior to understand the changes in health which occur when a population moves from its native habitat, in this case a remote Pacific island, to an industrialized society, in this case New Zealand (Wessen 1992). Cultural transition can, of course, take place without migration. The resulting increase in CHD frequency expected to occur in Third World countries falls in this category.

Epidemiological pathology has great potential but is hampered by the difficulties in obtaining adequate numbers of autopsies of deceased persons which are reasonably representative. Nevertheless, there are notable examples. The International Atherosclerosis Project showed marked differences in the extent of atherosclerotic lesions, comparing South American countries, the USA, and Europe (Geographic pathology of atherosclerosis 1968). These differences could be correlated with differences in diet and serum cholesterol. While the extent of arterial lesions and the frequency of CHD differed, severe lesions had to be present for death due to coronary disease to occur. A WHO project in several countries provided similar data, especially on geographical differences in young persons (Atherosclerosis of the aorta and coronary arteries in five towns 1976). A number of studies, though not cross-cultural, have provided data on the correlation between lesions and risk factors (Oslo, Bogalusa, Framingham, Hawaii). A community-based study in New Orleans has given insight into differences in the extent and type of lesions in black and white people (Strong *et al.* 1980). An important study of the evolution of lesions at younger ages is under way in the USA and other countries. These studies have strengthened the view that the geographical differences in mortality are real since they reflect structural changes in the coronary and other arteries.

2.5 Predicting CHD

The outstanding single achievement of CHD epidemiology is no doubt the development of the risk factor concept. When the first wave of prospective studies was started in the late 1940s, it could hardly be anticipated that 20 years later it would be possible to predict the disease in overtly healthy people with such accuracy and power. It is often said that individual prediction lacks precision, but is there any other chronic disease, with the exception of lung cancer in smokers, which can be predicted with anything like the precision attainable for CHD? In fact, two of the three major risk factors, serum cholesterol and blood pressure, were already firmly established within less than 10 years, while the evidence for smoking was strongly suggestive (Measuring the risk of coronary heart disease 1957). The term 'risk factor' first appeared in a Framingham publication in 1961 (Kannel *et al.* 1961). There were two more waves of prospective studies, not counting a considerable number of cross-sectional studies during the earlier years. The second wave started around 1960, while the third wave, consisting in part of follow-up observations on persons initially screened for participation in the large primary prevention trials, has covered the last 10–15 years. The prospective studies carried out over the years are very numerous. There are about 30 such studies in Europe and the Mediterranean area, around 25 in the USA, and some 5 in other parts of the world.

Considering the diversity of the populations included in these approximately 60 studies and the differences in their methodology, it is most remarkable that they all tell essentially the same story. Serum cholesterol, blood pressure, and smoking stand out as the major risk factors and carry the largest population-attributable risk. The importance of other risk factors, when measured, has also been generally confirmed; while the relative risk they carry may be relatively slight or their prevalence in the population comparatively low, their accumulated risk may approach that of the major risk factors. It would not have been possible to evaluate the many interacting and competing risk factors without powerful new biostatistical techniques, and great credit is due to those responsible for their development.

What are the limits of predictive power? It is now possible to identify 20% of the population in which close to 60% of the future events of CHD will occur. Perhaps this latter percentage, which is already very high, can be improved with the inclusion of new risk factors, in particular those related to thrombogenesis and genetic markers. Improvement of prediction for individuals would also require the development of more effective screening techniques. However desirable even more powerful prediction of disease would be, it could never replace the need for a population strategy of prevention because, amongst other reasons, the ultimate aim of prevention must be to create a new future generation of people in whom risk factors are less common.

Epidemiology has not only contributed the methods of predicting CHD, but has also developed the concept of 'tracking' risk factors, which aims to identify as early as possible in life those who will develop elevated risk factor levels in adulthood. Powerful methods of tracking would permit the institution of preventive measures before risk factors have already become too high, instead of waiting until they attain a level which should never have been reached in the first place and then lowering them when it is already too late. Efforts to improve tracking methods are under way. The matter of atherosclerosis as a childhood disorder and of early prevention will be touched upon in the next section.

2.6 **Preventing CHD**

The advent of the era of intervention studies, defined earlier, is tied closely to the emergence of risk factors and their power of prediction. When there remained no doubt in the 1960s that risk factors did indeed predict disease risk, it became urgently necessary to test whether lowering of risk factor level would lower the risk of CHD – whether, in fact, the relation between risk factors and risk was causal. A number of preliminary studies, notably the National Diet–Heart

Study (1968) in the USA, were carried out in the 1960s, followed by full-scale intervention studies in the 1970s, as reviewed elsewhere (Epstein and Pyörälä 1987). Researchers expected with confidence that these controlled trials would give a decisive and definitive answer, not fully realizing at first that a number of unforeseen practical problems may reduce their power in providing unequivocal results. The fact that the primary prevention trials taken as a whole, whether viewed singly or in terms of a meta-analysis, have yielded positive results in the face of problems apt to limit their power gives added confidence in the validity of the results. There is no evidence at the present time that preventive measures, while lowering the risk of CHD, increase the risk of other disorders. Furthermore, the case for the primary prevention of CHD does not rest on the results of preventive trials alone, but derives, in addition, from collateral evidence, such as the observations on cross-cultural differences and their relation to lifestyles, the solid indications from clinical, pathological, and experimental investigations that CHD risk factors and the disease are causally related, and the remarkable consistency of the data from observational studies. The results of the large number of secondary prevention studies likewise support the concept of the cause and effect relationship between risk factors and risk.

Trials like those considered so far, in which individuals are randomized to experimental and comparison groups, lend themselves best to drawing inferences on causality. On the other hand, intervention projects in which the comparison is between entire communities with and without intervention programmes reflect better the impact of preventive measures on the population as a whole and, as such, also suggest causal links. A halfway house between the two designs are trials in which circumscribed social or occupational groups are randomized, like the WHO European Trial (WHO 1989). In community projects, it generally takes longer for risk factor changes to show a demonstrable effect on mortality and morbidity because it takes time to mobilize the population to take part in the prevention effort. Evaluation is also made more difficult in countries where CHD is already declining 'naturally'. Nevertheless, the results of ongoing projects to date indicate the effectiveness of community-wide programmes in lowering risk factors and demonstrate, in some, a decline in mortality. Even in randomized trials, it may take longer than anticipated for effects on mortality to become evident (Multiple Risk Factor Intervention Trial Research Group 1990).

Over the years, increasing attention is being given to the fact that atherosclerosis starts early in life and therefore that prevention must also begin early. The matter has already been considered in connection with identifying risk carriers in youth. However, the ultimate aim must be to establish lifestyles in youth which will ensure optimal risk factor levels throughout life. Projects with these aims are underway (WHO 1990).

2.7 Contributions from epidemiological methodology

Standardization of methods is a prerequisite for the conduct of epidemiological studies and intervention trials, to ensure consistency of measurement over the course of the study and comparability between studies. Furthermore, methods used in clinical research may not be feasible in field studies, so that they have to be adapted for epidemiological purposes or it may be necessary to develop new methods. This is part and parcel of epidemiological research, but it could not be anticipated that these standardized methods would also find wide application in cardiological investigations. Major examples are the Minnesota Code for reading electrocardiograms, the Rose Questionnaire for the interpretation of chest pain and the diagnosis of angina pectoris, and methods for the unbiased measurement of blood pressure. Epidemiological studies have drawn attention to laboratory variation and error, leading, amongst others, to Lipid Standardization Programmes which have influenced clinical chemistry. Questionnaires have been developed for the assessment of psychosocial factors, the measurement of physical activity, and a variety of other purposes which have been found useful outside epidemiological research. A milestone along this road has been the 'Rose–Blackburn Manual', published by the WHO, which has provided guidelines for the application and use of standardized epidemiological methods in cardiovascular epidemiology (Rose and Blackburn 1968).

Epidemiological terms like specificity, sensitivity, and predictive power are now being used in clinical research for comparing, say, invasive and non-invasive methods of detecting coronary artery lesions. Clinical investigators have also been influenced by epidemiologists in the design of experiments, paying attention to the problem of choosing experimental and control subjects from comparable populations, or in the use of multivariate biostatistical techniques. These examples serve to illustrate the extent to which epidemiological and clinical research have moved closer together.

2.8 Impact on medical practice and public policy

Over the course of the years, cardiologists and medical practitioners in general in many countries have become increasingly aware of the importance of CHD risk factors and their significance for the prevention of the disease. At the same time, the public has become increasingly aware of this message. Heart associations, cardiac societies, and other professional organizations have helped in the dissemination of this knowledge. Governmental agencies in a number of countries have joined in the effort by appointing expert committees to prepare official reports and issuing recommendations. The WHO has played a key role during the last four decades in calling together experts to issue scientific progress reports, and major studies have been and are being conducted under its aegis. At the present time, hardly any argument exists about the need to detect and protect persons at increased risk, but there remains some opposition to the view, shared by most workers in the field, that preventive measures, especially those concerned with nutritional habits, must be extended to the entire population. There is still a long road to travel, more in some countries than others, in order to establish healthier lifestyles in the population and preventive cardiology in the daily practice of medicine, but the basic foundations have been solidly laid.

2.9 Understanding CHD: insights from epidemiology

The outstanding single message provided by epidemiology consists in having established a scientific basis for the recognition that CHD, as an epidemic condition in the population, is mostly due to environmental influences, thus opening the way for prevention. This is not to belittle the importance of genetic predispositions in modifying individual susceptibility. However, on both the community and individual levels, the disease is caused as much or more by what we do than by what we are. The view is crystallized in the concept of 'lifestyle', a component of the social environment. Lifestyle is the first step in the chain which leads over the risk factors to the clinical events. Lifestyle determines risk factor levels against the background of genetic variation. It is the confluence of clinical, pathological, experimental, and, last but not least, epidemiological evidence which attests to the causal relation between risk factors and the diseases primarily due to atherosclerosis. Furthermore, evaluation of the epidemiological data permits an estimate of how much of the disease is 'explained' by the known risk factors and how much remains to be discovered, with the conclusion that a larger proportion is known than unknown. All this reasoning is mostly based on epidemiological findings because only population-based data allow extrapolations which reflect the general validity of the results.

The entire risk factor concept is derived from epidemiological observations. It has been instrumental in bringing cardiovascular epidemiology to the attention of the medical profession and the public. There is a good reason, because the concept is not merely theoretical but has immediate applications in the practice of medicine both for the individual and on the community level. Its acceptance is gratifying since risk factors provide the key to prevention. Guidelines for the reduction of risk factors have been derived from epidemiological and clinical studies, including indications for pharmacological treatment when lifestyle alterations have been shown to be insufficient. Data on the distribution and prevalence of risk factors in different populations and social groups, essential for health planning and as a background for the practice of preventive cardiology, quite apart from their bearing on aetiology, come from epidemiological research.

Cardiovascular epidemiology has had a marked impact on cardiologists and practising physicians in general. To an increasing degree, curative and preventive practice are being seen as a continuum. Population-based studies have provided a picture of how CHD in its various stages, from latent to clinically overt manifestations, presents itself in the community, making it possible to detect and treat the disease earlier and to give more effective emergency care. Although it sounds strange today, one of the truly outstanding American cardiologists, some 25 years ago during a meeting at the National Heart Institute in Bethesda, expressed great surprise when told by the epidemiologist present that over half of CHD deaths occur outside the hospital; he knew only how many deaths occurred after admission! This illustrates, as an example, how the intense current preoccupation with sudden death was influenced by epidemiological findings. It has already been mentioned how epidemiological approaches and methods have been useful to clinical investigators in the design of studies and their interpretation. The amazing phenomenon of the rise and fall of CHD mortality in various countries has also attracted much attention amongst cardiologists and provided common ground with epidemiologists.

The understanding of CHD epidemiology has been greatly furthered by primary and secondary prevention studies, including clinical trials in their classical form, large unifactorial and multifactorial intervention studies, and community projects. The results, seen as a whole, have been encouraging, have yielded estimates of the effectiveness of preventive measures, and have made decisive contributions towards understanding their determinants. The trials have also helped clinicians and epidemiologists to understand each other and, as in other areas of mutual interest, to bring them closer together.

2.10 Conclusion

In this bird's-eye review, very few persons have been mentioned by name. The temptation to give credit to all the many workers primarily responsible for specific achievements was great, but it seemed impossible to be selective and fair at the same time. The problem was somewhat reduced because so many of the investigators are contributors to this book, though a good many more regrettably remain anonymous. It would not be inappropriate, however, to single out the man to whom this book is dedicated. Geoffrey Rose has carried out observational studies, conducted preventive trials, contributed to methodology, assumed leadership in applying research findings to prevention in the community, deliberately built bridges between epidemiology and clinicians, and has been a teacher of epidemiology. Thus he himself has covered most of the spectrum of epidemiological endeavour. His unique stature derives from having added to new knowledge a profound understanding of its scientific and social significance.

In the beginning, reference was made to epidemiology as an 'attitude of mind'. In closing, an early example of this attitude may be mentioned. Eighty-five years ago, Sir James Mackenzie, a founding father of modern cardiology, wrote on arteriosclerosis: 'In recent articles on this subject there is one very important aspect which has not been considered – that is the beginning of the conditions that lead on to arteriosclerosis. The case is generally considered when already the mischief is done, and the cause can usually be attributed to an agency that suits the particular fancy of the examining medical man' (Mackenzie 1906). To remedy the situation, Mackenzie attempted, towards the end of his life in 1921, the first long-term investigation of CHD (Mackenzie 1926). It gives reason for satisfaction that his vision is how being turned into action, based on better understanding.

References

Atherosclerosis of the aorta and coronary arteries in five towns (1976). *World Health Organization Bulletin*, **53**, 485–645.

Deuxième conférence internationale de pathologie géographique, Utrecht (1934). Oosthoek, Utrecht.

Dudley, S. F. (1936–37). The ecological outlook on epidemiology. *Proceedings of the Royal Society of Medicine*, **30**, 57–70.

Epstein, F. H. (1990). Die historische Entwicklung des Cholesterin-Atherosklerose-Konzepts. *Therapeutische Umschau*, **47**, 435–42.

Epstein, F. H. and Holland, W. W. (1983). Prevention of chronic diseases in the community: one-disease versus multiple-disease strategies. *International Journal of Epidemiology*, **12**, 135–7.

Epstein, F. H. and Pyörälä, K. (1987). Perspectives for the primary prevention of coronary heart disease. *Cardiology*, **74**, 316–31.

Feinleib, M., Lambert, P. M., Zeiner-Henriksen, T., Rogot, E., Hunt, B. M., and Ingster-Moore, L. (1982). The British–Norwegian migrant study: analysis of parameters of mortality differentials associated with angina. *Biometrics* (Suppl.), **38**, 55–71.

Geographical pathology of atherosclerosis (1968). *Laboratory Investigations*, **18**, 465–653.

Kannel, W. B., Dawber, T. R., Kagan, A., Revotskie, N., and Stokes III, J. (1961). Factors of risk in the development of coronary heart disease: six-year follow-up experience. *Annals of Internal Medicine*, **55**, 33–50.

Keys, A. (1953). Atherosclerosis: a problem in newer public health. *Journal of Mount Sinai Hospital*, **20**, 118–39.

Keys, A. (1975). Coronary heart disease: the global picture. *Atherosclerosis*, **22**, 149–92.

Keys, A. (1980). *Seven countries: a multivariate analysis of death and coronary heart disease*. Harvard University Press.

Keys, A. (1983). From Naples to seven countries: a sentimental journey. *Progress in Biochemical Pharmacology*, **19**, 1–30.

Mackenzie, J. (1906). Arterio-sclerosis. *British Medical Journal*, **1**, 319.

Mackenzie, Sir James (1926). *The basis of vital activity, being a review of five years' work at the St. Andrew's Institute for Clinical Research*. Faber and Gwyer, London.

Measuring the risk of coronary heart disease in adult population groups: a symposium (1957). *American Journal of Public Health*, **47** (4, Part 2), 1–64.

Morris, J. A. (1951). Recent history of coronary disease. *Lancet*, **i**, 1–7, 69–73.

Multiple Risk Factor Intervention Trial Research Group (1990). Mortality rates after 10.5 years for participants in the Multiple Risk Factor Intervention Trial. *Journal of the American Medical Association*, **263**, 1795–801.

National Diet–Heart Study (1968). *Circulation*, **37** (Suppl. 1).

Robertson, T. L., Kato, H., Rhoads, G. G., Kagan, A., Marmot, M., Syme, S. L. *et al.* (1977). Epidemiologic studies of coronary heart disease and stroke in Japanese men living in Japan, Hawaii and California: incidence of myocardial infarction and death from coronary heart disease. *American Journal of Cardiology*, **39**, 239–49.

Rose, G. A. and Blackburn, H. (1968). *Cardiovascular survey methods.* World Health Organization, Geneva.

Strong, J. P., Johnson, W. D., Oalman, M. C., Tracy, W. P., Newman III, W. P., Rock, W. A. *et al.* (1980). Community pathology of atherosclerosis and coronary heart disease in New Orleans: relationship of risk factors to atherosclerotic lesions. In *Atherosclerosis V* (ed. A. M. Gotto, Jr, L. C. Smith, and B. Allen), pp. 719–24. Springer Verlag, New York.

Wessen, A. F. (ed.) (1992). *Tokelau: migration and health in a small Polynesian society.* Oxford University Press.

WHO (World Health Organization) (1989). *WHO European Collaborative Trial in the multifactorial prevention of coronary heart disease.* WHO, Copenhagen.

WHO (World Health Organization) (1990). *Prevention in childhood and youth of adult cardiovascular disease: time for action.* Report of a WHO Expert Committee. Technical Report Series, 792. WHO, Geneva.

Chapter 3

Established major coronary risk factors: historical overview

J. Stamler

Knowledge and Human power are synonymous, since ignorance of the cause frustrates the effect . . . Now the true and lawful goal of the sciences is none other than this: that human life be endowed with new discoveries and powers.

Francis Bacon, Novum Organum 1620

Don't crowd diseases point everywhere to deficiencies of society? One may adduce atmospheric or cosmic conditions or similar factors. But never do they alone make epidemics. They produce them only where due to bad social conditions people have lived for some time in abnormal situations.

Epidemics of a character unknown so far appear, and often disappear without traces when a new culture period has started. Thus did leprosy and the English sweat. The history of artificial epidemics is therefore the history of disturbances of human culture. Their changes announce to us in gigantic signs the turning points of culture in new directions.

Epidemics resemble great warning signs on which the true statesman is able to read that the evolution of his nation has been disturbed to a point which even a careless policy is no longer allowed to overlook . . .

Rudolf Virchow (Ackerknecht 1953)

There are no such things as pure and applied science – there are only science and the application of science.

Louis Pasteur (Dubos 1960)

[I am] . . . a man whose invincible belief is that Science and Peace will triumph over Ignorance and War, that nations will unite not to destroy, but to build, and that the future will belong to those who will have done most for suffering humanity.

Louis Pasteur (Dubos 1960)

3.1 Introduction

The focus of this historical overview chapter is on six established major risk factors: adverse diet, diet-related above-optimal levels of serum total cholesterol (TC) and blood pressure (BP), overweight/obesity, diabetes mellitus (DM), and cigarette smoking. These have been shown to be centrally involved in the multifactorial causation of severe atherosclerotic disease, its complications, and its multiple clinical manifestations – first and foremost the epidemic of CHD in Western industrialized countries. The extensive scientific knowledge on these risk factors and their aetiological role is the solid foundation of the combined population-wide and high-risk strategy for the primary prevention and control of this epidemic (American Heart Association

1961, 1980, 1998, 2000; Department of Health 1994; Dietary Guidelines Advisory Committee 1995, 2000; International Task Force for Prevention of Coronary Heart Disease 1998; Inter-Society Commission for Heart Disease Resources (ISCHDR), Atherosclerosis Study Group and Epidemiology Study Group 1970; JNC 1993, 1997, 2003; Katz *et al.* 1958; National Cholesterol Education Program 1988, 1990, 1991, 2001, 2002; National Heart, Lung, and Blood Institute 1998*a, b*; National High Blood Pressure Education Program Working Group 1993; National Research Council 1989; Stamler 1966, 1967, 1978, 1979, 1992, 1995, 2003; Stamler and Shekelle 1988; Stamler *et al.* 1993, 1999; USDA, USDHHS 1995, 2000; USDHHS 1988, 1991, 1996, 1998, 1999; Whelton *et al.* 2002, 2003; White *et al.* 1959; WHO 1982, 1990*a, b*, 1997).

Of the six established major risk factors, two – adverse diet and cigarette smoking – are aspects of lifestyle that became mass phenomena in the twentieth century in Western industrialized countries. The other four are traits common in the adult population of these countries as a result of mass consumption of an adverse diet abetted by sedentary lifestyle. Thus, *a population-wide adverse eating pattern is the key aetiologically for five of these six established major risk factors.*

All these risk factors are designated *established* because substantial amounts of data from many disciplines have demonstrated their significant role in the aetiology of epidemic CHD. They are designated *major* for three reasons: their high prevalence in populations, particularly in Western industrialized countries and nowadays often also in other countries; their strong impact on coronary risk; and their preventability and reversibility, primarily by safe improvements in population lifestyles, from conception, gestation, and infancy on. (Age and male gender are known risk factors, but are not amenable to influence and hence are not designated major.)

Adverse diet is pivotal – the primary and essential cause of the coronary epidemic. Without it there is no epidemic even with high prevalence of smoking. Only in populations consuming an adverse diet and exhibiting its metabolic consequences does the important adjuvant (secondary) role of smoking in the aetiology of severe atherosclerotic disease become manifest on a large scale. Adverse diet is habitual fare high in animal products and processed animal products; high in total fat, hydrogenated fat, and separated (visible) fat; high in cholesterol, saturated and trans fatty acids; high in refined and processed sugars; high in salt; high in alcohol for many in the population; high in caloric density, empty calories, and ratio of calories to essential nutrients; relatively low in whole grain products, fruits, vegetables, legumes; hence, relatively low in potassium, magnesium, phosphorus, fibre, and often other essential nutrients, and high in total calories for the low level of energy expenditure in the era of the automobile, television, and mechanized work. This eating pattern and smoking, along with sedentary lifestyle, are unprecedented twentieth-century mass exposures – 'disturbances of human culture' (Virchow) (Ackerknecht 1953) – to which the human species is not adapted by evolution. Habitual adverse diet with little physical activity at work and leisure produces above-optimal population average levels of TC and its adverse components (low-density lipoprotein cholesterol (LDL-C), intermediate-density lipoprotein cholesterol (IDL-C), and very low-density lipoprotein cholesterol (VLDL-C)), of glycaemia, systolic blood pressure/diastolic blood pressure (SBP/DBP), body mass, and below-optimal average levels of HDL from childhood on; for most people a rise in TC, BP, body mass index (BMI), and plasma glucose from youth through middle age; low prevalence of optimal levels in the middle-aged and older population; and high prevalence (progressively through adulthood) of dyslipidemia, overweight/obesity, DM, and adverse BP levels. Along with sedentary habit, adverse diet accounts at the societal level for the pandemic of obesity from childhood on. This pandemic relates importantly – along with adverse diet composition – to dyslipidemia and adverse SBP/DBP levels, and is the main known risk factor for mounting rates of hyperglycaemia/DM (also for hyperuricaemia), including waxing prevalence of non-insulin-dependent diabetes mellitus in young adult, as well as in middle-aged and older, population strata. Moreover, in part because of its high cholesterol content, adverse diet is significantly and independently related to long-term risk of mortality from coronary, cardiovascular, and all causes over and above its unfavourable effects on TC, BP, BMI, and DM.

3.2 Historical overview

Most of the research leading to identification of the major risk factors and elucidation of their role in the aetiology of the atherosclerotic diseases was done in the nineteenth and twentieth centuries, but there are roots reaching back to the 1700s. Thus, in 1727 Brunner described the necropsy findings in the aorta of his 75-year-old father-in-law, Johann Jakob Wepfer (1620–95), discoverer of the relationship of cerebral haemorrhage to apoplexy. Wepfer's aorta was severely atherosclerotic, and Brunner noted: 'The internal coat in several places was ruptured, lacerated and rotten like fruit' (Stamler 1967, p. 42). In 1755 Albrecht von Haller, in a brief essay, also commented on aortic plaques (Stamler 1967, p. 42). On opening into these at autopsy he found a yellow mush effusing between the muscular fibres and the intima. He described this material as soft and pultaceous, not dissimilar to that seen in atheromata. (The word 'atheroma' is derived from the Greek *athere*, meaning mush or gruel. It had been in use since the ancient Greek writers to describe any closed sac or cyst of non-inflammatory origin filled with gruel-like material.) Von Haller noted that the same aorta exhibited multiple plaques, some harder and drier, that is, undergoing fibrotic, cartilaginous, and osseous metaplasia. He inferred that a gradual progression took place from the soft state of atheroma to final bone-like plaque. Thus his special contribution was to focus attention on the softening process (accumulation of 'mush') as of primary significance in atherosclerosis.

In the latter half of the eighteenth century, 'The coronary arteries entered medical thought and literature with the belief held by a brilliant group of English medical men, Jenner, Hunter, Fothergill, and Parry, that those vessels were closely associated with angina pectoris' (Dock 1939; Moriyama *et al.* 1971, p. 326). Jenner described the findings at post-mortem examination of Hunter, who died suddenly at St George's Hospital in 1793 after a 20-year history of recurrent anginal episodes. (At least one of them was too persistent to be called stable angina nowadays – possibly unstable angina or myocardial infarction?) The undersurface of the left auricle and ventricle revealed two areas nearly an inch and a half square which were of a white colour, with an opaque appearance, and entirely distinct from the general surface of the heart. These two areas were covered by an 'exudation of coagulating lymph . . . The coronary arteries had their branches which ramify through the substance of the heart in the state of bony tubes' (Moriyama *et al.* 1971, p. 327). In 1740, Krell had published a treatise on hardening of the coronary arteries (Moriyama *et al.* 1971, p. 323). He stated that the incrustations generally spoken of as ossifications were not bony but of a tophaceous nature, and were derived from atheromatous matter. He made the further point that this induration was not confined to senility but might occur at any period in life.

In the eighteenth century also the compound now known as cholesterol was first described, having been precipitated in crystalline form from alcoholic extracts of gallstones

(Stamler 1967, p. 44). In 1816, Chevreul named it, again from the Greek *chole*, bile, and *steros*, solid. In 1838 Lecanu showed that it was present in human blood, and in 1843 Vogel showed that it was present in atherosclerotic plaques (Stamler 1967, p. 44). In 1857 Mettenheimer noted that the lipoidal 'mush' was doubly refractive because of the presence of cholesterol esters (Stamler 1967, p.44).

During the second half of the nineteenth century, the microscopic studies of cellular pathology, initiated by Virchow and his colleagues, led to the delineation of atherosclerosis as a specific pathological entity in the generic grouping of the arterioscleroses (Katz and Stamler 1953; Marchand 1904; Windaus 1910). This advance stemmed from the elucidation of the unique morphological characteristics of the atherosclerotic plaque, that is, the demonstration that the mushy gruel-like material – the hallmark of the lesion – was an accumulation of lipids, including free and esterified cholesterol. This delineation in turn led to the posing of critical questions: At what stage of atherogenesis does cholesterol–lipid deposition occur? Is this an early primary event or a late secondary event? What is the source of this cholesterol–lipid? Is it derived from blood cholesterol–lipid? What are the relationships among cholesterol–lipid in the diet, the circulating blood, and the lesion? All these questions were posed with more or less clarity by the early years of the twentieth century, and theories of pathogenesis were formulated (Stamler 1967, p. 44).

In the first decade of the twentieth century, the biochemist Windaus demonstrated that atherosclerotic aortas contained six to seven times more free cholesterol, and 20–26 times more cholesterol esters than normal aortas. Over the course of a quarter-century, he also carried out decisive work on the chemical formula and structure of cholesterol (Stamler 1967, p. 44).

Late in the nineteenth and early in the twentieth century, clinical investigators went a step further in elucidating relationships. They showed that several disparate diseases – hypothyroidism, the nephrotic syndrome, essential familial xanthomatosis (as it was then called – now genetic hyperbetalipoproteinaemia), diabetes mellitus – were all characterized by prolonged hypercholesterolaemia and premature severe atherosclerosis (Stamler 1967, p. 47). These observations linked level of blood cholesterol and atherogenesis. In the 1920s, with the emergence of clinical cardiology as a medical specialty and the diagnosis in living patients of myocardial infarction (MI), this link was reinforced and extended by studies showing that people who had recovered from MI had higher mean serum cholesterol levels than controls (Stamler 1967, pp. 47, 49). These reports also noted that hypertension and diabetes were more common in post-MI patients than in controls, and that the great majority of MI cases were men. A related important advance during these early 20th century decades was the demonstration by clinicians in France and the USA that severe high blood pressure and its complications could be controlled with diets markedly reduced in salt (NaCl) (Allen and Sherrill 1922; Ambard and Beaujard 1904; Kempner 1948; Stamler 1997).

In 1908–12, Ignatowski, Anitschkow, and their colleagues serendipitously achieved the experimental production of atherosclerosis (Anitschkow 1933), accomplished initially by feeding rabbits animal products, in an experiment on the effect of dietary animal protein on the kidney. They noted that the sera of their rabbits fed eggs, milk, and meat were grossly hyperlipidaemic and that the arterial lesions were laden with cholesterol and fat. They inferred that the high cholesterol–lipid content, rather than the high protein content, of their experimental diets might be primarily responsible and verified this in subsequent studies by feeding diets supplemented with pure cholesterol plus fat. In the 1920s this group also showed that atherosclerosis could be produced by long-term feeding of diets supplemented with only small amounts of cholesterol, inducing only slight elevations of serum cholesterol; that is, massive hypercholesterolaemia and organ cholesterolosis were not prerequisites for experimental atherogenesis (Anitschkow 1933). Anitschkow emphasized that the critical offending dietary ingredient – the 'materia peccans', as he designated it – was the cholesterol (not the neutral fat or protein) in animal foods.

Late in the nineteenth century and early in the twentieth century 'geographical pathology' – that is, epidemiology – also emerged as a research discipline. Reports were published on populations in Africa, Asia, and Latin America with much less atherosclerotic disease than was prevalent in Europeans. These were, in the main, studies by European investigators discharging medical responsibilities in the colonies. In the early 1930s Rosenthal (1934) reviewed 28 such papers then extant and formulated the inference: 'In no race for which a high cholesterol intake (in the form of eggs, butter and milk) and fat intake are recorded is atherosclerosis absent . . . Where a high protein diet is consumed, which naturally contains small quantities of cholesterol, but where the neutral fat is low, atherosclerosis is not prevalent.' Raab (1932) arrived at similar conclusions based on his survey of this literature. Snapper (1941), describing his experience in China, also emphasized the association between a habitual diet of mainly vegetarian foods, low in cholesterol and fat, and rarity of atherosclerotic disease. Kuczynski (1925) reported on an Asian population at the opposite end of the dietary spectrum – nomadic Kirghiz plainsmen who habitually consumed large amounts of meat and milk. He noted high incidence of obesity, premature extensive atherosclerosis, contracted kidney, apoplexy, and arcus senilis. Their urbanized kinsmen, subsisting on more varied fare, did not exhibit such severe vascular disease. In relation to the famine and severe shortage of dietary fats in Germany immediately after the First World War, Aschoff (1924) noted post-mortem evidence for regression of atherosclerosis. During the early decades of the twentieth century, several reports also appeared on isolated preliterate populations (e.g. in Africa and Asia) with low BPs and with little or no rise in BP with age, high blood pressure (HBP), or hypertensive cardiovascular disease (Shaper 1974). Common characteristics of these populations were leanness and predominantly vegetarian diets low in salt.

In summary, by the 1930s seminal contributions had been published by investigators from all over the world using every method of medical research – gross and microscopic pathology, biochemical pathology, clinical investigation, animal experimentation, and epidemiology (geographical pathology). Nutritional factors, particularly dietary cholesterol–fat and also caloric imbalance with consequent obesity, had been implicated in the aetiology of atherosclerotic disease, and at least in experimental animals had been shown to influence serum lipids, although this relationship remained obscure for the human species. The scientific roots for the rapid growth of knowledge were deep and varied. Once the constraints of the Great Depression and the Second World War were removed, a resurgence of research quickly developed, relying on all that had gone before and rapidly going beyond it. Again, it involved every methodology. The scope of this investigative effort during the first post-war decade is reflected, at least in part, by the bibliographies of two monographs of the 1950s – the first with 713 references and the second with 787 references, the great majority of them original papers published during those years (Katz and Stamler 1953; Katz et al. 1958).

In animal experimental studies, hypercholesterolemia and atherosclerosis of all grades of severity, coronary as well as aortic, were induced by cholesterol–fat feeding (either alone, or in combination with another intervention, e.g. methionine deficiency, hypothyroidism) in virtually every species available to the laboratory: avian and mammalian, omnivorous, herbivorous, or carnivorous, including primates. Lesions were produced in young animals, data that helped lay to rest the notion – widely current for decades – that atherosclerosis was an inevitable consequence of 'normal' (whatever that meant) ageing (Katz and Stamler 1953). In the presence of the nutritional prerequisites for atherogenesis, that is, a cholesterol–fat-supplemented diet, other traits, exogenous and endogenous, were shown to influence the atherosclerotic process significantly (Katz and Stamler 1953; Katz et al. 1958). For example, in chickens with minimal hypercholesterolaemia due to feeding mash containing 0.25% cholesterol plus 5% fat, but not in chickens fed plain mash, BP elevation induced by adding salt to feed resulted in intensified atherogenesis. Also, both exogenous and endogenous oestrogens were shown to prevent and reverse coronary atherosclerosis induced by cholesterol–fat feeding. Such findings underscored both the key role of dietary cholesterol–fat and the multifactorial nature of the aetiology of atherosclerotic disease, including (as in the experiments on feeding both cholesterol–fat and salt) the importance of multiple nutritional factors. The experiments on combined cholesterol and salt feeding had their roots in data from several reports early after the Second World War showing that high salt intake (e.g. in chickens, rats) raised BP – a finding subsequently extended to other species, including chimpanzees, the primate most closely related to the human species (Denton et al. 1995; Laragh and Pecker 1983; Lenel et al. 1948; Meneely 1967; Meneely and Batterbee 1976; Stamler 1997; Tobian 1991).

These years also witnessed the demonstration in several species that arterial plaques gradually regressed after discontinuation of an atherogenic diet. Possible implications for humans of all these advances were virtually self-evident. To deny them either required evidence – not available – that humans were exceptional and hence that the animal findings were not relevant, or rejection of the principles of experimental medicine established by the work of Claude Bernard, Charles Darwin, Louis Pasteur, and other nineteenth-century giants on the unity of the animal kingdom and the relevance of animal research for the aetiology, pathogenesis, prevention, and treatment of human disease.

During this period, important developments also came from biochemical and biophysical laboratories. The ultracentrifuge method for the study of proteins was modified to accomplish flotation of plasma lipoproteins, their separation into several classes, and their quantification. Extensive data were published on their patterns, on factors influencing them, both exogenous (including nutrition) and endogenous, and on their relationships to atherosclerosis in experimental animals and humans (Katz and Stamler 1953; Katz et al. 1958).

The demonstration with isotopes that the characteristic of living organisms is a dynamic equilibrium, that is, a steady state achieved by constant turnover of molecular constituents and not a static state, and the development of tracer methodology with use of multiple isotopes, were extensively applied in atherosclerosis research. Results included the demonstration that cholesterol in atherosclerotic plaques was significantly derived from the circulating cholesterol-bearing lipoproteins of plasma. The painstaking task was accomplished of identifying the sequential steps in the biological synthesis of cholesterol from acetate, and their enzymatic regulation (Bloch 1965).

Clinical investigation demonstrated that serum total cholesterol, S_f 12–20 (low-density) lipoproteins (LDL), and S_f 20–100 (very low-density) lipoproteins (VLDL) were higher in men with a history of MI than in healthy controls, with differences in mean levels greater at younger ages (Lawry et al. 1957). In metabolic ward studies, it was shown that, with maintained weight loss, serum TC, LDL, intermediate-density lipoprotein (IDL), and VLDL all underwent marked sustained reduction (Katz et al. 1958, pp. 48–9, 82–3). This also resulted when people were isocalorically fed diets low in total fat and cholesterol. It was also shown that dietary neutral fats differed in their influences on serum cholesterol; that is saturated fats raised TC whereas unsaturated fats did not, and polyunsaturated fats from both plant and fish sources lowered TC (Katz *et al.* 1958, pp. 50–60). Short-term clinical studies in those years also indicated that high-fat meals induced decreased fibrinolysis and increased blood coagulability, measured *in vitro* (Katz *et al.* 1958, pp. 48–9, 82–3).

Finally, this period witnessed the emergence of cardiovascular epidemiology as a robust independent discipline, fruitfully linked with clinical medicine, physiology, biochemistry, pathology, and anthropology. Early on, several reports were published relating mass nutritional deprivation and other lifestyle changes during the Second World War (e.g. in the Low Countries, Scandinavia, and the USSR) to changes in population serum lipids, blood pressure, thromboembolic disease, atherosclerosis at autopsy, and/or national mortality rates from cardiovascular diseases (Katz and Stamler 1953; Katz *et al.* 1958, p. 30). By the time of the Second World Congress of Cardiology in 1954, sufficient work was in progress in several countries to make possible an international symposium, with published *Proceedings* edited by Ancel Keys and Paul Dudley White (Keys and White 1956). Papers reported on the rarity of severe coronary atherosclerosis and the low incidence of CHD throughout adulthood in both men and women in Japan, in contrast with the USA, and on the low mean serum cholesterol levels in Japanese farmers, industrial workers, and clerks, in contrast with Japanese physicians and Japanese-Americans in Hawaii and Los Angeles. These findings were related to the habitual diet of most Japanese, which was high in vegetable products and low in total lipid. The data on social class differences and on migrants, consonant with old and new findings in other populations (Katz *et al.* 1958, pp. 24–6; Rosenthal 1934), indicated that population genetics could not be a crucial determinant of large inter-population differences in mean TC levels and in atherosclerotic disease.

Japan was quickly recognized to be remarkable among industrialized countries for low CHD rates, and became a focus of research endeavour. Its high death rates from stroke also received attention, and were related to high salt intake and consequent high BP levels. Contrasting group mean levels of TC were also reported for healthy young adult and middle-aged southern Italian men compared with English, Swedish, and American men, and again were shown to correlate with mean dietary lipid intake (Katz *et al.* 1958, pp. 24–6). Striking contrasts – confirming those reported by classical geographical pathology – were also found in studies of Bantu compared with Europeans in South Africa and with Americans, and in rural Guatemalan handicraft and agricultural workers compared with urban Guatemalan and American business and professional men (Katz *et al.* 1958, pp. 20–4). The mean percentage of calories from total fat and from animal fat and the mean serum TC were all much lower in the Bantu and the rural Guatemalans compared with the others; mean serum TC was low at both age 30 and age 45 among the Bantu (167 and 179 mg/dl) in contrast with the higher levels of Americans (192 and 236 mg/dl) and the greater slope with age. Correspondingly, based either on clinical or post-mortem findings, atherosclerotic CHD was rare in the Bantu and the rural Guatemalans, but common in the other groups.

In agreement with these international cross-population findings, it was found that in the USA pure vegetarians – habitually eating fare devoid of cholesterol, lower in saturated fat, and higher in unsaturated fat than omnivores – had a mean serum cholesterol level much lower than that of omnivores, and lower BP (Sacks *et al.* 1974, 1975).

In 1953, data were published on the high prevalence of coronary atherosclerosis in young American soldiers killed in Korea, in contrast with its rarity in Koreans (Enos *et al.* 1953). Later in the decade, in relation to the establishment of the US National Heart Institute and the transformation of the American Heart Association (AHA) from a professional organization to a voluntary health agency, attention was focused on the increase in cardiovascular mortality rates for middle-aged white American men in the period from 1920 to 1955, despite declines in mortality from stroke and from the infectious heart diseases (Moriyama *et al*. 1958). It was concluded that this trend was due to rising CHD mortality rates, and environmental exposures which may have been responsible were noted.

In these years also, four reports were published on international ecological analyses using data from the Food and Agricultural Organization (FAO) on national per capita nutrients and from the WHO on national CHD mortality rates for industrialized countries (Katz *et al*. 1958, pp. 28–30). Several dietary constituents had significant positive correlations with CHD death rates in univariate analyses, including total calories and percentage of calories from total fat, animal fat, and animal protein; percentage of calories from vegetable fat, vegetable protein, and carbohydrate had significant inverse correlations with CHD death rates. None of these initial reports gave data on dietary cholesterol and CHD death rates, despite the compelling evidence from animal experimentation on the critical role of dietary cholesterol in the aetiology of severe atherosclerosis. When such analyses were performed in subsequent years, a significant positive relationship was shown in not only univariate but also bivariate (controlled for other dietary constituents) analyses and in trend analyses (Byington *et al*. 1979; Liu *et al*. 1982; Stamler 1979).

During this post-war period, there was a completely new development in cardiovascular epidemiology of major importance: the undertaking of long-term prospective within-population studies. In the latter 1950s, these investigation reported their first findings, relating several characteristics of individuals at baseline to CHD incidence and/or mortality during the next 3–5 years – in particular, in one or more studies, high serum TC, high LDL, high BP, obesity, cigarette smoking, and sedentary occupation (American Journal of Public Health 1957; Gofman *et al*. 1956; Hammond and Horn 1958; Katz *et al*. 1958; Morris *et al*. 1953). These data on the prognostic implications of these traits focused attention on their high prevalence in the middle-aged population, and in the USA it was noted that high mean values of serum cholesterol, SBP and DBP, and body mass (relative weight) were present in middle-aged men and women from all samples of the general population under study, irrespective of geographical locale, ethnicity, or socio-economic status. Relative weight was shown to be related to both BP and TC, but it was clear that the high cholesterol, high saturated fat *composition* of the habitual diet was playing a key role in determining population serum lipid–lipoprotein patterns. The prospective data also led to the recognition that observed values in populations of apparently healthy people – their means ±2.0 standard deviations – were not a sound basis for identifying 'normal' values. In addition, they stimulated interest in the definition of *optimal* values associated with low probabilities of developing cardiovascular disease over the years.

Based on all these concordant findings and discussions about their implications for coping with rising CHD rates, publicly described as epidemic in onslaught, the term *risk factor* began to be used in the late 1950s to describe traits assessed to be aetiologically significant in predisposing people to heart attack and stroke (Stamler *et al*. 1959). Concurrently, researchers in the UK, Finland, and the USA undertook the first trials on ability to achieve primary or secondary prevention of CHD by diet means, and the present author initiated the first trial involving multifactorial intervention to control all the major risk factors (Katz *et al*. 1958; Stamler 1967). All these, with small sample sizes (due mainly to limited funding) and with other design flaws, were in retrospect pilot projects, but they were also pioneering undertakings that set the stage for later trials and for population-wide preventive efforts. At the end of this eventful decade, in 1959, the first statement was addressed to the public on the risk factors – (1) obesity, (2) elevated blood cholesterol, (3) elevated blood pressure, (4) cigarette smoking, and (5) heredity – and the possibility of safely influencing the first four of them and thereby of preventing heart attacks and strokes (White *et al.* 1959). The initiators of this statement were senior American cardiologists, cardiovascular researchers, and medical statesmen, several of them past presidents of the AHA.

Not long after this 'Statement on Arteriosclerosis', the AHA published its first reports on the possibility of preventing the atherosclerotic diseases by not smoking and by improving eating habits. Its statement, 'Dietary fat and its relation to heart attacks and strokes' summarized the research evidence on the major risk factors, and then reviewed dietary recommendations – decreased intake of cholesterol, saturated fat, and (for overweight people) calories, and partial replacement of saturated fats by unsaturates, including polyunsaturates – aimed at 'a considerable alteration in the cholesterol level in the blood with the use of acceptable diets' (American Heart Association 1961). In paragraphs under the heading 'Who in particular should modify fat content of his diet?', this report concluded:

> Most persons in the United States who are overweight . . . Men with a strong family history of atherosclerotic heart or blood vessel disease, who have elevated blood cholesterol levels, an increase in blood pressure, are overweight and/or who lead sedentary lives of relentless frustrations . . . Those people who have had one or more atherosclerotic heart attacks . . .

Thus, this was a recommendation directed at tens of millions of higher-risk American adults. It was a fitting culmination of more than a decade of major research that led to the initial explicit pinpointing of major risk factors as important causes of the epidemic atherosclerotic diseases. It launched nationwide efforts in the USA for their prevention, primary and secondary, with reliance first and foremost on safe improvements in lifestyles.

These first two statements on prevention of the atherosclerotic diseases did not explicitly present a population-wide approach. That came a few years later, when the AHA updated its statements; in the 'Report on the Primary Prevention of the Atherosclerotic Diseases by the Inter-Society Commission for Heart Disease Resources'; in Scandinavian public health statements (ISCHDR 1970; National Heart, Lung, and Blood Institute 1981; Stamler 1979, 1981), and – under the leadership of Geoffrey Rose – as a fully developed **combined population-wide and high-risk strategy** in the report of the WHO Expert Committee on the Prevention of Coronary Heart Disease (WHO 1982).

Postscript: 2004

This up-dated chapter for the second edition of this monograph was completed in draft on 11 April 2004 – almost 13 months into the Iraq War launched by George W. Bush on 19 March 2003, and almost 12 months after he declared major combat operations in Iraq at an end on 1 May 2003. Today, Easter Sunday, 11 April 2004, the front-page headline on columns 1 and 2 of *The New York Times* is, '**U.S. Prepares a Prolonged Drive To Suppress the Uprisings in Iraq**'. The eight-column headline across page 1 of *Week in Review* is '**War's Full Fury is Suddenly Everywhere**'. As American Major General David H. Petraeus put it repeatedly to reporter Rick Atkinson in the field a year earlier, 'Tell me how this ends?' – the unanswered question before and since this war was launched.

In this situation, the original Postscript – for the first edition – remains all too relevant.

Postscript: 1991

The chapter was completed on 9 February 1991 – 24 days into the Gulf War. Leaders of the major powers, focused on waging war, have even less time than heretofore – and even less resources – to devote to prevention and control of epidemic diseases. Their will is elsewhere. But humanitarianism, and the goal of Bacon and Pasteur that science be applied to benefit mankind, can and must prevail, just as peace can and must prevail. The unremitting and skilful pursuit of these goals is the highest sign of objectivity and dedication in a medical scientist. Precisely because Geoffrey Rose epitomizes these qualities, it is a signal honour to write a chapter in this volume celebrating him.

Bibliography

Ackerknecht, E. H. (1953). *Rudolf Virchow: doctor, statesman, anthropologist*. University of Wisconsin Press, Madison, WI.

Allen, F. M. and Sherrill, J. W. (1922). The treatment of arterial hypertension. *Journal of Metabolic Research*, **2**, 429–545.

Ambard, L. and Beaujard, E. (1904). Causes of arterial hypertension. *Archives of General Medicine*, I, 520–33.

American Heart Association (1961). Dietary fat and its relation to heart attacks and strokes. *Circulation*, **23**, 133–6.

American Heart Association (1980). American Heart Association Committee Report. Risk factors and coronary diseases: a statement for physicians. *Circulation*, **62**, 449A–455A.

American Heart Association (1998). American Heart Association call to action: obesity as a major risk factor for coronary heart disease. *Circulation*, **97**, 2099–100.

American Heart Association (2000). AHA dietary guidelines. Revision 2000. A statement for healthcare professionals from the Nutrition Committee of the American Heart Association. *Circulation*, **102**, 2284–99.

American Journal of Public Health (1957). Measuring the risk of coronary heart disease in adult population groups: a symposium. *American Journal of Public Health*, **Part 2**, 1–63.

Anitschkow, N. (1933). Experimental arteriosclerosis in animals. In *Arteriosclerosis* (ed. E. V. Cowdry), pp. 271–322. Macmillan, New York.

Aschoff, L. (1924). *Lectures in pathology*. Hoeber, New York.

Bloch, K. (1965). The biological synthesis of cholesterol. *Science*, **150**, 19–28.

Byington, R., Dyer, A. R., Garside, D., Liu, K., Moss, D., Stamler, J., and Tsong, Y. (1979). Recent trends of major coronary risk factors and CHD mortality in the United States and other industrialized countries. In *Proceedings of the Conference on the Decline in Coronary Heart Disease Mortality* (ed. R. J. Havlik and M. Feinleib), pp. 340–80. National Institutes of Health publication 79-1610. National Institutes of Health, Washington, DC.

Denton, D., Weisinger, R., Mundy, N. I., Wickings, E. J., Dixon, A., Moisson, P. *et al.* (1995). The effect of increased salt intake on blood pressure of chimpanzees. *Nature Medicine*, **1**, 1009–16.

Department of Health (1994). *Nutritional aspects of cardiovascular disease: report of the Cardiovascular Review Group, Committee on Medical Aspects of Food Policy*. Report on Health and Social Subjects No. 46. HMSO, London.

Dietary Guidelines Advisory Committee (1995). *Report of the Dietary Guidelines Advisory Committee on the dietary guidelines for Americans*. US Government Printing Office, Washington, DC.

Dietary Guidelines Advisory Committee (2000). *Scientific rationale: dietary guidelines for Americans*. US Government Printing Office, Washington, DC.

Dock, G. (1939). Historical notes on coronary occlusion: from Heberden to Osler. *Journal of the American Medical Association*, **113**, 563–8.

Enos, W. F. Jr., Holmes, R. H., and Beyer, J. (1953). Coronary disease among United States soldiers killed in action in Korea. *Journal of the American Medical Association*, **152**, 1090–3.

Gofman, J. W., Andrus, E. C., Hanig, M., Jones, H. B., Lauffer, M. A., Lawrey, E. Y. *et al.* (1956). Evaluation of serum lipoprotein and cholesterol measurements as predictors of clinical complications of atherosclerosis: report of a cooperative study of lipoproteins and atherosclerosis. *Circulation*, **144** (2), 691–744.

Hammond, E. G. and Horn, D. (1958). Smoking and death rates: report on 44 months of follow-up of 187,783 men. *Journal of the American Medical Association*, **166**, 1159–72.

International Task Force for Prevention of Coronary Heart Disease in Cooperation with the International Atherosclerosis Society (1998). Coronary heart disease: reducing the risk. The scientific background for primary and secondary prevention of coronary heart disease. *Nutrition, Metabolism and Cardiovascular Disease*, **8**, 205–71.

ISCHDR (Inter-Society Commission for Heart Disease Resources, Atherosclerosis Study Group and Epidemiology Study Group) (1970). Primary prevention of the atherosclerotic diseases. *Circulation*, **42**, A55–A95.

JNC-V. National High Blood Pressure Education Program (1993). The Fifth Report of the Joint National Committee on Detection, Evaluation, and Treatment of High Blood Pressure (JNC-V). *Archives of Internal Medicine*, **153**, 154–83.

JNC-VI. National High Blood Pressure Education Program (1997). The Sixth Report of the Joint National Committee on Detection, Evaluation, and Treatment of High Blood Pressure (JNC-VI). *Archives of Internal Medicine*, **157**, 2413–46.

JNC-VII. Chobanian, A.V., Bakris, G. L., Black, H. R., Cushman, W. C., Green, L. A., Izzo, J. L. Jr *et al.* (2003). The Seventh Report of the Joint National Committee on Detection, Evaluation, and Treatment of High Blood Pressure (JNC-VII). National High Blood Pressure Education Program. *Hypertension*, **42**, 1206–52.

Katz, L. N. and Stamler, J. (1953). *Experimental atherosclerosis*. C. Thomas, Springfield, IL.

Katz, L. N., Stamler, J., and Pick. R. (1958). *Nutrition and atherosclerosis*. Lea and Febiger, Philadelphia.

Kempner, W. (1948). Treatment of hypertensive vascular disease with a rice diet. *American Journal of Medicine*, **4**, 545–77.

Keys, A. and White, P. D. (eds) (1956). *World trends in cardiology: cardiovascular epidemiology*. Selected papers from the Second World Congress and Twenty-Seventh Annual Scientific Sessions of the American Heart Association. Hoeber-Harper, New York.

Kuczynski, B. (1925). Pathologische-geographische untersuchungen in der kirgesisch-dsungarischen steppe. *Klinische Wochenschrift*, **4**, 39.

Laragh, J. H. and Pecker, M. S. (1983). Dietary sodium and essential hypertension: some myths, hopes and truths. *Annals of Internal Medicine*, **98** (2), 735–43.

Lawry, E. Y., Mann, G. V., Peterson, A., Wysocki, A. P., O'Connell, R., and Stare, F. J. (1957). Cholesterol and betalipoproteins in the serum of Americans: well persons and those with coronary heart disease. *American Journal of Medicine*, **22**, 605–23.

Lenel, R., Katz, L. N., and Rodbard, S. (1948). Arterial hypertension in the chicken. *American Journal of Physiology*, **152**, 557–62.

Liu, K., Stamler, J., Trevisan, M., and Moss, D. (1982). Dietary lipids, sugar, fiber and mortality from coronary heart disease: bivariate analysis of international data. *Arteriosclerosis*, **2**, 221–7.

Marchand, F. (1904). Über arteriosklerose (athersklerose). *Verhandelingen der Deutschen Gesellschaft fur Innere Medizin*, **21**, 23.

Meneely, G. R. (1967). The experimental epidemiology of sodium chloride toxicity in the rat. In *The epidemiology of hypertension* (ed. J. Stamler, R. Stamler, and T. N. Pullman), pp. 240–6. Grune and Stratton, New York.

Meneely, G. R. and Battarbee, H. D. (1976). High sodium-low potassium environment and hypertension. *American Journal of Cardiology*, **38**, 768–85.

Moriyama, I., Woolsey, T., and Stamler, J. (1958). Observations on possible causative factors responsible for the sex and race trends in cardiovascular-renal disease mortality in the United States. *Journal of Chronic Diseases*, **7**, 401–12.

Moriyama, I., Krueger, D. E., and Stamler, J. (1971). *Cardiovascular diseases in the United States*. Harvard University Press, Cambridge, MA.

Morris, J. N., Heady, J. H., Raffle, P. A. B., Roberts, C. G., and Parks, J. W. (1953). Coronary heart disease and physical activity of work. *Lancet*, **265** (6795), 1053–7, 1111–20.

National Cholesterol Education Program (1988). Report of the NCEP Expert Panel on Detection, Evaluation, and Treatment of High Blood Cholesterol in Adults. *Archives of Internal Medicine*, **148**, 36–69.

National Cholesterol Education Program (1990). *Report of the NCEP Expert Panel on Population Strategies for Blood Cholesterol Reduction*. NIH Publication No. 90-3046. US Department of Health and Human Services, Public Health Services, Washington, DC.

National Cholesterol Education Program (1991). *Report of the NCEP Expert Panel on Cholesterol Levels in Children and Adolescents*. NIH Publication No. 91-2732. National Institutes of Health, National Heart, Lung and Blood Institute, Bethesda, MD.

National Cholesterol Education Program (2001). Adult Treatment Panel III (ATP III). Executive Summary of the third report of the NCEP Expert Panel on Detection, Evaluation and Treatment of High Blood Cholesterol in Adults. *Journal of the American Medical Association*, **285**, 2486–97.

National Cholesterol Education Program (2002). *Third Report of the NCEP Expert Panel on Detection, Evaluation and Treatment of High Blood Cholesterol in Adults (Adult Treatment Panel III)*. NIH Publication No. 02-5215. National Institutes of Health, Washington, DC.

National Heart, Lung, and Blood Institute (1981). Working Group on Arteriosclerosis of the National Heart, Lung, and Blood Institute. *Arteriosclerosis*, Vol. 2, National Institutes of Health, Bethesda, MD.

National Heart, Lung, and Blood Institute (1998a). *The DASH diet*. NIH Publication No. 01-4082. US Department of Health and Human Services, Public Health Service, National Institutes of Health. National Heart, Lung, and Blood Institute, Bethesda, MD.

National Heart, Lung, and Blood Institute (1998b). NHLBI Obesity Education Initiative Expert Panel on the Identification, Evaluation, and Treatment of Overweight and Obesity in Adults. *Clinical guidelines on the identification, evaluation and treatment of overweight and obesity in adults: the evidence report*. NIH Publication No. 98-4083. National Institutes of Health, Bethesda, MD.

National High Blood Pressure Education Program Working Group (1993). National High Blood Pressure Education Program Working Group Report on Primary Prevention of Hypertension. *Archives of Internal Medicine*, **153**, 186–208.

National Research Council (1989). Committee on Diet and Health, Food and Nutrition Board, Commission on Life Sciences. *Diet and health: implications for reducing chronic disease*. National Academy Press, Washington, DC.

Raab, W. (1932). Alimentare faktoren in der enstehung von arteriosklerose und hypertonie. *Medizinische Klinik*, **28**, 487–521.

Rosenthal, S. R. (1934). Studies in atherosclerosis: chemical, experimental and morphologic. *Archives of Pathology*, **18**, 473–506, 660–98, 827–42.

Sacks, F. M., Rosner, B., and Kass, E. H. (1974). Blood pressure in vegetarians. *American Journal of Epidemiology*, **100**, 390–8.

Sacks, F. M., Castelli, W. P., Donner, A., and Kass, E. H. (1975). Plasma lipids and lipoproteins in vegetarians and controls. *New England Journal of Medicine*, **292**, 1148–51.

Shaper, A. G. (1974). Communities without hypertension. In *Cardiovascular disease in the tropics* (ed. A. G. Shaper, M. S. R. Hutt, and Z. Fejfar), pp. 77–83. British Medical Association, London.

Snapper, I. (1941). *Chinese lessons to Western medicine*. Interscience, New York.

Stamler, J. (1966). Nutrition, metabolism and atherosclerosis: a review of data and theories, and a discussion of controversial questions. In *Controversy in internal medicine* (ed. F. J. Inglefinger, A. L. Relman, and M. Finland), pp. 27–59. Saunders, Philadelphia.

Stamler, J. (1967). *Lectures on preventive cardiology*. Grune and Stratton, New York.

Stamler, J. (1978). George Lyman Duff Memorial Lecture: lifestyles, major risk factors, proof and public policy. *Circulation*, 58, 3–19.

Stamler, J. (1979). Population studies. In *Nutrition, lipids, and coronary heart disease: a global view* (ed. R. I. Levy, B. M. Rifkind, B. H. Dennis, and N. D Ernst), pp. 25–88, Raven Press, New York.

Stamler, J. (1981). Primary prevention of epidemic premature atherosclerotic coronary heart disease. In *Progress in Cardiology*, vol. 19 (ed. P. M. Yu and J. F. Goodwin), pp. 63–100, Rea and Febiger, Philadelphia, PA.

Stamler, J. (1992). Established major coronary risk factors. In *Coronary heart disease epidemiology: from aetiology to public health* (ed. M. Marmot and P. Elliott), pp. 35–66. Oxford University Press, New York.

Stamler, J. (1995). Potential for prevention of major adult cardiovascular disease. In *Lessons for science from the Seven Countries Study: a 35-year collaborative experience in cardiovascular disease epidemiology*. (ed. H. Toshima, Y. Koga, H. Blackburn, and A. Keys), pp. 195–235. Springer-Verlag, Tokyo.

Stamler, J. (1997). The INTERSALT Study: background, methods, findings, and implications. *American Journal of Clinical Nutrition*, 65, 626S–642S.

Stamler, J. (guest ed.) (2003). Special Issue: INTERMAP: International study of macro- and micronutrients and blood pressure. *Journal of Human Hypertension*, 17, 585–775.

Stamler, J. and Shekelle, R. (1988). Dietary cholesterol and human coronary heart disease: the epidemiologic evidence. *Archives of Pathology and Laboratory Medicine*, 112, 1032–40.

Stamler, J., Lindberg, H. A., Berkson, D. M., Shaffer, A., Miller, W., and Poindexter, A. (with the assistance of M. Colwell and Y. Hall) (1959). Epidemiological analysis of hypertension and hypertensive disease in the labor force of a Chicago utility company. In *Hypertension*, Vol. VII, *Drug action, epidemiology and hemodynamics: Proceedings of the Council for High Blood Pressure Research, American Heart Association* (ed. F. R. Skelton), pp. 23–50. American Heart Association, New York.

Stamler, J., Dyer, A. R., Shekelle, R. B., Neaton, J., and Stamler, R. (1993). Relationship of baseline major risk factors to coronary and all-cause mortality, and to longevity: findings from long-term follow-up of Chicago cohorts. *Cardiology*, 82, 191–222.

Stamler, J., Stamler, R., Neaton, J., Wentworth, D., Daviglus, M. L., Garside, D. *et al.* (1999). Low risk factor profile and long-term cardiovascular and non-cardiovascular mortality and life expectancy: findings for five large cohorts of young adult and middle-aged men and women. *Journal of the American Medical Association*, 282, 2012–18.

Thannhauser, S. J. (1950). *Lipidoses: diseases of the cellular lipid metabolism*. 2nd edn (ed. H. A. Christian), Oxford University Press, New York.

Tobian, L. (1991). Salt and hypertension: lessons from animal models that relate to human hypertension. *Hypertension*, 17 (Suppl. I), I-52–I-58.

USDA, USDHHS (US Department of Agriculture, US Department of Health and Human Services) (1995). *Dietary guidelines for Americans*, 4th edn. US Government Printing Office, Washington, DC.

USDA, USDHHS (US Department of Agriculture, US Department of Health and Human Services) (2000). *Dietary guidelines for Americans*. US Government Printing Office, Washington, DC.

USDHHS (US Department of Health and Human Services) (1988). *The Surgeon General's report on nutrition and health*. US Government Printing Office. Washington, DC.

USDHHS (US Department of Health and Human Services) (1991). *Healthy people 2000: national health promotion and disease prevention objectives (summary report)*. DHSS Publication No. (PHS) 91-50213. US Government Printing Office, Washington, DC.

USDHHS (US Department of Health and Human Services) (1996). *Physical activity and health: a Report of the Surgeon General.* US Department of Health and Human Services, Centers for Disease Control and Prevention, National Center for Chronic Disease Prevention and Health Promotion, Atlanta, GA.

USDHHS (US Department of Health and Human Services) (1998). Office of Public Health and Science. *Healthy people 2010 objectives: draft for public comment.* US Government Printing Office, Washington, DC.

USDHHS (US Department of Health and Human Services) (1999). *Healthy people 2000 review, 1998–1999.* Publication Number (PS) 99-1256. Department of Health and Human Services, Centers for Disease Control and Prevention, National Center for Health Statistics, Hyattsville, MD.

Whelton, P. K., He, J., and Louis, G. T. (eds) (2003). *Lifestyle modifications for the prevention and treatment of hypertension.* Marcel Dekker, New York.

Whelton, P. K., He, J., Appel, L. J., Cutler, J. A., Havas, S., Kotchen, T. A. *et al.* for the National High Blood Pressure Education Program Coordinating Committee (2002). Primary prevention of hypertension: clinical and public health advisory from the National High Blood Pressure Education Program. *Journal of the American Medical Association,* **288**, 1882–8.

White, P. D., Sprague, H. B., Stamler, J., Stare, F. J., Wright, J. S., Katz, L. N. *et al.* (1959). *A statement on arteriosclerosis, main cause of 'heart attacks' and 'strokes'.* National Health Education Council, New York.

Windaus, A. (1910). Über den gehalt normaler und atheromatoser aorten an cholesterin und cholesterinester. *Zeitschrift für Physiologische Chemie,* **67**, 174.

WHO (World Health Organization) (1982). WHO Expert Committee on the Prevention of Coronary Heart Disease. *Prevention of coronary heart disease.* World Health Organization Technical Report Series, 678. WHO, Geneva.

WHO (World Health Organization) (1990a). WHO Expert Committee on the Prevention in Childhood and Youth of Adult Cardiovascular Disease. *Prevention in childhood and youth of adult cardiovascular diseases – time for action: report of a WHO Expert Committee.* World Health Organization Technical Report Series, 792. WHO, Geneva.

WHO (World Health Organization) (1990b). WHO Study Group. *Diet, nutrition, and the prevention of chronic diseases.* World Health Organization Technical Report Series, 797. WHO, Geneva.

WHO (World Health Organization) (1997). *Obesity: preventing and managing the global epidemic.* WHO, Geneva.

Chapter 4

Current status: six established major risk factors – and low risk

J. Stamler, J. D. Neaton, D. B. Garside, and M. L. Daviglus

4.1 Introduction

This chapter has two interrelated purposes:

1 To update information on the six established major coronary heart disease–cardiovascular disease (CHD–CVD) risk factors, their impact and importance, singly and especially in combination.

2 To highlight the decisive role of low risk, that is, favourable findings for all major risk factors – decisive for individuals and for populations. In our judgement, the data now available on the benefits of low risk (see below) are the culmination of the decades-long research on risk factors. The concept of low risk and its decisive significance looms larger even than the concept of major risk factors. It is a concept epitomizing the basic thrust set down in Geoffrey Rose's seminal 1992 monograph *The strategy of preventive medicine* (Rose 1992). To grasp this concept and to apply it successfully in medical care and public health is to 'reach for the jugular' of the CHD–CVD epidemic.

Space limitations preclude even a brief survey of the prodigious research output during the last decades, right up to the present. Such a survey would not be feasible even if the writers were to ignore the important contributions of animal experimentation, pathological investigation, clinical research, and molecular and cell biology, and confine themselves to epidemiology. Suffice it here to highlight findings from cross-population and within-population epidemiological research, standing on the shoulders of prior ground-breaking contributions (see Chapter 3), and to call attention to more recent extensive bibliographies (generally not all-encompassing), in monographs and reviews (American Heart Association 1980, 2000; Barker 1998; Berenson 1986; Chobanian *et al.* 2003; Clarke *et al.* 1997; Department of Health 1994; Dietary Guidelines Advisory Committee 1995, 2000; Fraser 1986; International Task Force for Prevention of Coronary Heart Disease 1998; JNC-V 1993; JNC-VI 1997; Lauer *et al.* 2005; McGill *et al.* 2000; National Cholesterol Education Program 1988, 1990, 1991, 2002; National Heart, Lung, and Blood Institute 1981, 1998*a*, *b*; National High Blood Pressure Education Program Working Group 1993; National Research Council 1989; Pearson 1984; Prospective Studies Collaboration 2002; Stamler 1989, 1994, 1995, 1997, 2003; Stamler and Shekelle 1988; Stamler *et al.* 1993*a*, *b*, 1994, 1997*a*, *b*, *c*, 1999; USDHHS 1988, 1991, 1996, 1998, 1999, 2000; Whelton *et al.* 2002, 2003; WHO 1982, 1990*a*, *b*, 1997).

4.2 **Cross-population studies**

The literature includes reports on five types of cross-population (ecological) investigations:

1 Multiple analyses of FAO–WHO data on relationships between national nutritional and mortality patterns.

2 Analyses of autopsy findings from different countries, and factors related to these findings, including comprehensive data from the International Atherosclerosis Project on over 31000 decedents from 15 cities and countries, two of them highly industrialized (New Orleans and Oslo), and the other 13 non-industrialized low-income areas in Africa, the Far East, and Latin America.

3 Field investigations of population samples in different countries, including the Seven Countries Study led by Ancel Keys and the INTERSALT Study.

4 International studies on effects of migration, including the Ni-Hon-San Study and the INTERLIPID Study on Japanese in Japan and Japanese-Americans in Hawaii and California.

5 Comparisons of populations within countries.

These reports are consistent in finding relationships among population nutritional patterns (particularly dietary cholesterol–lipid), population mean serum lipids, and population CHD rates. Some also encompassed data on such variables as cigarette use, blood pressure–high blood pressure (BP–HBP), and diabetes, and found them to be associated with CHD rates across populations.

An important advance in this recent period has been expansion of the focus of international cross-population research, to go beyond work on the three-way relation among dietary lipids, serum lipids, and atherosclerotic disease, and address the long-neglected problem of nutritional factors as they influence systolic/diastolic BP (SBP/DBP), and possibly account for the rise in BP from youth through middle age, common in most populations. For example, with 52 population samples aged 20–59 (each ~200 people) from 32 countries worldwide, the INTERSALT Study showed that sample median 24-h sodium excretion (measure of dietary salt – NaCl – intake) was significantly related to five SBP/DBP variables independent of age, gender, body mass index (BMI), and alcohol intake: sample median SBP and DBP, sample upward slope of SBP and DBP from youth through middle age (e.g. over the 30 years from ages 25 to 55), and sample prevalence of high BP (Table 4.1) (Elliott *et al.* 1996; INTERSALT 1988; Stamler 1997).

A comment on this ecological aspect of epidemiological research may be useful. It has been asserted that such investigations serve only the purpose of formulating hypotheses for further research, with the implication that they have no other relevance in regard to central issues of causation. This is unsound, since *every* analysis relating one variable to another is by its nature based on a question; that is, at that stage it is already the exploration of a hypothesis. Studies of this type, like *all* other studies using whatever methodology, have their strengths and weaknesses, their possibilities and limitations, as discussed elsewhere (Stamler 1989). They should no more be 'put down' than any other type of investigation. In judging the crucial issue of aetiology of major chronic diseases, one must assess the *totality* of the data; nothing else suffices.

Specifically as to cross-population ecological studies, the judgement has been advanced by a senior colleague that when cross-population data show significant positive relationships and within-population data based on individuals do not, it is likely that the former, rather than the latter, are valid reflections of the real world (Hegsted 1985). When *within*-population studies are conducted in a way to minimize methodological limitations in *that* type of research, findings of

Table 4.1 Multiple linear regression coefficients for relation of sample median 24 h sodium excretion to sample BP indices: tests of the INTERSALT prior ecologic hypotheses[a]

Dependent variable	Adjusted for age and sex	Adjusted for age, sex, BMI, and alcohol
SBP slope with age (mmHg over 30 years with 100 mmol/day greater Na intake)	+9.0***	+10.2***
DBP slope with age (mmHg over 30 years with 100 mmol/day greater Na intake)	+6.3***	+6.3***
Median SBP (mmHg with 100 mmol/day greater Na intake)	+7.1***	+4.5***
Median DBP (mmHg with 100 mmol/day greater Na intake)	+3.8**	2.3[b]
Hypertension prevalence with 100 mmol/day greater Na intake[c]	+6.2**	4.8*

[a] n = all 52 INTERSALT population samples. (From Stamler 1997.)

[b] $p = 0.08$; *$p < 0.05$; **$p < 0.01$; ***$p < 0.001$.

[c] Hypertension is defined as SBP $\geq$ 140 mmHg, DBP $\geq$ 90 mmHg, or receiving antihypertensive drugs. Units of prevalence are percentage points.

cross- and within-population studies are likely to be concordant. A case in point is the relation of dietary lipid to serum total cholesterol (TC). A significant positive association was demonstrated decades ago in ecological studies across populations (as well as in animal experiments and clinical intervention studies), but not for individuals in within-population studies. For years this seemingly irreconcilable contradiction was emphasized by some to cast doubt on the validity of the relationship – until it was shown that there was marked within-individual day-by-day variation in eating patterns making it difficult to characterize individuals validly within more or less homogeneous groups and to rank them in regard to nutrient intake (Liu *et al.* 1978). It was soon recognized that this was at the root of the 'non-significant' findings in within-population studies. Lack of appreciation of this problem and of other sources of bias accounts for several false negative reports from within-population studies on dietary lipid and serum cholesterol, and on dietary lipid and CHD. As is now more widely understood, this methodological problem is soluble by in-depth procedures for assessing diets of individuals and/or by study designs involving large sample sizes (Elliott 1989; INTERSALT 1988; Stamler 1997, 2003).

4.3 Within-population studies

A review published in 1981 cited 57 papers on within-population studies reporting multivariate analyses on the combined impact of the major risk factors on CHD risk (National Heart, Lung, and Blood Institute 1981). It presented prospective data from more than 65 cohorts in 23 countries on four continents, reflecting a remarkable worldwide expansion of epidemiological research during the 1960s and 1970s. In the last 20+ years, many of these studies have contiued long-term surveillance of their cohorts and have reported additional results, including data based on 15, 25, 30, or more years of follow-up. In addition, other within-population investigations have been undertaken and have presented findings, for example on the MONICA cohorts in 20 countries; the ARIC Study cohorts in the USA; Chinese cohorts, for example, from the PRC-USA Cooperative Study on Cardiovascular and Cardiopulmonary Epidemiology; INTERSALT and INTERMAP population samples. The Prospective Studies Collaboration recently published a meta-analysis dealing with almost 1 000 000 adults from 61 longitudinal investigations, a comprehensive but not all-inclusive set (Prospective Studies Collaboration 2002).

Most of the studies reporting multivariate analyses on baseline traits and CHD risk have dealt with only five of the six established major risk factors, that is, serum cholesterol, blood pressure, cigarette smoking, body mass, and diabetes, but not diet. Only a small minority of these studies, far too few unfortunately, had resources permitting them to undertake assessments of the eating patterns of their individual participants. Some did this several years after their baseline examination, with consequent possible bias, for example due to change in diet by participants made aware at entry of high serum cholesterol and/or high BP (Shekelle et al. 1982). Some used only a single 24-h dietary recall with consequent sizeable error in classification (arraying) of individuals (e.g. on dietary cholesterol–fat intake) and marked attenuation in observed associations (e.g. between dietary lipids and TC, CHD) (Liu et al. 1978). Only a few studies evaluated eating habits of their participants at entry, hence at a relatively bias-free point and with in-depth methodology, for example multiple 24-h dietary recalls or Burke-type comprehensive standardized interviews on usual dietary pattern with cross-checks (Burke 1947; Shekelle et al. 1981; Stamler 2003; Stamler and Shekelle 1988), to permit reasonably valid ranking of individuals with regard to nutrient intake.

Among the within-population prospective investigations reporting data on four or five major risk factors, two are of special value because of their large sample sizes: the Multiple Risk Factor Intervention Trial (MRFIT) primary screenee cohort of 361 662 men aged 35–57 years at baseline, who were screened by standardized methods in 18 US cities in 1973–75 (Daviglus et al. 2004b; Neaton et al. 1984; Stamler et al. 1986, 1993a) and the Chicago Heart Association Detection Project in Industry (CHA) cohort totalling almost 40 000 men and women aged 18–74. (No diet data were collected.) Prospective findings on the mortality of these cohorts are now available based on 25 and 30 years of follow-up. The particular merit of these data – especially the MRFIT data – is their precision; owing to very large sample size, confidence intervals (CIs) around mortality rates are narrow.

4.4 Relation of each major risk factor considered singly to CHD mortality

Table 4.2 gives detailed data on the relation of major risk factors considered singly to long-term CHD risk, for MRFIT men baseline ages 35–44 (mean age 39.6, follow-up 25 years), and CHA men and women baseline ages 18–39 (mean ages 29.7 and 26.8, follow-up 30 years). Concurrent analyses show similar findings for MRFIT men baseline ages 45–57 and CHA men and women baseline ages 40–59 (see below).

4.4.1 Serum total cholesterol

For both male cohorts, the multivariate-adjusted relationship of baseline serum total cholesterol to CHD mortality is continuous (from <160 through 280+ mg/dl), graded (exponential), strong, independent, statistically significant ($p < 0.001$). Particularly for the younger CHA cohort, the relationship is stronger, as reflected in the Cox proportional hazards regression coefficient of 0.0132, than generally reported for middle-aged men, that is, about double in size (cf. Table 4.3 below). With a level 35 mg/dl higher (~1 standard deviation (SD)), hazard ratio (HR) is 1.59 for CHA men and 1.30 for MRFIT men. For the cohort of 6741 younger CHA women, with only 35 CHD deaths in 30 years, caution is in order in interpretation of the data on risk factor–CHD relationships. Thus, while the quantile data indicate a continuous, graded, strong, independent TC–CHD relationship and the Cox coefficient – hence also the HR – is almost the same quantitatively as for the MRFIT men, it is not statistically significant.

Table 4.2 Relationship of major risk factors considered singly to long-term risk of CHD death, for men and women aged 18–44 at baseline

Major risk factor level	CHA men aged 18–39[a]			CHA women aged 18–39[a]			MRFIT men aged 35–44[b]		
	n	Death rate[c]	HR[d]	n	Death rate[c]	HR[d]	n	Death rate[c]	HR[e]
Baseline serum cholesterol (mg/dl)[f]									
<160	2070	3.2	1.00	1919	1.1	1.00	11850	3.4	1.00
160–79	2297	5.5	1.89*	1857	0.6	0.64	21522	4.7	1.31*
180–99	2378	8.2	2.55***	1613	2.7	2.48	29936	6.2	1.67***
200–19	1891	8.2	2.58***	1050	2.1	2.31	32165	7.2	1.90***
220–39	1173	14.2	4.04***	537	2.3	2.14	24077	11.0	2.73***
240–59	533	21.3	4.32***	201	0.9	1.21	15009	14.1	3.31***
260–79	245	29.3	6.83***	95	5.2	4.33	8370	21.0	4.74***
280+	165	41.6	9.09***	63	6.0	4.01	6410	28.9	5.93***
<200	6745	5.8	1.00	5389	1.3	1.00	63308	5.2	1.00
200–39	3064	10.4	1.63	1587	2.1	1.57	56242	8.8	1.57***
240+	943	26.5	2.96***	359	3.1	1.80	29789	19.2	2.99***
Cox coefficient (SE)	0.0132*** (0.0015)			0.0072 (0.0046)			0.0074*** (0.0002)		
HR: +35 mg/dl	1.59			1.29			1.30		
95% CI	1.44–1.76			0.94–1.77			1.28–1.31		
Baseline SBP (mmHg)									
≤120	2707	5.4	1.00	4066	1.5	1.00	51344	5.2	1.00
121–9	–	–	–	–	–	–	39260	7.3	1.34***
121–39	3436	8.0	1.31	2073	1.3	0.77			
130–9	–	–	–	–	–	–	33445	10.2	1.78***
140–59	3681	9.5	1.35	1029	3.2	1.46	21857	17.6	2.82***
160+	928[g]	19.4	2.19***	167[g]	1.1	0.52	3433	34.8	5.43***
Cox coefficient (SE)	0.0124*** (0.0037)			−0.0003 (0.0121)			0.0280*** (0.0009)		
HR: +15 mmHg	1.20			1.00			1.52		
95% CI	1.08–1.34			0.70–1.42			1.48–1.56		
Baseline SBP/DBP: JNC-VII criteria									
Normotensive	2592	5.4	1.00	3978	1.5	1.00	39885	4.8	1.00
Prehypertensive	3232	7.3	1.20	1966	1.3	0.71	66265	7.2	1.40***
Hypertension stage 1	3861	9.6	1.39	1162	3.1	1.38	33556	13.4	2.45***
Hypertension stage 2	1067	18.7	2.15***	229	0.7	0.34	9633	29.1	4.89***

p 0.05 < 0.10; *< 0.05; **< 0.01;***< 0.001.

[a] Excludes persons with history of MI or major ECG abnormalities at baseline.

[b] Excludes men with history of MI at baseline. Length of follow-up: CHA cohorts: 30 years; MRFIT: 25 years. Number of CHD deaths: CHA men: 271; CHA women: 35; MRFIT men: 3,345.

Table 4.2 (continued)

Major risk factor level	CHA men aged 18–39[a]			CHA women aged 18–39[a]			MRFIT men aged 35–44[b]		
	n	Death rate[c]	HR[d]	n	Death rate[c]	HR[d]	n	Death rate[c]	HR[e]
Baseline cigarette smoking (cigarettes/day)									
Never	3074	4.5	1.00	2832	0.6	1.00	–	–	–
Non-smoker	–	–	–	–	–	–	90551	5.3	1.00
Former	2583	5.9	1.22	1215	1.2	1.85	–	–	–
<20	1475	9.4	2.14***	1577	2.6	3.92	28643	11.9	1.70***
20–39	3301	14.9	2.77***	1606	3.1	5.14	26145	19.3	2.95***
40+	319	14.9	2.76***	105	0.0	0.00	4000	23.6	3.74***
Cox coefficient (SE)	0.0222*** (0.0041)			0.0423*** (0.0123)			0.0288*** (0.0009)		
HR: 20/day	1.56			2.33			1.75		
95% CI	1.33–1.83			1.44–3.77			1.72–1.83		
Baseline BMI (kg/m²)									
<23.0	2063	6.1	1.00	4532	1.1	1.00	h	–	–
23.0–24.9	2419	7.0	1.13	1240	1.6	1.38	–	–	–
25.0–29.9	4978	8.9	1.20	1142	2.4	1.94	–	–	–
30.0–34.9	1084	16.2	1.91**	293	5.0	3.31	–	–	–
35.0+	208	20.3	1.82	128	3.7	3.53	–	–	–
<25.0	4482	6.5	1.00	5772	1.2	1.00	h	–	–
25.0–29.9	4978	8.9	1.11	1142	2.4	1.75	–	–	–
30.0+	1292	16.9	1.76**	421	4.6	3.04*	–	–	–
Cox coefficient (SE)	0.0465** (0.0164)			0.0826* (0.0331)			–		
HR: 4.0 kg/m²	1.20			1.39			–		
95% CI	1.06–1.37			1.07–1.81			–		
Baseline history of diabetes – No, Yes									
No	10636	8.8	1.00	7271	1.7	1.00	148204	9.1	1.00
Yes	116	22.1	2.37	64	0.0	0.00	1135	40.6	2.95***
Cox coefficient (SE)	0.8635* (0.3844)			i			1.0829 (0.1021)***		
HR: yes	2.37						2.95		
95% CI	1.12–5.04						2.42–3.61		

[c] Age adjusted, per 10 000 person years.
   Crude CHD death rate: CHA men: 25.2/1000 in 30 years; CHA women: 4.8/1000 in 30 years; MRFIT men: 22.2/1000 in 25 years.

[d] Adjusted for age, education, race, minor ECG abnormality, and other major risk factors.

[e] Adjusted for age, race, and other major risk factors.

[f] 100 mg/dl = 2.6 mmol/l.

[g] Includes people on antihypertensive drug treatment.

[h] Height and weight were not measured at MRFIT first screen.

[i] No CHD deaths in small subgroup with diabetes at baseline, hence not estimable.

4.4.2 **Blood pressure**

For the two male cohorts, the relationship of baseline systolic pressure to CHD mortality is continuous (from <120 through 160+ mmHg), graded (exponential), strong, independent, statistically significant ($p < 0.001$), with HRs 1.20 (CHA) and 1.52 (MRFIT) for SBP 15 mmHg higher ($\sim$1 SD) (Table 4.2). In contrast, for younger CHA women there is no apparent relation of SBP to CHD mortality. For these three cohorts findings similar to the foregoing were recorded with diastolic pressure as BP variable (data not shown). With use of both SBP and DBP to stratify the cohorts, per Joint National Committee on Prevention, Detection, Evaluation and Treatment of High Blood Pressure (JNC) VII Report criteria (Chobanian *et al.* 2003), results were again similar (Table 4.2).

The seemingly different findings for women and men almost certainly are artefactual, that is, due to few CHD deaths among the CHA younger women. This inference is powerfully supported by the extensive data on SBP and CHD in women amassed in a recent meta-analysis of 61 studies (Prospective Studies Collaboration 2002). This meta-analysis involves 958 074 participants aged 40–89, with 12.7 million person-years of follow-up, 33 867 CHD deaths in age–gender-specific analyses (8713 female and 25 154 male CHD deaths). For each of five 10-year age groups, CHD HR with 20 mmHg lower usual SBP (i.e., SBP corrected for regression-dilution bias) is sizeably lower for both genders; the tendency is for HRs to be lower for women than men (0.40–0.64 compared to 0.50–0.69) (Fig. 4.1) (Prospective Studies Collaboration 2002).

4.4.3 **Cigarette smoking**

For all three cohorts, there is a strong, graded, independent, significant relation of current cigarette smoking at baseline – that is, number of cigarettes per day – to risk of CHD death (Table 4.2). Based on the Cox multivariate analyses, for smokers of 20 (vs. 0) cigarettes/day, HR is 1.56 (CHA) and 1.75 (MRFIT) for men and even larger for women: 2.33. As to risk for former smokers compared to never smokers (data available only for two CHA cohorts), HR is 1.22 for men and 1.85 for women, considerably less than for current smokers and not significant statistically – consistent with extensive other data on the benefits of smoking cessation as well as never smoking.

4.4.4 **Body mass index (BMI)**

For the two CHA cohorts, with data on this major risk factor, its relation to CHD risk is generally continuous, graded (from levels of <23.0 through 35.0 kg/m^2), strong, independent (Table 4.2). For men and women classified by current criteria as obese, that is, BMI 30.0+ kg/m^2, HR for men is 1.76 compared to those with BMI < 25.0 (i.e., not overweight), and for women it is even stronger: 3.04. Both Cox multivariate coefficients are significant, with HR for BMI 4.0 kg/m^2 higher being 1.20 for men and 1.39 for women. It is relevant to emphasize that these relations of BMI to CHD death are independent of – that is, over and above – the adverse effects of overweight/obesity on SBP, DBP, TC, risk of diabetes, *et al.* (see also Daviglus *et al.* 2003*b*, 2004*c*, and Chapter 20).

4.4.5 **Diabetes**

While baseline prevalence of diabetes was only 1.1%, 0.9%, and 0.8% for these three younger cohorts, for CHA and MRFIT men a significant independent relation of this major risk factor to CHD death is evident: HR 2.37 (CHA) and 2.95 (MRFIT), 95% CI of 2.42–3.61 for the larger MRFIT cohort.

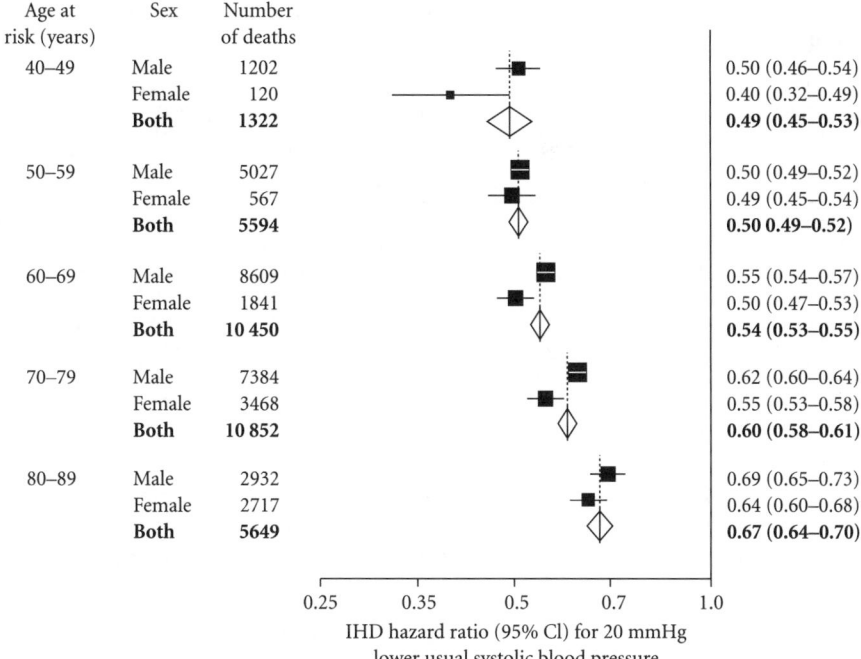

Age at risk (years)	Sex	Number of deaths		
40–49	Male	1202		0.50 (0.46–0.54)
	Female	120		0.40 (0.32–0.49)
	Both	**1322**		**0.49 (0.45–0.53)**
50–59	Male	5027		0.50 (0.49–0.52)
	Female	567		0.49 (0.45–0.54)
	Both	**5594**		**0.50 0.49–0.52)**
60–69	Male	8609		0.55 (0.54–0.57)
	Female	1841		0.50 (0.47–0.53)
	Both	**10 450**		**0.54 (0.53–0.55)**
70–79	Male	7384		0.62 (0.60–0.64)
	Female	3468		0.55 (0.53–0.58)
	Both	**10 852**		**0.60 (0.58–0.61)**
80–89	Male	2932		0.69 (0.65–0.73)
	Female	2717		0.64 (0.60–0.68)
	Both	**5649**		**0.67 (0.64–0.70)**

IHD hazard ratio (95% CI) for 20 mmHg
lower usual systolic blood pressure

Fig. 4.1 CHD mortality: sex-specific HRs for 20 mmHg lower usual SBP. The values plotted are the HRs in each decade of age associated with 20 mmHg lower usual SBP at the start of that decade; each square has an area inversely proportional to the effective variance of the log HR. In parallel analyses of the large MRFIT study, a 20 mmHg lower usual SBP at the start of the decade for deaths at ages 40–49, 50–59, and 60–69 years, respectively, was associated with HRs of (i) stroke: 0.30 (95% CI 0.23–0.40), 0.33 (0.29–0.38), and 0.35 (0.31–0.40); (ii) IHD: 0.42 (0.38–0.47), 0.44 (0.42–0.46), and 0.46 (0.44–0.48); and (iii) other vascular: 0.35 (0.30–0.42), 0.42 (0.39–0.46), and 0.44 (0.41–0.48). (From Prospective Studies Collaboration 2002, reprinted with permission from Elsevier, from *The Lancet*, 2002, **360**, 1903–13.)

HRs for these major risk factors are multiplicative; for example, for combinations of three of them HRs are: (CHA men) TC + SBP ∼1 SD higher + 20 cigarettes/day (vs. 0): HRs $1.59 \times 1.20 \times 1.56 = 2.98$, and (CHA women) TC + BMI ∼1 SD higher +20 cigarettes/day (vs. 0): HRs $1.29 \times 1.39 \times 2.33 = 4.08$, that is, CHD risks about three and four times higher. The corresponding estimates for lower levels of these combinations are: (CHA men) TC + SBP ∼1 SD lower and non-smoking (vs. 20 cigarettes/day): $0.63 \times 0.83 \times 0.64 = 0.33$, and (for CHA women) TC + BMI ∼1 SD lower and non-smoking (vs. 20 cigarettes/day): $0.78 \times 0.72 \times 0.43 = 0.24$ that is, CHD risks are lower by 67% and 76% (see below).

Most of these HRs are underestimates since they are based on only one measurement per person of each risk factor, and for traits except BMI there is limited reliability (reproducibility) with only one measurement – the regression-dilution bias problem (Liu *et al.* 1978; MacMahon *et al.* 1990; Prospective Studies Collaboration 2002).

Table 4.3 gives corresponding data for CHA men and women of baseline ages 40–59 and MRFIT men of ages 45–57. Findings are generally similar to those for the three younger cohorts. For all three middle-aged cohorts, baseline TC, SBP, cigarettes/day, and diabetes are significantly

Table 4.3 Relationship of major risk factors considered singly to long-term risk of CHD death, for men and women aged 40–59 at baseline

Major risk factor level	CHA men aged 40–59[a]			CHA women aged 40–59[a]			MRFIT men aged 45–57[b]		
	n	Death rate[c]	HR[d]	n	Death rate[c]	HR[d]	n	Death rate[c]	HR[e]
Baseline serum cholesterol (mg/dl)[f]									
<160	464	30.6	1.00	327	18.1	1.00s	9427	15.5	1.00
160–79	1013	36.2	1.24	670	25.7	0.98	20754	16.8	1.08
180–99	1686	40.6	1.37	1221	22.1	0.94	35399	20.8	1.34***
200–19	1896	45.5	1.49*	1403	20.0	0.88	43995	24.5	1.55***
220–39	1537	55.7	1.84**	1249	30.8	1.27	37132	30.7	1.90***
240–59	993	56.6	1.77**	832	27.9	1.09	25610	35.9	2.16***
260–79	457	70.3	2.09***	547	30.7	1.30	14775	41.5	2.40**
280+	361	97.9	3.23***	492	47.5	1.64[g]	11547	54.7	3.07***
<200	3163	37.8	1.00	2218	22.6	1.00	65580	18.8	1.00
200–39	3433	50.0	1.27**	2652	25.4	1.13	81127	27.3	1.42***
240+	1811	67.6	1.63***	1871	33.3	1.37**	51932	41.6	2.01***
Cox coefficient (SE)	0.0067*** (0.0008)			0.0037*** (0.0010)			0.0060*** (0.0002)		
HR: +35 mg/dl	1.26			1.14			1.23		
95% CI	1.20–1.34			1.06–1.22			1.22–1.24		
Baseline SBP (mmHg)									
≤120	1487	32.0	1.00	1989	17.4	1.00	51413	14.6	1.00
121–9	–	–	–	–	–	–	44276	19.7	1.31***
121–39	2189	39.6	1.16	1731	18.9	1.05			
130–9	–	–	–	–	–	–	45863	27.2	1.75***
140–59	2997	48.4	1.32*	1831	32.8	1.79***	44008	41.4	2.59***
160+	1734	78.2	2.11***	1190	43.7	2.07***	13079	72.1	4.23***
Cox coefficient (SE)	0.0135***(0.0015)			0.0125*** (0.0023)			0.0235*** (0.0004)		
HR: +15 mmHg	1.22			1.21			1.42		
95% CI	1.17–1.28			1.13–1.29			1.40–1.44		
Baseline SBP/DBP: JNC-VII criteria									
Normo-tensive	1403	30.0	1.00	1903	17.7	1.00	39797	13.6	1.00
Prehyper-tensive	1890	39.2	1.24	1628	18.4	0.99	79945	21.3	1.48***
Hypertension stage 1	3189	47.0	1.37***	1942	31.8	1.67***	56459	35.3	2.40***
Hypertension stage 2	1925	77.6	2.23***	1268	43.3	2.00***	22438	62.5	4.08***

[a] Excludes persons with history of MI or major ECG abnormalities at baseline.

[b] Excludes men with history of MI at baseline. Length of follow-up: CHA cohorts: 30 years; MRFIT: 25 years. Number of CHD deaths: CHA men: 1025; CHA women: 479; MRFIT men: 12 354.

Table 4.3 (continued)

Major risk factor level	CHA men aged 40–59[a]			CHA women aged 40–59[a]			MRFIT men aged 45–57[b]		
	n	Death rate[c]	HR[d]	n	Death rate[c]	HR[d]	n	Death rate[c]	HR[e]
Baseline cigarette smoking (cigarettes/day)									
Never	2023	36.0	1.00	3211	18.9	1.00	–	–	–
Non-smoker	–	–	–	–	–	–	130801	21.0	1.00
Former	2935	39.4	1.03	1067	22.9	1.30	–	–	–
<20	742	49.8	1.37*	1059	34.5	2.22***	34060	36.7	1.46***
20–39	2322	71.8	2.09***	1319	44.3	3.02***	29250	50.0	2.18***
40+	385	85.1	2.46***	85	41.8	4.83***	4528	60.5	2.63***
Cox coefficient (SE)	0.0230*** (0.0021)			0.0431*** (0.0039)			0.0230*** (0.0005)		
HR: 20/day	1.58			2.37			1.58		
95% CI	1.46–1.72			2.03–2.76			1.55–1.62		
Baseline BMI (kg/m²)									
<23.0	847	43.2	1.00	2349	20.0	1.00	*i*	–	–
23.0–24.9	1432	42.3	0.97	1483	22.7	1.15	–	–	–
25.0–29.9	4599	49.0	1.04	2063	28.4	1.34*	–	–	–
30.0–34.9	1326	56.2	1.07	611	43.9	2.07***	–	–	–
35.0+	203	81.0	1.47*	235	65.2	2.92***	–	–	–
<25.0	2279	42.6	1.00	3832	21.0	1.00	*i*	–	–
25.0–29.9	4599	49.0	1.05	2063	28.4	1.26*	–	–	–
30.0+	1529	59.3	1.14	846	49.5	2.16***	–	–	–
Cox coefficient (SE)	0.0190* (0.0087)			0.0583 *** (0.0096)			–		
HR: +4.0 kg/m²	1.08			1.26			–		
95% CI	1.01–1.16			1.17–1.36			–		
Baseline history of diabetes – No, Yes									
No	8117	47.2	1.00	6584	25.8	1.00	194611	26.9	1.00
Yes	290	103.0	2.33	157	69.3	2.22	4028	94.9	3.08***
Cox coefficient (SE)	0.8459*** (0.1238)			0.7993*** (0.2051)			1.1232*** (0.0381)		
HR: yes	2.33			2.22			3.08		
95% CI	1.83–2.97			1.49–3.32			2.85–3.31		

[c] Age adjusted, per 10 000 person years.
Crude CHD death rate: CHA men: 121.9/1000 in 30 years; CHA women: 71.1/1000 in 30 years; MRFIT men: 62.2/1000 in 25 years.

[d] Adjusted for age, education, race, minor ECG abnormality, and other major risk factors.

[e] Adjusted for age, race, and other major risk factors.

[f] 100 mg/dl = 2.6 mmol/l.

[g] p 0.10 > 0.05; *$p < 0.05$; **$p < 0.01$; ***$p < 0.001$.

[h] Includes people on antihypertensive drug treatment.

[i] Height and weight were not measured at MRFIT first screen.

and independently related to long-term risk of CHD death ($p < 0.001$). For the two CHA cohorts with BMI data, BMI is also significantly and independently related to CHD risk.

As noted above, for the two middle-aged male cohorts, Cox coefficients for the TC–CHD relationship (0.0067 and 0.0060 – Table 4.3) are about half as large as for CHA men baseline ages 18–39 (0.0132 – Table 4.2), that is, HRs for TC higher by 35 mg/dl are 1.26 and 1.23 (compared with 1.59 for younger men). Given the considerably higher CHD death rates for middle-aged than for younger adult men (e.g. 122/1000 compared to 25/1000 in 30 years for the two CHA cohorts), the less marked increase in HR for middle-aged men translates into absolute excess risks as high or higher than for younger adult men.

In contrast to the above-noted less strong TC–CHD relation in middle-aged compared to younger adult men, coefficient and HR sizes for the relations of SBP, cigarette smoking, and diabetes are no less large for middle-aged than for younger men, and this is the case also for women for cigarette smoking, BMI, and diabetes (Tables 4.2 and 4.3).

For the CHA cohort of middle-aged women, with 479 CHD deaths in 30 years, SBP is significantly related to CHD risk (Table 4.3), consistent qualitatively with the massive data from the Prospective Studies Collaboration (2002) (Fig. 1.1). This finding lends further support to the inference that the apparent absence of a SBP–CHD relation for the younger CHA female cohort is artefactual, due to few CHD deaths. For the CHA middle-aged female cohort, Cox coefficients for current cigarette smoking and for BMI are sizeably larger than for middle-aged men. Correspondingly, HRs are sizeably larger; their 95% CIs do not overlap with those for middle-aged men. These data indicate that for middle-aged women adverse impact on long-term CHD risk of these two major risk factors is even greater than for middle-aged men.

As noted above, risk factor HRs are multiplicative. For example (MRFIT men aged 45–57) TC + SBP + smoking: $1.23 \times 1.42 \times 1.58 = 2.76$, and (CHA women aged 40–59): $1.14 \times 1.21 \times 2.37 = 3.27$, that is, increases in long-term CHD risk of almost three-fold and greater than three-fold. For middle-aged women, BMI higher by 4 kg/m^2 increases the foregoing HR to 4.12. The markedly increased risk for all middle-aged diabetic subcohorts – compounded by all too frequent co-presence of one, two, or more other major risk factors – merits emphasis, especially given rising incidence/prevalence rates of diabetes due to the waxing obesity epidemic (see Chapter 20).

Again, for those with lower levels of multiple major risk factors, favourable effects on HRs are multiplicative; for example (MRFIT men aged 45–57) TC and SBP lower by ~1 SD and non-smoking (vs. 20 cigarettes/day): $0.81 \times 0.70 \times 0.63 = 0.36$, and (CHA women aged 40–59): $0.88 \times 0.83 \times 0.42 = 0.31$, $\times 0.79$ (BMI 4 kg/m^2 lower) $= 0.24$, that is, CHD risks are lower by 64%, 69%, and 76% (see below).

4.5 Relation of combinations of major risk factors to CHD mortality

Tables 4.4 and 4.5 give in-depth 50-cell analyses, made possible by the extraordinary sample sizes plus long-term follow-up of the MRFIT cohorts, that is, age–race–diabetes-adjusted HRs for 25-year CHD mortality for the two MRFIT cohorts stratified by baseline cigarette use and five levels each of TC and SBP. The upper left cell – non-smokers with TC < 180 mg/dl (<4.6 mmol/l) and SBP ≤ 120 mmHg – is set at 1.00. Only 6.2% of men baseline ages 35–44 and 3.2% of men ages 45–57 meet these criteria. Due to impact of prevailing unhealthy lifestyles, the problem of increased risk involves practically the whole population – it is not 'just' a problem for the 20 or 30% of people at very high risk, it is a population-wide problem (Rose 1992; WHO 1982).

Table 4.4 Serum cholesterol (SC), SBP strata, smoking, and HR[a] for CHD death, for 149 339 MRFIT men aged 35–44 at baseline

SC (mg/dl)[b]	SBP (mmHg)				
	≤120	121–9	130–9	140–59	160+
Non-smokers at baseline					
<180	1.00	1.38	2.45***	4.09***	10.25***
180–99	1.78*	2.50***	2.95***	4.79***	12.64***
200–19	1.96**	2.26***	3.14***	5.63***	8.57***
220–39	2.68***	2.84***	5.47***	7.61***	21.72***
240+	3.66***	6.64***	8.65***	13.18***	26.77***
Cigarette Smokers at baseline					
<180	3.35***	3.10***	7.55***	10.32***	37.61***
180–99	5.78***	6.86***	7.82***	12.82***	24.74***
200–19	5.69***	7.28***	10.22***	18.99***	22.25***
220–39	7.94***	10.74***	14.74***	23.16***	41.23***
240+	14.53***	19.09***	20.36***	34.46***	52.26***

All analyses exclude persons with history of MI at baseline; follow-up 25 years; 3345 CHD deaths.

* $p < 0.05$; ** $p < 0.01$; *** $p < 0.001$.

[a] HR, adjusted for age, race, and diabetes; substratum of non-smokers with TC < 180 mg/dl and SBP ≤ 120 mmHg set at 1.00.

[b] 100 mg/dl = 2.6 mmol/l.

Table 4.5 Serum cholesterol (SC), SBP strata, smoking, and HR[a] for CHD death, for 198 639 MRFIT men aged 45–57 at baseline

SC (mg/dl)[b]	SBP (mmHg)				
	≤120	121–9	130–9	140–59	160+
Non-smokers at baseline					
<180	1.00	1.32	2.09***	2.64***	5.31***
180–99	1.38*	1.79***	2.30***	3.95***	6.87***
200–19	1.43**	2.02***	2.89***	3.88***	7.69***
220–39	1.97***	2.33***	3.32***	5.42***	8.36***
240+	2.75***	3.57***	4.81***	7.07***	12.05***
Cigarette smokers at baseline					
<180	2.50***	3.32***	3.79***	6.74***	10.30***
180–99	2.77***	3.95***	5.45***	7.98***	11.80***
200–19	3.64***	4.86***	6.47***	9.24***	17.55***
220–39	4.72***	6.05***	7.28***	11.83***	18.09***
240+	5.65***	7.30***	9.59***	13.09***	19.28***

All analyses exclude persons with history of MI at baseline; follow-up 25 years; 12 354 CHD deaths.

* $p < 0.05$; ** $p < 0.01$; *** $p < 0.001$.

[a] Hazard ratio, adjusted for age, race, and diabetes; substratum of non-smokers with TC < 180 mg/dl and SBP ≤ 120 mmHg set at 1.00.

[b] 100 mg/dl = 2.6 mmol/l.

At every level of TC–SBP, smokers are at much higher CHD risk than non-smokers. Even with TC < 180 mg/dl and SBP ≤ 120 mmHg, smokers are at much higher risk than non-smokers – 3.35 times higher (ages 35–44) and 2.50 times higher (ages 45–57). In combination, higher levels of these major risk factors have markedly adverse influences on probability of CHD death; for example, TC 200–19 mg/dl and SBP 130–9 mmHg (centre of the distributions) for non-smokers ages 35–44, a more than 3-fold increase in risk (Table 4.4), and for smokers a more than 10-fold increase. For men of baseline ages 45–57, these increases in risk are almost 3-fold and more than 6-fold (Table 4.5). For men aged 35–44, across the 25 cells for non-smokers, range from lowest to highest risk is almost 27-fold; across the 50 cells, more than 52-fold (Table 4.4); for men aged 45–57, 12-fold and 19-fold (Table 4.5). These marked ranges in risk based on these three major risk factors considered together are despite the limitations – underestimations – due to one-time measurements only (regression-dilution bias).

In regard to the 'bottom-line' challenge, population-wide CHD prevention and control, the data of critical importance are the inverse of those in Tables 4.4 and 4.5, that is, the **lower** estimated risk for the all-too-few men in the upper left cell, with TC < 180 mg/dl, SBP ≤ 120 mmHg, non-smokers at baseline (only 6.2% and 3.2% of their cohorts). Compared to non-smokers in the centre of the TC–SBP distribution, their risk of CHD death in 25 years is lower by 68% (men aged 35–44) and 65% (men aged 45–57); compared to non-smokers with TC–SBP in stratum 5, 96% and 92% lower; compared to smokers in this same high TC–SBP stratum, 98% and 95% lower.

Data from the Chicago Western Electric Study (WE) (Paul *et al.* 1963; Shekelle *et al.* 1981; Stamler and Shekelle 1988; Stamler *et al.* 1993*a*) add meaningfully to the foregoing for two reasons. First, they include high-quality data on the major risk factor adverse diet, dietary lipid in particular, unlike most other studies. Second, since WE baseline was 1957–58, they portray the major risk factor status for employed middle-aged American men at the height of the CHD epidemic, before the decline in national CHD death rates that began in the 1960s. Data on the right in column 2 of Table 4.6 demonstrate the adverse average levels of all major risk factors prevailing for this whole cohort (saturated fat intake was also high: 16.4% of total calories; polyunsaturated fat was low: 4.0%). Diet cholesterol, serum cholesterol, systolic pressure, BMI, and cigarettes/day all relate significantly and independently to 24 year risk of CHD death; all of these major risk factors except BMI also relate significantly and independently to long-term risk of all-cause mortality. Compared to optimal levels for these risk factors (left, column 2, Table 4.6), adverse prevailing values are associated with substantially higher HRs for long-term CHD and all causes of death (columns 5 and 7, Table 4.6). For an absolute majority of these men, levels of two or more of these risk factors were high. Presence of any two only of these adverse traits was associated with an estimated doubling of CHD risk (HR 1.99 – unweighted average); any three only, almost a trebling (HR 2.87); any four only, almost a quadrupling (HR 3.89); all five, HR 5.41 times greater. Given sample size and prevailing lifestyles, there were few men in this cohort with favourable levels of all these risk factors, too few to serve as an actual comparison group; the foregoing HRs therefore are statistical estimates, similar to others made with such 'first generation' data (Pooling Project Research Group 1978; Stamler *et al.* 1993*a*). Their validity has stood the test of time, as shown by the similar HRs estimated from actual observed data on the MRFIT cohort (see above).

Again, perhaps the critically important statistics are the estimated lower risk with all major risk factors favourable: from the WE cohort data, HR for CHD death is 0.18; for all-cause mortality, it is 0.34; that is, compared to the whole cohort, CHD is lower by 82%, with all-causes

Table 4.6 Chicago Western Electric Study Cohort, 1903 men aged 41–57 in 1959: relation of major risk factors, including adverse dietary lipid intake, to 24 year risk of mortality from CHD and all causes, and to life expectancy

Baseline variable	Comparison	Cox multivariate coefficient (t-value)		Hazard Ratio		Life expectancy difference (years)	
		CHD	All causes	CHD	All causes	CHD	All causes
Dietary cholesterol (mg/1000 kcal)	50, 237	0.0028 (2.86)	0.0014 (2.10)	1.69[a] 0.59[b]	1.30[a] 0.77[b]	−2.6[c]	+2.8[d]
Saturated fat (% kcal)	–	0.0002 (0.73)	0.00007 (0.36)	– –	– –	–(NS)	–(NS)
Polyunsaturated fat (% kcal)	–	−0.0014 (1.77)	−0.0005 (−0.97)	– –	– –	–(NS)	–(NS)
Serum cholesterol (mg/dl)[e]	170, 242	0.0055 (4.98)	0.0024 (2.90)	1.49	1.19	−1.8	+1.8
SBP (mmHg)	112, 132	0.0191 (5.65)	0.0160 (6.83)	1.47	1.38	−3.2	+3.4
BMI (kg/m²)	22.0, 26.0	0.0380 (2.17)	0.0087 (0.71)	1.16	1.04	–(NS)	–(NS)
Cigarettes/day	0, 10[f]	0.0230 (4.38)	0.0289 (8.17)	1.26	1.34	−2.9	+3.1
Age (years)	50, 55	0.0519 (6.18)	0.0823 (8.88)	1.30	1.51	–	–

Also in analyses: past smoking (no, yes: $t = -0.54, +0.32$); alcohol intake (ml/day: $t = -0.78, +0.54$ and NS (not significant statistically) in quadratic analyses); past drinking (no, yes: $t = +2.01, +2.46$); BMI quadratic: NS; heart rate (beats/min: $t = +1.17, +2.57$); major ECG abnormality (no, yes: $t = +3.58, +2.24$); minor (but not major) ECG abnormality (no, yes: $t = +0.97, +1.33$); men with baseline diabetes, MI history excluded; life expectancy for 49-year-old US men, 1990 Life Table, 27.2 years.

[a] HR with higher value (see column 2).

[b] HR with lower value (see column 1).

[c] Estimated reduced life expectancy with higher value (see column 2).

[d] Estimated increased life expectancy with lower value (see column 1).

[e] 100 mg/dl = 2.6 mmol/l.

[f] Average for whole cohort; 53% were smokers; i.e., on average smokers consumed about 20 cigarettes/day.

death lower by 66% over the years from average age ~49 to average age 73. This more favourable estimated mortality translates into estimates of greater years of life expectancy with favourable levels of each risk factor (last column, Table 4.6) (Stamler *et al.* 1993*a*) – estimates that are additive, 2.8 + 1.8 + 3.4 + 3.1 = 11.1 more years, on top of the estimated 27.2 years average life expectancy for American men aged 49 (1990 US Life Table), that is, 38.3 years, a 41% enhancement of longevity, to age 87.3 instead of age 76.2 – a substantial gain especially if achievable with health (see below).

In the last decade, long-term follow-up of large cohorts – MRFIT, CHA, others – has made possible the accumulation (beyond the limited, albeit important, information above and in the first edition of this monograph; Stamler 1992) of extensive data on the multiple advantages of such *low risk* status. These newer data are ***actual findings*** on low risk people – young adult and middle-aged men and women – ***not*** results of statistical extrapolation down a smoothed risk function, the only kind of data previously available on low risk, given its rarity in American and other similar populations with adverse lifestyles (Pooling Project Research Group 1978). ***Their strategic importance merits a shift in attention and emphasis*** – from the adverse effects of unfavourable/higher levels of the major risk factors to the ***healthful influences that come with having favourable levels of all major risk factors.***

4.6 **Low risk**

4.6.1 **Definition and prevalence**

Subcohorts designated ***low risk (LR)***, as defined here, are made up of persons free of heart attack (myocardial infarction (MI)) history at baseline and with ***favourable levels of all readily measured major risk factors***, that is, SBP ≤ 120 *and* DBP ≤ 80 mmHg (physicians' classical cut-points for normal BP), *and* TC < 200 mg/dl, *and* BMI < 25.0 kg/m^2, *and* non-diabetic (Tables 4.7 and 4.8). To re-emphasize, as a consequence of virtually population-wide adverse lifestyles (adverse dietary and smoking patterns, little or no exercise at work or leisure: the fast food–automobile–TV culture), only a small proportion of each cohort is low risk, <10% of young adult and middle-aged men, ~20% of young adult women, and 5% of middle-aged women.

4.6.2 **Major risk factor levels**

In accordance with criteria for low risk, baseline average values of BP, TC, and BMI are much lower for LR subcohorts compared to all others (Tables 4.7 and 4.8). These contrasts are even more marked for middle-aged than for young adult cohorts (e.g. CHA 40–59 compared to 18–39, with average ages ~49 and 28 years), reflecting the lifestyle-driven rises in these variables experienced by most people in Western societies from youth through middle age. Also by definition, the contrast is marked between LR and other subcohorts in prevalence of cigarette smoking. (Diabetes was still a relatively low prevalence trait in the baseline years of the CHA and MRFIT Studies, 1967–73 and 1973–75, before the still waxing obesity epidemic took off.)

4.6.3 **Mortality rates**

For all three tabulated mortality end points, age-standardized rates were much lower for LR than other subcohorts (Tables 4.7 and 4.8). For example, for CHD, focus of this chapter, the

Table 4.7 Younger adult subcohorts, baseline ages 18–44 – low risk and others: number of people, average major risk factor levels, numbers of deaths by cause, and percentage deceased by cause

Cohort and variables	Low risk	All others: not low risk	Any two or more RF unfavourable or high[a]	Any two or more RF high[b]
No. of people				
CHA men	582	10170	9144	3491
CHA women	1479	5856	4701	1062
MRFIT men	13028	136311	91040	31387
% of cohort				
CHA men	5.4	94.6	85.0	32.5
CHA women	20.2	79.8	64.1	14.5
MRFIT men	8.8	91.2	61.0	21.4
Age (years)				
CHA men	27.9	29.8	29.9	30.2
CHA women	25.3	27.1	27.3	28.8
MRFIT men	39.2	39.6	39.7	39.9
Serum cholesterol (mg/dl)				
CHA men	162.9	191.3	193.2	204.4
CHA women	163.5	184.9	186.0	198.8
MRFIT men	172.8	212.8	225.0	242.0
SBP (mmHg)				
CHA men	115.6	135.4	136.8	145.0
CHA women	113.3	125.8	126.7	138.0
MRFIT men	112.4	128.6	131.1	137.5
Current cigarette smoking (%)				
CHA men	0.0	50.0	56.0	79.6
CHA women	0.0	56.0	70.0	85.3
MRFIT men	0.0	43.1	56.5	78.1
Cigarettes/day				
CHA men	0	10.6	11.8	17.3
CHA women	0	9.5	11.8	15.5
MRFIT men	0	11.1	14.7	20.7
BMI (kg/m^2)				
CHA men	22.6	26.2	26.4	27.9
CHA women	20.9	23.3	23.6	26.5
MRFIT men	–	–	–	–
Diabetes history (%)				
CHA men	0.0	1.1	1.3	2.5
CHA women	0.0	1.1	1.4	4.0
MRFIT men	0.0	0.8	1.2	1.8
CHD deaths (n)				
CHA men	1	270	264	165
CHA women	2	33	32	15
MRFIT men	48	3297	2901	1841

Table 4.7 (continued)

Cohort and variables	Low risk	All others: not low risk	Any two or more RF unfavourable or high[a]	Any two or more RF high[b]
CVD deaths (n)				
CHA men	4	383	372	232
CHA women	6	71	67	27
MRFIT men	70	4555	3953	2510
All deaths (n)				
CHA men	33	1130	1073	567
CHA women	46	383	347	103
MRFIT men	404	11263	9134	5039
% deceased, CHD				
CHA men	0.3	2.6	2.9	4.6
CHA women	0.2	0.5	0.6	1.2
MRFIT men	0.4	2.4	3.2	5.8
% deceased, CVD				
CHA men	0.9	3.7	4.0	6.4
CHA women	0.4	1.2	1.3	2.1
MRFIT men	0.5	3.3	4.3	7.9
% deceased, all causes				
CHA men	6.4	11.0	11.6	15.7
CHA women	3.4	6.4	7.1	8.2
MRFIT men	3.1	8.3	10.0	15.8

Serum cholesterol unit: mg/dl; SBP unit: mmHg; RF: risk factor.

For CHA men and women, aged 18–39 at baseline, percentage deceased are age adjusted.

Follow-up: for CHA men and women, average 30 years; for MRFIT men, median 25 years.

Criteria for low risk: *All* of SBP ≤ 120 mmHg, DBP ≤ 80 mmHg, TC < 200 mg/dl, no diabetes, no smoking, BMI < 25.0 kg/m² (CHA cohorts only).

[a] Criteria for unfavourable or high risk (i.e., not low risk): any one or more of baseline SBP 121+ mmHg, DBP 81+ mmHg, TC 200+ mg/dl, diabetes, smoking, BMI 25.0+ kg/m² (CHA cohorts only).

[b] Cut points for high risk: SBP 140+ mmHg, DBP 90+ mmHg, TC 240+ mg/dl (6.1 mmol/l), diabetes, smoking, BMI 30.0 + kg/m² (CHA cohorts only).

percentage deceased in 30 years was only 0.3 for CHA LR men aged 18–39 compared to 2.6 for all others, 2.9 for those with any two or more risk factors unfavourable or high (85% of the cohort), and 4.6 for those with any two or more risk factors high, that is, LR CHD death rates lower by 88%, 90%, and 93%. Corresponding CHD mortality rates for CHA young adult female subcohorts are: for LR 0.2%, and for the other three subcohorts 0.5%, 0.6%, and 1.2%; that is, rates lower for LR women by 60%, 67%, and 83%.

For all LR subcohorts, mortality rates are also much lower from all CVD and all-causes (Tables 4.7 and 4.8), reflecting rates lower also from stroke, cancers, other medical causes (data not tabulated, see earlier detailed MRFIT data in the first edition of this monograph; Stamler 1992). *All-causes mortality* is a 'bottom line' touchstone societal statistic: for example, for CHA LR men 18–39 it is 6.4% in 30 years, lower by 42% compared to all others, and by 59% compared to those with any two or more risk factors high (Table 4.7).

Table 4.8 Adult subcohorts, baseline ages 40–59 – low risk and others: number of people, average major risk factor levels, numbers of deaths by cause, and percentage deceased by cause

Cohort and variables	Low risk	All others: not low risk	Any two or more RF unfavourable or high[a]	Any two or more RF high[b]
No. of people				
CHA men	164	8243	7818	3886
CHA women	311	6430	5809	2585
MRFIT men	10437	188202	135850	53542
% of cohort				
CHA men	2.0	98.0	93.0	46.2
CHA women	4.6	95.4	86.2	38.3
MRFIT men	5.3	94.7	68.4	27.0
Age (years)				
CHA men	47.6	48.5	48.6	48.9
CHA women	46.4	49.4	49.6	50.4
MRFIT men	50.2	50.6	50.7	50.7
Serum cholesterol (mg/dl)				
CHA men	173.5	212.7	214.2	224.7
CHA women	176.1	220.5	223.1	238.6
MRFIT men	176.6	219.9	230.2	244.1
SBP (mmHg)				
CHA men	115.3	141.0	142.2	149.2
CHA women	114.2	136.4	138.1	146.4
MRFIT men	112.2	133.2	135.8	143.1
Current cigarette smoking (%)				
CHA men	0.0	41.8	44.1	63.6
CHA women	0.0	38.3	42.4	57.9
MRFIT men	0.0	36.0	45.9	67.6
Cigarettes/day				
CHA men	0	9.9	10.4	15.3
CHA women	0	6.8	7.5	10.0
MRFIT men	0	9.3	11.9	17.6
BMI (kg/m²)				
CHA men	22.9	27.2	27.4	28.4
CHA women	22.0	25.3	25.5	27.0
MRFIT men	–	–	–	–
Diabetes history (%)				
CHA men	0.0	3.5	3.7	6.5
CHA women	0.0	2.4	2.7	5.1
MRFIT men	0.0	2.1	2.9	4.8
CHD deaths (n)				
CHA men	7	1018	999	635
CHA women	5	474	456	308
MRFIT men	137	12217	10584	6252

Table 4.8 (continued)

Cohort and variables	Low risk	All others: not low risk	Any two or more RF unfavourable or high[a]	Any two or more RF high[b]
CVD deaths (n)				
CHA men	16	1539	1512	943
CHA women	8	799	762	495
MRFIT men	207	17425	14916	8852
All deaths (n)				
CHA men	39	3738	3643	2166
CHA women	45	2194	2085	1192
MRFIT men	972	40474	33210	18161
% deceased, CHD				
CHA men	4.5	12.3	12.7	16.1
CHA women	1.7	7.3	7.7	11.3
MRFIT men	1.3	6.5	7.8	11.7
% deceased, CVD				
CHA men	10.9	18.7	19.2	23.8
CHA women	2.7	12.3	12.8	18.1
MRFIT men	2.0	9.3	11.0	16.5
% deceased, all causes				
CHA men	25.7	45.3	46.3	54.7
CHA women	16.0	33.8	35.3	43.9
MRFIT men	9.3	21.5	24.5	33.9

Serum cholesterol unit: mg/dl; SBP unit: mmHg; RF: risk factor.

For CHA men and women, aged 40–59 at baseline, percentage deceased are age adjusted.

Follow-up: for CHA men and women, average 30 years; for MRFIT men, median 25 years.

Criteria for low risk: *All* of SBP ≤ 120 mmHg, DBP ≤ 80 mmHg, TC < 200 mg/dl, no diabetes, no smoking, BMI < 25.0 kg/m² (CHA cohorts only).

[a] Criteria for unfavourable or high risk (i.e., not low risk): any one or more of baseline SBP 121+ mmHg, DBP 81+ mmHg, TC 200+ mg/dL, diabetes, smoking, BMI 25.0+ kg/m² (CHA cohorts only).

[b] Cut points for High Risk: SBP 140+ mmHg, DBP 90+ mmHg, TC 240+ mg/dl (6.1 mmol/l), diabetes, smoking, BMI 30.0 + kg/m² (CHA cohorts only).

4.6.4 **Lives saved**

Probably the most important statistic for consideration here is the ***difference in rates, that is, lives saved per 100 people in 30 years*** by virtue of low risk status: for CHA men aged 18–39, it is 11.0−6.4 = 4.6 fewer deaths per 100 for LR compared to all other men, and 15.7 − 6.4 = 9.3 fewer deaths per 100 for LR compared to high risk men (about one-third of the total cohort). Findings are similar for the MRFIT LR subcohort aged 35–44: 5.2 and 12.7 fewer deaths per 100 in 25 years. These are ***large differences***; for example, per 100 000 (the usual demographic base for national mortality data), 5200 fewer premature deaths per 100 000 men over the 25 year span from average age ~39 to 64 for MRFIT LR men compared to all others, and 12 700 fewer compared to high risk men. See also below as to the implications for greater longevity with health. Data on absolute savings of lives are similar for CHA younger adult women; LR compared to all others: 6.4 − 3.4 = 3.0 fewer premature deaths per 100 over the 30 years from average age ~27 to 57; LR compared to high risk women: 8.2 − 3.4 = 4.8 fewer premature deaths per 100 (Table 4.7).

Findings on lives saved are even more impressive for LR subcohorts of baseline ages 40–59 (CHA) and 45–57 (MRFIT) (Table 4.8): For example, CHA LR men compared to all others: $45.3 - 25.7 = 19.6$ lives saved per 100 over the 30 years from average age ~49 to 79; LR compared to high risk men (46% of the whole cohort): $54.7 - 25.9 = 28.8$ lives saved per 100. For LR CHA women: $33.8 - 16.0 = 17.8$, and $43.9 - 16.0 = 27.9$ fewer deaths per 100.

4.6.5 Benefits by socio-economic status and ethnicity

For decades in the USA, the UK, and many other countries, lower socio-economic strata (SES) of the population have experienced higher mortality rates from major diseases and all causes, shorter life expectancies, and more morbidity and disability than higher SES strata (Davey Smith 2003; Davey Smith et al. 1996a, b; Marmot et al. 1991; Stamler and Hazuda 1996; Stamler et al. 1996c). In the USA, these SES-related findings prevail for all main ethnic groups (e.g. African-Americans, Hispanic-Americans, Non-Hispanic White Americans). Overcoming such inequalities in health is one of three primary health goals for the USA (USDHHS 1991, 1998). Substantial progress toward accomplishment of this goal requires a prioritized effective strategic focus. Data on the benefits of LR status for lower (as well as higher) SES Americans serve as the scientific foundation for such a focus (Table 4.9). For both Non-Hispanic White Men and African-American men of lower SES (lower income) in the MRFIT cohort, for both the CHD and all-cause mortality end points, LR status is associated with markedly lower 25 year death rates (Table 4.9, data column 2) compared to the rates for all men not LR, whether higher or lower SES (Table 4.9, data columns 3 and 4). For example, for Non-Hispanic White American men (the largest ethnic group in the MRFIT cohort), the LR and lower-income subcohort has a 25 year age-standardized CHD death rate of 4.4/10 000 person years, almost as low as that for the LR higher-income subcohort (3.5/10 000 person years); much lower than that of the higher income subcohort not LR (18.7/10 000 person years); and lower still compared to the subcohort not LR and with lower income (23.5/10 000 person years – the highest rate). For these LR lower-income men, compared to other (not LR) lower-income men, the 25 year CHD death rate is lower by 82% (HR 0.18), and compared to other (not LR) higher-income men lower by 78% (HRs 0.18/0.80). Findings are similar for LR lower-SES African-American men (Table 4.9). They are also similar for LR lower-SES Asian-American and Hispanic American men (MRFIT), and for LR lower-SES younger adult and middle-aged men and women of the four CHA cohorts (data not tabulated).

Absolute savings of lives are substantial for these LR lower-income subcohorts (as well as for LR higher-income subcohorts). For example, for the LR lower-income MRFIT men, compared to not-LR lower-income men, there were 45 fewer deaths per 10 000 person years; compared to not-LR higher income men the figure is 30/10 000 person years ($60.9 - 31.1$, Table 4.9).

4.6.6 Benefits summated

As shown in Table 4.10, for all four CHA and both MRFIT LR subcohorts, HRs for long-term CHD–CVD mortality are much lower than for other persons (not LR). For example, for the two MRFIT subcohorts, they are lower by 79% or more (HRs 0.16–0.21). Differences in CHD–CVD mortality risk are even more marked for LR compared to those with any two or more major risk factors unfavourable or high, and compared to those with any two or more major risk factors high; for example, for the two MRFIT LR subcohorts risks of CHD–CVD death are lower by 89% to 93% (HRs 0.07–0.11). Again, all these are underestimates of the benefits of LR due to regression-dilution bias and other limitations, for example, lack of data on BMI and dietary patterns. These findings underscore the falsity of the assertion, made

Table 4.9 Low risk and 25-year mortality by income and ethnicity, MRFIT men, baseline ages 35–57

Variable	Risk and income subcohort			
	Low risk, higher income	Low risk, lower income	All others, higher income	All others, lower income
Non-Hispanic white American men				
Number of men	11827	8983	136167	139101
% of cohort	4.0	3.0	46.0	47.0
CHD mortality[a]	3.5	4.4	18.7	23.5
Difference in CHD mortality[b]	−20.0	−19.1	−4.8	0.0
CHD HR[b]	0.15***	0.18***	0.80*	1.00
All causes mortality[a]	25.2	31.1	60.9	76.1
Difference in all causes mortality[b]	−50.9	−45.0	−15.2	0.0
All causes HR[b]	0.34***	0.41***	0.82***	1.00
African-American men				
Number of men	464	381	9251	9842
% of cohort	2.3	1.9	46.4	49.4
CHD mortality[a]	4.1	5.1	20.4	25.4
Difference in CHD mortality[b]	−21.3	−20.3	−5.0	0.0
CHD HR[b]	0.18**	0.16**	0.79	1.00
All causes mortality[a]	45.7	62.5	86.6	111.3
Difference in all causes mortality[b]	−65.6	−48.8	−24.7	0.0
All causes HR[b]	0.38***	0.52***	0.78***	1.00

Excludes men with baseline history of heart attack (MI).

Low risk: baseline SBP ≤ 120 *and* DBP ≤ 80 mmHg *and* TC < 200 mg/dl (5.2 mmol/l) *and* non-smoker *and* no history of drug treatment for diabetes.

Cut points for higher income: family income, zipcode of residence, 1980 US Census: for White Americans ≥ \$24 059 per year; for African-Americans ≥ \$14 300 per year.

* $p < 0.05$; ** $p < 0.01$; *** $p < 0.001$.

[a] Age adjusted rate per 10 000 person years.

[b] Per 10 000 person years, compared to the subcohort All others, lower income.

repeatedly over the years and still being reiterated, that the readily measured major risk factors account for no more than 50% of CHD cases. In fact, they are responsible for most cases (Greenland *et al.* 2003; Magnus and Beaglehole 2001; Stamler *et al.* 1999).

Correspondingly, reflecting lower risks of long-term non-CVD as well as CVD death, HRs for all-causes mortality are much lower for all LR subcohorts than for other subcohorts not LR; for example, for the two MRFIT LR subcohorts they are lower by 57% and 60% compared to all others (HRs 0.40 and 0.43), and lower by 75% and 80% compared to those with any two or more risk factors high (Table 4.10).

These substantial differences in long-term risk of death translate into several additional years of life expectancy; for example, for the two MRFIT LR subcohorts estimates of longevity are greater by 7.2 and 7.8 years compared to all others, and by 12.0 and 13.3 years compared to those with

Table 4.10 Low risk and long-term mortality: HR by cause of death and estimated greater longevity

Cause of death	HR[a] and estimated greater longevity								
	Low risk vs. all others			Low risk vs. those with any two or more RF unfavourable or high			Low risk vs. those with any two or more RF high		
	CHA men	CHA women	MRFIT men	CHA men	CHA women	MRFIT men	CHA men	CHA women	MRFIT men
Younger adult subcohorts (baseline ages 18–44)									
CHD	0.08	0.30	0.16	0.07	0.25	0.12	0.04	0.13	0.07
CVD	0.22	0.40	0.17	0.20	0.34	0.13	0.12	0.21	0.07
All causes	0.59	0.55	0.40	0.56	0.49	0.32	0.40	0.40	0.20
Greater longevity (years)	+7.9	+6.4	+7.8	+8.6	+7.8	+9.5	+12.3	+11.4	+13.3
Adult subcohorts (baseline ages 40–59)									
CHD	0.31	0.26	0.20	0.30	0.24	0.16	0.21	0.15	0.10
CVD	0.46	0.25	0.21	0.46	0.24	0.18	0.33	0.15	0.11
All causes	0.45	0.48	0.43	0.44	0.45	0.37	0.34	0.33	0.25
Greater longevity (years)	+5.8	+5.8	+7.2	+6.1	+6.3	+8.7	+8.2	+8.7	+12.0

Excludes people with baseline history of heart attack (MI) and – for two CHA cohorts – baseline major ECG abnormality.

For subcohort criteria, number of people, baseline average RF levels, number and % of death by cause, see Tables 4.7 and 4.8; CHA men and women aged 18–39 and 40–59 at baseline, follow-up 30 years; MRFIT men aged 35–44 and 45–57 at baseline, follow-up 25 years.

[a] Controlled for age and race, and – for two CHA cohorts – education and minor ECG abnormality.

any two or more risk factors high (Table 4.10). With average ages of the two MRFIT cohorts of ~40 and 51, and – from the 1990 US Life Table – expectation for additional years of life of 35.1 and 25.5 years (uncorrected for 'healthy worker' effect), the estimates here of several further additional years of life resulting from LR status are large both absolutely and percentage-wise. Thus, for the MRFIT LR subcohort aged 45–57 at baseline, the estimated increase in life expectancy of 7.2 years compared to all others (not LR) is a 28.2% enhancement in longevity (7.2/25.5 × 100).

Data on the benefits of LR have also been reported by the Nurses Health Study, based on 14 year follow-up of 84 129 US women aged 30 to 55 at baseline in 1976 (Stampfer *et al.* 2000). Since data were collected by questionnaire only (resulting in no measured data on serum TC, BP, or BMI), alternative criteria were used to define LR, that is, *all of the following*: not smoking; *and* BMI < 25.0 kg/m² (based on reported weight and height); *and* engaged in moderate-to-vigorous physical activity for at least one-half hour per day; *and* scored in the highest 40% of the cohort for diet high in cereal fibre, marine omega-3 fatty acids, folate, ratio of polyunsaturated to saturated fatty acids; *and* low intake of trans fatty acids, low glycaemic load; *and* average alcohol intake at least half a drink per day. Only 3% of the cohort met these criteria. For these LR women compared to all other women, relative risk of a major CHD event (1128 events total, 296 fatal and 832 non-fatal) was 0.17 (95% CI 0.07 to 0.41), with control for age, family history, diagnosed high BP or serum TC, and menopausal status. The percentage reduction in CHD risk, 83%, is similar to the findings for the CHA and MRFIT cohorts.

A further implication of these data from the Nurses Health Study is that LR status is highly protective against the risk of non-fatal as well as fatal CHD events. Data on CHA LR male and female subcohorts followed for 30 years show that at older ages (65+ years) they do indeed have less coronary artery calcification, and lower morbidity from CHD and other major causes of illness (Daviglus *et al.* 2004*a*). LR subcohorts also score significantly better in older age on multiple indices measuring health-related quality of life (Daviglus *et al.* 2003*a*). They also incur significantly lower costs for medical care in older age: lower average annual costs at ages 65+, cumulative costs, and costs in the last year of life (Daviglus *et al.* 1998, 2004, 2005).

From the research evidence accrued to date, it is reasonable to infer that these several long-term benefits – into older age – of LR status for younger adult and middle-aged men and women prevail across the board, that is, for all socioeconomic-ethnic strata of the population.

4.7 Improving major risk factor levels and the proportion of the population at low risk – scientific foundations

Extensive knowledge has been available for decades demonstrating that eating habits of populations determine their average levels of serum TC and the extent of the TC rise with age from youth through middle age. Dietary variables influencing these levels directly include saturated fatty acids (SFA) and cholesterol, trans fatty acids (TFA) (effects shown more recently), and positive caloric balance with consequent weight gain; dietary variables lowering TC include polyunsaturated fatty acids (PFA) and water-soluble fibre (Clarke *et al.* 1997; Hegsted *et al.* 1993; Katz *et al.* 1958; Keys *et al.* 1965; Stamler 1967, 1978, 1979, 1994, 1995). Effects are combinative; together they are large; for example, achievement of an optimal mean TC for the adult population of 160 mg/dl (down 20%) from an average level of 200 mg/dl (currently the approximate mean for adult Americans – see Table 4.11). Each and every one of these dietary improvements contributes importantly, including lower dietary cholesterol as well as neutral fat intake – a fact overlooked in some policy statements and deliberately obscured by the egg industry. TC lower by 1% is estimated to produce CHD risk lower by ~5% for young adult men and 2% for middle-aged persons, hence the importance of every percentage improvement in TC, including that resulting from lower dietary cholesterol intake. The role of dietary cholesterol looms even larger given other key facts: its role as a *sine qua non* for atherogenesis in

Table 4.11 Improved nutrition: estimated serum cholesterol effects

Dietary variable	Improvement	Serum Cholesterol effect	
		(mg/dl)	(%)
Saturated fats (% kcal)	12→6	−12	−6.0[a]
Cholesterol (mg/1000 kcal)	130→65	−3	−1.5
Polyunsaturated fats (% kcal)	6→9	−3	−1.5
Trans fatty acids (% kcal)	2→0	−4	−2.0
H₂0 soluble fibre (g/day)	4→8	−6	−3.0
Reduction of overweight (kg)	6	−12	−6.0
Total		−40	−20.0

Based on Stamler J. and Neaton, J. D. May/June, (1994). *Scientific American Science in Medicine*, **1**, 28–37. Clarke, R. *et al.* (1997). *British Medical Journal*, **314**, 112–17.

[a] From an adult population average of 200 mg/dl.

experimental animals, including non-human primates; its adverse influences on human atherogenic low-density lipoproteins (LDL); its possible unfavourable relations to intermediate-density lipoproteins (IDL, remnant particles), lipoprotein particle size, high-density lipoproteins (HDL) and BP; its adverse relation to risk of mortality over and above its adverse influences on TC (see Table 4.6).

Especially given the still waxing obesity epidemic in many countries, the favourable influence on TC of preventing and controlling overweight/obesity needs greater attention. Intervention data from the National Diet–Heart Study (ND–HS) and MRFIT clearly show that for overweight men consuming a fat-modified diet to lower TC, weight loss significantly and sizeably enhances TC fall, over and above the favourable effects of improved lipid composition (National Diet–Heart Study Research Group 1968; Stamler *et al.* 1997*a, b*). It also markedly reduces serum triglycerides, raises high-density lipoprotein cholesterol (HDL-C), and lowers plasma glucose and uric acid (Diabetes Prevention Program Research Group 2002; Farinaro *et al.* 1977; Hu *et al.* 2001; Stamler *et al.* 1997*c*).

When the first edition of this chapter was written in 1991, there were still doubters and nay-sayers (albeit few) in regard to the aetiological significance of the three-way relationship between dietary lipid, serum lipid, and CHD, and the possibility of preventing CHD by sustained sizeable improvement in dietary lipid intake and resultant sustained reduction in TC to favourable levels. Ironically, to dispel this residual scepticism on both sides of the Atlantic required the impressive consistent results in the 1990s of the several drug trials with statins for the primary and secondary prevention of CHD. Nowadays a main refrain of medical policy is the need for physicians to be more vigorous in treating patients with unfavourable TC levels.

Since the 1980s, important research knowledge has been accrued – from both population-based observational studies and randomized controlled feeding trials – on the *influences of multiple dietary factors on blood pressure* (see Chapter 43 for a detailed review).

In this regard, data from the INTERSALT (Elliott 1989; Elliott *et al.* 1996; INTERSALT 1988; Stamler *et al.* 1996*b*), MRFIT (Stamler *et al.* 1996*a*, 1997*c*), and Western Electric studies (Miura *et al.* 2004; Stamler *et al.* 2002) served as the foundation for the 'combination diet' evaluated in the two DASH (Dietary Approaches to Stop Hypertension) feeding trials (Appel *et al.* 1997; Sacks *et al.* 2001). This DASH diet (a) emphasizes fruits, vegetables, and low-fat and fat-free dairy products; (b) includes whole grains, legumes, nuts, fish, and poultry; (c) contains small amounts of red meat, eggs, visible fats, sweets, and sugar-containing beverages (Table 4.12 and Fig. 4.2) (National Heart, Lung, and Blood Institute 1998*a*; Nutrition Action Health Letter 2003). Compared to usual American fare, this DASH diet is higher relatively in total protein, complex carbohydrate, fibre, dietary PFA/SFA, magnesium, calcium, phosphorus, and potassium, and lower in total fat (~25% of total kcal), SFA (~6% of total kcal), monounsaturated fatty acids (MFA), cholesterol (but not PFA), and lower also in dietary Na/K. In the second DASH trial, in addition to random assignment to create the two parallel groups (control and combination diet), a crossover design was used to test the independent effect on BP of two reduced levels of salt (NaCl) intake. Both DASH trials were feeding studies; that is, participants ate lunch or dinner prepared for them at the research centre on every weekday, and received from the centre all other meals, plus packets of salt and instructions on use of caffeinated and alcoholic beverages. Therefore, adherence was excellent. Weight was kept stable based on daily weighing of each participant and immediate calorie adjustment where needed. Participants were men and women ages 22+, middle-aged on average, with average BPs in the prehypertensive or Stage 1 hypertensive range (SBP 120–59 and DBP 80–95 mm Hg) not taking antihypertensive drugs. About half were women; more than half were African-Americans. Altogether, 459 participated in the first and

Table 4.12 Foods and nutrients, DASH combination diet compared to control diet[a]

Variable	Control diet	Combination diet
Food groups: menu analysis (servings/day)		
Fruits and juices	1.6	5.2
Vegetables	2.0	4.4
Grains	8.2	7.5
Nuts, seeds, legumes	0.0	0.7
Low-fat + fat-free dairy	0.1	2.0
Regular-fat dairy	0.4	0.7
Poultry	0.8	0.6
Fish	0.2	0.5
Beef, pork, ham	1.5	0.5
Fats, oils, salad dressing	5.8	2.5
Snacks and sweets	4.1	0.7
Nutrients: menu analysis		
Protein (% kcal)	13.8	17.9
Carbohydrate (% kcal)	50.5	56.5
Total fat (% kcal)	35.7	25.6
SFA (% kcal)	14.1	7.0
MFA (% kcal)	12.4	9.9
PFA (% kcal)	6.2	6.8
Cholesterol (mg/day)	233	151
Fibre (g/day)	9[b]	31[b]
Magnesium (mg/day)	176	480
Calcium (mg/day)	443	1265
Potassium (mg/day)	1752	4415
Nutrients: 24 h urinary excretion		
Potassium (mmol)	39	75
Magnesium (mg)	70	98
Calcium (mg)	137	146
Phosphorus (mg)	739	851
Urea nitrogen (mg)	9026	11583
Sodium: DASH-1 (mmol)	138	136
Sodium: DASH-Na (mmol)		
Higher	141	144
Intermediate	106	107
Lower	64	67

From DASH-Na, total daily calorie intake averages 2576 (SD 493) and 2576 (SD 511) (Sacks *et al.* 2001).

In both trials, during the 8-week (Appel *et al.* 1997) and 90-day (Sacks *et al.* 2001) intervention periods, weight was stable in both groups, in accordance with the design provision for isocaloricity; average BMI values were about 28–9 kg/m² (SD 4–5 kg/m²). Also by design, participants were either non-users of alcoholic beverages or light drinkers; e.g. in the DASH-Na trial 43–4% were drinkers, who reported an average of 0.4–0.5 drinks/day (SD 0.4).

[a] Data are from the first DASH feeding trial (Appel *et al.* 1997) unless otherwise specified.

[b] Not available from DASH-1 menu analyses; data are nutrient targets; DASH-Na reported values were 17.3 and 35.0 g/day (Sacks *et al.* 2001).

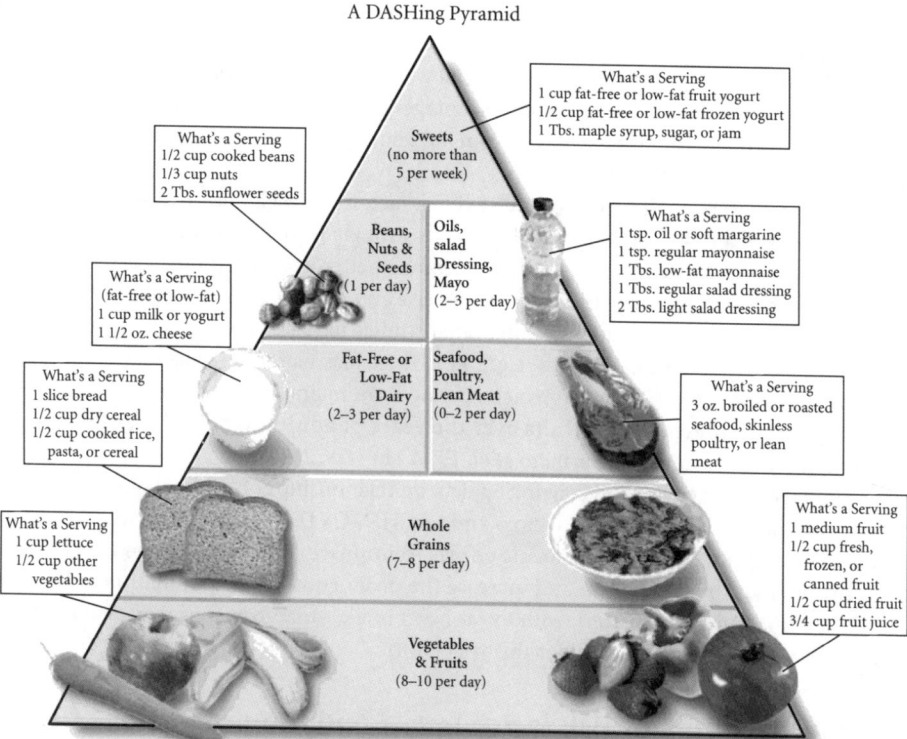

A DASHing Pyramid

What's a Serving
1 cup fat-free or low-fat fruit yogurt
1/2 cup fat-free or low-fat frozen yogurt
1 Tbs. maple syrup, sugar, or jam

What's a Serving
1/2 cup cooked beans
1/3 cup nuts
2 Tbs. sunflower seeds

Sweets
(no more than
5 per week)

What's a Serving
1 tsp. oil or soft margarine
1 tsp. regular mayonnaise
1 Tbs. low-fat mayonnaise
1 Tbs. regular salad dressing
2 Tbs. light salad dressing

What's a Serving
(fat-free ot low-fat)
1 cup milk or yogurt
1 1/2 oz. cheese

Beans,
Nuts &
Seeds
(1 per day)

Oils,
salad
Dressing,
Mayo
(2–3 per day)

What's a Serving
1 slice bread
1/2 cup dry cereal
1/2 cup cooked rice,
pasta, or cereal

Fat-Free or
Low-Fat
Dairy
(2–3 per day)

Seafood,
Poultry,
Lean Meat
(0–2 per day)

What's a Serving
3 oz. broiled or roasted
seafood, skinless
poultry, or lean
meat

What's a Serving
1 cup lettuce
1/2 cup other
vegetables

Whole
Grains
(7–8 per day)

What's a Serving
1 medium fruit
1/2 cup fresh,
frozen, or
canned fruit
1/2 cup dried fruit
3/4 cup fruit juice

Vegetables
& Fruits
(8–10 per day)

Note: Choose salt-free and low-salt foods from all categories.

Fig. 4.2 Food pyramid based on DASH eating pattern. (From *Nutrition Action Health Letter* 2003, reproduced with permission.)

412 in the second trial. In both trials, the DASH combination diet significantly and sizeably lowered SBP and DBP – casual and ambulatory – of both prehypertensive and hypertensive men and women, including SBP of people with isolated systolic hypertension. The second trial – Dash-Na – showed augmented SBP/DBP reduction with the combination diet plus reduced salt intake, especially with Na at the lower level of ~65 mmol/day (~1500 mg Na, 3800 mg NaCl).

In both DASH trials, participants were on average overweight, and – given the isocaloric design – remained overweight during the trials. It is a reasonable inference – given the established relationship of BMI to BP – that weight loss would have further enhanced these reductions in BP with the DASH combination diet plus lower NaCl intake.

As expected in view of its improved lipid and fibre composition, the DASH combination diet also significantly lowers TC and low-density lipoprotein cholesterol (LDL-C) (Harsha *et al.* 2004). For example, in the DASH-Na trial, with a baseline mean TC of 203 mg/dl, reductions were 15–19 mg/dl (7–9%); LDL-C decreased by 12–15 mg/dl (9–11%) from baseline mean of 132 mg/dl. These declines with the combination diet prevailed at each of the three levels of Na intake; that is, reduced Na intake did not interfere with these favourable effects on serum TC and LDL-C.

As data from the INTERMAP study indicate (Van Horn *et al.* 2004), a further positive aspect of the DASH combination diet is that its composition can favour avoidance of the third major risk factor, obesity. INTERMAP data include four 24 h dietary recalls, two timed 24 h urine collections, and eight BP measurements at four visits by 4680 men and women aged 40–59 from 17 population samples in China, Japan, UK, and USA (Stamler 2003). Thus, these INTERMAP data show that UK and US men and women with lower BMI—compared to those with higher BMI—tend to report higher percentages of calories from complex carbohydrates and vegetable protein, lower percentages from fat, and higher fibre intakes per 1000 kcal – all features of the DASH combination diet.

As to diabetes, the fourth major diet-related risk factor: it is well known that the far-more-common form of this disease – type 2 diabetes – is strongly related aetiologically to obesity, as are other traits of the so-called 'metabolic syndrome' (better designated the 'obesity constellation'), that is, hypertriglyceridaemia, prehypertensive and hypertensive BP, low serum HDL-C, and hyperuricaemia) (see Chapter 21). Repeated studies have shown that with a DASH-type eating pattern even modest weight loss (e.g. 5 kg) lowers plasma fasting glucose, etc., and raises HDL-C for obese people with hyperglycaemia; long-term maintenance of weight loss prevents or blunts rises in these adverse traits over the years of adulthood (Diabetes Prevention Program Research Group 2002; Farinaro *et al.* 1977; Hu *et al.* 2001).

In summary, the extensive and convincing data on relationships of habitual dietary/nutrient patterns to major CHD–CVD risk factors and to CHD–CVD risks serve as a solid scientific foundation for priority societal strategic efforts to improve progressively major risk factor levels throughout the population and increase the proportion of the population at LR. The DASH combination eating pattern with lower NaCl intake, adapted calorie-wise to deal with overweight/obesity, is a pivotal tool for this vital effort.

4.8 Improving major risk factor levels and the proportion of the population at low risk – feasibility

During the last five decades, extensive experience accrued in many countries has shown that it is feasible – based on sound public policy and reasonable resources for its sustained implementation – to improve population lifestyles and thereby shift major risk factor distributions to less adverse levels. This experience demonstrates both the interest and readiness of tens of millions to respond to sustained effective leadership, and also the obstacles that need to be overcome to achieve long-term, continuous, large-scale success. From the late 1950s on, official public policies for CHD primary prevention were developed at the national level in several countries with the support of professional organizations, voluntary health agencies, etc., and efforts at implementation were undertaken (American Heart Association 1961; ISCHDR 1970; National Cholesterol Education Program 1988, 1990, 1991; National Heart, Lung, and Blood Institute 1981; National Research Council 1989; Stamler 1978, 1979, 1992, 1995; Stamler *et al.* 1993*a, b*, 1994; White *et al.* 1959; WHO 1982, 1990*a, b*). These are based generally on lessons of the last 150 years demonstrating that the solution of mass public health problems requires multifaceted sustained effective public health efforts *based on national government leadership and support*, reaching into every corner of the nation. Therefore, the national public policies promulgated for CHD prevention are important prerequisites for progress. Their scientific foundation is the knowledge of the established major risk factors, and their cornerstone is the application of that knowledge. These public health endeavours were given an important boost by the 1982 *Report on the prevention of coronary heart disease* by a WHO Expert Committee under Geoffrey Rose's leadership, and by subsequent related WHO activity at the international and regional level (WHO 1982). Recently, at least in the USA, the focus of these efforts has by the National Heart, Lung, and Blood Institute's declaring a key policy strategic goal to be the task of progressively increasing the proportion of the population at LR. Unfortunately, these efforts have been and continue to be woefully underfunded in every country, and are impeded by many-sided persistent opposition from special commercial interests – butter councils, egg boards, fast-food marketers, salt institutes, tobacco institutes, etc. (Brownell and Horgen 2004; Hausman 1981; Nestle 2002; Schlosser 2002; Sims 1998). Nevertheless, progress has been made in several countries, reflected in trends of general national statistics. In the USA, for example, national data show declines in per capita availability of foods high in cholesterol and/or saturated fats. They indicate that the per capita dietary cholesterol intake of adult men decreased from ~750 mg/day in the late 1950s to ~350 mg/day in the late 1990s (−53%), SF decreased from ~17% of kcal to ~11% (−35%), and polyunsaturated fats increased from ~4% of kcal to ~7% (+75%). Trends for women are similar. Data are available indicating that decreases in dietary cholesterol and SF intakes have been greater among more educated than among less educated population strata.

In accordance with these trends in nutrient intake, multiple data sets, including those from serial national health surveys, show declines in mean TC levels of American adults, again differentially; that is, greater decreases for more educated than for less educated strata. Overall, the decline has been from a mean level of ~235 mg/dl in the late 1950s to ~200 mg/dl at the turn of the century. A national health goal was achieved, due mainly to improved diet composition (not drug treatment), despite the countervailing influence of the obesity epidemic.

Mean BP levels and rates of HBP were lower in successive surveys than in 1960–62 (Manolio 2004). Evidence is available from recent National Health and Nutrition Examination Surveys (NHANES) analyses that improvements in lifestyle (not just antihypertensive drug treatment) have played a role in producing this favourable trend.

Favourable trends in food intake for Americans, possibly contributing to declines in TC and BP, also include increased intakes of fruits, vegetables, legumes, soy products, and nuts. On the other hand, adverse trends are evident, for example, in daily kilocalories and percentage of kilocalories from total visible fats and oils, from sugars and sweeteners, and from grain products, together estimated to be supplying at the turn of the century 2530 kcal/person of the mounting total of kilocalories available for consumption (estimated to be 3900/person, up 18% from 3300 in 1970, when 1850 kcal were available from the three cited sources; that is, these three together are up 27%). No wonder epidemic obesity!

Prevalence of cigarette smoking also declined considerably in the USA during these decades. Whereas in 1965, the year after the landmark *Report to the Surgeon General on Smoking and Health* (Advisory Committee to the Surgeon General 1964), 50% of adult men were cigarette smokers, by 2000 this proportion had declined to 25% (50% fall). Of all adult women 32% were smokers in 1965, and 21% in 2000 (34% decrease). These trends also vary considerably by educational attainment. Thus, for persons who did not complete high school, little decrease in smoking prevalence was recorded for either non-Hispanic White Americans or African-Americans. In contrast, declines for college-educated persons were considerable.

These decades also witnessed sizeable increases in regular leisure time physical activity among American adults, once again more so among the more educated than among the less educated.

Of key importance, the proportion of the population at LR has been rising over these decades, at least based on the original set of criteria to define LR, that is, TC < 200 mg/dl *and* SBP < 120 mmHg *and* DBP < 80 mmHg *and* non-smoking, and no history of diabetes or MI (Manolio 2004; Stamler *et al.* 1999). This is evident from serial data of four successive

NHANES on random samples of the US adult population ages 25–74. In 1971–75, overall prevalence of LR was 6%; in 1976–80, 8%; in 1988–94, 17%; and in 1999–2000, 17% (Manolio *et al.* 2004). This rise was registered for men and women, African-Americans and White Americans, younger and older adults, less and more educated strata. It was greater for women than men, for younger than older, and for more than less educated. These findings document feasibility of the pivotal strategic goal for ending the CHD epidemic: achievement of progressive increases in proportion of the population at LR; this is their particular importance. At the same time, they highlight the challenges: there was no increase in LR prevalence in the latest survey; even with the rises recorded, only a small proportion of the population were LR; there were significant differentials in increase in LR prevalence by age, gender, and SES (with men, middle-aged and older persons, and lower-SES strata faring more adversely); and in all probability, with inclusion of BMI in the definition of LR there will be smaller increases in LR prevalence.

Extensive data reported recently from the MONICA Study afford a broad international perspective on late twentieth-century distributions and the trend of major risk factors and CHD, and thereby illuminate the key issues of what can be achieved and what needs to be done (Tunstall-Pedoe 2003). The MONICA Study involves 38 population samples, baseline ages 25–64, in 21 countries – 31 samples in Europe (east, north, south, west) and 7 others (in Australia, Canada, China, New Zealand, Russian central Asia, USA) – originally surveyed in the mid-1980s and followed for up to 10 years. Base populations varied from <100 000 to almost one million persons, with random sampling to assess risk factors. Actual sample sizes were most commonly 1000–2000, but up to 3000 in some populations (with generally a minimum sample size of 200 for each 10 year age-gender stratum, with surveys of 25–34-year-olds optional). Baseline data showed sizeable differences across populations in gender-specific prevalence rates of cigarette smoking, in average levels of BP, TC, and BMI, and in CHD risk score based on Cox coefficients for these four major risk factors. For men: smoking (no, yes) 0.807, SBP (mmHg) 0.014, TC (mg/dl) 0.0075, BMI (kg/m^2) 0.049; for women: 0.851, 0.020, 0.0065, and 0.007. CHD rates also varied considerably across populations, with sample baseline major risk factor levels significantly related to CHD incidence as expected in accordance with extensive findings from earlier studies. Of direct relevance here, 10 year changes in major risk factors varied in direction across populations and by gender. Thus, the age-standardized prevalence of cigarette smoking declined for men in 32 (of 38) samples, but for women in only 12 (in 25, it increased). Results varied also in different age groups. Average SBP decreased in a majority of populations, more so for women than men, but a few populations registered a higher mean SBP. For both men and women, about two-thirds of the populations registered 10 year decreases in average TC, but some showed increases. In confirmation of multiple data sets on the burgeoning epidemic of obesity on most continents, a majority of MONICA populations – male and female – showed average BMI to be higher in the mid-1990s than the mid-1980s. For men, only six registered lower mean BMI; for women, 15. In keeping with the favourable trends across a majority of populations for three of the four major risk factors (smoking, SBP, TC – all but BMI), the four-factor combined risk score was lower at 10 year follow-up than at baseline for 32 (men) and 29 (women) populations, but 6 (men) and 9 (women) had higher scores.

These 10 year trend data demonstrate that: (a) population mean levels of major risk factors, considered singly and in combination (risk score), are amenable to improvement; (b) reductions are not inevitable, trends can be – have been – adverse in some populations; (c) the sizeable cross-population differences in population average risk factor levels, and the extent and variety of 10 year change patterns indicate – in accordance with many other data sets (including on migrants) – that environmental factors are crucial determinants of these population average differences and trends (not population genetics).

The cited population-wide experiences in the USA and other countries show that it is possible, even with only limited resources and in the face of serious obstacles, to effect and sustain nationwide favourable trends in lifestyles and lifestyle-related major risk factors. It is a reasonable inference that these trends have contributed in an important way to the declines in CHD, CVD, and all-cause mortality in these countries. This inference is supported statistically by not only the above-cited MONICA data but also by analyses of international data for industrialized nations, showing significant correlations between national *trends* of per capita dietary lipid (including dietary cholesterol) and *trends* of CHD mortality, and between national *trends* of per capita cigarette use and *trends* of CHD mortality (Byington *et al.* 1979). It is further supported in a particular way by the American experience. As noted above, trends of nutritional pattern, serum cholesterol, cigarette use, and leisure time exercise have all been more favourable for more educated than for less educated Americans. If changes in these traits have played a significant aetiological role in the marked decline in CHD, stroke, CVD, and all-cause mortality in the USA since the late 1960s, then the declines should be greater in the more educated than in the less educated. Five papers have been published on this matter, all of them with data showing greater decreases in mortality for the more educated (Stamler 1992). This is further evidence for the crucial role of the established major risk factors, in the *ultimately decisive area: CHD prevention in the general population.*

4.9 **Summary and conclusions**

The evidence presented here builds on a huge body of research amassed over many years and from many scientific disciplines, testifying to the strength of the relationships of the established major risk factors to coronary risk. Adverse diet is pivotal among the risk factors and plays a primary and overwhelming role in the causation of epidemic CHD and CVD. The low prevalence in the population of truly LR people poses a vital challenge and points to the large possibilities for prevention through substantial shifts downwards in the population levels of these risk factors by safe improvements in population lifestyles, especially dietary habits from early childhood on. Geoffrey Rose's concept of the 'sick' population neatly elaborates this idea and illustrates the essentiality of a strategy of prevention which combines both population-wide and high-risk components (Rose 1985, 1992).

Large problems persist on both sides of the Atlantic in regard to scope and consistency of government efforts to implement policies including food and nutrition policies, recognized as vital for the control and prevention of CHD, CVD, and other chronic diseases. In the USA, intakes of saturated fat and cholesterol, despite the declines, are still above recommended levels, total fat intake remains high, and prevalence of obesity has risen. At the national level, some industrialized countries have registered little or no decline in CHD mortality, or increases. In several countries – the UK, USA, and others – there is the further gnawing problem, so far essentially unaddressed, of the particularly unfavourable findings for the less educated and less affluent, noted above for the USA. Clearly, systematic application in the population of knowledge on the established major risk factors and on the key strategic challenge of increasing the proportion of the population at LR is still limited everywhere. Much remains to be done at every level, from the top of government downwards, by public health and medical communities everywhere. Despite downturns in several countries, the CHD epidemic continues; on a world scale it is vast and mounting.

As the *British Medical Journal* commented in a news article on the problems of the world's children: 'The sad fact is that 40,000 children die every day from easily preventable diseases. *The solution is one of will not of technology*' (Logie 1990, emphasis added). This is also true for CHD–CVD prevention.

Acknowledgements

It is a pleasure to express appreciation to the many colleagues who collected the baseline data on the 361 662 men who were screened for MRFIT (see Bibliography for references with a listing), to colleagues at the MRFIT Coordinating Center who collected and analysed the data on the vital status of these men, particularly Joanna Shih MS and Deborah Wentworth MS, and to fellow members of the MRFIT Editorial Committee, Marcus Kjelsberg PhD (past Chairman), Jerome Cohen MD, Lewis Kuller MD, and Judith Ockene PhD. It is also gratifying to acknowledge the contribution of the many staff members and volunteers who accomplished the Chicago Heart Association Detection Project in Industry, particularly James A. Schoenberger MD, Richard B. Shekelle PhD, and Sue Shekelle MSW. It is likewise a pleasure to acknowledge the role of Oglesby Paul MD, founder and for many years leader of the Western Electric Study, Mark Lepper MD, and Ann MacMillan Shryock MS, who played a decisive role in collecting the baseline nutrition data in 1957–59. We are grateful to Ms Bonnie Liebman, The Center for Science in the Public Interest, and the Nutrition Action Health Letter for assistance and permission to use Fig. 2 here, and to the Prospective Studies Collaboration Research Group and *The Lancet* for permission to use Fig. 1 here. The research data reported here were collected with support from the American Heart Association and its Illinois and Chicago affiliates, the Chicago Health Research Foundation, the Illinois Regional Medical Program, the National Heart, Lung, and Blood Institute, and many private donors.

Bibliography

Advisory Committee to the Surgeon General (1964). *Smoking and health*. US Department of Health, Education and Welfare, Washington, DC.

American Heart Association (1961). Dietary fat and its relation to heart attacks and strokes. *Circulation*, **23**, 133–6.

American Heart Association (1980). American Heart Association Committee Report. Risk factors and coronary diseases: a statement for physicians. *Circulation*, **62**, 449A–455A.

American Heart Association (1998). American Heart Association call to action: obesity as a major risk factor for coronary heart disease. *Circulation*, **97**, 2099–100.

American Heart Association (2000). AHA Dietary Guidelines. Revision 2000: a statement for healthcare professionals from the Nutrition Committee of the American Heart Association. *Circulation*, **102**, 2284–99.

American Journal of Public Health (1957). Measuring the risk of coronary heart disease in adult population groups: a symposium. *American Journal of Public Health*, **2**, 1–63.

Appel, L. J., Moore, T. J., Obarzanek, E., Vollmer, W. M., Svetkey, L. P., Sacks, F. M. *et al.* for the DASH Collaborative Research Group (1997). A clinical trial of the effects of dietary patterns on blood pressure. *New England Journal of Medicine*, **336**, 1117–24.

Barker, D. J. P. (1998). *Mothers, babies, and health in later life*, Churchill Livingstone, Edinburgh.

Berenson, G. S. (ed.). (1986). *Causation of cardiovascular risk factors in children: perspective on cardiovascular risk in early life.* Raven Press, New York.

Berenson, G. S., McMahan, C. A., Voors, A. W., Webber, L. S., Srinivasan, S. R., Frank, G. C. *et al.* (eds). (1980). *Cardiovascular risk factors in children: the early natural history of atherosclerosis and essential hypertension.* Oxford University Press, New York.

Brownell, K. D. and Horgen, K. B. (2004). *Food fight: the inside story of the food industry, America's obesity crisis, and what we can do about it.* McGraw Hill, New York.

Burke, B. S. (1947). The dietary history as a tool in research. *Journal of the American Dietetic Association,* **23**, 1041–6.

Byington, R., Dyer, A. R., Garside, D., Liu, K., Moss, D., Stamler, J., and Tsong, Y. (1979). Recent trends of major coronary risk factors and CHD mortality in the United States and other industrialized countries. In *Proceedings of the Conference on the Decline in Coronary Heart Disease Mortality* (ed. R. J. Havlik and M. Feinleib), pp 340–80. NIH Publication 79-1610. National Institutes of Health, Washington, DC.

Clarke, R., Frost, C., Collins, R., Appleby, P., and Peto, R. (1997). Dietary lipids and blood cholesterol: quantitative meta-analysis of metabolic ward studies. *British Medical Journal,* **314**, 112–17.

Davey Smith, G. (2003). *Health inequalities: lifecourse approaches.* Policy Press, Bristol.

Davey Smith, G., Neaton, J. D., Wentworth, D., Stamler, R., and Stamler, J. (1996a). Socioeconomic differentials in mortality risk among men screened for the Multiple Risk Factor Intervention Trial: I. White men. *American Journal of Public Health,* **86**, 486–96.

Davey Smith, G., Neaton, J. D., Wentworth, D., Stamler, R., and Stamler, J. (1996b). Socioeconomic differentials in mortality risk among men screened for the Multiple Risk Factor Intervention Trial: II. Black men. *American Journal of Public Health,* **86**, 497–504.

Daviglus, M. L., Liu, K., Greenland, P., Dyer, A. R., Garside, D. B., Manheim, L. *et al.* (1998). Benefit of a favorable cardiovascular risk factor profile in middle age with respect to Medicare costs. *New England Journal of Medicine,* **339**, 1122–9.

Daviglus, M. L., Liu, K., Pirzada, A., Yan, L. L., Garside, D. B., Feinglass, J. *et al.* (2003a). Favorable cardiovascular risk factor profile in middle age and health-related quality of life in older age. *Archives of Internal Medicine,* **163**, 2460–8.

Daviglus, M. L., Liu, K., Yan, L. L., Pirzada, A., Garside, D. B., Schiffer, L. *et al.* (2003b). Body mass index in middle age and health-related quality of life in older age: The Chicago Heart Association Selection Project in Industry Study. *Archives of Internal Medicine,* **163**, 2448–55.

Daviglus, M. L., Pirzada, A., Liu, K., Yan, L. L., Garside, D. B., Dyer, A. R. *et al.* (2004a). Comparison of low risk and higher risk profiles in middle age to frequency and quantity of coronary artery calcium years later. *American Journal of Cardiology,* **94**, 367–9.

Daviglus, M. L., Stamler, J., Pirzada, A., Yan, L. L., Garside, D. B., Liu, K. *et al.* (2004b). Favorable cardiovascular risk profile in young women and long-term risk of cardiovascular and all-cause mortality. *Journal of The American Medical Association,* **292**, 1588–92.

Daviglus, M. L., Liu, K., Pirzada, A., Manheim, L., and Manning, W. *et al.* (2004c). Relation of body mass index in young adulthood and middle age to Medicare expenditures in older age. *Journal of The American Medical Association,* **292**, 2743–9.

Daviglus, M. L., Liu, K., Pirzada, A., Yan, L. L., Garside, D. B., Greenland, P. *et al.* (2005). Cardiovascular risk profile early in life and Medicare costs in the last year of life. *Archives of Internal Medicine,* in press.

Denton, D., Weisinger, R., Mundy, N. I, Wickings, E. J., Dixon, A., Moisson, P. *et al.* (1995). The effect of increased salt intake on blood pressure of chimpanzees, *Nature Medicine,* **1**, 1009–16.

Department of Health (1994). *Nutritional aspects of cardiovascular disease.* Report of the Cardiovascular Review Group, Committee on Medical Aspects of Food Policy. (Report on Health and Social Subjects No. 46). HMSO, London.

Diabetes Prevention Program Research Group (2002). Reduction in the incidence of Type 2 diabetes with lifestyle intervention or metformin. *New England Journal of Medicine*, **346**, 393–403.

Dietary Guidelines Advisory Committee (1995). *Report of the Dietary Guidelines Advisory Committee on the dietary guidelines for Americans*. US Government Printing Office, Washington, DC.

Dietary Guidelines Advisory Committee (2000). *Scientific rationale: dietary guidelines for Americans*. US Government Printing Office, Washington, DC.

Elliott, P. (guest ed.) (1989). INTERSALT Cooperative Research Group. The INTERSALT Study – an international cooperative study of electrolyte excretion and blood pressure – further results. *Journal of Human Hypertension*, **3**, 279–407.

Elliott, P., Stamler, J., Nichols, R., Dyer, A. R., Stamler, R., Kesteloot, H., and Marmot, M. for the INTERSALT Cooperative Research Group (1996). INTERSALT revisited: further analyses of 24-hour sodium excretion and blood pressure within and across populations. *British Medical Journal*, **312**, 1249–53.

Farinaro, E., Stamler, J., Upton, M., Mojonnier, L., Hall, Y., Moss, D., and Berkson, D. M. (1977). Plasma glucose levels: long-term effect of diet in the Chicago Coronary Prevention Evaluation Program. *Annals of Internal Medicine*, **86**, 147–54.

Fraser, G. E. (1986). *Preventive cardiology*. Oxford University Press, New York.

Greenland, P., Knoll, M., Stamler, J., Neaton, J. D., Dyer, A. R., Garside, D. B., and Wilson, P. W. (2003). Major risk factors as antecedents of fatal and nonfatal coronary heart disease events. *Journal of the American Medical Association*, **290**, 891–7.

Harsha, D. W., Sacks, F. M., Obarzanek, E., Svetkey, L. P., Lin, P. H., Bray, G. A. *et al.* (2004). Effect of dietary sodium intake on blood lipids: results from the DASH-Sodium Trial. *Hypertension* **43 (2)**, 393–8.

Hausman, P. (1981). *Jack Sprat's legacy: the science and politics of fat and cholesterol*. Richard Marak, New York.

Hegsted, D. M. (1985). An overview of nutrition research. In *NIH Workshop on Nutrition and Hypertension*. (ed. M. J. Horan, M. Blaustein, J. B. Dunbar, W. Kachadorian, N. M. Kaplan, and A. P. Simopoulos), pp. 9-16. Biomedical Information, New York.

Hegsted, D. M., Austman, L. M., Johnson, J. A., and Dallal, G. E. (1993). Dietary fat and serum lipids: an evaluation of the experimental data. *American Journal of Clinical Nutrition*, **57**, 875–83.

Hu, F. B., Manson, J. A. E., Stampfer, M. J., Colditz, G., Liu, S., Solomon, C. G., and Willett, W. C. (2001). Diet, lifestyle and the risk of Type 2 diabetes mellitus in women. *New England Journal of Medicine*, **345**, 790–7.

International Task Force for Prevention of Coronary Heart Disease in Cooperation with the International Atherosclerosis Society (1998). Coronary heart disease: reducing the risk. The scientific background for primary and secondary prevention of coronary heart disease. *Nutrition and Metabolism in Cardiovascular Disease*, **8**, 205–71.

INTERSALT Cooperative Research Group (1988). INTERSALT: an international study of electrolyte excretion and blood pressure. Results for 24-hour urinary sodium and potassium excretion. *British Medical Journal*, **297**, 319–28.

ISCHDR (Inter-Society Commission for Heart Disease Resources, Atherosclerosis Study Group and Epidemiology Study Group) (1970). Primary prevention of the atherosclerotic diseases. *Circulation*, **42**, A55–A95.

JNC-V. National High Blood Pressure Education Program (1993). The Fifth Report of the Joint National Committee on Detection, Evaluation, and Treatment of High Blood Pressure (JNC-V). *Archives of Internal Medicine*, **153**, 154–83.

JNC-VI. National High Blood Pressure Education Program (1997). The Sixth Report of the Joint National Committee on Detection, Evaluation, and Treatment of High Blood Pressure (JNC-VI). *Archives of Internal Medicine*, **157**, 2413–46.

JNC-VII (2003). The Seventh Report of the Joint National Committee on Detection, Evaluation, and Treatment of High Blood Pressure (JNC-VII). National High Blood Pressure Education Program. *Hypertension*, **42**, 1206–52.

Katz, L. N. and Stamler, J. (1953). *Experimental atherosclerosis*. C. Thomas, Springfield, IL.

Katz, L. N., Stamler, J., and Pick. R. (1958). *Nutrition and atherosclerosis*. Lea and Febiger, Philadelphia.

Keys, A. and White, P. D. (eds) (1956). *World trends in cardiology: cardiovascular epidemiology*. Selected papers from Second World Congress and Twenty Seventh Annual Scientific Sessions of the American Heart Association. Hoeber-Harper, New York.

Keys, A., Anderson, J. T., and Grande, F. (1965). Serum cholesterol response to changes in the diet. *Metabolism*, **14**, 747–87. [Four papers.]

Kimura, N. (1956). Analysis of 10,000 postmortem examinations in Japan. In *World trends in cardiology: cardiovascular epidemiology* (ed. A. Keys and P. D. White), pp. 22–33. Hoeber-Harper, New York.

Klag, M. J., Ford, D. E., Mead, L. A., He, J., Whelton, P. K., Liang, K. Y., and Levine, D. M. (1993). Serum cholesterol in young men and subsequent cardiovascular disease. *New England Journal of Medicine*, **328**, 313–18.

Lasser, N. L., Grandits, G., Caggiula, A. W., Cutler, J. A., Grimm, R. H., Jr., Kuller, L. H. *et al.* (1984). Effects of antihypertensive therapy on plasma lipids and lipoproteins in the Multiple Risk Factor Intervention Trial. *American Journal of Medicine*, **76** (Suppl. 2A), 52–66.

Lauer, R. M. and Shekelle, R. B. (eds) (1980). *Childhood prevention of atherosclerosis and hypertension*. Raven Press, New York.

Lauer, R. M., Connor, W. E., Leaverton, P. E., Reiter, M. A., and Clarke, W. R. (1975). Coronary heart disease risk factors in school children. *Journal of Pediatrics*, **86**, 697–706.

Lauer, R. M., Burns, T. L., and Daniels, S. R. (2005). *Paediatric prevention of adult cardiovascular disease*. Oxford University Press, in press.

Liu, K., Stamler, J., Dyer, A., McKeever, J., and McKeever, P. (1978). Statistical methods to assess and minimize the role of intra-individual variability in obscuring the relationship between dietary lipids and serum cholesterol. *Journal of Chronic Diseases*, **31**, 399–418.

Logie, D. (1990). The world summit for children. *British Medical Journal*, **301**, 625.

MacMahon, S., Peto, R., Cutler, J., Collins, R., Sorlie, P., Neaton, J. *et al.* (1990). Blood pressure, stroke, and coronary heart disease. Part 1. Prolonged differences in blood pressure: prospective observational studies corrected for the regression dilution bias. *Lancet*, **335**, 765–74.

Magnus, P. and Beaglehole, R. (2001). The real contribution of the major risk factors to the coronary epidemics: time to end the 'only 50%' myth. *Archives of Internal Medicine*, **161**, 2657–60.

Mancilha-Carvalho, J. J., Baruzzi, R. G., Howard, P. F., Poulter, N., Alpers, M. P., Franco, L. J. *et al.* (1989). Blood pressure in four remote populations in the INTERSALT Study. *Hypertension*, **14**, 238–46.

Manolio, T. (2004). Personal Communication.

Marmot, M. G., Smith, G. D., Stansfeld, S., Patel, C., North, F., Head, J. *et al.* (1991). Health inequalities among British civil servants: the Whitehall II study. *Lancet*, **337**, 1387–93.

McGill, H. C., Jr, MacMahon, C. A., Herderick, E. E., Malcom, G. T., Tracy, R. E., and Strong, J. P. for the Pathobiological Determinants of Atherosclerosis in Youth (PDAY). Research Group (2000). Origins of atherosclerosis in childhood and adolescence. *American Journal of Clinical Nutrition*, **72** (Suppl.), 1037S–1315S.

Miura, K., Greenland, P., Stamler, J., Liu, K., Daviglus, M. L., and Nakagawa, H. (2004). Relation of vegetable, fruit, and meat intake to 7-year blood pressure change in middle-aged men: the Chicago Western Electric Study. *American Journal of Epidemiology*, **159**, 572–80.

National Cholesterol Education Program (1988). Report of the NCEP Expert Panel on Detection, Evaluation, and Treatment of High Blood Cholesterol in Adults. *Archives of Internal Medicine*, **148**, 36–69.

National Cholesterol Education Program (1990). Report of the NCEP Expert Panel on Population Strategies for Blood Cholesterol Reduction. National Institutes of Health Publication No. 90-3046. US Department of Health and Human Services, Public Health Services, Bethesda, MD.

National Cholesterol Education Program (1991). Report of the NCEP Expert Panel on Cholesterol Levels in Children and Adolescents. NIH Publication No. 91-2732. National Institutes of Health, National Heart, Lung and Blood Institute, Bethesda, MD.

National Cholesterol Education Program (2001). Adult Treatment Panel III (ATP III). Executive Summary of the Third Report of the NCEP Expert Panel on Detection, Evaluation and Treatment of High Blood Cholesterol in Adults. *Journal of the American Medical Association*, **285**, 2486–97.

National Cholesterol Education Program (2002). Third Report of the NCEP Expert Panel on Detection, Evaluation and Treatment of High Blood Cholesterol in Adults (Adult Treatment Panel III). NIH Publication No. 02-5215. National Institutes of Health, Bethesda, MD.

National Diet-Heart Study Research Group (1968). The National Diet-Heart Study Final Report. *Circulation*, **37** (Suppl. 1), I-1–I-428.

National Heart, Lung, and Blood Institute (1981). Working Group on Arteriosclerosis of the National Heart, Lung, and Blood Institute. *Arteriosclerosis*, Vol. 2. National Institutes of Health, Bethesda, MD.

National Heart, Lung, and Blood Institute (1998*a*). *The DASH diet*. US Department of Health and Human Services, Public Health Service, National Institutes of Health. NIH Publication No. 01-4082. National Heart, Lung, and Blood Institute, Bethesda, MD.

National Heart, Lung, and Blood Institute (1998*b*). NHLBI Obesity Education Initiative Expert Panel on the Identification, Evaluation, and Treatment of Overweight and Obesity in Adults. Clinical Guidelines on the Identification, Evaluation and Treatment of Overweight and Obesity in Adults. The Evidence Report, NIH Publication No. 98-4083. National Institutes of Health, Bethesda, MD.

National High Blood Pressure Education Program Working Group (1993). National High Blood Pressure Education Program Working Group Report on Primary Prevention of Hypertension. *Archives of Internal Medicine*, **153**, 186–208.

National Research Council (1989). Committee on Diet and Health, Food and Nutrition Board, Commission on Life Sciences. *Diet and health: implications for reducing chronic disease*. National Academy Press, Washington, DC.

Neaton, J. D., Kuller, L. H., Wentworth, D., and Borhani, N. O. for the Multiple Risk Factor Intervention Trial Research Group (1984). Total and cardiovascular mortality in relation to cigarette smoking, serum cholesterol concentration, and diastolic blood pressure among black and white males followed for five years. *American Heart Journal*, **108**, 759–69.

Nestle, M. (2002). *Food politics: How the food industry influences nutrition and health*. University of California Press, Berkeley and Los Angeles.

Nutrition Action Health letter (2003). May Issue, p. 8. Center for Science in the Public Interest, Washington, DC.

Paul, O., Lepper, M. H., Phelan, W. H., Dupertuis, G. W., MacMillan, A., McKean, H., and Park, H. (1963). A longitudinal study of coronary heart disease. *Circulation*, **28**, 20–31.

Pearson, T. A. (1984). Coronary arteriography in the study of the epidemiology of coronary artery disease. *Epidemiologic Reviews*, **6**, 140–66.

Pooling Project Research Group (1978). Relationship of blood pressure, serum cholesterol, smoking habit, relative weight and ECG abnormalities to incidence of major coronary events: final report of the Pooling Project. *Journal of Chronic Diseases*, **31**, 201–306.

Prospective Studies Collaboration (2002). Age-specific relevance of usual blood pressure to vascular mortality: a meta-analysis of individual data for one million adults in 61 prospective studies. *Lancet*, **360**, 1903–13.

Rose, G. (1985). Sick individuals and sick populations. *International Journal of Epidemiology*, **14**, 32–8.

Rose, G. (1992). *The strategy of preventive medicine*. Oxford University Press.

Sacks, F. M., Rosner, B., and Kass, E. H. (1974). Blood pressure in vegetarians. *American Journal of Epidemiology*, **100**, 390–8.

Sacks, F. M., Castelli, W. P., Donner, A., and Kass, E. H. (1975). Plasma lipids and lipoproteins in vegetarians and controls. *New England Journal of Medicine*, **292**, 1148–51.

Sacks, F. M., Svetkey, L. P., Vollmer, W. M., Appel, L. J., Bray, G. A., Harsha, D. *et al.* for the DASH-Sodium Collaborative Research Group (2001). Effects on blood pressure of reduced sodium and the Dietary Approaches to Stop Hypertension (DASH). diet. *New England Journal of Medicine*, **344**, 3–10.

Schlosser, E. (2002). *Fast food nation: the dark side of the all American meal*. Perennial–Harper Collins, New York.

Shaper, A. G. (1974). Communities without hypertension. In *Cardiovascular disease in the tropics* (ed. A. G. Shaper, M. S. R. Hutt, and Z. Fejfar), pp. 77–83. British Medical Association, London.

Shekelle, R. B., Shryock, A. M., Paul, O., Lepper, M., Stamler, J., Liu, S., and Raynor, W. J., Jr (1981). Diet, serum cholesterol, and death from coronary heart disease. *New England Journal of Medicine*, **304**, 65–70.

Shekelle, R. B., Stamler, J., Paul, O., Shyrock, A. M., Liu, S., and Lepper, M. (1982). Dietary lipids and serum cholesterol level: change in diet confounds the cross-sectional association. *American Journal of Epidemiology*, **115**, 506–14.

Sims, L. S. (1998). *The politics of fat: food and nutrition policy in America*, Armonk, New York.

Sinha, R., Fisch, G., Teague, B., Tamboriane, W. V., Banyas, B., Allen, K. *et al.* (2002). Prevalence of impaired glucose tolerance among children and adolescents with marked obesity. *New England Journal of Medicine*, **346**, 802–10.

Stamler, J. (1966). Nutrition, metabolism and atherosclerosis: a review of data and theories, and a discussion of controversial questions. In *Controversy in internal medicine* (ed. F. J. Inglefinger, A. L. Relman, and M. Finland), pp. 27–59. Saunders, Philadelphia.

Stamler, J. (1967). *Lectures on preventive cardiology*. Grune and Stratton, New York.

Stamler, J. (1978). George Lyman Duff Memorial Lecture. Lifestyles, major risk factors, proof and public policy. *Circulation*, **58**, 3–19.

Stamler, J. (1979). Population studies. In *Nutrition, lipids, and coronary heart disease: a global view* (ed. R. I. Levy, B. M. Rifkind, B. H. Dennis, and N. D. Ernst), pp. 25–88. Raven Press, New York.

Stamler, J. (1989). Opportunities and pitfalls in international comparisons related to patterns, trends and determinants of CHD mortality. *International Journal of Epidemiology*, **18**, S3–S18.

Stamler, J. (1992). Established major coronary risk factors. In *Coronary heart disease epidemiology: from aetiology to public health* (ed. M. Marmot and P. Elliott), pp. 35–66. Oxford University Press, New York.

Stamler, J. (1994). Assessing diets to improve world health: nutritional research on disease causation in populations. *American Journal of Clinical Nutrition*, **59**, 146S–156S.

Stamler, J. (1995). Potential for prevention of major adult cardiovascular disease. In *Lessons for science from the seven countries study: a 35-year collaborative experience in cardiovascular disease epidemiology* (ed. H. Toshima, Y. Koga, H. J. Blackburn, A. Keys), pp. 195–235. Springer-Verlag, Tokyo.

Stamler, J. (1997). The INTERSALT Study: background, methods, findings, and implications. *American Journal of Clinical Nutrition*, **65**, 626S–642S.

Stamler, J. (Guest Editor) (2003). Special Issue: INTERMAP: International study of macro- and micronutrients and blood pressure. *Journal of Human Hypertension*, **17**, 585–775.

Stamler, J. and Hazuda, H. P. (1996). Executive summary. In *Report of the Conference on Socioeconomic Status and Cardiovascular Health and Disease*, 6–7 November 1995, pp. 3–10. National Institutes of Health; National Heart, Lung, and Blood Institute. Bethesda, MD. Reprinted in *Circulation* (1996), **94**, 2041–4 with an introduction by C. Lenfant. Also reprinted at <http://www.nhlbi.nih.gov/nhlbi/sciinf/other/othdocs.htm> as of 8 December 1996.

Stamler, J. and Shekelle, R. (1988). Dietary cholesterol and human coronary heart disease: the epidemiologic evidence. *Archives of Pathology and Laboratory Medicine*, **112**, 1032–40.

Stamler, J., Wentworth, D., and Neaton, J. D. (1986). Is the relationship between serum cholesterol and risk of premature death from coronary heart disease continuous and graded? Findings in 356,222 primary screenees of the Multiple Risk Factor Intervention Trial (MRFIT). *Journal of the American Medical Association*, **256**, 2823–8.

Stamler, J., Dyer, A. R., Shekelle, R. B., Neaton, J., and Stamler, R. (1993a). Relationship of baseline major risk factors to coronary and all-cause mortality, and to longevity: findings from long-term follow-up of Chicago cohorts. *Cardiology*, **82**, 191–222.

Stamler, J., Stamler, R., Brown, W. V., Gotto, A. M., Greenland, P., Grundy, S. *et al.* (1993b). Serum cholesterol: doing the right thing. *Circulation*, **88**, 1954–60.

Stamler, J., Stamler, R., Brown, W. V., Gotto, A. M., Greenland, P., Grundy, S. *et al.* (1994). Reply to Letters to Editor on Editorial, 'Doing the right thing'. *Circulation*, **90**, 2573–7.

Stamler, J., Caggiula, A. W., Grandits, G. A., Kjelsberg, M., and Cutler, J. A. for the MRFIT Research Group (1996a). Relationship to blood pressure of combinations of dietary macronutrients: findings of the Multiple Risk Factor Intervention Trial. *Circulation*, **94**, 2417–23.

Stamler, J., Elliott, P., Kesteloot, H., Nichols, R., Claeys, G., Dyer, A. R., and Stamler, R. for the INTERSALT Cooperative Research Group (1996b). Inverse relation of dietary protein markers with blood pressure: findings for 10,020 men and women in the INTERSALT Study. *Circulation*, **94**, 1629–34.

Stamler, J., Stamler, R., Garside, D., Greenlund, K., Archer, S., Neaton, J. D., and Wentworth, D. N. (1996c). Socioeconomic status, cardiovascular risk factors, and cardiovascular disease: findings on US working populations. In *Report of the Conference on Socioeconomic Status and Cardiovascular Health and Disease*, 6–7 November 1995, pp. 109–18. National Institutes of Health; National Heart, Lung and Blood Institute. Reprinted at <http://www.nhlbi.nih.gov/nhlbi/sciinf/other/othdocs.htm> as of 8 December 1996.

Stamler, J., Briefel, R. R., Milas, C., Grandits, G. A., and Caggiula, A. W. (1997a). Relation of changes in dietary lipids and weight, trial years 1–6, to changes in blood lipids in the special intervention and usual care groups in the Multiple Risk Factor Intervention Trial. *American Journal of Clinical Nutrition*, **65** (Suppl. 1), 272S–288S.

Stamler, J., Caggiula, A. W., Cutler, J. A., Dolccek, T. A., Grandits, G. A., Kjelsberg, M. O., and Tillotson, J. L. (guest scientific eds) (1997b). Dietary and nutritional methods and findings: the Multiple Risk Factor Intervention Trial (MRFIT). *American Journal of Clinical Nutrition*, **65** (Suppl. 1), 183S–402S.

Stamler, J., Caggiula, A. W., and Grandits, G. A. (1997c). Relation of body mass and alcohol, nutrient, fiber, and caffeine intakes to blood pressure in the special intervention and usual care groups in the Multiple Risk Factor Intervention Trial. *American Journal of Clinical Nutrition*, **65** (Suppl. 1), 338S–365S.

Stamler, J., Stamler, R., Neaton, J. D., Wentworth, D., Daviglus, M. L., Garside, D. *et al.* (1999). Low risk factor profile and long-term cardiovascular and non-cardiovascular mortality and life expectancy: findings for five large cohorts of young adult and middle-aged men and women. *Journal of the American Medical Association*, **282**, 2012–18.

Stamler, J., Daviglus, M. L., Garside, D. B., Dyer, A. R., Greenland, P., and Neaton, J. D. (2000). Relationship of baseline serum cholesterol levels in three large cohorts of younger men to long-term coronary cardiovascular, and all-cause mortality and to longevity. *Journal of the American Medical Association*, **284**, 311–18.

Stamler, J., Liu, K., Ruth, K. J., Pryer, J., and Greenland, P. (2002). Eight-year blood pressure change in middle-aged men: relationship to multiple nutrients. *Hypertension*, **39**, 1000–6.

Stamler, J., Elliott, P., Appel, L., Chan, Q., Buzzard, M., Dennis, B. *et al.* for the INTERMAP Research Group (2003). Higher blood pressure in middle-aged American adults with less education – role of multiple dietary factors: the INTERMAP Study. *Journal of Human Hypertension*, **17**, 655–64.

Stamler, J., Elliott, P., Chan, Q., Archer, S., Daviglus, M. L., Dyer, A. R. *et al.* for the INTERMAP Research Group (2004). Dietary amino acids – their relation to vegetable/animal protein intake and to blood pressure: The INTERMAP Study. *44th Annual Conference on Cardiovascular Disease Epidemiology and Prevention*, 3–6 March 2004. American Heart Association, San Francisco. [Abstract.]

Stamler, R., Shipley, M., Elliott, P., Dyer, A., Sans, S., and Stamler, J. (1992). Higher blood pressure in adults with less education: some likely explanatory factors. Findings of the INTERSALT Study. *Hypertension*, **19**, 237–41.

Stampfer, M. J., Hu, F. B., Manson, J. E., Rimm, E. B., and Willett, W. C. (2000). Primary prevention of coronary heart disease in women through diet and lifestyle. *New England Journal of Medicine*, **343**, 16–22.

Tunstall-Pedoe, H. (ed.) for the WHO MONICA Project (2003). *MONICA monograph and multimedia sourcebook*. World Health Organization, Geneva.

USDA, USDHHS (US Department of Agriculture, US Department of Health and Human Services) (1995). *Dietary guidelines for Americans*, 4th edn. US Government Printing Office, Washington, DC.

USDA, USDHHS (US Department of Agriculture, US Department of Health and Human Services) (2000). *Dietary guidelines for Americans*. US Government Printing Office, Washington, DC.

USDHHS (US Department of Health and Human Services) (1988). *The Surgeon General's report on nutrition and health*. US Government Printing Office, Washington, DC.

USDHHS (US Department of Health and Human Services) (1991). *Healthy People 2000: national health promotion and disease prevention objectives*. [Summary Report]. DHSS publication No. (PHS) 91-50213. US Government Printing Office, Washington, DC.

USDHHS (US Department of Health and Human Services) (1996). *Physical activity and health: a report of the Surgeon General*. US Department of Health and Human Services, Centers for Disease Control and Prevention, National Center for Chronic Disease Prevention and Health Promotion, Atlanta, GA.

USDHHS (US Department of Health and Human Services) (1998). Office of Public Health and Science. *Healthy people 2010 objectives: draft for public comment*. US Government Printing Office, Washington, DC.

USDHHS (US Department of Health and Human Services) (1999). *Healthy people 2000 review, 1998–1999*. Publication Number (PS) 99-1256. Department of Health and Human Services, Centers for Disease Control and Prevention, National Center for Health Statistics, Hyattsville, MD.

USDHHS (US Department of Health and Human Services). (2000). *Healthy people 2010: Understanding and improving health, 2nd edn*. US Government Printing Office, Washington DC.

Van Horn, L., Dyer, A. R., Liu, K., Garside, D., Greenland, P., Archer, S. *et al.* for the INTERMAP Research Group (2004). Relation of diet composition and physical activity to body mass index: the INTERMAP study. *44th Annual Conference on Cardiovascular Disease Epidemiology and Prevention*, 3–6 March 2004. American Heart Association, San Francisco. [Abstract.]

Whelton, P. K., He, J., Appel, L. J., Cutler, J. A., Havas, S., Kotchen, T. A. *et al.* for the National High Blood Pressure Education Program Coordinating Committee (2002). Primary prevention of hypertension: clinical and public health advisory from the National High Blood Pressure Education Program. *Journal of the American Medical Association*, **288**, 1882–8.

Whelton, P. K., He, J., and Louis, G. T. (eds) (2003). *Lifestyle modifications for the prevention and treatment of hypertension*. Dekker, New York.

White, P. D., Sprague, H. B., Stamler, J., Stare, F. J., Wright, J. S., Katz, L. N. *et al.* (1959). *A statement on arteriosclerosis, main cause of 'heart attacks' and 'strokes'*. National Health Education Council, New York.

WHO (World Health Organization) (1982). WHO Expert Committee on the Prevention of Coronary Heart Disease. *Prevention of Coronary Heart Disease.* WHO Technical Report Series, 678. WHO, Geneva.

WHO (World Health Organization) (1990a). WHO Expert Committee on the Prevention in Childhood and Youth of Adult Cardiovascular Disease. *Prevention in childhood and youth of adult cardiovascular diseases – time for action: Report of a WHO Expert Committee.* WHO Technical Report Series, 792. WHO, Geneva.

WHO (World Health Organization) (1990b). WHO Study Group. *Diet, nutrition, and the prevention of chronic diseases.* WHO Technical Report Series, 797. WHO, Geneva.

WHO (World Health Organization) (1997). *Obesity: preventing and managing the global epidemic.* WHO, Geneva.

Worth, B. M., Kato, H., Rhoads, G. G., Kagan, K., and Syme, S. L. (1975). Epidemiologic studies of coronary heart disease and stroke in Japanese men living in Japan, Hawaii, and California: mortality. *American Journal of Epidemiology,* **102,** 485–90.

Zhao, L., Stamler, J., Yan, L. L., Zhou, B., Wu, Y., Liu, K. *et al.* (2004). Blood pressure differences between northern and southern Chinese: role of dietary factors. *Hypertension,* **43,** 1332–7.

Section II

Global picture of coronary heart disease

II.I Worldwide trends

Chapter 5

US trends

R. V. Luepker

5.1 Introduction

Coronary heart disease (CHD), the leading cause of death in the United States in the twentieth century, began to decline in the mid-1960s. Age-adjusted rates of CHD continued to fall through the 1990s, although crude mortality changed more modestly and CHD remains the largest single cause of death and disability in the United States (Fig. 5.1). Infectious disease epidemics are well recognized and described as they appear and recede. The patterns for CHD, a major chronic disease, show many similarities, and have risen and fallen with associated changes in the environment, exposures, health behaviours, diagnosis, and treatment. The difference between CHD and infectious disease epidemics lies in the length of time during which these diseases progress as they emerge and disappear.

The United States provides a good example of the dynamic aspects of a chronic disease epidemic. The first half of the century saw a steady rise in CHD rates, while the last third had falling rates with resulting longer life spans. As with any population disease trend within a quarter of a billion people, we recognize that all subgroups that comprise the trend do not change equally. It is also important for epidemiologists to look for reasons for these trends in order to improve public health. In this effort, we are fortunate to have substantial CHD surveillance data available through projects supported by the National Heart, Lung, and Blood Institute and the National Center for Health Statistics (American Heart Association 2001; US Department of Health and Human Services 2000).

5.2 Mortality trends

The current decline in CHD mortality beginning in the 1960s in the United States is clear and unmistakable (Fig. 5.1). When first observed in the late 1970s, many wondered if the trend was

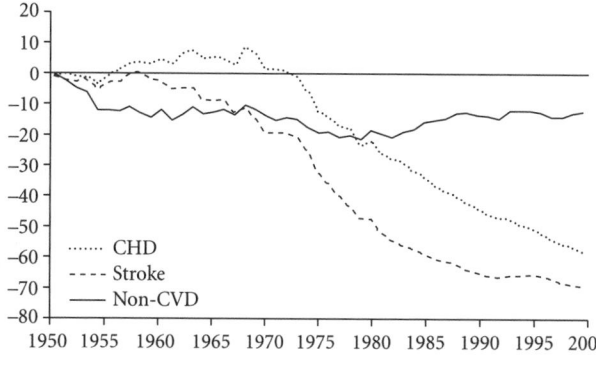

Fig. 5.1 Change in age-adjusted death rates, 1950–2000. (Reproduced from NHLBI Morbidity and Mortality 2002 Chart Book.)

the result of changes in diagnostic fashion, but subsequent analysis of death certificates suggests little systematic classification bias over time (Iribarren *et al.* 1998; US Department of Health and Human Services 1980). However, while age-adjusted mortality has fallen dramatically, an ageing population with extended longevity has seen only modest changes in crude or absolute mortality. As shown in Fig. 5.2, crude mortality from diseases of the heart rose steadily from 1900, peaking in the 1970s and then falling only slightly. These diseases are still common in the United States, but are appearing at older ages.

Crude mortality trends from 1979 to 1999 show a decline in mortality for men balanced by a gradual increase in mortality among women. While CHD continues to be a disease found first among younger men, the growing population of older women is experiencing increasing CHD mortality. Closer analysis of cardiovascular disease mortality trends demonstrates differing rates by gender and ethnic group. As shown in Table 5.1, men had greater decreases in CHD than women and these changes occurred across racial lines. At the same time as CHD mortality was falling, congestive heart failure (CHF) as a cause of death rose, particularly among whites. Hispanic Americans are less studied than other ethnic groups and many are recent

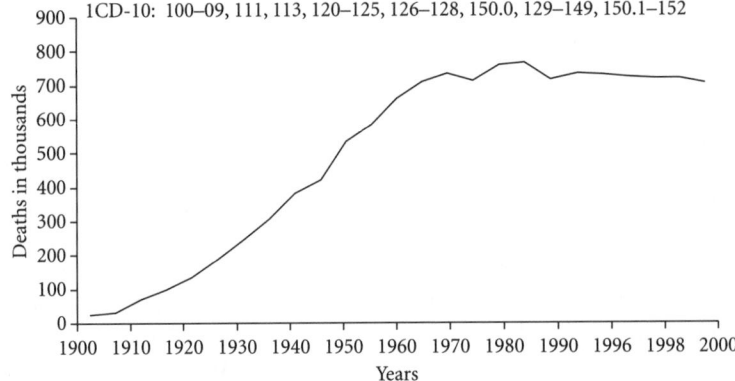

ICD-10: 100–09, 111, 113, 120–125, 126–128, 150.0, 129–149, 150.1–152

Fig. 5.2 Deaths from diseases of the heart, 1900–2000. (Reproduced from Heart Disease and Stroke Statistics—2003 update, American Heart Association.)

Table 5.1 Average annual percentage change in age-adjusted death rates[a] for all causes and cardiovascular diseases by race and sex, 1990–98

	Total	White male	White female	Black male	Black female
All causes	−0.7	−1.3	0.0	−1.9	−0.5
CVD[b]	−1.7	−2.2	−1.3	−2.1	−1.4
Heart disease	−1.9	−2.4	−1.6	−2.4	−1.9
CHD	−2.7	−3.1	−2.5	−2.7	−1.9
CHF[b]	+1.8	+1.6	+2.3	−0.6	+0.4
Stroke	−0.7	−1.0	−0.3	−2.0	−1.1
All non-CVD[b]	0.0	−0.6	+0.9	−1.8	+0.1

Source: National Institutes of Health 2000.

[a] Age-adjusted to the 2000 standard.

[b] 1990–97.

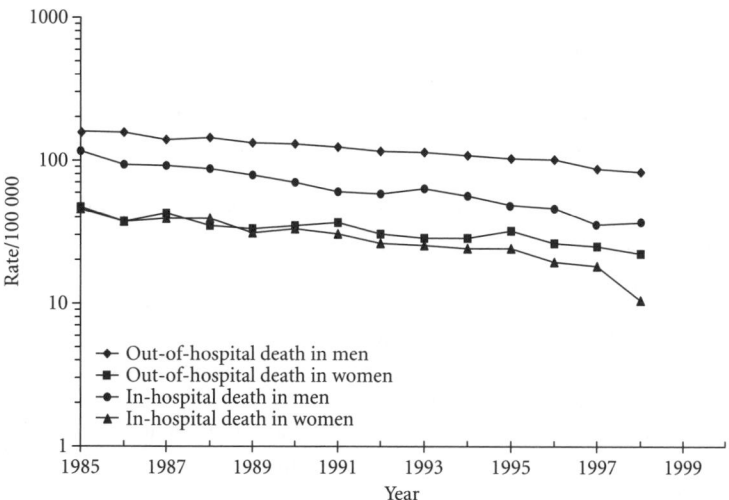

Fig. 5.3 In- and out-of-hospital trends in death from CHD in men and women aged 30–74 in Minnesota, adjusted to the 1990 US population.

immigrants. However, there are growing indications that Hispanics who are born in the United States or have lived there for a major portion of their lives assume similar CHD patterns to the majority population (Pandey *et al.* 2001).

In addition to racial and ethnic diversity, CHD mortality rates differ significantly within geographical areas in the United States. In 1996–98, age-adjusted CHD mortality ranged from 128.4 to 259.9 per 100 000 population, a two-fold difference. Generally, the lowest rates were found in the western parts of the country and the highest rates in the eastern half. Interestingly, the highest stroke rates are concentrated in the south-eastern states, the so-called 'stroke belt', which differs from CHD distributions (American Heart Association 2001).

Also of interest, particularly in relation to medical care and prevention, are the trends of in- and out-of-hospital mortality. The majority of CHD deaths (approximately two-thirds) occur outside of hospitals, most commonly as sudden death. In- and out-of-hospital mortality trends are shown in Fig. 5.3. CHD mortality is falling for both men and women and for in- and out-of-hospital death. However, the rates of decline are substantially greater for in-hospital death than for out-of-hospital death. Some have suggested that these observations are the result of improved in-hospital medical care with less progress in prevention and outpatient care (McGovern *et al.* 1996).

5.3 **Morbidity trends**

Acute myocardial infarction (AMI) is the most common and frequently fatal event in CHD. Although some cases are silent or unrecognized, the majority are hospitalized (McGovern *et al.* 1996; Shlipak *et al.* 2001). Most population-based studies are hospital based. Several observe a decline in incidence of hospitalized AMI over the past two decades.

As shown in Table 5.2 for the Minnesota Heart Survey, AMI incidence declined. The changes observed correspond to an annual rate of 1.2% for men and 0.5% for women (McGovern *et al.* 2001). Data from the Worcester Heart Attack Study showed a decline in the incidence of transmural

Q-wave infarctions (McGovern *et al.* 2001). At the same time, the incidence of non-Q-wave infarctions increased, blunting a decreasing incidence trend. Other studies such as the Olmsted County/Mayo Clinic experience also show mixed results in incidence (Roger *et al.* 1999) and the Atherosclerosis Risk in Communities Study (ARIC) observes no change in incidence (Rosamond *et al.* 1998). AMI incidence, like mortality, also shows differing patterns by age, gender, and ethnic group (Fig. 5.4). Black men had the highest rate at all ages followed by white men, black women, and white women. Black women have AMI incidence rates more similar to those in men than to white women.

A subsequent event or recurrent AMI presents a more consistent picture. It is declining in most population studies. As shown in the Minnesota Heart Survey, recurrent AMI fell by 2.4% for men and 3.3% for women annually from 1985 to 1995 (McGovern *et al.* 2001). Similar observations are found in the ARIC study where recurrent AMI fell by 2.6% for men and 1.9% for women annually (Rosamond *et al.* 1998).

Along with changes in incident and recurrent AMI admitted to hospital, the likelihood of dying during an AMI in hospital has declined substantially. As shown in Table 5.2, 28-day mortality among those hospitalized in the Minnesota Heart Survey with incident or recurrent AMI fell from 13 to 7% among men and 16 to 10% among women (McGovern *et al.* 2001). This absolute rate difference translates to an annual fall of 4.6% for men and 8.8% for women. Similar improvements were noted in the ARIC study where death in hospital fell by 4.1% for men and 9.8% for women annually (Rosamond *et al.* 1998). Long-term mortality at 3 years showed similar improvement in Minnesota among both men and women (Table 5.2).

Table 5.2 Age-adjusted rates of acute CHD in the Minneapolis–St Paul metropolitan region, 1985–95[a]

Hospitalized definite AMI	Men			Women		
	1985	1990	1995	1985	1990	1995
Attack rate (*n* per 100 000)	469	438	394	163	155	137
Incident	309	289	272	111	106	105
Recurrent	161	149	122	53	49	32
28-day mortality (%)	13	11	7	16	12	10
3-year mortality (%)	28	23	19	34	28	20

[a] Age adjusted to 1990 population.

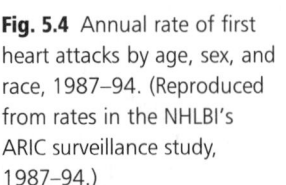

Fig. 5.4 Annual rate of first heart attacks by age, sex, and race, 1987–94. (Reproduced from rates in the NHLBI's ARIC surveillance study, 1987–94.)

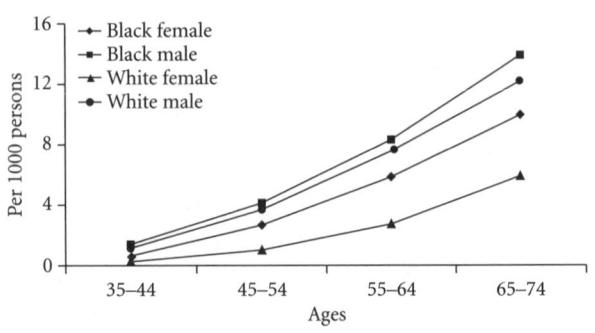

Overall mortality and case fatality in-hospital of AMI victims fell at a substantially greater rate than either incidence or recurrent AMI. Several reasons for this are considered. First, medical care for acute AMI has improved substantially in the United States. Cardiac defibrillation for ventricular fibrillation is now a routine procedure. Reperfusion of ischaemic myocardium with thrombolytic agents or acute coronary angioplasty has been routine for many years. These commonly used procedures are demonstrated in clinical trials to reduce mortality in AMI.

Additional data suggest that the diagnosis and severity of AMI is changing, leading both to ascertainment bias and the hospitalization of milder cases which have better prognosis. The Worcester study described above suggests that smaller myocardial infarctions, which do not produce a classical pattern of Q-waves, are becoming more common (Furman *et al.* 2001). Studies of peak creatine kinase-myocardial band (CK–MB) enzyme levels are also declining as observed in the Olmstead County/Mayo Clinic study and the ARIC study (Roger *et al.* 1999; Rosamond *et al.* 1998). A pattern of decreasing transmural infarctions and declining CK–MB levels suggest smaller infarctions with less muscle damage, resulting in a better prognosis. More recently, new and more sensitive biomarkers such as troponins have become widely available (Wu *et al.* 1999). With great sensitivity and specificity for damaged myocardium, these markers allow detection of smaller and less damaging infarctions. Some estimate that these markers will increase hospitalized AMI diagnoses from 30 to 40% (Wu *et al.* 1999).

One of the associated and evolving trends in hospitalized CHD in the United States is the dramatic increase in recent years in the diagnosis of unstable angina (American College of Cardiology and American Heart Association 2001). Unstable angina is a much debated diagnosis, but generally describes patients with signs of acute ischaemia related to CHD in a changing, increasing pattern without evidence of permanent muscle damage. This diagnosis is a common reason for hospitalization and invasive diagnostic procedures with therapeutic interventions in the United States. Rates of unstable angina (International Classification of Diseases (ICD)-9 411) have increased by more than 50% in some areas over the past decade. While some suggest changing disease patterns, increased clinical sensitivity to symptoms of CHD and an insurance reimbursement which provides greater physician and hospital fees for unstable angina may be one cause of this clinical epidemic (Assaf *et al.* 1993).

Modest changes in incidence, greater diagnostic sensitivity, and decreased case fatality in an ageing population result in increasing prevalence of diagnosed CHD in the population. This is manifest partly by increased rates of hospitalization for CHD in both men and women, as shown in Fig. 5.5. Figure 5.6 demonstrates the effect of age, as the increased hospitalization rate is due largely to those 65 years of age and older. While the mortality picture for CHD has improved, the disease burden in the population remains high and is growing. This population prevalence is also manifest in the rates of common outcomes of CHD other than AMI. Increased angina pectoris, or chest pain due to myocardial ischaemia, is now estimated to affect 6 400 000 adults in the United States (American Heart Association 2001). Similarly, survival from acute myocardial infarction may lead to chronically scarred and damaged heart muscle. Congestive heart failure is the common outcome of dysfunctional cardiac muscle resulting from acute and chronic CHD. As shown in Fig. 5.7, hospital discharges from congestive heart failure are rising steadily in the United States population. This severe and late complication of CHD affects a growing proportion of the population and is manifest by symptomatic disability and increased burden on the healthcare system.

Among the many unique characteristics of healthcare in the United States is the common use of invasive cardiovascular operations and procedures for the treatment of AMI and CHD. As shown in Fig. 5.8, there has been a steady rise in cardiocatherization, percutaneous transluminal

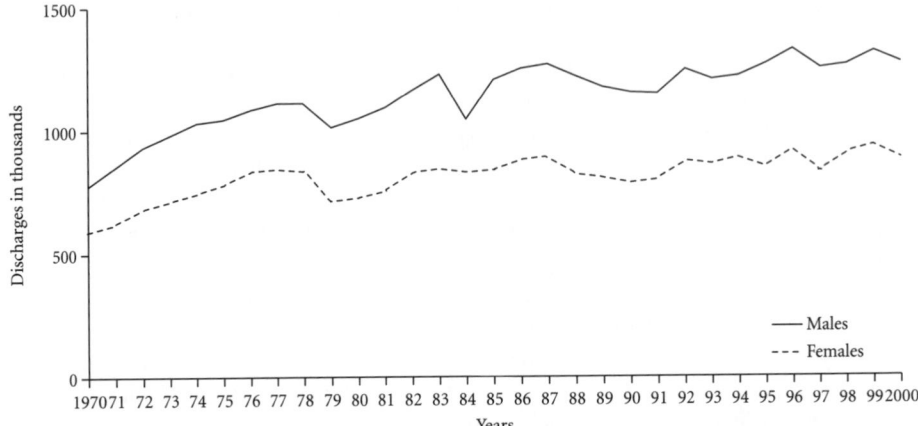

Fig. 5.5 Hospital discharges (including people both living and dead) for coronary heart disease by sex, 1970–2000. (Reproduced from Heart Disease and Stroke Statistics—2003 Update, American Heart Association.)

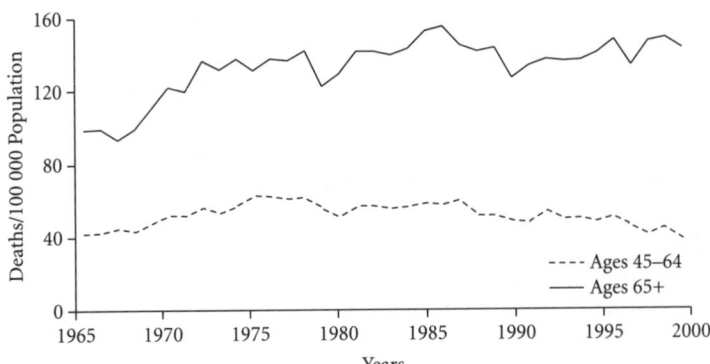

Fig. 5.6 Hospitalization rates for AMI, ages 45–64 and 65+, 1965–2000. (Reproduced from NHLBI Chartbook, 2002.)

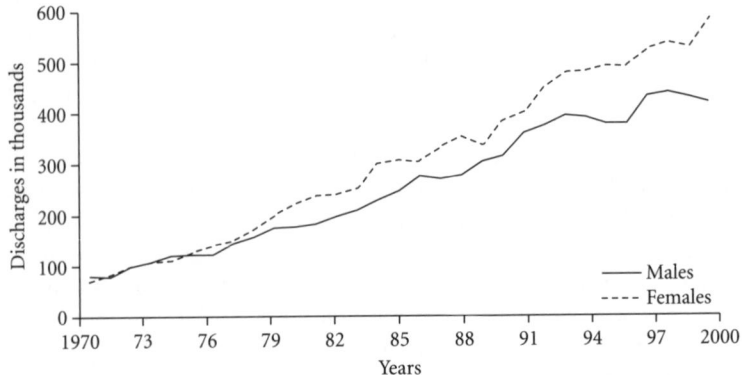

Fig. 5.7 Hospital discharges (including people both living and dead) for congestive heart failure by sex, 1970–2000. (Reproduced from Heart Disease and Stroke Statistics—2003 Update, American Heart Association.)

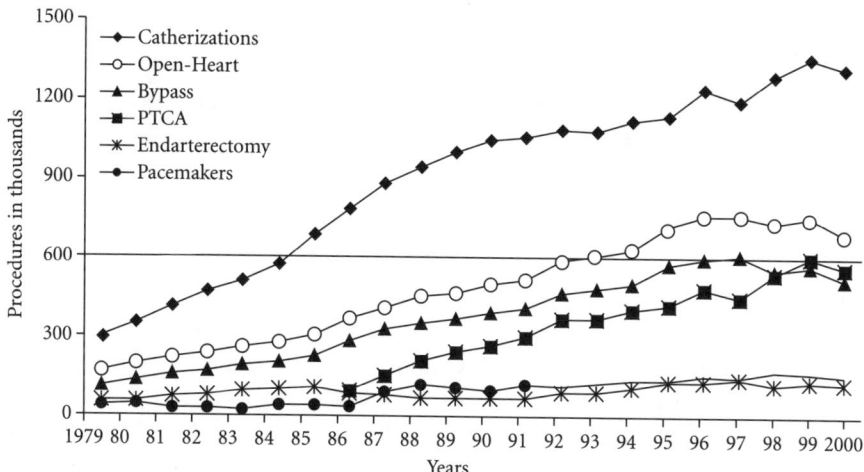

Fig. 5.8 Trends in cardiovascular operations and procedures, 1979–2000.

coronary angioplasty (PTCA), and bypass surgery. Over 1.3 million catherizations were performed in 1999, principally for coronary angiography. There were nearly 800 000 PTCA procedures performed. This aggressive intervention approach is demonstrated to improve outcomes and prolong life in clinical trials. However, comparisons with other advanced nations suggest similar outcomes are possible with less invasive strategies (McGovern *et al.* 1997).

5.4 **Factors associated with temporal CHD trends**

Changing CHD morbidity and mortality patterns are associated with changes in the risk factors known to be causal for CHD. Currently, within the United States, there is mass expression of the classical risk factors with hypertension affecting 25%, hyperlipidaemia 20–50%, and cigarette smoking 25% of the adult population. While these classical risk factors improved steadily in the 1970s and 1980s, their prevalence remains high. The most progress has been made in cigarette smoking, where tobacco consumption per capita for adults rose steadily from the 1900s until the late 1960s and then steadily declined (Centers for Disease Control 1998). The National Health Interview Survey found 25.7% of adult men and 21.5% of adult women were active smokers in the year 2000 (American Heart Association 2001). This compares to rates in the 35–40% range in 1980. There is significant regional variability within the United States. In 1999, the percentage of adults who smoked ranged from a high of 29.7% in Kentucky to a low of 13.9% in Utah (Centers for Disease Control 1998). In states such as California and Massachusetts, where increased taxes have been used for smoking prevention, cessation, and research, some of the lowest smoking rates in the country are observed among adults (19%). (See chapter 45.)

There has also been significant improvement in blood cholesterol levels in the United States. In the National Health and Nutrition Examination Survey (NHANES), mean cholesterol among adults fell from 220 mg/dl (mmol/l) to 205 mg/dl (mmol/l) between the 1976–80 NHANES survey and the 1988–91 survey. Similar trends were observed in Minnesota from 1980–82 to 1995–97 (Table 5.3). During this time, an increasing number of individuals were actively treated with medication (Table 5.3). However, the population-wide changes are more

Table 5.3 Trends in blood cholesterol in the Minneapolis–St Paul metropolitan region

Serum total cholesterol	Men				Women			
	1980–82	1985–87	1990–92	1995–97	1980–82	1985–87	1990–92	1995–97
mg/dl	212.2	208.9[a]	203.2[a]	204.8	207.6	204.2[a]	200.6[a]	200.5
mm/l	5.48	5.40	5.25	5.29	5.36	5.28	5.18	5.18
Lipid medication use (%)	1.0	1.4	2.7	6.0	0.6	0.5	2.8	3.9

[a] $p < 0.001$ compared to prior level.

likely due to the shifts in type of dietary fat intake from animal to vegetable which has occurred widely over the same period (American Heart Association 2001).

During these years, prevalence of hypertension in the United States fell 42.5% in men and 38.9% in women between the two NHANES studies (Burt *et al.* 1995). Although there is still considerable progress to be made, the same NHANES study showed substantial improvements in the detection, treatment, and control of high blood pressure (Burt *et al.* 1995; McGovern *et al.* 1999).

While the classical risk factors of smoking, hyperlipidaemia, and hypertension have shown improvement in the United States, other known risk characteristics remain unchanged or are moving in unhealthy directions. Leisure-time physical activity is unchanged in past decades, while work-related physical labour has declined (American Heart Association 1999). Among adult Americans, 25% report no leisure-time physical activity and only 23% report vigorous sustained physical activity lasting 30 minutes or more five times a week. The prevalence of obesity (body mass index greater than 30 kg/m^2) increased substantially in the NHANES and other studies (Flegal *et al.* 1998). Increasing obesity affects both genders and all race groups, but is particularly apparent among black women. Associated with increasing obesity is type 2 diabetes, also increasing in prevalence in the population (American Heart Association 2001). These risk factors are covered in more detail in later chapters.

Secondary prevention, as evidenced by long-term pharmacological therapy, has improved and may play an important role in recurrent AMI. For example, approximately 70% of those discharged with AMI are prescribed beta-blockers and over 90% aspirin (McGovern *et al.* 2001). In addition, hyperlipidaemia and hypertension are aggressively managed with cigarette cessation strongly encouraged post-AMI.

5.5 **Summary**

CHD mortality adjusted for age continues to decline in the United States. However, crude mortality, unadjusted for age, has changed more modestly, with CHD being postponed, and manifesting at progressively older ages. Incidence of AMI, defined to include both first hospitalized event and out-of-hospital death as first CHD manifestation, is declining modestly, mainly due to a decline in out-of-hospital mortality. Recurrent or second AMI is declining at a rate greater that incident AMI, particularly in the 1990s, as is case fatality for hospitalized AMI. There is also evidence that the severity of hospitalized AMI is declining.

Primary prevention, through population risk factor lowering, is associated with reduced incidence and severity. The decline in cigarette smoking is substantial and continues. Population levels of blood cholesterol are falling. Hypertension detection and control have improved significantly in the past two decades. But obesity, physical inactivity, and diabetes mellitus are all increasing. Furthermore, risk factor trends are not consistent across ethnic groups and regions.

Diagnosis and treatment for CHD is significantly improving and cases admitted to hospitals are less severe, leading to decreasing hospital fatality and improved prognosis. Similarly, secondary prevention through aggressive medical treatment in patients with known CHD has improved long-term survival.

These patterns taken in totality indicate improved CHD patterns in the United States in recent decades. However, as with any epidemic, continued progress is not assured and careful surveillance is needed to detect changing trends.

References

American College of Cardiology and American Heart Association (2001). *Management of patients with unstable angina and non-st-segment elevation myocardial infarction.* A report of the American College of Cardiology/American Heart Association Task Force on Practice Guidelines. Bethesda, MD.

American Heart Association (1999). *Physical inactivity biostatistical fact sheets.* American Heart Association, Dallas.

American Heart Association (2001). *2002 heart and stroke statistical update.* American Heart Association, Dallas.

American Heart Association (2002). *Heart disease and stroke statistics: 2003 update.* American Heart Association, Dallas.

Assaf, A. R., Lapane, K. L., McKenney, J. L., and Carleton, R. A. (1993). Possible influence of the prospective payment system on the assignment of discharge diagnoses for coronary heart disease. *New England Journal of Medicine*, **329**, 931–5.

Burt, V. L., Whelton, P., Roccella, E. J., Brown, C., Cutler, J. A., Higgins, M., Horan, M. J., and Labarthe, D. (1995). Prevalence of hypertension in the U.S. adult population. Results from the Third National Health and Nutrition Examination Survey, 1988–1991. *Hypertension*, **25**, 305–13.

Centers for Disease Control (1998). *Chronic diseases and their risk factors.* Centers for Disease Control, Atlanta, GA.

Flegal, K. M., Carroll, M. D., Kuczmarski, R. J., and Johnson, C. L. (1998). Overweight and obesity in the United States: prevalence and trends, 1960–1994. *International Journal of Obesity Related Metabolic Disorders*, **22**, 39–47.

Furman, M. I., Dauerman, H. L., Goldberg, R. J., Yarzebski, J., Lessard, D., and Gore, J. M. (2001). Twenty-two year (1975 to 1997) trends in the incidence, in-hospital and long-term case fatality rates from initial Q-wave and non-Q-wave myocardial infarction: a multi-hospital, community-wide perspective. *Journal of the American College of Cardiology*, **37**, 1571–80.

Iribarren, C., Crow, R. S., Hannan, P. J., Jacobs, D. R. Jr, Luepker, R. V. (1998). Validation of death certificate diagnosis of out-of-hospital sudden cardiac death. *American Journal of Cardiology*, **82**, 50–3.

McGovern, P. G., Pankow, J. S., Shahar, E., Doliszny, K. M., Folsom, A. R., Blackburn, H., and Luepker, R. V. (1996). Recent trends in acute coronary heart disease: mortality, morbidity, medical care, and risk factors. *New England Journal of Medicine*, **334**, 884–90.

McGovern, P. G., Herlitz, J., Pankow, J. S., Karlsson, T., Dellborg, M., Shahar, E., and Luepker, R. V. (1997). Comparison of medical care and one- and 12-month mortality of hospitalized patients with acute myocardial infarction in Minneapolis-St. Paul, Minnesota, United States of America and Göteborg, Sweden. *American Journal of Cardiology*, **80**, 557–62.

McGovern, P. G., Arnett, D. K., Shahar, E., and Luepker, R. V. (1999). Trends in serum cholesterol levels, 1980–1997: The Minnesota Heart Survey. *Circulation*, **99**, 1104.

McGovern, P. G., Jacobs, D. R. Jr, Shahar, E., Arnett, D. K., Folsom, A. R., Blackburn, H., and Luepker, R. V. (2001). Trends in acute coronary heart disease mortality, morbidity, and medical care from 1985 through 1997: the Minnesota Heart Survey. *Circulation*, **104**, 19–24.

NHLBI (National Heart, Lung, and Blood Institute) (2002). *National Heart, Lung, and Blood Institute Morbidity and Mortality: 2002 Chart Book on Cardiovascular, Lung and Blood Diseases.* National Heart, Lung, and Blood Institute. Bethesda, MD.

National Institutes of Health (2000). *National Heart, Lung, and Blood Institute Morbidity and Mortality: 2000 Chart Book on Cardiovascular, Lung and Blood Diseases.* National Heart, Lung, and Blood Institute. Bethesda, MD.

Pandey, D. K., Labarthe, D. R., Goff, D. C., Chan, W., and Nichaman, M. Z. (2001). Community-wide coronary heart disease mortality in Mexican Americans equals or exceeds that in non-Hispanic whites: the Corpus Christ Heart Project. *American Journal of Medicine*, **110**, 81–7.

Roger, V. L., Jacobsen, S. J., Weston, S. A., Bailey, K. R., Kottke, T. E., and Frye, R. L. (1999). Trends in heart disease deaths in Olmsted County, Minnesota, 1979–1994. *Mayo Clinical Proceedings*, **74**, 651–7.

Rosamond, W. D., Chambless, L. E., Folsom, A. R., Cooper, L. S., Conwill, D. E., Clegg, L., Wang, C. H., and Heiss, G. (1998). Trends in the incidence of myocardial infarction and in mortality due to coronary heart disease, 1987 to 1994. *New England Journal of Medicine*, **339**, 861–7.

Shlipak, M. G., Elmouchi, D. A., Herrington, D. M., Lin, F., Grady, D., and Hlatky, M. A. (2001). The incidence of unrecognized myocardial infarction in women with coronary heart disease. *Annals of Internal Medicine*, **134**, 1043–7.

US Department of Health and Human Services (1980). *NHLBI Proceedings of the Conference on the Decline in Coronary Heart Disease.* Publication No. 79-1610. Washington, DC.

Wu, A. H. B., Apple, F. S., Gibler, W. B., Jesse, R. L., Warshaw, M. M., and Valdes, R. Jr (1999). National Academy of Clinical Biochemistry Standards of Laboratory Practice: recommendations for use of cardiac markers in coronary artery disease. *Clinical Chemistry*, **45**, 1104–21.

Chapter 6

Coronary heart disease in Central and Eastern Europe and the former Soviet Union

M. Bobak and M. Marmot

6.1 Introduction

In the late 1980s and early 1990s, a picture of the former Communist countries of Central and Eastern Europe (CEE) and the former Soviet Union (FSU) started emerging in the literature that was characterized by relatively low and stagnating life expectancy and high rates of chronic non-communicable diseases. The most prominent aspect of the health crisis in CEE was the high rates of cardiovascular diseases (CVD) and coronary heart disease (CHD) in middle-aged men.

There had been little research on CHD and its determinants in CEE/FSU prior to 1990, but the literature has grown rapidly since then. There is now enough material for a review of the epidemiological features of CHD in the region and for identification of the most salient aspects of this, in many respects, unprecedented epidemic.

This chapter has three parts. First, we describe the levels and trends of mortality from CHD in CEE/FSU. Second, we review the possible explanations for the high rates and for the trends. Finally, we will touch upon a few aspects of CHD in CEE/FSU that provide important findings or hypotheses relevant for the rest of the world, such as socio-economic inequalities, impact of societal transformation, and binge drinking.

6.2 Description of CHD mortality in CEE/FSU

6.2.1 Cross-sectional view

Until the 1980s, little was known about CHD rates in CEE/FSU. During preparations for the WHO MONICA Project, designed to monitor trends in, and risk factors for, CVD in selected populations around the world (http://www.ktl.fi/monica), it became apparent that most countries with high CHD mortality were clustered in CEE/FSU. The same pattern persisted in Europe in the late 1990s (Fig. 6.1). Mortality was highest in the FSU, somewhat lower in central European countries (Hungary, Poland, Czech Republic), and lowest in south-western Europe. There was little overlap between the former Communist countries and the rest of Europe, except for Ireland and the UK with high mortality, and Albania where the lifestyle of the population can be characterized as Mediterranean (Gjonca and Bobak 1997).

There has been a debate as to whether the large differences in CHD rates between populations are real or whether they could be attributed to differences in coding of causes of death. The MONICA study showed a good agreement between official mortality rates and rates based

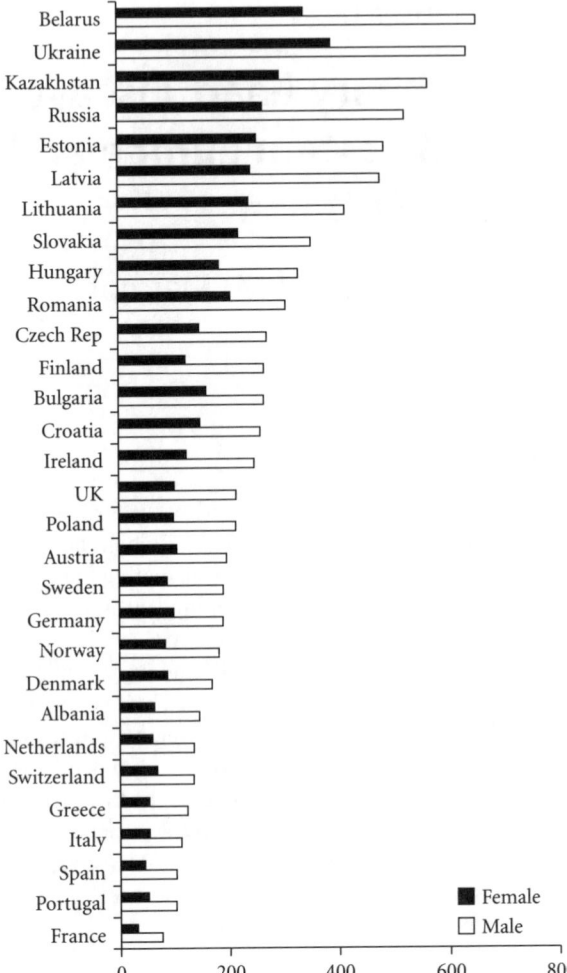

Fig. 6.1 Age-standardized mortality from CHD per 100 000 in European countries in 2000 or the latest available year. (Data from the WHO Health for All database.)

on standardized registration of fatal events, though there were some exceptions, from both Eastern and Western countries (WHO MONICA Project *et al.* 1994). The validated CHD mortality rates in the MONICA centres in the early 1990s are shown in Fig. 6.2. As in the official statistics, rates in MONICA centres in CEE/FSU are high though there is some overlap with Western Europe (e.g. with Glasgow, UK). Overall, available data strongly suggest that the high rates of CHD and other vascular diseases in CEE/FSU are a real phenomenon, and not an artefact caused by inaccurate coding of death certificates.

6.2.2 CHD mortality in CEE/FSU: trends

Figures 6.3 to 6.6 show trends in CHD mortality in the former Communist countries between the mid-1950s and 2000 in men and women aged 45–54 years. (Trends in other age groups are similar, see below). For comparison, we also included Sweden as a country with one of the lowest rates in Europe.

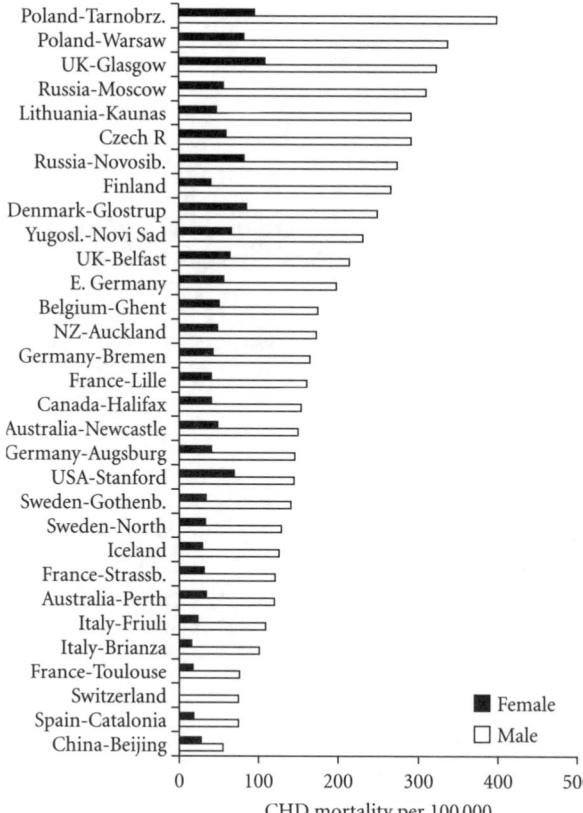

Fig. 6.2 Age-standardized mortality from validated CHD events in the MONICA centres, age group 35–64 years, early 1990s, rates per 100 000. (Data from the WHO MONICA Project.)

In men in CEE, CHD mortality rates were similar to those in Sweden in the 1950s. The increase in rates in the 1960s and 1970s was relatively small in Sweden, but rates more than doubled in CEE during this period (Fig. 6.3). CHD rates started declining in all countries of CEE some time in the late 1980s or in the 1990s. In some countries, for example Poland and the Czech Republic, the decline in male mortality since 1990 was considerable, by some 30% and 40%, respectively.

Long-time series of CHD mortality for the FSU were not available before 1990 (Uemura and Pisa 1988). The longest data series we are aware of are the Russian data reconstructed subsequently (Mesle *et al.* 1996). In Figs 6.4 and 6.6 we have included these estimates, labelled as 'Russia(2)', as well as data published retrospectively by the European WHO for Russia ('Russia(1)') for the period 1980–2000 in the Health for All database (http://www.euro.who.int/hfadb). Latvia is also shown to represent the Baltics, and Poland is shown to provide comparison with CEE. There is a discrepancy between the two Russian datasets for CHD mortality, caused mainly by different coding of causes of death, but it is likely that within each dataset the trends are roughly correct (Fig. 6.4). In 1965, Russian mortality from CHD was 50% higher than in Sweden, and the Russian rates approximately doubled by mid-1980s. The trends between 1985 and 1994 are typical for all countries of the FSU (and for most major causes of death except cancer): a small decline between 1985 and 1987, relatively stable between 1987 and 1991, and a sharp rapid increase between 1991 and 1994. After 1994, trends diverged

Fig. 6.3 Trends in male mortality from CHD in CEE between the mid-1950s and 2000, age group 45–54 years. (Data from the WHO Health for All database.)

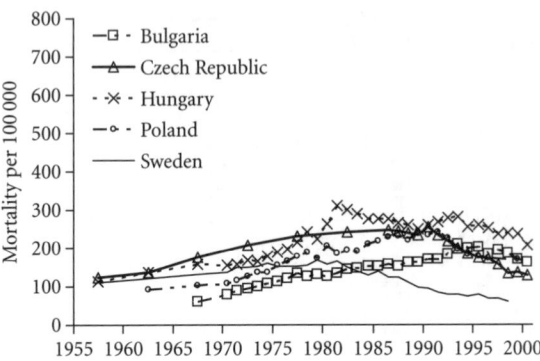

Fig. 6.4 Trends in male mortality from CHD in the FSU between the mid-1950s and 2000, age group 45–54 years. (Data from the WHO Health for All database.)

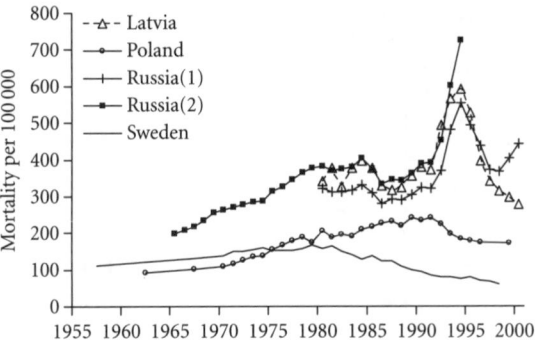

Fig. 6.5 Trends in female mortality from CHD in CEE between mid-1950s and 2000, age group 45–54 years. (Data from the WHO Health for All database.)

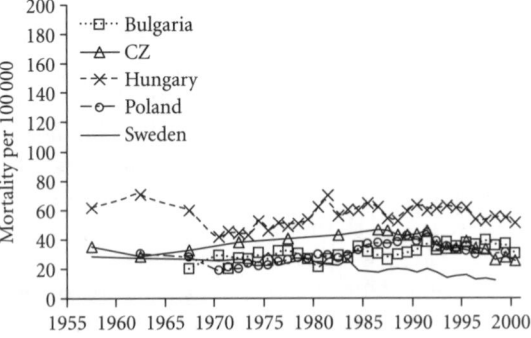

between Latvia (and other Baltic countries, see Section 3.2.2) and Russia: mortality has been declining in the Baltics, but started to rise again in Russia in 1998.

Among women in CEE, the increase in CHD mortality was less pronounced in absolute terms, but it was roughly similar in relative terms (Fig. 6.5). In the late 1990s mortality in Hungary was almost three times higher than in Sweden. In FSU, female CHD mortality was almost four times higher in Russia than in Sweden in the late 1960s; the trends in the 1980s and 1990s were analogous to those in men (Fig. 6.6).

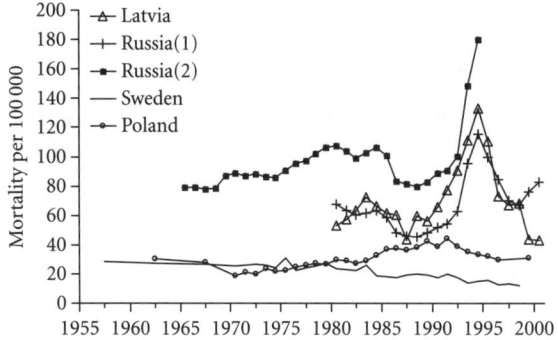

Fig. 6.6 Trends in female mortality from CHD in the FSU between mid-1950s and 2000, age group 45–54 years. (Data from the WHO Health for All database.).

The rates of CVD and CHD in CEE/FSU in the 1970s and 1980s were high by international standards, but they were not the highest rates ever recorded. In the 1950s and 1960s, rates in Finland, Ireland, and the UK were of similar magnitude (WHO data compiled by John Powles, unpublished). However, the rates seen in the FSU in the 1990s are unprecedented: the male CVD mortality rates in Russia and Latvia in 1994 were about 40% higher than the highest rates ever seen elsewhere (Finland in 1971) (Powles, unpublished).

Trends in CVD and in all-cause mortality are similar to those in CHD. Vascular diseases have been driving the trends in overall mortality in the region, at least in the post-war period. Therefore understanding determinants of CVD sheds light on the overall health experience of these countries.

6.3 Explanations for differences in CHD rates

A number of explanations have been put forward to account for the trends in CHD mortality in CEE/FSU. Some time ago, when we reviewed the East–West gap in life expectancy, we divided the potential explanations into several categories (Bobak and Marmot 1996). We still find these categories helpful, and they are reviewed below.

6.3.1 Conventional coronary risk factors

The simplest explanation is that high levels of classical coronary risk factors (smoking, cholesterol, blood pressure, and body mass index) described in Chapters 3 and 4 are the main causes for the high rates of CHD in CEE/FSU. The MONICA data provide the most reliable data on CHD rates and risk factors to test this proposition. The data show that while the levels of risk factors tended to be, in general, higher in CEE/FSU centres than in Western centres, the division between Eastern and Western European centres in terms of risk factors was far less clear cut than for CHD rates. An ecological analysis of the MONICA centres found that only a part (23% in men and 14% in women) of the variation in CHD mortality between centres in the late 1980s could be explained by the four main risk factors (WHO MONICA Project 1994) (see also Chapters 48 and 49).

We have conducted a similar analysis on the MONICA data from the early 1990s available on the web (http://www.ktl.fi/monica/index.html); some data were published recently (Kuulasmaa *et al.* 2000; Tunstall-Pedoe *et al.* 2000). Contemporary mean levels of systolic blood pressure, body mass index and total cholesterol and prevalence of smoking explained 30% of CHD mortality variation in men and 45% in women. These risk factors also contributed to the differences

Table 6.1 Mortality rates in MONICA centres in CEE/FSU and Western countries, East/West mortality rate ratios after controlling for risk factors (RF) and medical care. Age band 35–64, data from the MONICA Project

	Rates in CEE/FSU	Rates in Western countries	East/West rate ratio
Men			
(Number of centres)	(10)	(26)	
Age adjusted	274	162	1.81
Adjusted for risk factors	245	173	1.42
Adjusted for care	257	167	1.54
Adjusted for RF + care	269	165	1.63
Women			
(Number of centres)	(10)	(24)	
Age adjusted	75	44	1.70
Adjusted for risk factors	66	45	1.47
Adjusted for care	67	46	1.46
Adjusted for RF + care	72	45	1.59

between CEE/FSU and Western centres, when all Eastern European and Western centres were aggregated into two groups. The age-adjusted male CHD mortality rates were 81% higher in CEE/FSU than in Western centres; after controlling for the four risk factors the excess in CEE was almost halved, to 42% (Table 6.1). Smoking made the largest contribution to this reduction. Among women, however, the contribution of risk factors to the East–West differences was smaller: the age-adjusted rates were 70% higher in CEE/FSU than in Western centres; this was reduced to 47% after adjustment of risk factors (Table 6.1).

Powles and Sanz 1996 used indirect estimation (Peto *et al.* 1992, 1994) to assess the role of smoking in CVD mortality in selected countries. The method used cancer rates to estimate prevalence of smoking; relative risks of CVD death from the US Cancer Prevention Study (CPS) were then halved (in order to avoid overestimation) and used to calculate the proportion of CVD deaths attributable to smoking. The results suggest that in Poland, Hungary, and Bulgaria in the mid-1990s tobacco accounted for about a third of CVD deaths in men; the contribution of tobacco to CVD mortality in women was negligible. Deaths from CHD have not been analysed separately, but the results would be similar because the relative risks for CVD and CHD in the CPS study were similar.

The MONICA data also allowed analysis of determinants of trends in CHD mortality over the 10 years of the MONICA Project, roughly from mid-1980s to mid-1990s. Changes in risk factors were associated with 10-year trends in CHD event rate and mortality, but the results depended on time lag, model specification, and age group (Kuulasmaa *et al.* 2000). Powles and Sanz (1996) also examined the contribution of smoking to temporal trends in CVD mortality. Their results suggest that tobacco contributed substantially to the increase in CVD mortality in men, at least in Poland and Hungary. In women, tobacco did not contribute to temporal trends in CVD mortality.

There are obvious problems with the analyses of both cross-sectional and temporal variation in CHD. The MONICA-based analyses were ecological and other factors, associated with both risk factors and CHD, can confound the association. In addition, the results of the MONICA data depended on selection of centres and time period (see more details in section on medical care). There may also be problems with specifying the lag time between exposure and disease which may differ for different risk factors. All this would lead to underestimation of the contribution of risk factors to variation in CHD between populations. The indirect method also has problems. It assumes that the temporal relationship (latency period) between smoking and CVD is similar to that for lung cancer, and that the strength of the association between smoking and CVD is the same in all populations. If these assumptions are not met, the estimates of death attributable to tobacco become unreliable. Nevertheless, it is probable that the conventional risk factors provide a partial explanation for the differences in CHD risk between populations and for the trends in CHD and CVD mortality. Classical coronary risk factors, and particularly smoking, made a sizeable contribution to the East–West gap in CHD mortality.

6.3.2 Quality of medical care

It has been widely believed in Eastern Europe that the mortality disadvantage from CVD and other chronic diseases is primarily due to poor quality of medical care. The lack of objective information did not allow direct test of this proposition until data from the MONICA study became available. The MONICA study collected data on the quality of treatment in the participating centres, based on the use of beta-blockers, antiplatelet drugs, coronary-artery reperfusion procedures, and angiotensin converting enzyme (ACE) inhibitors (Tunstall-Pedoe *et al.* 2000).

Cross-sectional association between case-fatality rates and treatment quality score (constructed from the four treatments listed above) in the early 1990s is shown in Figs 6.7 (men) and 6.8 (women). There was a strong inverse association between treatment quality and case-fatality rates (correlation coefficients were 0.74 in men and 0.75 in women). Centres in CEE/FSU had higher case-fatality rates than Western centres, although this pattern was somewhat exaggerated by the outlier Tarnobrzeg, Poland. Even after excluding Tarnobrzeg, the mean male and female case-fatality rates in Eastern European centres were 15% and 11%, respectively, higher than in Western centres. Controlling for treatment quality score reduced these differences to 6% and 3%, respectively.

It is apparent that treatment quality is strongly associated with case-fatality rates. We have further investigated whether it is also associated with CHD mortality rates. CHD mortality was correlated with treatment quality score (r 0.49 in men and 0.52 in women). Male CHD mortality in Eastern European centres was 81% higher than in Western centres, and adjustment for treatment quality reduced this excess to 54% (Table 6.1). Results in women were broadly similar (Table 6.1). Exclusion of Tarnobrzeg from the analyses made little difference.

These results should be viewed as merely indicative of the potential contribution of medical care. The same caveats mentioned in relation to analyses of risk factors apply here. In addition, since not all MONICA centres had all data on CHD mortality and survival, risk factors, and medical care, the East/West mortality ratio depended on selection of centres and time periods used in the analyses. However, while the East/West rate ratio differed by the choice of units for the analysis, the proportional reductions of the rate ratios were similar. Adjustment for quality of treatment reduced the rate ratio by 39% in the smaller dataset and 43% in the larger dataset,

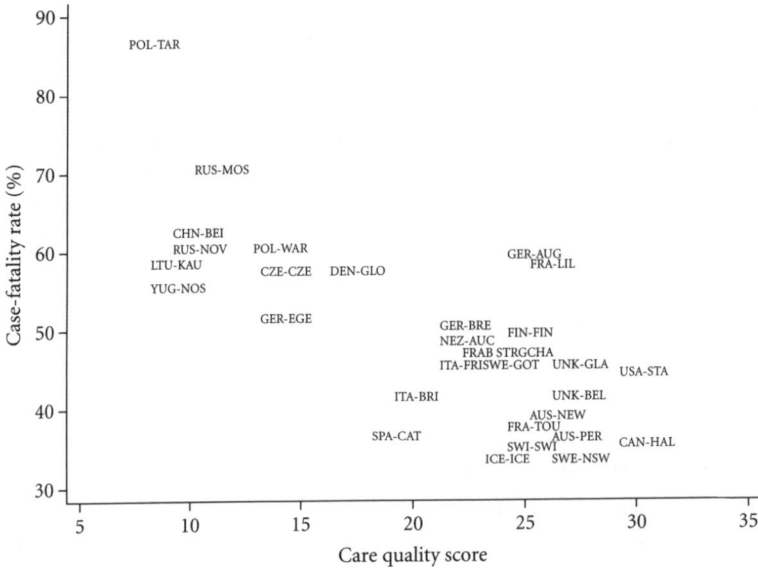

Fig. 6.7 Age-standardized case-fatality rates (percentage) by the treatment quality score in men 35–64 years old ($r = -0.74$). Abbreviations: AUS-NEW: Australia Newcastle; AUS-PER: Australia Perth; BEL-GCH: Belgium Ghent; CAN-HAL: Canada Halifax; CHN-BEI: China Beijing; CZE-CZE: Czechoslovakia; DEN-GLO: Denmark Glostrup; FRA-LIL: France Lille; FRA-STR: France Strassbourg; FRA-TOU: France Toulouse; FIN-FIN: Finland; GER-AUG: Germany Augsburg; GER-BRE: Germany Bremen; GER-EGE: East Germany; ITA-BRI: Italy Brianza; ICE-ICE: Iceland; LTU-KAU: Lithuania Kaunas; NEZ-AUC: New Zealand Auckland; POL-TAR: Poland Tarnobrzeg; POL-WAR: Poland Warsaw; RUS-MOS: Russia Moscow; RUS-NOV: Russia Novosibirsk; SPA-CAT: Spain Catalonia; SWE-GOT: Sweden Gothenburg; SWE-NSW: Sweden North; SWI-SWI: Switzerland; UNK-BEL: United Kingdom Belfast; UNK-GLA: United Kingdom Glasgow; USA-STA: USA Stanford; YUG-NOS: Yugoslavia Novi Sad. (Data from the MONICA project.)

and adjustment for risk factors reduced the rate ratio by 49% in the larger dataset and by 44% in the smaller dataset.

It is likely that quality of treatment is associated with a number of factors, such as prosperity, socio-economic development, or inequality, which are also associated with mortality. This has been shown in analyses of trends in CHD mortality. The results suggested that improvement in treatment score over time was associated with reduction in case-fatality rate in the MONICA centres (Tunstall-Pedoe *et al.* 2000). However, the changes in treatment were associated with changes not only in CHD mortality and case-fatality (where effects would be expected), but also with coronary event rates and prehospital mortality where a causal relation is less likely. While there is no doubt that the quality of coronary medical care is associated with CHD mortality and case fatality, the quantification of this association has yet to be clarified.

The fact that the combination of risk factors and treatment quality explained less of the East/West rate ratio than each of them alone is intriguing. The most likely reason is that both risk factors and care – while important – are associated with some underlying feature of society, such as socio-economic development, adoption of Western lifestyles and values, or the stage of the society in the epidemiological transition. Separating the effects of mutually

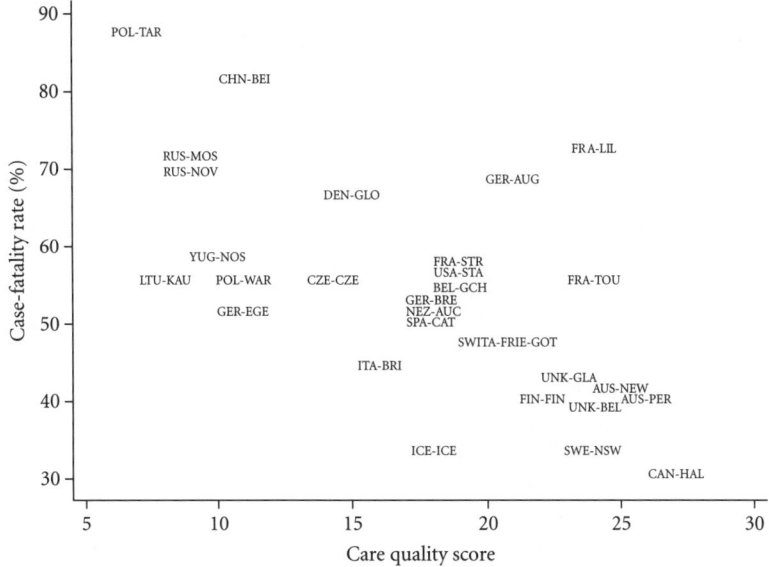

Fig. 6.8 Age-standardized case-fatality rates (percentage) by the treatment quality score in women 35–64 years old ($r = -0.63$). For abbreviations, see Fig. 6.7. (Data from the MONICA project.)

associated variables is notoriously difficult; the conclusions often depend on the choice of a causal model.

6.3.3 Dietary risk factors

A vast number of coronary risk factors other than smoking, cholesterol, blood pressure, and body mass index have been proposed, and many of them have been confirmed as genuinely linked to CHD (see the chapters in Section III). Some of them may contribute to the high rates of CHD in CEE/FSU. Below we consider the evidence on two of the most widely discussed dietary factors: dietary fat intake and dietary intake of fresh fruits and vegetables.

Dietary fat

Dietary intake of fats and its biological correlates has long been suspected to play a major role in the international differences in mortality from CVD. Mortality is higher in countries with higher intake of saturated fats (of animal origin) (Kesteloot 1992). It is believed that high dietary intake of animal fat acts through plasma lipids which in turn are related to increased risk of CVD.

This is probably true for studying CHD within populations, but the contribution of dietary intake of saturated fats to explaining the East–West gap has not been confirmed. Non-specific biomarkers of high saturated fat intake, such as elevated total and LDL serum cholesterol and triglycerides have not been found in CEE populations. In the MONICA study there was no clear East–West divide in total cholesterol (Principle investigators 1989). Two small but detailed studies also did not find any support for the saturated fat hypothesis. The Czech–Bavarian study, which compared random samples of middle-aged men in two towns, Pardubice in the Czech Republic and Augsburg in Bavaria, did not discover any major differences in blood lipids (Bobak et al. 1999a). The LiViCordia study, using similar design, also did not report any differences in blood lipids between middle-aged men in Vilnius (Lithuania) and Linkoping (Sweden) (Kristenson *et al.* 1997). Moreover, there were no differences between Lithuanian and Swedish men in the concentrations of specific fatty acids in abdominal tissue samples, which are relatively specific indicators for long-term intake of different types of fat (Kaminskas *et al.* 1999). In general, it seems unlikely that fat intake played a major role in the East–West divide in mortality.

Dietary intake of fresh fruits and vegetables

Intake of fresh fruits and vegetables offers more promise. Numerous observational studies suggest that persons with low dietary intakes or plasma levels of antioxidant vitamins (carotenoids, vitamins A, E, C) have an increased risk of CVD (Kardinaal *et al.* 1993; Knekt *et al.* 1994; Kohlmeier *et al.* 1997; Kushi *et al.* 1996; Riemersma *et al.* 1991; Rimm *et al.* 1993; Stampfer *et al.* 1993). Several mechanisms have been discussed for the protective role of carotenoids, including their *in vitro* and *in vivo* antioxidant activity. Aside from their antioxidant properties, plasma levels of carotenoids may be markers of dietary intakes of their food sources, most notably fruits and vegetables. These foods contain many other biologically important substances (e.g. ferulic acid, glutathione, folic acid, non-starch polysaccharide fibres, or other antioxidants such as flavonoids). A beneficial effect of high dietary consumption of fresh fruits and vegetables has been shown repeatedly in epidemiological studies (Ness and Powles 1997).

Available data show large East–West differences in consumption of fresh fruits and vegetables, and at the ecological level there is a good correlation between consumption of fresh fruits and vegetables (as recorded in the FAO Food Balance Sheets) and national cardiovascular mortality of both men and women (Ginter 1995, 1996). The optional study of dietary antioxidants in the MONICA Project provided further ecological evidence; there was a strong correlation between serum levels of alpha-tocopherol and beta carotene and mortality (Gey *et al.* 1991). Several smaller ecological studies examined and compared fruit intakes and/or blood vitamin concentration in population samples in Eastern and Western Europe. A study of men in Finnish North Karelia and in the Russian Republic of Karelia found large differences in dietary intakes of fruits and vegetables between these two populations, and these differences were confirmed by biomarkers levels: virtually all men in the Russian Karelia were classified as vitamin C deficient (Fig. 6.9) (Matilainen *et al.* 1996).

The LiViCordia Study reported large differences in antioxidant concentrations between Lithuanian and Swedish men; in addition, blood lipids of Swedish men were much more resistant

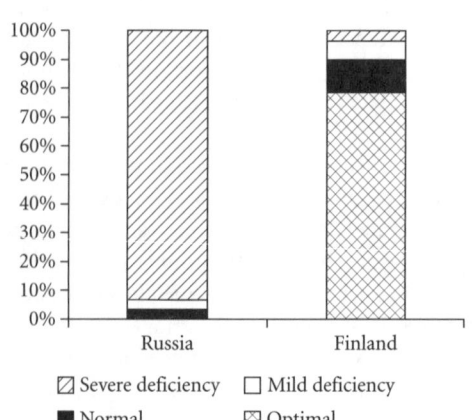

Fig. 6.9 Plasma vitamin C concentrations in Republic of Karelia, Russia and in North Karelia, Finland. (Adapted from Matilainen *et al.* 1996.)

to oxidation (Kristenson *et al.* 1997). The Czech–Bavarian study produced similar results: there were large differences in plasma concentration of carotenoids and vitamin E between these two populations (Bobak *et al.* 1999*a*). In addition, Czech men had higher levels of plasma homo-cysteine, another potential risk factor for vascular disease.

The most prominent finding of all these studies – the very low antioxidant concentrations – can most plausibly be explained by low dietary intake of their dietary sources. Consumption of fresh fruits and vegetables has been very low in CEE, particularly in winter and spring. It was suggested that this highly pronounced seasonality contributed to the high mortality in Eastern Europe where very low dietary intakes of fresh fruits and vegetables are common over a large part of each year (Powles *et al.* 1996). Consistent with this observation, Albania has had high consumption of fresh fruits and vegetables (Gjonca and Bobak 1997).

There is a wealth of studies that link dietary intake of fruits and vegetables, and their bio-markers, with reduced cardiovascular mortality in individuals in Western populations, but we are aware of only one such study in CEE. In a small case-control study of non-fatal myocardial infarction in the Czech Republic, men with below median concentrations of beta-carotene and alpha-tocopherol plasma concentrations had 3 times and 1.5 times higher risk of heart attack, respectively, compared to men in the upper half of the distribution (Bobak *et al.* 1998*a*).

On balance, there is good evidence of low dietary intakes of fresh fruits and vegetables in CEE/FSU, but direct evidence that it contributes to high rates of CHD in the region, and the quantification of such contribution, has yet to be established.

6.3.4 Psychosocial factors

Geographical distribution of CHD mortality copied the political East–West division of Europe. This observation led to a speculation that CHD risk is at least partly caused by the unfavourable psychosocial factors associated with living under oppressive regimes. Since 1990, evidence has emerged that distribution of psychosocial factors in CEE/FSU (such as perceived control, depression, mastery, hopelessness) was indeed less favourable than in Western countries (Carlson 1998; Pikhart *et al.* 2004; Steptoe and Wardle 2001). Ecologically, CHD mortality was found to be associated with low perceived control (Carlson 1998). There are only few pub-lished studies of CHD and psychosocial factors within countries in CEE/FSU. Risk of CHD was found to be related to job strain (Bobak *et al.* 1998*b*) and unmarried status, a marker of low social networks (Broda *et al.* 1994; Hajdu *et al.* 1995; Malyutina *et al.* 2004). All-cause mortality in Russia and Hungary is associated, geographically, with markers of low social capital (Kennedy *et al.* 1998; Skrabski *et al.* 2003). Unpublished cohort analyses of the follow-up of the MONICA samples in Kaunas, Lithuania, and Novosibirsk, Russia found strong relationships between mortality and job strain and depression (Pikhart, unpublished; Gafarov, personal communication). Although direct evidence that psychosocial factors contributed to the differ-ences in CHD risk between Eastern and Western Europe remains limited, the results of studies published so far implicate psychosocial factors in the high rates of CHD in CEE and FSU.

6.3.5 Birth cohort effect

There is now good evidence that factors operating in early life contribute to CHD risk at adult ages (Barker 1995) (Chapter 31). It might be argued that the sharp increase in CHD rates in the 1960s in CEE/FSU may have resulted from a particular susceptibility of some subpopulations, perhaps due to exposure to war, poverty, or nutritional scarcity earlier in their life. In such cases it would be expected that the rise in CHD mortality would be limited to, or at least more pronounced in persons born in certain periods (birth cohorts). We have examined this possibility in data from Poland and Hungary; since both these countries recorded a sharp rise in male CHD mortality in the 1960s and both countries have data on age-specific CHD mortality rates going back to the 1950s. There is little evidence of a birth cohort effect; the increase started in all age groups at approximately the same time (about mid-1960s in Poland and end of 1960s in Hungary), and was not confined to any particular birth cohort (Figs 6.10 and 6.11).

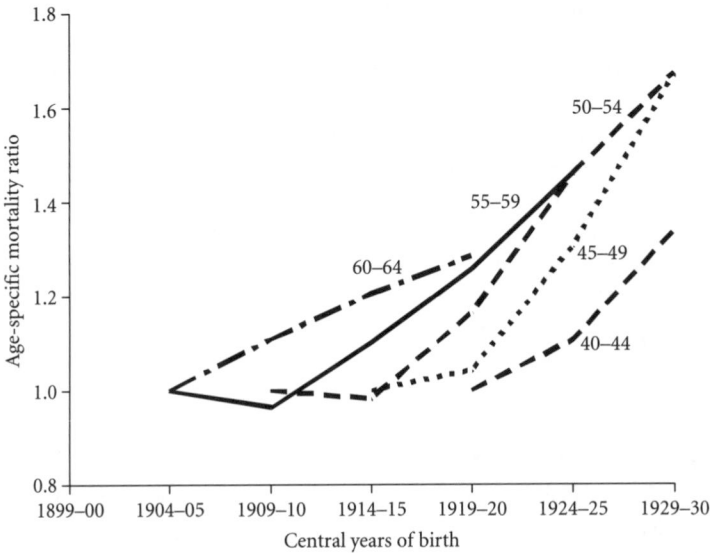

Fig. 6.10 Age-specific CHD mortality ratio (relative to the first birth cohort available) by year of birth in Hungarian men. (Data from WHO.)

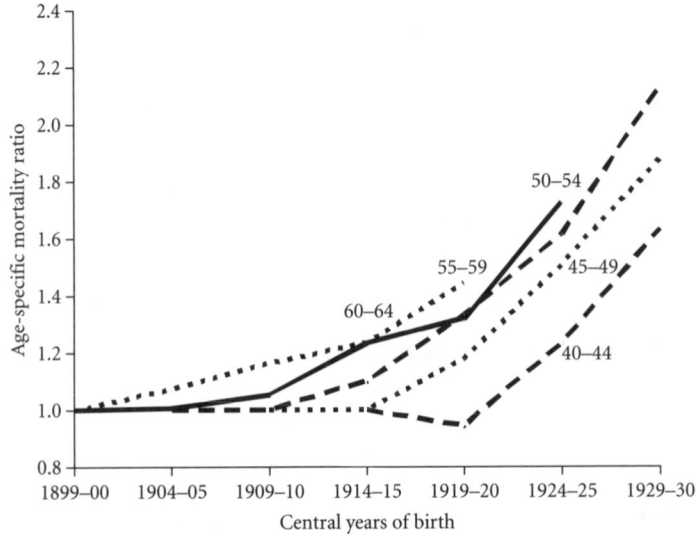

Fig. 6.11 Age-specific CHD mortality ratio (relative to the first birth cohort available) by year of birth in Polish men. (Data from WHO).

6.3.6 Air pollution

In the early 1990s, there was a widespread belief in the CEE/FSU, and to a lesser extent in the West, that the high levels of environmental pollution in Eastern Europe made a substantial contribution to the high mortality in the region (Hertzman 1994). The initial claims were exaggerated, but several estimates suggested that air pollution played a role in mortality. For example, on the basis of time-series studies it was estimated that about 3% of all deaths in the Czech Republic in 1989 – about 9% of the mortality gap between the Czech Republic and Austria – could have been caused by air pollution (Bobak and Feachem 1995). Other estimates were similar (Jakubowski 1991) or even higher (Ostro 1996). Later, as the time-series methodology was criticized as inadequate for providing reliable estimates of long-term effects (McMichael *et al.* 1998), such calculations of the contribution of air pollution to long-term mortality rates were considered as probable overestimates.

However, there is now solid evidence from longitudinal studies that air pollution is indeed associated with cardiorespiratory mortality (Dockery *et al.* 1993; Hoek *et al.* 2002; Pope III *et al.* 1995, 2002) (Chapter 28). The relative risk is relatively low (around 1.07 per each 10 $\mu g/m^3$ increase in concentration of particulate matter with particle diameters less than 10 μm), but larger than that estimated in time-series studies. However, applying small relative risk to a common exposure may result in non-negligible attributable risk fraction. In the case of the Czech Republic, using exposures in the late 1980s and relative risk estimates from the follow-up of the US Cancer Prevention Study (the largest of the three cohort studies, by Pope III *et al.* 2002) up to 7% of all-cause mortality and up to 13% of coronary mortality could have been attributed to air pollution. These may be overestimates, but the results illustrate that air pollution may account for a non-negligible proportion of CHD deaths in severely polluted countries, such as the Czech Republic or Poland before 1990. It has been argued that the 10% decline in CVD mortality observed in Dublin after a ban of coal sales in 1990 was caused by the decline in air pollution (Clancy *et al.* 2002). It is not entirely implausible that some of the rapid decline in CVD mortality in Poland and the Czech Republic after 1989 was due to the substantial decline in air pollution caused by the falling industrial production in the early years of transition.

6.4 Lessons from CEE/FSU

Studies of CHD in CEE/FSU have produced several findings or hypotheses which may require further confirmation or research, but which are important for the understanding of CHD determinants in general. We will describe in more detail three issues that we consider the most significant.

6.4.1 Socio-economic inequalities in CHD

A recent review of studies of non-communicable diseases in CEE/FSU concluded that social differences in mortality in the post-Communist countries are pervasive, and are of similar or larger magnitude to those in Western societies (Bobak and Powles 2001). This is surprising, since social equity was a proclaimed and, to a large extent, pursued goal of the Communist regimes prior to 1990. Income inequalities were, on average, substantially smaller than in Western countries (Atkinson and Micklewright 1992). To give some guidance, the Gini coefficient of income inequality is typically around 0.35 in Western countries and over 0.5 in Latin America; it was around 0.2 in CEE/FSU before 1990. (The Gini coefficient approximately indicates the proportion of the overall income in a country that would need to be redistributed so that everybody has the same income.)

Thus the Communist regimes in CEE/FSU succeeded in compressing income inequalities. However, this did not eliminate or reduce social inequalities in health. There are no reliable data on health inequalities by income, but there is ample evidence on differentials in total, CVD and CHD mortality by education, with education being the best available socio-economic predictor of health in CEE/FSU (Bobak and Powles 2001).

This observation has two implications. First, since better education was not associated with material advantage before 1990, data from CEE/FSU allow us to break the confounding due to mutual correlation of different socio-economic indicators in Western countries. For this reason, the effects of education on CHD and other health outcomes cannot be ascribed to confounding by material factors. This is an important contribution to the current debate on the materialist vs. psychosocial explanations for social inequalities in health (Lynch et al. 2000; Marmot and Wilkinson 2001).

Second, the Eastern European experience shows that reducing inequalities in income does not necessarily reduce general inequalities in health. Health inequalities may not be seen by income (we do not have good data on this), but they were pronounced by education. This may be of importance for designing policies aiming to reduce inequalities within countries (Acheson 1998).

6.4.2 Effect of societal transition on CHD mortality

The second unique observation from CEE/FSU is the powerful effect of societal transformation on health in general and CHD specifically. The fall of Communist regimes in 1989 brought about profound political, economic, and social changes that affected whole populations. The impact on mortality differed between CEE and FSU.

In CEE, several countries (Czech Republic, Poland, former East Germany) recorded a short-term increase in all-cause and CVD mortality in the first post-revolution year (1991), but this was followed by declining mortality. Death rates from CHD are now declining in virtually all CEE. The exact reasons for the decline are not fully understood, but they probably include changing dietary habits (increased consumption of fresh fruits and vegetables and vegetable fats, and reduced consumption of animal products) accompanied by a fall in blood lipids (Bobak et al. 1997; Zatonski et al. 1998).

In the FSU, the changes went less well. Figure 6.12 shows trends in CHD in Russia and the three Baltic countries; the pattern was similar for all-cause mortality. After Gorbachev come to power in 1985, mortality declined slightly until 1991, and rose dramatically after the break-up of the Soviet Union (the Soviet Union ceased to exist on 31 December 1991). Mortality started to decline in 1995, but increased again after the rouble crisis in 1998 (and crude mortality was still rising in 2002 (J. Shapiro, personal communication)). Interestingly, mortality in Estonia and Latvia also increased in 1998 before continuing to decline; only Lithuania was not affected by the Russian economic crisis in 1998.

It is widely believed that the underlying causes of the massive and rapid changes in death rates in FSU are social. There is less consensus as to the factors mediating the effects of transformation on CHD. A number of factors have been proposed which can be divided into three broad categories: poverty, stress, and alcohol and other health behaviours. There is no doubt that material conditions of most people in FSU deteriorated during the transformation. Gross domestic product and real wages declined between one-third and two-thirds in the first few

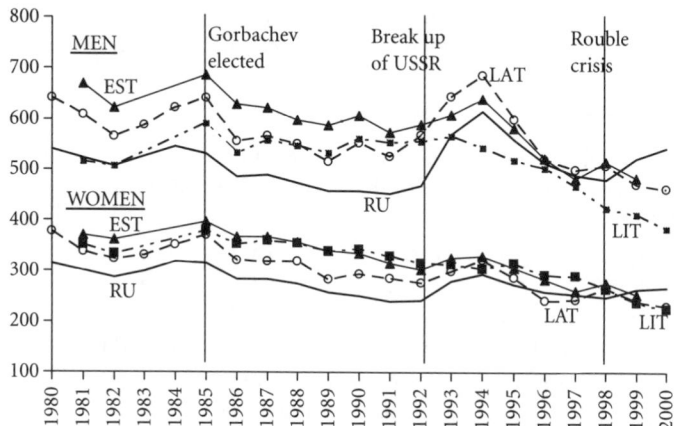

Fig. 6.12 Trends in mortality from CHD in Russia and the Baltic states, 1980–2000, per 100 000 Abbreviations: EST: Estonia; LAT: Latvia; LIT: Lithuania; RU: Russia. (Data from the WHO Health for All database.)

years of transition (UNICEF 2003). In a panel study of households, income fell substantially between 1992 and 1996 and the proportion of households under 50% of the poverty line increased from 3 to 20% (Zohoori *et al.* 1998). On the other hand, infant mortality, usually seen as a sensitive indicator of material deprivation, did not increase during the 1990s (UNICEF 2003). Parallel to economic difficulties was social disruption characterized by a rapid rise in job insecurity, crime and corruption, lawlessness, divorces, and income inequalities (Cornia 1997; Klein and Pomer 2001; Zohoori *et al.* 1998). It has been shown that mortality increase by Russian regions was directly associated with 'stress caused by unexpected situations' (Cornia 1997; Walberg *et al.* 1998). There were also alarming reports about the rise in alcoholism and its consequences on health (Shkolnikov and Nemtsov 1997).

6.4.3 **Alcohol and CHD**

There is indirect evidence that alcohol could provide at least a partial link between the societal changes and trends in mortality. The temporal changes in estimated alcohol consumption corresponded, at least until mid-1990s, to both social changes and to fluctuations in mortality by age group and cause of death (Leon *et al.* 1997; Nemtsov 2000). The similarity of changes in mortality from alcohol poisoning, injuries, and CVD lead to the hypothesis that they have a similar proximal cause – alcohol. It has been proposed that the hypothesized adverse effect of alcohol on cardiac deaths in Russia (which is the opposite of the generally accepted cardio-protective effect seen elsewhere and described in Chapter 16) has been ascribed to the binge-drinking pattern common in Russia (Britton and McKee 2000). The biological mechanisms proposed may involve blood lipids and arrhythmia, possibly leading to sudden death (McKee and Britton 1998).

There are several observations that contradict the hypothesis, most notably the fact that the increase was, in relative terms, similar in men and women, but all data so far have shown very low levels of drinking in women, both before and during the transition period (Bobak and Marmot 1999; Bobak *et al.* 1999*b*; Malyutina *et al.* 2001; Simpura *et al.* 1997). The hypothesis remains to be debated, but it already had a significant impact. Firstly, it has attracted considerable attention to the Russian mortality crisis and stimulated a debate on its causes. Secondly, it re-emphasized the importance of drinking patterns for population health and it gave a fresh impetus to new research into the relation between binge and heavy drinking and CHD.

6.4 Conclusions

CHD rates are now falling in most countries of CEE, but are still rising or unstable in Russia and several other countries of FSU, and the CHD rates in FSU remain among the highest ever recorded. Factors responsible for the CHD epidemic in CEE/FSU in the last third of the twentieth century are only partly understood. Classical risk factors and medical care made a substantial contribution to the high mortality, but they do not provide a complete explanation. Psychosocial factors, nutrition, and alcohol (in FSU) also seem to be implicated. All risk factors, conventional, dietary, or psychosocial, are strongly influenced by social condition. As a whole, the Eastern European experience provides unique evidence of the powerful effect of societal forces on both long-term and short-term trends in CHD.

References

Acheson, D. (1998). *Great Britain Independent Inquiry into Inequalities in Health.* The Stationary Office, London.

Atkinson, A. B. and Micklewright, J. (1992). *Economic transformation in Eastern Europe and the distribution of income.* Cambridge University Press.

Barker, D. J. P. (1995). Fetal origins of coronary heart disease. *British Medical Journal,* **311,** 171–4.

Bobak, M. and Feachem, R. G. A. (1995). Air pollution and mortality in Central and Eastern Europe: an estimate of the impact. *European Journal of Public Health,* **5,** 82–6.

Bobak, M. and Marmot, M. (1996). East-west mortality divide and its potential explanations: proposed research agenda. *British Medical Journal,* **312,** 421–5.

Bobak, M. and Marmot, M. (1999). Alcohol and mortality in Russia: is it different than elsewhere? *Annals of Epidemiology,* **9,** 335–8.

Bobak, M. and Powles, J. (2001). *Poverty and non-communicable diseases in Central and Eastern Europe and the former Soviet Union: a report for the Non-Communicable Diseases and Mental Health Cluster, WHO Geneva.* University College London.

Bobak, M., Skodova, Z., Pisa, Z., Poledne, R., and Marmot, M. (1997). Political changes and trends in cardiovascular risk factors in the Czech Republic 1985–1992. *Journal of Epidemiology and Community Health,* **51,** 272–7.

Bobak, M., Brunner, E., Miller, N. J., Skodova, Z., and Marmot, M. (1998a). Could antioxidants play a role in the high rates of coronary heart disease in the Czech Republic? *European Journal of Clinical Nutrition,* **52,** 632–6.

Bobak, M., Hertzman, C., Skodova, Z., and Marmot, M. (1998b). Association between psychosocial factors at work and non-fatal myocardial infarction in a population based case-control study in Czech men. *Epidemiology,* **9,** 43–7.

Bobak, M., Hense, H. W., Kark, J. D., Kuch, B., Vojtisek, P., Sinnreich, R. *et al.* (1999a). An ecological study of determinants of cardiovascular disease rates: a comparison of Czech, Bavarian and Israeli men. *International Journal of Epidemiology,* **28,** 437–44.

Bobak, M., McKee, M., Rose, R., and Marmot, M. (1999b). Alcohol consumption in a national sample of the Russian population. *Addiction,* **94,** 857–66.

Britton, A. and McKee, M. (2000). The relation between alcohol and cardiovascular disease in Eastern Europe: explaining the paradox. *Journal of Epidemiology and Community Health,* **54,** 328–32.

Broda, G., Rywik, S., and Piotrowski, W. (1994). 10-year mortality from all causes and cardiovascular disease in relation to education level and marital status on Polish MONICA Warsaw population. National Institute of Cardiology, Warsaw.

Carlson, P. (1998). Self-perceived health in East and West Europe: another European health divide. *Social Science in Medicine*, **46**, 1355–66.

Clancy, L., Goodman, P., Sinclair, H., and Dockery, D. W. (2002). Effect of air-pollution control on death rates in Dublin, Ireland: an intervention study. *Lancet*, **360**, 1210–14.

Cornia, G. A. (1997). *Labour market shocks, psychosocial stress and the transition's mortality crisis: research in Progress 4 Working Paper*. United Nations University World Institute for Development Economics Research, Helsinki.

Dockery, D. W., Pope III, C. A., Xu, X., Spengler, J. D., Ware, J. H., Fay, M. E. *et al.* (1993). An association between air pollution and mortality in six U.S. cities. *New England Journal of Medicine*, **329**, 1753–9.

Gey, K. F., Puska, P., Jordan, P., and Moser, U. K. (1991). Inverse correlation between plasma vitamin E and mortality from ischemic heart disease in cross-cultural epidemiology. *American Journal of Clinical Nutrition*, **53** (Suppl.), 326S–334S.

Ginter, E. (1995). Cardiovascular risk factors in the former communist countries: analysis of 40 European MONICA populations. *European Journal of Epidemiology*, **11**, 199–205.

Ginter, E. (1996). High cardiovascular mortality in postcommunist countries: participation of oxidative stress? *International Journal of Vitamins and Nutrition Research*, **66**, 183–9.

Gjonca, A. and Bobak, M. (1997). Albanian paradox, another example of protective effect of Mediterranean lifestyle? *Lancet*, **350**, 1815–17.

Hajdu, P., McKee, M., and Bojan, F. (1995). Changes in premature mortality differentials by marital status in Hungary and in England and Wales. *European Journal of Public Health*, **5**, 259–64.

Hertzman, C. (1994). *Environment and health in Central and Eastern Europe*. World Bank, Washington.

Hoek, G., Brunekreef, B., Goldbohm, S., Fischer, P., and van den Brandt, P. A. (2002). Association between mortality and indicators of traffic-related air pollution in the Netherlands: a cohort study. *Lancet*, **360**, 1203–9.

Jakubowski, M. (1991). Ambient air pollution and health effects. In *Air pollution in Central and Eastern Europe: health and public policy* (ed. B. S. Levy), pp. 47–58. Edited proceedings of the Second Annual Symposium on Environmental and Occupational Health during Societal Transition in Central and Eastern Europe, Frydek-Mistek, Czechoslovakia, 14–19 June 1991. Management Sciences for Health, Boston.

Kaminskas, A., Zieden, B., Elving, B., Kristenson, M., Abaravicius, A., Bergdahl, B. *et al.* (1999). Adipose tissue fatty acids in men from two populations with different cardiovascular risk: the LiVicordia Study. *Scandinavian Journal of Clinical Laboratory Investigation*, **59**, 227–32.

Kardinaal, A. F. M., Kok, F. J., Ringstad, J., Gomez-Aracena, J., Mazaev, V. P., Kohlmeier, L. *et al.* (1993). Antioxidants in adipose tissue and risk of myocardial infarction: the EURAMIC study. *Lancet*, **342**, 1379–84.

Kennedy, B. P., Kawachi, I., and Brainerd, E. (1998). The role of social capital in the Russian mortality crisis. *World Development*, **26**, 2029–43.

Kesteloot, H. (1992). Nutrition and health. *European Heart Journal*, **13**, 120–8.

Klein, L. R. and Pomer, M. (2001). *The new Russia: transition gone awry*. Stanford University Press.

Knekt, P., Reunanen, A., Jarvinen, R., Seppanen, R., Heliovaara, M., and Aromaa, A. (1994). Antioxidant vitamin intake and coronary mortality in a longitudinal population study. *American Journal of Epidemiology*, **139**, 1180–9.

Kohlmeier, L., Kark, J. D., Gomez-Gracia, E., Martin, B. C., Steck, S. E., Kardinaal, A. F. M. *et al.* (1997). Lycopene and myocardial infarction risk in the EURAMIC Study. *American Journal of Epidemiology*, **146**, 618–26.

Kristenson, M., Zieden, B., Kucinskiene, Z., Schafer Elinder, L., Bergdahl, B., Elwing, B. *et al.* (1997). Antioxidant state and mortality from coronary heart disease in Lithuanian and Swedish men: concomitant cross-sectional study of men aged 50. *British Medical Journal*, **314**, 629–33.

Kushi, L. H., Folsom, A. R., Prineas, R. J., Mink, P. J., Wu, Y., and Bostick, R. M. (1996). Dietary antioxidant vitamins and death from coronary heart disease in postmenopausal women. *New England Journal of Medicine*, **334**, 1156–62.

Kuulasmaa, K., Tunstall-Pedoe, H., Dobson, A., Fortmann, S. P., Sans, S., Tolonen, H. *et al.* (2000). Estimation of contribution of changes in classic risk factors to trends in coronary-event rates across the WHO MONICA Project populations. *Lancet*, **335**, 675–87.

Leon, D. A., Chenet, L., Shkolnikov, V., Zakharov, S., Shapiro, J., Rakhmanova, G. *et al.* (1997). Huge variation in Russian mortality rates 1984–94: artefact, alcohol, or what? *Lancet*, **350**, 383–8.

Lynch, J. W., Davey Smith, G., Kaplan, G. A., and House, J. S. (2000). Income inequality and mortality: importance to health of individual income, psychosocial environment, or material conditions. *British Medical Journal*, **320**, 1200–4.

Malyutina, S., Bobak, M., Kurilovitch, S., Ryizova, E., Nikitin, Y., and Marmot, M. (2001). Alcohol consumption and binge drinking in Novosibirsk, Russia, 1985–95. *Addiction*, **96**, 987–95.

Malyutina, S., Bobak, M., Simonova, G., Gafarov, V., Nikitin, Y., and Marmot, M. (2004). Education, marital status and all-cause and cardiovascular mortality in Novosibirsk, Russia: a prospective cohort study. *Annals of Epidemiology*, **14**, 244–9.

Marmot, M. G. and Wilkinson, R. G. (2001). Psychosocial and material pathways in the relation between income and health: a response to Lynch *et al. British Medical Journal*, **322**, 1233–6.

Matilainen, T., Vartiainen, E., Puska, P., Alfthan, G., Pokusajeva, S., Moisejeva, N., and Uhanov, M. (1996). Plasma ascorbic concentrations in the Republic of Karelia, Russia, and in North Karelia, Finland. *European Journal of Clinical Nutrition*, **50**, 115–20.

McKee, M. and Britton, A. (1998). The positive relationship between alcohol and heart disease in eastern Europe: potential physiological mechanisms. *Journal of the Royal Society of Medicine*, **91**, 402–7.

McMichael, A. J., Anderson, H. R., Brunekreef, B., and Cohen, A. J. (1998). Inappropriate use of daily mortality analyses to estimate longer-term mortality effects of air pollution. *International Journal of Epidemiology*, **27**, 450–3.

Mesle, F., Shkolnikov, V. M., Hertrich, V., and Vallin, J. (1996). *Tendances recentes de la mortalite par cause en Russie 1965–1994* [Recent trends in mortality by cause in Russia 1965–1994]. INED, Paris.

Nemtsov, A. (2000). Estimates of total alcohol consumption in Russia, 1980–1994. *Drugs and Alcohol Dependence*, **58**, 133–43.

Ness, A. R. and Powles, J. W. (1997). Fruit and vegetables and cardiovascular disease: a review. *International Journal of Epidemiology*, **26**, 1–13.

Ostro, B. (1996). Air pollution and mortality in Central and Eastern Europe. In *East-west life expectancy gap in Europe: environmental and non-environmental determinants* (ed. C. Hertzman, S. Kelly, and M. Bobak), pp. 85–96. Kluwer, Dordrecht.

Peto, R., Lopez, A. D., Boreham, J., Thun, M., and Heath, C. Jr. (1992). Mortality from tobacco in developed countries: indirect estimation from national vital statistics. *Lancet*, **339**, 1268–78.

Peto, R., Lopez, A. D., Boreham, J., Thun, M., and Heath, C. Jr. (1994). Mortality from smoking in developed countries 1950–2000: indirect estimates from national vital statistics. Oxford University Press.

Pikhart, H., Bobak, M., Pajak, A., Malyutina, S., Kubinova, R., Topor, R. *et al.* (2004). Psychosocial factors at work and depression in three countries of Central and Eastern Europe, *Social Science in Medicine*, **58**, 1475–82.

Pope III, C. A., Thun, M. J., Namboodiri, M. M., Dockery, D. W., Evans, J. S., Speizer, F. E., and Heath, C. W. (1995). Particulate air pollution as a predictor of mortality in a prospective study of US adults. *American Journal of Respiratory Critical Care Medicine*, **151**, 669–74.

Pope III, C. A., Burnett, R. T., Thun, M. J., Calle, E. E., Krewski, D., Ito, K., and Thurston, G. D. (2002). Lung cancer, cardiopulmonary mortality, and long-term exposure to fine particulate air pollution. *Journal of the American Medical Association*, **287**, 1132–41.

Powles, J. W. and Sanz, M. A. (1996). Vascular mortality not attributable to smoking: trends in European populations since the 1950s. In *The XIV International Scientific Meeting of the International Epidemiological Association: global health in a changing environment*, p. 189. Program and abstracts. International Epidemiological Association, Nagoya.

Powles, J. W., Day, N. E., Sanz, M. A., and Bingham, S. A. (1996). Protective foods in winter and spring: a key to lower vascular mortality? [Letter.] *Lancet*, **348**, 898–9.

Principle investigators (1989). The MONICA project: a worldwide monitoring system for cardiovascular diseases. *World Health Statistics Annual*, 27–149.

Riemersma, R. A., Wood, D. A., MacIntyre, C. C. A., Elton, R., Gey, K. F., and Oliver, M. F. (1991). Risk of angina pectoris and plasma concentrations of vitamins A, C, and E and carotene. *Lancet*, **337**, 1–5.

Rimm, E. B., Stampfer, M. J., Ascherio, A., Giovannucci, E., Colditz, G. A., and Willett, W. C. (1993). Vitamin E consumption and the risk of coronary heart disease in men. *New England Journal of Medicine*, **328**, 1450–6.

Shkolnikov, V. M. and Nemtsov, A. (1997). The anti-alcohol campaign and variations in Russian mortality. In *Premature death in the New Independent States* (ed. J. L. Bobadilla, C. A. Costello, and F. Mitchell), pp. 239–61. National Academy Press, Washington, DC.

Simpura, J., Levin, B. M., and Mustonen, H. (1997). Russian drinking in the 1990s: patterns and trends in international comparison. In *Demystifying Russian drinking: comparative studies from the 1990s* (ed. J. Simpura and B. M. Levin), pp.79–107. STAKES, Helsinki.

Skrabski, A., Kopp, M., and Kawachi, I. (2003). Social capital in a changing society: cross sectional associations with middle aged female and male mortality rates. *Journal of Epidemiology and Community Health*, **57**, 114–19.

Stampfer, M. J., Hennekens, C. H., Manson, J. E., Colditz, G. A., Rosner, B., and Willett, W. C. (1993). Vitamin E consumption and the risk of coronary heart disease in women. *New England Journal of Medicine*, **328**, 1444–9.

Steptoe, A. and Wardle, J. (2001). Health behaviour, risk awareness and emotional well-being in students from Eastern Europe and Western Europe. *Social Science & Medicine*, **53**, 1621–30.

Tunstall-Pedoe, H., Vanuzzo, D., Hobbs, M., Mahonen, M., Cepaitis, Z., Kuulasmaa, K., and Keil, U. (2000). Estimation of contribution of changes in coronary care to improving survival, event rates, and coronary heart disease mortality across the WHO MONICA project populations., *Lancet*, **355**, 688–700.

Uemura, K. and Pisa, Z. (1988). Trends in cardiovascular disease mortality in industrialized countries since 1950, *World Health Statistics Quarterly*, **41**, 155–178.

UNICEF (2003). *Social Monitor 2003. Social trends in transition* Florence: UNICEF Innocenti Research Centre.

Walberg, P., McKee, M., Shkolnikov, V., Chenet, L., and Leon, D. A. (1998). Economic change, crime, and the Russian mortality crisis: a regional analysis, *British Medical Journal*, **317**, 312–318.

WHO (World Health Organization) MONICA Project (1994). Ecological analysis of the association between mortality and major risk factors of cardiovascular disease. *International Journal of Epidemiology*, **23**, 505–16.

WHO MONICA Project, Tunstall-Pedoe, H., Kuulasmaa, K., Amouyel, P., Arveiler, D., Rajakangas, A.-M., and Pajak, A. (1994). Myocardial infaction and coronary deaths in the World Health Organization MONICA Project: registration procedures, event rates, and case-fatality rates in 38 populations from 21 countries in four continents. *Circulation*, **90**, 583–612.

Zatonski, W. A., McMichael, A. J., and Powles, J. W. (1998). Ecological study of reasons for sharp decline in mortality from ischaemic heart disease in Poland since 1991. *British Medical Journal*, **316**, 1047–51.

Zohoori, N., Mroz, T. A., Popkin, B. M., Glinskaya, E., Lokshin, M., Mancini, D. *et al.* (1998). Monitoring the economic transition in the Russian Federation and its implications for the demographic crisis: the Russian longitudinal monitoring survey. *World Development*, **26**, 1977–93.

Chapter 7

Trends in Asia

H. Ueshima

7.1 Mortality studies

Mortality statistics are available in some Asian countries from the World Health Statistics Annual and government statistics (Department of Health, Republic of China; WHO). Based on these statistics, age-adjusted (35–74 years old) mortality from coronary heart disease (CHD) was calculated. Fig. 7.1 shows that a specific feature of most of the Asian countries except for Singapore is that they have lower CHD mortality but higher stroke mortality compared to Western countries (Department of Health, Republic of China 1981–99; Uemura and Pisa 1988; Ueshima 1990; WHO). CHD mortality rates in Westernized Asian populations such as Singapore and Hong Kong, with higher serum total cholesterol (TC) levels, are relatively higher compared to other Asian populations. Japan showed the lowest mortality from CHD among industrialized countries (Fig. 7.1) (Uemura and Pisa 1988; Ueshima 1990). In China, mortality statistics were available only for some selected populations in urban and rural areas in 1990. Although CHD mortality for both of them was lower than those of Western populations, those of rural Chinese populations were lower than those of urban ones. Korea and Taiwan also showed similar mortality rates to Japan. Thailand showed the lowest mortality from CHD among all the Asian countries.

Mortality from CHD started to decline from approximately 1970–1980 worldwide, although in some east European countries it increased (Uemura and Pisa 1988; Ueshima 1990; Ueshima et al. 1987). This is also true in most Asian countries including Japan, Singapore, and Hong Kong (Fig. 7.1). In Singapore, Hong Kong, and Japan, age-adjusted CHD mortality showed an increasing trend until approximately 1970 (Emmanuel 1989; Huges 1986; Ng et al. 1999; Uemura and Pisa 1988; Ueshima 1990; Ueshima et al. 1987; Yu et al. 1995). Thereafter, it has shown a decline similar to that observed in Western countries (Fig. 7.1). In South Korea, age-adjusted CHD mortality increased until 1990 and thereafter levelled off (Suh 2001). In Taiwan, CHD mortality also increased until approximately 1990, but since then has started to decline (Department of Health, Republic of China 1981–99).

In China there are no nationally representative trend data available that have been reported to WHO. However, some epidemiological studies have shown that CHD mortality remains low with no definite increasing trends (Tao et al. 1989; Wu et al. 1996; Wu et al. 2001; Zhou et al. 1998).

As shown in Fig. 7.1, the mortality rate for Japanese people in 1997 remained at one-forth to one-fifth of that of America and England and Wales, despite the increase in fat intake and serum TC levels in Japan. On the other hand, mortality from CHD in Singapore was higher than in other Asian countries, although it has declined.

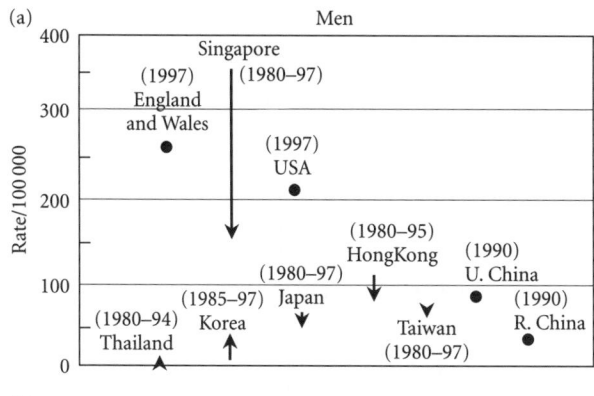

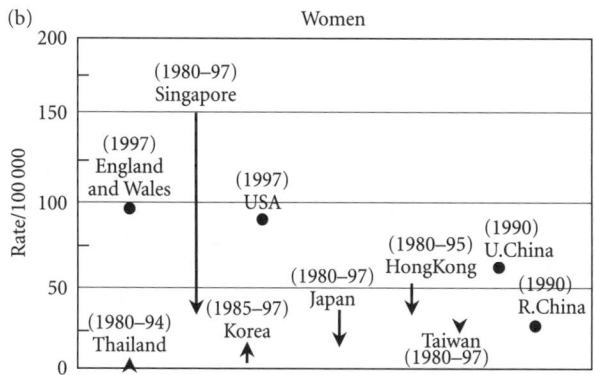

Fig. 7.1 Age-adjusted (35–74 years old) mortality trends in CHD, 1980–97, among Asian countries, USA, and England/Wales. Mortality rates from CHD for men and women in Singapore were the highest among selected Asian countries, followed by Hong Kong. CHD mortality rates in Japan, Singapore, and Hong Kong declined from 1980–97. Those of Korea and Thailand increased. (From WHO 1981–99, and data from Department of Health, Executive Yan, Republic of China 1981–99). Age-adjusted rates were calculated using the European standard population.

7.2 Information on incidence

The incidence rates of acute myocardial infarction in Chinese and several Japanese populations were determined in 1985–93 by the WHO MONICA project and similar criteria (Tunstall-Pedoe *et al.* 1994). These findings show that the incidence rates of acute myocardial infarction in several Chinese and Japanese populations were well below those found in the other countries that were examined (Fig. 7.2). Therefore, the specific feature that explains the lowest mortality rates from CHD in Asian populations is the low incidence rates of acute myocardial infarction.

In addition to this, some Japanese cohort studies in Hiroshima and Nagasaki, Hisayama, the northern part of Japan, and Osaka have also shown declining or stable trends in the incidence rate of myocardial infarction (Fujishima *et al.* 1992; Kodama *et al.* 1990; Shimamoto *et al.* 1989). These findings are compatible with CHD mortality trends in Japan.

The Sino-MONICA Project has monitored incidence rates from coronary events for men and women of 35–64 years of age in various Chinese populations from north to south of the country, and found that 9 of 12 populations showed declining trends during 1987–93, although these trends were not significant (Lee *et al.* 2001). In Singapore, the mortality and incidence rate for CHD was higher than in other Asian countries (Woo *et al.* 1997). The incidence rate of CHD was obtained from the Singapore Myocardial Infarction Registry, and it was found that the age-adjusted (20–64 years) incidence rate of CHD had declined during the period 1988–96.

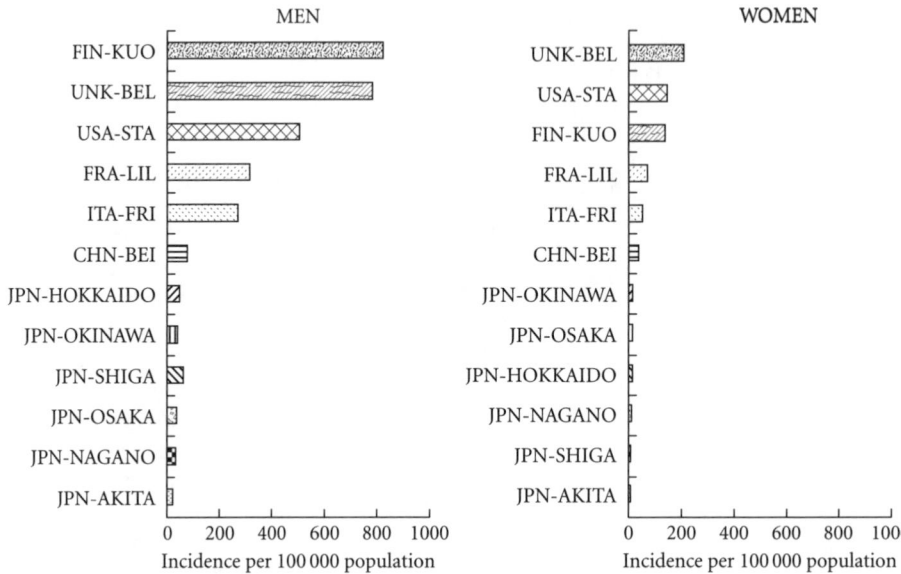

Fig. 7.2 Age-adjusted incidence rate of acute myocardial infarction for men and women aged 35–64 years in China, Japan, and selected industrialized countries in Europe and USA, 1985–93. The survey years of the MONICA Project and a Japanese study were from 1985–87 and 1989–99, respectively. Except for Japanese findings, all incidence rates were based on the MONICA Project. The MONICA criteria were used for the registration of acute myocardial infarction in all Japanese populations. Incidence rates of six Japanese populations and of China were far lower than those of selected industrialized countries. The world standard population was used for the calculation of age-adjusted rates of 35–64 years old. Abbreviations: Fin-KUO: Finland-Kuopio; UNK-BEL: UK-Belfast; USA-STA: USA-Stanford; FRA-LIL: France-Lille; ITA-FRI: Italy-Friuli; CHN-BEI: China-Beijing; JPN: Japan. (From WHO MONICA Project (Tunstall-Pedoe *et al.* 1994) and Isomura 1994.)

Considered together with the mortality from CHD and the incidence rate of myocardial infarction in several countries, we could reasonably conclude that it is essential to reduce the incidence rate of acute myocardial infarction in order to reduce CHD mortality.

7.3 Explaining the trends

7.3.1 Serum total cholesterol

Risk factors for CHD in Asian countries are not different from those found in Western countries (Fujishima *et al.* 1992; Kodama *et al.* 1990; Lee *et al.* 2001; Shimamoto *et al.* 1989; Ueshima 1997; Wang *et al.* 2001; Woo *et al.* 1997). Conventional risk factors such as hypertension, hypercholesterolaemia, smoking, and diabetes mellitus have been found to be the major risk factors for CHD in Asian populations by many epidemiological cohort studies.

The specific feature apparent among these risk factors in Asian populations is that the serum TC level was far lower than in Western populations (Fig. 7.3) (Chan *et al.* 1999; Chen *et al.* 1999; Chou *et al.* 1992; Chu *et al.* 2000; Huges *et al.* 1989; Janus *et al.* 1997; Johnson *et al.* 1993; Lee *et al.* 2000; Lyu *et al.* 1993; Ministry of Health and Welfare (Koseisho) 1993; Ministry of Health, Labour and Welfare (Kosei-Roudousho) 2002; Pan and Chiang 1995; Suh *et al.* 2001;

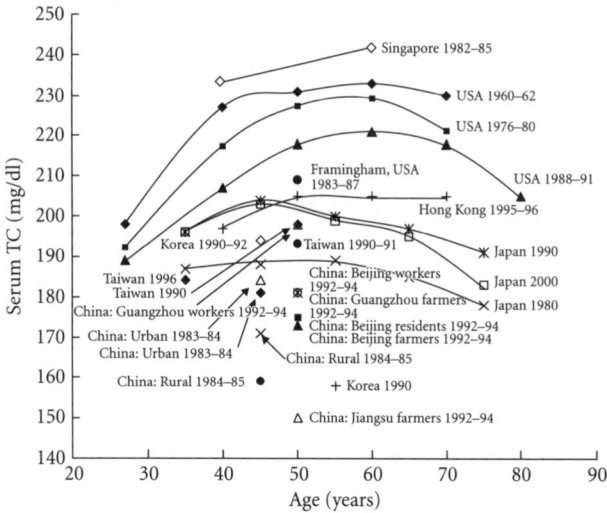

Fig. 7.3 Serum TC levels for men among Asian populations in 1980–2000, and in the USA in 1960–91. The serum TC level in Singapore was the highest among the selected Asian populations, followed by Hong Kong and Japan. That of Japanese people increased from 1980–2000 and currently young people show levels similar to their American counterparts. However, there remains a 20 mg/dl difference in those of the elderly Japanese and Americans. The levels of Taiwanese and Korean populations were between those of the Japanese and Chinese. Chinese and some Korean populations show lower serum TC levels than those of other industrialized Asian populations. The serum TC level in the USA declined significantly from 1960–91.

Wu *et al.* 1996; Wu *et al.* 2001). The serum TC level of Japanese people has increased in recent years and has become greater than 200 mg/dl in middle-aged men. However, the serum TC level of elderly Japanese people is still significantly lower than those of their Western counterparts. Therefore, the difference in the serum TC levels between the elderly people of Japan and the USA remains at approximately 20 mg/dl, although those of American people declined significantly between 1960 and 1991.

In Asian countries, Singapore and Hong Kong show similarly high levels of serum TC to those of Americans (Fig. 7.3). Levels in Singapore reported in the 1982–85 survey, as shown in Fig. 7.3, may be the highest among Asian populations, and are also compatible with the highest mortality rate from CHD among the Asian countries (Fig. 7.1). The serum TC levels in Singapore and in the elderly people of Hong Kong were higher than those of the Japanese. Therefore, it is also explicable that CHD mortality rates in Singapore and Hong Kong were higher than in Japan. In Singapore the prevalence of hypercholesterolaemia during 1992–98 increased despite the introduction of the National Healthy Lifestyle Programme (Cutter *et al.* 2001).

In China, Taiwan, and Korea serum TC levels were lower than in Japan, although these levels increased recently due to lifestyle changes, especially with respect to an increase in fat consumption (Pan and Chiang 1995; Okayama *et al.* 1993; Suh 2001; Tao *et al.* 1989; Ueshima 1990; Ueshima *et al.* 1987). The Sino-MONICA study found that there was a large difference in serum TC levels among populations (Zhou *et al.* 1998). In general, rural and farming populations had lower serum TC levels than urban populations (Fig. 7.3). This phenomenon was also previously observed in Japan, although recently the difference has almost disappeared (Okayama *et al.* 1995).

The serum TC level is well correlated with body mass index (BMI) and Keys' dietary lipid factor (Choudhury *et al.* 1994; Liu *et al.* 1999; Ueshima *et al.* 1982; Yoshida *et al.* 1998). In most Asian countries, including Japan, there is a specific dietary feature such as low fat and high carbohydrate intake (Cutter *et al.* 2001; Okayama *et al.* 1993, 1995; Pan and Chiang 1995; Suh 2001; Tao *et al.* 1989; Ueshima 1990; Ueshima *et al.* 1982; Yoshida *et al.* 1998; Zhou *et al.* 1998). In addition to this, low saturated fatty acid intake maintains a high polyunsaturated/saturated fatty acid (P/S) ratio. These specific dietary features in Asian countries keep serum TC lower than that of Western people. In Japan, high fish consumption, that is, 100 g/day, and rice eating habits keep serum TC lower than that of other industrialized countries. Therefore, energy intake from fat is around 10–30% in China, Taiwan, and Korea, and less than 30% in the young generation of Japan (Pan and Chiang 1995; Suh 2001; Tao *et al.* 1989; Ueshima *et al.* 1982; Yoshida *et al.* 1998).

7.3.2 Explanation for the declining trends in Japan, Singapore, and Hong Kong

In some industrialized Asian countries such as Japan, Singapore, and Hong Kong, CHD mortality and incidence increased until approximately 1980 and then started to decline, as observed in other industrialized countries (Emmanuel 1989; Huges 1986; Ng *et al.* 1999; Uemura and Pisa 1988; Ueshima 1990; Ueshima *et al.* 1987; Yu *et al.* 1995). The decline since 1980 was observed despite the increase in the serum TC level in these populations. These were different phenomena from that of other industrialized countries, that is, a declining trend in serum TC levels in the USA (Fig. 7.3). The serum TC level of Japanese people at approximately 1960 was 160–70 mg/dl (Okayama *et al.* 1995). This has increased steadily since the Second World War and currently approaches the level of its American counterparts, especially in the young generation.

One possible explanation for the declining trends in CHD mortality in Japan is that serum TC in the elderly remains significantly lower than in their counterparts in the USA even in 2000, and they had lower serum cholesterol levels in the past than those presently observed (Fig. 7.3). This arises from still lower fat consumption (around 23% of total energy from fat) compared to that of the young to middle-aged generation. In addition, the increase in the population average of serum TC levels in Japan was mostly due to increases in the rural population (Ueshima *et al.* 1982). The serum cholesterol levels of people living in urban areas have been relatively stable during the past 20 years or so (Ueshima *et al.* 1982). As people in rural areas who had low serum TC increased their levels, the relative increase did not cause any adverse effect on the declining trend in mortality from CHD. In contrast, people living in large metropolitan areas such as Tokyo and Osaka caused a slow down of the declining trend in mortality from CHD (Okayama *et al.* 2001). Therefore, a very important question is raised as to whether the middle-aged people of the post-Second World War generation, who have similar serum TC levels to their US counterparts, have similar coronary artery atherosclerosis rates (Sekikawa *et al.* 2000).

There are two other major possible explanations for the reason why Japanese people could reduce CHD mortality and also maintain a low incidence rate for CHD among industrialized countries. The most important changes in CHD risk factors are the reduction of population blood pressure levels and the prevalence of hypertension after 1965. Figure 7.4 shows the trends in systolic blood pressure (SBP) for men and women by 10-year age group. The National Nutrition Survey in Japan has been carried out every year and includes blood pressure measurement for 8–10 000 representative people. The average SBP level of men aged 60–9 years has been

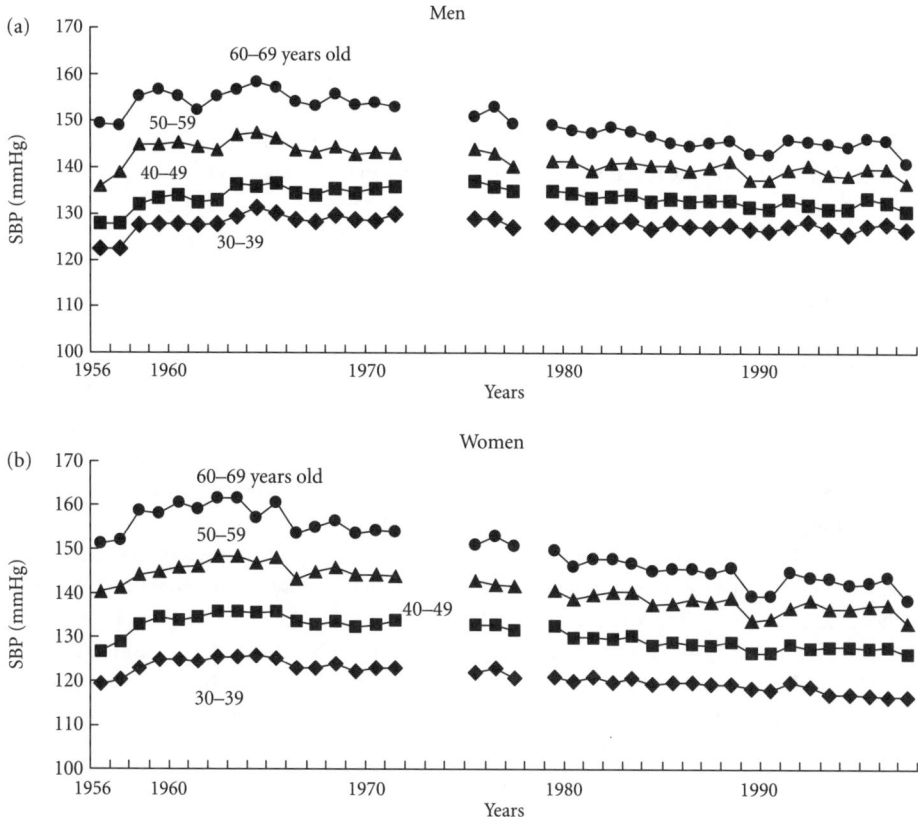

Fig. 7.4 Trends in age-specific SBP levels during 1956–97 in Japan, based on the National Nutrition Survey in Japan. SBP levels for men and women increased until 1965, but since then have started to decline. Men aged 60–7 years old showed an ~15 mmHg decline in SBP during 1965–90. Similar trends were observed in every age group for both genders except men aged 30–9 years and 40–9 years. The National Nutrition Survey has been carried out every year for around 8000–10000 representative Japanese.

reduced by about 15 mmHg during the period 1965–90 (see Fig. 7.4a). The reduction in blood pressure level occurred in every age group and in both genders.

It is estimated, based on US and UK cohort studies, that a 1 mmHg reduction in population SBP could reduce CHD by 2% and strokes by 3% (Stamler *et al.* 1989).

A similar estimate was obtained from Japanese cohort studies: a 2.4% reduction in CHD and a 3.2% reduction in strokes by a decrease of 1 mmHg of SBP in the population (Health Japan). Therefore, it could be expected that a 36% reduction would accompany a 15 mmHg fall in SBP in men aged 60–9 years in Japan. The second major change was the great decrease in smoking rates in Japanese men. The smoking rate was very high in Japanese men, greater than 70% in 1980 and approaching 50% in 2000 (Ministry of Health, Labour and Welfare (Kosei-Roudousho) 2002; Ministry of Health and Welfare (Koseisho) 1993), although it is still higher than other industrialized countries and also that of Singapore and Hong Kong. In Asian countries smoking rates for women were significantly lower than those for Western populations in the years 1990–2000; with only a few percent in Singapore, Hong Kong, Korea, Taiwan, and China, and

15% in Japan. Therefore, the decrease in smoking rates for men could also contribute to the reduction in CHD mortality for men in Japan.

Again, a 1% CHD reduction associated with a 1% decrease in the smoking rate of the population was expected in the US and UK cohort studies and also Japanese cohort studies (Health Japan; Stamler *et al.* 1989). In Japan, the average reduction of SBP in men aged 30–69 years during 1965–90 was approximately 7.4 mmHg and that of the smoking rate was approximately 20%. Combining the effect of the reduction in SBP and smoking rate, a 44% CHD reduction in Japanese men aged 30–69 years old was expected based on these estimates, and a 51% actual reduction was observed during the period 1965–90. Therefore, most of the reduction in CHD mortality in men could be explained by the reduction in blood pressure levels and smoking rates.

In Singapore and Hong Kong, declining trends in CHD mortality were observed without a decrease in the serum TC level (Cutter *et al.* 2001; Janus *et al.* 1997; Ng *et al.* 1999). However, smoking rates were reduced in these populations. There was no conclusive evidence showing the declining trends in blood pressure levels or a prevalence of hypertension during these few decades in Singapore and Hong Kong. Some evidence in Singapore actually shows an increasing trend in the prevalence of hypertension during 1992–98 (Cutter *et al.* 2001). The number of cases who received a primary prevention by coronary artery bypass graft (CABG) or percutaneous transluminal coronary angioplasty (PTCA) increased during 1991–96 in Singapore (Ng *et al.* 1999). Therefore, the primary prevention by PTCA and CABG may in part have contributed to the reduction in CHD morality and morbidity in Singapore (Ng *et al.* 1999). A similar increase in PTCA and CABG cases in Japan was reported during the short observation period of 1997–99 (Tuchihashi *et al.* 2001). Since ischaemic heart disease mortality has declined slowly in Japan since 1980, it is unlikely that primary intervention by PTCA and CABG has contributed greatly to the reduction in CHD incidence and mortality.

The case-fatality rate is expected to have improved in Japan (Watanabe *et al.* 2001), Singapore (Ng *et al.* 1999), and Hong Kong; however, it is very difficult to estimate to what extent the improvement of case-fatality rate contributed to the decline in CHD mortality. Improvements in diagnostic procedures and early treatment for CHD may increase the number of patients with mild CHD in hospitals and clinics. This may lead to an improved case-fatality rate. In this situation, a reduction in CHD mortality may not be explained by the improvement in the case-fatality rate and may rather be due to the decrease in severe cases of acute myocardial infarction by primary prevention through the control of hypertension, hypercholesterolaemia, and smoking.

7.3.3 Explanation for the increasing trends in some periods and countries

Among Asian industrialized countries CHD mortality rates in Singapore, Hong Kong, and Japan increased until approximately 1980, although they have since started to decline (Emmanuel 1989; Huges 1986; Ng *et al.* 1999; Ueshima 1990; Ueshima *et al.* 1987; Yu *et al.* 1995). These findings are partly explained by the increased serum TC levels through higher fat consumption and increased BMI than those of previous years found among these countries (Emmanuel 1989; Huges 1986; Ng *et al.* 1999; Ueshima 1990; Ueshima *et al.* 1987; Yu *et al.* 1995). A similar increasing trend in CHD mortality was observed in Korea between 1984 and 1993, and since then CHD mortality has levelled off (Suh 2001). In Taiwan, CHD mortality also increased from 1971 to 1992 (Department of Health, Republic of China), and has since then started to decline, as observed in Japan, Singapore, and Hong Kong. These increasing trends in CHD mortality in Asian countries are related to lifestyle changes, especially from traditional Asian diets to more Westernized diets, resulting in an increase in the serum TC level (Fig. 7.3) (Emmanuel 1989; Huges 1986; Ng *et al.* 1999; Okayama *et al.* 1993; Pan and Chiang 1995; Ueshima *et al.* 1987; Yu *et al.* 1995).

The Sino-MONICA study on 17 selected populations in China monitored the cardiovascular mortality and incidence rate using standardized methods during 1987–93 (Wu *et al.* 2001). It found a large difference in CHD mortality and morbidity among populations and also increasing and decreasing trends in different populations during the 7-year observation period, although they did not reach significant levels (Wu *et al.* 1996; Wu *et al.* 2001; Zhou *et al.* 1998). As a whole, Chinese CHD mortality and morbidity did not show a clear trend, even when considered together with results from other epidemiological studies in China. The reasons why CHD mortality and morbidity are stable in China is that the prevalence of hypertension shows a stable or rather increasing trend, and the smoking rate did not decrease during these periods. In addition, more long-term observational data to allow comparison of the trends are needed in China (Wu *et al.* 1996; Wu *et al.* 2001; Zhou *et al.* 1998).

7.3.4 Impact of smoking and hypertension control on mortality trends in CHD

Conventional risk factors for CHD in Asian countries are similar to those of Western countries. The major determinant of CHD mortality and morbidity among populations is the population level of serum TC, which is related to the levels of fat intake, Keys score, and BMI in populations (Liu *et al.* 1999; Pan and Chiang 1995; Suh 2001; Ueshima 1990; Ueshima *et al.* 1982, 1987; Yoshida *et al.* 1998). The reasons why CHD mortality and morbidity have started to decline or have levelled off after the early phase of increase in Japan, Singapore, Hong Kong, Taiwan, and Korea that are common to these countries are the declining trends in smoking and the prevalence of hypertension and/or blood pressure levels (Cutter *et al.* 2001; Johnson *et al.* 1993; Pan and Chiang 1995; Ueshima 1990; Ueshima *et al.* 1987). In all of these countries, it has been observed that smoking rates are decreasing steadily for men. A large decline in the prevalence of hypertension is observed for both men and women in Japan; those of men and women aged 60–9 years defined by SBP was 180 mmHg and was greater than 20% in 1965; this has reduced to less than 5% since 1990 (Ueshima 1990).

Therefore, in addition to moderate fat intake, it is very important for Asian developing and developed countries to further reduce their smoking rates, to control hypertension, and to lower the population blood pressure level to help prevent increases in CHD.

References

Chan, W. K., Chiu, A., Ko, G. T. C. *et al.* (1999). Ten-year cardiovascular risk in a Hong Kong population. *Journal of Cardiovascular Risk*, **6**, 163–9.

Chen, K. L., Lee, Y. T., Sung, F. C., Hsu, H. C., Su, T. C., and Lin, R. S. (1999). Hyperinsulinemia and related atherosclerotic risk factors in the population at cardiovascular risk: a community-based study. *Clinical Chemistry*, **45**, 838–46.

Chou, P., Hsiao, K. J., Lin, J. W., and Chen, S. T. (1992). Community-based survey on blood pressure, blood biochemistry and dietary habits in Pu-Li, Taiwan. *Chinese Medical Journal*, **50**, 279–87.

Choudhury, S. R., Ueshima, H., Kita, Y., Kobayashi, K. M., Okayama, A., Yamakawa, M. *et al.* (1994). Alcohol intake and serum lipids in a Japanese population. *International Journal of Epidemiology*, **23**, 940–7.

Chu, N. F., Wang, D. J., Liou, S. H., and Shieh, S. M. (2000). Relationship between hyperuricemia and other cardiovascular disease risk factors among adult men in Taiwan. *European Journal of Epidemiology*, **16**, 13–17.

Cutter, J., Tan, B. Y., and Chew, S. K. (2001). Levels of cardiovascular disease risk factors in Singapore following a national intervention programme. *Bulletin of WHO*, **79**, 908–15.

Department of Health (1981–99). *Health and Vital Statistics: (2) Vital Statistics, Taiwan area, ROC*. Executive Yuan, Taipei, Republic of China.

Emmanuel, S. C. (1989). Trends in coronary heart disease mortality in Singapore. *Singapore Medical Journal*, **30**, 17–23.

Fujishima, M., Kiyohara, Y., Ueda, K., Hasuo, Y., Kato, I., and Iwamoto, H. (1992). Smoking as cardiovascular risk factor in low cholesterol population: the Hisayama study. *Clinical and Experimental Hypertension. Part A, Theory and Practice*, **A14** (1 and 2): 99–108.

Health Japan 21. <http://www.kenkounippon21.gr.jp/kenkounippon21/intro/index_menu1.html> [in Japanese].

Huges, K. (1986). Trends in mortality from ischemic heart disease in Singapore, 1959 to 1983. *International Journal of Epidemiology*, **15**, 44–50.

Huges, K., Yeo, P. P. B., Lun, K. C. *et al.* (1989). Ischemic heart disease and its risk factors in Singapore in comparison with other countries. *Annals of Academy of Medicine*, **18**, 245–9.

Isomura, K. (1994). 3A-1 *Study on the development of the community based long-term follow-up system for cardio-cerebrovascular diseases*. 1993 Annual Report of the Research on Cardiovascular Diseases, Osaka, National Cardiovascular Center.

Janus, E. D., Cockram, C. S., Fielding, R. *et al.* (1997). *Hong Kong Cardiovascular Risk Factor Prevalence Study, 1995–1996*. Department of Clinical Biochemistry, Queen Mary Hospital of Hong Kong.

Johnson, C. L., Rifkind, B. M., Sempos, C. T., Carroll, M. D., Bachorik, P. S., Briefel, R. R. *et al.* (1993). Declining serum total cholesterol levels among US adults: the National Health and Nutrition Examination Surveys. *Journal of the American Medical Association*, **269**, 3002–8.

Kodama, K., Sasaki, H., and Shimizu, Y. (1990). Trend of coronary heart disease and its relationship to risk factors in a Japanese population: a 26-year follow-up, Hiroshima/Nagasaki study. *Japanese Circulation Journal*, **54**, 414–21.

Lee, J., Heng, D., Chia, K. S., Chew, S. K., Tan, B. Y., and Hughes, K. (2001). Risk factors and incident coronary heart disease in Chinese, Malay and Asian Indian males: the Singapore cardiovascular cohort study. *International Journal of Epidemiology*, **30**, 983–8.

Lee, Y. T., Lin, R. S., Sung, F. C., Yang, C., Chien, K., Chen, W. *et al.* (2000). Chin-Shan community cardiovascular cohort in Taiwan-baseline data and five-year follow-up morbidity and mortality. *Journal of Clinical Epidemiology*, **53**, 838–46.

Liu, L., Choudhury, S., Okayama, A., Hayakawa, T., Kita, Y., Ueshima, H. (1999). Changes in body mass index and its relationships to other cardiovascular risk factors among Japanese population: results from the 1980 and 1990 national cardiovascular surveys in Japan. *Journal of Epidemiology*, **9**, 163–74.

Lyu, L. C., Shieh, M. J., Ordovas, J. M., Lichtenstein, A. H., Wilson, P. W., and Schaefer, E. J. (1993). Plasma lipoprotein and apolipoprotein levels in Taipei and Framingham. *Arteriosclerosis and Thrombosis*, **13**, 1429–40.

Ministry of Health and Welfare (Koseisho) (1993). *National Survey of Circulatory Disorders 1990*. Foundation of Cardiovascular Research Promotion and Japanese Society of Cardiovascular Disease Control, Tokyo.

Ministry of Health, Labour and Welfare (Kosei-Roudousho) (2002). *National Cardiovascular Survey 2000*. Cardiovascular Disease Control, Tokyo.

Ng, T. P., Mak, K. H., Phua, K. H., and Tan, C. H. (1999). Trends in mortality, incidence, hospitalization, cardiac procedures and outcomes of care for coronary heart disease in Singapore, 1991–1996. *Annals Academy of Medicine Singapore*, **28**, 395–401.

Okayama, A., Ueshima, H., Marmot, M. G., Nakamura, M., Kita, Y., and Yamakawa, M. (1993). Changes in total serum cholesterol and other risk factors for cardiovascular disease in Japan 1980–1989. *International Journal of Epidemiology*, **22**, 1038–47.

Okayama, A., Ueshima, H., Marmot, M. G., Elliott, P., Yamakawa, M., and Kita, Y. (1995). Different trends in serum cholesterol levels among rural and urban populations aged 40–59 in Japan from 1960 to 1990. *Journal of Clinical Epidemiology*, **48**, 329–37.

Okayama, A., Ueshima, H., Marmot, M. G., Elliott, P., Choudhury S. R., and Kita, Y. (2001). Generational and regional differences in trends of mortality from ischemic heart disease in Japan from 1969 to 1992. *American Journal of Epidemiology*, **153**, 1191–8.

Pan, W. H. and Chiang, B. N. (1995). Plasma lipid profile and epidemiology of atherosclerotic diseases in Taiwan: a unique experience. *Atherosclerosis*, **118**, 285–95.

Sekikawa, A., Ueshima, H., Saitoh, T., and Kuller, L. H. (2000). Rise in mortality from coronary heart disease among post-World War II birth cohorts in Japan? *Epidemiology*, **11**, 738.

Shimamoto, T., Komachi, Y., Inada, H., Doi, M., Iso, H., Sato, S. *et al.* (1989). Trends for coronary heart disease and stroke and their risk factors in Japan. *Circulation*, **79**, 503–15.

Stamler, J., Rose, G., Stamler, R., Elliott, P., Dyer, A. R., and Marmot, M. G. (1989). INTERSALT study findings: public health and medical care implications. *Hypertension*, **14**, 570–7.

Suh, I. (2001). Cardiovascular mortality in Korea: a country experiencing epidemiologic transition. *Acta Cardiologica*, **56**, 75–81.

Suh, I., Jee, S. H., Kim, H. C., Nam, C. M., Kim, J. S., and Appel, L. J. (2001). Low serum cholesterol and haemorrhagic stroke in men: Korea Medical Insurance Cooperation Study. *Lancet*, **357**, 922–5.

Tao, S., Huang, Z., Xiao, Z. K., Hao, J. S., Li, Y. H., Cen, R. C., and Rao, X. X. (1989). CHD and its risk factors in the People's Republic of China. *International Journal of Epidemiology*, **18** (Suppl. 1), s159–s163.

Tuchihashi, M., Tsutui, H., *et al.* (2001). Coronary revascularization in Japan – Part 2: comparison of facilities between 1997 and 1999. *Japanese Circulation Journal*, **65**, 1011–16.

Tunstall-Pedoe, H., Kuulasmass, K., Amouyel, P., Arveiler, D., Rajakangas, A. M., and Pajak, A. (1994). Myocardial infarction and coronary deaths in the World Health Organization MONICA Project: registration procedures, event rates, and case-fatality rates in 38 populations from 21 countries from 4 continents. *Circulation*, **90**, 583–612.

Uemura, K. and Pisa, Z. (1988). Trends in cardiovascular disease mortality in industrialized countries since 1950. *World Health Statistics Quarterly*, **41**, 155–78.

Ueshima, H. (1990). Changes in dietary habits, cardiovascular risk factors and mortality in Japan. *Acta Cardiologica*, **45**, 311–27.

Ueshima, H. (1997). A follow-up study on 1980 National Cardiovascular Disease Survey (NIPPON DATA). *Nihon Junnkanki Kanri Kenkyu Kyougikai Zasshi*, **31**, 231–7. [In Japanese.]

Ueshima, H., Iida, M., Shimamoto, T., Konishi, M., Tanigaki, M., Doi, M. *et al.* (1982). Dietary intake and serum total cholesterol level: their relationship to different lifestyles in several Japanese populations. *Circulation*, **66**, 519–26.

Ueshima, H., Tatara, K., and Asakura, S. (1987). Declining mortality from ischemic heart disease and changes in coronary risk factors in Japan, 1956–1980. *American Journal of Epidemiology*, **125**, 62–72.

Wang, T. D., Chen, W. J., Chien, K. L., She-Yi Su, S. S., Hsu, H. C., Chen, M. F. *et al.* (2001). Efficacy of cholesterol levels and ratios in predicting future coronary heart disease in a Chinese population. *American Journal of Cardiology*, **88**, 737–43.

Watanabe, J., Iwabuchi, K., Koseki, Y., Fukuchi, M., Shinozaki, T., Miura, M. *et al.* (2001). Declining trend in the in-hospital case-fatality rate from acute myocardial infarction in Miyagi Prefecture from 1980 to 1999. *Japanese Circulation Journal*, **65**, 941–6.

Woo, K. S., Chook, P., Young, R. P., and Sanderson, J. E. (1997). New risk factors for coronary heart disease in Asia. *International Journal of Cardiology*, **62** (Suppl. 1), s39–s42.

WHO (World Health Organization). (1982–2002). Causes of Death. World Health Statistics Annual 1982–1996 and WHO Statistics Information System <http://www3.who.int/whosis/menu.cfm> (2002).

Wu, X., Huang, Z., Stamler, J., Wu, Y., Li, Y., Folsom, A. R. *et al.* (1996). Changes in average blood pressure and incidence of high blood pressure 1983–1984 in four population cohorts in the People's Republic of China. *Journal of Hypertension*, **14**, 1267–74.

Wu, Z., Yao, C., Zhao, D., Wu, G., Wang, W., Liu, J. *et al.* (2001). Sino-MONICA project: a collaborative study on trends and determinants in cardiovascular diseases in China. Part I: Morbidity and mortality monitoring. *Circulation*, **103**, 462–8.

Yoshida, Y., Okayama, A., Mikawa, K. *et al.* (1998). Dietary intake and its relationship to serum total cholesterol concentrations among Japanese populations in the early 1990s: INTERSALT II study in Japan. *Journal of Shiga University of Medical Science*, **13**, 63–79.

Yu, T. S., Wong, S. L., Lloyd, O. L., and Wong, T. W. (1995). Ischemic heart disease: trends in mortality in Hong Kong, 1970–89. *Journal of Epidemiology and Community Health*, **49**, 16–21.

Zhou, B., Zhang, H., Wu, Y. *et al.* (1998). Ecological analysis of the association between incidence and risk factors of coronary heart disease and stroke in Chinese populations. *CVD Prevention*, **1**, 207–16.

Chapter 8

Developing countries

K. S. Reddy

8.1 **Overview**

The rising burdens of cardiovascular diseases (CVD) as a group, and coronary heart disease (CHD) in particular, have been highlighted in several publications in the last decade (Murray and Lopez 1996; Reddy and Yusuf 1998; WHO 2001; Yusuf *et al.* 2001). These have profiled the estimates of CVD and CHD-related mortality and disability in 1990 as well as the projections for 2020. The key messages emerging from these estimates and projections are:

1 The developing countries, even in 1990, had a high burden of CVD and CHD in terms of the absolute number of deaths and disability adjusted life years (DALYs) lost.

2 The proportional mortality rates of CHD-related deaths as a fraction of total deaths will rise sharply by 2020.

3 CVD will become the leading cause of death in most developing countries by 2020, with CHD as the main contributor in many of them.

4 A much larger proportion of CHD-related deaths occur below 70 years of age in the developing countries than in the industrially developed countries.

These estimates and projections are limited by inadequate data and uncertainty about data quality. Cause-specific mortality data are not routinely gathered in a standardized and systematic manner by many developing countries. The estimates of CHD-related deaths are, therefore, based on approximations derived from multiple data sources in a country. The projections for 2020 are based on demographic and econometric models, which also accommodate time trends, where available. While the dimensions of CHD-related disease burdens might be imprecise because of these factors, the upward direction of the epidemic is very clearly discernible in the developing countries (Table 8.1).

According to the Global Burden of Disease Study (Murray and Lopez 1996), the developing countries contributed 3.5 million of the 6.2 million global deaths attributable to CHD in 1990. The projections envisage that these countries will account for 7.8 million of the 11.1 million deaths related to CHD in 2020. Nearly half of these deaths will occur below the age of 70 years, in contrast to less than a quarter of CHD deaths in the rich industrial countries. Because of the early onset of the disease and early age of death, the developing countries contributed to 66% of the global DALY loss related to CHD in 1990 and will contribute to 78% of that global estimate in 2020 (Chapters 10 and 11 discuss data from the WHO Global Burden of Disease Study).

While these large absolute burdens reflect the large population sizes of developing countries, proportional mortality rates of deaths attributable to CVD have also risen in these countries, from 24.5% in 1990 to 28.5% in 1998 (WHO 2001). The relative importance of CHD and

Table 8.1 Deaths due to CVD and CHD in 2000 and 2020 (as % of total deaths)

Year	World	India	China	OAI	LAC	MEC	SSA
Deaths due to CVD							
2000	32.2	31.7	32.1	30.0	30.6	34.4	11.2
2020	36.3	41.8	32.5	36.0	36.7	44.7	16.9
Deaths due to CHD							
2000	14.3	16.8	9.6	11.0	13.7	16.9	3.0
2020	16.3	22.6	9.8	14.0	16.7	23.2	4.6

Source: Murray and Lopez 1996.

OAI: other Asia and Islands; LAM: Latin America and the Caribbean; MEC: Middle Eastern Crescent; SSA: sub-Saharan Africa.

stroke varies across regions and from country to country. For example, more than twice as many deaths from stroke occurred in the developing countries as in the developed countries. CHD is the dominant form of CVD in the developed countries, Latin America, and India, while stroke is the leading cause of cardiovascular death in sub-Saharan Africa, China, and other parts of Asia. Developing countries such as Argentina, Colombia, and China now have CVD mortality rates higher than most other countries. The CVD mortality rate in Argentina currently exceeds that in many European and North American countries.

The rising rates of death due to CVD and CHD have been documented in several developing countries (AHA 1999). The increase in standardized mortality rate (SMR) for acute myocardial infarction in Mexico was 53% over the period 1980–98 (Rivera *et al.* 2002). Death rates in China due to CHD rose from 18.64/100 000 in 1980 to 30.58.100 000 in 1999 (Ministry of Health, China 2000). In countries where cause-specific mortality data are not available, community-based prevalence studies of CHD as well as hospital-based CHD admission and mortality data have provided surrogate measures of rising CHD burdens (Gupta and Gupta 1996; Noor 2002). It has been estimated that the urban prevalence of CHD in Indian adults rose from 1% in 1960 to 9.6% in 1995, while the prevalence of CHD in rural Indian adults rose from 2 to 3.7% during 1974–95 (Gupta and Gupta 1996). There is a clear need to establish sound and sustainable mortality surveillance systems in the developing countries in order to track the advancing epidemics of CHD.

8.2 The model of epidemiological transition

This model has been widely used to explain as well as predict CHD trends in the developing countries (Olshansky and Ault 1986; Omran 1971). It was originally described by Omran with three phases (the age of pestilence and famine; the age of receding pandemics; the age of degenerative and man-made diseases) and was later modified to include a fourth phase (the age of delayed degenerative diseases). Life expectancy progressively increases from around 30 years in the first phase to over 70 years in the fourth phase. The shift to a dominant chronic disease profile occurs in the third phase. As average life expectancy exceeds 50–55 years, the proportionate mortality due to CVD begins to exceed that of infectious diseases. CHD is the leading cause of death in the third and fourth phases, with a shift to older ages in the fourth phase. Many countries of Central and South America, the Middle East, and urban India are currently in the third phase of the epidemic.

The transition to the atherothrombotic phase of the epidemic may be preceded by a sharp fall in the burden of haemorrhagic strokes, which characterize the second phase. The recent decline in CVD mortality reported from South Korea reflects such a fall in the contribution from haemorrhagic strokes, while thrombotic stroke and CHD burdens have just begun to rise (Suh 2001). It remains to be studied whether adherence to traditional diets will result in a continued decline of CVD in South Korea or CHD rates will further rise to push up CVD mortality rates. The model of 'health transition', while very useful, is not immutable and is likely to vary according to both levels of development and the nature of public health responses to social transition. The challenge of preventive cardiology is to telescope the transition, to prevent or abbreviate the third phase of high mid-life burdens, and reduce the impact of atherothrombotic vascular disease in countries which ascend the ladder of economic development.

The well-documented trends in coronary risk factors in developing country populations constitute a strong reason to believe that CHD-related mortality and morbidity would indeed rise sharply in the developing countries. Increase in body weight (adjusted for height), blood pressure and cholesterol levels in Chinese population samples aged 35–64 years, between the two phases of the Sino-MONICA study (1984–86, 1988–89) and the substantially higher levels of most CVD risk factors in urban population groups compared to rural population groups in India, provide evidence of such trends (Reddy 1993; Yao et al. 1993). While only 3.5% of Chinese adults aged 20–45 years had a body mass index above 25 in 1982, over 40% of urban residents in Beijing were overweight and obese in 1992 (Du et al. 2002).

8.3 Increased fat consumption

The global availability of cheap vegetable oils and fats has resulted in greatly increased fat consumption among low-income countries in recent years (Drewnowski and Popkin 1997). The transition now occurs at lower levels of gross national product than previously and is further accelerated by rapid urbanization. In China, for example, the proportion of upper income persons who were consuming a relatively high fat diet (>30% of daily energy intake) rose from 22.8 to 66.6% between 1989 and 1993 (Drewnowski and Popkin 1997). The lower and middle-income groups also showed a rise (from 19 to 36.4% in the former and from 19.1 to 51.0% in the latter). The Asian countries, traditionally high in carbohydrates and low in fat, have shown an overall decline in the proportion of energy from complex carbohydrates along with an increase in the proportion of fat (Drewnowski and Popkin 1997). The globalization of food production and marketing is also contributing to the increasing consumption of energy dense foods that are poor in dietary fibre and several micronutrients.

8.4 Other primary contributors to CHD

The rising tobacco consumption patterns in most developing countries contrast sharply with the overall decline in the industrial nations (Peto 1996). Projections from the WHO suggest that by the year 2020 tobacco will become the largest single cause of death, accounting for 12.3% of global deaths (Peto 1996; WHO 1996). India, China, and countries in the Middle Eastern crescent will by then have tobacco contributing to more than 12% of all deaths. A large proportion of these deaths will be related to CHD.

The developing countries are currently contributing to three-quarters of the global burden attributable to diabetes. The anticipated rise in the number of diabetics in the world, from 135 million in 1995 to 300 million in 2025, would principally be related to a sharp rise in diabetes prevalence in the developing countries, exemplified by a 195% rise in India (King *et al.* 1998). This, in turn, would impact adversely on the CHD-attributable burden of disease in the developing countries.

The importance of blood pressure as a major contributor to global mortality and disability has been highlighted in the *World Health Report* of 2002 (WHO 2002). Sub-optimal blood pressure has been identified as a major risk factor in low-mortality developing countries as well as high-mortality developing countries. The report also projects that blood pressure, tobacco, and cholesterol, as well as other risk factors such as overweight and a low intake of fruits and vegetables, will progressively add higher burdens to the developing countries by 2020.

Tobacco consumption, even in the developing countries, is much more common among the poor and less literate sections of the population. As epidemiological transition advances, other risk factors also demonstrate a reversal of the social gradient. This would place the highest burdens of CHD on the poor among nations and the poor within nations, as the global epidemic matures. Studies in India and Brazil are suggestive of a progressive reversal of the social gradient for CHD and its risk factors (Monteiro *et al.* 2002; Pais *et al.* 1996). These trends and projections portend a huge burden of CHD in the developing countries with unaffordable demands on healthcare systems and unacceptable consequences for development. The need for CHD prevention in these countries is clear and urgent.

References

AHA (American Heart Association) (1999). *2000 heart and stroke statistical update.* American Heart Association, Dallas.

Drewnowski, A. and Popkin, B. M. (1997). The nutrition transition: new trends in the global diet. *Nutrition Reviews*, **55**, 31–43.

Du, S., Lu, B., Zhai, F., and Popkin, B. M. (2002). A new stage of the nutrition transition in China. *Public Health Nutrition*, **5** (IA), 169–74.

Gupta, R. and Gupta, V. P. (1996). Meta-analysis of coronary heart disease prevalence in India. *Indian Heart Journal*, **48**, 241–5.

King, H., Aubert, R. E., and Herman, W. H. (1998). Global burden of diabetes, 1995–2025: prevalence, numeric estimates and projections. *Diabetes Care*, **21**, 1414–31.

Ministry of Health (2000). *Annual statistical reports of death, injuries and causes of death in China, 1979–2000.* Ministry of Health, Beijing.

Monteiro, C. A., Conde, W. L., and Popkin, B. M. (2002). Is obesity replacing or adding to undernutrition? Evidence from different social classes in Brazil. *Public Health Nutrition*, **5** (IA), 105–12.

Murray, C. J. L. and Lopez, A. D. (1996). *The global burden of disease: a comprehensive assessment of mortality and disability from disease, injuries and risk factors in 1990 and projected to 2020.* Harvard University Press, Boston.

Noor, M. I. (2002). The nutrition and health transition in Malaysia. *Public Health Nutrition*, **5** (1A), 191–5.

Olshansky, S. J. and Ault, A. B. (1986). The fourth stage of the epidemiologic transition: the age of delayed degenerative diseases. *Milbank Memorial Fund Quarterly*, **4**, 355–91.

Omran, A. R. (1971). The epidemiologic transition: a key of the epidemiology of population change. *Milbank Memorial Fund Quarterly*, **49**, 509–38.

Pais, P., Pogue, J., Gerstein, H., *et al.* (1996). Risk factors for acute myocardial infarction in Indians: a case control study. *Lancet*, **348**, 358–63.

Peto, R. (1996). Tobacco: the growing epidemic in China. *Journal of the American Medical Association*, **275**, 1683–4.

Reddy, K. S. (1993). Cardiovascular disease in India. *World Health Statistics Quarterly*, **46**, 101–7.

Reddy, K. S. and Yusuf, S. (1998). The emerging epidemic of cardiovascular disease in developing countries. *Circulation*, **97**, 596–601.

Rivera, J. A., Barquera, S., Campirano, F., Campos, I., Safdie, M., and Tovar, V. (2002). Epidemiological and nutritional transition in Mexico: rapid increase of non-communicable chronic disease and obesity. *Public Health Nutrition*, **5** (IA), 113–22.

Suh, I. (2001). Cardiovascular mortality in Korea: a country experiencing epidemiologic transition. *Acta Cardiologica*, **56**, 75–81.

WHO (World Health Organization) (2001). *The world health report 2001*. WHO, Geneva.

WHO (World Health Organization) (1996). *Tobacco or health: first global status report*. WHO, Geneva.

WHO (World Health Organization) (2002). *World health report 2002*. WHO, Geneva.

Yao, C., Wu, Z, and Wu, J. (1993). The changing pattern of cardiovascular diseases in China. *World Health Statistics Quarterly*, **46**, 113–18.

Yusuf, S., Reddy, S., Ounppuu, S., and Anand, S. (2001). Global burden of cardiovascular diseases. Part I: General considerations, the epidemiological transition, risk factors, and impact of urbanisation. *Circulation*, **104**, 2746. Part II: Variations in cardiovascular disease by specific ethnic groups and geographic regions and prevention strategies. *Circulation*, **104**, 2855.

Chapter 9

Coronary heart disease burden among persons of African origin

R. S. Cooper

I very early got the idea that what I was going to do was prove to the world the Negroes were just like other people.

W. E. B. DuBois

9.1 Introduction

The epidemiology of cardiovascular disease (CVD) among black populations has been the subject of numerous controversies. The force of this assertion is apparent in the difficulty that arises in even identifying the populations that should be included in a comparative analysis. The definition of 'black' varies in different societies and becomes even more inadequate as an inclusive category for the heterogeneous population groups in Africa. For historical reasons the designation in this discussion will apply to sub-Saharan countries, primarily on the west coast, and their descendants in the Americas and Europe. The largest black population outside Africa resides in Brazil, followed by the US and the black majority island nations in the Caribbean. Secondary recent migrations from the Caribbean and Africa have created growing black populations in Europe, particularly in the UK. Enormous diversity exists among contemporary African populations, and blacks in the Caribbean and Brazil have distinctive health status compared to those in the US. In general, however, there is a graded increase in the burden of CVD as one moves from West Africa, to the Caribbean, to the US (Fig. 9.1). Since the knowledge base about CVD is very unevenly distributed, this chapter will focus primarily on what has been learned in the US, while noting the contrasts with West Africa and the Caribbean.

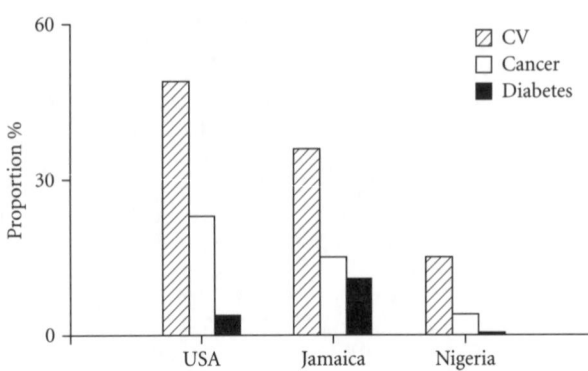

Fig. 9.1 Proportion of deaths from CVD, cancer, and diabetes in US blacks, Jamaicans, and Nigerians.

Africa entered the modern world through a very distinctive route. Having given birth to our species and provided the foundational ideas of 'Western culture' by way of Egypt to Greece (Bernal 1987), the development of technologically based societies languished in Africa. Reunited with the mainstream of Western history through the slave trade and colonialism, blacks remain subject to domination by a persistently hostile culture wherever they live (Gilroy 2000). Consequently, Africans on the continent have not shared the benefits of the capitalist economy and the modern nation state, while their descendants abroad have been excluded from full citizenship in those countries that they did so much to create. This historical framework determines not only the current health status of black populations, but also the way in which this health status is studied and explicated.

Without taking account of the history of the European encounter with Africa and its accompanying intellectual and ideological justification, an analysis of health status of African-Americans risks repeating the mistake of substituting justification for explanation. The concept of race has been the primary framework used to examine health disparities in the US and other industrialized societies, introducing serious distortions, and the political vulnerability of blacks has hampered efforts to definitively counter racialist notions. Molecular genetics has now begun to reframe some of these questions regarding genetic variation in our species (Cooper et al. 2003; Rosenberg et al. 2002). Whether the beliefs held by the public or scientists will be overturned by this knowledge is, of course, a more complicated social question. What is new and exciting, however, is the opportunity to bring an entirely new source of information to bear on these vexing problems.

9.2 **Africa**

The burden of CVD in Africa is largely unmeasured (Cooper et al. 1998). Data imputation projects, most notably the Global Burden of Disease Study, have published estimates for Africa (Murray and Lopez 1996), giving the impression that information exists. In some regards this impression is unfortunate, implying as it does that these countries have vital registration systems, which is universally untrue, or that public health policy can be effectively developed without surveillance systems, which is equally open to question (Cooper et al. 1998). The only widespread risk factor for stroke or CHD in sub-Saharan Africa (SSA) is hypertension (Cooper et al. 1996; Kaufman et al. 1996). The majority of Africans below the Sahara still live in rural areas and rely on subsistence agriculture. Life is physically demanding and there is only a modest intrusion of mass-produced consumer goods, including cigarettes and manufactured food based on animal products. Although current data are limited, the diet in SSA most likely provides more than 65% of calories from carbohydrate, compared to less than 50% in the US, with 18–20% and 35–40% of calories from fat, respectively. The pattern of lipids and lipoproteins in populations of the African diaspora has not been well characterized in a standardized protocol as yet. However, information from a set of small samples from West Africa, the Caribbean, and the US reflect the pattern one would anticipate with the accompanying dietary change (Luke et al. 2001) (Table 9.1). It should be noted, however, that large, more representative samples from the US black population generally demonstrate somewhat higher levels of total cholesterol.

Given the favourable lipid status in SSA, CHD is exceedingly rare, except among the elite. On the other hand, with a hypertension prevalence of ~15% and the absence of effective treatment, stroke is a serious threat to the health of older adults in Africa. A large prospective study in Tanzania demonstrated rates of stroke that were apparently higher than those observed in

Table 9.1 Plasma lipids and lipoproteins in Nigerians, Jamaicans, and US blacks

	Nigeria		Jamaica		US blacks	
	Men (n = 52)	Women (n = 43)	Men (n = 456)	Women (n = 683)	Men (n = 159)	Women (n = 337)
Age	42 (9)	46 (9)	47 (15)	45 (13)	47 (13)	48 (14)
BMI	21 (2)	24 (4)	24 (4)	28 (7)	30 (6)	32 (7)
TC	142 (37)	168 (37)	177 (40)	188 (43)	193 (35)	196 (41)
HDL-C	33 (14)	41 (11)	45 (11)	45 (11)	45 (14)	54 (14)
LDL-C	94 (27)	112 (33)	128 (39)	134 (40)	116 (34)	119 (37)
Triglycerides	82 (34)	72 (38)	71 (33)	70 (31)	159 (100)	117 (81)
Lipoprotein(a)	13 (7)	13 (7)	N/A	N/A	16 (10)	21 (12)

BMI: body mass index; TC: total cholesterol.

n = 139; US, n = 99.

the UK (Walker *et al.* 2000). In a rural cohort of 5000 persons in Nigeria over the age of 25 CVD accounted for 25% of deaths; infection was thought to be the direct cause of 36% of these deaths (Kaufman *et al.* 1996).

Despite the low risk of atherosclerosis in these populations, concern remains for the future. Increases in average levels of LDL-C are unlikely to occur in the near term, although the intrusion of the multinational food industry has wreaked havoc in other regions after only modest progress on the road to economic development. Poor countries have also been subjected to the scourges of tobacco and obesity in the immediate stages of release from abject poverty. Unfortunately these countries have limited resources with which to resist these epidemics and treatment of established disease is virtually non-existent. A sober prediction, therefore, based on the forces that are currently at play, includes a major epidemic of CVD in West Africa over the coming decades.

Geographic comparison of cardiovascular (CV) risk factors across the diaspora clearly implicates the changing social environment as the determinant of CV disease patterns in black populations. In 1990 the International Collaborative Study on Hypertension in Blacks (ICSHIB) was initiated to provide standardized survey data on population samples from West Africa, the Caribbean, and the US (Cooper *et al.* 1997). A highly consistent pattern has emerged demonstrating a gradient in risk status that is strongly correlated with the relevant CV exposures. After rank ordering the sampled communities by the average gross national product a monotonic increase in the prevalence of hypertension is observed (Fig. 9.2). This pattern closely follows the increase in risk factors (Fig. 9.3).

9.3 The Caribbean

The black nations of the Caribbean occupy a precarious dependent niche at the periphery of the US economy and their CV risk profile is determined by the resulting mix of desperate poverty, as in Haiti, and rapid adoption of the US commercial culture, as in Barbados. In the mid-1990s the age-adjusted CV mortality rate in Barbados was reported as 259/100 000, compared to 228 in the US and 180 in Canada (PAHO 1998); comparable data were not available for Jamaica or Haiti.

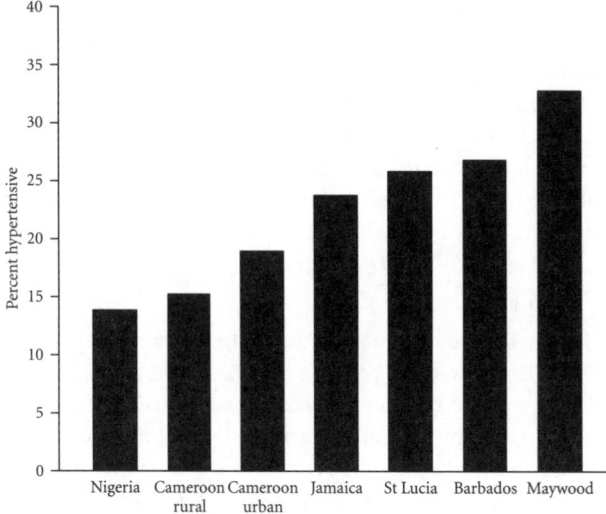

Fig. 9.2 Prevalence of hypertension (defined as blood pressure ≥140/90, or taking antihypertension medication) among seven populations of West African origin. (From the ICSHIB Study 1995.)

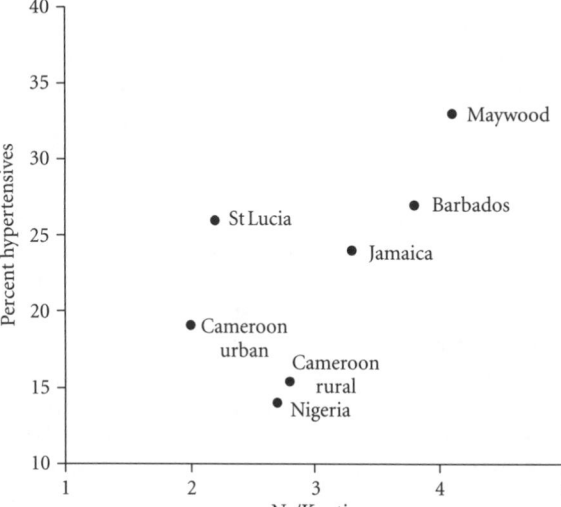

Fig. 9.3 Prevalence of hypertension (defined as blood pressure ≥140/90, or taking antihypertension medication) by mean Na/K ratio in seven populations of West African origin. (From the ICSHIB Study 1995.)

Jamaica, the largest of the primarily black nations of the Caribbean, occupies a middle position in the epidemiological transition to CV disease (Forrester *et al.* 1998). Much of the population, both in the rural and urban areas, has not obtained sufficient affluence to acquire coronary disease, and stroke is still the most common CV cause of death. A novel aspect of the emerging CVD epidemic in Jamaica is the unusual gender pattern. In the most recent vital statistics, CHD accounted for 7.4% of deaths among Jamaican women, compared to 5.7% among men, while stroke accounted for 16.4% in women and 12.2% in men (Statistical Institute of Jamaica 2001). An ongoing longitudinal epidemiological study in Spanish Town, Jamaica, will provide specific data on this pattern (Sargeant *et al.* 2002). Competing causes among men reduce the opportunity to die from CVD; however, the risk factor status is consistent with this relative female disadvantage. Diabetes and hypertension are much more frequent in women, and, most striking of all, high-density lipoprotein cholesterol (HDL-C) levels are identical in the two sexes (Table 9.1). Gender equality of HDL-C has not been observed in any other population sample, to my knowledge. As among other island nations, the epidemic of diabetes is resulting in high rates of peripheral vascular disease, amputation, blindness, and renal failure. The relative prominence of diabetes in Jamaica, and the unusual gender balance, has for the moment muted the male predominance of CHD. Hypertension rates in this black population are the same as those among whites in the US (Cooper *et al.* 1997).

9.4 United States

Awareness of the burden of CHD for the US black population has evolved over a complicated, circuitous route (Francis *et al.* 1994). Clinical wisdom through the 1970s held that CHD was rare in blacks and that as a group they enjoyed resistance to the disease. A series of seminal papers and conferences in the 1980s by Gillum brought the light of more objective scrutiny to bear on this question (Johnson and Payne 1984). A host of studies have now filled the void in clinical epidemiology. Despite the small samples enrolled in population surveys and cohort studies, a reasonably complete picture has also emerged in the community setting.

Two primary themes are intertwined in the story of CHD in blacks. The first theme is built on the history of the black experience in the US – from slavery, to the era of 'Jim Crow' legal discrimination, to the 'great migration' from the rural South and the creation of isolated communities in the urban centres. The second theme involves race as a construct to categorize geographical populations, and its influence on the theory and practice of epidemiology. These historical determinants provide the framework for understanding the evolving description of CHD among US blacks.

In the first 200 years of their experience in North America the vast majority of blacks lived in conditions of grinding rural poverty. High rates of hypertension were apparent with the first field surveys in the 1930s, yet CHD was less common. The urban migration to industrial jobs transformed the social status of these communities, and in the last half century brought them fully into the consumer culture of food, cigarettes, and other lifestyle factors that provide the basis for widespread atherosclerosis. As the health-destroying properties of these lifestyle factors have been more fully recognized, the affluent have sought protection from their effects while exploitative marketing has been less successfully curbed among blacks and the working class in general. Rates of all forms of CVD are now more common in blacks. Attempts to provide a biological accounting of this story have been hampered by incorporation of a serious epistemological flaw into the analysis strategy. This flaw consists of the belief in a concept of race that lacks biological validity (Cooper 1984; Cooper *et al.* 2003). Like alchemy in eighteenth-century chemistry or 'vitalism' in nineteenth-century medicine, the operative notion of race in biomedicine has frequently led to inconsistent and biased interpretation of the experimental findings (Cooper *et al.* 2003; Cooper and Kaufman 1998).

9.4.1 Trends in mortality

In the late 1960s mortality rates in the US began to decline at 2–3% per year for all race/ethnic groups. In the last two decades, however, the decline has slowed for all groups except white men (Cooper *et al.* 2000) (Fig. 9.4). CHD rates for black women are now substantially higher than for white women, while black men have slightly higher mortality than their white counterparts. In comparison to other race/ethnic groups, blacks have much higher rates of both

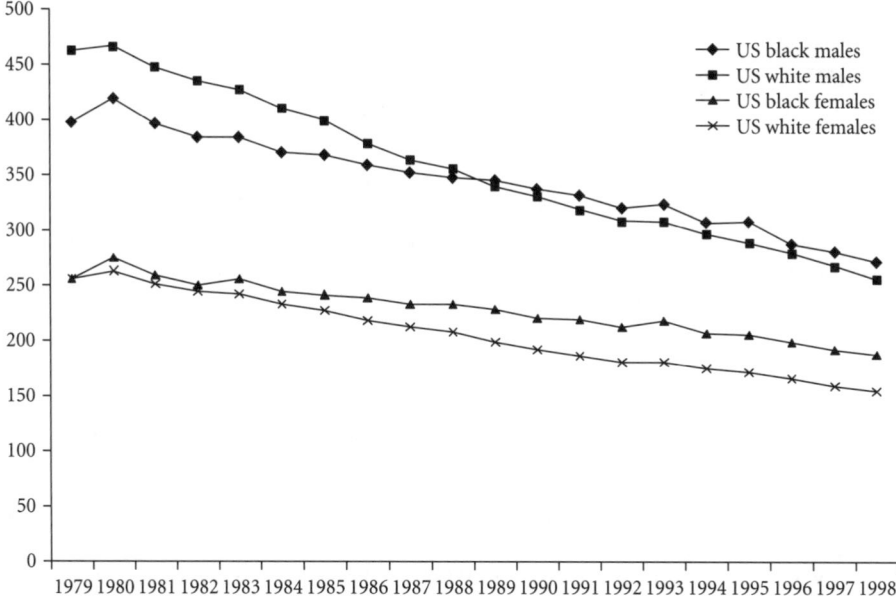

Fig. 9.4 CHD mortality by race and gender, US, 1979–98 (per 100 000). (Data from CDC Wonder 2003.)

Table 9.2 Age-adjusted death rates from heart disease and stroke in racial/ethnic groups in the US, 1998 (per 100 000)

Cause of death	White	Black	Hispanic	Asian
Heart disease	121.9	183.3	84.2	67.4
CHD	79.2	92.5	54.7	42.9
Stroke	23.3	41.4	19.0	22.7

Source: CDC.

CHD and stroke (Table 9.2). Age-adjusted comparisons are not fully revealing about the racial contrasts, however; the greatest disparity is at younger ages (Roig *et al.* 1987).

However, mortality rates are not a particularly sensitive surveillance tool for CHD, and numerous biases exist in comparisons among population groups. In the US census undercount reaches 10% in young black men and age estimation of the very elderly has been unreliable. Even more problematic, the assignment of cause of death can be biased. For example, heart disease death among whites is overwhelmingly assigned to CHD, while hypertensive heart disease and other less well-defined causes account for a much larger proportion among blacks. Heart disease mortality, which is a more robust category for black:white comparisons, is therefore substantially higher in blacks than whites (Fig. 9.5). Competing mortality from other CV conditions, such as stroke, heart failure, and renal disease, may also decrease the pool of susceptible elderly, thereby reducing the age-adjusted rate. Fully characterizing the force of CV mortality in these two contrasting populations in fact has never been adequately solved as an epidemiological problem.

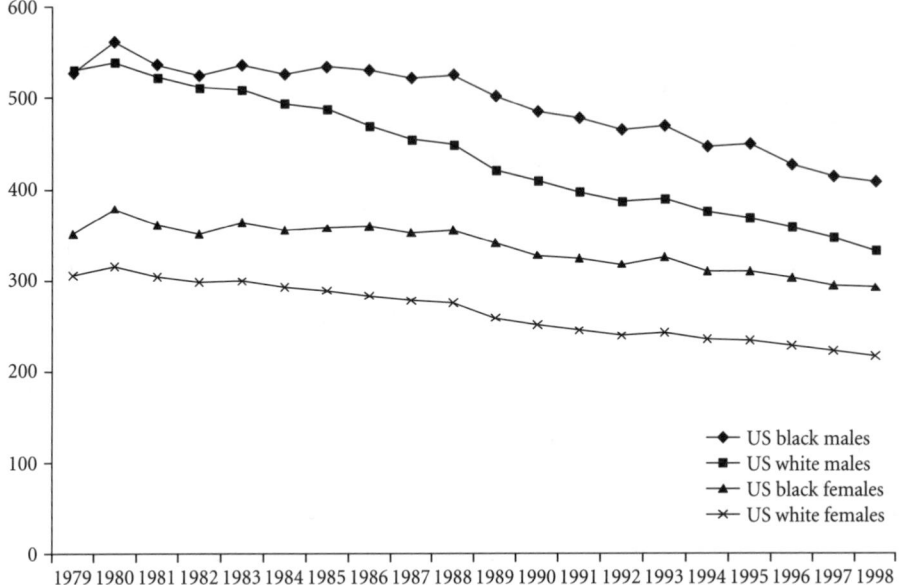

Fig. 9.5 Heart disease mortality by race and gender, US, 1979–98 (per 100 000). (Data from CDC Wonder 2003.)

Regional trends in heart disease are prominent in the US, with rising rates in blacks in Mississippi and other mid-South states (Jones *et al.* 2000; Rosamond *et al.* 2001). High CV mortality is also found in core neighbourhoods in large cities, and life expectancy for black men was less than 60 years in 1992 in cities like Atlanta, Baltimore, St. Louis, and Los Angeles (Good 1998). The current stage of the CHD epidemic in blacks is thus consistent with the consequences of full integration into the US consumer culture over the last generation and continued economic disadvantage.

9.4.2 Risk factors

In the rural South blacks were less likely to smoke than whites and had lower serum cholesterols. At the present time blacks suffer a modestly worse coronary risk profile (Table 9.3). Men smoke more, but black women less, compared to whites, while total cholesterol levels are similar. High-density lipoprotein (HDL) levels are substantially higher, particularly among black men, with the correspondingly opposite pattern for triglycerides (Table 9.3). As noted above, HDL levels are much lower in Nigeria, and in men and women in Jamaica they are identical.

The complex gender–race pattern seen in the US is therefore intriguing and suggests that the influences on HDL are more responsive to environmental conditions than is generally thought. Lp(a) is substantially higher in US blacks than whites, although its role in atherogenesis is still not well defined; in Nigeria Lp(a) levels are substantially lower, particularly in women (Table 9.1). The two-fold higher prevalence of hypertension has been the primary cause of higher CV mortality in the past, although the rapid increase in diabetes will make a substantial impact in the coming decades. Individually the coronary risk factors predict clinical events among blacks to the same degree as among whites; however, the summary risk from the

Table 9.3 Cardiovascular risk factors in US whites and blacks, NHANES III

	Men		Women	
	White (mean)	Black (mean)	White (mean)	Black (mean)
Risk factor				
Age	47.67	44.29	49.85	45.71
BMI	26.92	26.54	26.26	28.97
SBP	123.24	127.12	119.50	123.83
DBP	76.30	78.61	70.51	73.28
Cholesterol	206.06	201.06	210.69	204.54
HDL-C	44.77	52.41	55.66	57.42
LDL-C	133.60	128.64	127.69	124.97
Triglycerides	162.46	126.91	137.66	109.22
Smoking	30%	42%	25%	30%
Disease prevalence				
Hypertension	26%	33%	25%	34%
Diabetes	8%	9%	7%	11%
Heart disease	6%	5%	4%	5%

DBP: diastolic blood pressure; SBP: systolic blood pressure.

Framingham model overpredicts the absolute rate in black men (Cooper and Ford 1992; Liao *et al.* 1999).

9.4.3 Clinical aspects

It has been recognized for a number of years that survival among black patients with CHD is shorter than among whites (Castaner *et al.* 1988). The extent of coronary artery disease at the time of the first myocardial infarction is similar in the two groups (Cooper *et al.* 1989), although left ventricular hypertrophy (LVH), as a consequence of hypertension, is much more common in blacks (Ghali *et al.* 1992). The co-occurrence of other forms of heart disease, such as left ventricular dysfunction and hypertrophy, increase the case-fatality rate among blacks with CHD (Liao *et al.* 1995). In a clinical series of patients with heart disease the attributable risk for mortality associated with LVH was considerably more than that for obstructive coronary disease (Liao *et al.* 1995); this feature of the epidemiology of heart disease among blacks likely explains much of black:white differentials presented in Fig. 9.3.

Medical care, both secondary prevention and invasive therapy, is playing an increasingly important role in reductions of mortality. An important emerging issue in the clinical epidemiology of CHD in the US is the limited access to these forms of care that is experienced by blacks. In the early 1980s investigators found that blacks were half as likely to receive bypass after angiography, with adjustment for patient characteristics and disease severity (Johnson and Payne 1984). This general finding was quickly confirmed by the database from a clinical trial (Maynard *et al.* 1986). Based on that evidence alone the assumption could not be made that these samples were sufficiently representative, or that bias did not exist in the reporting or analysis. Gillum *et al.* used the National Hospital Discharge Survey, a representative sample of US hospitals, to examine the use of services, relative to the frequency of acute myocardial infarction, in blacks and whites. Large differentials were found for both catheter-based procedures and bypass surgery (Ford *et al.* 1989; Gillum 1987). Although detailed case information was not available, mortality rates for blacks were comparable to whites in the peri-infarct period, suggesting that disease severity was similar. The differential use of surgical treatment has since been shown not to be a result of payment source. In a study of physician practice patterns it was demonstrated that blacks were less likely to be recommended for referral to surgery than were whites with identical clinical histories (Schulman *et al.* 1996).

Based on an extensive set of recent studies, remarkable consistency has emerged in terms of the racial differentials in the use of cardiac services. All catheter-based and surgical procedures – up to and including transplant – are used less often in the treatment of black patients, with an average black: white ratio of 0.67 for angiography, 0.62 for angioplasty, and 0.54 for bypass (Ford and Cooper 1995). These effects are usually cumulative; that is, beginning with 100 black patients for whom a procedure is indicated at the rate received by whites, one first takes into account the decrement for angiography (i.e. 0.67), then that figure is further reduced by 0.62 for angioplasty, or 0.54 for bypass surgery. Thus, the final bias against receiving a therapeutic procedure may be in the range of 0.4.

The report by Hannan *et al.* from New York is one of the most sophisticated studies to be published to date and provides a useful summary. A weighted random sample of 56 hospitals that provide angiography services was selected (Hannan *et al.* 1999). Using the RAND criteria for 'appropriateness' and 'necessity', 4905 cases from the selected hospitals were reviewed. Among those patients for whom surgery was judged to be 'appropriate', 57% of whites, 45% of blacks, and 46% of Hispanics actually received the procedure. Based on the criterion that surgery was 'necessary', the operation was performed 65% of the time in whites, 49% in blacks, and 57% in Hispanics. After adjustment for insurance status, coronary anatomy, and other covariates, the odds ratio associated with black race was 0.6 for both the 'appropriate' and 'necessary' indications ($p < 0.02$). To evaluate the role of patient decision-making, questionnaire data were obtained from 717 'gatekeeper' physicians who provided care for a subset of patients who did not go on to receive warranted surgery. These additional data demonstrated that patient refusal was not the cause of these differentials, since physicians recommended surgery even less often for black patients than for whites.

9.5 Seeking explanations

The contrasting experience of blacks and whites in the US with regard to CHD has provoked widespread speculation about potential causes. It comes as no surprise, given the high prevalence of hypertension and social disadvantage, that blacks have higher mortality. Several incongruent findings have been reported, however, including low rates of obstructive CHD at angiography and lower mortality among men than would be anticipated. Unfortunately, the epidemiological analyses that should provide the most useful answers have been hampered by the limited samples of blacks enrolled in prospective studies. The black sample in the Atherosclerosis Risk in Communities (ARIC) study, which forms the principal database (Rosamond *et al.* 2001), is drawn primarily from Mississippi and is not typical of the entire US population. The difficulty in assessing lifetime cumulative risk, which is the exposure measurement of interest when incidence rates between populations are being compared, has also undermined the usefulness of these analyses. Most likely the unexpectedly lower rates of CHD in the past reflect competing mortality, bias in cause of death assignment, and reduced cumulative lifetime risk for a generation that had low cholesterols in young adulthood. In the absence of an uncontested explanation, however, the debate has focused on the relative impact of causal exposures versus differentials in genetic susceptibility. Finally, a new element in this debate draws attention to 'macro-social' forces, like economic disadvantage and racism. A brief summary of these issues is presented below.

9.5.1 Genes

The genomic revolution has renewed speculation about the potential role of genetics in racial/ethnic variation in chronic disease (Cooper *et al.* 2003; Khoury 2000; Risch *et al.* 2002; Templeton 1999). Up until the last few years indirect methods – that is, those that did not rely on information about genotype – had been used by epidemiologists to examine this question. A common indirect method involves the attempt to partial out 'environmental' factors by adjusting for covariates and then arguing that 'what is left over', or the residual effect after subtracting external exposures, is likely to be genetic. For example, because a strong social class gradient exists for most CV risk factors, the data are routinely adjusted by educational level to examine whether a racial effect persists. Any residual difference has frequently been attributed to intrinsic attributes of the two races. The 'subtraction method' has been criticized, however, and the weak proxies for environmental factors that are being used cannot summarize the influence of lifestyle exposures (Kaufman *et al.* 1997). In particular, adjusting for education and income does not eliminate the effect of the social position of blacks and whites, since many other aspects of the social environment are unequally distributed. In practice this method tends to reinforce the essentialist concept of race.

Molecular data can now be brought to bear on this question in two ways. First, the degree of differentiation of the world's populations can be quantified (Rosenberg *et al.* 2002). Second, susceptibility genes can potentially be identified. Molecular evidence does not suggest that there has been significant variation among continental populations (Templeton 1999). The most recent estimates suggest that only ~3% of variation summarized by microsatellites is between populations, while the rest is within populations (Rosenberg *et al.* 2002). Primate evolution occurred over millions of years in Africa, yet modern humans migrated to other continents only 50–100 000 years ago, beginning from an original population of about 10 000 (Harpending *et al.* 1998). These migrations either involved small numbers of individuals, or were subject to severe demographic bottlenecks, as in the case of Europe (Reich *et al.* 2001). As a result the repository of human diversity within modern African populations is much greater than among those outside Africa (Harpending *et al.* 1998). Within a pattern that completely overlaps, the haplotypes and single nucleotide variants in populations outside of Africa are a subset of those found in Africa, that is to say, they are a sample of the African whole (Gabriel *et al.* 2002). It is deeply ironic, therefore, that the regional population which is the source of all other populations and today contains the most complete reservoir of human diversity has been repeatedly characterized as uniquely shaped by evolution and 'genetically susceptible' to the broad disease syndromes which now occur world-wide (Cooper *et al.* 2003).

Susceptibility genes for complex disorders, like CHD, hypertension, and diabetes, have been difficult to define. It is therefore premature to speculate on the distribution of mutations that create risk in different racial/ethnic populations. Because many genetic variants are likely to be responsible for susceptibility in a given individual, and because these common variants will be distributed broadly in human populations, it seems unlikely that genetic factors will be aggregated or 'lumped' in specific groups. This situation contrasts to monogenic disorders involving recent mutations, like Tay Sachs or cystic fibrosis, that do vary markedly among groups. Hopefully the findings emerging from population genetics, where current tools have found their most effective application, will inform the debate about racial differences and moderate to some extent the exaggerated emphasis on genetic factors in inter-ethnic variation in chronic disease.

In the renin–angiotensin system (RAS), where there do appear to be several variants within the same gene that influence blood pressure, the older, more common variants are shared by all populations (Zhu *et al.* 2003*a*, *b*). Among the RAS genes it is also clear that more genetic diversity, including more frequent polymorphisms and shorter haplotypes, is present in blacks (Zhu *et al.* 2003*b*), while non-Africans are a sub-sample of this 'African whole'. Fine mapping of causal variants is therefore much more efficient in African-origin populations since the information content is higher (Zhu *et al.* 2000).

What is at stake in the genetic hypothesis of racial susceptibility is whether evolutionary selection has taken place among geographically regional human populations since the dispersion from Africa. The classic example of this process is of course the development of sickle cell disease and thalassaemia in response to the emergence of endemic malaria within the last 10 000 years. However, this imprint of evolution was inferred indirectly from the geographical prevalence rather than from direct molecular evidence. Based on analysis of haplotype patterns, molecular analyses have now been able to identify the 'positive signature of selection' for genes that confer protection against malaria (Sabeti *et al.* 2002). However, studying the same question in relation to chronic disease will be much more difficult, given the weaker selective forces, and no evidence is yet available. Therefore, any inferences regarding racial susceptibility offered at the present time are mere speculation based on prior beliefs.

9.5.2 Social and economic inequality

Black Americans experience significant social and economic disadvantage that undoubtedly makes a large contribution to the excess CHD. The income ratio between blacks and whites has not changed since 1900 and purchasing power for most blacks has actually declined in the last two decades. It is difficult, however, with current epidemiological methods to make quantitative estimates of the impact of social disadvantage. Cardiovascular epidemiology has traditionally focused on physical risk factors that can be measured at the individual level. While this approach has obviously produced very effective preventive strategies, it may not be sufficient to explain residual differences across social class or racial/ethnic groups.

Table 9.4 Correlation between income equality[a] and heart disease mortality, 1990, US big cities

Population	Correlation ($n = 47$)	p
Total population	−0.41	0.006
White men	−0.28	0.063
White women	−0.20	0.196
Black men	−0.55	0.002
Black women	−0.27	0.093

[a] Percentage of income to bottom half of the distribution.

Racial discrimination and social inequality are conceptualized as causes of excess CV mortality that cannot be measured at the individual level. A recent analysis used metropolitan statistical areas and measures of inequality and residential segregation to examine this question (Cooper 2001). All-cause mortality was 81% higher in blacks compared to whites and median household income was 40% lower. Income inequality across cities was significantly correlated with mortality (Gini coefficient vs. mortality, $r = 0.33$) and residential segregation was significantly related to mortality and income inequality for blacks. Income equality and racial segregation were also independently correlated with heart disease mortality (Table 9.4; $r = -0.4$; $p = 0.006$) (Cooper *et al.* 2002).

9.6 Conclusions

For all forms of heart disease combined death rates are 50% higher in US blacks compared to whites. The risk factor pattern that underlies this differential has evolved over the course of the African diaspora and reflects the severe social and economic disadvantage currently experienced by US blacks. The classic finding of a positive association of CVD and economic development across countries, with a negative association between socio-economic strata and risk within industrialized countries, is apparent in this sample of populations. Overall, the anticipated risk factor–outcome relationships for CHD are observed in blacks, although rates had been lower up through the 1990s than would have been anticipated. These lower rates are probably a combination of the effect of competing cause, differences in classification of cause of death, and the lag time to develop this condition after populations become fully exposed to the full range of the atherogenic lifestyle factors. In general, the genetic hypothesis regarding unusual black predisposition or resistance to CVD has been grossly overstated and has deflected efforts to define the relevant environmental effects. Despite considerable progress, black Americans are not currently enjoying the full benefit of the ongoing rapid decline in CV mortality.

Acknowledgement

This work was supported by grants from the National Heart, Lung and Blood Institute (HL 45508 and HL 47910) and the Reynolds Cardiovascular Clinical Research Center at the University of Texas Southwestern, Dallas, TX.

References

Bernal, M. (1987). *Black Athena: the Afroasiatic roots of classical civilization*. Rutgers University Press, New Brunswick, NJ.

Castaner, A., Simmons, B. E., Mar, M., and Cooper, R. (1988). Poor prognosis after hospital discharge for myocardial infarction among blacks. *Annals of Internal Medicine*, **109**, 33–5.

CDC Wonder <http://wonder.cdc.gov>, accessed 2003.

Cooper, R. S. (1984). A note on the biological concept of race and its application in epidemiological research. *American Heart Journal*, **108**, 715–23.

Cooper, R. S. (2001). Social inequalities, ethnicity and cardiovascular disease. *International Journal of Epidemiology*, **30**(Suppl. 1), S48–S52.

Cooper, R. and Ford, E. (1992). Comparability of risk factors for coronary heart disease among blacks and whites in the NHANES-I Epidemiologic Follow-up Study. *Annals of Epidemiology*, **2**, 637–45.

Cooper, R. S. and Kaufman, J. S. (1998). Race and hypertension: science or nescience? *Hypertension*, **32**, 813–16.

Cooper, R., Castaner, A., Campo, A., Islam, N., and Simmons, B. (1989). Severity of coronary artery disease among blacks with acute myocardial infarction. *American Journal of Cardiology*, **63**, 788–91.

Cooper, R. S., Muna, W., Kingue, S., Osotimehin, B., Kadiri, S., Rotimi, C., and Kaufman, J. (1996). The burden of hypertension in rural Africa: results from the International Collaborative Study on Hypertension in Blacks. *Tropical Cardiology*, **22**, 69–75.

Cooper, R., Rotimi, C., Ataman, S., McGee, D., Osotimehin, B., Kadiri, S. *et al.* (1997). Hypertension prevalence in seven populations of African origin. *American Journal of Public Health*, **87**, 160–8a.

Cooper, R., Osotimehin, B., Kaufman, J., and Forrester, T. (1998). Disease burden in sub-Saharan Africa: what should we conclude in the absence of data? *Lancet*, **351**, 208–10.

Cooper, R., Cutler, J., Desvigne-Nickens, P., Fortmann, S. P., Friedman, L., Havlik, R. *et al.* (2000). Trends and disparities in coronary heart disease, stroke, and other cardiovascular diseases in the United States. *Circulation*, **102**, 3137–47.

Cooper, R. S., Kennelly, J. F., Durazo-Arvizu, R., Oh, H-J., Kaplan, G., and Lynch, J. W. (2002). The relationship between mortality and socioeconomic factors in blacks and whites in US metropolitan areas. *Public Health Reports*, **116**, 464–73.

Cooper, R. S., Kaufman, J., and Ward, R. (2003). Race and genomics. *New England Journal of Medicine*, **348**, 1166–70.

Ford, E. S. and Cooper, R. S. (1995). Racial/ethnic differences in health care utilization of cardiovascular procedures: a review of the evidence. *Health Services Research*, **30**, 237–52.

Ford, E., Cooper, R., Castaner, A., Simmons, B., Mar, M. (1989). Coronary arteriography and coronary bypass surgery among whites and blacks relative to hospital-based incidence rates for coronary artery disease: findings from the National Hospital Discharge Survey. *American Journal of Public Health*, **79**, 437–40.

Forrester, T., Cooper, R. S., and Weatherall, D. (1998). Emergence of western diseases in the tropical world: the experience with chronic cardiovascular diseases. *British Medical Bulletin*, **54**, 463–73.

Francis, C. K., Grant, A. O., Cooper, R. S., and the Working Group Members (1994). *Report of the Working Group on Research in Coronary Heart Disease in Blacks*. National Heart, Lung and Blood Institute, Public Health Service, Bethesda, MD.

Gabriel, S. B., Schaffner, S. F., Nguyen, H., Moore, J. M., Roy, J., Blumensteil, B. *et al.* (2002). The structure of haplotype blocks in the human genome. *Science*, **296**, 2225–9.

Ghali, J. K., Liao, Y., Simmons, B., Castaner, A., Cao, G., and Cooper, R. S. (1992). The prognostic role of left ventricular hypertrophy in patients with or without coronary artery disease. *Annals of Internal Medicine*, **117**, 831–6.

Gillum, R. F. (1987). Coronary artery bypass surgery and coronary angiography in the United States. *American Heart Journal*, **113**, 1255–60.

Gilroy, P. (2000). *Against race: imagining political culture beyond the color line*. Harvard University Press, Cambridge, MA.

Good, G. (1998). *Life expectancy in big cities in the United States, 1992*. City of Chicago Department of Public Health.

Hannan, E. L., van Ryn, M., Burke, J., Stone, D., Kumar, D., Arani, D. *et al.* (1999). Access to coronary artery bypass surgery by race/ethnicity and gender among patients who are appropriate for surgery. *Medical Care*, **37**, 68–77.

Harpending, H. C., Batzer, M. A., Gurven, M., Jorde, L. B., Rogers, A. R., and Sherry, S. T. (1998). Genetic traces of ancient demography. *Proceedings of the National Academy of Sciences, USA*, **95**, 1961–7.

Johnson, K. W. and Payne, G. H. (1984). Report of a working conference on coronary heart disease in black populations. *American Heart Journal*, **108**, 633–862.

Jones, D. W., Sempos, C. T., Thom, T. J., Harrington, A. M., Taylor, H. A. Jr., Fletcher, B. W. *et al.* (2000). Rising levels of cardiovascular mortality in Mississippi, 1979–1995. *American Journal of Medical Science*, **319**, 131–7.

Kaufman, J. S., Rotimi, C. N., Brieger, W. O., Oladokun, M. A., Osotimehin, B., Kadiri, S., and Cooper, R. S. (1996). The mortality risk associated with hypertension: preliminary results of a prospective study in rural Nigeria. *Journal of Human Hypertension*, 10, 461–4.

Kaufman, J. S., Cooper, R. S., and McGee, D. (1997). Socioeconomic status and health in blacks and whites: the problem of residual confounding and the resiliency of race. *Epidemiology*, 6, 621–8.

Khoury, M. J. Burke, W., and Thomson, E. J. (eds) (2000). *Genetics and public health in the 21st century: using genetic information to improve health and prevent disease.* Oxford University Press.

Liao, Y., Cooper, R., McGee, D. L., Mensah, G. A., and Ghali, J. K. (1995). The relative effects of left ventricular hypertrophy, coronary artery disease, and ventricular dysfunction on survival among black adults. *Journal of the American Medical Association*, 273, 1592–7.

Liao, Y., McGee, D. L., and Cooper, R. S. (1999). Prediction of coronary heart disease mortality in blacks and whites: pooled data from two national cohorts. *American Journal of Cardiology*, 84, 31–6.

Luke, A., Cooper, R. S., Forrester, T., Adeyemo, A., and Prewitt, E. (2001). The nutritional consequences of the African diaspora. *Annual Review of Nutrition*, 21, 47–71.

Maynard, C., Fisher, L. D., Passamani, E. R., and Pullum, T. (1986). Blacks in the Coronary Artery Surgery Study (CASS): race and clinical decision making. *American Journal of Public Health*, 76, 1446–8.

Statistical Institute of Jamaica (2001). *Mortality statistics.* Statistical Institute of Jamaica, Kingston.

Murray, C. J. L. and Lopez, A. D. (eds) (1996). *The global burden of disease: a comprehensive assessment of mortality and disability from diseases, injuries, and risk factors in 1990 and projected to 2020.* Harvard University Press, Cambridge, MA.

PAHO (Pan American Health Organization) (1998). *Health in the Americas.* PAHO, Washington, DC.

Reich, D. E., Cargill, M., Bolk, S., Ireland, J., Sabeti, P. C., Richter, D. J. *et al.* (2001). Linkage disequilibrium in the human genome. *Nature*, 444, 199–204.

Risch, N., Burchard, E., Ziv, E., and Tang, H. (2002). Categorization of humans in biomedical research: genes, race and disease. *Genome Biology*, 3 (7), comment 2007.

Roig, E., Castaner, A., Simmons, B., Patel, R., and Cooper, R. (1987). In-hospital mortality rates from acute myocardial infarction by race in U. S. hospitals: findings from the National Hospital Discharge Survey. *Circulation*, 76, 280–8.

Rosamond, W. D., Folsom, A. R., Chambless, L. E., and Wang, C. H. (2001). ARIC investigators: coronary heart disease trends in four United States communities. *International Journal of Epidemiology*, 30(Suppl. 11), S17–S22.

Rosenberg, N. A., Pritchard, J. K., Weber, J. L., Cann, H. M., Kidd, K. K., Zhivotovsky, L. A., and Feldman, M. W. (2002). Genetic structure of human populations. *Science*, 298, 2381–5.

Sabeti, P., Reich, D. E., Higgins, J. M., Platko, J. V., Richter, D. J., Schaffner, S. F. *et al.* (2002). Detecting recent positive selection in the human genome from haplotype structure: two genes associated with malaria resistance. *Nature*, 419, 832–7.

Sargeant, L. A., Bennett, F. I., Forrester, T. E., Cooper, R., and Wilks, R. J. (2002). Incident diabetes in Jamaican adults: the role of obesity and fat distribution. *Obesity Research*, 10, 792–8.

Schulman, K. A., Berlin, J. A., Kerner, J. F., Sistrunk, S., Gersh, B. J., Dube, R. *et al.* (1996). The effect of race and sex on physician's recommendations for cardiac catheterization. *New England Journal of Medicine*, 340, 618–26.

Templeton, A. R. (1999). Human races: a genetic and evolutionary perspective. *American Anthropologist*, 100, 632–50.

Walker, R. W., McLarty, D. G., Kitange, H. M., Whiting, D., Masuki, G., Mtasiwa, D. M. *et al.* (2000). Stroke mortality in urban and rural Tanzania: Adult Morbidity and Mortality Project. *Lancet*, 355, 1684–7.

Zhu, X., McKenzie, C., Forrester, T., Nickerson, D. A., Cooper, R. S., and Rieder, M. J. (2000). Localization of a small genomic region associated with elevated ACE. *American Journal of Human Genetics*, **67**, 1144–53.

Zhu, X., Chang, C., Yan, D., Weder, A., Cooper, R. S., Luke, A., Kan, D., and Chakravarti, A. (2003*a*). Associations between hypertension and genes in the renin-angiotensin system. *Hypertension*, **41**, 1027–34.

Zhu, X., Yan, D., Cooper, R. S., Luke, A., Ikeda, M. A., Chang, Y-P. C. *et al.* (2003*b*). Linkage disequilibrium and haplotype diversity in the genes of the renin-angiotensin system: findings from the Family Blood Pressure Program. *Genomic Research*, **13**, 173–81.

Section II

Global picture of coronary heart disease

II.II Global patterns and the burden of disease

Chapter 10

Coronary heart disease mortality attributable to smoking: global and regional estimates for 2000

M. Ezzati and A. D. Lopez

10.1 Introduction

Smoking has been one of the most extensively studied human health risks, with detailed epidemiological research dating back to the 1930s (see table 1 in Doll 1986 for a summary of early studies). The sample size, data, and methods have improved in subsequent studies in a number of countries, leading to a growing list of more than 60 000 publications on the hazards of smoking. The evidence for the causal relationship between smoking and all-cause and cause-specific mortality, as well as the mechanisms of disease causation, have been extensively reviewed in a number of works (Doll 1986; 1998; Lopez 1999; US Department of Health and Human Services 1989, 2004). Added to these are a number of recent studies from developing countries, including China and India (Gajalakshmi *et al.* 2003; Liu *et al.* 1998). Given the substantially increased risk of premature mortality from a number of medical causes as a result of smoking (Doll *et al.* 1994; Liu *et al.* 1998; Thun *et al.* 1997a, 2000; US Department of Health and Human Services 1989, 2004; Zaridze and Peto 1986), in populations where smoking has been common for many decades, tobacco use accounts for a considerable proportion of premature mortality, as illustrated by estimates of smoking-attributable deaths in industrialized countries (Peto *et al.* 1992). These initial estimates also illustrate that, although lung cancer is the disease with the highest *fraction* due to smoking, vascular diseases are those which account for the largest absolute number of deaths due to smoking (together with chronic obstructive pulmonary disease (COPD), in some developing countries).

The specific evidence on smoking and vascular disease first became evident in the early 1950s based on the initial follow-up years of the male British doctors cohort (Doll and Hill 1954, 1956) and has been subsequently confirmed in numerous studies. A key feature of these studies is the marked age gradient of the relative risk of coronary heart disease (CHD) for smokers, as illustrated by the International Studies of Infarct Survival (ISIS) in the UK (Parish *et al.* 1995). This age gradient is also illustrated in Table 10.2, based on the results of the American Cancer Society's (ACS) Cancer Prevention Study, Phase II (CPS-II). This study found that, at young adult ages (<55 years), smokers have up to 6–7 times the risk of CHD mortality compared to non-smokers, decreasing to less than two at the oldest ages.

Many of the health effects of smoking depend on the exposure history, including the age at which smoking began, the number of cigarettes smoked per day, and cigarette characteristics such as tar and nicotine content or filter type (Fletcher and Peto 1977; Liu *et al.* 1998; Peto 1986). Therefore, current smoking prevalence alone would be an insufficient indicator of accumulated risk from smoking, even if detailed (i.e. age–sex specific) prevalence data were available in all countries. We extended the indirect Smoking Impact Ratio (SIR) method of Peto *et al.* (1992) for estimating excess mortality due to smoking, to provide estimates of premature mortality from CHD caused by smoking in all regions of the world.

10.1.1 Environmental tobacco smoke and CHD

In addition to the direct effects of smoking on CHD and stroke, environmental tobacco smoke (ETS) is a risk factor for vascular disease in otherwise healthy non-smokers. Given the importance of CHD as a cause of death in almost all populations, even a slight increase in risk of CHD from ETS can have a substantial impact on mortality. A feature of the relationship between ETS and CHD risk has been a dose–response relationship suggested by epidemiological studies, which indicates a very rapid increase in risk at very low levels of exposure to tobacco smoke (Law *et al.* 1997). Allowing for possible confounding, Law *et al.* (1997) concluded from a systematic review of available studies that ETS increases the risk of CHD in non-smokers by 23%, a level similar to that reported in other studies (Glantz and Parmeley 1995; Steenland 1992). It has been suggested that the rapid increase in risk is due to the effect of small doses on platelet aggregation (Blache *et al.* 1992; Davis *et al.* 1989). While this evidence strongly supports a significant impact of ETS on CHD mortality, further corroborative evidence on the sharp dose–response relationship, such as the mechanisms of impact on cardiac function and damage (Pope *et al.* 2001), would increase the confidence in the extrapolation of risk to other populations.

10.2 Methods and data

10.2.1 Mortality statistics

For the analysis described in this chapter, the age–sex-specific mortality statistics for the 191 World Health Organization (WHO) member states were taken from WHO's Global Burden of Disease (GBD) database. The 191 WHO member states are divided into 14 sub-regions based on a combination of the WHO regional breakdown and epidemiological characteristics (child and adult mortality) (Table 10.1). The sources of mortality data for each region include vital registration and sample registration, incidence registries, and epidemiological studies. Details of mortality and cause-of-death analysis methods are provided elsewhere (Mathers *et al.* 2002), and summarized below as relevant. Mortality statistics by cause, region, and broad age groups are provided in the annexes of the *World Health Report* on an annual basis.

The reliability of the Smoking Impact Ratio (SIR), described below, is determined by the reliability of lung cancer mortality estimates. In countries with good vital registration and medical certification of deaths (~75 countries), lung cancer mortality is diagnosed with a high degree of accuracy. For example, microscopic confirmation of diagnosis against the cause reported on death certificates has suggested a 95% or higher confirmation rate in these settings (Percy and Muir 1989; Percy *et al.* 1990). In approximately another 50 countries, vital registration of mortality is incomplete and medical certification of the cause much less reliable. Standard demographic techniques (Bennett and Horiuchi 1984; Hill 1981; Preston *et al.* 2000) are used in the GBD project to correct all-cause death rates by age for these populations, and lung cancer rates are adjusted accordingly. In the absence of evidence for bias in mortality recording, the same correction factor is applied for all causes of death. Finally, for countries without vital registration, overall age-specific death rates are first determined using model life-tables (Lopez *et al.* 2002). Total cancer death rates are then estimated based on models and regional information about proportionate cancer mortality. Within this death rate, the distribution by site is based on regional

Table 10.1 World sub-regions used in analysis

WHO region	Mortality stratum[a]	Countries	Population in 2000 (thousands)
AFR	D	Algeria, Angola, Benin, Burkina Faso, Cameroon, Cape Verde, Chad, Comoros, Equatorial Guinea, Gabon, Gambia, Ghana, Guinea, Guinea-Bissau Liberia, Madagascar, Mali, Mauritania, Mauritius, Niger, Nigeria, Sao Tome and Principe, Senegal, Seychelles, Sierra Leone, Togo	294 078
	E	Botswana, Burundi, Central African Republic, Congo, Côte d'Ivoire, Democratic Republic of the Congo, Eritrea, Ethiopia, Kenya, Lesotho, Malawi, Mozambique, Namibia, Rwanda, South Africa, Swaziland, Uganda, United Republic of Tanzania, Zambia, Zimbabwe	345 515
AMR	A	Canada, Cuba, United States of America	325 183
	B	Antigua and Barbuda, Argentina, Bahamas, Barbados, Belize, Brazil, Chile, Colombia, Costa Rica, Dominica, Dominican Republic, El Salvador, Grenada, Guyana, Honduras, Jamaica, Mexico, Panama, Paraguay, Saint Kitts and Nevis, Saint Lucia, Saint Vincent and the Grenadines, Suriname, Trinidad and Tobago, Uruguay, Venezuela	430 932
	D	Bolivia, Ecuador, Guatemala, Haiti, Nicaragua, Peru	71 230
EMR	B	Bahrain, Cyprus, Iran (Islamic Republic of), Jordan, Kuwait, Lebanon, Libyan, Arab Jamahiriya, Oman, Qatar, Saudi Arabia, Syrian Arab Republic, Tunisia, United Arab Emirates	139 059
	D	Afghanistan, Djibouti, Egypt, Iraq, Morocco, Pakistan, Somalia, Sudan, Yemen	342 576
EUR	A	Andorra, Austria, Belgium, Croatia, Czech Republic, Denmark, Finland, France, Germany, Greece, Iceland, Ireland, Israel, Italy, Luxembourg, Malta, Monaco, Netherlands, Norway, Portugal, San Marino, Slovenia, Spain, Sweden, Switzerland, United Kingdom	411 889
	B	Albania, Armenia, Azerbaijan, Bosnia and Herzegovina, Bulgaria, Georgia, Kyrgyzstan, Poland, Romania, Slovakia, Tajikistan, The Former Yugoslav Republic of Macedonia, Turkey, Turkmenistan, Uzbekistan, Yugoslavia	218 458
	C	Belarus, Estonia, Hungary, Kazakhstan, Latvia, Lithuania, Republic of Moldova, Russian Federation, Ukraine	243 184
SEAR	B	Indonesia, Sri Lanka, Thailand	293 819
	D	Bangladesh, Bhutan, Democratic People's Republic of Korea, India, Maldives, Myanmar, Nepal	1 241 806
WPR	A	Australia, Brunei Darussalam, Japan, New Zealand, Singapore	154 354
	B	Cambodia, China, Cook Islands, Fiji, Kiribati, Lao People's Democratic Republic, Malaysia, Marshall Islands, Micronesia (Federated States of), Mongolia, Nauru, Niue, Palau, Papua New Guinea, Philippines, Republic of Korea, Samoa, Solomon Islands, Tonga, Tuvalu, Vanuatu, Vietnam	1 532 933

Source: WHO 2002.

[a] **A**: very low child mortality and very low adult mortality; **B**: low child mortality and low adult mortality; **C**: low child mortality and high adult mortality; **D**: high child mortality and high adult mortality; **E**: high child mortality and very high adult mortality.

incidence patterns from cancer registries reporting to the International Agency for Research on Cancer, IARC (Parkin *et al.* 1992, 1997). While this indirect procedure has considerable uncertainty (see below), it is preferable to estimating mortality directly from reports of deaths to cancer registries, which would be very likely to substantially underestimate mortality from lung and other cancers. Further, for the majority of populations to which this indirect procedure is applied, lung cancer mortality is still low, hence constraining the estimate.

10.2.2 **ACS Cancer Prevention Study, Phase II (CPS-II)**

The ACS Cancer Prevention Study, Phase II (CPS-II) is a prospective study of smoking and death in more than 1 million Americans aged 30 and older when they completed a questionnaire in 1982, with the latest follow-up in 1998. A complete description of the study is provided elsewhere (Garfinkel 1985; Peto *et al.* 1992; Thun *et al.* 1995, 1997a, b, 2000). In 1992, when the first 6-year (1982–88) results were obtained, mortality follow-up was virtually complete for the first 2 years, and about 98–9% complete for the next four. Because some conditions that cause death in the first 2 years may have affected smoking habits at entry (e.g. those diagnosed with lung cancer may have stopped smoking because of their disease or related symptoms), analysis was restricted to years 3–6 inclusive (1984–88) (Peto *et al.* 1992). The analysis related deaths (subdivided by cause, sex, and 5-year age groups at the time of death) to person years (with accounting for incompleteness) for those who in 1982 had never smoked regularly, and for those who were then current cigarette smokers. Most of the CPS-II current smokers were lifelong cigarette smokers with a mean consumption of about 20 cigarettes/day. Relative risks for CHD mortality among smokers in the CPS-II population without adjustment are provided in Table 10.2, and show a strong age gradient. Relatively small numbers of CHD deaths at

Table 10.2 Cigarette smokers versus non-smokers (never smoked regularly): CHD mortality relative risks for years 3–6 inclusive (approximately 1984–88) of ACS CPS-II prospective study of 1 million American adults

Age	Male	Female
35–9	3.3	1.0
40–4	6.3	1.5
45–9	5.5	7.2
50–4	3.8	5.7
55–9	2.7	3.2
60–4	2.4	2.6
65–9	1.9	2.4
70–4	1.7	1.9
75–9	1.4	1.6
80+	1.4	1.3

Source: Thun *et al.* 1997*a*.

younger adult ages distort the age pattern below the age of 40, but the important impact of smoking on CHD risk in younger adults can be seen. Indeed, these numbers suggest that if a smoker at ages 40–54 dies of CHD, there is an ~80% probability that the death was caused by smoking.

10.2.3 Lung cancer mortality as indicator of accumulated hazards of smoking

Peto *et al.* (1992) observed that the level of lung cancer mortality in a population compared with non-smokers is an indicator of the 'maturity' of the smoking epidemic, confirmed by the observed relationship between cumulative smoking and lung cancer (Peto 1986; Yamaguchi *et al.* 2000). Based on this observation, the smoking impact ratio, *SIR*, is defined as population lung cancer mortality in excess of that of never-smokers, relative to excess lung cancer mortality for a known reference group of smokers. Formally, the ratio in eqn 10.1 measures the *absolute* 'maturity' of lung cancer mortality due to smoking (i.e. excess lung cancer mortality) in the study population, relative to the *absolute* 'maturity' of lung cancer mortality in life-long smokers of the reference population.

$$SIR = \frac{C_{LC} - N_{LC}}{S_{LC}^{*} - N_{LC}^{*}} \tag{10.1}$$

C_{LC}: age–sex specific lung cancer mortality rate in the study population (e.g. country of analysis); N_{LC}: age–sex specific lung cancer mortality rate of never-smoker in the same population; and S_{LC}^{*} and N_{LC}^{*}: age–sex specific lung cancer mortality rates for smokers and never-smokers in a reference population.

Liu *et al.* (1998) found that in China, the relative risk of mortality from lung cancer as a result of smoking is approximately constant in different cities whose non-smoker lung cancer mortality rates varied by a factor of 10 (see fig. 4 in Liu *et al.* 1998). A constant relative risk means that smoking results in a larger absolute excess mortality (i.e. the numerator of eqn 10.1) where never-smoker lung cancer mortality is higher (and smaller absolute excess mortality where never-smoker lung cancer mortality is lower). Therefore, to be converted to an indicator of the maturity of the smoking epidemic, the numerator and denominator of eqn 10.1 need to be normalized with the respective never-smoker lung cancer mortality rates. We define the background-adjusted Smoking Impact Ratio, *SIR*, by the following relationship:

$$SIR = \frac{C_{LC} - N_{LC}}{S_{LC}^{*} - N_{LC}^{*}} \times \frac{N_{LC}^{*}}{N_{LC}} \tag{10.2}$$

where C_{LC}, N_{LC}, S_{LC}^{*}, and N_{LC}^{*} are defined as above (Ezzati and Lopez 2003a).

It is straightforward to show that *SIR* equals the proportion of reference-population (i.e. CPS-II) smokers in a mix of smokers and never-smokers which has the same lung cancer mortality rate as the study population (Peto *et al.* 1992). This provides a convenient interpretation of *SIR*: using excess lung cancer mortality over never-smokers, *SIR* captures the accumulated hazards of smoking by converting the smokers in the study population into equivalents of smokers in the reference population, where hazards for other diseases have been measured (Peto *et al.* 1992).

Following Peto *et al.* (1992), we used the CPS-II study population as the reference population. This is because among the various studies of smoking and cause-specific mortality (US

Department of Health and Human Services 1989), CPS-II is one of the very few conducted when the smoking epidemic was at its highest, especially for men. The vast majority of (male) CPS-II current smokers had been lifelong cigarette smokers. Further, the estimates of increased risk of mortality among smokers are available for both men and women and in finer age groups than in other studies of smoking and mortality, such as the male British doctors cohort (Doll *et al.* 1994).

SIR values were calculated for individual countries and then averaged (population-weighted) in each of the 14 GBD sub-regions, for each age group and sex. No CHD deaths before the age of 35 were attributed to smoking. *SIR* values larger than 1.0 were set to 1.0. This occurred in the case of males in the 30–44 age group in 17 European countries and one Western Pacific island, and in the 45–59 age group in three countries in Eastern Europe. Relatively low lung cancer mortality in younger ages is one factor which can lead to unstable *SIR* values. This is particularly the case if the never-smoker rates are estimated with error, which is more likely in younger ages when lung cancer is relatively rare. Further, although an *SIR* larger than 1.0 may seem to imply that a population which consists of some smokers and some never-smokers had higher lung cancer mortality than CPS-II life-long smokers, factors such as the type and number of cigarettes, or the age at which smoking began can result in such a pattern, especially where prevalence of smoking is high. The age of smoking initiation is particularly important for *SIR* values in earlier ages, such as those affected in this analysis. For example, historical lung cancer mortality data show an *SIR* larger than 1.0 for British males under age 60 in some years between 1950 and 1970, and among American males between 1968 and 1976. We nonetheless set the *SIR* for these groups to 1.0 to avoid any potential overestimation of risk.

To estimate mortality due to smoking from causes other than lung cancer (e.g. CHD), a mixture of CPS-II smokers and non-smokers was taken to give an *SIR* equal to that of the study population (it is simple to show that the fraction of smokers in the mixture equals the *SIR* of the study population). This mixture was then used together with the cause-specific relative risks from CPS-II to estimate the smoking-attributable fraction of mortality.

Before using the hazard estimates from CPS-II, Peto *et al.* (1992) reduced the excess risk attributed to smoking using constant correction factors. As explained by Peto *et al.* (1992), a constant correction factor, although arbitrary, avoided overestimating mortality due to confounding in the ACS CPS-II relative risk estimates (which were initially adjusted for age and sex only) as well as extrapolation of relative risk values from CPS-II to other populations, where exposure to other risk factors could modify the effects of smoking in a non-multiplicative way. The correction factor used by Peto *et al.* (1992) was 50% of excess risk because relative risks had not been adjusted for covariates other than age. In studies other than CPS-II, the overall impact of confounding has been found to be considerably less than half of the excess risk for vascular diseases (including evidence of negative confounding for some causes) (Hirayama 1990; Kawachi *et al.* 1997; LaCroix *et al.* 1991; Law *et al.* 1997). The Chinese prospective study of Liu *et al.* (1998) also provides some evidence that background disease rates do not change the proportion of mortality attributable to smoking (figs 4 and 5 in Liu *et al.* 1998), as confirmed in studies which stratified on serum cholesterol (Jee *et al.* 1999).

In response to criticism about the lack of empirical evidence for confounding correction (Lee 1996; Sterling *et al.* 1993), CPS-II data were re-analysed together with adjustment for potential confounding (Malarcher *et al.* 2000; Thun *et al.* 2000). In the analysis of

Table 10.3 Relative risk (RR) of mortality from CHD for CPS-II current smokers relative to non-smokers from re-analysis of CPS-II data. Relative risks were estimated from Cox proportional hazard models, with non-smokers as the reference group (RR = 1.0 for non-smokers). Numbers in brackets show the 95% confidence intervals. All risks were adjusted for age, race, education, marital status, 'blue collar' employment in most recent or current job, weekly consumption of vegetables and citrus fruit, vitamin (A, C, and E) use, alcohol use, aspirin use, BMI, exercise, and dietary fat consumption. Details of re-analysis are described elsewhere

Age (years)	Male	Female
30–44[a]	5.49 (2.46–12.25)	2.28 (0.83–6.23)
45–59	3.05 (2.67–3.49)	3.77 (3.09–4.60)
60–9	1.87 (1.69–2.08)	2.47 (2.17–2.81)
70–9	1.40 (1.24–1.58)	1.57 (1.37–1.81)
80+	1.01 (0.75–1.37)	1.34 (1.04–1.72)

Source: Thun *et al.* 2000; Ezzati, M., Henley, S. J., Thun, M. J., Lopez, A. D. (2005). The role of smoking in global and regional cardiovascular mortality. *Circulation*. In press.

[a] No deaths before the age of 30 were attributed to smoking.

Malarcher *et al.* (2000), except for cerebrovascular disease among men (where the fraction attributable to smoking decreased from 0.16 to 0.10), adjustment for confounding had no or little effect on smoking-attributable mortality (the next largest decrease was for lung cancer among men from 0.91 to 0.89 and COPD among women from 0.70 to 0.68). In the case of CHD, adjustment even resulted in a slight increase in risk (Malarcher *et al.* 2000). In a more detailed analysis, Thun *et al.* (2000) adjusted for age, race, education, marital status, occupation ('blue collar' worker), and total weekly consumption of citrus fruits and vegetables in estimating the relative risk of mortality due to a range of neoplasms, vascular diseases, and respiratory diseases. The analysis for vascular diseases also adjusted for current aspirin use, alcohol consumption, body mass index (BMI), physical activity at work or leisure, and weekly consumption of fatty foods. Overall, Thun *et al.* (2000) found that adjustment for confounding reduced their estimates of mortality attributable to smoking in the United States by approximately 1%. Adjustment resulted in no or little change (both increasing and decreasing the estimated hazard) in CHD risk. Adjusted relative risks for CHD from a re-analysis of CPS-II data are shown in Table 10.3, and were used in this chapter to estimate smoking-attributable CHD mortality.

10.2.4 Choice of never-smoker lung cancer mortality

Peto *et al.* (1992) used the same lung cancer mortality for never-smokers in the study and reference populations (numerator and denominator of eqn 10.1). Figure 10.1 shows non-smoker lung cancer mortality for the US (from CPS-II) and China (divided into urban, coastal rural, and inland rural areas) (from Liu *et al.* 1998). The different non-smoker lung cancer mortality rates in Fig. 10.1 are explained by patterns of household energy use in China over the past few decades. Coal is a common household fuel in China, often burned in stoves and

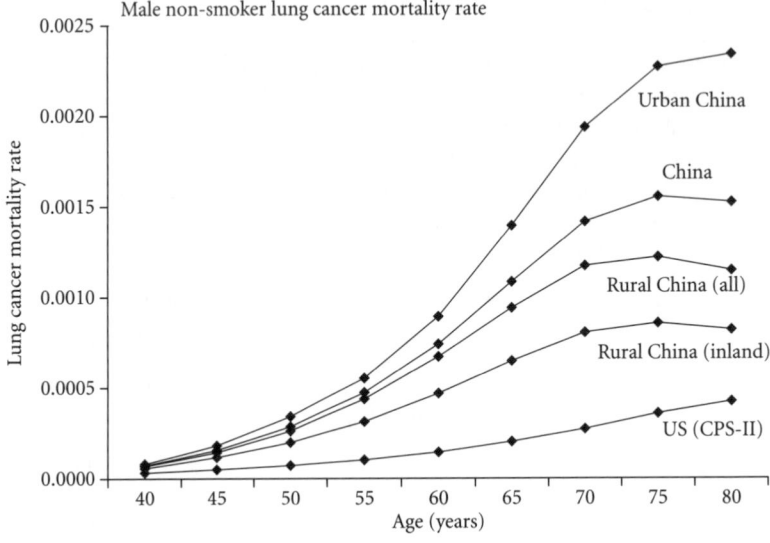

Male non-smoker lung cancer mortality rate

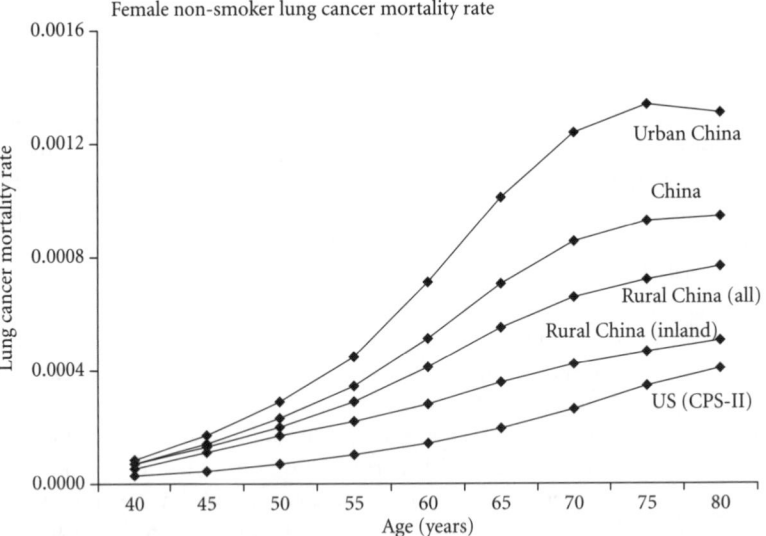

Female non-smoker lung cancer mortality rate

Fig. 10.1 Non-smoker mortality from lung cancer in US and China. Note that the scales on the female and male charts are different. (From Ezzati and Lopez 2003a.)

buildings without adequate ventilation (Du *et al.* 1996; Smith *et al.* 1993). Exposure to coal smoke and cooking fumes has been associated with increased lung cancer incidence in China (Du *et al.* 1996; Lan *et al.* 2002). Until recently, in inland rural regions of China, where incomes are low, biomass (including crop residues and wood) has been the dominant household fuel, compared to coastal villages and cities where coal was more commonly used.

The relationship between wood smoke and lung cancer has been absent or considerably smaller than that between coal and lung cancer in epidemiological studies (Bruce *et al.* 2000). Although urban air pollution has been linked to increased lung cancer mortality in some studies, the size of the risk is considerably smaller than the effects of smoking or direct exposure to coal smoke (Jedrychowski *et al.* 1990; Nyberg *et al.* 2000; Pope *et al.* 2002; Vena 1982). Further, the impact of ambient air pollution on lung cancer has been found to be smaller among non-smokers than among smokers, with one study finding increased risk of lung cancer as a result of urban air pollution among smokers only (Jedrychowski *et al.* 1990; Vena 1982). Because only a small fraction of national populations live in the most polluted urban areas, overall population lung cancer mortality is not expected to be greatly affected by urban air pollution.

Therefore, background (never-smoker) lung cancer rates for the different regions were based on the estimated use of coal for domestic energy in unvented stoves (Smith *et al.* 2004). We used Chinese non-smoker rates for China, a weighted average of Chinese and CPS-II non-smoker rates for the Indian sub-continent where coal is also used for household fuel (with weights for Chinese rates equal to the prevalence of coal use) (Smith *et al.* 2004), and CPS-II non-smoker rates for the remaining countries of the world where domestic coal use in unvented stoves is absent or negligible. The remaining risk factors for lung cancer mortality (ambient air pollution, occupational hazards, indoor air pollution from radon or biomass smoke, etc.) affect most populations to varying degrees. Therefore, the net impacts of these other risk factors were considered as sources of uncertainty in never-smoker lung cancer mortality, rather than in mean non-smoker lung cancer rates.

10.3 Analysis of uncertainty

Uncertainty for each of the variables and parameters in the analysis (population lung cancer mortality, never-smoker lung cancer mortality, reference population smoker and never-smoker lung cancer mortality, and relative risk) was estimated separately. Uncertainties of individual parameters were combined in a stratified sampling simulation to obtain overall uncertainty for the fraction of mortality due to smoking.

10.3.1 Population lung cancer mortality

To estimate uncertainty for population lung cancer mortality, we assigned each country to one of four uncertainty categories based on the quality of available mortality data. Lung cancer mortality information for the four categories were assigned uncertainty levels equal to 10%, 20%, 40%, and 80% of the best estimate, with the lowest level assigned to countries with good vital registration and medical certification. Since in countries with good vital registration, 95% or higher confirmation rates of the cause reported on death certificates have been found (Percy and Muir 1989; Percy *et al.* 1990), 10% is double the observed uncertainty level and hence a conservative estimate. 80% uncertainty for the least certain countries, those with no mortality reporting, implies that we have allowed nearly all of lung cancer mortality to be due to misclassification. Countries with less complete and/or less reliable data were assumed to have 20% or 40% uncertainty around the best estimate.

10.3.2 Never-smoker lung cancer mortality

For China, estimates of the uncertainty for non-smoker lung cancer mortality rates from the proportional mortality study were used (Liu *et al.* 1998). For all other countries, where never-smoker lung cancer mortality rates were assumed to be those of CPS-II, we assumed an uncertainty of 15% around CPS-II estimates plus the sampling uncertainty of the CPS-II estimates. Fifteen per cent is approximately equivalent to the whole (non-smoker) population being exposed to the highest levels of air pollution, such as that in the centre of the industrial city of

Cracow, Poland, which resulted in a 14% increase in lung cancer mortality (Jedrychowski *et al.* 1990), or equivalently, the whole population being exposed to an additional 20 mg/m^3 of PM$_{2.5}$ (particulates below 2.5 μm in diameter) (Pope *et al.* 2002). Given that the net difference between those exposed to these additional risk factors (radon, ambient air pollution, biomass smoke) in any two countries is less than the whole population, this assumption is likely to overestimate uncertainty of the never-smoker lung cancer mortality rates. For reference population smoker and never-smoker lung cancer mortality, the sampling uncertainty of CPS-II was used.

10.3.3 Relative risks

Uncertainty in relative risks were from the analysis of CPS-II, as described in Table 10.3. Other sources of uncertainty, which were not quantified, include:

1 the cigarette smoke characteristics that cause lung cancer may be different from those that cause CHD;

2 time-to-hazard may be different for lung cancer and CHD mortality caused by smoking; and

3 SIR estimates are likely to be affected by exposure to environmental tobacco smoke.

10.4 Results

10.4.1 Prevalence of smoking

While measures such as the *SIR* are better able to capture the cumulative effects of tobacco smoking on populations (Ezzati and Lopez 2003*a*), and are therefore more epidemiologically relevant than current smoking prevalence, they are not intuitively obvious. Prevalence is a more widely understood measure of the extent of tobacco use in a population and hence more policy relevant. Worldwide, about 30% of all adults smoke, being roughly the same in low- and middle-income countries, as a whole, as in high-income countries (Gajalakshmi *et al.* 2000; World Bank 1999). Globally, smoking is much more common among males (47%) than females (12%), although the sex differential in prevalence is much less apparent in high-income countries (39% prevalence for males, 22% for females), than in low- and middle-income populations (49% for males, 9% for females). In low- and middle-income countries, male smoking prevalence is particularly high in east Asia (60%) and Eastern Europe (60%), ranging from 33% to 44% in other regions. Typically, female prevalence is below 10%, with the exception of Latin America and the Caribbean (21%) and Eastern Europe (26%).

10.4.2 CHD mortality attributable to smoking

Table 10.4 provides the estimated number of smoking-attributable CHD deaths for different regions and age–sex groups using the methods described above. The results are reported in two age groups (30–69 and 70+) to be comparable with the previous estimates of mortality due to smoking (Ezzati and Lopez 2003*b*; Liu *et al.* 1998; Peto *et al.* 1992).

We have estimated that the number of adult (30+) CHD deaths attributable to smoking worldwide in 2000 was approximately 873 000 (95% CI 723 000–1 024 000), accounting for 15% of global adult CHD mortality. Some 674 000 (95% CI 530 000–762 000) of the smoking-attributable CHD deaths were among men (21% of adult male CHD mortality) and 199 000

Table 10.4 Coronary heart disease (CHD) mortality (in thousands of deaths) attributable to smoking in different regions of the world. No deaths below the age of 30 are attributed to smoking. The first number shows the number of deaths and the second the fraction of CHD mortality in the respective age-sex group. The discrepancies in the last significant digits between components and totals are due to rounding. PAF: population attributable fraction.

Region	Sex	30–69		70+		30+	
		number of deaths	PAF	number of deaths	PAF	number of deaths	PAF
Developing countries							
AFR D	M	4	10	1	2	4	6
	F	1	3	0	0	1	1
AFR E	M	7	16	1	2	8	11
	F	3	8	1	1	4	4
AMR B	M	22	26	3	5	25	17
	F	6	14	3	4	10	7
AMR D	M	0	5	0	1	1	3
	F	0	3	0	0	0	1
EMR B	M	15	26	2	6	16	19
	F	3	12	1	2	3	6
EMR D	M	24	22	3	3	27	14
	F	4	5	1	1	5	3
SEAR B	M	21	33	3	7	24	22
	F	2	5	0	0	3	3
SEAR D	M	141	26	18	5	159	18
	F	24	7	3	1	26	4
WPR B (excluding China)	M	18	40	3	9	20	28
	F	3	12	2	4	5	8
China	M	10	8	2	1	12	4
	F	3	3	2	1	5	2
All Developing	M	263	23	34	4	297	15
	F	50	7	12	1	62	4
Industrialized countries							
AMR A	M	42	40	14	10	56	23
	F	19	47	47	18	66	22
EUR A	M	49	40	20	11	69	22
	F	7	20	16	5	23	6
EUR B	M	58	46	9	9	67	30
	F	10	17	6	3	16	7
EUR C	M	151	52	25	12	176	36
	F	13	11	13	3	26	4
WPR A	M	6	23	3	9	8	15
	F	1	13	5	10	6	10
All Industrialized	M	305	46	72	11	377	28
	F	51	19	86	7	137	9
World	M	568	32	106	7	674	21
	F	101	10	98	4	199	6
	Both	669	24	204	5	873	13

(95% CI 147 000–284 000) among women (6% of adult female CHD mortality). There were 669 000 deaths among those aged 30–69, resulting in a large number of potential life years lost to premature mortality, and 204 000 among those above 69.

10.4.3 CHD mortality in industrialized countries

In year 2000, smoking resulted in an estimated 514 000 (95% CI 450 000-587 000) CHD deaths in industrialized countries for people over the age of 30, accounting for 18% of CHD mortality at these ages. Of these deaths, 377 000 (95% CI 388 000-459 000) were among men (28% of CHD mortality of adult males)[1] and 137 000 (95% CI 104 000-153 000) among women (9% of CHD mortality of adult females). The magnitude of the years of life lost due to premature mortality becomes more obvious when we note that 377 000, or over two-thirds, of these deaths occurred between the ages of 30 and 69, therefore accounting for a disproportionately larger loss of life years.

In these countries, CHD deaths caused by smoking accounted for 46% of CHD mortality among males aged 30–69 (305 000 deaths), 11% of CHD mortality among males above the age of 70 (72 000 deaths), 19% of CHD mortality among females aged 30–69 (51 000 deaths), and 7% of CHD mortality among females above the age of 70 (86 000 deaths).

The fraction of smoking-attributable mortality among men was highest in the EUR-C and EUR-B regions where the respective 176 000 and 67 000 smoking-attributable CHD deaths were 36% and 30% of all adult male CHD deaths (52% and 12% of CHD deaths for 30–69 and 70+ age groups, respectively, in EUR-C; 46% and 9% of CHD deaths for 30–69 and 70+ age groups, respectively, in EUR-B). This high attributable fraction in Eastern and Central European countries (compared to Western Europe and North America, for example) reflects the fact that these regions are at different stages of the tobacco epidemic, in which smoking prevalence and *SIR* values are particularly high among those aged 30–69 (Ezzati and Lopez 2003a). It is at these ages that CHD mortality due to smoking has the highest relative risks, as seen in Tables 10.2 and 10.3. Among women the highest fraction of smoking-attributable mortality was in the AMR-A region, where 66 000 CHD deaths, 22% of adult female CHD mortality (47% and 18% of CHD deaths for 30–69 and 70+ age groups, respectively) were caused by smoking. The lowest fraction of smoking-attributable mortality among men in the industrialized world was in WPR-A (15% of all CHD deaths; 23% and 8% of all deaths for 30–69 and 70+ age groups, respectively) and among women in EUR-C (4% of adult CHD deaths; 11% and 3% of CHD deaths for 30–69 and 70+ age groups, respectively).

10.4.4 CHD mortality in developing countries

The estimated number of CHD deaths attributable to smoking among those older than 30 years in developing countries in 2000 was approximately 359 000 (95% CI 247 000–470 000), accounting for 10% of CHD mortality in this group. Some 297 000 (95% CI 190 000–371 000) of the smoking-attributable CHD deaths were among men (15% of adult male CHD mortality) and 62 000 (95% CI 41 000–114 000) among women (4% of adult female CHD mortality). Eighty per cent (313 000) of smoking-attributable CHD deaths were among those aged 30–69 and 46 000 among those aged 70+. In these countries, CHD deaths caused by smoking accounted for 23% of CHD mortality among males aged 30–69 (263 000 deaths), 4% of CHD mortality among males above the age of 70 (34 000 deaths), 7% of CHD mortality among

---

[1] All fractions are based on mortality in the respective age group: 30–69, 70+, and 30+.

females aged 30–69 (50 000 deaths), and 1% of CHD mortality among females aged 70+ (12 000 deaths).

In general, there was larger variation in mortality due to smoking among different regions of the developing world than industrialized nations, due to the variability in the stages of the smoking epidemic. The fraction of adult CHD mortality due to smoking ranged from a low of 2–4% in AMR-D and AFR-D to a high of 12–13% in SEAR-D and SEAR-B, and 18% in WPR-B (excluding China). For males, the lowest fraction of CHD mortality due to smoking was in AMR-D (3%) and AFR-D (6%), reflecting the more recent status of the smoking epidemic in these regions. Given that the current prevalence of smoking among adult men is approximately 25–30% in AFR-D, this result also illustrates that current prevalence is a poor marker of accumulated smoking risks (Ezzati and Lopez 2003a). The highest fractions of adult male CHD mortality due to smoking were in WPR-B (excluding China) (28%), SEAR-B (22%), SEAR-D (18%), EMR-B (19%), and AMR-B (17%). For females, the fraction of CHD mortality due to smoking in 2000 was 1% in AFR-D and AMR-D, and 1–4% in AFR-E, EMR-D, SEAR-B, SEAR-D, and China. The highest fraction of female CHD mortality due to smoking was in AMR-B (7%) and WPR-B (excluding China) (8%), reflecting more recent increases in female smoking in these regions, especially with increasing urbanization and economic development.

10.5 **Discussion**

In this analysis we employed the indirect smoking impact ratio method (Peto *et al.* 1992), which uses absolute lung cancer mortality in a population as a marker for accumulated hazards of smoking, to estimate the global impact of smoking on CHD mortality. We chose the parameters of the model, such as relative risks and non-smoker lung cancer mortality, based on direct estimates or by extrapolation from other regions based on the best available evidence, explicitly stating the assumptions and reasons for this choice.

Using this method, we estimated that in 2000 approximately 873 000 (95% CI 723 000–1 024 000) people died from CHD in the world due to smoking, accounting for 15% of global adult CHD mortality. This figure represents a significant proportion of the more than 4.8 million smoking-attributable deaths in 2000 (Ezzati *et al.* 2002). Of these deaths, 359 000 (95% CI 247 000–470 000) were in developing countries, marking a transition to an era in which smoking kills a comparable number of people from CHD in developing countries as in industrialized nations.[2] In fact, even at these earlier stages of the tobacco epidemic, CHD deaths from smoking among men in the two regions were even closer (359 000 in developing countries and 377 000 in industrialized countries). Male CHD mortality due to smoking was considerably higher than female mortality, three times in industrialized countries and five times in developing nations. Over 70% (669 000) of global CHD deaths due to smoking were in the 30–69 age group. It is this relatively younger pattern of smoking-caused CHD mortality, compared to most other diseases caused by this risk factor, that further highlights the magnitude of the loss of life due to the global smoking epidemic.

Mortality due to smoking (in terms of the fraction of cause-specific or all-cause mortality) has been relatively stable in industrialized countries over the past decade. Conversely, CHD mortality due to smoking, including its share of total mortality by sex and age, exhibits large variation among different geographical regions of the developing world. This

---

[2] We have estimated elsewhere that when all causes of death are considered, developing and industrialized country mortalities due to smoking were practically identical in the year 2000, each at approximately 2.4 million deaths (Ezzati *et al.* 2002).

inter-regional variation, which is larger than that observed in industrialized countries, results from the fact that the shape and progress of the smoking epidemic is greatly affected by the varying economic and cultural determinants of smoking in developing nations. A few general statements can nonetheless be made about the health impacts of smoking in these countries. First, current CHD mortality due to smoking in developing countries is highly concentrated among men. Given that the prevalence of smoking among women is still low in developing countries (with the exception of countries in Latin America and the Caribbean, and some in Asia), the current magnitude of male mortality provides an indicator of the large health losses that can occur if female smoking increases over the next few decades. Second, relative to industrialized countries, developing countries have a higher proportion of smoking-attributable CHD mortality in the 30–69 age group than in the 70+ group (over 80% in developing countries versus about 70% in industrialized countries). This suggests that as people (mostly men) who began smoking over the past three decades in developing countries become older, mortality due to smoking will continue to rise.

Smoking prevalence in some developing countries has currently stabilized, albeit at very high levels. In others, it is still rising. Given shifting disease patterns and the fact that most of the growth in global population is expected to take place in the developing world, the health loss due to smoking, already an important global health hazard, will continue to grow (Peto and Lopez 2001) unless effective interventions and policies that curb and reduce smoking among males and prevent increases among females in these countries are implemented. At the same time, because the health benefits of smoking cessation occur faster for cardiovascular than other diseases, policies that prevent and reduce smoking will have immediate and large benefits for reducing CHD mortality.

Acknowledgement

This research was sponsored by the National Institute on Aging Grant PO1-AG17625. We thank R. Peto and J. Boreham for discussions on methodology and for additional re-analysis of data from CPS-II and the Chinese retrospective proportional mortality study, and M. Thun and J. Henley for additional re-analysis of data from CPS-II. The participants in the Global Burden of Disease (GBD) project Comparative Risk Assessment review meetings provided valuable comments on methods and assumptions.

References

Bennett, N. G. and Horiuchi, S. (1984). Mortality estimation from registered deaths in less developed countries. *Demography*, **21**, 217–34.

Blache, D., Bouthillier, D., and Davignon, J. (1992). Acute influence of smoking on platelet behaviour, endothelium and plasma lipids and normalisation by aspirin. *Atherosclerosis*, **93**, 179–88.

Bruce, N., Perez-Padilla, R., and Albalak, R. (2000). Indoor air pollution in developing countries: a major environmental and public health challenge. *Bulletin of the World Health Organization*, **78**, 1078–92.

Davis, J. W., Shelton, J., Watanabe, I. S., and Arnold, J. (1989). Passive smoking affects endothelium and platelets. *Archives of Internal Medicine*, **149**, 386–9.

Doll, R. (1986). Tobacco: an overview of health effects. In *Tobacco: a major international health hazard* (ed. D. G. Zaridze and R. Peto), pp. 11–22. IARC Scientific Publication No. 74. International Agency for Research on Cancer, Lyon.

Doll, R. (1998). Uncovering the effects of smoking: historical perspective. *Statistical Methods in Medical Research*, **7**, 87–117.

Doll, R. and Hill, A. B. (1954). The mortality of doctors in relations to their smoking habits: a preliminary report. *British Medical Journal*, **ii**, 1451–5.

Doll, R. and Hill, A. B. (1956). Lung cancer and other causes of death in relation to smoking. *British Medical Journal*, **ii**, 1071–81.

Doll, R., Peto, R., Wheatly, K., Gray, R., and Sutherland, I. (1994). Mortality in relation to smoking: 40 years' observation on male British doctors. *British Medical Journal*, **309**, 901–11.

Du, Y. X., Cha, Q., Chen, X. W. *et al.* (1996). An epidemiological study of risk factors for lung cancer in Guangzhou, China. *Lung Cancer*, **14**, S9–S37.

Ezzati, M. and Lopez, A. D. (2003*a*). Estimating the accumulated hazards of smoking: methods, data, and global and regional estimates for 2000. *Tobacco Control*, **12**, 79–85.

Ezzati, M. and Lopez, A. D. (2003*b*). Estimates of global mortality attributable to smoking in 2000. *Lancet*, **362**, 847–52.

Ezzati, M., Lopez, A. D., Rodgers, A., Vander Hoorn, S., and Murray, C. J. L., and the Comparative Risk Assessment Collaborative Group (2002). Selected major risk factors and global and regional burden of disease. *Lancet*, **360**, 1347–60.

Fletcher, C. M. and Peto, R. (1977). The natural history of chronic airflow obstruction. *British Medical Journal*, **i**, 1645–8.

Gajalakshmi, C. K., Jha, P., Ranson, K., and Nguyen, S. N. (2000). Global patterns of smoking and smoking-attributable mortality patterns. In *Tobacco control in developing countries* (ed. P. Jha and F. J. Chaloupka), pp. 11–39. Oxford University Press, New York.

Gajalakshmi, V., Peto, R., Kanaka, T. S., and Jha, P. (2003). Smoking and mortality from tuberculosis and other diseases in India: retrospective study of 43000 adult male deaths and 35000 controls. *Lancet*, **362**, 1243–4.

Garfinkel, L. (1985). Selection, follow-up, and analysis in the American Cancer Society prospective studies. In *Selection, follow-up, and analysis in prospective studies: a workshop*. NCI Monograph 67 (ed. L. Garfinkel, O. Ochs, and M. Mushinkski), pp. 49–52. National Cancer Institute, Bethesda, MD.

Glantz, S. A. and Parmeley, W. W. (1995). Passive smoking and heart disease: mechanisms and risks. *Journal of the American Medical Association*, **273**, 1047–53.

Hill, K. (1981). Estimating census and death registration completeness. *Asian and Pacific Population Forum*, **1**, 8–13.

Hirayama, T. (1990). *Life-style and mortality: a large-scale census-based cohort study in Japan*. Karger, Tokyo.

Jedrychowski, W., Becher, H., Wahrendorf, J., and Basa-Cierpialek, Z. (1990). A case-control study of lung cancer with special reference to the effect of air pollution in Poland. *Journal of Epidemiology and Community Health*, **44**, 114–20.

Jee, S. H., Suh, I., Kim, I. S., and Appel, L. J. (1999). Smoking and atherosclerotic cardiovascular disease in men with low levels of serum cholesterol: the Korea Medical Insurance Corporation Study. *Journal of the American Medical Association*, **282**, 2149–55.

Kawachi, I., Colditz, G. A., and Stampfer, M. J. *et al.* (1997). Smoking cessation and decreased risks of total mortality, stroke, and coronary heart disease incidence among women: a prospective cohort study. In *Changes in cigarette-related disease risks and their implications for prevention and control*. Smoking and Tobacco Control Monograph No. 8 (ed. National Cancer Institute), pp. 531–64. National Cancer Institute, Bethesda, MD.

LaCroix, A. Z., Lang, J., Scherr, P. *et al.* (1991). Smoking and mortality among older men and women in three communities. *New England Journal of Medicine*, **324**, 1619–25.

Lan, Q., Chapman, R. S., Schreinemachers, D. M., Tian, L., and He, X. (2002). Household stove improvement and risk of lung cancer in Xuanwei, China. *Journal of the National Cancer Institute*, **94**, 826–35.

Law, M. R., Morris, J. K., and Wald, N. J. (1997). Environmental tobacco smoke exposure and ischaemic heart disease: an evaluation of the evidence. *British Medical Journal*, **315**, 973–80.

Lee, P. N. (1996). Mortality from tobacco in developed countries: are indirect estimates reliable. *Regulatory Toxicology and Pharmacology*, **24**, 60–8.

Liu, B. Q., Peto., R., Chen, Z. M. *et al.* (1998). Emerging tobacco hazards in China: 1. Retrospective proportional mortality study of one million deaths. *British Medical Journal*, **317**, 1411–22.

Lopez, A. D. (1999). Alcohol and smoking as risk factors. In *Health and mortality: issues of global concern* (ed. J. Chamie and R. L. Cliquet), pp. 374–411. Proceedings of the United Nations Symposium on Health and Mortality, Brussels, 19–22 November 1997. United Nations Population Division, New York.

Lopez, A. D., Ahmad, O. B., Guillot, M. *et al.* (2002). *World mortality in 2000: life tables for 191 countries*. WHO, Geneva.

Malarcher, A. M., Schuman, J., Epstein, L. A. *et al.* (2000). Methodological issues in estimating smoking-attributable mortality in the United States. *American Journal of Epidemiology*, **152**, 573–84.

Mathers, C. D., Stein, C., Ma Fat, D. *et al.* (2002). *The global burden of disease 2000: version 2, methods and results*. GPE Discussion Paper No. 36. Global Programme on Evidence for Health Policy, WHO, Geneva (available online at <http://www.who.int/evidence>).

Nyberg, F., Gustavsson, P., Jarup, L. *et al.* (2000). Urban air pollution and lung cancer in Stockholm. *Epidemiology*, **11**, 487–95.

Parish, S., Collins, R., Peto, R. *et al.* (1995). Cigarette smoking, tar yields, and non-fatal myocardial infarction: 14000 cases and 32000 controls in the United Kingdom. *British Medical Journal*, **311**, 471–7.

Parkin, D. M., Muir, C. S., Whelan, S. L., Gao, Y. T., Ferlay, J., and Powell, J. (eds) (1992). *Cancer incidence in five continents: volume VI*. IARC Scientific Publications No. 120. International Agency for Research on Cancer, Lyon.

Parkin, D. M., Whelan, S. L., Ferlay, J., and Black, R. J. (eds) (1997). *Cancer incidence in five continents: volume VII*. IARC Scientific Publications No. 143. International Agency for Research on Cancer, Lyon.

Percy, C. and Muir, C. (1989). The international comparability of cancer mortality data: results of an international death certificate study. *American Journal of Epidemiology*, **129**, 934–46.

Percy, C., Miller, B. A., Gloeckler Reis, L. A. (1990). Effect of changes in cancer classification and the accuracy of cancer death certificates on trends in cancer mortality. *Annals of New York Academy of Sciences*, **609**, 87–97.

Peto, R. (1986). *Influence of dose and duration of smoking on lung cancer rates*. In Zaridze, D. and Peto, R. (1986), pp. 22–33. International Agency for Research on Cancer, Lyon.

Peto, R. and Lopez, A. D. (2001). Future world-wide health effects of current smoking patterns. In *Critical issues in global health* (ed. E. Koop, C. E. Pearson, and M. R. Schwarz), pp. 154–61. Wiley, San Francisco.

Peto, R., Lopez, A. D., Boreham, J., Thun, M., and Heath, C., Jr. (1992). Mortality from tobacco in developed countries. *Lancet*, **339**, 1268–78.

Pope III, C. A., Eatough, D. J., Gold, D. R. *et al.* (2001). Acute exposure to environmental tobacco smoke and heart rate variability. *Environmental Health Perspectives*, **109**, 711–16.

Pope III, C. A., Burnett, R. T., Thun, M. J. *et al.* (2002). Lung cancer, cardiopulmonary mortality, and long-term exposure to fine particulate air pollution. *Journal of the American Medical Association*, **287**, 1132–41.

Preston, S. H., Heuveline, P., and Guillot, M. (2000). *Demography: measuring and modelling population processes*. Blackwell, Oxford.

Smith, K. R., Shuhua, G., Kun, H., and Daxiong, Q. (1993). One hundred million improved cookstoves in China: how was it done? *World Development*, **21**, 941–61.

Smith, K. R., Metha, S., and Maeusezahl-Feuz, M. (2004). Indoor air pollution from household solid fuel use. In *Comparative quantification of health risk: global and regional burden of disease attributable to selected major risk factors* (ed. M. Ezzati, A. D. Lopez, A. Rodgers, and C. J. L. Murray), pp. 1435–93. World Health Organization, Geneva.

Steenland, K. (1992). Passive smoking and the risk of heart disease. *Journal of the American Medical Association*, **267**, 94–9.

Sterling, T. D., Rosenbaum, W. L., and Weinkam, J. J. (1993). Risk attribution and tobacco-related deaths. *American Journal of Epidemiology*, **138**, 128–39.

Thun, M. J., Day-Lally, C. A., Calle, E. E., Flanders, W. D., and Heath, C. W., Jr. (1995). Excess mortality among cigarette smokers: changes in a 20-year interval. *American Journal of Public Health*, **85**, 1223–30.

Thun, M. J., Day-Lally, C. A., Myers, D. G. *et al.* (1997a). Trends in tobacco smoking and mortality from cigarette use in Cancer Prevention Studies I (1959 through 1965) and II (1982 through 1988). In *Changes in cigarette-related disease risks and their implications for prevention and control*. Smoking and Tobacco Control Monograph No. 8 (ed. National Cancer Institute), pp. 305–82. National Cancer Institute, Bethesda, MD.

Thun, M. J., Myers, D. G., Day-Lally, C. *et al.* (1997b). Age and exposure-response relationships between cigarette smoking and premature death in Cancer Prevention Study II. In *Age and exposure-response relationships between cigarette smoking and premature death in Cancer Prevention Study II* (ed. National Cancer Institute), pp. 383–441. National Cancer Institute, Bethesda, MD.

Thun, M. J., Apicella, L. F., and Henley, S. J. (2000). Smoking vs other risk factors as the cause of smoking-attributable mortality: confounding in the courtroom. *Journal of the American Medical Association*, **284**, 706–12.

US Department of Health and Human Services (1989). *Reducing the consequences of smoking: 25 years of progress. A report of the Surgeon General, 1989*. USDHHS, Public Health Service, Centers for Disease Control, Center for Chronic Disease Prevention and Health Promotion, Office on Smoking and Health, Bethesda, MD.

US Department of Health and Human Services (2004). *The health consequences of smoking: a report of the Surgeon General, 2004*. USDHHS, Public Health Service, Centers for Disease Control, Center for Chronic Disease Prevention and Health Promotion, Office on Smoking and Health, Bethesda, MD.

Vena, J. E. (1982). Air pollution as a risk factor in lung cancer. *American Journal of Epidemiology*, **116**, 42–56.

World Bank (1999). *Curbing the epidemic: governments and the economics of tobacco control*. World Bank, Washington, DC.

WHO (World Health Organization) (2002). *World health report 2002: reducing risks, promoting healthy life*. WHO, Geneva.

Yamaguchi, N., Mochizuki-Kobayashi, Y., and Utsunomiya, O. (2000). Quantitative relationship between cumulative cigarette smoking and lung cancer mortality in Japan. *International Journal of Epidemiology*, **29**, 963–8.

Zaridze, D. and Peto, R. (eds) (1986). *Tobacco: a major international health hazard*. IARC Scientific Publication No. 74. International Agency for Research on Cancer, Lyon.

Chapter 11

Blood pressure and the burden of coronary heart disease

C. M. M. Lawes, S. Vander Hoorn, M. R. Law,
P. Elliott, S. MacMahon, and A. Rodgers

11.1 Introduction

Blood pressure is known to be a major risk factor for coronary heart disease (CHD) and other sorts of cardiovascular disease (CVD) and a leading cause of mortality and morbidity globally (WHO 2002). Development of strategies to improve health and reduce the impact of diseases such as CHD requires a focus not only on the distribution of the disease endpoints, but also on the causes of the disease or the risks to health. Reliable analyses of the risks to health are key to preventing disease (Ezzati *et al.* 2002; WHO 2002).

Despite high blood pressure being an accepted risk factor for diseases that cause substantial morbidity and mortality worldwide (Murray and Lopez 1996), there are no global overviews of blood pressure levels by age, sex, and region, and few estimates of how much CHD morbidity and mortality is attributable to blood pressure. These analyses, when undertaken on a global scale, quantify the blood pressure-related CHD burden across different population groups. The data also provide information that can be used to estimate the potential impact of prevention strategies in different populations.

This chapter aims to present estimates of blood pressure distributions by age, sex, and world region, and to estimate the burden of CHD attributable to raised blood pressure worldwide in the year 2000. It summarizes work produced for the WHO Global Burden of Disease 2000 study and the *World Health Report 2002* (Ezzati *et al.* 2002; Lawes *et al.* 2004; WHO 2002), which included estimates of the burden of disease attributable to a variety of risk factors including blood pressure.

11.2 Methods

11.2.1 Blood pressure levels by age, sex, and subregion globally

Blood pressure can be measured as systolic blood pressure (SBP), diastolic blood pressure (DBP), and various combinations such as mean arterial pressure or pulse pressure. Throughout this chapter blood pressure will be defined in terms of SBP, as the majority of analyses have demonstrated that the association between SBP and CVD is stronger than that of DBP (Asia Pacific Cohort Studies Collaboration 2003b; Franklin *et al.* 1999, 2001; Mitchell *et al.* 1997; Miura *et al.* 2001; Sesso *et al.* 2000; Stamler *et al.* 1989, 1993). Other measures such as mean arterial pressure and pulse pressure have not been shown to be conclusively superior to SBP in terms of cardiovascular risk (Asia Pacific Cohort Studies Collaboration 2003b; Benetos 1999; Franklin *et al.* 1999, 2001; Mitchell *et al.* 1997; Sesso *et al.* 2000).

All analyses have been presented in subregions defined by the World Health Organization (WHO 2000, 2002). These 14 subregions are defined by six geographical WHO world regions (Africa, The Americas, Eastern Mediterranean, Europe, South East Asia, and the Western Pacific), which have been further divided into strata based on mortality data. The strata range from 'low child and adult mortality' (A regions) to 'high child mortality and very high adult death rates' (E regions) (WHO 2000, 2002).

Data sources

Data to estimate global blood pressure levels were collated from three major sources. First, the MONICA (Anonymous 1989*b*) and INTERSALT (Anonymous 1989*a*) studies which collected blood pressure data from a variety of world regions between 1979 and 1987. While they do not present an entirely global overview of blood pressure distributions, these studies were the largest standardized assessments of blood pressure. Second, data were obtained through a literature search using MEDLINE and the key words 'blood pressure', 'hypertension,' 'survey', 'health survey', and 'cross sectional survey.' Studies were reviewed and included in analyses if they fulfilled the following criteria: conducted from 1980 onwards; included randomly selected or representative participants; included a sample size of over 1000 in developed regions (a smaller sample size was acceptable in other regions if other criteria were fulfilled); described sample size and age group of participants; presented mean values of blood pressure by age and sex; utilized a standard protocol for blood pressure measurement. Third, data were obtained via personal communications with researchers and study investigators. This included contacting authors of surveys, data from the Asia Pacific Cohort Studies Collaboration (a collaboration involving 37 cohorts in the Asia Pacific region) (Asia Pacific Cohort Studies Collaboration 1999), and data from a previous global review of blood pressure levels (Elliott *et al.* 1999) where it fulfilled the above criteria.

Methods to obtain age-, sex-, and region-specific estimates

Detailed methods used to estimate mean blood pressure levels by age, sex, and region from survey data have been presented elsewhere (Lawes *et al.* 2004). In brief, mean SBP values, standard deviation, sample size, and age ranges from all surveys were extracted. Exploratory analyses using non-parametric methods were utilized to assess the general shape of the age–SBP association for all data combined and for each subregion and sex separately. Based on the shape of the association, regression analyses were used to estimate age-specific mean SBP levels by country. Where multiple surveys were available, data were weighted by study size within each country. Country-specific data were then combined (weighted by country population size) to provide estimates of mean SBP by age, sex, and subregion (Lawes *et al.* 2004). A similar approach was used to estimate the standard deviations for each age, sex, and region category. Confidence intervals around the means and standard deviations were also estimated to allow for uncertainty due to real study differences within a country, and the little or no data in some countries.

11.2.2 Blood pressure and the burden of CHD

Input data

To calculate the burden of CHD attributable to blood pressure, it was necessary to define a counterfactual or alternative distribution of SBP (to which current levels could be compared), to obtain estimates of relative risk of CHD per mmHg change in blood pressure, and estimate CHD burden by age, sex, and WHO subregion.

The counterfactual distribution of blood pressure The counterfactual distribution of blood pressure is defined as the theoretical minimum distribution that would yield the lowest population risk of adverse health outcomes (Murray and Lopez 1999; WHO 2002). Data from prospective cohort studies and from populations with low rates of CHD were reviewed to make a judgement on the theoretical minimum blood pressure level (Lawes *et al.* 2004).

Two major overviews of prospective cohort studies in Asia Pacific (37 cohorts and over 425 000 participants) (Asia Pacific Cohort Studies Collaboration 2003*a*) and predominantly North American and European populations (61 cohorts and almost 1 million participants) (Prospective Studies Collaboration 2002) have confirmed a continuous log linear relationship between blood pressure and CHD. The lowest demonstrated relative risk for CHD occurred at ~115 mmHg. Data on a variety of populations with little or no CVD also suggests that these typically isolated populations have low blood pressure (mean SBP < 115 mmHg), and little or no increase in blood pressure with age (Barnes 1965; Carvalho *et al.* 1989; Connor *et al.* 1978; He *et al.* 1991*a, b*; Page *et al.* 1974; Poulter and Sever 1994). Recent experimental evidence has also confirmed the benefits of blood pressure lowering to around these levels (Progress Collaborative Group 2001). The level of SBP associated with a theoretical minimum risk was therefore set at 115 mmHg for all age, sex, and region subgroups.

Relative risk relationship Prospective cohort studies provide data from which the effects of prolonged blood pressure differences can be estimated (MacMahon *et al.* 1990); that is, risk accumulation. Trials provide data about the effects of short-term blood pressure reduction (Collins *et al.* 1990), or risk reversal. Overviews or meta-analyses of these studies provide the most reliable estimates of risk as they are based on greater sample size, more endpoints, and have the power to provide reliable estimates of associations for different population subgroups (MacMahon *et al.* 1990). In general, overviews of cohort studies have corrected for regression-dilution bias (Asia Pacific Cohort Studies Collaboration 2003*a*; Eastern Stroke and Coronary Heart Disease Collaborative Research Group 1998; MacMahon *et al.* 1990; Prospective Studies Collaboration 1995, 2002), the bias that occurs when associations are calculated from 'one-off' measures of blood pressure (i.e. measures taken once on one occasion) rather than 'usual' blood pressure. These overviews were, therefore, the source of estimates of risk.

There have been four major cohort study overviews of the association between blood pressure and CVD (Asia Pacific Cohort Studies Collaboration 1999; Eastern Stroke and Coronary Heart Disease Collaborative Research Group 1998; MacMahon *et al.* 1990; Prospective Studies Collaboration 1995, 2002). At the time analyses for the *World Health Report 2002* (WHO 2002) were undertaken, age-specific data on the association between blood pressure and risk of CHD were only available from the Asia Pacific Cohort Studies Collaboration (APCSC) (Asia Pacific Cohort Studies Collaboration 2003*a*), which comprised cohorts from mainland China, Hong Kong, Taiwan, Japan, Singapore, South Korea, Australia, and New Zealand. However, subsequent analyses from another overview presented very similar results (Prospective Studies Collaboration 2002).

Overall, the results of the cohort study overviews suggest that a 10 mmHg lower SBP (or 5 mmHg lower DBP) was associated with approximately a 20–5% lower risk of CHD (Asia Pacific Cohort Studies Collaboration 2003*a*; MacMahon *et al.* 1990). There were no detectable differences in the association for fatal and non-fatal CHD, or between men and women (Asia Pacific Cohort Studies Collaboration 2003*a*; MacMahon *et al.* 1990; Prospective Studies Collaboration 2002). These results are consistent with those from several major individual cohort studies not involved in these overviews (Cooper and Ford 1992; Franklin *et al.* 2001; Haheim *et al.* 1993; Jousilahti *et al.* 1999; Keil *et al.* 1993; Neaton and Wentworth 1992; Psaty

Table 11.1 Relative risk of CHD associated with 10 mmHg lower usual SBP

Age (years)	Relative risk (%)	95% confidence interval
30–44	48	(35–58%)
45–59	40	(36–43%)
60–9	25	(21–8%)
70–9	20	(16–24%)
>80	6	(1–12%)

APCSC data used for the Global Burden of Disease 2000 study (Ezzati *et al*. 2002; Lawes *et al*. 2004; WHO 2002).

et al. 2001). Age had an important influence on the size of the association (Table 11.1). The proportional relationship was steepest for those in younger age groups, but remained strong and continuous in older age groups (Asia Pacific Cohort Studies Collaboration 2003*a*; Prospective Studies Collaboration 2002). Regional analyses within APCSC suggested that the size and shape of the association between blood pressure and CHD was broadly similar within Asian regions (China, Japan, Korea, and Other Asia) and between Asia and Australasia (Australia and New Zealand) (Asia Pacific Cohort Studies Collaboration 2003*a*). Associations did not differ between regional or ethnic population subgroups in other individual cohort studies (Cooper and Ford 1992; Garcia-Palmieri M. R. and Jr 1986; Keil *et al*. 1993, 1995).

Data from overviews of randomized controlled trials have also confirmed the reversibility of CHD with blood pressure lowering (Blood Pressure Lowering Treatment Trialists' Collaboration 2003; Collins and Peto 1994; Collins *et al*. 1990; He and Whelton 1999; Lawes *et al*. 2002; MacMahon and Rodgers 1993*a, b*; Neal *et al*. 2000; Pahor *et al*. 2000; Psaty *et al*. 1997), and demonstrated that a reduction in SBP of about 10 mmHg (or 5 mmHg DBP) resulted in about a 20–5% lower risk of CHD. Overviews of clinical trials have demonstrated that this magnitude of blood pressure reduction is associated with about a 15–20% reduction in CHD. There is some evidence that benefit in the first year is not as great as in later years (Boutitie *et al*. 1998), so overall results may underestimate the long-term benefits of blood pressure lowering. Nonetheless, since the trials lasted about 4 years on average, their results suggest that most or all of the epidemiologically expected benefits for CHD are realized within 2–3 years of blood pressure treatment (Lawes *et al*. 2002). Meta-analyses also indicate that a more intensive blood pressure regimen is associated with a greater coronary risk reduction than a less intensive regimen (Blood Pressure Lowering Treatment Trialists' Collaboration 2003; Lawes *et al*. 2002; Neal *et al*. 2000). There is some uncertainty about the size of the benefits per mmHg with different blood pressure lowering agents (see Chapter 50), but overall, any differences between agents are likely to be small in comparison to the benefits of lowering blood pressure per se.

CHD mortality and morbidity Data on CHD mortality and morbidity by age, sex, and subregion were compiled for the WHO Global Burden of Disease study (Murray *et al*. 2001). Estimates were made of cause-specific deaths and disability-adjusted life years (DALYs). DALYs were developed for the WHO Global Burden of Disease study to quantify burden of disease and disability in populations by capturing both life expectancy (or years of life lost) and some measure of quality of life (Mathers *et al*. 2001). DALYs measure the gap between current health and a hypothetical ideal for health achievement by combining years of life lost due to premature mortality and years of life lost due to disability or non-fatal conditions adjusted for severity (Mathers *et al*. 2001).

Attributable burden analyses

Population-attributable risk is the proportion of disease burden (e.g. CHD) in an exposed population that can be attributed to a particular risk factor (e.g. blood pressure) (Murray and Lopez 1999; Northridge 1995). It is calculated using a 'potential impact fraction', which estimates the proportional reduction in the total number of new (incident) cases of a certain disease that would theoretically result from a specific change in the distribution of a risk factor in the population at risk. Calculation of the potential impact fraction requires information on the distribution of a risk factor, a counterfactual distribution (i.e. the theoretical minimum) and the relative risk of a disease outcome (for all levels of the risk factor and for reversibility to the counterfactual level) (Ezzati *et al.* 2002; Murray and Lopez 1999; Northridge 1995; WHO 2002). Further details on the methodology are given elsewhere (Vander Hoorn *et al.* 2004).

$$\text{Potential Impact Fraction} = \frac{\Sigma P_x RR_x - \Sigma P'_x RR_x}{\Sigma P_x RR_x}$$

These calculations, for each age, sex, and region subgroup, result in population-attributable fractions. Attributable burden is defined as the amount of current burden that would have been observed if past levels of exposure to a risk factor had been maintained at the counterfactual or theoretical minimum distribution. It is calculated by multiplying the population-attributable fraction by the disease burden.

11.3 Results

11.3.1 Blood pressure levels by age, sex, and subregion globally

Data from about 230 studies (total sample size of over 660 000 participants) have been included in analyses. A summary of studies by region is presented in Table 11.2. The regions with the most data—studies including a total of more than 50 000 participants—were North America, Western Europe, and the Western Pacific. All other regions had data on a total of more than 2000 participants.

Non-parametric analyses demonstrated an approximately linear association between age and SBP from the age of about 30 to 70 years in males and females. This was consistent in all regions despite variation in the overall slope and starting SBP level. There were few data over the age of 70 years, but in many cohorts the association appeared to level off. It was, therefore, assumed that in all regions SBP levels increased linearly to 70 years of age in both males and females, after which (i.e. the 70–9 and ≥80 year group) levels flattened out. This approach is appropriate given the limitations of the data for those aged >70 years; it is also more conservative than assuming that the levels of SBP continue to increase with age.

Separate country-level estimates using weighted linear regression analyses were possible on nationally representative surveys from Australia, Canada, Egypt, Germany, Japan, Paraguay, the UK, and the USA. There were also sufficient survey data to utilize this approach on an additional 61 countries. Country-level estimates were combined, weighting by population size, to estimate mean SBP levels by age, sex, and subregion (Table 11.3).

. . . .

P_x = proportion of the population in the risk factor category currently;

P'_x = proportion of the population in the risk factor category in a counterfactual scenario;

R_x = relative risk for the risk factor category compared to the counterfactual distribution (or per unit change for continuous data).

Table 11.2 Countries, studies,[a] and sample size by subregion, included in current blood pressure data review

Subregion[b]	Countries and studies included	Sample size
Africa D	Gambia (van der Sande et al. 1997), Ghana (Nyarko et al. 1994), Liberia (Giles et al. 1994), Mauritius (Nan et al. 1991), Nigeria (Bunker et al. 1992; Idahosa 1985, 1987; Idahosa and Ilawole 1984; Lang et al. 1988; Ogunlesi et al. 1991; Okesina et al. 1999; Oviasu and Okupa, 1980a, b; Professor Paul Elliott 2001), Senegal (Astagneau et al. 1992), Seychelles (Bovet et al. 1991; Sierra Leone (Lisk et al. 1999)	28 457
Africa E	Democratic Republic of the Congo (M'Buyamba-Kabangu et al. 1986, 1987), Ethiopia (Pauletto et al. 1994), Kenya (Anonymous 1989a; Poulter et al. 1984), Malawi (Simmons et al. 1986), South Africa (Professor Paul Elliott 2001; Seedat et al. 1982; Steyn et al. 1985, 1996), United Republic of Tanzania (Edwards et al. 2000; Kitange et al. 1993; Swai et al. 1993), Zimbabwe (Anonymous 1989a; Dr Therese Allain 2001; Hunter et al. 2000; Mufunda et al. 2000)	35 361
America A	Canada (Anonymous 1989a, b; Joffres et al. 1992), USA (Anonymous 1989a, b; Burt et al. 1995; Hutchinson et al. 1997; National Center for Health Statistics (NCHS) 2002; Sprafka et al. 1990)	57 875
America B	Argentina (Anonymous 1989a; Professor Paul Elliott 2001), Bahamas (Professor Paul Elliott 2001), Barbados (Foster et al. 1993; Professor Paul Elliott 2001), Belize (Simmons 1983), Brazil (Anonymous 1989a; Costa et al. 1990; Fuchs et al. 2001; Professor Flavio Dannii Fuchs 2001; Professor Paul Elliott 2001; Ribeiro and Ribeiro 1986; Ribeiro et al. 1981), Chile (Dr Liliana Jadue 2001; Jadue et al. 1999; Professor Paul Elliott 2001), Colombia (Anonymous 1989a), Jamaica (Professor Paul Elliott 2001; Professor Rainford Wilks 2001), Mexico (Anonymous 1989a; Dr Liria Yamamoto 2001; Gonzalez-Villalpando et al. 1999; Professor Clicerio Gonzalez 2001; Rosenthal 1989), Paraguay (Ramirez et al. 1995), St Lucia (Khaw and Rose 1982), Trinidad and Tobago (Anonymous 1989a; Professor Paul Elliott 2001), Uruguay (Professor Paul Elliott 2001)	36 858
America D	Ecuador (Cornejo et al. 2000)	10 605
Eastern Mediterranean B	Iran (SarrafZadegan and AminiNik 1997), Jordan (Professor Hashem Jaddou and Jordan University of Science and Technology 2001), Saudi Arabia (Khalid et al. 1994; Soyannwo et al. 1998), Tunisia (Ghannem and Hadj Fredj 1997; Ghannem et al. 2001; Professor Hassan Ghannem 2001)	17 732
Eastern Mediterranean D	Egypt (Ashour et al. 1995; Ibrahim et al. 1995)	6 600

Table 11.2 Continued

Subregion[b]	Countries and studies included	Sample size
Europe A	Belgium (Anonymous 1989a, b), Czechoslovakia (Professor Paul Elliott 2001), Denmark (Andersen 1994; Anonymous 1989a, b), Finland (Anonymous 1989a, b; Professor Paul Elliott 2001; Puska et al. 1993; Vartiainen et al. 2000), France (Anonymous 1989b), Germany (Anonymous 1989a, b; Heinemann et al. 1995; Hoffmeister et al. 1994), Iceland (Anonymous 1989a, b), Italy (Anonymous 1981, 1989a, b; Fogari et al. 1997; Vaccarino et al. 1995), Israel (Gofin et al. 1995; Professor Paul Elliott 2001), Malta (Anonymous 1989a, b), The Netherlands (Anonymous 1989a; Bosma et al. 1994), Norway (Professor Paul Elliott 2001), Portugal (Anonymous 1989a), Slovenia (Professor Paul Elliott 2001), Spain (Anonymous 1989a, b; Masia et al. 1998), Sweden (Anonymous 1989b; Asplund-Carlson and Carlson 1994), Switzerland (Anonymous 1989b), UK (Anonymous 1989a, b; Bajekal et al. 1999; MacAuley et al. 1996; Mann et al. 1988; Professor Paul Elliott 2001; Shelley et al. 1991, 1995; Smith et al. 1989)	191 304
Europe B	Poland (Anonymous 1989a, b; Davis et al. 1994), Uzbekistan (King et al. 1998), Yugoslavia (Anonymous 1989b)	7 306
Europe C	Hungary (Anonymous 1989a, b), Lithuania (Bosma et al. 1994), Russia (Anonymous 1989a, b; Puska et al. 1993)	14 626
South East Asia B	Sri Lanka (Professor Paul Elliott 2001; Mendis et al. 1988)	10 109
South East Asia D	India (Anonymous 1989a; Dr B. V. Babu 2001; Dr Y. S. Kusuma 2001; Gilberts et al. 1994; Gupta et al. 1995; Misra et al. 2001; Professor Anoop Misra 2001; Professor Paul Elliott 2001; Singh et al. 1997a, b, 1998)	19 408
Western Pacific A	Australia (Anonymous 1989b; Asia Pacific Cohort Studies Secretariat 2001; Gliksman et al. 1990; Jamrozik and Hockey 1989; Professor Paul Elliott 2001), Japan (Anonymous 1989a; Asia Pacific Cohort Studies Secretariat 2001; Baba et al. 1991; Okayama et al. 1993; Sakata and Labarthe 1996; Shimamoto et al. 1989), New Zealand (Anonymous 1989b; Asia Pacific Cohort Studies Secretariat 2001; Bullen et al. 1998; Flight et al. 1984; Ministry of Health 1999), Singapore (Asia Pacific Cohort Studies Secretariat, 2001; Hughes et al. 1990; Professor Paul Elliott 2001)	83 807
Western Pacific B	China (Anonymous 1989a, b; Asia Pacific Cohort Studies Secretariat 2001; He et al. 1991a; Huang et al. 1994; Klag et al. 1993; People's Republic of China–United States Cardiovascular and Cardiopulmonary Epidemiology Research Group 1992), South Korea (Anonymous 1989a; Kim et al. 1994), Papua New Guinea (Anonymous 1989a; King et al. 1985; Lindeberg et al. 1994), Pacific (Patrick et al. 1983; Professor Paul Elliott 2001), Taiwan (Anonymous 1989a; Asia Pacific Cohort Studies Secretariat 2001)	147 752

[a] References refer to studies used to estimate blood pressure levels by age, sex, and subregion in the Global Burden of Disease 2000 study (Ezzati et al. 2002; Lawes et al. 2004; WHO 2002).

[b] A regions = very low child and very low adult mortality stratum; B regions = low child and low adult mortality stratum; C regions = low child and high adult mortality stratum; D regions = high child and high adult mortality stratum; E regions = high child and very high adult mortality stratum.

Table 11.3 Estimated mean (standard deviation) of SBP by age, sex, and subregion

Subregion	Sex and age (years)							
	Females				Males			
	30–44	45–59	60–69	≥ 70[a]	30–44	45–59	60–69	≥ 70[a]
Africa D	123	136	146	150	127	135	141	144
	(20)	(25)	(29)	(31)	(17)	(21)	(25)	(27)
Africa E	121	131	140	143	124	130	135	137
	(13)	(18)	(22)	(23)	(13)	(16)	(19)	(20)
America A	114	127	138	143	122	129	137	141
	(14)	(19)	(22)	(24)	(14)	(17)	(20)	(21)
America B	115	130	142	147	122	131	138	141
	(15)	(21)	(26)	(28)	(16)	(20)	(23)	(24)
America D	117	129	139	143	123	131	136	139
	(15)	(19)	(23)	(24)	(15)	(18)	(21)	(22)
Eastern	126	137	147	150	125	132	139	143
Mediterranean B	(15)	(17)	(19)	(20)	(15)	(19)	(22)	(24)
Eastern	121	135	146	150	123	131	138	141
Mediterranean D	(15)	(19)	(23)	(24)	(15)	(18)	(21)	(22)
Europe A	122	136	147	151	130	138	144	147
	(15)	(19)	(22)	(23)	(14)	(18)	(21)	(23)
Europe B	122	141	154	161	128	140	149	153
	(16)	(23)	(28)	(31)	(16)	(21)	(26)	(28)
Europe C	125	143	158	164	129	138	146	149
	(17)	(23)	(29)	(31)	(16)	(21)	(25)	(27)
South East Asia B	120	130	139	142	122	131	138	141
	(15)	(20)	(23)	(25)	(13)	(18)	(22)	(24)
South East Asia D	117	126	132	135	118	127	134	137
	(14)	(18)	(20)	(21)	(14)	(19)	(23)	(24)
Western Pacific A	120	133	144	148	127	137	145	148
	(15)	(18)	(21)	(22)	(15)	(18)	(21)	(22)
Western Pacific B	115	127	137	141	117	126	133	136
	(16)	(22)	(27)	(29)	(14)	(19)	(24)	(25)

Data from the Global Burden of Disease 2000 study (Ezzati *et al.* 2002; Lawes *et al.* 2004; WHO 2002).
[a] Mean SBP levels for the age group ≥80 years were taken to be the same as that in the 70–9-year age group in all subregions except America A where nationally representative data were available. In America A the mean (standard deviation) for males was 144 (21) mmHg and for females 149 (24) mmHg.

Overall, the analyses demonstrated higher SBP levels in younger males than females (e.g. 30–44-year-olds), an age-related rise in SBP in both sexes, but a steeper gradient in females resulting in them tending to have higher mean SBP levels than males in old age. While absolute SBP levels varied at a given age across regions, this general pattern was consistent across the WHO world regions. The relative ranking of regional mean SBP levels differed slightly by age and sex subgroup; however, several themes were evident. All European regions, but in particular Europe B and C, had the highest mean SBP levels. Mean SBP levels from Africa D were also relatively high. In contrast, several Asian populations (particularly in South East Asia and Western Pacific B) tended to have the lowest mean SBP levels. The relative rankings of regions were maintained when age-specific SBP levels for males and females aged 30–80 years were age standardized to the Segi world population (Waterhouse *et al.* 1982).

11.3.2 **Blood pressure and the burden of CHD**

The population-attributable fraction is the proportion of CHD disease burden that would theoretically not have occurred if the population distribution of blood pressure had been equal to that of the theoretical minimum (mean SBP = 115 mmHg). Globally, 49% of CHD was attributable to SBP > 115 mmHg (range 40–64% by subregion) (Table 11.4). Subregions with the lowest attributable fractions included America A, America D South East Asia D, and Western Pacific B. In contrast, Europe B and Europe C had the highest values, reflecting current blood pressure levels.

When applied to mortality and morbidity data, these population-attributable fractions translated into about 3 million deaths and 28 million DALYs in the year 2000. The region with the highest attributable burden was South East Asia D (650 000 deaths, 7.1 million DALYs), followed by Europe C (603 000 deaths, 5.2 million DALYs), Europe A (290 000 deaths, 2.3 million DALYs), and Western Pacific B (291 000 deaths, 2.6 million DALYs).

The attributable deaths and DALYs were higher for males than females overall in most regions (Fig. 11.1), and between 30 and 69 years. In contrast, attributable deaths and DALYs were higher for females in the oldest age groups: 70–9 and 80+ years. This was because older females have higher mean SBP (and therefore greater attributable fraction) than males, and also a larger number of cardiovascular deaths occur in older females compared to older males.

The age group with the greatest number of attributable deaths for both males and females was 70–9 years, while for DALYs it was most often 45–59 years (Fig. 11.2). This reflects the incidence, mortality, and disability rates in different age groups, as well as the absolute numbers of people. The peak was sooner for DALYs as there are less years of life lost and years of life lived with disability with advancing age. For example, overall 48% of all attributable CHD deaths were in those aged ≥ 70 years, compared to 24% of attributable DALYs; the latter theoretically provides a better measure of attributable burden.

The attributable burden of blood pressure may also be examined with respect to the level of development in different world regions. The 'developed region' includes America A, Europe A, B, and C, and Western Pacific A. The 'low mortality developing region' includes America B, Eastern Mediterranean B, and South East Asia B and Western Pacific B. Finally, the 'high mortality developing region' includes Africa D and E, America D, Eastern Mediterranean D, and South East Asia D (Fig. 11.2). There were approximately 11.6 million attributable CHD DALYs in the most developed regions, 5.8 million in the low mortality developing regions, and ~10.8 million in high mortality developing regions. (Almost one-third of the attributable DALYs in the last region occurred in South East Asia D). Overall, these figures indicate that

Table 11.4 CHD-attributable deaths and DALYS for non-optimal blood pressure by subregion

	Africa		Americas			Eastern Mediterranean		Europe			South East Asia		Western Pacific		All
	D	E	A	B	D	B	D	A	B	C	B	D	A	B	
Attributable fraction	57	46	44	50	45	55	51	54	64	63	46	41	52	41	49
Attributable deaths (000s)	82	67	203	129	13	71	176	290	263	603	100	650	51	291	2991
Attributable DALYs (000s)	893	760	1548	1303	132	811	1922	2079	2320	5239	1050	7080	400	2664	28201

Data from the Global Burden of Disease 2000 study (Ezzati et al. 2002; Lawes et al. 2004; WHO 2002).

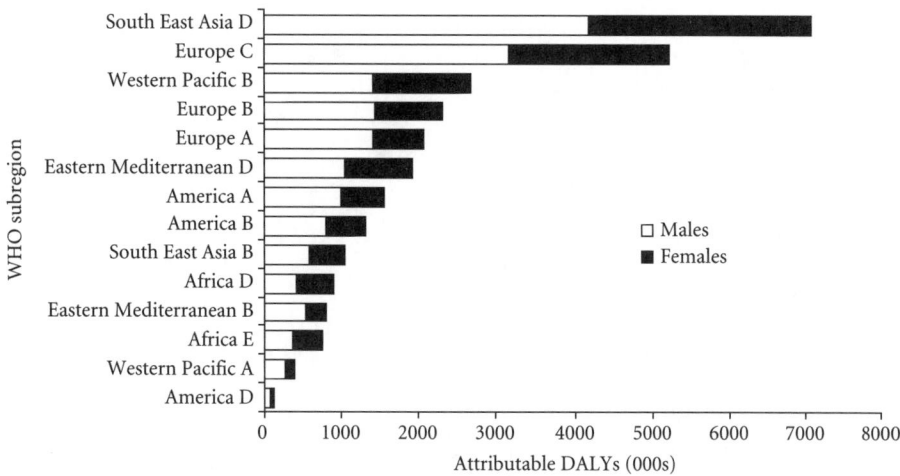

Fig. 11.1 CHD DALYS attributable to non-optimal SBP by sex and subregion. Plot based on data from the Global Burden of Disease 2000 study (Ezzati *et al.* 2002; Lawes *et al.* 2004; WHO 2002).

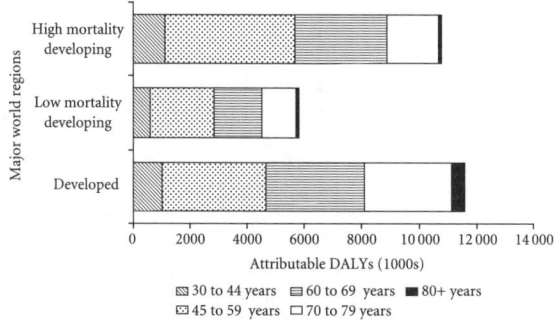

Fig. 11.2 Distribution of CHD DALYS attributable to non-optimal SBP by age and major world region. (For definition of major world regions, see text.) Plot based on data from the Global Burden of Disease 2000 study (Ezzati *et al.* 2002; Lawes *et al.* 2004; WHO 2002).

~40% of the CHD burden attributable to non-optimal blood pressure occurs in developed regions, another 40% in high mortality developing regions, and 20% in low mortality developing regions. The age distribution of the attributable burden differs across these three world regions, with a greater percentage of the burden occurring in younger age groups in developing regions. For example, ~70% of attributable CHD DALYs in developed regions occurred in 30–69-year-olds compared to ~78% in low mortality developing regions, and 82% in high mortality developing regions.

The distribution of attributable DALYs by SBP level is shown in Fig. 11.3. As can be seen, the attributable DALYS related to blood pressure are not limited to those with 'high' blood pressure, and occur over a range of blood pressure values, with about half of all DALYs occurring in those with a blood pressure of <140 mmHg (usual SBP).

The estimates amount to a large fraction of all-cause disease burden; ~5.4% of all DALYs in developed regions, 1.4% of all DALYS in the low mortality developing regions, and 1.3% of all

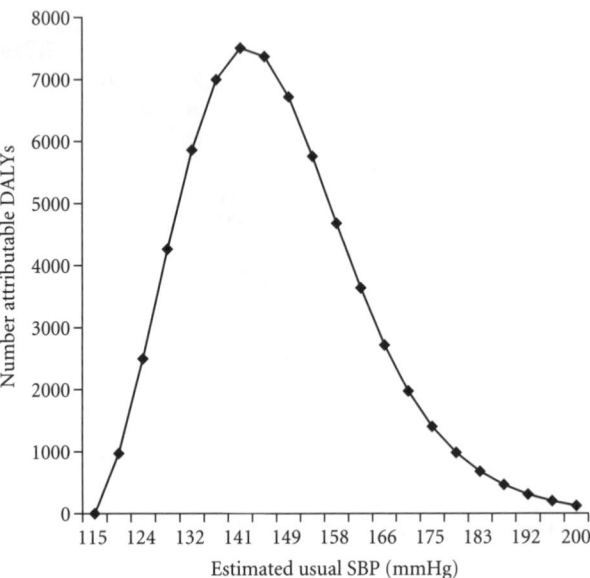

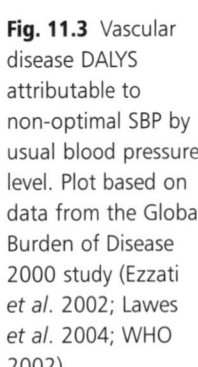

Fig. 11.3 Vascular disease DALYS attributable to non-optimal SBP by usual blood pressure level. Plot based on data from the Global Burden of Disease 2000 study (Ezzati *et al.* 2002; Lawes *et al.* 2004; WHO 2002).

DALYs in high mortality developing regions. Overall, ~5.4% of all deaths and 1.9% of DALYs in the year 2000 were estimated to be from CHD attributable to non-optimal blood pressure.

11.4 Discussion

The analyses presented in this chapter indicate that the range of mean SBP levels for any given age group was 0–25 mmHg across subregions. Estimates of the attributable burden suggested that globally about half of CHD burden was associated with non-optimal blood pressure distributions. This equated to about 3.0 million deaths and 28 million DALYs in the year 2000, and this disease burden was distributed over different age groups and world regions. Much of this CHD burden was in Eastern Europe (see Chapter 6) and Asia (see Chapter 7), and much of it was in those without hypertension.

11.4.1 Blood pressure levels by age, sex, and subregion globally

Several factors were taken into account in the analyses to improve the reliability of blood pressure distribution estimates. To minimize random error, a large number of blood pressure surveys were included, and over 70% of individual surveys had sample sizes of greater than 500. Only those surveys with random selection of participants, or collection of data from a representative sample were included. These estimates would be improved by further nationally representative surveys, especially in developing countries. At present there is still uncertainty around blood pressure estimates, particularly in those regions where limited data were available, and it is not possible to control for different methodologies used in surveys.

The shape of the age–blood pressure association demonstrated in all subregions for males and females is consistent with the literature (Franklin *et al.* 1997; Kannel 1996, 1999; Whelton 1994; Whelton *et al.* 1994). It has been suggested that the age-related changes in SBP and DBP are due to a predominance of increased peripheral vascular resistance within the blood vessels in the younger age groups (which leads to increases in both SBP and DBP), but a predominance of large artery stiffness and reduced compliance with ageing, which results in an increase in SBP, but a possible decrease in DBP (Domanski *et al.* 1999; Franklin *et al.* 1997). Reasons for the sex-related differences are unclear but shorter stature in women, and differential arterial stiffening (associated with menopause) have been suggested (London *et al.* 1995).

The results demonstrated relatively high mean SBP levels in European regions and parts of sub-Saharan Africa, which is also consistent with the literature (Cooper *et al.* 1998; Fuentes *et al.* 2000; Kaufman and Barkey 1993; Seedat 2000; Wolf *et al.* 1997). Both genetic and environmental factors are likely to play a role in determining blood pressure levels. Assessing the relative importance of each is difficult, and it is likely to vary between individuals and populations. There is evidence that differences in blood pressure levels in the same ethnic group living in different areas can be greater than those for different ethnic groups living in the same area (Ueshima *et al.* 2000) and that differences in blood pressure between populations are more marked in older age groups (Marmot 1984), possibly reflecting differences in lifetime exposures. There is also considerable evidence that mean blood pressure levels in a given population can change over time (Burt *et al.* 1995; Capewell *et al.* 1999; Garraway and Whisnant 1987; McGovern *et al.* 1996; Sakata and Labarthe 1996; Ueshima *et al.* 2000; Vartiainen *et al.* 1994; Wu *et al.* 1996) and with migration to more urbanized settings (He *et al.* 1991*a, b*; Joseph *et al.* 1983; Poulter and Sever 1994; Poulter *et al.* 1988, 1990; Salmond *et al.* 1985, 1989). These data all suggest that while genetics may play a role, more important determinants of population blood pressure level are likely to include body weight (Anonymous 1997; Appel *et al.* 1997; Leiter *et al.* 1999; National High Blood Pressure Education Program Working Group 1993; Whelton *et al.* 1998), physical activity (Anonymous 1997; Anonymous 1999; Arroll and Beaglehole 1993; Cleroux *et al.* 1999; National High Blood Pressure Education Program Working Group 1993), dietary sodium (Elliott *et al.* 1996; Law *et al.* 1991; Midgley *et al.* 1996; Whelton *et al.* 1998), intake of fruit and vegetables, dairy products, and saturated and total fat (Appel *et al.* 1997), and alcohol intake (Campbell *et al.* 1999; Kaplan 1995). Chapter 43 covers these factors in more detail than we can here. The differences in blood pressure demonstrated between regions are, therefore, likely to primarily reflect these environmental (including socio-cultural, demographic, and economic) factors, rather than predominantly genetic differences.

11.4.2 Blood pressure and the burden of CHD

The estimates of attributable burden required a variety of data in addition to estimates of mean blood pressure levels. The estimates of relative risk were taken from a large-scale overview of cohort studies, which is less likely to be biased than individual study data (Asia Pacific Cohort Studies Collaboration 1999). Estimates of CHD deaths and DALYs were made by WHO and whilst they may be sensitive to limited data in some regions, they are currently the most reliable and internally consistent estimates available.

The estimates of attributable burden presented have only focused on one of several cardiovascular outcomes affected by blood pressure. The Global Burden of Disease 2000 study (Ezzati *et al.* 2002; Lawes *et al.* 2004; WHO 2002) on which this chapter is based also estimated the burden of other CVD endpoints attributable to non-optimal blood pressure, and also the disease burden attributable to a variety of other risk factors. Overall, the analyses indicated that about two-thirds of stroke, one-half of CHD, and about one-sixth of other CVD was attributable to non-optimal blood pressure. Worldwide, 7.1 million deaths (about 12.8% of the total) and 64.3 million DALYs (4.4% of the total) were estimated to be due to non-optimal blood pressure (Ezzati *et al.* 2002; Lawes *et al.* 2004; WHO 2002). Globally, blood pressure ranked as the third most important risk factor (in terms of attributable DALYs), behind underweight and unsafe sex. It ranked second most important in developed regions (behind tobacco), and low mortality developing regions (behind alcohol). Of interest, it was also among the leading 10 selected risk factors in high mortality developing regions (Ezzati *et al.* 2002; Lawes *et al.* 2004; WHO 2002). Overall, the results suggest that a considerable proportion of CVD is related to non-optimal blood pressure and this translates into an important portion of all deaths and years of life lost to deaths and disability worldwide.

The analyses presented relate to individual risk factors and most diseases have multiple causal factors. Individual population-attributable fractions of multiple risk factors for a given endpoint often sum to greater than 100%. This is due to the 'overlapping,' or multi-causal aetiology of diseases. Preliminary analyses have estimated the joint contribution of a variety of risk factors to CVD (WHO 2002). These results suggest that ~80–90% of the global CHD burden is attributable to the impact of non-optimal levels of blood pressure, total cholesterol, body mass index, physical activity, fruit and vegetable intake, smoking, alcohol, and tobacco (Ezzati *et al.* 2003).

The current estimates are approximately double those of the Global Burden of Disease estimates for 1990 (Elliott *et al.* 1999; Murray and Lopez 1996, 1997). (Worldwide, 5.8% of deaths and 1.4% of DALYs were attributable to blood pressure in 1990 compared to 12.8% of deaths and 4.4% of DALYs in these analyses.) This is largely due to correction for regression-dilution bias in the current analyses. This bias occurs when relative risk estimates are based on one-off measures of blood pressure (i.e. taken at one point in time) which are subject to random fluctuations (MacMahon *et al.* 1990). Correcting for this bias with re-measurement data results in 'regression to the mean' of blood pressure values (MacMahon 1994), and a steeper association between blood pressure and disease outcomes (MacMahon *et al.* 1990). Without correction for this bias there will be systematic underestimation of risk of CVD by a factor of about two (MacMahon *et al.* 1990).

11.4.3 Implications of results

A primary objective of undertaking burden of disease analyses is to provide information to inform prevention, and ultimately, to improve population health (Ezzati *et al.* 2002; WHO 2002), and several key results have emerged from the analyses.

A major input into developing effective prevention strategies is an understanding of both the determinants of disease and the distribution of these risks within and across populations. Estimates of mean SBP by age, sex, and subregion have an important role in public health surveillance. Risk factor prevalence not only complements surveillance data on disease occurrence, but may also provide important health information where disease outcome data are limited, and/or contribute to predictions of future disease burden (Bonita *et al.* 2001; Buehler 1998). With standardization of the methodology used in blood pressure surveys, comparison across different regions is meaningful, and data may be available for a wide range of world regions, including those where data on disease rates may be scarce. There is a need for more standardized surveys, particularly in the developing world.

The results demonstrated that a substantial proportion of CHD (and all CVD) is attributable to non-optimal blood pressure levels. This blood pressure-related burden is not experienced by one specific subgroup of the population, as it occurs across all ages, world regions, and blood pressure levels. While there are some subgroups that experience a greater absolute amount or proportion of this burden, the results confirm the observations of Rose and others that, as with the majority of diseases, 'nature presents us with a process or continuum, but not a dichotomy' (Rose 1992). Labels such as 'hypertensive' and 'normotensive' do not adequately reflect where the burden of disease occurs, as about half of the burden of vascular disease is estimated to occur in those with a usual SBP of less than 140 mmHg. This reflects one of Rose's most fundamental axioms of preventive medicine: 'a large number of people exposed to a small risk may generate many more cases than a small number exposed to high risk' (Rose 1992). This was also apparent when the burden of disease across subregions was compared. The relative CHD burden attributable to non-optimal blood pressure was greatest in those regions with the highest blood pressure, but in absolute terms the greatest burden occurred in the most populous regions of the world.

This means that in terms of prevention, and reduction of the burden of CHD, blood pressure-lowering strategies should not dichotomize groups by blood pressure levels into 'hypertensive' and 'normotensive', as this gives the erroneous impression that those who are 'normal' have no cause for concern (Rose 1989, 1992). Strategies should aim to tackle underlying causes of disease and to reduce the risk profile in entire populations, as 'a relatively small downward shift in the distribution of a risk factor throughout the entire population might have unexpected large benefits by comparison with the identification and treatment of individuals in the upper tail of the distribution' (Strachan and Rose 1991). Strategies could include reduced salt and saturated fat in manufactured foods, environmental change promoting physical activity and weight reduction (Anonymous 1997, 1999; Cleroux et al. 1999; Fodor et al. 1999; Leiter et al. 1999; Ramsay et al. 1999).

The population-wide approaches should be coupled with attempts to identify and treat those at greatest absolute risk of a CHD event. An absolute risk-based strategy involves treating those over a threshold of absolute risk, and aims to prevent more events per unit of treatment provided. It can involve consideration of treatment of those with mild to moderate hypertension (Jackson et al. 1993), or even those with average or below average (but still non-optimal) blood pressure (Murray et al. 2003). A variety of equations to estimate absolute risk have been derived, most notably from the Framingham data (Anderson et al. 1991a, b; Jackson et al. 1993), but there are several other examples (Haq et al. 1999; Shaper et al. 1986; Tunstall-Pedoe 1991, see Chapter 39). These preventive approaches should be viewed as complementary as the population-wide approach effectively broadens the coverage of prevention strategies aimed at those at highest absolute risk of CHD.

Acknowledgements

Particular acknowledgements to The Asia Pacific Cohort Studies Collaboration secretariat, and all study collaborators for allowing us to access and analyse their data for estimates of mean blood pressure levels and relative risk; Sarah Lewington of the Prospective Studies Collaboration for assistance with analyses and helpful advice; Varsha Parag and Derrick Bennett for biostatistical support, including analyses of data from the Asia Pacific Cohort Studies Collaboration; Angela Hurley for research assistance; Clarissa Gould-Thorpe for secretarial support.

References

Andersen, L. B. (1994). Blood pressure, physical fitness and physical activity in 17-year-old Danish adolescents. *Journal of Internal Medicine*, **236**, 323–9.

Anderson, K. M., Odell, P. M., Wilson, P. W., and Kannel, W. B. (1991a). Cardiovascular disease risk profiles. *American Heart Journal*, **121**, 293–8.

Anderson, K. M., Wilson, P. W., Odell, P. M., and Kannel, W. B. (1991b). An updated coronary risk profile. A statement for health professionals. *Circulation*, **83**, 356–62.

Anonymous (1981). Distribution of some risk factors for atherosclerosis in nine Italian population samples. *American Journal of Epidemiology*, **113**, 338–46.

Anonymous (1989*a*). The INTERSALT Co-operative Research Group. Appendix tables. Centre-specific results by age and sex. *Journal of Human Hypertension*, **3**, 331–407.

Anonymous (1989*b*). The WHO MONICA Project. A worldwide monitoring system for cardiovascular diseases: cardiovascular mortality and risk factors in selected communities. *World Health Stat A*, 27–149.

Anonymous (1997). The sixth report of the Joint National Committee on prevention, detection, evaluation, and treatment of high blood pressure. *Archives of Internal Medicine*, **157**, 2413–46.

Anonymous (1999). 1999 World Health Organization–International Society of Hypertension Guidelines for the Management of Hypertension. *Journal of Hypertension*, **17**, 151–83.

Appel, L. J., Moore, T. J., Obarzanek, E., Vollmer, W. M., Svetkey, L. P., Sacks, F. M. *et al.* (1997). A clinical trial of the effects of dietary patterns on blood pressure. *New England Journal of Medicine*, **336**, 1117–24.

Arroll, B. and Beaglehole, R. (1993). Exercise for hypertension. *Lancet*, **341**, 1248–9.

Ashour, Z., Ibrahim, M. M., Appel, L. J., Ibrahim, A. S., and Whelton, P. K. (1995). The Egyptian National Hypertension Project (NHP). Design and rationale. *Hypertension*, **26**, 880–5.

Asia Pacific Cohort Studies Collaboration (1999). Determinants of cardiovascular disease in the Asia Pacific region: protocol for a collaborative overview of cohort studies. *CVD Prevention*, **2**, 281–9.

Asia Pacific Cohort Studies Collaboration (2003*a*). Blood pressure and cardiovascular disease in the Asia Pacific region. *Journal of Hypertension*, **21**, 707–16.

Asia Pacific Cohort Studies Collaboration (2003*b*). Blood pressure indices and cardiovascular disease in the Asia Pacific region: a pooled analysis. *Hypertension*, **42**, 69–75.

Asia Pacific Cohort Studies Secretariat (2001). Personal communication.

Asplund-Carlson, A., and Carlson, L. A. (1994). Studies in hypertriglyceridaemia. 1. Serum triglyceride distribution and its correlates in randomly selected Swedish middle-aged men. *Journal of Internal Medicine*, **236**, 57–64.

Astagneau, P., Lang, T., Delarocque, E., Jeannee, E., and Salem, G. (1992). Arterial hypertension in urban Africa: an epidemiological study on a representative sample of Dakar inhabitants in Senegal. *Journal of Hypertension*, **10**, 1095–101.

Baba, S., Pan, W. H., Ueshima, H., Ozawa, H., Komachi, Y., Stamler, R. *et al.* (1991). Blood pressure levels, related factors, and hypertension control status of Japanese and Americans. *Journal of Human Hypertension*, **5**, 317–32.

Bajekal, M., Boreham, R., Erens, B., Falaschetti, E., Hirani, V., Primatesta, P. *et al.* (1999). Health Survey for England 1998. London: The Department of Health, London.

Barnes, R. (1965). Comparisons of blood pressure and blood cholesterol levels in New Guineans and Australians. *Medical Journal of Australia*, **1**, 611–17.

Benetos, A. (1999). Pulse pressure and cardiovascular risk. *Journal of Hypertension*, **17**, S21–4.

Blood Pressure Lowering Treatment Trialists' Collaboration (2003). Effects of different blood-pressure-lowering regimens on major cardiovascular events: results of prospectively-designed overviews of randomised trials. *Lancet*, **362**, 1527–35.

Bonita, R., De Courten, M., Dwyer, T., Jamrozik, K. D., and Winkelmann, R. (2001). Surveillance of risk factors for non-communicable disease: the WHO STEPwise approach. Geneva: World Health Organization.

Bosma, H., Appels, A., Sturmans, F., Grabauskas, V., and Gostautas, A. (1994). Differences in mortality and coronary heart disease between Lithuania and The Netherlands: results from the WHO Kaunas-Rotterdam Intervention Study (KRIS). *International Journal of Epidemiology*, **23**, 12–19.

Boutitie, F., Gueyffier, F., Pocock, S. J., and Boissel, J. P. (1998). Assessing treatment-time interaction in clinical trials with time to event data: a meta-analysis of hypertension trials. *Statistics in Medicine*, **17**, 2883–903.

Bovet, P., Shamlaye, C., Kitua, A., Riesen, W. F., Paccaud, F., and Darioli, R. (1991). High prevalence of cardiovascular risk factors in the Seychelles (Indian Ocean). *Arteriosclerosis and Thrombosis*, **11**, 1730–6.

Buehler, J. W. (1998). In *Modern epidemiology* (ed. K. J. Rothman and S. Greenland), pp. 435–7. Philadelphia: Lippincott-Raven Publishers.

Bullen, C., Simmons, G., Trye, P., Lay-Yee, R., Bonita, R., and Jackson, R. (1998). Cardiovascular disease risk factors in 65–84 year old men and women: results from the Auckland University Heart and Health Study 1993–4. *New Zealand Medical Journal*, **111**, 4–7.

Bunker, C. H., Ukoli, F. A., Nwankwo, M. U., Omene, J. A., Currier, G. W., Holifield-Kennedy, L. *et al.* (1992). Factors associated with hypertension in Nigerian civil servants. *Preventive Medicine*, **21**, 710–22.

Burt, V. L., Culter, J. A., Higgins, M., Horan, M. J., Labarthe, D., Whelton, P. *et al.* (1995). Trends in the prevalence, awareness, treatment, and control of hypertension in the adult US population. Data from the health examination surveys, 1960 to 1991. *Hypertension*, **26**, 60–9.

Campbell, N. R., Ashley, M. J., Carruthers, S. G., Lacourciere, Y., and McKay, D. W. (1999). Lifestyle modifications to prevent and control hypertension. 3. Recommendations on alcohol consumption. *Canadian Medical Association Journal*, **160**, S13–20.

Capewell, S., Morrison, C. E., and McMurray, J. J. (1999). Contribution of modern cardiovascular treatment and risk factor changes to the decline in coronary heart disease mortality in Scotland between 1975 and 1994. *Heart*, **81**, 380–6.

Carvalho, J. J., Baruzzi, R. G., Howard, P. F., Poulter, N., Alpers, M. P., Franco, L. J. *et al.* (1989). Blood pressure in four remote populations in the INTERSALT Study. *Hypertension*, **14**, 238–46.

Cleroux, J., Feldman, R. D., and Petrella, R. J. (1999). Lifestyle modifications to prevent and control hypertension. 4. Recommendations on physical exercise training. *Canadian Medical Association Journal*, **160**, S21–8.

Collins, R. and Peto, R. (1994). Antihypertensive drug therapy: effects on stroke and coronary heart disease. In *Textbook of Hypertension*, (ed. J. D. Swales), pp. 11–21. Oxford: Blackwell Scientific Publications.

Collins, R., Peto, R., MacMahon, S., Hebert, P., Fiebach, N. H., Eberlein, K. A. *et al.* (1990). Blood pressure, stroke, and coronary heart disease. Part 2, short-term reductions in blood pressure: overview of randomised drug trials in their epidemiological context. *Lancet*, **335**, 827–38.

Connor, W. E., Cerqueira, M. T., Connor, R. W., Wallace, R. B., Malinow, M. R., and Casdorph, H. R. (1978). The plasma lipids, lipoproteins, and diet of the Tarahumara indians of Mexico. *American Journal of Clinical Nutrition*, **31**, 1131–42.

Cooper, R. S. and Ford, E. (1992). Comparability of risk factors for coronary heart disease among blacks and whites in the NHANES-I Epidemiologic Follow-up Study. *Annals of Epidemiology*, **2**, 637–45.

Cooper, R. S., Rotimi, C. N., Kaufman, J. S., Muna, W. F., and Mensah, G. A. (1998). Hypertension treatment and control in sub-Saharan Africa: the epidemiological basis for policy. *British Medical Journal*, **316**, 614–17.

Cornejo, C., Vinueza, R., Moscoso, F., Calero, E., Gonzalez, G., Perugachi, C. *et al.* (2000). Prevalence of arterial hypertension in the urban adult population of Ecuador: Quito, guayaquil, and Cuenca–the PREHTAE study. *Cvd Prevention*, **3**, 47–58.

Costa, E., Rose, G. A., Klein, C. H., Leal, M., Szwarcwald, C. L., Bassanesi, S. L. *et al.* (1990). Salt and blood pressure in Rio Grande do Sul, Brazil. *Bulletin of the Pan American Health Organization*, **24**, 159–76.

Davis, C. E., Pajak, A., Rywik, S., Williams, D. H., Broda, G., Pazucha, T., and Ephross, S. (1994). Natural menopause and cardiovascular disease risk factors. The Poland and US Collaborative Study on Cardiovascular Disease Epidemiology. *Annals of Epidemiology*, **4**, 445–8.

Domanski, M. J., Davis, B. R., Pfeffer, M. A., Kastantin, M., and Mitchell, G. F. (1999). Isolated systolic hypertension : prognostic information provided by pulse pressure. *Hypertension*, **34**, 375–80.

Dr B. V. Babu, Indian Council of Medical Research and India (2001). Personal communication.

Dr Liliana Jadue, Diagonal Paraguay and Santiago Chile (2001). Personal communication.

Dr Liria Yamamoto, Facultad de Medicina and Mexico (2001). Personal communication.

Dr Therese Allain, Southmead Hospital and England (2001). Personal communication.

Dr Y. S. Kusuma, Indian Council of Medical Research and India (2001). Personal communication.

Eastern Stroke and Coronary Heart Disease Collaborative Research Group (1998). Blood pressure, cholesterol, and stroke in eastern Asia. *Lancet*, **352**, 1801–7.

Edwards, R., Unwin, N., Mugusi, F., Whiting, D., Rashid, S., Kissima, J. *et al.* (2000). Hypertension prevalence and care in an urban and rural area of Tanzania. *Journal of Hypertension*, **18**, 145–52.

Elliott, P., Stamler, J., Nichols, R., *et al.* for the INTERSALT Cooperative Research Group (1996). INTERSALT revisited: Further analyses of 24 hour sodium excretion and blood pressure within and across populations. *BMJ*, **312**, 1249–53.

Elliott, P., Nichols, R., and Chee, D. (1999). Quantifying risk of death and disability associated with raised blood pressure. *Clinical and Experimental Hypertension (New York)*, **21**, 571–82.

Ezzati, M., Lopez, A. D., Rodgers, A., Vander Hoorn, S., Murray, C. J. L., and the Comparative Risk Assessment Collaborating Group (2002). Selected major risk factors and global and regional burden of disease. *Lancet*, **360**, 1347–60.

Ezzati, M., Vander Hoorn, S., Rodgers, A., Lopez, A. D., Mathers, C. D., Murray, C. J. L., and the Comparative Risk Assessment Collaborating Group (2003). Estimates of global and regional potential health gains from reducing multiple major risk factors. *Lancet*, **362**, 271–80.

Flight, R. J., McKenzie-Pollock, M., Hamilton, M. A., Salmond, C. E., and Stokes, Y. M. (1984). The health status of fourth form students in Northland. *New Zealand Medical Journal*, **97**, 1–6.

Fodor, J. G., Whitmore, B., Leenen, F., and Larochelle, P. (1999). Lifestyle modifications to prevent and control hypertension. 5. Recommendations on dietary salt. *Canadian Medical Association Journal*, **160**, S29–34.

Fogari, R., Zoppi, A., Marasi, G., Preti, P., Mugellini, A., Vanasia, A., and Lusardi, P. (1997). The epidemiology of resting heart rate in a male working population: association with blood pressure, age, smoking habits and other cardiovascular risk factors. *Journal of Cardiovascular Risk*, **4**, 209–13.

Foster, C., Rotimi, C., Fraser, H., Sundarum, C., Liao, Y., Gibson, E. *et al.* (1993). Hypertension, diabetes, and obesity in Barbados: findings from a recent population-based survey. *Ethnicity & Disease*, **3**, 404–12.

Franklin, S. S., Gustin, W. T., Wong, N. D., Larson, M. G., Weber, M. A., Kannel, W. B., and Levy, D. (1997). Hemodynamic patterns of age-related changes in blood pressure. The Framingham Heart Study. *Circulation*, **96**, 308–15.

Franklin, S. S., Khan, S. A., Wong, N. D., Larson, M. G., and Levy, D. (1999). Is pulse pressure useful in predicting risk for coronary heart Disease? The Framingham heart study. *Circulation*, **100**, 354–60.

Franklin, S. S., Larson, M. G., Khan, S. A., Wong, N. D., Leip, E. P., Kannel, W. B., and Levy, D. (2001). Does the Relation of blood pressure to coronary heart disease risk change with aging? The Framingham Heart Study. *Circulation*, **103**, 1245–9.

Fuchs, S. C., Petter, J. G., Accordi, M. C., Zen, V. L., Pizzol, A. D., Jr, Moreira, L. B., and Fuchs, F. D. (2001). Establishing the prevalence of hypertension. Influence of sampling criteria. *Arquivos Brasileiros de Cardiologia*, **76**, 445–52.

Fuentes, R., Ilmaniemi, N., Laurikainen, E., Tuomilehto, J., and Nissinen, A. (2000). Hypertension in developing economies: a review of population-based studies carried out from 1980 to 1998. *Journal of Hypertension*, **18**, 521–9.

Garcia-Palmieri M. R. and Jr, C. R. (1986). In *Progress in cardiology*, Vol. 14 (ed. P. N. Yu and J. F. Goodwin), pp. 101–90. Lea & Febiger, Philadelphia.

Garraway, W. M. and Whisnant, J. P. (1987). The changing pattern of hypertension and the declining incidence of stroke. *Journal of the American Medical Association*, **258**, 214–17.

Ghannem, H. and Hadj Fredj, A. (1997). Prevalence of cardiovascular risk factors in the urban population of Soussa in Tunisia. *Journal of Public Health Medicine*, **19**, 392–6.

Ghannem, H., Darioli, R., Limam, K., Harrabi, I., Gaha, R., Trabelsi, L. *et al.* (2001). Epidemiology of cardiovascular risk factors among schoolchildren in Sousse, Tunisia. *Journal of Cardiovascular Risk*, **8**, 87–91.

Gilberts, E. C., Arnold, M. J., and Grobbee, D. E. (1994). Hypertension and determinants of blood pressure with special reference to socioeconomic status in a rural south Indian community. *Journal of Epidemiology and Community Health*, **48**, 258–61.

Giles, W. H., Pacque, M., Greene, B. M., Taylor, H. R., Munoz, B., Cutler, M., and Douglas, J. (1994). Prevalence of hypertension in rural west Africa. *American Journal of the Medical Sciences*, **308**, 271–5.

Gliksman, M. D., Dwyer, T., and Wlodarczyk, J. (1990). Differences in modifiable cardiovascular disease risk factors in Australian schoolchildren: the results of a nationwide survey. *Preventive Medicine*, **19**, 291–304.

Gofin, J., Kark, J. D., Abramson, J. H., and Epstein, L. (1995). Trends in blood pressure levels over time in middle-aged and elderly Jerusalem residents. *European Heart Journal*, **16**, 1988–94.

Gonzalez-Villalpando, C., Stern, M. P., Haffner, S. M., Gonzalez-Villapando, M. E., Gaskill, S., and Rivera Martinez, D. (1999). Prevalence of hypertension in a Mexican population according to the Sixth Report of the Joint National Committee on Prevention, Detection, Evaluation and Treatment of High Blood Pressure. *Journal of Cardiovascular Risk*, **6**, 177–81.

Gupta, R., Guptha, S., Gupta, V. P., and Prakash, H. (1995). Prevalence and determinants of hypertension in the urban population of Jaipur in western India. *Journal of Hypertension*, **13**, 1193–200.

Haheim, L. L., Holme, I., Hjermann, I., and Leren, P. (1993). The predictability of risk factors with respect to incidence and mortality of myocardial infarction and total mortality. A 12-year follow-up of the Oslo Study, Norway. *Journal of Internal Medicine*, **234**, 17–24.

Haq, I. U., Ramsay, L. E., Yeo, W. W., Jackson, P. R., and Wallis, E. J. (1999). Is the Framingham risk function valid for northern European populations? A comparison of methods for estimating absolute coronary risk in high risk men. *Heart*, **81**, 40–6.

He, J. and Whelton, P. K. (1999). Elevated systolic blood pressure as a risk factor for cardiovascular and renal disease. *Journal of Hypertension*, **17** (Suppl.), S7–13.

He, J., Klag, M. J., Whelton, P. K., Chen, J. Y., Mo, J. P., Qian, M. C. *et al.* (1991a). Migration, blood pressure pattern, and hypertension: the Yi Migrant Study. *American Journal of Epidemiology*, **134**, 1085–101.

He, J., Tell, G. S., Tang, Y. C., Mo, P. S., and He, G. Q. (1991b). Effect of migration on blood pressure: the Yi People Study. *Epidemiology*, **2**, 88–97.

Heinemann, L., Barth, W., and Hoffmeister, H. (1995). Trend of cardiovascular risk factors in the East German population 1968–1992. *Journal of Clinical Epidemiology*, **48**, 787–95.

Hoffmeister, H., Mensink, G. B., and Stolzenberg, H. (1994). National trends in risk factors for cardiovascular disease in Germany. *Preventive Medicine*, **23**, 197–205.

Huang, Z., Wu, X., Stamler, J., Rao, X., Tao, S., Friedewald, W. T. *et al.* (1994). A north-south comparison of blood pressure and factors related to blood pressure in the People's Republic of China: a report from the PRC-USA Collaborative Study of Cardiovascular Epidemiology. *Journal of Hypertension*, **12**, 1103–12.

Hughes, K., Yeo, P. P., Lun, K. C., Thai, A. C., Sothy, S. P., Wang, K. W. *et al.* (1990). Cardiovascular diseases in Chinese, Malays, and Indians in Singapore. II. Differences in risk factor levels. *Journal of Epidemiology and Community Health*, **44**, 29–35.

Hunter, J. M., Sparks, B. T., Mufunda, J., Musabayane, C. T., Sparks, H. V., and Mahomed, K. (2000). Economic development and women's blood pressure: field evidence from rural Mashonaland, Zimbabwe. *Social Science & Medicine*, **50**, 773–95.

Hutchinson, R. G., Watson, R. L., Davis, C. E., Barnes, R., Brown, S., Romm, F. *et al.* (1997). Racial differences in risk factors for atherosclerosis. The ARIC Study. Atherosclerosis Risk in Communities. *Angiology*, **48**, 279–90.

Ibrahim, M. M., Rizk, H., Appel, L. J., el Aroussy, W., Helmy, S., Sharaf, Y. *et al.* (1995). Hypertension prevalence, awareness, treatment, and control in Egypt. Results from the Egyptian National Hypertension Project (NHP). *Hypertension*, 26, 886–90.

Idahosa, P. E. (1985). Blood pressure pattern in urban Edos. *Journal of Hypertension*, 3 (Suppl.), S379–81.

Idahosa, P. E. (1987). Hypertension: an ongoing health hazard in Nigerian workers. *American Journal of Epidemiology*, 125, 85–91.

Idahosa, P. E. and Ilawole, M. (1984). Towards Nigeria's first National Blood Pressure Survey: a pilot study of arterial blood pressure in members of the National Youth Service Corps. *Journal of Hypertension*, 2 (Suppl.), S209–11.

Jackson, R., Barham, P., Bills, J., Birch, T., McLennan, L., MacMahon, S., and Maling, T. (1993). Management of raised blood pressure in New Zealand: a discussion document. *British Medical Journal*, 307, 107–10.

Jadue, L., Vega, J., Escobar, M. C., Delgado, I., Garrido, C., Lastra, P. *et al.* (1999). Risk factors for non communicable diseases: methods and global results of the CARMEN program basal survey. *Revista Medica de Chile*, 127, 1004–13.

Jamrozik, K. and Hockey, R. (1989). Trends in risk factors for vascular disease in Australia. *Medical Journal of Australia*, 150, 14–18.

Joffres, M. R., Hamet, P., Rabkin, S. W., Gelskey, D., Hogan, K., and Fodor, G. (1992). Prevalence, control and awareness of high blood pressure among Canadian adults. *Canadian Medical Association Journal*, 146, 1997–2005.

Joseph, J. G., Prior, I. A., Salmond, C. E., and Stanley, D. (1983). Elevation of systolic and diastolic blood pressure associated with migration: the Tokelau island migrant study. *Journal of Chronic Diseases*, 36, 507–16.

Jousilahti, P., Vartiainen, E., Tuomilehto, J., and Puska, P. (1999). Sex, age, cardiovascular risk factors, and coronary heart disease: a prospective follow-up study of 14 786 middle-aged men and women in Finland. *Circulation*, 99, 1165–72.

Kannel, W. B. (1996). Blood pressure as a cardiovascular risk factor: prevention and treatment. *Journal of the American Medical Association*, 275, 1571–6.

Kannel, W. B. (1999). Historic perspectives on the relative contributions of diastolic and systolic blood pressure elevation to cardiovascular risk profile. *American Heart Journal*, 138, 205–10.

Kaplan, N. M. (1995). Alcohol and hypertension. *Lancet*, 345, 1588–9.

Kaufman, J. and Barkey, N. (1993). Hypertension in Africa: an overview of prevalence rates and causal risk factors. *Ethnicity & Disease*, 3, S83–101.

Keil, J. E., Sutherland, S. E., Knapp, R. G., Lackland, D. T., Gazes, P. C., and Tyroler, H. A. (1993). Mortality rates and risk factors for coronary disease in black as compared with white men and women. *New England Journal of Medicine*, 329, 73–8.

Keil, J. E., Sutherland, S. E., Hames, C. G., Lackland, D. T., Gazes, P. C., Knapp, R. G., and Tyroler, H. A. (1995). Coronary disease mortality and risk factors in black and white men. Results from the combined Charleston, SC, and Evans County, Georgia, heart studies. *Archives of Internal Medicine*, 155, 1521–7.

Khalid, M. E., Ali, M. E., Ahmed, E. K., and Elkarib, A. O. (1994). Pattern of blood pressures among high and low altitude residents of southern Saudi Arabia. *Journal of Human Hypertension*, 8, 765–9.

Khaw, K. T. and Rose, G. (1982). Population study of blood pressure and associated factors in St Lucia, West Indies. *International Journal of Epidemiology*, 11, 372–7.

Kim, J. S., Jones, D. W., Kim, S. J., and Hong, Y. P. (1994). Hypertension in Korea: a national survey. *American Journal of Preventive Medicine*, 10, 200–4.

King, H., Collins, A., King, L. F., Heywood, P., Alpers, M., Coventry, J., and Zimmet, P. (1985). Glucose intolerance and associated factors in the Fergana Valley, Uzbekistan. *Journal of Epidemiology and Community Health*, 39, 215–19.

King, H., Abdullaev, B., Djumaeva, S., Nikitin, V., Ashworth, L., and Dobo, M. G. (1998). Blood pressure in Papua New Guinea: a survey of two highland villages in the Asaro Valley. *Diabetic Medicine*, 15, 1052–62.

Kitange, H. M., Swai, A. B., Masuki, G., Kilima, P. M., Alberti, K. G., and McLarty, D. G. (1993). Coronary heart disease risk factors in sub-Saharan Africa: studies in Tanzanian adolescents. *Journal of Epidemiology and Community Health*, 47, 303–7.

Klag, M. J., He, J., Whelton, P. K., Chen, J. Y., Qian, M. C., and He, G. Q. (1993). Alcohol use and blood pressure in an unacculturated society. *Hypertension*, 22, 365–70.

Lang, T., Pariente, P., Salem, G., and Tap, D. (1988). Social, professional conditions and arterial hypertension: an epidemiological study in Dakar, Senegal. *Journal of Hypertension*, 6, 271–6.

Law, M., Frost, C., and Wald, N. (1991). By how much does dietary salt reduction lower blood pressure? III--Analysis of data from trials of salt reduction. *British Medical Journal*, 302, 819–24.

Lawes, C. M. M., Bennett, D. A., Lewington, S., and Rodgers, A. (2002). Blood pressure and coronary heart disease: a review of the evidence. *Seminars in Vascular Medicine*, 2, 355–68.

Lawes, C. M. M., Vander Hoorn, S., Law, M. R., MacMahon, S., Elliott, P., and Rodgers, A. (2004). Blood pressure and the global burden of disease. In *Comparative Quantification of Health Risks: global and regional burden of disease attributable to selected major risk factors* (ed. M. Ezzati, A. Lopez, A. Rodgers, S. Vander Hoorn, and C. J. L. Murray). World Health Organization, Geneva. In press.

Leiter, L. A., Abbott, D., Campbell, N. R., Mendelson, R., Ogilvie, R. I., and Chockalingam, A. (1999). Lifestyle modifications to prevent and control hypertension. 2. Recommendations on obesity and weight loss. *Canadian Medical Association Journal*, **160**, S7–12.

Lindeberg, S., Nilsson-Ehle, P., Terent, A., Vessby, B., and Schersten, B. (1994). Cardiovascular risk factors in a Melanesian population apparently free from stroke and ischaemic heart disease: the Kitava study. *Journal of Internal Medicine*, **236**, 331–40.

Lisk, D. R., Williams, D. E., and Slattery, J. (1999). Blood pressure and hypertension in rural and urban Sierra Leoneans. *Ethnicity & Disease*, **9**, 254–63.

London, G. M., Guerin, A. P., Pannier, B., Marchais, S. J., and Stimpel, M. (1995). Influence of sex on arterial hemodynamics and blood pressure. Role of body height. *Hypertension*, **26**, 514–19.

MacAuley, D., McCrum, E. E., Stott, G., Evans, A. E., McRoberts, B., Boreham, C. A. *et al.* (1996). Physical activity, physical fitness, blood pressure, and fibrinogen in the Northern Ireland health and activity survey. *Journal of Epidemiology and Community Health*, **50**, 258–63.

MacMahon, S. (1994). Blood Pressure and Risks of cardiovascular Disease. In *Textbook of hypertension* (ed. J. Swales), pp. 46–57. Blackwell Scientific, Oxford.

MacMahon, S. and Rodgers, A. (1993*a*). The effects of anti-hypertensive treatment on vascular disease: reappraisal of the evidence in 1994. *Journal of Vascular Medicine and Biology*, **4**, 265–71.

MacMahon, S. and Rodgers, A. (1993*b*). The effects of blood pressure reduction in older patients: an overview of five randomized controlled trials in elderly hypertensives. *Clinical & Experimental Hypertension (New York)*, **15**, 967–78.

MacMahon, S., Peto, R., Cutler, J., Collins, R., Sorlie, P., Neaton, J. *et al.* (1990). Blood pressure, stroke, and coronary heart disease. Part I, prolonged differences in blood pressure: prospective observational studies corrected for the regression dilution bias. *Lancet*, **335**, 765–74.

Mann, J. I., Lewis, B., Shepherd, J., Winder, A. F., Fenster, S., Rose, L., and Morgan, B. (1988). Blood lipid concentrations and other cardiovascular risk factors: distribution, prevalence, and detection in Britain. *British Medical Journal Clinical Research Edition*, **296**, 1702–6.

Marmot, M. G. (1984). Geography of blood pressure and hypertension. *British Medical Bulletin*, **40**, 380–6.

Masia, R., Pena, A., Marrugat, J., Sala, J., Vila, J., Pavesi, M. *et al.* (1998). High prevalence of cardiovascular risk factors in Gerona, Spain, a province with low myocardial infarction incidence. REGICOR Investigators. *Journal of Epidemiology and Community Health*, **52**, 707–15.

Mathers, C. D., Vos, T., Lopez, A. D., Salomon, J., and Ezzati, M. (2001). *National Burden of Disease Studies: a practical guide.* Geneva: *Global program on evidence for health policy.* WHO, Geneva.

M'Buyamba-Kabangu, J. R., Fagard, R., Lijnen, P., Staessen, J., Ditu, M. S., Tshiani, K. A., and Amery, A. (1986). Epidemiological study of blood pressure and hypertension in a sample of urban Bantu of Zaire. *Journal of Hypertension*, **4**, 485–91.

M'Buyamba-Kabangu, J. R., Fagard, R., Staessen, J., Lijnen, P., and Amery, A. (1987). Correlates of blood pressure in rural and urban Zaire. *Journal of Hypertension*, **5**, 371–5.

McGovern, P. G., Pankow, J. S., Shahar, E., Doliszny, K. M., Folsom, A. R., Blackburn, H., and Luepker, R. V. (1996). Recent trends in acute coronary heart disease – mortality, morbidity, medical care, and risk factors. *New England Journal of Medicine*, **334**, 884–90.

Mendis, S., Ranasinghe, P., and Dharmasena, B. D. (1988). Prevalence of hypertension in Sri Lanka. A large population study in the central province. *Public Health*, **102**, 455–62.

Midgley, J. P., Matthew, A. G., Greenwood, C. M., and Logan, A. G. (1996). Effect of reduced dietary sodium on blood pressure: a meta-analysis of randomized controlled trials. *Journal of the American Medical Association*, **275**, 1590–7.

Ministry of Health (1999). NZ Food: NZ People. Key results of the 1997 National Nutrition Survey. Ministry of Health, Wellington.

Misra A., Sharma R., Pandey, R. M., and Khanna, N. (2001). Adverse profile of dietary nutrients, anthropometry and lipids in urban slum dwellers of northern India. *European Journal of Clinical Nutrition*, **55**, 727–34.

Mitchell, G. F., Moye, L. A., Braunwald, E., Rouleau, J. L., Bernstein, V., Geltman, E. M. *et al.* (1997). Sphygmomanometrically determined pulse pressure is a powerful independent predictor of recurrent events after myocardial infarction in patients with impaired left ventricular function. *Circulation*, **96**, 4254–60.

Miura, K., Dyer, A. R., Greenland, P., Daviglus, M. L., Hill, M., Liu, K. *et al.* (2001). Pulse pressure compared with other blood pressure indexes in the prediction of 25-year cardiovascular and all-cause mortality rates: The Chicago Heart Association Detection Project in Industry Study. *Hypertension*, **38**, 232–7.

Mufunda, J., Scott, L. J., Chifamba, J., Matenga, J., Sparks, B., Cooper, R., and Sparks, H. (2000). Correlates of blood pressure in an urban Zimbabwean population and comparison to other populations of African origin. *Journal of Human Hypertension*, **14**, 65–73.

Murray, C. J. L. and Lopez, A. D. (1996). *The global burden of disease: a comprehensive assessment of mortality and disability from diseases, injuries, and risk factors in 1990 and projected to 2020.* Harvard University Press, Cambridge, MA.

Murray, C. J. and Lopez, A. D. (1997). Global mortality, disability, and the contribution of risk factors: Global Burden of Disease Study. *Lancet*, **349**, 1436–42.

Murray, C. J. and Lopez, A. D. (1999). On the comparable quantification of health risks: lessons from the Global Burden of Disease Study. *Epidemiology*, **10**, 594–605.

Murray, C. J. L., Lopez, A. D., Mathers, C. D., and Stein, C. (2001). *Global program on evidence for health policy*. WHO, Geneva. Global Program on Evidence for Health Policy. World Health Organization.

Murray, C. J. L., Lauer, J. A., Hutubessy, R. C. W., Niessen, L., Tomijima, N., Rodgers, A. *et al.* (2003). Reducing the risk of cardiovascular disease: effectiveness and costs of interventions to reduce systolic blood pressure and cholesterol – a global and regional analysis. *Lancet*, **361**, 717–25.

Nan, L., Tuomilehto, J., Dowse, G., Zimmet, P., Gareeboo, H., Chitson, P. *et al.* (1991). Prevalence and medical care of hypertension in four ethnic groups in the newly-industrialized nation of Mauritius. *Journal of Hypertension*, **9**, 859–66.

National Center for Health Statistics (NCHS) (2002). The National Health and Nutrition Examination Survey (NHANES) III. Vol. 2002 <http://www.cdc.gov/nchs/nhanes.htm>.

National High Blood Pressure Education Program Working Group Report on Primary Prevention of Hypertension, o. (1993). National High Blood Pressure Education Program Working Group report on primary prevention of hypertension. *Archives of Internal Medicine*, **153**, 186–208.

Neal, B., MacMahon, S., and Chapman, N. (2000). Effects of ACE inhibitors, calcium antagonists, and other blood-pressure-lowering drugs: results of prospectively designed overviews of randomised trials. *Lancet*, **356**, 1955–64.

Neaton, J. D. and Wentworth, D. (1992). Serum cholesterol, blood pressure, cigarette smoking, and death from coronary heart disease. Overall findings and differences by age for 316 099 white men. *Archives of Internal Medicine*, **152**, 56–64.

Northridge, M. E. (1995). Public health methods–attributable risk as a link between causality and public health action. *American Journal of Public Health*, **85**, 1202–4.

Nyarko, N. K., Adubofour, K. O., Ofei, F., Pobee, J. O., and Owusu, S. K. (1994). Serum lipids and lipoprotein in adult Ghanaians. *Journal of Internal Medicine*, **236**, 251–3.

Ogunlesi, A., Osotimehin, B., Abbiyessuku, F., Kadiri, S., Akinkugbe, O., Liao, Y. L., and Cooper, R. (1991). Blood pressure and educational level among factory workers in Ibadan, Nigeria. *Journal of Human Hypertension*, **5**, 375–80.

Okayama, A., Ueshima, H., Marmot, M. G., Nakamura, M., Kita, Y., and Yamakawa, M. (1993). Changes in total serum cholesterol and other risk factors for cardiovascular disease in Japan 1980-1989. *International Journal of Epidemiology*, **22**, 1038–47.

Okesina, A. B., Oparinde, D. P., Akindoyin, K. A., and Erasmus, R. T. (1999). Prevalence of some risk factors of coronary heart disease in a rural Nigerian population. *East African Medical Journal*, **76**, 212–16.

Oviasu, V. O. and Okupa, F. E. (1980*a*). Arterial blood pressure and hypertension in Benin in the equatorial forest zone of Nigeria. *Tropical and Geographical Medicine*, **32**, 241–4.

Oviasu, V. O. and Okupa, F. E. (1980*b*). Relation between hypertension and occupational factors in rural and urban Africans. *Bulletin of the World Health Organization*, **58**, 485–9.

Page, L. B., Damon, A., and Moellering, R. C., Jr. (1974). Antecedents of cardiovascular disease in six Solomon Islands societies. *Circulation*, **49**, 1132–46.

Pahor, M., Psaty, B. M., Alderman, M. H., Applegate, W. B., Williamson, J. D., Cavazzini, C., and Furberg, C. D. (2000). Health outcomes associated with calcium antagonists compared with other first-line antihypertensive therapies: a meta-analysis of randomised controlled trials. *Lancet*, **356**, 1949–54.

Patrick, R. C., Prior, I. A., Smith, J. C., and Smith, A. H. (1983) Relationship between blood pressure and modernity among Ponapeans. *International Journal of Epidemiology*, **12**, 36–44.

Pauletto, P., Caroli, M., Pessina, A. C., and Dal Palu, C. (1994). Hypertension prevalence and age-related changes of blood-pressure in semi-nomadic and urban Oromos of Ethiopia. *European Journal of Epidemiology*, **10**, 159–64.

People's Republic of China–United States Cardiovascular and Cardiopulmonary Epidemiology Research Group (1992). An epidemiological study of cardiovascular and cardiopulmonary disease risk factors in four populations in the People's Republic of China. *Circulation*, **85**, 1083–96.

Poulter, N., Khaw, K. T., Hopwood, B. E., Mugambi, M., Peart, W. S., Rose, G., and Sever, P. S. (1984). Blood pressure and associated factors in a rural Kenyan community. *Hypertension*, **6**, 810–13.

Poulter, N. R., Khaw, K. T., and Sever, P. S. (1988). Higher blood pressures of urban migrants from an African low-blood pressure population are not due to selective migration. *American Journal of Hypertension*, **1**, 143S–145S.

Poulter, N. R., Khaw, K. T., Hopwood, B. E., Mugambi, M., Peart, W. S., Rose, G., and Sever, P. S. (1990). The Kenyan Luo migration study: observations on the initiation of a rise in blood pressure. *British Medical Journal*, **300**, 967–72.

Poulter, N. and Sever, P. (1994). Blood Pressure in Other Populations. A. Low Blood Pressure Populations and the Impact of Rural-Urban Migration. In *Textbook of hypertension* (ed. J. Swales), pp. 22–36. Blackwell Scientific, Oxford.

Professor Anoop Misra, All India Institute of Medical Sciences and New Delhi (2001). Personal communication.

Professor Clicerio Gonzalez, Centro de Estudios en Diabetes and Mexico (2001). Personal communication.

Professor Flavio Dannii Fuchs, Hospital de Clinicas de Porto Algre and Brazil (2001). Personal communication.

Professor Hashem Jaddou and Jordan University of Science and Technology (2001). Personal communication.

Professor Hassan Ghannem, University Hospital Farhat Hached and Tunisia (2001). Personal communication.

Professor Paul Elliott, Imperial College School of Medicine and London (2001). Personal communication.

Professor Rainford Wilks, L. Sargent, F. Bennett, R. Cooper, T. Forrester, The University of the West Indies and Jamaica (2001). Personal communication.

Progress Collaborative Group (2001). The lowering of blood-pressure after stroke. *Lancet*, **358**, 1994–5.

Prospective Studies Collaboration (1995). Cholesterol, diastolic blood pressure, and stroke: 13 000 strokes in 45 000 people in 45 prospective cohorts. *Lancet*, **346**, 1647–53.

Prospective Studies Collaboration (2002). Age-specific relevance of usual blood pressure to vascular mortality: a meta-analysis of individual data for one million adults in 61 prospective studies. *Lancet*, **360**, 1903–13.

Psaty, B. M., Furberg, C. D., Kuller, L. H., Cushman, M., Savage, P. J., Levine, D. *et al.* (2001). Association between blood pressure level and the risk of myocardial infarction, stroke, and total mortality: the cardiovascular health study. *Archives of Internal Medicine*, **161**, 1183–92.

Psaty, B. M., Smith, N. L., Siscovick, D. S., Koepsell, T. D., Weiss, N. S., Heckbert, S. R. *et al.* (1997). Health outcomes associated with antihypertensive therapies used as first-line agents. A systematic review and meta-analysis. *Journal of the American Medical Association*, **277**, 739–45.

Puska, P., Matilainen, T., Jousilahti, P., Korhonen, H., Vartiainen, E., Pokusajeva, S. *et al.* (1993). Cardiovascular risk factors in the Republic of Karelia, Russia, and in North Karelia, Finland. *International Journal of Epidemiology*, **22**, 1048–55.

Ramirez, M. O., Pino, C. T., Furiasse, L. V., Lee, A. J., and Fowkes, F. G. (1995). Paraguayan National Blood Pressure Study: prevalence of hypertension in the general population. *Journal of Human Hypertension*, **9**, 891–7.

Ramsay, L., Williams, B., Johnston, G., MacGregor, G., Poston, L., Potter, J. *et al.* (1999). Guidelines for management of hypertension: report of the third working party of the British Hypertension Society. *Journal of Human Hypertension*, **13**, 569–92.

Ribeiro, A. B. and Ribeiro, M. B. (1986). Epidemiological and demographic considerations. Hypertension in underdeveloped countries. *Drugs*, **31**, 23–8.

Ribeiro, M. B., Ribeiro, A. B., Neto, C. S., Chaves, C. C., Kater, C. E., Iunes, M. *et al.* (1981). Hypertension and economic activities in Sao Paulo, Brazil. *Hypertension*, **3**, II-233–7.

Rose, G. (1989). High-risk and population strategies of prevention: ethical considerations. *Annals of Medicine*, **21**, 409–13.

Rose, G. (1992). *The strategy of preventive medicine*. Oxford University Press.

Rosenthal, J. (1989). The epidemiology of blood pressure in young Mexican adults. *Journal of Hypertension*, **7**, 355–60.

Sakata, K. and Labarthe, D. R. (1996). Changes in cardiovascular disease risk factors in three Japanese national surveys 1971–1990. *Journal of Epidemiology*, **6**, 93–107.

Salmond, C. E., Joseph, J. G., Prior, I. A., Stanley, D. G., and Wessen, A. F. (1985). Longitudinal analysis of the relationship between blood pressure and migration: the Tokelau Island Migrant Study. *American Journal of Epidemiology*, **122**, 291–301.

Salmond, C. E., Prior, I. A., and Wessen, A. F. (1989). Blood pressure patterns and migration: a 14-year cohort study of adult Tokelauans. *American Journal of Epidemiology*, **130**, 37–52.

SarrafZadegan, N. and AminiNik, S. (1997). Blood pressure pattern in urban and rural areas in Isfahan, Iran. *Journal of Human Hypertension*, **11**, 425–8.

Seedat, Y. K. (2000). Hypertension in developing nations in sub-Saharan Africa. *Journal of Human Hypertension*, **14**, 739–47.

Seedat, Y. K., Seedat, M. A., and Hackland, D. B. (1982). Prevalence of hypertension in the urban and rural Zulu. *Journal of Epidemiology and Community Health*, **36**, 256–61.

Sesso, H. D., Stampfer, M. J., Rosner, B., Hennekens, C. H., Gaziano, J. M., Manson, J. E., and Glynn, R. J. (2000). Systolic and diastolic blood pressure, pulse pressure, and mean arterial pressure as predictors of cardiovascular disease risk in Men. *Hypertension*, **36**, 801–7.

Shaper, A. G., Pocock, S. J., Phillips, A. N., and Walker, M. (1986). Identifying men at high risk of heart attacks: strategy for use in general practice. *British Medical Journal Clinical Research Edition*, **293**, 474–9.

Shelley, E., Daly, L., Kilcoyne, D., Graham, I., and Mulcahy, R. (1991). Risk factors for coronary heart disease: a population survey in County Kilkenny, Ireland, in 1985. *Irish Journal of Medical Science*, **160**, 22–8.

Shelley, E., Daly, L., Collins, C., Christie, M., Conroy, R., Gibney, M. *et al.* (1995). Cardiovascular risk factor changes in the Kilkenny Health Project. A community health promotion programme. *European Heart Journal*, **16**, 752–60.

Shimamoto, T., Komachi, Y., Inada, H., Doi, M., Iso, H., Sato, S. *et al.* (1989). Trends for coronary heart disease and stroke and their risk factors in Japan. *Circulation*, **79**, 503–15.

Simmons, D. (1983). Blood pressure, ethnic group, and salt intake in Belize. *Journal of Epidemiology and Community Health*, **37**, 38–42.

Simmons, D., Barbour, G., Congleton, J., Levy, J., Meacher, P., Saul, H., and Sowerby, T. (1986). Blood pressure and salt intake in Malawi: an urban rural study. *Journal of Epidemiology and Community Health*, **40**, 188–92.

Singh, R. B., Beegom, R., Ghosh, S., Niaz, M. A., Rastogi, V., Rastogi, S. S. *et al.* (1997a). Epidemiological study of hypertension and its determinants in an urban population of North India. *Journal of Human Hypertension*, **11**, 679–85.

Singh, R. B., Sharma, J. P., Rastogi, V., Niaz, M. A., and Singh, N. K. (1997b). Prevalence and determinants of hypertension in the Indian social class and heart survey. *Journal of Human Hypertension*, **11**, 51–6.

Singh, R. B., Beegom, R., Mehta, A. S., Niaz, M. A., De, A. K., Haque, M. *et al.* (1998). Prevalence and risk factors of hypertension and age-specific blood pressures in five cities: a study of Indian women. NKP Salve Institute of Medical Sciences, Nagpur, India. *International Journal of Cardiology*, **63**, 165–73.

Smith, W. C., Tunstall-Pedoe, H., Crombie, I. K., and Tavendale, R. (1989). Concomitants of excess coronary deaths – major risk factor and lifestyle findings from 10,359 men and women in the Scottish Heart Health Study. *Scottish Medical Journal*, **34**, 550–5.

Soyannwo, M. A., Kurashi, N. Y., Gadallah, M., Hams, J., el-Essawi, O., Khan, N. A. *et al.* (1998). Blood pressure pattern in Saudi population of Gassim. *African Journal of Medicine and Medical Sciences*, **27**, 107–16.

Sprafka, J. M., Burke, G. L., Folsom, A. R., Luepker, R. V., and Blackburn, H. (1990). Continued decline in cardiovascular disease risk factors: results of the Minnesota Heart Survey, 1980-1982 and 1985-1987. *American Journal of Epidemiology*, **132**, 489–500.

Stamler, J., Neaton, J. D., and Wentworth, D. N. (1989). Blood pressure (systolic and diastolic) and risk of fatal coronary heart disease. *Hypertension*, **13**, I2–12.

Stamler, J., Stamler, R., and Neaton, J. D. (1993). Blood pressure, systolic and diastolic, and cardiovascular risks. US population data. *Archives of Internal Medicine*, **153**, 598–615.

Steyn, K., Jooste, P. L., Langenhoven, M. L., Benade, A. J., Rossouw, J. E., Steyn, M. *et al.* (1985). Hypertension in the black community of the Cape Peninsula, South Africa. *South African Medical Journal*, **67**, 619–25.

Steyn, K., Fourie, J., Lombard, C., Katzenellenbogen, J., Bourne, L., and Jooste, P. (1996). Coronary risk factors in the coloured population of the Cape Peninsula. *East African Medical Journal*, **73**, 758–63.

Strachan, D. and Rose, G. (1991). Strategies of prevention revisited: effects of imprecise measurement of risk factors on the evaluation of 'high-risk' and 'population-based' approaches to prevention of cardiovascular disease. *Journal of Clinical Epidemiology*, **44**, 1187–96.

Swai, A. B., McLarty, D. G., Kitange, H. M., Kilima, P. M., Tatalla, S., Keen, N. *et al.* (1993). Low prevalence of risk factors for coronary heart disease in rural Tanzania. *International Journal of Epidemiology*, **22**, 651–9.

Tunstall-Pedoe, H. (1991). The Dundee coronary risk-disk for management of change in risk factors. *British Medical Journal*, **303**, 744–7.

Ueshima, H., Zhang, X. H., and Choudhury, S. R. (2000). Epidemiology of hypertension in China and Japan. *Journal of Human Hypertension*, **14**, 765–9.

Vaccarino, V., Borgatta, A., Gallus, G., and Sirtori, C. R. (1995). Prevalence of coronary heart disease risk factors in northern-Italian male and female employees. *European Heart Journal*, **16**, 761–9.

Vander Hoorn, S., Ezzati, M., Rodgers, A., Lopez, A., and Murray, C. J. L. (2004). Estimating attributable burden of disease from exposure and hazard data. In *Comparative quantification of health risks: global and regional burden of disease attributable to selected major risk factors* (ed. M. Ezzati, A. Lopez, A. Rodgers, S. Vander Hoorn, and C. J. L. Murray). WHO, Geneva. World Health Organization.

van der Sande, M. A., Bailey, R., Faal, H., Banya, W. A., Dolin, P., Nyan, O. A. *et al.* (1997). Nationwide prevalence study of hypertension and related non-communicable diseases in The Gambia. *Tropical Medicine & International Health*, **2**, 1039–48.

Vartiainen, E., Puska, P., Pekkanen, J., Tuomilehto, J., and Jousilahti, P. (1994). Changes in risk factors explain changes in mortality from ischaemic heart disease in Finland. *British Medical Journal*, **309**, 23–7.

Vartiainen, E., Jousilahti, P., Alfthan, G., Sundvall, J., Pietinen, P., and Puska, P. (2000). Cardiovascular risk factor changes in Finland, 1972-1997. *International Journal of Epidemiology*, **29**, 49–56.

Waterhouse, J., Muir, C., and Shanmugaratnam, K. (1982). *Cancer Incidence in Five Continents IV*. Lyon: IARC, Scientific Publications.

Whelton, P. K. (1994). Epidemiology of hypertension. *Lancet*, **344**, 101–6.

Whelton, P., He, J., and Klag, M. (1994). Blood pressure in westernised populations. In *Textbook of hypertension* (ed. J. Swales), pp. 11–21. Oxford: Blackwell Scientific Publications.

Whelton, P. K., Appel, L. J., Espeland, M. A., Applegate, W. B., Ettinger, W. H., Jr, Kostis, J. B. *et al.* (1998). Sodium reduction and weight loss in the treatment of hypertension in older persons: a randomized controlled trial of nonpharmacologic interventions in the elderly (TONE). *Journal of the American Medical Association*, **279**, 839–46.

Wolf, H. K., Tuomilehto, J., Kuulasmaa, K., Domarkiene, S., Cepaitis, Z., Molarius, A. *et al.* (1997). Blood pressure levels in the 41 populations of the WHO MONICA Project. *Journal of Human Hypertension*, **11**, 733–42.

WHO (World Health Organization) (2000). *The World Health Report 2000. Health Systems: Improving Performance*. Geneva: World Health Organisation.

WHO (World Health Organisation) (2002). *The World Health Report 2002. Reducing risks, promoting healthy life*. Geneva: World Health Organisation.

Wu, X., Huang, Z., Stamler, J., Wu, Y., Li, Y., Folsom, A. R. *et al.* (1996). Changes in average blood pressure and incidence of high blood pressure 1983–1984 to 1987–1988 in four population cohorts in the People's Republic of China. *Journal of Hypertension*, **14**, 1267–74.

Chapter 12

Lipids and cholesterol

M. R. Law and A. Rodgers

12.1 Introduction

Coronary heart disease (CHD) became common only in the twentieth century. Rare in the Victorian era, it reached a peak in Western countries around 1970, when it accounted for 25–30% of all deaths in older (50+) adults. It still accounts for over 20%. The high fat diet typical of many Western countries during the greater part of the twentieth century was a major underlying factor. Similar dietary patterns are emerging in developing countries, in which CHD is increasing (Murray and Lopez 1996; WHO 2002). In reversing this epidemic, modern cholesterol-lowering drugs can reduce risk by more than any other single intervention. Dietary change has the potential to achieve benefits of similar magnitude, but would need to be radical and involve changes by the food industry in the saturated fat content and price of foods, as well as individual behavioural changes.

12.2 Serum total and low-density lipoprotein cholesterol

Typical values of serum total and low-density lipoprotein (LDL) cholesterol in Western countries are high in comparison to those in agricultural and hunter-gatherer communities, because of the high saturated fat content of the Western diet. Average serum cholesterol concentration (in people aged 45–60) is 3.0–3.5 mmol/l in hunter-gatherer societies with traditional diets and lifestyle (where heart disease is rare). It is ~3.5 mmol/l in rural China, ~5.0 mmol/l in Japan, 5.5 mmol/l in Mediterranean populations, and a little higher in the United States, and 6.0 mmol/l in Britain and other northern European countries (Law and Wald 1994). There is a strong and continuous cross-country correlation between average serum cholesterol and heart disease mortality (Law and Wald 1994). Use of the term 'normal' in reference to usual or average Western cholesterol values may therefore be misleading (Law and Wald 2002).

Of the average total serum cholesterol of ~6 mmol/l in Western populations, two-thirds is LDL cholesterol and one-quarter is high-density lipoprotein (HDL) cholesterol. Across countries average levels of LDL cholesterol are ~2 mmol/l lower than total cholesterol levels (Law and Wald 1994). The atherogenic properties lie in the LDL fraction (sometimes measured as its carrier protein, apolipoprotein B, with which it is highly correlated). Many of the large cohort studies and some of the randomized trials measured only total serum cholesterol, and results based on total serum cholesterol have been taken to estimate effects of LDL cholesterol. Fortuitously the approximation is a good one. Observational differences between individuals in total cholesterol are close to the corresponding differences in LDL cholesterol (Pocock *et al.* 1989; Law *et al.* 1994a), and the absolute reduction in total serum cholesterol produced by diet and by most drugs is similar to the reduction in LDL cholesterol. Much epidemiological and clinical trial data are therefore available in estimating quantitatively the effect of lowering serum LDL cholesterol on the risk of CHD.

12.3 **Serum cholesterol and CHD**

Evidence from genetics, animal studies, experimental pathology, epidemiological studies, and clinical trials indicates conclusively that increasing serum cholesterol is an important cause of CHD and that lowering serum cholesterol reduces the risk. There is now widespread acceptance of this, though as many as nine large randomized placebo controlled trials of statins and cardiovascular disease events were conducted (Scandinavian Simvastatin Survival Study Group 1994; Shepherd *et al.* 1995; Sacks *et al.* 1996; Downs *et al.* 1998; LIPID Study Group 1998; Heart Protection Study Collaborative Group 2002; PROSPER Study Group 2002; ALLHAT-LLT Trial 2002; Sever *et al.* 2003). In this chapter we address important practical questions: the nature of the dose–response relationship, the size of the effect, the speed of the reversal of risk, and who should be treated with statins. To answer such questions from trial data alone (which many attempt to do) is misleading. Data from both observational epidemiology (cohort studies) and randomized controlled trials are necessary; the two are complementary (MacMahon *et al.* 1990).

12.4 **The nature of the dose–response relationship: is there a threshold?**

Cohort (or prospective observational) studies (in which serum cholesterol is measured in a large number of individuals and subsequent CHD events are recorded), best show the dose–response relationship, because they examine the effect of cholesterol differences across the entire range of values in a population. Figure 12.1 shows CHD mortality plotted according to fifths of the serum cholesterol distribution in the largest cohort study (Neaton and Wentworth 1992). With heart disease mortality plotted on a logarithmic scale, the relationship is described almost perfectly by a straight line (Law and Wald 2002), linking the *proportional* change in CHD to the *absolute* difference in serum cholesterol. The 95% confidence limits of the risk estimates in each group do not overlap, establishing that there is no threshold below which a further decrease in serum cholesterol is not associated with a further decrease in risk of CHD. The exponential relationship indicated by the straight line means that a given absolute difference in serum cholesterol concentration from *any* point on the cholesterol distribution is associated with a constant percentage difference in the incidence of CHD events (Law and Wald 2002).

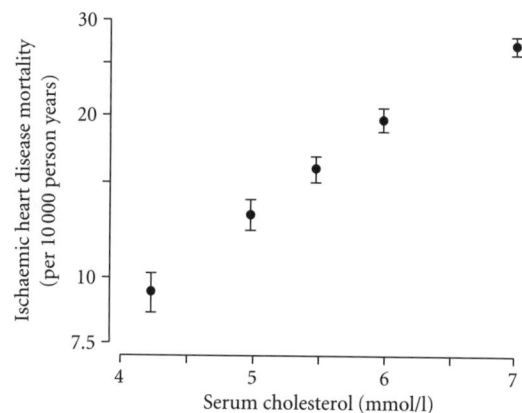

Fig. 12.1 Mortality from CHD (with 95% confidence interval) according to serum cholesterol in a large cohort study. (Data from Neaton and Wentworth 1992.)

This absence of a threshold has been contentious: published guidelines on lowering serum cholesterol have invoked one. There was never evidence in favour, and the evidence is now firmly against any threshold across the range of values seen in Western populations. The data in Fig. 12.1 (which alone are conclusive), are supported by data from other large cohort studies (Law et al. 1994b), including one from China which shows that the continuous relationship extends below serum cholesterol values of 4 mmol/l (Chen et al. 1991). Large trials also confirm the continuous dose–response relationship. Randomized trials show that statins are beneficial with low pre-treatment levels of LDL cholesterol (LIPID Study Group 1998; ALLHAT-LLT Trial 2002; Heart Protection Study Collaborative Group 2002), especially two trials of intensive versus moderate lipid lowering with statins (Cannon et al. 2004; Nissen et al. 2004). The postulated thresholds have steadily declined in value over time from those advocated 20 years ago, but even recommendations to use statins in high-risk patients only if pre-treatment serum cholesterol exceeds 5 mmol/l should be abandoned. The trial data show that the *proportional* reduction in risk from lowering serum cholesterol is similar in persons with and without previous myocardial infarction or other clinical evidence of coronary artery disease (Law and Wald 2002; Law et al. 2003). This 'primary secondary-distinction' is somewhat arbitrary; extensive atherosclerotic disease in the coronary arteries will necessarily be common among people with previous myocardial infarction and less common in the general population, and there is no reason why this should influence the effect of cholesterol reduction on atherosclerotic disease. It is clear that the constant proportional reduction in risk for a specified cholesterol reduction applies to high and low risk as well as high and low cholesterol levels.

Most of the cohort studies and the earlier trials of cholesterol and CHD recruited men – for reasons of economy since CHD events are more common in men. But the large statin trials show a similar proportional effect of cholesterol reduction on coronary risk in women and men.

12.5 The size of the effect

Cohort studies provide the best estimates in quantifying the maximum long-term effect of a specified serum cholesterol reduction on the incidence of CHD events according to age. This is because they cover a wide age range and because the serum cholesterol differences between individuals recorded on entry to a cohort study will have been present on average for decades beforehand (so cohort studies show long-term associations) (Law et al. 1994b). Trials, on the other hand, show the effect of short-term cholesterol differences.

Table 12.1 shows estimates of the long-term percentage decrease in the risk of CHD according to the decrease in serum cholesterol concentration and age at death. The estimates are taken from an analysis of the 10 largest cohort studies in Western populations, corrected for the regression-dilution bias and for the minor distinction between differences in total and in LDL cholesterol discussed above (Law et al. 1994a, b). At age 60 a 1 mmol/l decrease in total or LDL cholesterol reduces risk by an estimated 41%. The *proportional* decrease in risk decreases with age, but the *absolute* benefit increases because the disease becomes more common with age. The increasing reduction in risk with greater reduction in serum cholesterol shown in Table 12.2 follows from the exponential dose–response relationship described above. For a 0.6 mmol/l cholesterol reduction at age 60, for example, the reduction in risk is 27% and the relative risk is therefore 0.73; with a serum cholesterol reduction three times as great (1.8 mmol/l) the relative risk is 0.73 cubed ($0.73 \times 0.73 \times 0.73$), which is 0.39, so the reduction in risk is 61%.

Table 12.1 Estimates (based on an overview of 10 large cohort studies in Western populations) of the percentage decrease in risk of CHD events according to serum LDL cholesterol reduction and age

Age (years)	Reduction in LDL cholesterol (mmol/l)						
	0.6	1.0	1.4	1.8	2.2	2.6	3.0
50	39	56	68	77	84	88	91
60	27	41	52	61	68	74	79
70	20	31	41	49	56	62	67

Source: Law et al. 1994b.

Table 12.2 Reduction in incidence of CHD events[a] for a 1.0 mmol/l decrease in serum LDL cholesterol, according to duration of treatment[b]

Years in trial	Risk reduction (%)	95% CI
1st	11	4–18
2nd	24	17–30
3rd–5th	33	28–37
6th and subsequent	36	26–45
Long term[c]	41	38–43

CI: confidence interval.

[a] Relative odds reduction in coronary heart death and non-fatal myocardial infarction.

[b] From analysis of 58 randomized trials (Law et al. 2003).

[c] From cohort studies (Table 12.1).

12.6 Speed of reversal, and consistency of observational and trial data

Figure 12.2 shows the reduction in incidence of CHD events according to time since entry (standardized to an LDL cholesterol reduction of 1.0 mmol/l), from an analysis of 58 randomized trials of serum cholesterol reduction and disease events (Law et al. 2003), and compares the trend with the estimate of the long-term decrease in risk from the cohort studies. Table 12.2 summarizes the results. There was little reduction in risk in the first year (10% per 1 mmol/l LDL cholesterol reduction), and 23% in the second year. From the third to fifth years the average reduction in risk was 33%, and after 5 years it was 36%. The CHD events in these trials mostly occurred at an average age of ~60, and at this age the estimate of the long-term effect from the cohort studies is 41% (Table 12.2). This is a striking effect; there is relatively little reduction in risk in the first year, but by the third year the reduction approximates the long-term value. The similarity of the estimates from the cohort studies and from the trial data from the third year onwards validate the accuracy of the cohort study estimates, and show that the reduction of risk is near maximal after 2 years – a surprisingly rapid effect.

Subdivision of the 58 cholesterol trials according to the LDL cholesterol reduction attained, into three groups with average reduction around 0.5 mmol/l, 1.0 mmol/l, and 1.6 mmol/l,

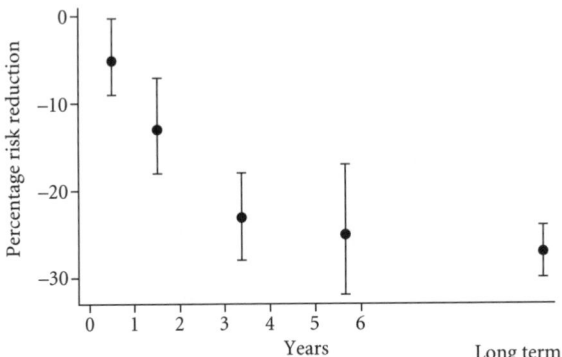

Fig. 12.2 Reduction in the incidence of CHD per 1.0 mmol/l (~10%) decrease in serum cholesterol, as estimated from randomized trials according to time since entry, and from cohort studies (which reflect the long-term association). (Data from Law *et al.* 2003.)

confirmed the dose–response relationship shown by the cohort studies. In each group the observed reduction in incidence of CHD events (from the third year onwards) was similar to the expected long-term reduction from the cohort studies according to the LDL cholesterol reduction (Law *et al.* 2003). In trials attaining an LDL cholesterol reduction of around 1.6 mmol/l, the reduction in risk was over 50%.

The close consistency of the observational (cohort study) and trial data indicate that all, or almost all, of the reduction in CHD events from statins is attributable to the LDL cholesterol reduction and not to other mechanisms such as anti-inflammatory properties of the drugs. Similarly, the more modest effects of other interventions (such as fibrates or dietary change) are attributable to their smaller effects on LDL cholesterol.

12.7 Global disease burden due to serum cholesterol

The foregoing evidence on the association between serum cholesterol and CHD risk can be combined with data on population cholesterol levels to estimate the fraction of CHD events occurring in a population that is attributable to high cholesterol. A recent analysis on behalf of the WHO estimated that 3.6 million deaths per year worldwide (~8% of global deaths) were attributable to 'non-optimal' serum cholesterol (taken as exceeding 3.8 mmol/l) (Ezzati *et al.* 2002; WHO 2002). See Table 12.3.

The estimates for different WHO regions in developed countries indicated that about two-thirds of CHD can be attributed to cholesterol levels exceeding 3.8 mmol/l (that is, about two-thirds of CHD events would be prevented if population cholesterol levels were this low). Non-optimal cholesterol was a leading cause of death in all developed regions, and of emerging importance in middle-income countries. About half the healthy life years lost occurred in middle age, and the burden was equally shared among the sexes.

12.8 Dietary fat and serum cholesterol

The relationship between dietary saturated fat and serum cholesterol is shown by the data from Japan and Britain in Table 12.4. This comparison is a useful one because dietary saturated fat differs greatly, yet dietary polyunsaturated fat and cholesterol are similar in the two countries.

Table 12.3 Estimates of the annual global disease burden attributable to non-optimal (>3.8 mmol/l) serum cholesterol

WHO subregion(s)[a]	Population (millions)	Attributable mortality (thousands)				Life years lost (disability adjusted) thousands			
		Males		Females		Males		Females	
		No. of deaths	% of total[b]	No. of deaths	% of total[b]	No.	% of total[b]	No.	% of total[b]
Developed									
Western Europe (Eur A)	412	228	13	223	14	1670	7	930	5
Eastern Europe including Russia (Eur B&C)	461	449	18	515	25	4608	10	3060	10
North America (Amr A)	325	150	12	168	14	1264	6	822	5
Japan, Australia, and other Western Pacific (Wpr A)	154	30	6	28	8	252	4	136	3
Developing									
Central and South America (Amr B&D)	502	82	6	69	7	934	2	641	2
Sub-Saharan Africa (Afr D&E)	640	57	1	80	2	647	1	850	1
North Africa, Middle East, and Pakistan (Emr B&D)	482	149	8	114	7	1699	3	1178	2
South East Asia including India (Sear B&D)	1536	490	7	456	8	5591	3	4998	3
Western Pacific including China (Wpr B)	1533	146	4	174	5	1481	2	1339	2
World	6045	1781	7.2	1827	8.6	18146	3.9	13953	2.6

Source: Ezzati et al. 2002; WHO 2002.

[a] Full details of member states in 14 WHO epidemiological subregions given in Ezzati et al. 2002 and WHO 2002.

[b] Denominator of percentages is all-cause deaths or disability-adjusted life years (DALYs).

Table 12.4 Serum cholesterol and dietary saturated fat in Japan and Britain

Age (years)	Japan	Britain	Difference
Dietary saturated fat (% calories)			
All ages	6	16	10
Serum cholesterol (mmol/l)			
20–9	4.5	5.0	0.5
30–9	5.0	5.6	0.6
40–9	5.1	6.0	0.9
50–9	5.2	6.2	1.0
60–9	5.0	6.2	1.2

Data compiled from national surveys in each country (Law and Wald 1994).

The size of the association varies with age, yet there has been a tendency to generalize to older age groups the results of studies conducted in younger age groups. Most dietary trials, for example, have been conducted in people under 30, few in people over 50. In older people a reduction in dietary saturated fat equivalent to 10% of calories would lower serum cholesterol by ~1 mmol/l, which in turn would reduce CHD mortality in the long-term by ~40%.

The chain lengths of saturated fatty acids influence the extent to which they increase blood cholesterol. Palmitic ($C_{16:0}$) and myristic ($C_{14:0}$) acids have the major effect, lauric acid ($C_{12:0}$) some effect, while stearic acid ($C_{18:0}$) and medium chain fatty acids have little or no effect.

Trans-unsaturated fatty acids are also important: randomized trials show that they increase serum total and LDL cholesterol by about as much as longer chain saturated fatty acids (Mensink and Katan 1990; Nestel *et al.* 1992). They are scanty in naturally occurring fats, but are generated by the hydrogenation of vegetable oils for use as hardening agents in manufactured foods. They constitute 6–8% of dietary fat, or 2% of calories, in Western diets. Naturally occurring *cis*-unsaturated fatty acids reduce serum cholesterol by approximately half as much as longer chain saturated fatty acids increase it. Reduction in dietary cholesterol has a small effect on blood cholesterol concentration (AHA 1990). Substitution of *cis*-unsaturated for saturated fats in the Western diet is thus the most appropriate change in lowering the high levels of blood cholesterol in Western populations.

The reduction in serum cholesterol that can easily be attained by an individual trying to reduce dietary fat in isolation from family, friends, and workmates is relatively small (~0.3 mmol/l, or 5%). A larger reduction may be feasible when a family undertakes to change its diet. A reduction of ~0.6 mmol/l (10%) is realistic on a community basis if demand for palatable low fat food ensured a change in the food supply. A reduction in saturated fat consumption by ~7% of calories, a realistic target for a high fat population, would lower serum cholesterol by 0.6 mmol/l. Reductions in average serum cholesterol of ~0.6 mmol/l through dietary change have occurred over less than two decades in entire Western communities, in the United States and Finland for example (Law and Wald 1994). Measures that facilitate such a change include wider public education, labelling of foods sold in supermarkets, provision of information on the fat content of restaurant meals, and use of food technology to provide palatable and inexpensive manufactured foods with low saturated fat content. Implementing national and international policies on food subsidies that are linked to health priorities is also important (see Chapter 46).

12.9 The efficacy of different interventions in lowering LDL cholesterol and reducing risk of CHD events

Table 12.5 shows estimates of the reduction in LDL cholesterol attainable with various interventions, and the corresponding expected long-term reduction in the incidence of CHD events at age 60 (from Table 12.1). Dietary change in a population might reduce LDL cholesterol by 0.6 mmol/l, as discussed above; this would be expected to reduce CHD events by about a quarter. Adding plant stanols to margarine or other foods is also effective (Katan *et al.* 2003).

The different statins vary in their efficacy in lowering LDL cholesterol (Law *et al.* 2003). Fluvastatin and pravastatin, even at the highest doses tested in trials (80 mg/day), are less effective than simvastatin or lovastatin. Simvastatin or lovastatin at 40 mg/day reduce LDL cholesterol by 1.8 mmol/l on average, a change that would reduce the risk of CHD events by ~60%. These drugs have the advantages that they are now off patent and therefore could be inexpensive, and that they are extensively tested in randomized trials and clinical practice and known to be effective and safe. Rhabdomyolysis and liver failure from hepatitis are recognized complications, but both are extremely rare: the death rate from rhabdomyolysis and the incidence of liver failure are each about one per million person years of use (Law *et al.* 2003). Atorvastatin and rosuvastatin produce even greater reductions in LDL cholesterol. The expected reduction in CHD events in the long term, albeit not confirmed in randomized trials, is ~70%.

Table 12.5 Interventions to lower serum LDL cholesterol by diet or drugs, the typical reduction in LDL cholesterol that they can produce, and the corresponding expected long-term reduction in CHD events at age 60 (from the analysis of cohort studies in Table 12.1)

Intervention	Reduction in LDL cholesterol		Expected reduction in CHD events (%)
	Percentage	Absolute (mmol/l)[a]	
Dietary change by an individual	6	0.3	15
Dietary change in a population	12	0.6	27
Plant stanols or sterols added to margarines and other foods (Katan *et al.* 2003)	8	0.4	19
Older cholesterol-lowering drugs (Law *et al.* 2003)	12	0.6	27
Modern fibrates (Law *et al.* 2003)	10	0.5	23
Statins (Law *et al.* 2003):			
Fluvastatin or pravastatin 40 mg/day	28	1.3	49
Simvastatin or lovastatin 20 mg/day or atorvastatin 5 mg/day	30	1.5	54
Simvastatin or lovastatin 40 mg/day or atorvastatin 10 mg/day or rosuvastatin 5 mg/day	37	1.8	61
Atorvastatin 40 mg/day or rosuvastatin 20 mg/day	48	2.3	70

[a] From a pre-treatment LDL cholesterol of 4.8 mmol/l.

These statins are still on patent and therefore more expensive, and they are as yet less widely tested. With these relative disadvantages it might be reasonable that they be used only for patients at particularly high risk, with simvastatin or lovastatin the drugs of choice in routine clinical use. Table 12.5 also shows that cholesterol-lowering drugs other than statins are much less effective than statins. Fibrates or other drugs have been used in combination with statins to produce larger cholesterol reductions, but increasing the dose of a statin is as effective (and cheaper). It is also safer, since the risk of rhabdomyolysis, albeit low, is increased by using different cholesterol-lowering drugs in combination. Drugs other than statins, therefore, have little or no place in modern clinical practice.

12.10 Safety of cholesterol reduction

The uncertainty concerning the excess mortality from haemorrhagic stroke at low serum cholesterol concentration shown in cohort studies is unresolved. There are too few trial data on haemorrhagic stroke to be informative (Law *et al.* 2003). This uncertainty should not preclude the use of statins in the prevention of cardiovascular disease; any possible excess of haemorrhagic stroke is greatly outweighed by the protective effect against CHD events and thromboembolic stroke. Haemorrhagic stroke apart, concern over hazard has been resolved (Law *et al.* 1994c), and the statin trials, particularly informative on safety because of the large reduction in serum cholesterol, showed no excess mortality from non-circulatory causes (Scandinavian Simvastatin Survival Study Group 1994; Shepherd *et al.* 1995; Sacks *et al.* 1996; Downs *et al.* 1998; LIPID Study Group 1998; ALLHAT-LLT Trial 2002; Heart Protection Study Collaborative Group 2002; PROSPER Study Group 2002; Law *et al.* 2003). The condition of heterozygous familial hypobetalipoproteinaemia, in which total serum cholesterol levels are as low as 2–3 mmol/l, provides an important natural experiment. Life expectancy is prolonged because coronary artery disease is avoided, and no adverse effects from the low cholesterol are recognized (Glueck *et al.* 1976; Linton *et al.* 1993).

12.11 Why was cholesterol reduction contentious until recently?

Few medical issues over recent decades have been so controversial and seemingly difficult to resolve as lipids and cardiovascular disease. Many clinicians regarded serum cholesterol reduction with uncertainty or suspicion. Until 10 years ago, apparently unfavourable evidence had been reported at regular intervals over many years. The earliest trials used toxic agents to lower serum cholesterol, notably oestrogen (in men) and thyroxine, and the benefit from the modest cholesterol reduction was exceeded by the hazards. Some trials were short in duration, and showed little reduction in risk because little occurs in the first year after lowering cholesterol (Table 12.2). Cross-sectional studies of dietary saturated fat and serum cholesterol showed little association, an observation that was wrongly interpreted as indicating that lowering dietary saturated fat did not reduce cholesterol; the weak observational association was in fact due to regression-dilution bias (the error in measuring individual dietary saturated fat consumption is large in relation to the small degree of variation between individuals in their true saturated fat consumption (Jacobs *et al.* 1979)). The notion that the average serum cholesterol in entire Western populations is high, and that nearly all people have non-optimal levels, appeared counterintuitive against a culture of defining dichotomous cut points in medicine (such as hypertension, obesity) (Law and Wald 2002). The issue of safety caused concern, as discussed above. Lastly, it has seemed inconsistent that serum cholesterol is a poor screening test and yet an important cause of heart disease. These issues are now satisfactorily resolved, but it has taken an enormous (and expensive) body of randomized trial data (Scandinavian Simvastatin Survival Study Group 1994; Shepherd *et al.* 1995; Sacks *et al.* 1996; Downs *et al.* 1998; LIPID Study Group 1998; ALLHAT-LLT Trial 2002; Heart Protection Study Collaborative Group 2002; PROSPER Study Group 2002; Sever *et al.* 2003) to overcome entrenched suspicions and encourage clinicians to use statins widely, despite their unusually high degree of efficacy and safety.

12.12 Triglycerides

Serum triglyceride concentration was associated with the risk of CHD in many cohort studies, but the association is subject to confounding by serum LDL and HDL cholesterol, diabetes, and other factors (Pocock *et al.* 1989; Wald *et al.* 1994; Ezzati *et al.* 2002). Whether an independent association exists is contentious. Very high serum levels of triglyceride caused by genetic defects (familial lipoprotein lipase deficiency, for example) are not associated with atheroma or coronary artery disease. These observations suggest that a material cause and effect relationship between serum triglyceride and heart disease is unlikely.

12.13 High-density lipoprotein (HDL) cholesterol

Cohort studies show an inverse association between HDL cholesterol (or apolipoprotein A1) and CHD. A randomized trial showing regression of coronary artery atheroma with administration of recombinant apo A1 has strengthened the evidence on causality (Nissen *et al.* 2003). In the cohort studies an absolute increase corresponding to 0.12 mmol/l ($\sim$10% of the average value) is associated with about a 15% decrease in the risk of CHD at age 60 (Pocock *et al.* 1989; Wald *et al.* 1994), or a 20% decrease with adjustment for the regression-dilution bias (Wald *et al.* 1994). Statins increase HDL cholesterol by $\sim$5%; the effect of this on risk of CHD events is relatively small. Other cholesterol-lowering drugs (such as fibrates and niacin) increase HDL cholesterol more, but their overall protective effect is smaller because they reduce LDL cholesterol much less (Table 12.5), so there is no case for using them in preference to statins. Effects on HDL cholesterol are important contributions to the effect of alcohol in protecting against CHD (Gaziano *et al.* 1993), and to the effect of smoking in causing it.

12.14 Appropriate policy

Dietary measures should be directed at the entire population. Serum cholesterol reductions of 0.6 mmol/l (10%), as discussed above, have occurred in entire Western communities, facilitated by health education, food labelling, widespread availability of palatable, affordable low fat foods in restaurants and supermarkets, and a positive image of healthy eating. Measures to promote these changes should be encouraged.

In persons with familial hypercholesterolaemia, the absolute risk of death from CHD at a young age is so great that affected persons should be identified and treated, even though the condition is rare and accounts for few of the heart disease deaths in a population. The most appropriate screening strategy has not yet been devised: measuring lipids in first-degree relatives of known cases will not identify all cases.

The most important high-risk group, however, are patients who have had a myocardial infarction. About half of all deaths from CHD occur in this group (Law *et al.* 2002). Without preventive treatment they face an annual risk of death from CHD of ~5% per year, a risk that persists indefinitely (and probably for the rest of a person's life), and varies little with age or sex (Law *et al.* 2002). Other high-risk groups include patients with angina, ischaemic stroke, peripheral arterial disease, and diabetes. All these patients with clinically recognized disease should receive statins; serum cholesterol measurements should not be used to impose artificial thresholds. Moreover, the reasons for treating all high-risk patients with statins irrespective of lipid levels apply equally to other cardioprotective drugs; all risk factors should be reduced in people at high risk (Law and Wald 2002), so there are virtually no patients who should receive statins alone.

Among persons without known occlusive arterial disease, it is not possible to identify a minority of the population who will experience the majority of the heart disease deaths (Wald *et al.* 1994; Law and Wald 2002). Population screening based on cardiovascular risk factors cannot do so, nor can it identify a group who would *not* benefit from a reduction in serum cholesterol (Wald *et al.* 1994; Law and Wald 2002). The most discriminatory predictor of risk is age. With the expiry of patents, statins and other cardioprotective drugs have become cheap, and trials and extensive clinical use have established their safety. This supports the case for a combination of such drugs to be recommended for widespread use among all persons in Western populations judged to be at sufficiently high risk – those above a specified age, for example (Wald and Law 2003). Simvastatin is now available over the counter in Britain to persons at higher risk, risk being determined mostly on the basis of existing disease and age.

12.15 Conclusions

The high levels of serum cholesterol found in Western populations are a major cause of the high mortality from CHD. Realistic dietary change in a community can lower serum cholesterol by 0.6 mmol/l (10%) and reduce heart disease mortality by ~25% among middle-aged individuals. Cholesterol-lowering drugs (statins) can lower cholesterol by 1.8 mmol/l (30%), and reduce the risk of heart disease death by ~60% from the third year onwards. Statins are inexpensive and safe, and their widespread use should be encouraged.

Acknowledgement

The authors would like to acknowledge the assistance of Dr Carlene Lawes in preparing the estimates in Table 12.3.

References

AHA (American Heart Association), National Heart, Lung, and Blood Institute (1990). The cholesterol facts: a summary of the evidence relating dietary fats, serum cholesterol, and coronary heart disease. *Circulation*, 81, 1721–33.

ALLHAT-LLT (The Antihypertensive and Lipid-Lowering Treatment to Prevent Heart Attack) Trial (2002). Major outcomes in moderately hypercholesterolemic, hypertensive patients randomized to pravastatin vs usual care. *Journal of the American Medical Association*, 288, 2998–3007.

Cannon, C. P., Braunwald, E., McCaben, C. H., Rader, D. J., Rouleau, J. L., Belder, R. *et al.* (2004). Intensive versus moderate lipid lowering with statins after acute coronary syndromes. *N Engl J Med*, 350, 1495–504.

Chen, Z., Peto, R., Collins, R., MacMahon, S., Lu, J., and Li, W. (1991). Serum cholesterol concentration and coronary heart disease in a population with low cholesterol concentrations. *British Medical Journal*, 303, 276–82.

Downs, R. J., Clearfield, M., Weis, S., Whitney, E., Shapiro, D. R., Beere, P. A. *et al.* (1998). Primary prevention of acute coronary events with lovastatin in men and women with average cholesterol levels. *Journal of the American Medical Association*, **279**, 1615–22.

Ezzati, M., Lopez, A. D., Rodgers, A., Vander Hoorn, S., Murray, C. J. L., and the Comparative Risk Assessment Collaborating Group (2002). Selected major risk factors and global and regional burden of disease. *Lancet*, **360**, 1347–60.

Gaziano, J. M., Buring, J. E., Breslow, J. L., Goldhaber, S. Z., Rossner, B., VanDenburgh, M., *et al.* (1993). Moderate alcohol intake, increased levels of high-density lipoprotein and its subfractions, and decreased risk of myocardial infarction. *New England Journal of Medicine*, **329**, 1829–34.

Glueck, C. J., Gartside, P., Fallat, R. W. W., Sielski, J., and Steiner, P. M. (1976). Longevity syndromes: familial hypobeta and familial hyperalpha lipoproteinemia. *Journal of Laboratory Clinical Medicine*, **88**, 941–57.

Heart Protection Study Collaborative Group (2002). MRC/BHF Heart Protection Study of cholesterol lowering with simvastatin in 20 536 high-risk individuals: a randomised placebo-controlled trial. *Lancet*, **360**, 7–22.

Jacobs, D. R., Anderson, J. T., and Blackburn, H. (1979). Diet and serum cholesterol. *American Journal of Epidemiology*, **110**, 77–87.

Katan, M. B., Grundy, S. M., Jones, P., Law, M., Miettinen, T., and Paoletti, R. (2003). Efficacy and safety of plant stanols and sterols in the management of blood cholesterol levels. *Mayo Clinic Proceedings*, **78**, 965–78.

Law, M. R. and Wald, N. J. (1994). An ecological study of serum cholesterol and ischaemic heart disease between 1950 and 1990. *European Journal of Clinical Nutrition*, **48**, 305–25.

Law, M. R. and Wald, N. J. (2002). Risk factor thresholds: their existence under scrutiny. *British Medical Journal*, **324**, 1570–6.

Law, M. R., Wald, N. J., Wu, T., Hackshaw, A., and Bailey, A. (1994a). Systematic underestimation of association between serum cholesterol concentration and ischaemic heart disease in observational studies: data from the BUPA study. *British Medical Journal*, **308**, 363–6.

Law, M. R., Wald, N. J., and Thompson, S. G. (1994b). By how much and how quickly does reduction in serum cholesterol concentration lower risk of ischaemic heart disease? *British Medical Journal*, **308**, 367–72.

Law, M. R., Wald, N. J., Wu, T., and Bailey, A. (1994c). Assessing possible hazards of reducing serum cholesterol. *British Medical Journal*, **308**, 373–9.

Law, M. R., Watt, H. C., and Wald, N. J. (2002). The underlying risk of death after myocardial infarction in the absence of treatment. *Archives of Internal Medicine*, **162**, 2405–10.

Law, M. R., Wald, N. J., and Rudnicka, A. R. (2003). Quantifying the effect of statins on LDL cholesterol, ischaemic heart disease and stroke: systematic review and meta-analysis. bmj.com, **326**, 1423.

Linton, M. F., Farese, R. V., and Young, S. G. (1993). Familial hypobetalipoproteinemia. *Journal of Lipid Research*, **34**, 521–41.

LIPID (The Long-Term Intervention with Pravastatin in Ischaemic Heart Disease) Study Group (1998). Prevention of cardiovascular events and death with pravastatin in patients with coronary heart disease and a broad range of initial cholesterol levels. *New England Journal of Medicine*, **339**, 1349–57.

MacMahon, S., Peto, R., Cutler, J., Collins, R., Sorlie, P., Neaton, J. *et al.* (1990). Blood pressure, stroke and coronary heart disease. Part 1, prolonged differences in blood pressure: prospective observational studies corrected for the regression dilution bias. *Lancet*, **335**, 765–74.

Mensink, R. P. and Katan, M. B. (1990). Effect of dietary trans fatty acids on high-density and low-density lipoprotein cholesterol levels in healthy subjects. *New England Journal of Medicine*, **323**, 439–45.

Murray, C. J. L. and Lopez, A. D. (1996). *Global health statistics: a compendium of incidence, prevalence and mortality estimates for over 200 conditions*. Harvard University Press, Cambridge, MA.

Neaton, J. D. and Wentworth, D. (1992). Serum cholesterol, blood pressure, cigarette smoking, and death from coronary heart disease. *Archives of Internal Medicine*, **152**, 56–64.

Nestel, P., Noakes, M., Belling, B., McArthur, Clifton, P., Janus, E. *et al.* (1992). Plasma lipoprotein lipid and Lp[a] changes with substitution of elaidic acid for oleic acid in the diet. *Journal of Lipid Research*, **33**, 1029–36.

Nissen, S. E., Tsunoda, T., Tuzcu, E. M., Schoenhagen, P., Cooper, C. J., Yasin, M. *et al.* (2003). Effect of recombinant ApoA-I Milano on coronary atherosclerosis in patients with acute coronary syndromes. *Journal of the American Medical Association*, **290**, 2292–300.

Nissen, S. E., Tuzcu, E. M., Schoenhagen, P., Brown, B. G., Ganz, P., Vogel, R. A., *et al.* (2004). Effect of intensive compared with moderate lipid-lowering therapy on progression of coronary atherosclerosis. *JAMA*, **291**, 1071–80.

Pocock, S. J., Shaper, A. G., and Phillips, A. N. (1989). Concentrations of high density lipoprotein cholesterol, triglycerides, and total cholesterol in ischaemic heart disease. *British Medical Journal*, **298**, 998–1002.

PROSPER (PROspective Study of Pravastatin in the Elderly at Risk) Study Group (2002). Pravastatin in elderly individuals at risk of vascular disease (PROSPER): a randomised controlled trial. *Lancet*, **360**, 1623–30.

Sacks, F. M., Pfeffer, M. A., Moye, L. A., Rouleau, J. L., Rutherford, J. D., Cole, T. G. *et al.* (1996). The effect of pravastatin on coronary events after myocardial infarction in patients with average cholesterol levels. *New England Journal of Medicine*, **335**, 1001–9.

Salomaa, V., Rasi, V., Pekkanen, J., Jauhiainen, M., Vahtera, E., Peitinen, P. *et al.* (1993). The effects of saturated fat and n-6 polyunsaturated fat on postprandial lipema and hemostatic activity. *Atherosclerosis*, **103**, 1–11.

Scandinavian Simvastatin Survival Study Group (1994). Randomised trial of cholesterol lowering in 4444 patients with coronary heart disease: the Scandinavian Simvastatin Survival Study (4S). *Lancet*, **344**, 1383–9.

Sever, P. S., Dahlöf, B., Poulter, N. R., Wedel, H., Beevers, G., Caulfield, M. *et al.* (2003). Prevention of coronary and stroke events with atorvastatin in hypertensive patients who have average or lower-than-average cholesterol concentrations, in the Anglo-Scandinavian Cardiac Outcomes Trial – Lipid Lowering Arm (ASCOT-LLA): a multicentre randomised controlled trial. *Lancet*, **361**, 1149–58.

Shepherd, J., Cobbe, S. M., Ford, I., Isles, C. G., Lorimer, A. R., Macfarlane, P. W. *et al.* (1995). Prevention of coronary heart disease with pravastatin in men with hypercholesterolemia. *New England Journal of Medicine*, **333**, 1301–7.

Wald, N. J. and Law, M. R. (2003). A strategy to reduce cardiovascular disease by over 80%. bmj.com, **326**, 1419.

Wald, N. J., Law, M., Watt, H. C., Wu, T., Bailey, A., Johnson, A. M. *et al.* (1994). Apolipoproteins and ischaemic heart disease: implications for screening. *Lancet*, **343**, 75–9.

WHO (World Health Organization) (2002). *World health report 2002: reducing risks, promoting healthy life*. WHO, Geneva.

Chapter 13

Trends in all-cause and cardiovascular mortality: a comparison between Belgium, the Netherlands, and Denmark, 1950–99

J. V. Joossens and H. Kesteloot

13.1 Introduction

Valuable insights can be gained from analysing differences in mortality rates worldwide (Kesteloot 1994). This can be especially useful when data from neighbouring countries are compared (Kesteloot 1999). Many factors influence mortality, and to eliminate some of these it is valuable to compare countries where these factors are similar.

In this chapter we compare mortality trends and possible explanatory factors in three developed affluent countries: Belgium (B) (population 10.2 million, with 1 million in Brussels), the Netherlands (NL) (pop. 15.8 million) and Denmark (DK) (pop. 5.3 million). These countries have similar socio-economic systems, and each has a social healthcare system covering the whole population, but they have important differences in employment. Relevant data on nutrition and smoking are available from 1960 onwards for the Netherlands (Kromhout *et al.* 1990; Anonymous 1998) and Belgium, including data from Flanders (FL) (North, pop. 5.9 million) and Wallonia (W) (South, pop. 3.3 million) (Joossens *et al.* 1966, 1985; BIRNH 1989; Den Hond *et al.* 1994). Data from Denmark (FAO 1998; Pietinen 1998) are more limited. Important differences in mortality rates exist between Belgium, its regions, the Netherlands, and Denmark (Joossens *et al.* 1977, 1985; BIRNH 1989; Kesteloot *et al.* 1995; Joossens and Kesteloot 1996). In this chapter all-cause mortality is used as the 'gold standard' against which to validate cardiovascular mortality.

To explore which factors might explain the observed changes in mortality in the three countries, levels and time-related changes in mortality rates in both sexes are compared with changes in lifestyle and in socio-economic factors, primarily unemployment. Socio-economic factors have separately been shown to influence mortality within and possibly between countries (Marmot 1999). Ecological studies cannot prove causality, but they may generate hypotheses and can indicate where certain relationships are not valid. As changes in mortality can differ between the sexes, a separate analysis for men and women is reported.

13.2 Mortality in Belgium, the Netherlands, and Denmark, 1950–2000

13.2.1 Methods

All-cause, cardiovascular and cancer mortality data in 5-year age groups for Belgium were obtained from the World Health Organization (WHO), Geneva, for 1954–94. Similar data for

1995 were obtained from the National Institute of Statistics, Brussels, which also provided all-cause mortality data for Belgium, Flanders, and Wallonia for 1996 to 2000. Mortality data for Flanders and Wallonia were also obtained for 1971–95. Data for the Netherlands were available for 1950–99 and for Denmark for 1952–96. The mortality data were age-adjusted to ages 45 and 74 years using the old European population standard (Doll *et al.* 1970). These age limits were chosen as the most reliable for the study of mortality from chronic diseases as well as having enough events to reduce random error. Belgian regional data are presented for six major causes of death: all-cause (AC) (1971–2000), total cardiovascular (TCV), coronary heart disease (CHD), cerebrovascular accidents (CVA), non-cardiovascular (AC–TCV) and lung cancer mortality rates (all 1971–95).

The yearly data in the Figures are smoothed over 5 years in order to reduce random variation and to increase readability. Differences in death rates and in percentage of the most remote year are calculated between 1969–71 and 1954–56, and between 1993–95 and 1969–71.

The significance of positive or negative differences between pairs of observations is calculated using the non-parametric sign-test (Lentner 1982). The intercorrelations of cardiovascular, site-specific cancer mortality rates and sex are studied among 40 countries worldwide using univariate linear regression.

13.2.2 Mortality data

The time trends from 1950 to 2000 of AC and TCV mortality rates are illustrated for each sex in Figs 13.1 and 13.2. AC and TCV mortality generally follow a similar pattern. In the 1950s Belgium had the highest mortality for AC and TCV in each sex, although by the end of the period Denmark had the highest rates (Figs 13.1, 13.2). However, there are two major differences between the sexes: in men both AC and TCV mortality increase from the 1950s to the 1970s and decrease thereafter, with a large mortality gradient across the countries during the period 1950–70; in women mortalities decrease during the same period and the differences in

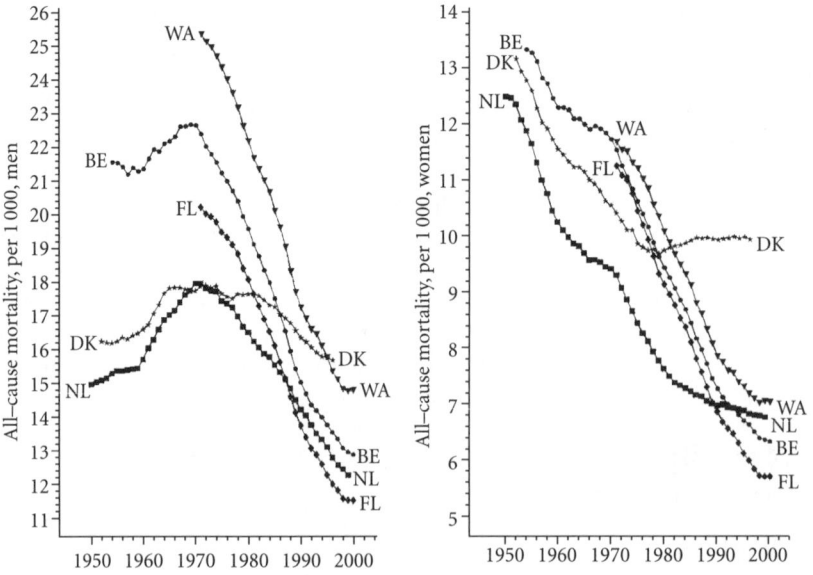

Fig. 13.1 All-cause mortality in men and women. Age adjusted 45–74 years. (BE: Belgium, WA: Wallonia.) Data are yearly-smoothed over 5 years.

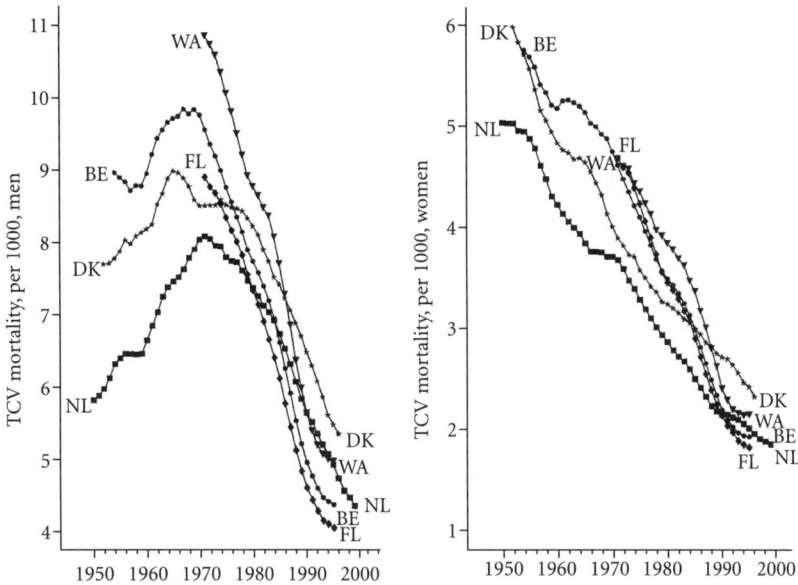

Fig. 13.2 Total cardiovascular mortality in men and women. (As in Fig. 13.1.)

mortality across countries are smaller. Danish women are the only exception. Their AC mortality rate increases slightly ($p < 0.05$) from the late 1970s (Fig. 13.1).

In 1971 Wallonia, followed by Belgium and Flanders, had the highest AC and TCV mortality in each sex. Subsequently, the largest decrease in male AC and TCV mortality was seen in Wallonia and the smallest in Denmark (Figs 13.1, 13.2). In women the largest decrease was seen in Flanders and the smallest in Denmark (Figs 13.1, 13.2).

For male AC–TCV mortality, an increase up to 1970 is followed by a decrease. The latter is more marked in Belgium and its regions, but less so in the Netherlands. However, in Denmark an important increase occurs (Table 13.1). For female AC–TCV mortality a decrease is seen in Belgium and its regions, especially Flanders, whereas in the Netherlands the decrease is fastest up to 1970 and is followed by a more moderate decrease (Table 13.2). In Denmark there is a marked increase after 1970 (Table 13.2), such that Danish women have a higher AC–TCV mortality in 1995 (759/100 000/year) than in 1955 (698/100 000/year) (Table 13.2).

The increasing pattern of male AC mortality in the period 1950–70 (Figs 13.1, 13.2) is mostly due to lung cancer (Fig. 13.3) and other smoking-attributable non-lung cancer mortality, including part of TCV mortality. According to Peto *et al.* (1992) total mortality related to smoking is 3.6 times lung cancer mortality in men and 2.5 times in women. For TCV mortality the factors are 1.4 times lung cancer mortality in men and 1.0 times for women (Peto *et al.* 1992). When subtracting smoking-attributable deaths from AC and TCV, the increasing/decreasing pattern is changed to a decreasing one from start to end of the observations, again decreasing faster after 1970. Therefore, smoking-adjusted male AC and TCV mortality rates were already decreasing from the 1950s until the 1970s. In that period drug treatment of hypertension and hypercholesterolaemia was less effective than currently and only used in a minority of the population.

Table 13.1 Mean mortality for men (per 100 000/year) for 3 years (around 1955, 1970, 1994), and difference between two periods and percentage of most remote year. Age adjusted 45–74 years

Cause	Belgium		The Netherlands		Denmark		Belgium		The Netherlands		Denmark	
	Mean 1955	Δ (1970–55) (%)	Mean 1955	Δ (1970–55) (%)	Mean 1955	Δ (1970–55) (%)	Mean 1970	Δ (1994–70) (%)	Mean 1970	Δ (1994–70) (%)	Mean 1970	Δ (1994–70) (%)
AC	2158	112 (5)	1551	253 (16)	1622	154 (9)	2270	−861 (−38)	1804	−461 (−26)	1776	−183 (−10)
TCV	894	80 (9)	652	153 (24)	783	60 (8)	974	−540 (−55)	805	−298 (−37)	843	−284 (−34)
CHD	324	167 (52)	395	142 (36)	454	146 (32)	491	−279 (−57)	537	−259 (−48)	600	−252 (−42)
CVA			156	−24 (−16)	168	−41 (−25)	210	−136 (−65)	131	−57 (−44)	127	−39 (−31)
TCA	453	127 (28)	426	127 (30)	430	55 (13)	580	−26 (−4)	553	−41 (−7)	485	38 (8)
Lung cancer[a]	104	160 (153)	115	141 (123)	79	105 (133)	264	−38 (−14)	257	−62 (−24)	184	−19 (−10)
Stomach cancer	98	−34 (−35)	105	−39 (−37)	90	−43 (−47)	64	−42 (−65)	66	−36 (−55)	48	−29 (−61)
Rectal cancer	28	−3 (−10)	20	−1 (−7)	37	−7 (−19)	25	−13 (−52)	18	−7 (−36)	30	−6 (−20)
Colon cancer	30	6 (21)	25	5 (20)	32	−1 (−2)	36	0 (0)	31	6 (19)	31	8 (27)
Prostate cancer	30	−1 (−4)	24	3 (15)	29	−0 (−1)	28	4 (14)	27	5 (20)	29	15 (52)
Oesophagus ca.	11	0 (1)	9	−1 (−13)	10	−1 (−9)	11	7 (62)	8	12 (153)	9	11 (121)
Cirrhosis	25	11 (46)	11	2 (17)	14	8 (57)	36	−3 (−8)	13	1 (10)	22	27 (122)
AC-TCV	1264	32 (3)	900	100 (11)	839	94 (11)	1296	−321 (−25)	999	−163 (−16)	933	101 (11)
AC-TCA	1705	−16 (−1)	1126	126 (11)	1191	99 (8)	1689	−835 (−49)	1251	−419 (−34)	1291	−221 (−17)
AC-TCV-TCA	811	−95 (−12)	474	−28 (−6)	409	39 (9)	715	−295 (−41)	446	−122 (−27)	448	63 (14)

TCA = total cancer

[a] For lung cancer the mid-period is 1980.

Table 13.2 Mean mortality for women (per 100 000/year) for 3 years (around 1955, 1970, 1994), and difference between two periods and percentage of most remote year. Age adjusted 45–74 years

Cause	Belgium		The Netherlands		Denmark		Belgium		The Netherlands		Denmark	
	Mean 1955	Δ (1970–55) (%)	Mean 1955	Δ (1970–55) (%)	Mean 1955	Δ (1970–55) (%)	Mean 1970	Δ (1994–70) (%)	Mean 1970	Δ (1994–70) (%)	Mean 1970	Δ (1994–70) (%)
AC	1333	−154 (−12)	1161	−209 (−18)	1246	−194 (−16)	1179	−492 (−42)	951	−256 (−27)	1052	−45 (−4)
TCV	574	−98 (−17)	494	−120 (−24)	548	−153 (−28)	477	−286 (−60)	374	−169 (−45)	395	−147 (−37)
CHD	150	20 (14)	213	−41 (−19)	227	−5 (−2)	170	−99 (−58)	171	−81 (−47)	221	−96 (−44)
CVA			174	−69 (−39)	177	−81 (−46)	147	−100 (−68)	105	−57 (−54)	95	−35 (−37)
TCA	351	−21 (−6)	353	−20 (−6)	398	−13 (−3)	330	−35 (−11)	332	−19 (−6)	386	50 (13)
Lung cancer[a]	11	9 (84)	10	10 (103)	13	40 (300)	21	11 (55)	19	27 (139)	53	44 (83)
Stomach cancer	54	−27 (−49)	58	−30 (−52)	48	−27 (−55)	28	−20 (−71)	28	−17 (−62)	22	−13 (−59)
Rectal cancer	18	−4 (−24)	14	−2 (−15)	21	−2 (−11)	14	−7 (−54)	12	−5 (−40)	18	−5 (−27)
Colon cancer	31	5 (17)	30	2 (7)	34	2 (4)	36	−12 (−32)	32	−4 (−13)	36	−4 (−11)
Breast cancer	61	8 (14)	73	10 (13)	75	5 (7)	69	10 (14)	83	−3 (−3)	81	8 (10)
Endometrium	33	−12 (−36)	15	−2 (−11)	28	−13 (−47)	21	−12 (−56)	13	−7 (−50)	15	−3 (−24)
Oesophagus ca.	3	−1 (−22)	3	−0 (−11)	3	−0 (−9)	3	0 (13)	3	3 (92)	3	2 (74)
Cirrhosis	11	6 (49)	8	−1 (−14)	18	−4 (−22)	17	0 (2)	6	1 (16)	14	10 (74)
AC-TCV	759	−56 (−7)	667	−89 (−13)	698	−40 (−6)	703	−206 (−29)	578	−88 (−15)	657	102 (16)
AC-TCA	983	−133 (−14)	808	−189 (−23)	848	−181 (−21)	849	−456 (−54)	619	−237 (−38)	667	−96 (−14)
AC-TCV-TCA	408	−35 (−9)	314	−69 (−22)	299	−28 (−9)	373	−171 (−46)	245	−69 (−28)	272	52 (19)

TCA = total cancer.
[a] For lung cancer the mid-period is 1980.

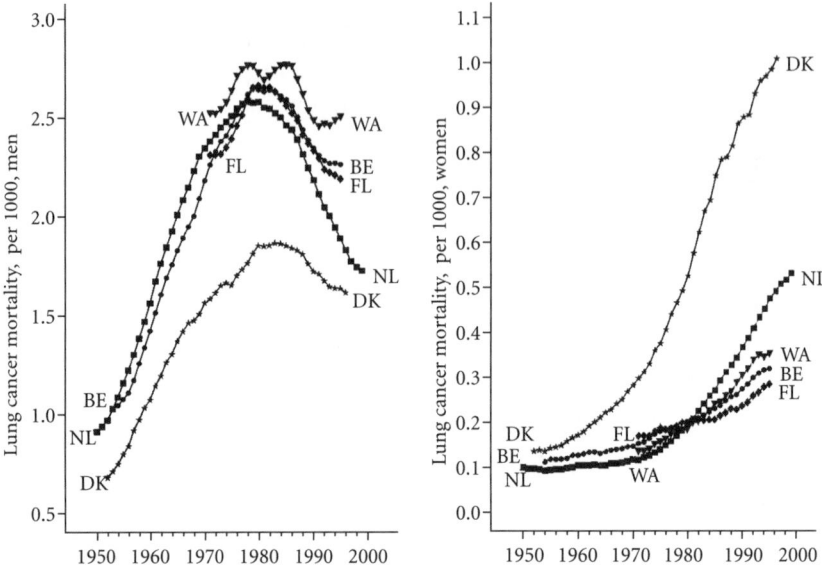

Fig. 13.3 Lung cancer mortality. (As in Fig. 13.1.)

The decrease in mean male AC mortality between 1993–95 and 1954–55 as a percentage of 1954–55 was −35% in Belgium, −13% in the Netherlands, and −2% in Denmark. In women it was −48, −40, and −19%, respectively. Similarly for TCV in men, the changes were −52, −22, and −29%; in women −67, −59, and −55%, respectively.

For men in 1955 the mortality ratio B/NL from AC was 1.39, in B/DK 1.33, and in NL/DK 0.96. In 1994 these ratios were 1.05, 0.88, and 0.84, respectively. For women in 1955 the ratios were 1.15, 1.07, and 0.93, while in 1994 the ratios were 0.99, 0.68, and 0.69, respectively. These changes essentially reflect a worsening of relative mortality in Danish women.

The sex ratio (male/female) of AC in 1955 was 1.6 in Belgium, 1.3 in the Netherlands, and 1.3 in Denmark. In 1994 it was 2.0, 1.9, and 1.6, respectively. Danish women benefited the least from the ongoing changes (Fig. 13.1, Tables 13.1, 13.2). The increasing mortality sex ratio in Belgium is due to a relatively faster decrease in AC mortality in women.

CHD mortality behaved as for AC and TCV in men from the three countries: increasing up to 1970 and decreasing afterwards (Fig. 13.4). In women CHD continuously decreased in the Netherlands. The current rates are lowest in Flanders and highest in Denmark for both sexes.

Mortality from CVA decreased in the Netherlands and Denmark from the mid-1950s to the end of the period (Fig. 13.5). Similar changes in CVA were observed in the western world (Sans *et al.* 1997; Joossens 2000). However, CVA markedly increased in Belgium in both men and women up to 1970. This was an artefact resulting from misclassification of CVA as diseases of the arteries (Joossens 1980) and disappeared with the eighth revision of the international classification of diseases. In 1971 Belgium and its regions had the highest CVA levels, while the rates are now slightly higher in Denmark for both sexes (Fig. 13.5).

For lung cancer mortality there are major differences in relative mortality ranking between the sexes (Fig. 13.3). In men the lowest lung cancer mortality over the whole period is seen in Denmark and the highest in Wallonia. The largest increase is seen in Belgium during the

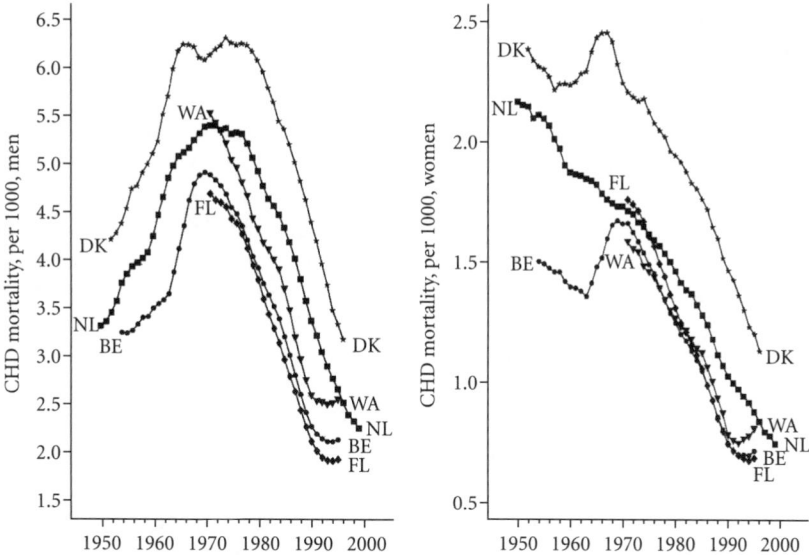

Fig. 13.4 CHD mortality. (As in Fig. 13.1.)

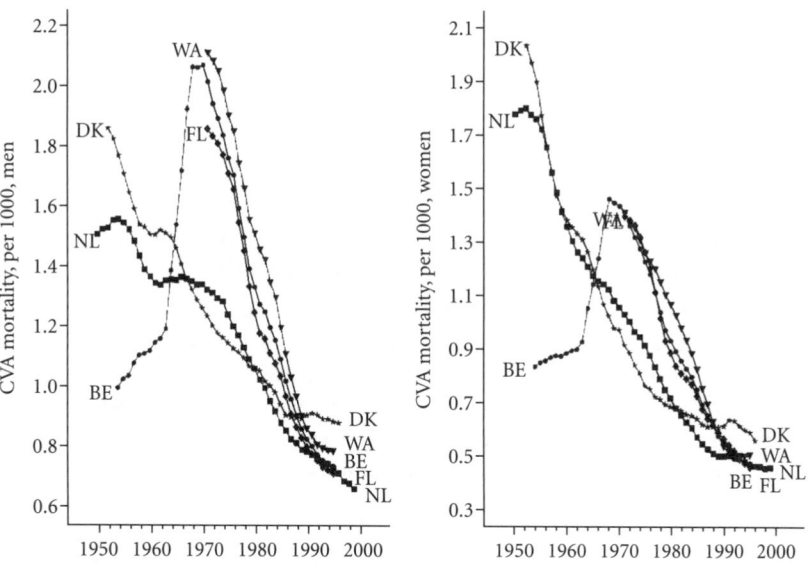

Fig. 13.5 Cerebrovascular accidents mortality. (As in Fig. 13.1.)

period 1955–80. From 1980–94 the smallest decrease in lung cancer mortality is seen in Denmark and the largest in the Netherlands (Table 13.1). In women the situation is different and the smallest increase in lung cancer mortality is seen in Belgium and the largest in Denmark during both time periods (Table 13.2). The level of female lung cancer in Denmark is now three times higher than in Belgium. The sex ratio (male/female) of lung cancer mortality is now 7.1 in Belgium, 4.2 in the Netherlands, and 1.7 in Denmark.

13.2.3 Changes and levels of mortality in Belgium, the Netherlands, and Denmark

Levels of mortality

Mortality levels in Belgium in 1955 and 1970 were higher than in the Netherlands and Denmark for nearly all major causes of death (Tables 13.1, 13.2). After 1970 the differences between Belgium and the Netherlands gradually narrowed and nearly disappeared in women (Tables 13.1, 13.2). This is even more evident when comparing Belgium to Denmark. Danish men in 1994 had higher mortality rates than Belgian men in 12 out of 15 causes of death (Table 13.1) (sign-test of paired differences: $p < 0.05$). Female mortality rates were higher for all 16 causes of death (sign-test: $p < 0.001$) (Table 13.2). This resulted in a reversal of the ranking for AC mortality in women between 1970 and 1994.

Time-related changes in mortality

Mortality differences and the percentage changes for 15 causes of death in men and 16 in women were estimated for the three countries (Tables 13.1, 13.2). The changes were measured between identical years (1970–55 and 1994–70). In the first period the paired differences in percentage changes between Belgium and the Netherlands and between Belgium and Denmark are not significant (sign-test: $p > 0.2$). After 1970 Belgium has better results in men in 13 out of 15 paired differences than the Netherlands (sign-test: $p < 0.002$) and they are better than Denmark for all 15 paired differences ($p < 0.0001$). For women the results are better for 15 out of 16 paired differences ($p < 0.001$) between Belgium and the Netherlands and for all paired differences between Belgium and Denmark ($p < 0.0001$).

The lowest AC and TCV mortality rates are seen in Flanders and the highest in Denmark (Figs 13.1, 13.2). For all major causes of death Flanders has lower mortality rates than Wallonia (Figs 13.1–5).

13.2.4 Correlations between cardiovascular mortality and selected cancers in 40 countries worldwide

In 1965 it was shown that stomach cancer and CVA were strongly correlated (Joossens 1965). This correlation persisted over many years, yielding highly significant regression coefficients of stomach cancer on CVA of the same order of magnitude both between and within countries (Joossens 2000; Joossens and Kesteloot 1998), making a spurious association unlikely. A significant positive correlation was also found between levels and time-related changes of rectal cancer and of CHD and CVA mortality (Joossens and Geboers 1985; Joossens and Kesteloot 1990). These findings are confirmed by recent data from 40 countries worldwide (Table 13.3).

Stomach cancer mortality has the strongest relation with CVA, but it also significantly relates to TCV in each sex. For TCV, CHD, and CVA from each sex the best correlations are seen with rectal and endometrial cancer and with male lung cancer mortality. All the significant correlations between cardiovascular mortality and stomach, rectal, endometrial, and lung cancer in a given sex yield similar values within and between sexes (Table 13.3), showing that the intercorrelations are not markedly influenced by sex-linked factors. No positive significant correlation is obtained between cardiovascular disease mortality and female breast cancer, prostate cancer, and colon cancer mortality in univariate analysis. Prostate, female breast, and colon cancer are generally significantly intercorrelated across the 40 countries (Table 13.3).

Table 13.3 Intercorrelations between cardiovascular and cancer mortality. Mean of three last available years. Age adjusted 45–74 years between 1995 and 1997 from 40 countries worldwide

	Cancer from								
	Lung		Stomach		Rectum		Endometrium	Prostate	Breast
	M	F	M	F	M	F			F
TCV M	0.55	−0.07	0.45	0.46	0.62	0.72	0.55	0.01	0.05
TCV F	0.47	−0.11	0.49	0.52	0.55	0.66	0.60	−0.12	−0.08
CHD M	0.45	0.12	0.25	0.27	0.56	0.63	0.35	0.18	0.25
CHD F	0.37	0.09	0.27	0.31	0.50	0.57	0.41	0.07	0.15
CVA M	0.40	−0.29	0.74	0.77	0.49	0.59	0.55	−0.31	−0.28
CVA F	0.36	−0.27	0.72	0.76	0.43	0.56	0.56	−0.34	−0.30
Prostate	−0.05	0.36	−0.52	−0.56	0.07	0.06	0.08		0.63
Breast	0.20	0.43	−0.52	−0.55	0.11	0.05	−0.01	0.63	
Colon M[a]	0.46	0.40	−0.32	−0.33	0.56	0.40	0.01	0.28	0.54
Colon F[a]	0.27	0.50	−0.41	−0.41	0.42	0.38	−0.01	0.39	0.58

$r \geq 0.31$, $p < 0.05$; $r \geq 0.40$, $p < 0.01$; $r \geq 0.50$, $p < 0.001$; $r \geq 0.57$, $p < 0.0001$.

M: male mortality; F: female mortality.

[a] Colon cancer of either sex is not significantly related to cardiovascular mortality.

13.2.5 Factors potentially influencing the observed variation in mortality

Medical, socio-economic, and genetic factors

The level of medical care and coverage by social security at the population level is high in the three countries. In Belgium the number of doctors and the global costs of medical care are higher in Wallonia than in Flanders, while as shown, Wallonia has higher mortality.

No comparable data are available on levels of physical activity in the 45–74-year age group between the three countries. Cycling is more common in the Netherlands and Denmark than in Belgium.

The three countries are affluent as indicated by the yearly gross national product (GNP). The most affluent is Denmark ($32 100/person), followed by Belgium ($26 440), and the Netherlands ($25 990) (World Bank 1998). The percentage of unemployment in the three countries and two regions in 1982 and 1998 is given for each sex in Table 13.4. The lowest values are seen in the Netherlands in 1998 and the highest in Wallonia, both in 1982 and 1998.

In a recent study the observed male all-cause mortality data in the 42 Belgian counties, at ages 40–60 years, were corrected for eight socio-economic factors as found in the national census of 1991. The mortality gradient between Flanders and Wallonia did not change substantially after correction. The seven counties with the highest corrected mortality risk in Belgium were rural areas in Wallonia; that is, the least polluted ones (Deboosere and Gadeyne 2000).

The number of cars per square kilometre and population density are lowest in Denmark. It is nearly entirely surrounded by the sea and, therefore, pollution resulting from industrialization and from the use of cars can be assumed to be lowest in Denmark and highest in the Netherlands, Flanders, and two industrial areas in Wallonia (Liège and Charleroi).

Table 13.4 Percentage of unemployed subjects

	Men		Women	
	1982	1998	1982	1998
Netherlands	12.3	3.7	0.3	4.8
Flanders	11.3	6.1	24.7	12.4
Denmark		7.8		9.9
Belgium (including Brussels)	11.8	10.6	23.1	17.8
Wallonia	14.0	17.8	26.9	26.9

Note: data are ranked according to levels in men in 1998. Data were obtained from the Central Bureau of Statistics, the Netherlands, Rijksdienst voor Arbeidsvoorziening (Federal Department of Employment), Belgium, and from the World Bank for 1996, Denmark. Data from NSY 1999: unemployment, both sexes combined 1999: 5.3%.

Genetic factors at the population level cannot explain the substantial decrease or increase in mortality rates over short periods of time (Figs 13.1–5; Tables 13.1, 13.2) (Kesteloot 1991; Marmot 1992).

Lifestyle factors: nutrition

Nutrition has potentially both harmful and beneficial components (NRC 1989; Renaud and de Lorgeril 1989; Kesteloot 1991; Kesteloot *et al.* 1991; WCRF 1997). There are considerable qualitative similarities between the three countries in terms of nutrition, but also marked quantitative differences.

The intake of fatty acids is best documented in Belgium, its regions, and in the Netherlands (Table 13.5). A higher saturated fat intake and a lower polyunsaturated fat intake were observed in Flanders compared to the Netherlands in 1960, gradually equalizing in the 1990s after a peak in the 1970s for polyunsaturated fat in Belgium (Table 13.5). A higher saturated and a lower polyunsaturated fat intake in Wallonia compared to Flanders is observed in all other surveys, which is consistent with the higher AC and TCV mortality in Wallonia (Figs 13.1, 13.2; Table 13.5). Olive oil has become more popular in Belgium since 1990, but quantitative data are not available.

Less information is available from Denmark. According to the Food and Agricultural Organization (FAO) total fat intake in Denmark provided around 43% of energy from 1965–95, higher than in Belgium and the Netherlands (FAO 1998). Vegetable fat intake was nearly 50% lower in Denmark (1965–95) (FAO 1998). A 37% total fat intake and a polyunsaturated/saturated fat (P/S) ratio of 0.33 was found in Denmark in a 1995 survey (Pietinen 1998). The health situation in Denmark has been improving since then. From 1995 to 1999 life expectancy, mean of both sexes, increased by 1.2 years in Denmark, compared to 0.6 years from 1980 to 1995.

Salt intake was slightly lower in Denmark than in the other two countries in the INTERSALT study (Elliott *et al.* 1988). Salt intake in Belgium decreased by 25% from 1966 to 1986. Systolic blood pressure and prevalence of hypertension decreased markedly in Belgium between 1968 and 1986. Severe systolic hypertension in the elderly (>220 mmHg), present in 1967 and 1972, disappeared completely from 1975 onwards. The mean rise of blood pressure with age, mean of both sexes, between 25 and 55 years, decreased from 22 mmHg to 10 mmHg over the same time period (Joossens and Kesteloot 1991).

Table 13.5 Fat intake in % energy (mean of both sexes)

	N	Total fat	Saturated FA*	Polyunsaturated FA	P/S ratio
The Netherlands					
1960	1049	42	17.5	5.8	0.33
1987/88	5898	41	16.6	7.0	0.42
1992	6218	39	14.8	6.4	0.43
1997/98	5958	38	16.3	7.2	0.44
Belgium					
1974	2613	42	18.2	8.3	0.46
1979	2600	42	17.9	7.7	0.43
1982	10981	42	17.2	7.8	0.45
1991/92	563	40	17.4	6.3	0.36
Flanders					
1960	769	38.2	19.7	3.9	0.20
1974		42	17.2	9.3	0.54
1979		42	17.3	8.1	0.47
1982	6947	42	16.5	8.5	0.52
1991/92	492	40	16.6	6.9	0.42
Wallonia					
1974		43	20.0	6.8	0.34
1979		43	19.2	7.1	0.37
1982	4034	43	18.5	6.5	0.35
1991/92	71	41	18.9	5.1	0.26

References: data from Anonymous 1998; Joossens and Kesteloot 1996; Joossens et al. 1966, 1985; Kornitzer and Bara 1989; Kromhout et al. 1996.

The values for 1974 and 1979 for Belgium are distributed proportionally for Flanders (+60%) and Wallonia (+40%).

* FA = fatty acids

Worldwide, salt intake is an important determinant for hypertension, stroke (Joossens and Kesteloot 1998; Joossens 2000) and most likely also for stomach cancer mortality. Stomach cancer mortality is a rough indicator of mean salt intake at the population level (Joossens *et al.* 1996). The similar levels and trends of stomach cancer suggest no major differences in levels and trends of salt intake in the three countries since the 1950s (Tables 13.1, 13.2). Hence they do not explain the marked differences in AC and cardiovascular mortality. While hypertension plays an important role in haemorrhagic stroke mortality, saturated fat intake, especially when combined with hypertension, is also an important risk factor for thromboembolic stroke and n-6 polyunsaturated fat could decrease its risk (Hornstra 1980). The decreasing salt intake (Joossens and Kesteloot 1991) and the differences in fat intake in the three countries (Table 13.5) are consistent with the observed time-related changes in stroke mortality since 1970 (B > NL > DK) (Fig. 13.5). The influence of fat and salt intake is also suggested by the significant correlation of stroke with both stomach and rectal cancer (Table 13.3). This correlation remains significant after adjustment by multiple regression analysis. Rectal cancer correlates strongly with CHD (Table 13.3), suggesting a similar detrimental influence of saturated fat and a beneficial one for polyunsaturated fat.

According to FAO data fruit and vegetable intake (g/day/10.5 MJ) increased most in Belgium from 1965 to 1995 (340 to 482), followed by the Netherlands (350 to 435) and Denmark (220 to 280) (FAO 1998).

Fish fat consumption in 1980–82 was highest in Denmark (1.9% of energy), followed by Belgium (0.9%), and the Netherlands (0.6%). Non-fish animal fat provided 35% of energy in Denmark, 26% in Belgium, and 23% in the Netherlands (Zhang *et al.* 1999).

Nutrition plays an important role in obesity. However, the body mass index was similar in the three countries in the INTERSALT study (Elliott *et al.* 1988) and could not explain the differences in mortality observed at that time.

Lifestyle factors: smoking and drinking habits

Smoking habits, as percentage of adult smokers (18+ years), are documented in the three countries. Around 1969 74% of men in Belgium were smokers and in 1982 40% of men and 28% of women. This declined further to 31% and 19%, respectively, in 1993 and has since increased to 36% (90% cigarette smokers) and 26%, respectively, in 2000. In 1982 39% were smokers in Flanders and 42% in Wallonia. This changed to 28% and 33%, respectively, in 2000. In the age group 35–64 years 39% of Belgian men were daily smokers and 30% of women in the year 2000 (CRIOC 2001). Data from the Netherlands are available from 1958 to 1998. In 1958 90% and 29% of men and women, respectively, were smokers; in 1982 the figures were 41% and 34%, and in 1998, 37% and 30% for men and women, respectively. Data from 1998 for the Netherlands only indicate that 18% of all smokers were cigar or pipe smokers in men and 1% in women (STIVORO 1999). In 1964 68% of Danish men and 55% of Danish women were smokers, of which 78% of men and 74% of women inhaled (Chenet *et al.* 1996). The percentage smoking rates decreased in 1980 to 59% and 43%, respectively, and to 49% and 41% in 1990 (Prescott *et al.* 1998).

According to FAO data, alcohol consumption in Belgium (g/day/10.5 MJ) was 23 g in 1965 and 28 g in 1980, decreasing to 21 g in 1995. In the Netherlands it was 8 g, increasing to 18 g in 1995, and in Denmark it increased from 15 to 22 g (1965–95) (FAO 1998). The level of cirrhosis mortality in 1994 was highest in Denmark and increasing fastest in both sexes, whereas it was lowest in the Netherlands (Tables 13.1, 13.2). The most favourable changes in cirrhosis mortality have occurred in Belgium (Tables 13.1, 13.2).

13.3 Discussion

13.3.1 Medical and socio-economic factors

Medical and surgical treatment, available in the three countries at a high-quality level, may reduce death rates, but cannot explain why male AC mortality in the 1950s was much higher in Belgium. It does not explain why mortality rates in Belgium and the Netherlands are now nearly identical in each sex and much lower than in Denmark (Fig. 13.1, Tables 13.1, 13.2). Medical care was not able to improve the health situation of Danish men, where AC mortality decreased by only 2% between 1955 and 1994 (Fig. 13.1). Neither could it prevent a rise in AC mortality from 1980 to 1996 in Danish women (Fig. 13.1). Medical care influences only the treated group and cannot explain the significant correlations between cancer and cardiovascular mortality in either the same or different sex (Table 13.3). Similar conclusions about medical care have been reached previously (Marmot 1992).

Although unemployment may influence mortality (Marmot 1999), it does not explain why since 1971 AC mortality has decreased more in Wallonia than in Denmark (Fig. 13.1), although Wallonia had the highest unemployment rates in each sex and time period (Table 13.4). Available data on income levels, pollution, and obesity do not help explain the differences in mortality between the three countries.

13.3.2 Reliability of cardiovascular mortality data

During the period 1983–90 the values for CHD mortality in Ghent, Belgium were artefactually too low by 25% (De Backer 1996) and this was also the case in 1990 for Belgium (−30%) and the Netherlands (− 15%) (Murray and Lopez 1997). Since 1990 CHD mortality has improved in Belgium and its regions (Fig. 13.4). Only in Denmark was the absolute decrease in CHD mortality since 1970 in each sex similar to that of TCV and higher than the change in AC mortality (Tables 13.1, 13.2). This is unlikely and again raises the question of the reliability of CHD mortality data. Looking at AC–TCV mortality, where the highest levels are now seen in Wallonia and the lowest in the Netherlands and Flanders, can partially solve the problem. Male AC–TCV mortality has been decreasing in the Netherlands, in Belgium, and its regions since 1970 and increasing in Denmark since 1955 (Tables 13.1, 13.2). This makes it plausible that TCV mortality statistics are slightly underestimated but accuracy is improving in Belgian men, and are underestimated and accuracy is deteriorating in Denmark. Cardiovascular mortality is likely too low in Wallonia, but the accuracy of its classification is improving (Fig. 13.2).

13.3.3 Nutrition, smoking habits, and mortality

The sharp increase in polyunsaturated fat (mostly linoleic acid) intake in Belgium from 1960 to 1974 and the decrease after 1982 (Table 13.5) is related to the influence of Belgian universities in promoting a prudent diet since 1960 and a mass media campaign in the 1970s (Joossens *et al.* 1977). In 1968 a media campaign was started in Belgium in order to reduce salt intake (Joossens 2000). A higher intake of fruits, vegetables, and olive oil has been promoted since the 1980s.

These dietary changes since 1970 were associated in Belgium with a sharp decrease in all-cause mortality and in TCV, CHD, CVA, and stomach cancer mortality (B > NL > DK; Figs 13.1, 13.2, 13.4, 13.5; Tables 13.1,13.2). This was also observed in Flanders and Wallonia.

The largest decrease in stroke and stomach cancer mortality since 1970 in the three countries is seen in Belgium (Tables 13.1, 13.2). There is no evidence that treatment of hypertension is better in Belgium and treatment of stomach cancer has made no progress over recent decades. Other associations with the dietary changes in Belgium were fast decreasing rectal and endometrial cancer mortality since the 1950s (B > NL > DK). Generally increasing patterns were observed for breast and male colon cancer rates between 1995 and 1970, whereas changes in prostate cancer were more limited (Tables 13.1, 13.2). After 1970 breast, prostate, and male colon cancer rates increased in Denmark, whereas the female colon cancer rate decreased in the three countries. After 1970 prostate cancer increased in Belgium until 1980 (until 1985 in the Netherlands) and decreased afterwards. Breast cancer increased until 1986 and decreased afterwards in Belgium and the Netherlands (figure not shown). In 1994 Denmark had the highest mortality for prostate, breast, endometrial, male and female colon, and rectal cancer. This evolution is generally consistent with the time-related changes in saturated and polyunsaturated fat intake in Belgium and the Netherlands (Table 13.5). An ecological study of breast cancer mortality showed that polyunsaturated fat had a multiplicative influence on the promoting effect of saturated fat (Sasaki *et al.* 1993). Both saturated and n-6 polyunsaturated fat increase the risk for breast cancer in animals (Carroll 1985). These observations also are consistent with the lack of correlation between cardiovascular and breast, prostate, or colon cancer mortality rates in 40 countries worldwide (section 13.2.4 and Table 13.3).

Male lung cancer mortality is highest in Belgium from around 1980 (Table 13.1, Fig. 13.3). Male lung cancer mortality has decreased least in Denmark since 1980, but it has nevertheless the lowest mortality rates of the three countries since 1952 (Table 13.1, Fig. 13.3). Male smoking rates are now lowest in Belgium and the Netherlands, and highest in Denmark. This paradox cannot be explained by a possible enhancing influence of total and saturated fat intake (Wynder *et al.* 1987; Xie *et al.* 1991), which is highest in Denmark, nor by the known important lag period between smoking and lung cancer (Xie *et al.* 1991), since smoking rates decreased earlier in Belgium than in Denmark. It could, however, be related to other nutritional factors such as n-6 polyunsaturated fat intake, which could increase the influence of saturated fat intake (Beems and van Beek 1984) and fish fat intake which could decrease it (Zhang *et al.* 2000). In the 10-year follow-up of the Seven Countries Study it was found that for the same amount of cigarette smoking the level and slope of lung cancer and total cancer was much higher in Northern Europe than Southern Europe. Lung cancer mortality, for those who smoked ≥20 cigarettes daily, was four times higher in Northern Europe and total cancer mortality was 1.6 times higher (Keys 1980). Fat intake, especially saturated fat, was higher in Northern than in Southern Europe at that time. The level of total fat intake increased the risk of lung cancer mortality in a 10-year prospective follow-up study of the BIRHN study (1979–84) in Belgium (Stam-Moraga and Kornitzer 1998). Japanese men have a much higher smoking level compared to men from the three countries considered here and yet have a two times lower lung cancer mortality (Kesteloot *et al.* 1995). More research is needed in this field. On the other hand, female lung cancer mortality rates from the three countries fit with their smoking patterns. A possible explanation for the relatively high female smoking rates in Denmark has been proposed recently, namely the influence of the smoking habits of a highly popular public figure, Queen Margrethe II of Denmark (Kesteloot 2001).

The changes in nutrition, especially concerning fat intake, resulted in a progressively greater similarity in the intake of these nutrients between Belgium and the Netherlands (Table 13.5). This could offer, when combined with the changes in smoking habits, an explanation for the growing similarity between Belgium and the Netherlands for many mortality rates including AC, TCV, CHD, CVA, stomach cancer, and rectal cancer (Figs 13.1–5, Tables 13.1, 13.2). Denmark, with a less healthy fat intake and worse smoking habits, especially in women, now has generally higher mortality rates for these causes of death (Figs 13.1–5; Tables 13.1, 13.2).

13.4. Conclusions

Marked changes in nutrition and smoking habits have been observed in Belgium, the Netherlands, and Denmark over the years: decreasing saturated fat and salt intake, increasing n-6 polyunsaturated fat (more so in Belgium 1966–80, later decreasing), fruit, vegetables, fish, and olive oil intake. Current levels are similar in Belgium and the Netherlands and less favourable in Denmark. These lifestyle changes are consistent with trends observed for AC, TCV, CHD, CVA, and stomach cancer mortality (Fig. 13.1, 13.2, 13.4, 13.5; Tables 13.1, 13.2), which cannot be explained by improvements in medical care.

The current recommended nutrition for the prevention of cardiovascular diseases (Simopoulos *et al.* 2000) – less saturated fat, n-6 polyunsaturated fat, and salt, but more monounsaturated fat, n-3 polyunsaturated fat, fish, fruit, and vegetables – when combined with improving smoking habits and more exercise could further decrease AC, TCV, CHD, and CVA mortality. It is to be hoped that the same could happen to lung, stomach, rectal, endometrial, breast, prostate, and colon cancers.

Acknowledgement

The grants for research to H. Kesteloot from the Unilever Chair of Nutritional Epidemiology and the support of the Belgian Federation against Cancer are gratefully acknowledged.

References

Anonymous (1998). *Eating in The Netherlands 1987–1998* [in Dutch]. Nutrition Centre, The Hague.

Beems, R. B. and van Beek, L. (1984). Modifying effect of dietary fat on benzo[a]pyrene-induced respiratory tract tumours in hamsters. *Carcinogenesis*, 5, 413–17.

BIRNH (Belgian Interuniversity Research on Nutrition and Health) (1989). *Acta Cardiologica*, 2, 89–194.

Carroll, K. K. (1985). Diet and breast cancer: experimental approaches. In *Diet and human carcinogenesis*, International Congress Series 685 (ed. J. V. Joossens, M. J. Hill, and J. Geboers), pp. 265–73. Excerpta Medica, Amsterdam.

CBS (Central Bureau for Statistics), Voorburg, 1999. <http://neon.vb.cbs.nl/statweb>.

Chenet, L., Osler, M., McKee, M., and Krasnik, A. (1996). Changing life expectancy in the 1980s: why was Denmark different from Sweden? *Journal of Epidemiology and Community Health*, 50, 404–7.

CRIOC (Centre for Research and Information from Consumers Organizations). Press release [in Dutch], Brussels, 8 March 2001, pp. 1–5.

De Backer, G. (1996). Study of the incidence and development of acute coronary attacks in the Ghent population, 1983–1990 [in Dutch]. *Verhandelingen van de Koninklijke Academie voor Geneeskunde van België*, 58, 61–92.

Deboosere, P. and Gadeyne, S. (2000). May regional mortality pattern in Belgium be explained by individual socio-economic determinants? [in Dutch], Working Paper 2000–3 <http://www.vub.ac.be/SOCO>.

Den Hond, E., De Schryver, M., Muylaert, A., Lesaffre, E., and Kesteloot, H. (1994). The Inter-regional Belgian Bank Employee Nutrition Study (IBBENS). *European Journal of Clinical Nutrition*, 48, 106–17.

Doll, R., Muir, C., and Waterhouse, J. (1970). *Cancer incidence in five continents*, Vol. II. Springer-Verlag, Berlin.

Elliott, P., Dyer, A., and Stamler, R., on behalf of the INTERSALT Co-operative Research Group (1988). The INTERSALT Study: results for 24-hour sodium and potassium by age and sex. Appendix tables A1 to A38. *Journal of Human Hypertension*, 3, 323–30.

FAO (Food and Agriculture Organization) (1998). *Food balance sheets, 1994–1996 average* [data from 1964, 1980, and 1995]. United Nations, Rome.

Hornstra, G. (ed.) (1980). *Dietary fats and arterial thrombosis*. University Maastricht, The Netherlands.

Joossens, J. V. (1965). Het probleem van de kankersterfte. *Verhandelingen van de Koninklijke Academie voor Geneeskunde van België*, 27, 489–545.

Joossens, J. V. (1980). Stroke, stomach cancer and salt: a possible clue to the prevention of hypertension? In *Epidemiology of arterial blood pressure* (ed. H. Kesteloot and J. V. Joossens), pp. 489–508. Martinus Nijhoff, The Hague.

Joossens, J. V. (2000). Community control of hypertension in Belgium. In *Handbook of hypertension*, Vol. 20: *Epidemiology of hypertension* (ed. C. J. Bulpitt), pp. 645–60. Elsevier, Amsterdam.

Joossens, J. V. and Geboers, J. (1985). Diet, cancer and other diseases. In *Diet and human carcinogenesis*, International Congress Series 685 (eds. J. V. Joossens, M. J. Hill, and J. Geboers), pp. 277–97. Excerpta Medica, Amsterdam.

Joossens, J. V. and Kesteloot, H. (1990). Fats, cancer and cardiovascular diseases. In *Lipids and health* (ed. G. Ziant), pp. 93–157. Excerpta Medica, Amsterdam.

Joossens, J. V. and Kesteloot, H. (1991). Trends in systolic blood pressure, 24-hour sodium excretion, and stroke mortality in the elderly in Belgium. *American Journal of Medicine*, **90** (Suppl. 3A), 5S–11S.

Joossens, J. V. and Kesteloot, H. (1996). Forty years of evolution of mortality in Belgium and The Netherlands. *Verhandelingen van de Koninklijke Academie voor Geneeskunde van België*, **58**, 439–77.

Joossens, J. V. and Kesteloot, H. (1998). Nutrition in relation to stomach cancer and stroke mortality. In *Current perspectives on nutrition and health* (ed. K. K. Carroll), pp. 227–36. McGill-Queen's University Press, London, Ontario, Canada.

Joossens, J. V., Verdonk, G., and Pannier, R. (1966). 'Normal' serum cholesterol values in Belgium as related to age and diet. *Acta Cardiologica*, **21**, 431–45.

Joossens, J. V., Geboers, J., and Kesteloot, H. (1985). Regional trends in nutrition and mortality in Belgium. *Verhandelingen van de Koninklijke Academie voor Geneeskunde van België*, **47**, 207–44.

Joossens, J. V., Brems-Heyns, E., Claes, J. H., Graffar, M., Kornitzer, M., Pannier, R. *et al.* (1977). The pattern of food and mortality in Belgium. *Lancet*, **1**, 1069–72.

Joossens, J. V., Hill, M. J., Elliott, P., Stamler, R., Lesaffre, E., Dyer, A. *et al.* (1996). Dietary salt, nitrate and stomach cancer mortality in 24 countries. *International Journal of Epidemiology*, **25**, 494–504.

Kesteloot, H. (1991). Nutrition and health: epidemiological considerations. *Archives of Public Health*, **49**, 107–26.

Kesteloot, H. (1994). Nutrition and the aging process: a population study. *American Journal of Geriatric Cardiology*, **3**, 8–19.

Kesteloot, H. (1999). Regional differences in mortality: a comparison between Austria, Hungary and Switzerland. *Acta Cardiologica*, **54** (6), 299–309.

Kesteloot, H. (2001). Queen Margrethe II and mortality in Danish women. *Lancet*, **357**, 871–2.

Kesteloot, H., Lesaffre, E., and Joossens, J. V. (1991). Dairy fat, saturated animal fat, and cancer risk. *Preventive Medicine*, **20**, 226–36.

Kesteloot, H., Sasaki, S., Zhang, X., and Joossens, J. (1995). Mortality trends: a comparison between Denmark, Hungary and Japan. *Acta Cardiologica*, **50**, 343–67.

Keys, A. (ed.) (1980). *Seven countries.* Harvard University Press, Cambridge, MA.

Kornitzer, M. and Bara, L. (1989). Differences between North and South in coronary risk factors, food habits and mortality in Belgium. *Acta Cardiologica*, **44**, 145–55.

Kromhout, D., de Lezenne-Coulander, C., Obermann-de Boer, G. L., van Kampen-Donker, M., Goddijn, E., and Bloemberg, B. P. (1990). Changes in food and nutrient intake in middle-aged men from 1960 to 1985 (the Zutphen Study). *American Journal of Clinical Nutrition*, **51**, 123–9.

Lentner, C. (ed.) (1982). *Geigy scientific tables*, Vol. 2: *Introduction to statistics. Statistical tables. Mathematical formulae*, pp. 104–7. Ciba-Geigy, Basle, Switzerland.

Marmot, M. (1992). Coronary heart disease: rise and fall of a modern epidemic. In *Coronary heart disease epidemiology* (ed. M. Marmot and P. Elliott), pp. 3–19. Oxford University Press.

Marmot, M. (1999). Epidemiology of socio-economic status and health: are determinants within countries the same as between countries? *Annals of the New York Academy of Sciences*, **896**, 16–29.

Murray, C. and Lopez, A. (1997). Mortality by cause for eight regions of the world: Global Burden of Disease Study. *Lancet*, **349**, 1269–76.

NRC (National Research Council) (1989). *Diet and health.* National Academy Press, Washington, DC.

NSY (Nordic Statistical Yearbook) (1999). Nordic Council of Ministers. <http://www.dst.dk/siab.asp?frame=right2ando_id=788>.

Peto, R., Lopez, A. D., Boreham, J. *et al.* (1992). Mortality from tobacco in developed countries: indirect estimation from national vital statistics. *Lancet*, **339**, 1268–78.

Pietinen, P. (1998). Diet and cardiovascular diseases: the Nordic experience. In *Current perspectives on nutrition and health* (ed. K. K. Carroll), pp. 40–7. McGill-Queen's University Press, Montreal and Kingston.

Prescott, E., Osler, M., Hein, H. O. *et al.* (1998). Life expectancy in Danish women and men related to smoking habits: smoking may affect women more. *Journal of Epidemiology and Community Health*, 52, 131–2.

Renaud, S. and de Lorgeril, M. (1989). Dietary lipids and their relation to ischemic heart disease: from epidemiology to prevention. *Journal of Internal Medicine*, 225 (Suppl. 1), 39–46.

Sans, S., Kesteloot, H., and Kromhout, D. (1997). The burden of cardiovascular diseases mortality in Europe. *European Heart Journal*, 18, 1231–48.

Sasaki, S., Horacsek, M., and Kesteloot, H. (1993). An ecological study of the relationship between dietary fat intake and breast cancer mortality. *Preventive Medicine*, 22, 187–202.

Simopoulos, A. P., Leaf, A., and Salem, N., Jr (2000). Workshop on the essentiality of and recommended dietary intakes for omega-6 and omega-3 fatty acids. *Nutrition Today*, 35, 166–7.

Stam-Moraga, M. C. and Kornitzer, M. (1998). Nutrition and cancer mortality in Belgium. Ten-year follow-up of the BIRNH Study (1980–84). Congress Report, Brussels.

STIVORO (1999). *Smoking, the hard facts: adults 1958–1998* [in Dutch]. Stichting Volksgezondheid en Roken. The Hague.

WCRF (World Cancer Research Fund and American Institute for Cancer Research) (1997). *Food, nutrition and the prevention of cancer: a global perspective*, pp. 384. AICR, Washington, DC.

World Bank (1998). *World development indicators*. World Bank, Washington, DC.

Wynder, E. L., Hebert, J. R., and Kabay, G. C. (1987). Association of dietary fat and lung cancer. *Journal of the National Cancer Institute*, 79, 631–7.

Xie, J., Lesaffre, E., and Kesteloot, H. (1991). The relationship between animal fat intake, cigarette smoking, and lung cancer. *Cancer Causes and Control*, 2, 79–83.

Zhang, J. J., Sasaki, S., Amano, K., and Kesteloot, H. (1999). Fish consumption and mortality from all causes, ischemic heart disease, and stroke: an ecological study. *Preventive Medicine*, 28, 520–9.

Zhang, J., Temme, E. H. M., and Kesteloot, H. (2000). Fish consumption is inversely associated with male lung cancer mortality in countries with high levels of cigarette smoking or animal fat consumption. *International Journal of Epidemiology*, 29, 615–21.

Section III

Aetiology

III.I Risk factors

Chapter 14

Dietary patterns and coronary heart disease risk

T. P. Erlinger and L. J. Appel

14.1 Introduction

A confluence of evidence from observational and experimental studies strongly supports the hypothesis that multiple dietary factors determine coronary heart disease (CHD) risk and that modification of diet can have powerful, beneficial effects. In view of the striking worldwide differences in CHD mortality and the equally striking differences in diet, it is now well-accepted that lifestyle factors, particularly diet, account for a substantial portion of the variation in CHD risk.

In this setting, the purpose of this chapter is to describe and compare selected dietary patterns, each of which has been associated with reduced CHD risk. The dietary patterns include those consumed by free-living persons (i.e. a traditional Mediterranean diet consumed in Crete, vegetarian diets, diets consumed in rural China, and a traditional Okinawan diet) and diets tested in clinical trials (i.e. Lyon Diet Heart Study, Indo-Mediterranean Diet Heart Study, and the DASH clinical trial). In the process, we describe the nutrient and food composition of the diets (Table 14.1) and highlight their effects on CHD and its risk factors.

Still, several limitations are noteworthy. First, dietary patterns are exceedingly difficult to describe, in part, because of substantial heterogeneity of the diets that fall under a common rubric (e.g. Mediterranean diets) and because of secular trends. Traditional diets known for their health benefits are being supplanted by contemporary versions of these diets that often reflect Western culture. Hence this chapter will focus, to the extent possible, on pre-transition dietary patterns. Second, with the exception of the Seven Countries Study (Keys 1980), which applied standardized methods to compare diets in its surveyed countries, comparisons of the diets described in this chapter rely on available sources of data, which are quite heterogeneous. Third, health outcomes such as CHD mortality are often unavailable and, when available, are not directly comparable across studies.

14.2 The Mediterranean diet

In view of the numerous cultures and agricultural patterns of the Mediterranean region, the 'Mediterranean' diet is a not a single dietary pattern. Rather, this term applies to a dietary pattern that emphasizes fruits, vegetables, bread, cereals, potatoes, beans, nuts, and seeds; that includes olive oil, dairy products, fish, poultry, wine, and eggs; and that is reduced in red meat (Kris-Etherton *et al.* 2001). Despite the difficulties of characterizing a 'Mediterranean-style' diet, interest in traditional Mediterranean-style diets is considerable because of their apparent health benefits, particularly a reduced risk of CHD. Results from observational studies and

Table 14.1 Characteristics of selected dietary patterns that are associated with reduced CHD risk

Pattern	Mediterranean		Indo-Mediterranean Diet Heart Study (Singh et al. 2002)	US vegetarians (Kennedy et al. 2001)	DASH/Prudent American (Appel et al. 1997)	Rural Chinese diets (Campbell and Junshi 1994)	Okinawan, 1919 (Sho 2001)[a]
	Crete, 1960 (Kromhout et al. 1989)	Lyon Diet Heart Study (de Lorgeril et al. 1994)					
Source of diet information	Food record	Unspecified diet survey	7-day detailed food diary	Interviewer-administered 24-h recall	Analyses of composited meals and from menus	3-day diet surveys administered to households	Unspecified food survey of public officials
Fat, % kcal	41.9	30.4	26.3	27	25.6	14.5	1.6
Saturated, % kcal	8.9	8	8.2	9	7		
n-3 polyunsaturated, % kcal		0.84	1.79				
n-6 polyunsaturated, % kcal		3.6					
Total polyunsaturated, % kcal	4.4	4.6	8.1	6	6.8		
Monounsaturated, % kcal	26.8	17.8	10	9	9.9		
Protein, % kcal	12.5	16.2	14.2	11	17.9	9.6	5.3
% protein from plant				100	35	89	

Carbohydrates, % kcal	43	53.4	59.5	62	56.5	76	93.1
Fibre, g/1000 kcal	15.2	9.6	23.9		14.8	12.6	
Cholesterol, mg/1000 kcal	74.5	104	62		72		
Alcohol, % kcal	2.7	5.8					
Red meat and poultry, g/1000 kcal	12.4	21.1		0		2.1	
Description	Emphasizes fruits, vegetables, bread, cereals, potatoes, beans, nuts, and seeds; includes olive oil, dairy products, fish, poultry, wine, and eggs; reduced in red meat	Emphasizes bread, root vegetables, green vegetables, fish, poultry; reduced in red meat. Butter and cream replaced with margarine rich in ALA	Emphasizes fruits, vegetables, nuts, whole grains, and oils rich in ALA (mustard seed or soybean oil). Reduced in total fat, saturated fat, and cholesterol	Notable for the absence of dietary meat (red meat, poultry, and fish). Often includes consumption of dairy and eggs	Emphasizes fruits, vegetables, and low-fat dairy products; includes whole grains, poultry, fish, and nuts; reduced in red meat, sweets, and sugar-containing beverages	Emphasizes plant-based cereal staples, typically rice and in some instances wheat. Vegetable consumption can be high. Although diets differ by region, diets within a region are extremely limited in variety	Emphasizes the Satsamu sweet potato, tofu, and a variety of seaweeds and herbaceous plants; includes some pork and fish

[a] Survey of common diet in Okinawa in 1919 (Sho 2001).

clinical trials suggest that consumption of a Mediterranean diet, similar to that of Crete in the 1960s, is associated with one of the lowest risks of CHD in the world. In this context, we describe this dietary pattern, which was extensively studied in the Seven Countries Study, and then describe two variations of this diet which were tested in clinical trials, specifically, the Lyon Diet Heart Study (de Lorgeril *et al.* 1994) and the Indo-Mediterranean Diet Heart Study (Singh *et al.* 2002).

14.2.1 The Seven Countries Study

The Seven Countries Study, which began in the mid-1950s, was the first study that systematically examined the relationship between diet and risk of cardiovascular disease across geographically and culturally distinct populations. The countries were the United States, Finland, the Netherlands, Italy, Yugoslavia, Greece, and Japan. Over the course of 10 years of follow-up, CHD mortality varied widely among these countries, with the highest age-adjusted incidence occurring in East Finland (68/1000) and the US (42/1000), and the lowest in Greece (0/1000) and Japan (7/1000) (Keys 1980). These striking differences can be attributed, in part, to differences in dietary patterns.

Compared to the diet of the US cohort in the Seven Countries Study, the Cretan diet in 1960 was higher in bread, legumes, fruit, olive oil, and wine. Smaller differences were observed for vegetables, cereals, and potatoes. In contrast, the diet in Tanushimaru, Japan was substantially higher in cereals, soy products, rice, and legumes, and lower in bread and fruit compared to the US diet. In addition, consumption of fish was much higher in Tanushimaru than in both Crete and the US. One common finding was the low consumption of non-fish meats in both Crete and Tanushimaru compared to the US.

Over time, the diet of Crete has changed remarkably and is now characterized by higher intake of saturated fat and cholesterol, and reduced intake of monounsaturated fats. At the same time, total fat consumption has fallen. These trends have been accompanied by a steady rise in CHD risk during 25 years of follow-up of the Cretan cohort (Menotti *et al.* 1999). Hence, as the Cretan diet increasingly resembles a Western diet, there has been a concurrent rise in CHD risk.

14.2.2 The Lyon Diet Heart Study

The Lyon Diet Heart Study was designed to evaluate the impact of a Mediterranean diet on the risk of cardiovascular mortality in persons at high risk for CHD. The diet was based on the 1960 Cretan diet as defined by the Seven Countries Study, but the intervention also included supplementation with margarine rich in alpha-linolenic acid (ALA). Participants were advised to eat more bread, root vegetables, green vegetables, fish, and fruit. In addition, participants were asked to reduce their intake of red meat and pork. Finally, participants were asked to replace butter and cream with the supplemental margarine rich in ALA that was provided by the study. Estimated energy intake (% kcal) from fats was 30.5% from total fat, 8.3% from saturated fats, 0.8% from n-3 fatty acids, and 3.6% from n-6 fatty acids. Mean cholesterol intake was 217 mg/day. After a mean follow-up of 27 months, there was a 70% reduction in total mortality (20 deaths in control group vs. 8 deaths in experimental group) and a 73% reduction in the combined endpoint of cardiovascular deaths and non-fatal myocardial infarctions among persons assigned to the Mediterranean diet intervention compared to the control group (33 events in control group vs. 8 events in experimental group) (de Lorgeril *et al.* 1994, 1998).

While the results of this trial were impressive, several issues deserve comment. First, a beneficial effect of the intervention was observed very early in the trial, well before significant regression of atherosclerotic plaque might occur. This would suggest that mechanisms other than prevention of atherosclerosis, per se, might be responsible for the beneficial effects of the study diet. Experimental evidence suggests that ALA could have anti-thrombotic and anti-arrythmogenic effects (Freese *et al.* 1994; Renaud and Lanzmann-Petithory 2002). Hence, the impact of the intervention in preventing atherosclerosis is uncertain. A second and related issue is whether the Lyon Diet Heart Study diet can prevent CHD to the same extent as a traditional Mediterranean diet and other diets associated with a very low incidence of CHD. Despite the impressive relative risk reductions associated with the Lyon Diet Heart Study diet, it is quite possible that the absolute risk of CHD might still exceed that associated with other dietary patterns. Third, the study diet had no significant impact on blood lipids and blood pressure (BP). The emphasis on unsaturated fatty acids rather than saturated or trans-fatty acids would be expected to beneficially affect serum lipid levels (Sacks 1999). Likewise, dietary patterns emphasizing fruits and vegetables have been shown to substantially lower BP (Appel *et al.* 1997). Fourth, it is difficult to separate the effects of the diet from the effects of the ALA supplements that were provided to participants. Dietary advice was given infrequently in the trial, whereas the ALA-rich oils were supplied free of charge to participants. Behavioural intervention studies suggest that the frequency of dietary advice provided in the Lyon Diet Heart Study was insufficient to substantially change diet. In contrast, provision of the free ALA supplements might have been sufficient to accomplish this aspect of the intervention.

14.2.3 Indo-Mediterranean Diet Heart Study

A recently completed trial conducted in India complements findings from the Lyon Diet Heart Study (Singh 2002). The study population consisted primarily of men (~90%) who were at high risk for either a first myocardial infarction or a recurrence; approximately 60% had a history of myocardial infarction at baseline, and 35% had a recent (<4 weeks) myocardial infarction. In contrast to the Lyon Diet Heart Study, two-thirds of participants were vegetarian at baseline. All participants were given advice to reduce their intake of fat, saturated fat, and cholesterol (<30% kcal from fat, <10% kcal from saturated fat, and <300 mg cholesterol/day). Those participants in the intervention arm were also advised to increase their consumption of fruits, vegetables, and nuts and to use mustard seed and soybean oil (3–4 servings per day), both of which are rich in ALA.

It is noteworthy that approximately 60% of calories came from carbohydrates, of which a substantial proportion was presumably from fruit, vegetable, and grain consumption. In contrast to the Lyon Diet Heart Study, consumption of the Indo-Mediterranean diet resulted in significant reductions in total and low-density lipoprotein (LDL) cholesterol, and an increase in high-density lipoprotein (HDL) cholesterol. In addition, BP and body mass index were reduced with the Indo-Mediterranean diet compared to controls. A common feature of both the Lyon and Indo-Mediterranean studies was the emphasis on ALA consumption. In the latter study, increased consumption was achieved by emphasizing foods and oils rich in ALA (nuts, soybean oil, and mustard seed oil).

After 2 years of follow-up, there was a 50% reduction in total cardiovascular endpoints (fatal myocardial infarction, non-fatal myocardial infarction, and sudden cardiac death) in the intervention group (39 events) compared to the control group (76 events). Both non-fatal myocardial infarction and sudden death were reduced in the intervention group; however, there was no significant difference in fatal myocardial infarction. These results are consistent with those from the Lyon Diet Heart Study, where there were significant reductions in sudden death and non-fatal myocardial infarctions. Still, these impressive results are somewhat surprising, because, at baseline, two-thirds of participants were vegetarians.

14.3 **Vegetarian diets**

Observational studies from Europe and the US have consistently documented that vegetarian diets are associated with a reduced risk of CHD. Several prospective studies have examined the effects of meat consumption on CHD risk (Table 14.2). A recent study that combined results from five large prospective studies among vegetarians documented that vegetarians have about a 25% lower risk of heart disease than non-vegetarians (Key *et al.* 1999). In the Seven Countries Study, after 25 years of follow-up, meat consumption remained one of the key factors explaining the variation in CHD risk between countries after adjusting for other factors, including smoking (Menotti *et al.* 1999). Interestingly, very-low-fat diets such as those consumed by vegans do not clearly reduce total or cause-specific mortality below the rates seen in the more liberal vegetarians; however, evidence is scant (Key *et al.* 1999).

In the US, approximately 6% of the population can be classified as vegetarian (Kennedy *et al.* 2001). Strict vegetarians, that is vegans, do not consume any animal products while other types of vegetarians, for example lacto-ovo vegetarians, consume milk and eggs. Despite the wide variation in vegetarian diets, it is noteworthy that the average vegetarian does not consume a low fat diet. In studies of Seventh-Day Adventists, average fat consumption was 100.5 mg/day in vegetarians and 102.2 mg/day in non-vegetarians (Key *et al.* 1999). In the Oxford Study of vegetarians, total fat consumption comprised 36% of total energy intake (Burr and Butland 1988). In the US as a whole, vegetarians derive somewhat fewer calories from fat than non-vegetarians (27 vs. 33%, respectively), particularly saturated fat, and have a higher consumption of carbohydrates than non-vegetarians (Kennedy *et al.* 2001). In addition, vegetarians tend to consume fewer overall calories and have a lower body mass index than non-vegetarians. These characteristics, in addition to the dietary pattern per se, may contribute to lower BP and a more optimal lipid profile among vegetarians (Appleby *et al.* 2002; Thorogood *et al.* 1987).

While reduced meat consumption is generally associated with reduced CHD risk, there is a clear potential for confounding, particularly from other dietary factors. Hence, the improved health experience of vegetarians may not only result from reduced consumption of saturated fats, but also from greater consumption of vegetables, fruit, nuts, and grains. These foods contain phytosterols and unsaturated fats that have favourable effects on blood lipids. Among Seventh-Day Adventists, many of whom are vegetarians, increased nut consumption was associated with reduced CHD risk (Fraser 1999). Vegetarian diets are also rich in nutrients, including antioxidants (e.g. tocopherols, ascorbate, carotenoids, saponins, and flavonoids) that may prevent oxidation of LDL cholesterol.

14.4 **The DASH diet**

The well-established, dietary determinants of BP are salt, weight, and alcohol. The Dietary Approaches to Stop Hypertension (DASH) trial tested whether modification of whole dietary patterns might also affect BP (Appel *et al.* 1997). In contrast to most diet–BP trials, the DASH trial was a feeding study. Participants ($n = 459$, 29% hypertensive, 60% African-American) were randomized to (a) a control diet, (b) a 'fruits and vegetables' diet, or (c) the DASH diet.

Table 14.2 Prospective studies of meat intake and risk of cardiovascular disease

	Exposure	Comparison	Findings
Burr and Sweetnam 1982[a]	Any meat	Vegetarian vs. non-vegetarian	SMR 0.97 (0.81, 1.16)
Burr and Burland 1988	Any meat	Vegetarian vs. non-vegetarian	SMR 0.43
Snowdon et al. 1984	Beef	Vegetarian vs. beef >3 times/week	> two-fold risk reduction (men only)
Frentzel-Beyme et al. 1988	Any meat	Vegetarian vs. non-vegetarian	SMR 0.45 (0.22, 0.95)
Snowdon 1988 [a]	Any meat	Vegetarian vs. non-vegetarian	SMR 0.74 (0.63, 0.88)
Beeson et al. 1989	Any meat	Vegetarian vs. non-vegetarian	SMR 0.62 (0.53, 0.73)
Chang-Claude et al. 1992	Any meat	Vegetarian vs. non-vegetarian	SMR 0.39 (0.29, 0.51) (men) SMR 0.46 (0.35, 0.60) (women)
Thorogood et al. 1994	Any meat	Vegetarian vs. non-vegetarian	Unadjusted SMR, 0.38 (0.30, 0.46) Adjusted SMR, 0.72 (0.47, 1.10)
Mann et al. 1997	Any Meat	Vegetarian and vegan vs. non-vegetarian	Adjusted SMR, 0.63 (0.42, 0.93)
Hu et al. 1999	Red Meat	RR per 1 serving/day	Age-adjusted RR, 1.43 (1.35–1.65) Multivariate adjusted RR, 1.09 (0.91, 1.30)
Key et al. 1999[b]	Any Meat	Vegetarian vs. non-vegetarian	SMR 0.66 (0.55–0.79)

SMR = standardized mortality ratio; RR = relative risk.

[a] Results included in study by Key et al. 1999.

[b] This study was a meta-analysis of five separate studies evaluating the impact of vegetarian diets on CHD risk.

The DASH diet emphasizes fruits, vegetables, and low-fat dairy products; includes whole grains, poultry, fish, and nuts; and is reduced in red meat, sweets, and sugar-containing beverages (Karanja *et al.* 1999). This diet is rich in potassium, magnesium, calcium, and fibre, and is reduced in total fat, saturated fat, and cholesterol; it is also slightly increased in protein. The control diet has a nutrient composition that is typical of that consumed by many Americans. Its potassium, magnesium, and calcium levels are comparatively low, while its macronutrient profile and fibre content correspond to average US consumption. The fruits and vegetables diet is rich in potassium, magnesium, and fibre, but otherwise similar to the control diet. All three diets contain similar amounts of sodium (~3000 mg/day).

Among all participants, the DASH diet significantly lowered mean systolic blood pressure (SBP) by 5.5 mmHg and mean diastolic blood pressure (DBP) by 3.0 mmHg. The fruits and vegetables diet also significantly reduced BP, but to a lesser extent: ~50% of the effect of the DASH diet. The effects occurred rapidly and were apparent after only 2 weeks (see Fig. 14.1). In subgroup analyses, the DASH diet significantly lowered BP in all major subgroups (men, women, African-Americans, non-African-Americans, hypertensives, and non-hypertensives). However, in the African-Americans, BP reductions (SBP/DBP) from the DASH diet (6.9/3.7 mmHg) were significantly greater than corresponding reductions in white participants (3.3/2.4 mmHg). The reductions in hypertensive individuals (11.6/5.3 mmHg) were striking and were significantly greater than the corresponding effects in non-hypertensive individuals (3.5/2/2 mmHg). In addition to BP reduction, the DASH diet also reduced serum homocysteine levels (Appel *et al.* 2000) and had favourable effects on blood lipids (Obarzanek *et al.* 2001).

Results from the DASH trial have important public health and clinical implications. It has been estimated that a population-wide reduction in BP of the magnitude observed in DASH could reduce stroke incidence by 27% and CHD by 15%. Further reduction in CHD risk might be anticipated from the net changes in lipids and homocysteine. Evidence from prospective observational studies corroborates this notion.

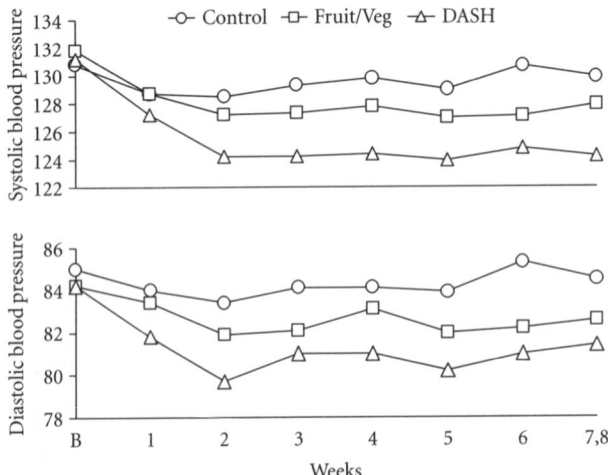

Fig. 14.1 Mean BP by week of feeding in a (a) typical American diet (control diet), (b) diet rich in fruits and vegetables, and (c) the DASH diet (rich in fruits, vegetables and low-fat dairy products, and reduced in cholesterol and fat). (Main results of the DASH trial, adapted with permission from Appel *et al.* 1997, p. 1122.)

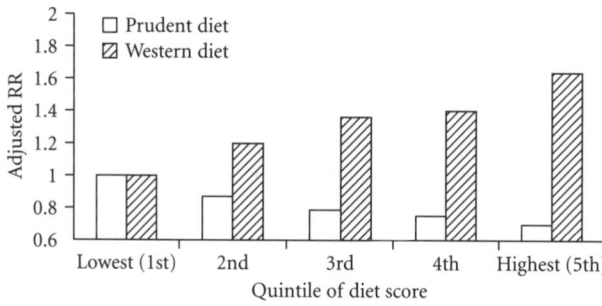

Fig. 14.2 Relative risk (RR) of ischaemic heart disease events by quintile of diet score in a Prudent diet and a Western diet, adjusted for age and cardiovascular risk factors, in the Health Professionals Follow-Up Study (Hu *et al.* 2000). (*p* (trend) <0.001 for each diet.)

In factor analyses of the Nurses Health Study (Fung *et al.* 2001) and the Health Professionals Follow-up cohort study (Hu *et al.* 2000), investigators identified two major dietary patterns. The dietary pattern termed 'prudent' was similar in several respects to the DASH diet, and characterized by a high intake of vegetables, fruit, legumes, whole grains, fish, and poultry. The other pattern, termed 'Western', was characterized by high intake of red meat, processed meat, refined grains, sweets and desserts, French fries, and high-fat dairy products. Scores for each diet were derived by adding the reported intake of food items weighted by factor loading. Individuals were then grouped by quintile of diet scores. Those in the lowest (first) quintile of the prudent diet score consumed a diet that was least consistent with this diet, whereas those in the highest (fifth) quintile consumed a diet that was most consistent with the prudent diet. Those who consumed a diet most consistent with the prudent diet had a reduced risk of CHD, while those who consumed a diet most consistent with a Western diet had an increased risk of CHD (Fig. 14.2).

14.5 **East Asian dietary patterns**

14.5.1 **Rural Chinese diets**

Rural China is extremely heterogeneous in terms of diet, geography, and also causes of mortality. Despite this heterogeneity, mortality from CHD has been relatively uncommon. According to a nationwide mortality survey in 1973–75, the age-specific annual death rates (per million) among men, ages 50–4, from CHD, stroke, and cancer were 109, 706, and 4401, respectively (Junshi *et al.* 1990). Corresponding mortality rates among women were 96, 622, and 2696.

A major ecological survey of 65 rural Chinese counties provides substantial insights into dietary patterns that were prevalent in 1983 and that might account for the low incidence of CHD (Junshi *et al.* 1990). The 65 counties accounted for 2.7% of the approximately 2400 counties and were widely dispersed throughout mainland China. Although the counties were selected to achieve a distribution in cancer mortality rates, results of the dietary survey should reflect the diversity of dietary patterns and habits of the broader population of rural Chinese.

The most striking aspect of these diets is the predominance of plant-based foods. This is evident from the distribution of protein sources; of the average 65 g/day in estimated total protein intake, 89% comes from plants. Another, but related characteristic is the source of energy: specifically, the staple food is typically a grain or cereal. However, the type of staple differs by region. Rice is the major staple in southern and eastern China, while wheat and other grains are the primary staple in several northern and central regions. In this context, the predominant source of energy is carbohydrate, which on average accounts for 76% of energy, while fat provides only 14.5%, and protein just 9.6%. Average vegetable intake was 312 g/day;

however, in a few counties, vegetable intake was negligible. Other interesting findings from the survey are the remarkable homogeneity of diets within each county and the extremely limited variety of foods. Both of these findings reflect consumption of just those foods that are either locally grown or locally available. In each surveyed region, the number of consumed foods was typically less than 25. Of final note, average estimated total calorie intake was high: 2641 kcal/day. Despite this high level of caloric intake, rural Chinese are extremely lean, as a result of routine physical activity.

14.5.2 Okinawan diet

Okinawa, with a population of 1.3 million in 2000, is the southernmost prefecture of Japan. The longevity of Okinawans is among the highest in the world. In 1995, the average life expectancy was 81.2 years in Okinawa and 76.8 in the United States (Suzuki *et al.* 2001). It has been estimated that CHD death rates in Okinawa are less than one-fifth of corresponding rates in the US (Suzuki *et al.* 2001). Interestingly, in contrast to the social gradient theory, which postulates the greatest health and longevity in the most affluent subpopulations of a country, Okinawa is the poorest prefecture in Japan (Cockerham and Yamori 2001).

Researchers attribute the longevity and health of Okinawans, in large part, to their diet. The traditional Okinawan diet has been described as a synthesis of foods derived from Chinese, Japanese, and other South East Asian cultures (Sho 2001). The indigenous Satsamu sweet potato, which is rich in nutrients, is the food staple that provides the bulk of energy intake. Other prominent foods in the diet are a wide variety of seaweeds, Okinawan tofu, and herbaceous plants. Okinawan food culture also includes a modest amount of fish and pork; however, the latter is prepared in such a fashion as to remove saturated fat. The most common oil used in cooking is a canola–soy oil blend, rich in monounsaturated fatty acids and to some extent n-3 PUFA. Salt intake is the lowest of all Japan. However, the traditional Okinawan diet has changed, such that fast foods and processed foods are increasingly consumed (Suzuki *et al.* 2001). As displayed in Table 14.1, the estimated carbohydrate content of this diet is extremely high at over 90% kcal.

14.6 Summary and conclusion

Several distinct dietary patterns are associated with lower CHD rates and with improved CHD risk factors. A common feature of these diets is an emphasis on plant-based foods. Accordingly, fibre intake is high while saturated fat intake is low, less than 10% kcal in all instances. When total fat intake is high, that is, over 30% kcal, the predominant fat is monounsaturated fats. N-3 polyunsaturated fats are frequently consumed in small quantities and in a variety of forms. Carbohydrate intake is typically high; the predominant forms appear to be complex carbohydrates, likely from whole grain products with minimal processing.

Still, few clinical trials have assessed the effect of dietary patterns on CHD outcomes, and there is no direct comparison of these diets on CHD risk. Moreover, the available trials are secondary prevention trials. From a public health perspective, the impact of these dietary patterns in the primary prevention of CHD is of paramount importance. Finally, in the interpretation of observational data, it is difficult to separate the effects of diet from other factors, for example smoking and physical inactivity, that likely account, in part, for observed differences in CHD risk. Nonetheless, the totality of evidence documenting a beneficial impact of plant-based dietary patterns on CHD risk is remarkable.

Overall, such findings have tremendously important public health implications. Despite broad variation in geography, lifestyle, and locally available foods, it is evident that for most populations, a diet that reduces CHD risk is readily available. The public health challenge is to achieve population-wide adoption of beneficial dietary patterns in the setting of powerful influences that promote unhealthy lifestyles.

References

Appel, L. J., Moore, T. J., Obarzanek, E., Vollmer, W. M., Svetkey, L. P., Sacks, F. M. *et al.* (1997). A clinical trial of the effects of dietary patterns on blood pressure. DASH Collaborative Research Group. *New England Journal of Medicine*, **336**, 1117–24.

Appel, L. J., Miller III, E. R., Jee, S. H., Stolzenberg-Solomon, R., Lin, P. H., Erlinger, T. *et al.* (2000). Effect of dietary patterns on serum homocysteine: results of a randomized, controlled feeding study. *Circulation*, **102**, 852–7.

Appleby, P. N., Davey, G. K., and Key, T. J. (2002). Hypertension and blood pressure among meat eaters, fish eaters, vegetarians and vegans in EPIC-Oxford. *Public Health Nutrition*, **5**, 645–54.

Beeson, W. L., Mills, P. K., Phillips, R. L., Andress, M., and Fraser, G. E. (1989). Chronic disease among Seventh-day Adventists, a low-risk group: rationale, methodology, and description of the population. *Cancer*, **64**, 570–81.

Burr, M. L. and Butland, B. K. (1988). Heart disease in British vegetarians. *American Journal of Clinical Nutrition*, **48** (Suppl. 3), 830–2.

Burr, M. L. and Sweetnam, P. M. (1982). Vegetarianism, dietary fiber, and mortality. *American Journal of Clinical Nutrition*, **36**, 873–7.

Campbell, T. C. and Junshi, C. (1994). Diet and chronic degenerative diseases: perspectives from China. *American Journal of Clinical Nutrition*, **59** (Suppl. 5), 1153S–1161S.

Chang-Claude, J., Frentzel-Beyme, R., and Eilber, U. (1992). Mortality pattern of German vegetarians after 11 years of follow-up [see comments]. *Epidemiology*, **3**, 395–401.

Cockerham, W. C. and Yamori, Y. (2001). Okinawa: an exception to the social gradient of life expectancy in Japan. *Asia Pacific Journal of Clinical Nutrition*, **10**, 154–8.

de Lorgeril, M., Renaud, S., Mamelle, N., Salen, P., Martin, J. L., Monjaud, I. *et al.* (1994). Mediterranean alpha-linolenic acid-rich diet in secondary prevention of coronary heart disease [see comments] [published erratum appears in *Lancet* 1995, 18 Mar, **345**: 738]. *Lancet*, **343**, 1454–9.

de Lorgeril, M., Salen, P., Martin, J. L., Monjaud, I., Boucher, P., and Mamelle, N. (1998). Mediterranean dietary pattern in a randomized trial: prolonged survival and possible reduced cancer rate [see comments]. *Archives of Internal Medicine*, **158**, 1181–7.

Fraser, G. E. (1999). Associations between diet and cancer, ischemic heart disease, and all-cause mortality in non-Hispanic white California Seventh-day Adventists. *American Journal of Clinical Nutrition*, **70** (Suppl. 3), 532S–538S.

Freese, R., Mutanen, M., Valsta, L. M., and Salminen, I. (1994). Comparison of the effects of two diets rich in monounsaturated fatty acids differing in their linoleic/alpha-linolenic acid ratio on platelet aggregation. *Thrombosis and Haemostasis*, **71**, 73–7.

Frentzel-Beyme, R., Claude, J., and Eilber, U. (1988). Mortality among German vegetarians: first results after five years of follow-up. *Nutrition and Cancer*, **11**, 117–26.

Fung, T. T., Willett, W. C., Stampfer, M. J., Manson, J. E., and Hu, F. B. (2001). Dietary patterns and the risk of coronary heart disease in women. *Archives of Internal Medicine*, **161**, 1857–62.

Hu, F. B., Stampfer, M. J., Manson, J. E., Ascherio, A., Colditz, G. A., Speizer, F. E. *et al.* (1999). Dietary saturated fats and their food sources in relation to the risk of coronary heart disease in women [see comments]. *American Journal of Clinical Nutrition*, **70**, 1001–8.

Hu, F. B., Rimm, E. B., Stampfer, M. J., Ascherio, A., Spiegelman, D., and Willett, W. C. (2000). Prospective study of major dietary patterns and risk of coronary heart disease in men. *American Journal of Clinical Nutrition*, 72, 912–21.

Junshi, C., Campbell, T. C., Li, J., and Peto, R. (1990). *Diet, life-style, and mortality in China: a study of the characteristics of 65 Chinese countries.* Oxford University Press, Oxford; Cornell University Press, Ithaca, NY; People's Medical Pub. House, People's Republic of China.

Karanja, N. M., Obarzanek, E., Lin, P. H., McCullough, M. L., Phillips, K. M., Swain, J. F. *et al.* (1999). Descriptive characteristics of the dietary patterns used in the Dietary Approaches to Stop Hypertension Trial. DASH Collaborative Research Group. *Journal of the American Dietetic Association*, 99 (Suppl. 8), S19–S27.

Kennedy, E. T., Bowman, S. A., Spence, J. T., Freedman, M., and King, J. (2001). Popular diets: correlation to health, nutrition, and obesity. *Journal of the American Dietetic Association*, 101, 411–20.

Key, T. J., Fraser, G. E., Thorogood, M., Appleby, P. N., Beral, V., Reeves, G. *et al.* (1999). Mortality in vegetarians and nonvegetarians: detailed findings from a collaborative analysis of 5 prospective studies. *American Journal of Clinical Nutrition*, 70 (Suppl. 3), 516S–524S.

Keys, A. (1980). *Seven countries: a multivariate analysis of death and coronary heart disease.* Harvard University Press, Cambridge, MA.

Kris-Etherton, P., Eckel, R. H., Howard, B. V., St Jeor, S., and Bazzarre, T. L. (2001). AHA Science Advisory: Lyon Diet Heart Study. Benefits of a Mediterranean-style, National Cholesterol Education Program/American Heart Association Step I Dietary Pattern on Cardiovascular Disease. *Circulation*, 103, 1823–5.

Kromhout, D., Keys, A., Aravanis, C., Buzina, R., Fidanza, F., Giampaoli, S. *et al.* (1989). Food consumption patterns in the 1960s in seven countries. *American Journal of Clinical Nutrition*, 49, 889–94.

Mann, J. I., Appleby, P. N., Key, T. J., and Thorogood, M. (1997). Dietary determinants of ischaemic heart disease in health conscious individuals. *Heart*, 78, 450–5.

Menotti, A., Kromhout, D., Blackburn, H., Fidanza, F., Buzina, R., and Nissinen, A. (1999). Food intake patterns and 25-year mortality from coronary heart disease: cross-cultural correlations in the Seven Countries Study. The Seven Countries Study Research Group. *European Journal of Epidemiology*, 15, 507–15.

Obarzanek, E., Sacks, F. M., Vollmer, W. M., Bray, G. A., Miller III, E. R., Lin, P. H. *et al.* for the DASH Research Group (2001). Effects on blood lipids of a blood pressure-lowering diet: the Dietary Approaches to Stop Hypertension (DASH) Trial. *American Journal of Clinical Nutrition*, 74, 80–9.

Renaud, S. and Lanzmann-Petithory, D. (2002). Dietary fats and coronary heart disease pathogenesis. *Current Atherosclerosis Reports*, 4, 419–24.

Sacks, F. (1999). *Dietary factors. Clinical trials in cardiovascular disease: a companion to Bruanwald's Heart Disease*, pp. 423–31. W. B. Saunders, Philadelphia.

Sho, H. (2001). History and characteristics of Okinawan longevity food. *Asia Pacific Journal of Clinical Nutrition*, 10, 159–64.

Singh, R. B., Dubnov, G., Niaz, M. A., Ghosh, S., Singh, R., Rastogi, S. S. *et al.* (2002). Effect of an Indo-Mediterranean diet on progression of coronary artery disease in high risk patients (Indo-Mediterranean Diet Heart Study): a randomised single-blind trial. *Lancet*, 360, 1455–61.

Snowdon, D. A. (1988). Animal product consumption and mortality because of all causes combined, coronary heart disease, stroke, diabetes, and cancer in Seventh-day Adventists. *American Journal of Clinical Nutrition*, 48 (Suppl. 3), 739–48.

Snowdon, D. A., Phillips, R. L., and Fraser, G. E. (1984). Meat consumption and fatal ischemic heart disease. *Preventive Medicine*, 13, 490–500.

Suzuki, M., Wilcox, B. J., and Wilcox, C. D. (2001). Implications from and for food cultures for cardiovascular disease: longevity. *Asia Pacific Journal of Clinical Nutrition*, 10, 165–71.

Thorogood, M., Carter, R., Benfield, L., McPherson, K., and Mann, J. I. (1987). Plasma lipids and lipoprotein cholesterol concentrations in people with different diets in Britain. *British Medical Journal (Clinical Research Edition)*, **295**, 351–3.

Thorogood, M., Mann, J., Appleby, P., and McPherson, K. (1994). Risk of death from cancer and ischaemic heart disease in meat and non-meat eaters [see comments]. *British Medical Journal*, **308**, 1667–70.

Chapter 15

Antioxidants and cardiovascular disease

E. R. Miller III and L. J. Appel

15.1 Introduction

Antioxidant vitamin supplements are regularly consumed by over one-third of all adults in the United States (Balluz *et al.* 2000*a*). While the health benefits of vitamin supplements are unproven, many lay persons and health professionals believe that pill supplementation with antioxidants is an effective strategy for the prevention and treatment of acute and chronic illnesses, including cardiovascular diseases (CVDs). In this setting, a large nutraceutical industry has developed to meet and promote this demand.

Contrary to the commonly held beliefs, recent large-scale randomized clinical trials have repeatedly documented no benefit from antioxidant vitamin supplements. In some trials, supplements appeared to be harmful. This chapter reviews evidence for biological plausibility; the major observational studies which linked antioxidant intake to reduced risk of cardiovascular and other chronic diseases; and finally reviews the large number of trials which, collectively, fail to show benefit of antioxidant vitamin supplement use in preventing CVD and mortality.

15.2 Biological plausibility

A substantial body of evidence, predominantly from laboratory-based studies, suggests that free radicals may be important in the pathophysiology of ageing as well as the development of CVDs, cancer, and other chronic diseases (Steinberg *et al.* 1989). Free radicals react easily with proteins, lipids, carbohydrates, DNA, and other biological molecules, triggering self-perpetuating chain reactions resulting in cell damage or death. Because the formation of free radicals is unavoidable in aerobic organisms, organisms have developed systems that protect against oxidative damage (Fig. 15.1). Anti-oxidant systems include endogenous systems (e.g. superoxide dismutases, bilirubin, albumin, etc.) and antioxidants derived from diet. Some antioxidants act by preventing the formation of free radicals, for example, by sequestering transition metal ions. More often, their mode of action involves a reaction with free radicals already formed. Through this process, antioxidant molecules act as acceptors or donors of electrons, and become oxidized in the process.

Hundreds of dietary antioxidants have been identified. These include tocopherols (including α-tocopherol – vitamin E, as well as other tocopherols (β, γ, and Δ)), carotenoids (including β-carotene – a provitamin A), and ascorbic acid (vitamin C) (McCall and Frei 1999). Vitamin E is a fat-soluble vitamin found in cell membranes as well as supramolecular assemblies including low-density lipoprotein (LDL) particles. Vitamin E's integration into the LDL particle makes

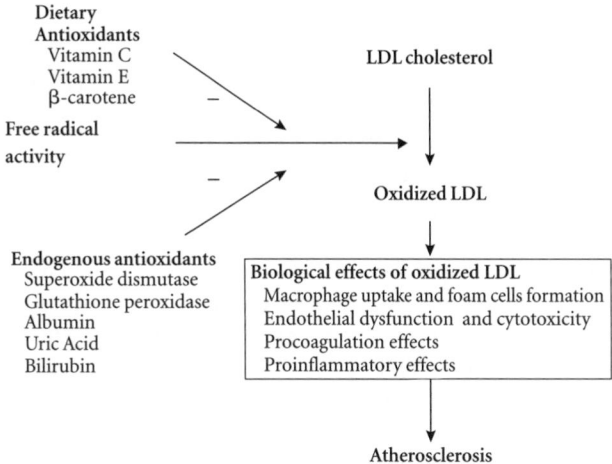

Fig. 15.1 Pathway of LDL oxidation and the potential role of antioxidants in preventing oxidative damage.

supplementation an appealing choice of therapy. There, it acts as a chain-breaking, free-radical trapping antioxidant, inhibiting non-enzymatic damage to polyunsaturated fatty acids. β-carotene is a fat-soluble precursor of vitamin A derived from vegetable sources that is both an efficient quencher of singlet oxygen and a radical-trapping antioxidant. Unlike vitamin E and β-carotene, vitamin C is a water-soluble vitamin that prevents peroxy radical formation in the aqueous domain. In certain *in vitro* systems, it appears to regenerate (i.e., reduce) 'oxidized' vitamin E formed during antioxidant reactions. However, recent studies in humans cast doubt on such synergistic effects (Huang *et al.* 2002).

Several lines of evidence suggest that oxidation of LDL is an important if not obligatory step in the pathogenesis of atherosclerosis (Steinberg and Witztum 2002). Oxidized LDL is a particularly atherogenic form of this cholesterol–lipid transport particle and intermediate steps in the formation of early atherosclerotic lesions have been identified. Specifically, oxidized LDL enhances migration (chemotaxis) of monocytes into the sub-endothelial space and inhibits efflux of tissue macrophages. Further, oxidative modification of LDL appears to be required for macrophage uptake of cholesterol and formation of the lipid-laden macrophage found in early lesions. Oxidized LDL is also toxic to endothelial cells (Parthasarathy *et al.* 1999).

Additional evidence suggests that these properties may have clinical relevance (reviewed by McCall and Frei 1999). First, oxidized LDL has been identified in atherosclerotic lesions. Further, antibodies to epitopes of oxidized LDL (but not to native LDL) have been isolated from patients with atherosclerosis. Third, the susceptibility of LDL to oxidation has been correlated with the severity of atherosclerosis. Finally, *in vivo* and *in vitro* studies of LDL oxidation have shown repeatedly that vitamin E supplementation reduces oxidation of LDL. Such mechanistic evidence supports the biological plausibility of antioxidants as a means to prevent atherosclerosis and/or its clinical complications, and in part provides supporting evidence to justify large-scale clinical trials.

15.3 Ecological, cross-sectional, and case-control studies

In ecological, cross-sectional, and case-control studies, the relationship between antioxidant vitamin intake (or blood levels) and vascular disease has been inconsistent. However, those studies with the strongest design and methods tended to demonstrate inverse relationships of vascular disease with vitamin E and β-carotene. In the Atherosclerosis Research In Communities (ARIC) cohort, low dietary β-carotene intake was associated with increased intima–media thickness (IMT) in men; dietary intake of vitamin E was inversely associated with IMT, most prominently in men with high LDL cholesterol (Kritchevsky *et al.* 1995). In addition, significant inverse associations between vitamin C intake and IMT were documented in both men and women. In a well-designed nested case-control study, there was a greater risk of myocardial infarction (MI) in persons in the lowest quintile of serum β-carotene (Street *et al.* 1991).

An indirect line of evidence also suggests that antioxidants might be beneficial. In cross-sectional studies, cigarette smokers who are at high risk for developing atherosclerotic CVDs have lower serum β-carotene levels than non-smokers (Stryker *et al.* 1988). Whether the lower serum level of β-carotene in smokers results from reduced dietary intake or from increased utilization as a consequence of metabolic effects of cigarette smoke is unclear.

The plausibility of greater turnover and utilization of β-carotene during antioxidant reactions is supported by findings from a cross-sectional study of US adults from the National Health and Nutrition Survey. In this survey of 30 000 people, serum β-carotene levels were inversely associated with markers of inflammation, including C-reactive protein and white blood cell counts, even after controlling for dietary intake of β-carotene (Erlinger *et al.* 2001). Inflammatory processes and oxidative stress deplete β-carotene and other antioxidants. Low serum levels of β-carotene in smokers were, in part, the rationale for trials of antioxidants that focused exclusively on smokers.

15.4 **Prospective observational studies**

Several longitudinal observational studies have examined the relationship between dietary intake of antioxidants measured at baseline and subsequent vascular diseases (Lonn and Yusuf 1997). A few points are noteworthy. First, there was no attempt to assign persons to diets or supplements high in antioxidant vitamins. Hence, the potential for uncontrolled confounding is a major concern in these reports. Examination of results from certain studies, specifically the Nurses Health Study (Stampfer *et al.* 1993), the Health Professionals Follow-Up Study (Rimm *et al.* 1993), the Massachusetts Elderly Cohort Study (Gaziano *et al.* 1992), and the First and Second National Health and Nutrition Examination Surveys (NHANES I (Enstrom *et al.* 1992) and NHANES II (Loria *et al.* 2000)) highlight the potential efficacy of antioxidant vitamins as well as inconsistencies in the existing database and the potential for confounding.

In the Nurses Health Study, 87 245 healthy female nurses (34–59 years of age), who were free of diagnosed CVD, completed food frequency questionnaires that assessed their average consumption of a wide range of nutrients, including vitamin E. During 8 years of follow-up, 552 cases of major coronary disease (437 non-fatal MIs and 115 deaths due to coronary disease) were documented (Stampfer *et al.* 1993). Those women in the top fifth of vitamin E consumption (mean = 208 IU/day) had a relative risk of major coronary disease of 0.66, adjusted for age and smoking, compared to the lowest quintile (mean = 2.8 IU/day) (95% CI: 0.50–0.87). Most of the reduction in risk was attributable to vitamin E consumed as vitamin supplements. In contrast, a study carried out in postmenopausal women (Kushi *et al.* 1996) documented that the reduced risk of CVD from vitamin E resulted from increased vitamin intake in foods rather than pill supplements.

Additional findings from the Nurses Health Study are relevant. First, women who took vitamin E supplements for short periods had little apparent benefit, but those who took them for 2 years or more had an adjusted relative risk of major coronary disease of 0.59 (95% CI: 0.38–0.91). Second, the authors reported the effects of multivitamin and vitamin E supplements separately. After women who used vitamin E in low doses were removed from the analyses, the following relative risks of coronary heart disease (CHD) were observed:

- 0.41 (95% CI: 0.18–0.93) for users of vitamin E supplements only;
- 0.87 (95% CI: 0.69–1.09) for users of multivitamins only;
- 0.50 (95% CI: 0.31–0.83) for users of both.

Despite these impressive findings, certain limitations of the data are noteworthy. First, while adjustment for a variety of other coronary risk factors and nutrients, including other antioxidants, had little effect on the results, users of vitamins were distinctly different from non-users. For instance, use of Vitamin E was associated with frequent exercise, postmenopausal hormone use, and non-smoking status. Second, β-carotene, not vitamin E, appeared to be most relevant in terms of reducing the risk of cerebrovascular disease (Stampfer *et al.* 1993).

In the Health Professionals Follow-up Study (Rimm *et al.* 1993), 39 910 US male health professionals (40–75 years of age) who were free of diagnosed CHD, diabetes, and hypercholesterolaemia at baseline completed food frequency questionnaires that assessed their usual intake of vitamin C, carotene, vitamin E, and other nutrients. During 4 years of follow-up, 667 cases of coronary disease were documented. Men in the top quintile for vitamin E consumption (mean = 419 IU/day) had an age-adjusted relative risk of coronary disease of 0.59 (95% CI: 0.47–0.75) in comparison to men in the lowest quintile (mean = 6.4 IU/day). As compared with men who did not take vitamin E supplements, men who took at least 100 IU/day for at least 2 years had a multivariate relative risk of coronary disease of 0.63 (95% CI: 0.47–0.84). Carotene intake was not associated with a lower risk of CHD among those who had never smoked, but was inversely associated with CHD risk among current smokers (relative risk, 0.30; 95% CI: 0.11–0.82) and former smokers (relative risk 0.60; 95% CI: 0.38–0.94). In contrast, a high intake of vitamin C was not associated with a lower risk of coronary disease. Similar to the Nurses Health Study, there is considerable concern over the possibility of residual confounding; specifically, users of vitamin E displayed a number of desirable health habits (i.e., less smoking, more frequent aspirin use, and exercise).

In the Massachusetts Elderly Cohort Study (Gaziano *et al.* 1992), the association between dietary consumption of β-carotene and CVD mortality was examined prospectively in a cohort of 1299 elderly Massachusetts residents followed for 4.75 years. Using six items on a food frequency questionnaire administered at baseline, a β-carotene fruit and vegetable score was derived corresponding to the number of servings per day of foods rich in this micronutrient. For CVD death, the age- and sex-adjusted relative risks among those in the highest quartile of β-carotene fruit and vegetable score compared with the lowest was 0.55 (95% CI: 0.34–0.87), with an inverse trend across quartiles (p (trend) = 0.002). Although data pertaining to dietary intake of vitamin E were not presented, the strong relationship between β-carotene and CHD stands in marked contrast to the previously cited studies.

NHANES I provides some evidence in support of a protective effect of vitamin C (Enstrom *et al.* 1992). In this cohort study, 11 348 non-institutionalized US adults, ages 25–74 years, were examined at baseline during 1971–74. During follow-up through 1984, a median of 10 years, 1809 deaths occurred. An index of vitamin C intake from diet measurements and use of vitamin supplements was developed. The relation of the standardized mortality ratio (SMR) for all causes of death to increasing vitamin C intake was strongly inverse for men and weakly inverse for women. Among those with the highest vitamin C intake, males had an SMR of 0.65

(95% CI: 0.52–0.80) for all-cause mortality and 0.58 (95% CI: 0.41–0.78) for CVD mortality; females had an SMR of 0.90 (95% CI: 0.74–1.09) for all-cause mortality and 0.75 (95% CI: 0.55–0.99) for CVD mortality. Comparisons were made relative to all US whites, for whom the SMR was defined to be 1.00. The relation with all-cause mortality among males persisted after adjustment for age, gender, and 10 potentially confounding variables (including cigarette smoking, education, race, and disease history). As in the previously mentioned studies, interpretation of these data is complicated by lack of adjustment for relevant covariates, including vitamin E.

The NHANES II Mortality Study further examined the relationship between Vitamin C and mortality (Loria *et al.* 2000). In this prospective study, serum vitamin C levels were measured at baseline and vital status was ascertained 12–16 years later. The relative risk of death in men in the lowest quartile (28.4 µmol/l) compared with the highest quartile of vitamin C levels (73.8 µmol/l) was 1.57 (95% CI: 1.21–2.03), adjusted for potential confounders. However, in subgroup analyses, this association was only found in non-smoking men. There was no increased risk of CVD mortality in men or women, or in total mortality in women in those in the lowest quartile of vitamin C (which included 1% vitamin C supplement users) compared with the highest intake (which included 19% vitamin C supplement users). Also, this study provides no evidence that vitamin C supplementation was effective at reducing risk of CVD or death.

15.5 Observational study results and clinical trial designs

As discussed above, dietary intake of vitamin C, vitamin E, and β-carotene in observational studies tends to be inversely associated with subsequent CVD, although the evidence is by no means consistent. In general, those with the highest intake or highest blood levels of antioxidants have lower rates of CVD compared to those with low levels. Individuals with higher intake of antioxidants include a large proportion of individuals who take vitamin supplements – usually at supra-physiological doses (Table 15.1). For example, vitamin E intake in the US adult population averages ~25.7 mg/day, while vitamin E supplements typically provide 300–600 mg/day.

Table 15.1 Dietary intake, antioxidant supplement use in the US populations, and US RDA recommended guidelines for intake of vitamin E, β-carotene, and vitamin C

	Vitamin E	β-carotene	Vitamin C
Mean daily intake from diet and supplements[a]	25.7 mg	2.9 mg	167 mg
US RDA recommended daily minimum dose[b]	15 mg (10 IU)	3–6 mg from food	90 mg (men) 75 mg (women)
Tolerable daily upper limit intake[b]	1000 mg	Not established	2000 mg
Typical daily supplement dose range used in clinical trial	400–800 IU	15–50 mg	500–1000 mg
Supplement use by US population[c]	23% of men 29% of women	No reliable estimates	31% of adults

[a] NHANES-II (Nebeling *et al.*1997). [c] Moss *et al.* 1989.

[b] Reported in the Institute of Medicine Report 2000.

Although one study (Kushi *et al.* 1996) suggests that vitamin E from food is more beneficial than vitamin E from supplements, the most persuasive evidence of benefit from antioxidants came from observational studies in which subgroups that benefited were those who consumed vitamin E supplements. This observation provided the rationale to test the efficacy of high-dose supplements in large-scale clinical trials for the prevention of cardiovascular and other diseases.

Observational studies also documented that patients with deficiencies in antioxidant intake were often those at highest risk for disease, that is, groups that most likely would benefit from antioxidant vitamin supplements. Hence, in clinical trials of antioxidant supplements, participants were selected to be at high risk for CVDs (i.e., those with established risk factors for CVD), those at risk for developing cancers (i.e., cigarette smokers at risk for lung cancer or adults with sunlight exposure at risk for developing skin cancers), or those with vitamin deficiencies (such as cigarette smokers or adults living in China). It was hypothesized that those at highest risk for disease would show the greatest benefit from supplements.

15.6 **Clinical trials of β-carotene supplementation**

Six large (>1000 patients) clinical trials published since 1990 tested the effects of β-carotene supplementation (Table 15.2).

The Alpha-tocopherol, β-Carotene (ATBC) Lung Cancer prevention study was a 2×2 factorial study in which 29 133 male Finnish smokers were randomly assigned to (a) β-carotene (20 mg/day) or corresponding placebo, and (b) *dl*-α-tocopherol (50 mg/day) or corresponding placebo (ATBC 1994). In this study, β-carotene was associated with an 18% increased risk of incident lung cancer (95% CI: 3–30%) and an 8% increased risk in total mortality (relative risk (RR) = 1.08; 95% CI: 1.01–1.16). Vascular outcomes were only presented as counts and rates without any reports of statistical significance. For nearly every vascular outcome, more events occurred in those assigned to β-carotene than those not assigned to β-carotene. In a subgroup analysis of the ATBC study that focused on men with previous MI, there were significantly more deaths from fatal CHD in the β-carotene alone group (multivariate RR = 1.75; 95% CI: 1.16–2.64; $p = 0.007$) and in the combined β-carotene and alpha-tocopherol group (RR = 1.58; 95% CI: 1.05–2.40; $p = 0.03$) compared to placebo group (Rapola *et al.* 1997).

The surprising results of increased mortality risk with β-carotene supplements in the ATBC study were replicated in the CARET (Combination of B-carotene and Vitamin A on lung cancer and cardiovascular disease) study (Omenn *et al.* 1996). Similar to the ATBC trial, CARET enrolled a cohort at high risk for lung cancer, specifically smokers, former smokers, and asbestos workers. In this trial, 18 314 adults were assigned to 30 mg/day of β-carotene (plus 25 000 IU/day of retinol) or placebo. After 4 years of supplementation, those assigned to β-carotene had a significantly higher incidence of lung cancer (RR = 1.28; 95% CI: 1.04–1.57), total mortality (RR = 1.17; 95% CI: 1.03–1.33), and borderline significantly higher mortality from CVD (RR = 1.26; 95% CI: 0.99–1.61) compared with placebo.

The results of the ATCB and CARET studies were not replicated in two primary prevention trials. In the Physicians Health Study, 22 071 healthy male physicians, a population at relatively low risk for cancer and CVD, were assigned to 20 mg of β-carotene every other day, or placebo. After 12 years of supplementation, total mortality (RR = 1.02, 95% CI: 0.93–1.11) and cardiovascular mortality (RR = 1.09; 95% CI: 0.93–1.27) were similar in the β-carotene and placebo groups (Hennekens *et al.* 1996). In the Women's Health Study (Lee *et al.* 1999) healthy women were randomized in a placebo-controlled clinical trial to aspirin, vitamin E, and/or β-carotene. Outcomes were incident cancers and CVD among 39 876 women aged

Table 15.2 Clinical trials of β-carotene with vascular outcomes and mortality

Study	n	Population	Men (%)	Mean age (years)	Antioxidant(s) (mg/day)	Duration (years)	Outcomes	Relative risk (±95% CI)*
Skin Cancer Prevention Study (Greenberg et al. 1990)	1805	Free of skin cancers	70	65	50 β-carotene	5	Total mortality	RR = 1.08 (0.98–1.19)
ATBC 1994	29 133	Finnish smokers	100	57	20 β-carotene	6.1	Total mortality CVD events IHD Hem-CVA Isc-CVA	RR = 1.08 (1.01–1.16) RR = 1.11 (NS) RR = 1.16 (NS) RR = 1.11 (NS)
CARET (Omenn et al. 1996)	18 314	Smokers, former smokers, asbestos workers	100	58	30 β-carotene + 25 000 IU retinol	4.0	Overall mortality CVD death	RR = 1.17 (1.03–1.33) RR = 1.26 (0.99–1.61)
PHS (Hennekens et al. 1996)	22 071	Healthy physicians	100	40–84	20 β-carotene every other day	12	Total mortality CVD events CVD death MI Stroke	RR = 1.02 (0.93–1.11) RR = 1.09 (0.93–1.27) RR = 0.96 (0.84–1.09) RR = 0.96 (0.83–1.11)
Skin Cancer Prevention Trial (Greenberg et al. 1999)	1383	Free of skin cancers	43	49	30 β-carotene	4.5	Total mortality CVD mortality	RR = 0.50 (0.24–1.03) RR = 0.51 (NS)
WHS (Lee et al. 1999)	39 876	Healthy women	0	>45	50 β-carotene every other day	4.1[a]	Total mortality CVD events	RR = 1.07 (0.74–1.56) RR = 1.14 (0.87–1.49)

Hem-CVA: haemorraghic cerebrovascular accident; Isc-CVA: ischaemic cerebrovascular accident.

* Relative risk (±95% confidence interval).

[a] Supplements stopped after 2 years.

45 years or older. The β-carotene arm was terminated after a median duration of 2.1 years and results were reported against placebo. Among women assigned to receive β-carotene (50 mg every other day), there were no statistically significant differences in incidence of cancers (RR = 1.03; 95% CI: 0.89–1.18), deaths from CVDs (RR = 1.17; 95% CI: 0.54–2.53; p = 0.69), or total mortality (RR = 1.07; 95% CI: 0.74–1.56) compared with placebo after a median of 4.1 years (2.1 years of treatment plus 2.0 years follow-up).

Finally, two small trials tested the efficacy of β-carotene supplementation for the prevention of skin cancer (Green et al. 1999; Greenberg et al. 1990). Neither trial documented benefit of β-carotene supplementation. In the skin cancer prevention study (Greenberg et al. 1990) elderly patients assigned to 50 mg/day of β-carotene had a non-significantly higher death rate (RR = 1.08; 95% CI: 0.98–1.19), with similar relative risk for developing skin cancer. In the Skin Cancer Protection Study (Green et al. 1999), there was a non-significant reduced risk (RR = 0.50; 95% CI: 0.24–1.03) in the group assigned to 30 mg/day of β-carotene. In this study, participants were young (~49 years old), free of known CVD or cancer at baseline, and there were few events (less than 2% of those randomized). Hence, in view of the results of other trials, the apparent protective effect of β-carotene in this study may be the result of chance (type I error). Still if this finding is true, a possible explanation is the possibility that β-carotene may help prevent atherosclerosis and its complications in young people, yet be harmful in those with subclinical disease or established atherosclerosis.

15.7 **Clinical trials of multivitamins**

Eight large clinical trials of multivitamin therapies for the prevention of cancers or CVD have been published – six of which included β-carotene as a component (Table 15.3).

Two cancer prevention trials conducted in Linxian, China highlight the potential benefits of antioxidant vitamin combinations. These studies were undertaken in an effort to determine whether the high mortality from oesophageal cancer in this region (100 × rate of US Caucasians) is related to certain nutritional factors, including a low dietary intake of fruits and vegetables (and accompanying antioxidant vitamins). In the general population study, 29 584 were assigned in a partial factorial design, which tested the following four factors (A–D) (Blot et al. 1993):

A   retinol (5000 IU) and zinc (22.5 mg)

B   riboflavin (3.2 mg) and niacin (40 mg)

C   ascorbic acid (120 mg) and molybdenum (30 μg)

D   β-carotene (15 mg), selenium (50 mg), and α-tocopherol (30 mg)

After 5.3 years of supplementation, total mortality was significantly lower in the D group, which contained β-carotene (RR = 0.91; 95% CI: 0.84–0.99) compared with the placebo group. While none of the four nutrient combinations led to statistically significant reductions in cerebrovascular mortality, the RR reduction from treatment D approached significance (RR = 0.90; 95% CI: 0.76–1.07).

In a separate study (Li et al. 1993), 3318 Chinese adults with oesophageal dysplasia were assigned to daily multivitamin therapy (β-carotene 15 mg, α-tocopherol 60 IU, ascorbic acid 180 mg, plus 11 other vitamins and 12 minerals) or placebo. After >6 years of follow-up, multivitamin therapy achieved a nearly significant reduced risk of cerebrovascular disease (RR = 0.62; 95% CI: 0.37–1.06; p = 0.08) and non-significant reductions in total mortality (RR = 0.93; 95% CI: 0.75–1.16). While encouraging, the applicability of the Linxian studies to

Table 15.3 Clinical trials of multivitamin supplements with vascular outcomes and mortality

Study	n	Population	Men (%)	Mean age	Antioxidant(s) (daily dose)	Duration (years)	Outcomes	Relative risk (±95% CI)*
Linxian Study A (Blot et al. 1993)	29 584	Adults 40–69	45	40–69	A Retinol 500 IU + zinc 22.5 mg B Riboflavin 3.2 mg + niacin 40 mg C Vitamin C 120 mg + molybdenum 30 µg D β-carotene 15 mg + α-tocopherol 30 mg + selenium 50 µg	5.3	Total mortality CVD events Stroke	RR = 0.91 (0.84–0.99) A: RR = 0.99 (0.84–1.18) B: RR = 0.93 (0.79–1.11) C: RR = 1.04 (0.88–1.24) D: RR = 0.90 (0.84–1.11)
Linxian Study B (Li et al. 1993)	3318	Oesophageal dysplasia	44	54	β-carotene 15 mg + vitamin E 60 IU + 12 vitamins and 11 minerals	6	Total mortality CVD events Stroke	RR = 0.93 (0.75–1.16) RR = 0.62 (0.37–1.06)
Girodon et al. 1999	725	Institutionalized elderly	34	84	Vitamin E 15 mg + vitamin C 120 mg + β-carotene 15 mg	2	Total mortality	RR = 0.94 (0.74–1.19)
AREDS 2001	4757	Elderly at risk for eye disease	44	68	Vitamin E 400 IU + β-carotene 15 mg + vitamin C 500 mg	6.3	Total mortality CVD events Chest pain	RR = 1.06 (0.84–1.33) RR = 0.87 (p = 0.01)
MRC/BHF-HPS (HPS 2002a, b)	20 536	CAD, arterial disease, or diabetes	75	40–80	Vitamin E 600 mg synthetic + vitamin C 250 mg + β-carotene 20 mg	5	Total mortality CVD events Coronary death, non-fatal MI Revascularization procedure Stroke	RR = 1.04 (0.97–1.12) RR = 1.02 (0.93–1.11) RR = 0.98 (0.90–1.06) RR = 0.99 (0.87–1.12)
REACT (Chylack et al. 2002)	297	Elderly with age-related cataracts	41	67	Vitamin E 600 mg + vitamin C 750 mg + β-carotene 18 mg	3–5	Total mortality	RR = 1.49 (1.06–2.11)
WAVE (Waters et al. 2002)	423	Postmenopausal women with CAD	0	65	Vitamin E 800 IU + vitamin C 1000 mg	2.8	Total mortality CVD events Death, non-fatal MI, stroke	RH = 2.8 (1.1–7.2) RH = 1.5 (0.80–2.9)
ASAP (Salonen et al. 2003)	520	Men and postmenopausal women	49	45–69	Vitamin E 272 IU + vitamin C 500 mg	6	Total mortality	RR = 1.15 (0.96–1.37)

CAD: coronary artery disease.

* Relative risk (RR) or relative hazard (RH) ±95% confidence interval.

the general US population remains a matter of speculation because of the distinctive nature of the study population. Serum levels of β-carotene were considerably lower than in the US population levels, suggesting nutritional deficiencies in the study population.

Subsequent to the Chinese trials, two large multivitamin studies have recently been conducted in the US. In the Age-Related Eye Disease Study (AREDS 2001), 4757 elderly at risk for retinal, lens, and corneal eye diseases were assigned to a multivitamin therapy (vitamin E 400 IU/day, β-carotene 15 mg/day, and vitamin C 500 mg/day) or placebo. After 6.3 years of intervention, total mortality was similar in both groups (RR = 1.06; 95% CI : 0.84–1.33). Although specific cardiovascular outcomes were not reported, there was a slight reduction in self-reported chest pain in the active vs. placebo groups (19.8 vs. 22.8%, respectively; $p = 0.01$).

In the MRC/BHF Heart Protection Study (HPS) trial, 20 536 British adults with established coronary artery disease, peripheral arterial disease, or diabetes were randomly assigned in a 2×2 factorial design to (a) a daily multivitamin (vitamin E 600 mg, β-carotene 20 mg, and vitamin C 250 mg) or placebo, and (b) 40 mg/day of a lipid-lowering medication (40 mg/day of simvastatin) or placebo, and followed for 5 years (HPS 2002a, b). There were no significant differences in total mortality, coronary death, non-fatal MI, or stroke between the vitamin and placebo groups (HPS 2002a). In addition, although the simvastatin group had significant reductions in cardiovascular and total mortality, there was no additive effect from multivitamin therapy (HPS 2002b).

Finally, a small trial ($n = 423$) of daily multivitamin therapy for the prevention of age-related cataracts, the Roche European American Cataract Trial (REACT) (Chylack et al. 2002) reported total mortality over 3–5 years. Participants, who were elderly, consumed a daily multivitamin (vitamin C 750 mg, β-carotene 18 mg, vitamin E 600 mg) or placebo. The RR for mortality was non-significantly increased in the multivitamin group (RR = 3.0; $p = 0.07$) compared with the placebo group.

15.8 Interpretation of β-carotene and multivitamin supplementation trials

Overall, the surprising results of the β-carotene trials, particularly the lack of any benefit from β-carotene supplementation and the possibility of harm, should be interpreted in the context of all the available evidence. For instance, results from numerous observational studies indicate that high intakes of β-carotene, at least from food sources, should be beneficial in terms of a reduced risk of lung cancer and of vascular disease. The mechanisms responsible for the increased cardiovascular deaths with supplements are unknown, but might be related to the supra-physiological doses of β-carotene used in these trials: levels which are far greater than could be achieved by diet. Consuming a diet rich in fruits and vegetables enriched with natural sources of dietary β-carotene may increase serum β-carotene levels by 50% (Miller et al. 1998). In contrast, in clinical trials of β-carotene supplementation, consumption of 15–50 mg of β-carotene daily results in substantially higher levels of serum β-carotene (4–20 times initial levels) over those who are not supplemented. β-carotene at these levels has been shown to have pro-oxidant effects under certain physiological conditions (Krinsky 1993).

The two Linxian studies of β-carotene supplementation were notable exceptions to the apparent trend of higher mortality with supplementation from β-carotene. Both studies reported reductions in overall mortality (~10%). However, the populations involved in these trials were distinctive from those studied in other supplementation trials. In the Linxian trials, participants had low levels of serum β-carotene at baseline – less than half the levels found in the European or American study populations. Hence, one plausible explanation is that the supplements may lower risk of mortality, but only in the setting of a diet deficient in β-carotene. An alternative explanation is that the selenium and vitamin E, also parts of the supplement, ameliorated the pro-oxidant effects of high dose β-carotene. What is quite apparent from the ATBC and CARET studies is that β-carotene supplementation provides no benefit and may in fact be harmful, at least in smokers, a population with greater free radical activity, inflammation and oxidative stress, and reduced serum β-carotene levels.

15.9 Clinical trials of vitamin E supplementation (clinical outcomes)

Of the available antioxidant vitamin supplements, vitamin E had the greatest appeal as a means to prevent CVD. In laboratory studies, vitamin E reduced oxidative damage to lipids. In addition, observational studies provided strong evidence for benefit from vitamin E supplementation in spite of the potential for residual confounding. Despite this promising evidence, several large, well-conducted clinical trials have documented that vitamin E supplementation does not prevent CVD and is ineffective for the treatment of established CVD (Table 15.4).

The first large trial of vitamin E supplementation was the ATBC study, completed in 1994. In this 2×2 factorial design clinical trial ((a) α-tocopherol or placebo, and (b) β-carotene or placebo), Finnish smokers assigned to 50 mg/day of α-tocopherol had similar deaths rates from ischaemic heart disease and ischaemic stroke than the placebo group and more deaths ($p < 0.05$) from haemorrhagic stroke than the placebo group after 5–8 years. The latter finding, if true, may be explained by the possibility of an antiplatelet effect of vitamin E. In a subgroup analysis of men in the ATBC trial with previous MI, vitamin E supplementation was associated with a significant reduction in non-fatal MI (RR = 0.62; 95% CI: 0.41–0.96), but a non-significant increase in fatal CHD (RR = 1.33; 95% CI: 0.86–2.05) (Rapola et al. 1997).

Another large trial of vitamin E supplementation was a secondary prevention trial of patients with previous MI, the Cambridge Heart Antioxidant Study (CHAOS) (Stephers et al. 1996). This study reported a significant reduction in non-fatal MI (RR = 0.23; 95% CI: 0.11–0.47) after only 1.4 years of supplementation of 400 or 800 IU of vitamin E. However, total mortality (RR = 1.24; $p = 0.31$) and cardiovascular mortality (RR = 1.18; 95% CI: 0.62–2.27) were higher in those assigned to vitamin E compared with placebo groups.

The GISSI–Prevenzionne trial (GISSI-Prevenzione Investigators 1999) was a secondary prevention trial of 11 324 men and women who had had a recent MI. In those assigned to 300 IU vitamin E, there were non-significant reductions in total mortality (RR = 0.86; 95% CI: 0.72–1.02) and death, non-fatal MI, and non-fatal stroke (RR = 0.88; 95% CI: 0.75–1.04) after 3.5 years of follow-up.

Two additional trials of vitamin E supplementation for the prevention of CVD in patients at high risk for disease were completed and published in 2000 and 2001. The HOPE (Heart Outcome Prevention Evaluation) ($n = 9541$) and PPP (Primary Prevention Project) ($n = 4495$) trials randomized adults at high risk for CVD to 400 and 300 IU/day, respectively (Collaborative Group of the Primary Prevention Program 2001; HOPE 2000). In both studies, vitamin E had no significant effect on total mortality, or fatal or non-fatal cardiovascular events. In both trials, the vitamin E supplemented groups had a non-significantly higher relative risk for stroke (RR = 1.17; 95% CI: 0.95–1.42) in HOPE and (RR = 1.56; 95% CI: 0.77–3.13) in PPP.

In a meta-analysis of vitamin E trials that included the ATBC, CHAOS, GISSI, and HOPE trials (Dagenais et al. 2000), the overall relative risks in those assigned to vitamin E were similar to those assigned to placebo for all cardiovascular outcomes, including total cardiovascular

Table 15.4 Clinical trials of vitamin E supplements and total mortality and cardiovascular events

Study	n	Population	Men (%)	Age (years)	Antioxidant (daily dose)	Duration (years)	Outcomes	Relative risk (±95% CI)*
ATBC 1994	29 133	Finnish Smokers	100	57	dl-α-tocopherol 50 mg	6.1	Total mortality	RR = 1.02 (0.95–1.09)
							CVD events	RR = 0.96 (0.90–1.03)
							IHD	RR = 1.50 (<0.05)
							Hem-CVA	RR = 0.84 (NS)
							Isc-CVA	
CHAOS (Stephers et al. 1996)	2002	Angiographic evidence of CAD	84	62	α-tocopherol 400 IU or 800 IU	1.4	Total mortality	RR = 1.24 (0.90–1.39)
							CVD events	RR = 0.23 (0.11–0.47)
							Non-fatal MI	RR = 1.18 (0.62–2.27)
							CVD death	RR = 0.53 (0.34–0.83)
							Any CVD event	
GISSI-Prevenzione Investigators 1999	11324	Recent MI	85	59	Vitamin E 300 mg	3.5	Total mortality	RR = 0.86 (0.72–1.02)
							CVD events	RR = 0.89 (0.77–1.03)
							Death, non-fatal MI, non-fatal stroke	RR = 0.88 (0.75–1.04)
							CVD death, non-fatal MI, stroke	RR = 1.02 (0.81–1.28)
							Non-fatal CVD events	
HOPE 2000	9541	High risk for CVD	73	66	Vitamin E 400 IU	4.5	Total mortality	RR = 1.00 (0.89–1.13)
							CVD events	RR = 1.05 (0.95–1.16)
							MI, stroke, CVD death	RR = 1.02 (0.90–1.15)
							CVD death	RR = 1.17 (0.95–1.42)
							Stroke	
SPACE (Boaz et al. 2000)	196	Dialysis patients with CVD	70	65	α-tocopherol 800 IU natural	1.4	Total mortality	RR = 1.09 (0.70–1.70)
							CVD events	RR = 0.54 (0.33–0.89)
							Total CVD events	RR = 0.35 (0.10–1.24)
							Non-fatal MI	RR = 0.61 (0.28–1.30)
							CVD death	RR = 0.85 (0.30–2.70)
							Stroke	

Table 15.4 (continued)

Study	n	Population	Men (%)	Age (years)	Antioxidant (daily dose)	Duration (years)	Outcomes	Relative risk (±95%CI)
PPP (Collaborative Group 2001)	4495	Risk factors for CVD	43	64	α-tocopherol 300 mg synthetic	3.6	Total mortality	RR = 1.07 (0.77–1.49)
							CVD events	
							CVD death,	
							non-fatal MI, stroke	RR = 1.07 (0.74–1.56)
							Non-fatal MI	RR = 1.01 (0.56–2.03)
							Non-fatal stroke	RR = 1.56 (0.77–3.13)
VEAPS (Hodis et al. 2002)	353	Healthy except for LDL > 130 mg/dl	80	56	dl-α-tocopherol 400 IU	3	Total mortality	RR = 1.36 (0.61–3.06)

CAD: coronary artery disease;
Hem-CVA: haemorraghic cerebrovascular accident;
Isc-CVA: ischaemic cerebrovascular accident.

* Relative risk (±95% confidence interval).

mortality (RR = 0.99; 95% CI: 0.92–1.06), fatal ischaemic heart disease (RR = 0.95; 95% CI: 0.87–1.03), and non-fatal MI (RR = 0.98; 95% CI: 0.91–1.07).

Since then, two small trials of vitamin E supplementation in unique populations have recently been published. The SPACE trial was a secondary prevention trial that tested the effects of vitamin E on CVD in patients with end-stage renal disease (ESRD). In this trial, 196 patients with ESRD on dialysis were assigned high-dose vitamin E (800 IU/day) or placebo (Boaz et al. 2000). This study reported a significant reduction in total CVD events which included non-fatal MI, stroke, and cardiovascular deaths (RR = 0.54; 95% CI: 0.33–0.89) at 1.4 years. However, overall mortality was non-significantly higher in the vitamin E group (RR = 1.09; 95% CI: 0.70–1.70). The WAVE (Women's Angiographic Vitamin and Estrogen) trial (Waters et al. 2002) reported an increased risk in total mortality in postmenopausal women with coronary artery stenosis assigned to high-dose vitamin E (800 IU/day) and 1000 mg/day of vitamin C (relative hazard (RH) = 2.8; 95% CI: 1.1–7.2), compared with those assigned placebo, and non-significant increases in cardiovascular events including death, non-fatal MI, and stroke (RH = 1.5; 95% CI: 0.8–2.9).

15.10 Clinical trials of vitamin E: radiographic markers of disease progression

Several studies examined the effects of vitamin E supplementation on intermediate vascular outcomes in selected populations, usually in those with pre-existing vascular diseases (Table 15.5). These clinical trials examined the efficacy of vitamin E on angiographic markers of coronary artery disease and on ultrasound measurements of carotid and coronary artery disease progression. In spite of the heterogeneity of these studies, including different study populations (primary and secondary prevention trials), differences in vitamin E dose (400–1200 IU/day, either alone or as a multivitamin), study duration (4 months to 4.5 years), and different imaging techniques (angiography and ultrasonography), the results were similar; that is, there was little evidence for a protective effect of vitamin E supplementation on progression of atherosclerotic disease.

A notable exception was a recent Scandinavian trial which reported reduced progression of carotid artery disease following 6 years of supplementation with vitamin E and vitamin C in combination in people with risk factors for atherosclerosis (the Antioxidant and Supplementation and Atherosclerosis Progression trial (ASAP)) (Salonen et al. 2003).

15.11 Interpretation of the vitamin E trials

Despite biological plausibility and strong evidence from observational studies that vitamin E supplements should be protective against CVDs, clinical trials do not support their use. A recent dose response meta-analysis of vitamin E supplementation and all-cause mortality in 19 randomized clinical trials (Figure 15.2) demonstrated a statistically significant relationship between vitamin E dosage and mortality, with increased risk mortality with dosages above 150 IU per day (Millet et al. 2005). There is no evidence for benefit and an apparent increased risk for mortality with higher doses. The trials which used higher vitamin E doses generally had patients at higher risk for mortality (REACT, WAVE, and CHAOS). In trials with sub-clinical outcomes, vitamin E likewise had no consistent benefit. Hence, available evidence from several large, well-designed trials are broadly consistent in documenting that vitamin E supplementation does not protect against CVD, particularly in high-risk populations.

Table 15.5 Clinical trial of antioxidant vitamin supplementation and angiographic markers of cardiovascular disease progression

Study	n	Population	Men (%)	Mean age (years)	Antioxidant(s) (daily dose)	Duration	Outcomes	Rate of progression
DeMaio 1992	100	Coronary angioplasty patients	82	54	dl-α-tocopherol 1200 IU	4 months	Restenosis	Vitamin group 35% Placebo group 50% (p = 0.06)
MVP (Tardif et al. 1997)	317	Angiographic evidence of CAD	81	59	dl-α-tocopherol 30 000 IU + β-carotene 700 IU + vitamin C 500 mg	6 months	Repeated angioplasty	Vitamin group 24.4% Placebo group 26.6% (p = 0.75)
SECURE (Lonn et al. 2001)	732	High risk for CVD (HOPE study subgroup)	77	65	Vitamin E 400 IU	4.5 years	Carotid artery progression (IMT by ultrasound: mean slope)	Vitamin group 0.0180 mm/year (0.0022) Placebo group 0.0174 mm/year (0.0020) (p = 'NS')
HATS (Brown et al. 2001)	160	Clinical CAD with low HDL levels	84	62	dl-α-tocopherol 800 IU + vitamin C 1000 mg + β-carotene 25 mg + selenium 100 μg	3 years	Carotid artery progression (Mean change in % stenosis (standard deviation))	Vitamin group 1.8 (4.2%) Placebo group 3.9 (5.2%) (p = 0.16)
VEAPS (Hodis et al. 2002)	353	Healthy except for LDL > 130 mg/dl	80	56	dl-α-tocopherol 400 IU	3 years	Carotid artery progression (IMT by ultrasound: mean slope)	Vitamin group 0.0040 mm/year (0.0007) Placebo group 0.0023 mm/year (0.0007) (p = 0.08)
WAVE (Waters et al. 2002)	423	Postmenopausal women with CAD	0	65	Vitamin E 800 IU + vitamin C 1000 mg	2.8 years	CAD progression (angiography) (IMT by ultrasound: mean slope)	Vitamin group 0.044 (0.15) mm/year Placebo group 0.028 (0.15) mm/year(p = 0.32)
Cardiac Transplant (Fang et al. 2002)	40	Cardiac transplant patients	87	51	Vitamin E 800 IU + vitamin C 1000 mg	1 year	CAD progression (intravascular ultrasonography: mean change in intimal index)	Vitamin group 0.8 (1) Placebo group 8.0 (2) (p = 0.008)
ASAP (Salonen et al. 2003)	520	Men and postmenopausal women	49	45–69	Vitamin E 272 IU + vitamin C 500 mg	6 years	Carotid artery progression (IMT thickness by ultrasound:mean slope)	Vitamin group 0.010 mm/year Placebo group 0.014 mm/year (p = 0.034)

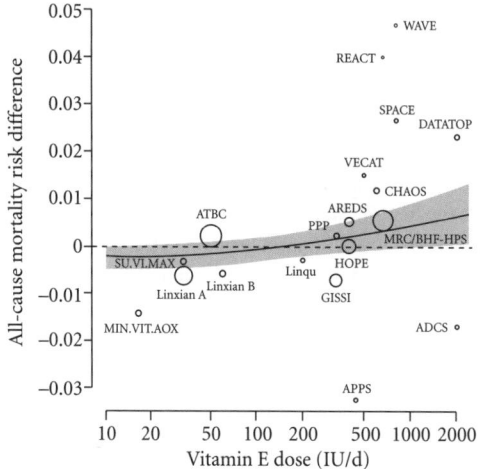

Fig. 15.2 All-cause mortality risk difference in clinical trials of vitamin E supplementation reported by vitamin E dose. Vertical lines show ±95% CI.

15.12 **Conclusions**

Trials of antioxidant vitamin supplements typically conducted in persons with, or at high risk for, CVD have conclusively and repeatedly documented no benefit from antioxidant supplements, either β-carotene or vitamin E. These results stand in contrast to observational studies, which often suggested benefit from a high intake of antioxidants. Some trials (de Lorgeril *et al.* 1994; Singh *et al.* 2002) documented benefit from diets rich in antioxidants. The potential for confounding from changes in other nutrients is substantial. One reason for these discrepancies is the possibility that antioxidants are effective only in persons without established disease, that is, the type of individuals enrolled in observational studies. Alternatively, the supra-physiological dose used in supplement trials not only exceeds typical dietary intake, but may also exert harmful, pro-oxidant effects. The form of antioxidants provided in supplements may also differ from that consumed in foods. Hence, policy-making bodies, including the American Heart Association (Tribble 1999) and the Institute of Medicine (2000), do not recommend antioxidant vitamin supplement use, either for the prevention or treatment of CVD.

Trials of multivitamins provide some evidence that these supplements might be beneficial in persons with vitamin deficiencies. However, trials conducted in Western countries among individuals without apparent vitamin deficiencies document no clear benefit. Because of the greater likelihood of benefit than harm in patients with subclinical vitamin deficiencies, some experts recommend that individuals take a daily multivitamin that does not exceed the recommended daily allowance (RDA) of its component vitamins. However, recommendations for high-dose supplementation are clearly unjustified.

References

AREDS (Age-Related Eye Disease Study) Research Group (2001). A randomized, placebo-controlled, clinical trial of high-dose supplementation with vitamins C and E and β carotene for age-related cataract and vision loss. AREDS report no. 9. *Archives of Ophthalmology*, **119**, 1439–52.

ATBC (The Alpha-Tocopherol, β-Carotene) Lung Cancer Prevention Study Group (1994). The effect of vitamin E and β carotene on the incidence of lung cancer and other cancers in male smokers. *New England Journal of Medicine*, **330**, 1029–35.

Blot, W. J., Li, J., Taylor, P. R. *et al.* (1993). Nutrition intervention trials in Linxian, China: supplementation with specific vitamin/mineral combinations, cancer incidence, and disease-specific mortality in the general population. *Journal of the National Cancer Institute*, **85**, 1483–92.

Boaz, M., Smetana, S., Weinstein, T. *et al.* (2000). Secondary prevention with antioxidants of cardiovascular disease in endstage renal disease (SPACE): randomized placebo-controlled trial. *Lancet*, **356**, 1213–18.

Brown, B. G., Zhao, X. Q., Chait, A. *et al.* (2001). Simvastatin and niacin, antioxidant vitamins, or the combination for the prevention of coronary disease. *New England Journal of Medicine*, **345**, 1583–92.

Balluz, L. S., Kieszak, S. M., Philen, R. M., and Mulinare, J. (2000). Vitamin and mineral supplement use in the United States. Results from the third National Health and Nutrition Examination Survey. *Archives of Family medicine*, **9**, 258–62.

Chylack, L. T., Brown, N. P., Bron, A. *et al.* (2002). The Roche European American Cataract Trial (REACT): a randomized clinical trial to investigate the efficacy of an oral antioxidant micronutrient mixture to slow progression of age-related cataract. *Ophthalmic Epidemiology*, **9**, 48–80.

Collaborative Group of the Primary Prevention Project (PPP) (2001). Low-dose aspirin and vitamin E in people at cardiovascular risk: a randomized trial in general practice. *Lancet*, **357**, 89–95.

Dagenais, G. R., Marchioli, R., Tognoni, G. *et al.* (2000). B-Carotene, vitamin C, and vitamin E and cardiovascular diseases. *Current Cardiology Reports*, **2**, 293–9.

de Lorgeril, M., Renaud, S., Mamelle, N. *et al.* (1994). Mediterranean alpha-linolenic acid-rich diet in secondary prevention of coronary heart disease. *Lancet*, **343**, 1454–9.

DeMaio, S. J., King, S. B., Lembo, N. J. *et al.* (1992). Vitamin E supplementation, plasma lipids and incidence or restenosis after percutaneous transluminal coronary angioplasty (PTCA). *Journal of the American College of Nutrition*, **11**, 68–73.

Enstrom, J. E., Kanim, L. E., Klein, M. A. (1992). Vitamin C intake and mortality among a sample of the United States population. *Epidemiology*, **3**, 194–202.

Erlinger, T. P., Guallar, E., Miller III, E. R. *et al.* (2001). Relationship between systemic markers of inflammation and serum-carotene levels. *Archives of Internal Medicine*, **161**, 1903–8.

Fang, J. C., Kinlay, S., Beltrame, J. *et al.* (2002). Effect of vitamins C and E on progression of transplant-associated atherosclerosis: a randomized trial. *Lancet*, **359**, 1108–13.

Gaziano, J. M., Manson, J. E., Branch, L. G. *et al.* (1992). Dietary β carotene and decreased cardiovascular mortality in an elderly cohort. *Journal of the American College of Cardiology*, **19** (3 Suppl. A), 337-A.

Girodon, F., Galan, P., Monget, A.-L. *et al.*, and the MIN.VIT.AOX.geriatric network (1999). Impact of trace elements and vitamin supplementation on immunity and infections in institutionalized elderly patients. *Archives of Internal Medicine*, **159**, 748–54.

GISSI-Prevenzione Investigators (1999). Dietary supplementation with n-3 polyunsaturated fatty acids and vitamin E after myocardial infarction: results of the GISSI-Prevenzione trial. *Lancet*, **354**, 447–55.

Green, A., Williams, G., Neale, R. *et al.* (1999). Daily sunscreen application and β-carotene supplementation in prevention of basal-cell and squamous-cell carcinomas of the skin: a randomized controlled trial. *Lancet*, **354**, 723–9.

Greenberg, E. R., Baron, J. A., Stukel, T. A. *et al.* (1990). A clinical trial of β carotene to prevent basal-cell and squamous-cell cancers of the skin. *New England Journal of Medicine*, **323**, 789–95.

HPS (Heart Protection Study) Collaborative Group (2002*a*). MRC/BHF heart protection study of cholesterol lowering with simvastatin in 20 536 high-risk individuals: a randomized placebo-controlled trial. *Lancet*, **360**, 7–22.

HPS (Heart Protection Study) Collaborative Group (2002*b*). MRC/BHF heart protection study of antioxidant vitamin supplementation in 20 536 high-risk individuals: a randomized placebo-controlled trial. *Lancet*, **360**, 23–33.

Hennekens, C., Buring, J. E., Manson, J. E. *et al.* (1996). Lack of effect of long-term supplementation with β carotene on the incidence of malignant neoplasms and cardiovascular disease. *New England Journal of Medicine,* **334,** 1145–9.

Hodis, H. N., Mack, W. J., Labree, L. *et al.* (2002). Alpha-Tocopherol supplementation in healthy individuals reduces low-density lipoprotein oxidation but not atherosclerosis: The Vitamin E Atherosclerosis Prevention Study (VEAPS). *Circulation,* **106,** 1453–9.

HOPE (The Heart Outcomes Prevention Evaluation Study Investigators) (2000). Vitamin E supplementation and cardiovascular events in high-risk patients. *New England Journal of Medicine,* **342,** 154–60.

Huang, H.-Y., Appel, L. J., Croft, K. D. *et al.* (2002). The effects of vitamin C and vitamin E on in vivo lipid peroxidation: results from a controlled clinical trial. *American Journal of Clinical Nutrition,* **76,** 549–55.

Institute of Medicine (2000). *Dietary reference intakes for vitamin C, vitamin E, selenium, and carotenoids.* National Academy Press, Washington, DC.

Krinsky, N. I. (1993). Actions of carotenoids in biological systems. *Annual Reviews in Nutrition,* **13,** 561–87.

Kritchevsky, S. B., Shimakawa, T., Tell, G. S. *et al.* (1995). Dietary antioxidants and carotid artery wall thickness: the ARIC study. *Circulation,* **92,** 2142–50.

Kushi, L. M., Folsom, A. R., Prineas, R. J. *et al.* (1996). Dietary antioxidant vitamins and death from coronary heart disease in postmenopausal women. *New England Journal of Medicine,* **334,** 1156–62.

Lee, I. M., Cook, N. R., Manson, J. E. *et al.* (1999). -carotene supplementation and incidence of cancer and cardiovascular disease: the Women's Health Study. *Journal of the National Cancer Institute,* **91,** 2101–6.

Li, J., Taylor, P. R., Li, B. *et al.* (1993). Nutrition intervention trials in Linxian, China: multiple vitamin/mineral supplementation, cancer incidence, and disease-specific mortality among adults with esophageal dysplasia. *Journal of the National Cancer Institute,* **85,** 1492–8.

Lonn, E. M., Yusuf, S., Dzavik, F. *et al.* (2001). Effects of ramipril and vitamin E on atherosclerosis. The study to evaluate carotid ultrasound changes in patients treated with ramipril and vitamin E (SECURE). *Circulation,* **103,** 919–925.

Lonn, E., Yusuf, S., Hoogwerf, B. *et al.* (2002). Effects of vitamin E on cardiovascular and microvascular outcomes in high risk patients with diabetes: results of the HOPE Study and MICRO-HOPE sub study. *Diabetes Care,* **25,** 1919–27.

Loria, C. M., Klag, M. J., Caulfield, L. E. *et al.* (2000). Vitamin C status and mortality in US adults. *American Journal of Clinical Nutrition,* **72,** 139–45.

McCall, M. R. and Frei, B. (1999). Can antioxidant vitamins materially reduce oxidative damage in humans? *Free Radical Biology and Medicine,* **26,** 1034–53.

Miller, E. R. III, Appel, L. J., and Risby, T, H. (1998). The effects of dietary patterns on measures of lipid peroxidation: results from a randomized clinical trial. *Circulation,* **98,** 2390–5.

Miller, E. R. III, Pastor-Barriuso, R., Dalal, D., Riemersma, R. A., Appel, L. J., and Guallar, E. (2005). Vitamin E supplementation may increase mortality: a dose response meta-analysis of randomized trials. *Annals of Internal Medicine,* **142,** 37–46.

Moss, A. J., Levy, A. S., Kim, I. *et al.* (1989). *Use of vitamins and mineral supplements in the United States: advance data, vital and health statistics of the National Center for Health Statistics.* Number 174. National Center for Health Statistics, Hyattsville, MD.

Nebeling, L. C., Forman, M. R., Graubard, B. I. *et al.* (1997). Changes in carotenoid intake in the United States: the 1987 and 1992 NHANES. *Journal of the American Dietetic Association,* **97,** 991–6.

Omenn, G. S., Goodman, G. E., Thornquist, M. D. *et al.* (1996). Effects of a combination of β carotene and vitamin A on lung cancer and cardiovascular disease. *New England Journal of Medicine,* **334,** 1150–5.

Parthasarathy, S., Santanam, N., Ramachandran, S., and Meihac, O. (1999). Oxidants and antioxidants in atherogenesis: an appraisal. *Journal of Lipid Research*, **40**, 2143–57.

Rapola, J. M., Virtamo, J., Ripatti, S. *et al.* (1997). Randomised trial of -tocopherol and -carotene supplements on incidence of major coronary events in men with previous myocardial infarction. *Lancet*, **349**, 1715–20.

Rimm, E. B., Stampfer, M. J., Ascherio, A. *et al.* (1993). Vitamin E consumption and the risk of coronary heart disease in men. *New England Journal of Medicine*, **328**, 1450–60.

Salonen, R. M., Nyyssonen, K., Kaikkonen, J. *et al.* (2003). Antioxidant Supplementation in Atherosclerosis Prevention Study. Six-year effect of combined vitamin C and E supplementation on atherosclerotic progression: the Antioxidant Supplementation in Atherosclerosis Prevention (ASAP) Study. *Circulation*, **107** (7), 947–53.

Singh, R. B., Dubnov, G., Niaz, M. A. *et al.* (2002). Effect of an Indo-Mediterranean diet on progression of coronary artery disease in high risk patients (Indo-Mediterranean Diet Heart Study): a randomized single-blind trial. *Lancet*, **360**, 1455–61.

Stampfer, M. J., Hennekens, C. H., Manson, J. E. *et al.* (1993). Vitamin E consumption and the risk of coronary disease in women. *New England Journal of Medicine*, **328**, 1444–9.

Steinberg, D. and Witztum, J. L. (2002). Is the oxidative modification hypothesis relevant to human atherosclerosis? Do the antioxidant trials conducted to date refute the hypothesis? *Circulation*, **105**, 2107–11.

Steinberg, D., Parthasarathy, S., Carew, T. E. *et al.* (1989). Modifications of low-density lipoprotein that increase its atherogenicity. *New England Journal of Medicine*, **320**, 915–24.

Stephers, N. G., Parsons, A., Schofield, P. M. *et al.* (1996). Randomised controlled trial of vitamin E in patients with coronary disease: Cambridge Heart Antioxidant Study (CHAOS). *Lancet*, **347**, 781–6.

Street, D. A., Comstock, G. W., Salkeld, R. M. *et al.* (1991). A population based case-control study of serum antioxidants and myocardial infarction. *American Journal of Epidemiology*, **134**, 719–70.

Stryker, W. S., Kaplin, L. A., Stein, A. *et al.* (1988). The relation of diet, cigarette smoking, and alcohol consumption to plasma beta-carotene and alpha-tocopherol levels. *American Journal of Epidemiology*, **127**, 114–23.

Tardif, J. C., Cote, G., Lesperance, J. *et al.* (1997). Probucol and multivitamins in the prevention of restenosis after coronary angioplasty: The Multivitamin and Probucol Study Group. *New England Journal of Medicine*, **337**, 365–72.

Tribble, D. L. (1999). Antioxidant consumption and risk of coronary heart disease: emphasis on vitamin C, vitamin E, and -carotene. *Circulation*, **99**, 591–5.

Waters, D. D., Alderman, E. L., Hsia, J. *et al.* (2002). Effects of hormone replacement therapy and antioxidant vitamin supplements on coronary atherosclerosis in postmenopausal women: a randomized controlled trial. *Journal of the American Medical Association*, **288**, 2432–40.

Chapter 16

Serum homocysteine and coronary heart disease

D. S. Wald, M. R. Law, N. J. Wald, and J. K. Morris

16.1 Introduction

In the 35 years since the link between serum homocysteine and cardiovascular disease was first made (McCully 1969) much evidence has accumulated on the subject. However, opinion on whether homocysteine causes cardiovascular disease remains divided. Resolving the uncertainty is important, as serum homocysteine levels can be lowered by taking additional folic acid, raising the prospect of a simple means of prevention (Homocysteine Lowering Trialists Collaboration 1998). This chapter examines the evidence for causality with respect to coronary heart disease (CHD).

16.2 Homocysteine and B vitamins

Homocysteine is an amino acid formed from the essential amino acid methionine. Methionine is the major methyl group donor in mammals and homocysteine is a by-product of this process. Homocysteine provides a reservoir for regenerating methionine (Fig. 16.1), thereby maintaining

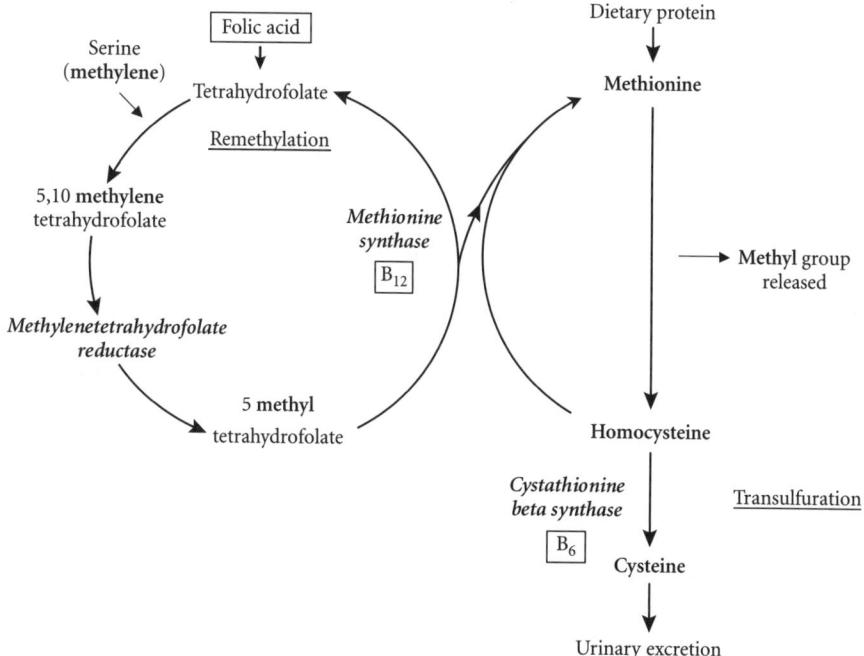

Fig. 16.1 Summary of the major pathways of homocysteine metabolism.

the methylation process throughout the body (Hankey and Eikelboom 1999). Otherwise it serves no known useful function and is thought to be toxic to vascular endothelial cells, to increase blood coagulability, and to promote smooth muscle cell proliferation – processes central to atherosclerosis (Brown *et al.* 1998; Fryer *et al.* 1993; Bellamy *et al.* 1998).

Homocysteine is metabolized in two ways (Fig. 16.1). It is remethylated to methionine, with 5-methyl tetrahydrofolate acting as the methyl group donor, a process dependent on vitamin B_{12} and the enzyme methionine synthase. Tetrahydrofolate is then remethylated to replenish 5-methyl tetrahydrofolate, a process dependent on the enzyme methylenetetrahydrofolate reductase (MTHFR) and the amino acid serine. Natural folate and folic acid (its synthetic analogue helps to replenish tetrahydrofolate). Homocysteine is also metabolized by transulfuration to cystathionine, a process dependent on vitamin B_6 and the enzyme cystathionine beta synthase. Impairment of either of these two processes can increase serum homocysteine concentrations.

The Homocysteine Trialists Collaboration (1998) showed that folic acid was the most effective of the B vitamins in lowering serum homocysteine. A dose of about 1 mg/day lowered serum homocysteine by 25% (or ~3 μmol/l from the population average level of 12 μmol/l); doses above 1 mg/day produced no additional benefit. Vitamin B_{12} (0.5 mg/day) produced only an additional 7% reduction and B_6 had no further detectable effect. Subsequent trials have shown that the full homocysteine-lowering effect of folic acid is achieved with about 0.8 mg folic acid per day, and most of the effect with 0.4 mg (van Oort *et al.* 2003; Wald *et al.* 2001). Folic acid lowers serum homocysteine from all pre-treatment levels in Western populations, though the reduction is greater from higher levels (Wald *et al.* 2001). Folic acid supplementation is more effective than dietary change; an unrealistically large amount of folate-containing foods (such as ~4 kg of broccoli per day) would need to be eaten to reach the equivalent homocysteine-lowering effect of a daily 0.8 mg folic acid supplement. This is because the folate concentration of foods is relatively low and the bioavailability of natural folate is about half that of folic acid.

16.3 The link between homocysteine and CHD: homocystinuria

The association between homocysteine and CHD was identified in 1969 by McCully, who described premature atherosclerotic disease at autopsy in two children who died with the rare autosomal recessive condition, homocystinuria (McCully 1969). Homocystinuria is a deficiency of one of three enzymes involved in homocysteine metabolism (Fig. 16.1), leading to three distinct disorders: cystathionine beta synthase deficiency, methylenetetrahydrofolate reductase deficiency, and the B_{12} metabolic defects that result in impaired methionine synthase activity. Heterozygotes for these three disorders have about three times the population average serum homocysteine concentration and a high risk of cardiovascular disease. Homozygotes have serum homocysteine levels 10–50 times the population average and a very high risk of premature cardiovascular disease; ~50% of them experience an arterial or venous disease event by the age of 30 (Mudd *et al.* 1985). A high homocysteine level is the only biochemical change common to all three disorders; no other substance is consistently high or low. It follows, therefore, that the high homocysteine causes the increased risk of cardiovascular disease. Two studies among homozygotes with homocystinuria treated with vitamins B_6, B_{12}, and folic acid indicate that risk can be reduced (Table 16.1). Treatment with these vitamins led to only 2 vascular events when 30 would have been expected (from previous observation in untreated patients) in one study (Kluijtmans *et al.* 1999), and 0 events when 29 would have been expected in the other (Yap and Naughten 1998). While these were not randomized trials, selection bias could not reasonably explain so large a difference with 2 events observed versus 59 expected.

Table 16.1 Observed numbers of vascular events in two studies of patients (homozygotes) with homocystinuria treated with B vitamins, and the expected numbers of events calculated by the authors of the two studies from age-specific rates in 629 untreated patients with homocystinuria

Study (first author)	No. of patients	Median age at diagnosis of homocystinuria	Mean follow-up (years)	Vascular events[a]		p value
				Observed	Expected	
Kluijtmans 1999	29	23	13	2	30	<0.001
Yap 1998	25	0 (newborn)	15	0	29	<0.001

[a] Deep vein thrombosis, pulmonary embolism, myocardial infarction, stroke, or peripheral arterial disease).

16.4 Retrospective and prospective epidemiological studies

Retrospective and prospective studies provide evidence of the dose–response relationship across the range of serum homocysteine in the population. There is about a two-fold risk gradient from the highest to the lowest fifth of serum homocysteine values.

In retrospective studies, homocysteine is measured after the diagnosis of CHD in cases (generally after a myocardial infarction) and in unaffected controls. Over 30 such studies have been published and all show a positive association between CHD and serum homocysteine. Figure 16.2 shows the results of a meta-analysis of the 12 published retrospective studies (combining data from 1517 cases of myocardial infarction) that reported the proportional difference in risk for a specified serum homocysteine difference, adjusted for age and, in some studies, other cardiovascular risk factors (or reported data from which this could be calculated) (Chao *et al.* 1999; Genest *et al.* 1990; Hoogeveen *et al.* 1998; Hopkins *et al.* 1995; Israelsson *et al.* 1988; Joubran *et al.* 1998; Loehrer *et al.* 1996; Malinow *et al.* 1996; Pancharuniti *et al.* 1994; Schwartz *et al.* 1997; Thögersen *et al.* 2001; Verhoef *et al.* 1996). The risk of a CHD event (odds ratio) for 3 μmol/l lower serum homocysteine (achievable by taking 0.8 mg folic acid) is shown for each study together with the summary estimate for all studies combined. The summary odds ratio was 0.78 (95% confidence interval: 0.72–0.85), or 0.75 (0.68–0.82) adjusted for regression-dilution bias (i.e., the diminution of an association because of imprecise measurement) (Clarke *et al.* 2001). This result is likely to overestimate the true effect, as some of the studies did not adjust for confounding by cardiovascular risk factors such as smoking, serum cholesterol, and blood pressure and possibly because atherosclerotic disease may increase homocysteine, due to reduced renal function (so-called 'reverse causality') (Wald *et al.* 2003).

Prospective studies, by their design, guard against an effect of disease on homocysteine. In these studies blood is taken from healthy subjects who are then followed up for several years. An efficient design used in many of the prospective studies of homocysteine and vascular disease, which avoids testing many thousands of samples at the outset, is to store the blood and test stored samples from those who later develop CHD events and from matched controls, a so-called nested case control design. Figure 16.3 shows the results of a meta-analysis of 16 published prospective studies of serum homocysteine and CHD events (death or non-fatal myocardial infarction, $n = 3144$) (Wald *et al.* 2002). The odds ratios shown were adjusted for age, sex, smoking habits, blood pressure, and serum cholesterol in all the studies except one, which was adjusted for age and sex alone (Stampfer *et al.* 1993). The summary odds ratio was 0.89 (0.85–0.92) for a 3 μmol/l lower serum homocysteine, or 0.85 (0.80–0.90) adjusted

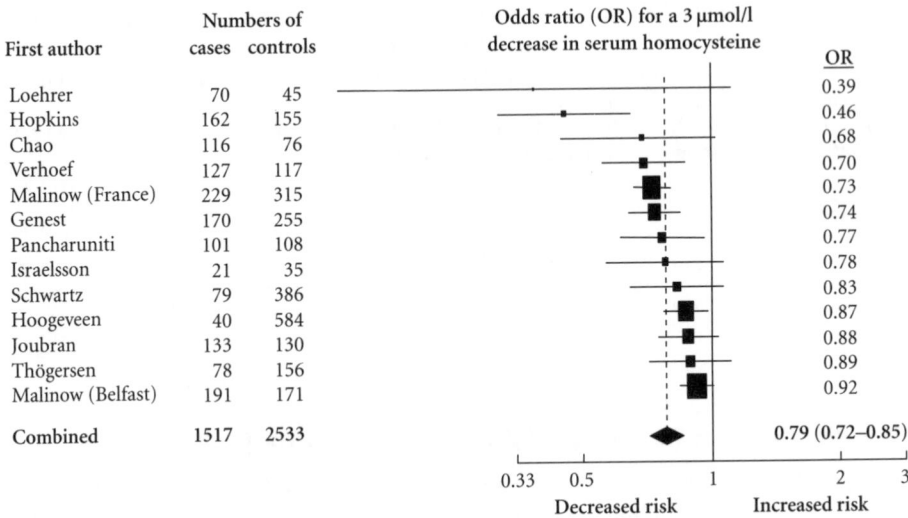

First author	Numbers of cases	controls		OR
Loehrer	70	45		0.39
Hopkins	162	155		0.46
Chao	116	76		0.68
Verhoef	127	117		0.70
Malinow (France)	229	315		0.73
Genest	170	255		0.74
Pancharuniti	101	108		0.77
Israelsson	21	35		0.78
Schwartz	79	386		0.83
Hoogeveen	40	584		0.87
Joubran	133	130		0.88
Thögersen	78	156		0.89
Malinow (Belfast)	191	171		0.92
Combined	1517	2533		0.79 (0.72–0.85)

Fig. 16.2 Results of 12 retrospective studies of serum homocysteine and CHD events: values are odds ratios (95% confidence intervals) for a 3 μmol/l lower serum homocysteine. Results are adjusted for age, sex, and, in some studies, other cardiovascular risk factors, but not for regression-dilution bias.

First author	Cohort size	Follow-up (years)	Number of events	OR
Knekt, disease	1641	13	240	0.72
Nygard	802	5	64	0.77
Vollset	4766	4	88	0.78
Arnesen	10963	4	122	0.81
Kark	1788	10	135	0.84
Bots	7983	3	104	0.84
Stampfer	14916	5	271	0.86
Wald	21520	9	229	0.87
Ridker	28263	3	85	0.88
Folsom	15792	3	232	0.89
Stehouwer	878	10	98	0.90
Whincup	7735	13	386	0.92
Fallon	2290	10	312	0.93
Alfthan	7424	9	191	1.00
Knekt, no disease	5309	13	347	1.02
Evans	12866	9	240	1.07
Combined	144936		3144	0.89 (0.85–0.92)

Fig. 16.3 Results of 16 prospective studies of serum homocysteine and CHD events: values are odds ratios (95% confidence intervals) for a 3 μmol/l lower serum homocysteine, adjusted for age, sex, smoking, serum cholesterol, and blood pressure (age and sex alone in one study (Stampfer et al. 1993)) but not for regression-dilution bias. Modified from Wald et al. 2002.

for regression-dilution bias. These results are similar to those published from another meta-analysis of 11 prospective studies (Homocysteine Studies Collaboration 2002).

The retrospective and prospective studies show a positive association between serum homocysteine and CHD. These studies on their own may be insufficient to determine whether the association is one of cause and effect but with the additional evidence from genetic epidemiological studies of the thermolabile C677T MTHFR polymorphism, the uncertainty can be resolved.

16.5 Genetic epidemiology: the MTHFR studies

Moderately raised serum homocysteine levels (about 25% above average levels) occur as a result of a single mutation in the MTHFR gene (cytosine to thymidine ($C \rightarrow T$) at base pair position 677) that renders the enzyme thermolabile with reduced activity (Frosst *et al.* 1995). The presence of this polymorphism in the population provides a natural experiment capable of testing whether moderately raised levels cause CHD. The $C \rightarrow T$ mutation is common (about 10% of individuals are homozygous (TT) and about 47% are heterozygous (CT)) such that it has been possible to conduct studies of the risk of CHD in persons with and without the mutation, and many are now available.

The estimated difference in homocysteine levels between persons homozygous for the abnormal allele (TT) and persons homozygous for the normal allele (CC), from a meta-analysis of 33 studies, is 2.7 µmol/l (Wald *et al.* 2002). The effect of the TT genotype on serum homocysteine levels varies between individuals and communities because it is subject to environmental influence, in particular serum folate (Kluijtmans *et al.* 1997). The variable differences in serum homocysteine mean that heterogeneity between studies is to be expected and has been observed. The heterogeneity and the relatively small difference in homocysteine between TT and CC mean that large numbers are needed to show a statistically significant association with CHD. It is only in 2002 that sufficient data have become available (through the publication of over 40 studies) to permit a meta-analysis with sufficient statistical power.

Figure 16.4 shows the odds ratios of CHD (95% confidence intervals) for CC homozygotes relative to TT homozygotes in order of increasing effect, from a meta-analysis of 46 studies combining data from 12 193 cases and 11 945 controls. The overall summary odds ratio is 0.83 (95% confidence interval: 0.72–0.94; $p = 0.01$), indicating that the risk of CHD is, on average, 17% lower in CC homozygotes than in TT homozygotes (Wald *et al.* 2002). Another meta-analysis yielded a similar result (0.86 (0.78–0.95)) (Klerk *et al.* 2002). The odds ratio of 0.83 for the average homocysteine difference of 2.7 µmol/l is equivalent to an odds ratio of 0.81 (0.69–0.88) for the 3 µmol/l decrease in homocysteine produced by folic acid (calculated by raising 0.83 to the power of 3/2.7). This is similar to the summary estimate from the prospective studies for the same difference in serum homocysteine (odds ratio 0.85 (0.80–0.90)).

16.6 Interpretation of the evidence on causality

The results from the prospective and the MTHFR studies can in principle be interpreted in one of two ways – a direct (or causal) explanation or an indirect (or non-causal) explanation. An indirect (non-causal) explanation would depend on the prospective and MTHFR studies both showing associations with homocysteine through confounding. In the MTHFR studies, the homocysteine difference arises from a single gene mutation effectively allocated at random throughout the population through the random segregation of alleles during gametogenesis and conception – known as Mendelian randomization. There is, therefore, no basis for expecting that persons with and without the mutant gene would systematically differ in other cardiovascular risk factors. The data from these studies confirm this; there were no statistically significant differences in serum cholesterol levels, blood pressure, or smoking habits between

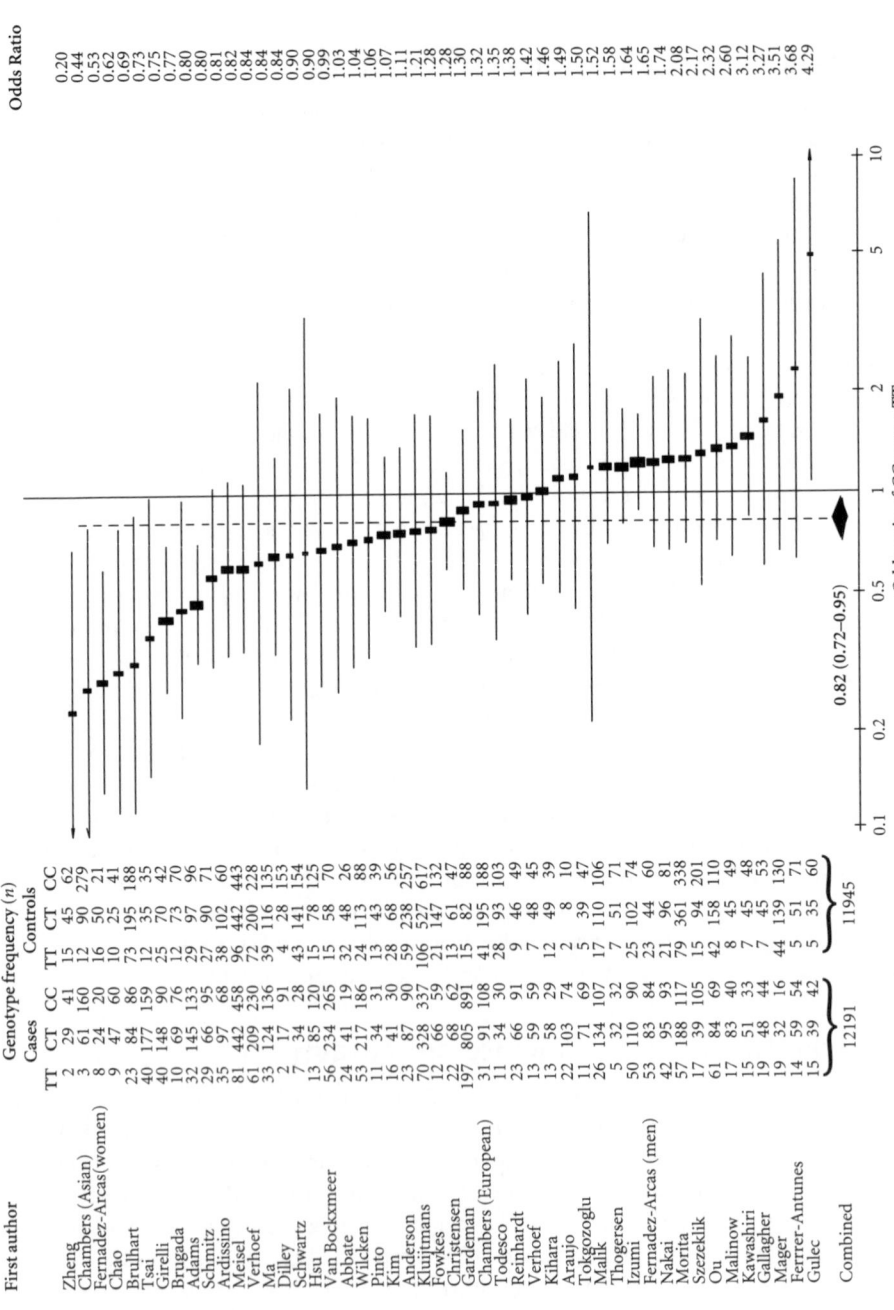

Fig. 16.4 Results of published studies of association between methylenetetrahydrofolate reductase (MTHFR) mutation and CHD events: values are odds ratios (95% confidence intervals) for homozygotes for mutant allele (TT) vs. wild type (CC). Modified from Wald et al. 2002.

persons with the TT and CC genotypes (Wald *et al.* 2002). The confounding would, therefore, have to involve some unknown cardiovascular risk factor, controlled by a gene linked to the MTHFR gene (i.e., at a neighbouring locus on the same chromosome). Importantly, the proposed genetic linkage could not account for confounding in the prospective studies because it would be too weak to do so, accounting for only one-quarter of the two-fold higher risk observed from the 10–90th centiles in the prospective studies. The indirect explanation relies on two separate explanations for the effects in the prospective and genetic epidemiological studies that produce nearly identical results for a given difference in serum homocysteine, even though any confounding would differ across the two types of study. This is so complex and improbable that it can be reasonably rejected, leaving the direct (causal) explanation as the simpler and more plausible interpretation of the results.

16.7 Dose-response relationship between homocysteine and CHD

Figure 16.5 shows dose-response plots of the incidence of CHD events against serum homocysteine. The figure shows plots of two prospective studies (Ridker *et al.* 1999; Wald *et al.* 1998), both of which reported summary estimates of risk close to the median for all prospective studies, a meta-analysis of retrospective studies (seven that published individual data on serum homocysteine in cases and controls – so permitting a plot of the combined results) (Genest *et al.* 1990; Hoogeveen *et al.* 1998; Joubran *et al.* 1998; Malinow *et al.* 1996; Pancharuniti *et al.* 1994; Thögersen *et al.* 2001; Verhoef *et al.* 1996) and a meta-analysis of the MTHFR studies (plots of relative risk over a narrower range of homocysteine in persons with the CC, CT, and TT genotypes) (Wald *et al.* 2002).

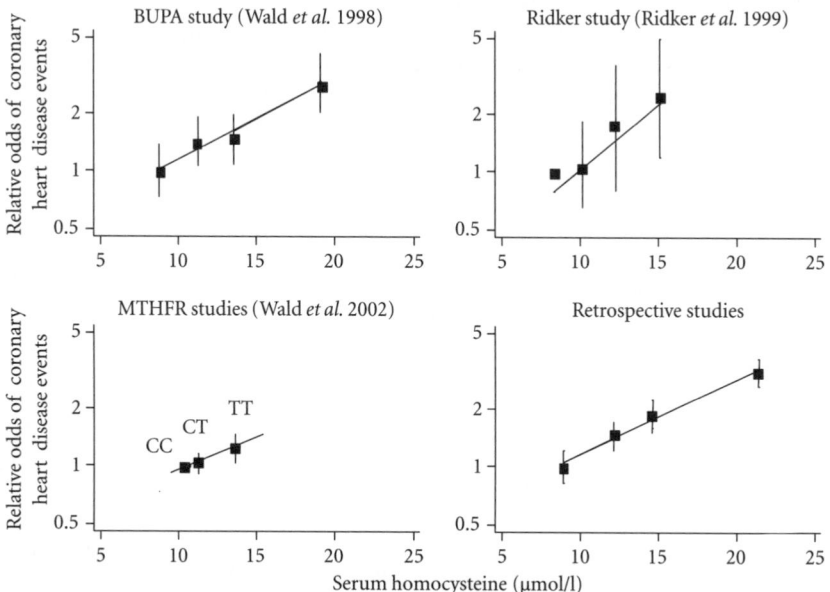

Fig. 16.5 Dose-response plots of the relative odds of CHD events against serum homocysteine from two prospective studies, a meta-analysis of 46 methylenetetrahydrofolate reductase (MTHFR) studies, and a meta-analysis of seven retrospective studies.

With relative odds of disease on the vertical axis using a proportional (or logarithmic) scale, the plots yield reasonably straight lines, indicating a constant proportional lower risk with lower serum homocysteine levels, from any starting point of serum homocysteine. It follows from the continuous dose-response plots in Fig. 16.5 that, as with the other cardiovascular risk factors, intervention to lower serum homocysteine should not be limited to people with a high serum homocysteine, but should be applicable to everyone at high risk whatever the reason for the high risk.

16.8 Implications for prevention

The summary results from the MTHFR and prospective studies are combined in Table 16.2. The effects on deep vein thrombosis and stroke are also shown (Wald *et al.* 2002). The overall (weighted average) odds ratio for CHD is 0.84 (0.80–0.89) for 3 μmol/l lower serum homocysteine – an expected reduction in risk of 16% (11–20%). This estimated risk reduction is relatively modest compared to the effect of treatments that lower serum cholesterol or blood pressure. Nonetheless, the public health impact would be large because CHD is so common (about 120 000 deaths in the UK and about 400 000 deaths in the USA each year).

16.9 The ongoing randomized trials of homocysteine reduction

It is widely felt that clinical practice should not change until there are randomized trials that show the effect of treatment on disease events. We believe that this is too simplistic. For example, there is no randomized trial evidence of the effect of giving up smoking on the risk of CHD, but causality is accepted. It is argued that we have previously been misled by associations in epidemiological studies (for example, the anti-oxidant, vitamin E, and CHD in the US Nurses Study and in the US male Health Professionals Study (Rimm *et al.* 1993; Stampfer *et al.* 1993)), but randomized trials showed otherwise (Heart Protection Study Collaborative Group 2002; The Heart Outcomes Evaluation Study Investigators 2000; see also the previous chapter). The inference from this that observational studies cannot be relied on is unjustified because in

Table 16.2 Summary results (95% confidence intervals) from the MTHFR studies and the prospective studies on CHD, deep vein thrombosis, and stroke[a]

Study type	No. of studies	No. of cases	OR for 3 μmol/l lower homocysteine		OR expressed as risk reduction
CHD					
MTHFR	46	12193	0.81 (0.69–0.88)	0.84 (0.80–0.89)	16% (11–20%)
Prospective[b]	16	3144	0.85 (0.80–0.90)		
Deep vein thrombosis					
MTHFR	26	3439	0.75 (0.62–0.92)		25% (8–38%)
Stroke					
MTHFR	7	1217	0.74 (0.43–1.28)	0.76 (0.67–0.85)	24% (15–33%)
Prospective[b]	8	676	0.76 (0.67–0.86)		

[a] Results taken from Wald *et al.* 2002.

[b] Prospective studies adjusted for regression-dilution bias, and for age, sex, blood pressure, and serum cholesterol in all studies, except age and sex only in one.

Table 16.3 Randomized trials of homocysteine reduction with folic acid, Vitamin B_6, and Vitamin B_{12} with vascular disease endpoints

Study	Population	Start	Primary outcome	Intervention	Size
Cambridge Heart Antioxidant Study, *UK*	MI/angina	1998	MI	Folic acid, 5 mg/day vs. placebo	4000
Oxford Study of the Effectiveness Of Additional Reductions in Cholesterol and Homocysteine, *UK*	MI	1998	MI	Folic acid 2 mg/day and vitamin B_{12} 1 mg/day vs. placebo; [SEARCH] Study	12000
Norwegian Study of Homocysteine Lowering with B Vitamins in Myocardial Infarction [NORVIT] Study, *Norway*	MI	1998	MI	Folic acid 5 mg/day for 2 weeks, then 0.8 mg vs. placebo; vitamin B_6, 40 mg/day vs. placebo	3000
Bergan Vitamin study, *Norway*	Stroke/TIA	1997	Stroke	Folic acid 5 mg/day for 2 weeks, then 0.8 mg vs. placebo; vitamin B_6 40 mg/day vs. placebo	2000
Prevention with a Combined Inhibitor and Folate in Coronary Heart Disease [PACIFIC] study, *Australia*	MI/angina and risk factors	1998	Peripheral vascular disease	Folic acid 0.2 or 2 mg/day, vs. placebo	10000
Vitamins To prevent Stroke [VITATOPS] study, *Australia*	Stroke/TIA	1999	Stroke	Folic acid 2 mg/day, B_6 25 mg/day, and B_{12} 0.4 mg/day, vs. placebo	5000
Vitamins in stroke prevention [VISP] study, *USA*	Stroke/TIA	1998	Stroke	Folic acid 2.5 mg/day, B_6 25 mg/day, and B_{12} 0.4 mg/day, vs. folic acid 0.2 mg/day and B_{12} 0.06 mg/day	3600
Womens Antioxidant and Cardiovascular disease Study, *USA*	Vascular disease and risk factors	1998	Vascular disease	Folic acid 2.5 mg/day, B_6 50 mg/day, and B_{12} 1 mg/day, vs. placebo.	8000
Heart Outcomes Prevention Evaluation Study [HOPE-2], *Canada*	Vascular disease	1999	Peripheral vascular disease	Folic acid 2.5 mg/day, B_6 50 mg/day, and B_{12} 1 mg/day	5000
Vitamin and Thrombosis Trial, *Netherlands*	DVT/PE	2000	Venous thrombosis	Folic acid 5 mg/day, B_{12} 0.4 mg/day, and B_6 50 mg/day	600

DVT: deep vein thrombosis; PE: pulmonary embolism; TIA: transient ischaemic attack.

Adapted from Clarke and Collins 1998.

these examples there was no basis to exclude confounding as the reason for the association in the observational studies, as acknowledged by the authors (Rimm *et al.* 1993; Stampfer *et al.* 1993). Also there was genuine uncertainty over whether hormone replacement therapy reduced cardiovascular risk, which is why randomized trials were needed (Grady *et al.* 2002). In the case of homocysteine and CHD the position is very different. As well as the evidence from prospective studies, there is genetic evidence from the MTHFR and the homocystinuria studies, the kind of corroboration which was lacking for vitamin E and hormone replacement therapy. In our view, randomized trials are not necessary to show that homocysteine levels are causally related to cardiovascular disease but, if sufficiently large, may provide an indication of the time required to realize the full potential 16% reduction in CHD risk, which is not known from current evidence.

Table 16.3 lists the ongoing large randomized trials of folic acid, vitamin B_6, and vitamin B_{12} in relation to cardiovascular disease events (Clarke and Collins 1998). Because the expected effect of homocysteine reduction on CHD prevention is modest, the trials need to be extremely large to have sufficient statistical power to show it. A trial of recurrent CHD events (a secondary prevention trial) would require about 15 000 participants followed for 5 years to demonstrate the expected 16% reduction in CHD events. None of the ongoing trials are this large. The introduction of folic acid fortification of flour (to prevent neural tube defects) in the US and other countries has, furthermore, reduced the statistical power by reducing the already small homocysteine difference between treated and control groups (since the control as well as the treated individuals groups are now receiving some folic acid).

Three small randomized trials have been published. There is a tendency for these to be interpreted as either positive or negative when, in fact, they lack the statistical power to be informative (Baker *et al.* 2002; Liem *et al.* 2003; Schnyder *et al.* 2001); their confidence intervals are consistent with no effect and with the expected modest effect. Over the next few years, evidence from other trials will emerge and it will be important to avoid interpreting non-significant results as negative – that is, to avoid concluding that no evidence of an effect is evidence of no effect. The focus should be on whether the confidence intervals include the expected relative risk of 0.84 for a 3 μmol/l homocysteine reduction. Only if they include 1.0 but exclude 0.84 would there be reason to question our expectation.

16.10 **Conclusions**

Four observations arise from the evidence summarized in this chapter:

1 The genetic (MTHFR) studies show a moderately higher risk of CHD for a moderately higher level of serum homocysteine.

2 The prospective studies show a positive association between serum homocysteine and cardiovascular disease after allowance for confounding.

3 These two types of study are susceptible to different sources of error, but show quantitatively similar associations, a result that is unlikely to have occurred through different potential sources of confounding acting independently.

4 The homocystinurias cause high serum homocysteine levels and high risks of premature cardiovascular disease, and lowering serum homocysteine reduces this high risk.

Together, these observations provide a compelling case for a cause and effect relationship between homocysteine and CHD and, therefore, a protective role for folic acid on CHD prevention.

References

Baker, F., Picton, D., Blackwood, S. *et al.* (2002). Blinded comparison of folic acid and placebo in patients with ischaemic heart disease: an outcome trial [Abstract]. *Circulation*, **106** (Suppl. II), 274.

Bellamy, M. F., McDowell, I. F., Ramsey, M. W. *et al.* (1998). Hyperhomocysteineia after an oral methionine load acutely impairs endothelial function in healthy adults. *Circulation*, **98**, 1848–52.

Brown, J. C., Rosenquist, T. H., and Monaghan, D. T. (1998). ERK2 activation by homocysteine in vascular smooth muscle cells. *Biochemical and Biophysical Research Communications*, **251**, 669–76.

Chao, C. L., Tsai, H. H., Lee, C. M. *et al.* (1999). The graded effect of hyperhomocysteinemia on the severity and extent of coronary atherosclerosis. *Atherosclerosis*, **147**, 379–86.

Clarke, R. and Collins, R. (1998). Can dietary supplements with folic acid or vitamin B6 reduce cardiovascular risk? Design of clinical trials to test the homocysteine hypothesis of vascular disease. *Journal of Cardiovascular Risk*, **5**, 249–55.

Clarke, R., Lewington, S., Donald, A. *et al.* (2001). Underestimation of the importance of homocysteine as a risk factor for cardiovascular disease in epidemiological studies. *Journal of Cardiovascular Risk*, **8**, 363–9.

Frosst, P., Blom, H. J., and Milos, R. (1995). A candidate genetic risk factor for vascular disease: a common mutation in methylenetetrahydrofolate reductase. *Nature Genetics*, **10**, 111–13.

Fryer, R. H., Wilson, B. D., Gubler, D. B. *et al.* (1993). Homocysteine, a risk factor for premature vascular disease and thrombosis, induces tissue factor activity in endothelial cells. *Arteriosclerosis and Thrombosis*, **13**, 1327–33.

Genest, J. J., McNamara, J. R., Salem, D. N. *et al.* (1990). Plasma homocysteine levels in men with premature coronary artery disease. *Journal of the American College of Cardiology*, **16**, 1114–19.

Grady, D., Herrington, D., Bittner, V. *et al.* (2002). Cardiovascular disease outcomes during 6.8 years of hormone therapy: Heart and Estrogen/progestin Replacement Study follow-up (HERS II). *Journal of the American Medical Association*, **288** (1), 49–57.

Hankey, G. J. and Eikelboom, J. W. (1999). Homocysteine and vascular disease. *Lancet*, **354**, 407–13.

Heart Protection Study Collaborative Group (2002). MRC/BHF Heart Protection Study of antioxidant vitamin supplementation in 20 536 high-risk individuals: a randomised placebo-controlled study. *Lancet*, **360**, 23–33.

Homocysteine Lowering Trialists Collaboration (1998). Lowering blood homocysteine with folic acid based supplements: meta-analysis of randomised trials. *British Medical Journal*, **316**, 894–8.

Homocysteine Studies Collaboration (2002). Homocysteine and risk of ischaemic heart disease and stroke. *Journal of the American Medical Association*, **288**, 2015–22.

Hoogeveen, E. K., Kostense, P. J., Beks, P. J. *et al.* (1998). Hyperhomocysteinemia is associated with an increased risk of cardiovascular disease, especially in non-insulin-dependent diabetes mellitus. *Arteriosclerosis, Thrombosis, and Vascular Biology*, **18**, 133–8.

Hopkins, P. N., Wu, L. L., Hunt, S. C. *et al.* (1995). Higher plasma homocysteine and increased susceptibility to adverse effects of low folate in early familial coronary artery disease. *Arteriosclerosis, Thrombosis, and Vascular Biology*, **15**, 1314–20.

Israelsson, B., Bratttstrom, L. E., and Hultberg, B. L. (1988). Homocysteine and myocardial infarction. *Atherosclerosis*, **71**, 227–33.

Joubran, R., Asmi, M., Busjahn, A. *et al.* (1998). Homocysteine levels and coronary heart disease in Syria. *Journal of Cardiovascular Risk*, **5**, 257–61.

Klerk, M., Verhoef, P., Clarke, R. *et al.* (2002). MTHFR 677C to T Polymorphism and risk of coronary heart disease. *Journal of the American Medical Association*, **288**, 2023–31.

Kluijtmans, L. A. J., Kastelein, J. J. P., Lindemans, J. *et al.* (1997). Thermolabile methylenetetrahydrofolate reductase in coronary artery disease. *Circulation*, **96**, 2573–7.

Kluijtmans, L. A. J., Boers, G. H. D., Kraus, J. P. *et al.* (1999). The molecular basis of cystathionine-synthase deficiency in Dutch patients with homocystinuria: effect of CBS genotype on biochemical and clinical phenotype and on response to treatment. *American Journal of Human Genetics*, **65**, 59–67.

Liem, A., Reynierse-Buitenwerf, G. H., Zwinderman, A. H. *et al.* (2003). Secondary prevention with folic acid: effects on clinical outcomes. *Journal of the American College of Cardiology*, **41**, 2105–13.

Loehrer, F. M., Angst, C. P., Haefeli, W. E. *et al.* (1996). Low whole-blood s-adenosylmethionine and correlation between 5-methylenetetrahydrofolate and homocysteine in coronary artery disease. *Arteriosclerosis, Thrombosis, and Vascular Biology*, **18**, 727–33.

Malinow, M. R., Ducimetiere, P., Luc, G. *et al.* (1996). Plasma homocysteine levels and graded risk for myocardial infarction: findings in two populations at contrasting risk for coronary disease. *Atherosclerosis*, **126**, 27–34.

McCully, K. S. (1969). Vascular pathology of homocyteinemia: implications for the pathogenesis of arteriosclerosis. *American Journal of Pathology*, **56**, 111–28.

Mudd, S. H., Skovby, F., Levy, H. L. *et al.* (1985). The natural history of homocystinuria due to cystathionine beta-synthase deficiency. *American Journal of Human Genetics*, **37**, 1–31.

Pancharuniti, N., Lewis, C. A., Sauberlich, H. E. *et al.* (1994). Plasma homocysteine, folate, vitamin B12 concentrations and risk for early onset coronary artery disease. *American Journal Clinical Nutrition*, **59**, 940–94.

Ridker, P. M., Manson, J. E., Buring, J. E. *et al.* (1999). Homocysteine and risk of cardiovascular disease among postmenopausal women. *Journal of the American Medical Association*, **281**, 1817–21.

Rimm, E. B., Stampfer, M. J., Ascherio, A. *et al.* (1993). Vitamin E consumption and the risk of coronary heart disease in men. *New England Journal of Medicine*, **328**, 1450–6.

Schnyder, G., Roffi, M., and Pin, R. (2001). Decreased rate of coronary restenosis after lowering of plasma homocysteine levels. *New England Journal of Medicine*, **345**, 1593–600.

Schwartz, S. M., Siscovick, D. S., Malinow, M. R. *et al.* (1997). Myocardial infarction in young women in relation to plasma total homocysteine, folate, and a common variant in the methylenetetrahydrofolate reductase gene. *Circulation*, **96**, 412–17.

Stampfer, M. J., Hennekens, C. H., Manson, J. E. *et al.* (1993). Vitamin E consumption and the risk of coronary disease in women. *New England Journal of Medicine*, **328**, 1444–9.

The Heart Outcomes Evaluation Study Investigators (2000). Vitamin E supplementation and cardiovascular events in high-risk patients. *New England Journal of Medicine*, **342**, 154–60.

Thögersen, A. M., Nilsson, T. K., Dahlen, G. *et al.* (2001). Homozygosity for the mutation C^{677T} of 5,10-methylenetetrahydrofolate reductase and total plasma homocysteine are not associated with greater than normal risk of a first myocardial infarction in northern Sweden. *Coronary Artery Disease*, **12**, 85–90.

van Oort, F. V. A., Melse-Boonstra, A., Brouwer, I. A. *et al.* (2003). Folic acid and reduction of plasma homocysteine concentrations in older adults: a dose-response study. *American Journal of Clinical Nutrition*, **77**, 1318–23.

Verhoef, P., Stampfer, M. J., Buring, J. E. *et al.* (1996). Homocysteine metabolism and risk of myocardial infarction: relation with vitamins B6, B12 and folate. *American Journal of Epidemiology*, **143**, 845–59.

Wald, D. S., Bishop, L., Wald, N. J. *et al.* (2001). Randomised trial of folic acid supplementation on serum homocysteine levels. *Archives of Internal Medicine*, **161**, 695–700.

Wald, D. S., Law, M., and Morris, J. (2002). Homocysteine and cardiovascular disease: evidence on causality from a meta-analysis. *British Medical Journal*, **325**, 1202–6.

Wald, D. S., Law, M. L., and Morris, J. (2003). Is serum homocysteine measurement of value in predicting the severity of coronary artery disease? *Thrombosis Research*, **111**, 55–7.

Wald, N. J., Watt, H. C., Law, M. R. *et al.* (1998). Homocysteine and ischaemic heart disease: results of a prospective study with implications regarding prevention. *Archives of Internal Medicine*, **158**, 862–7.

Yap, S. and Naughten, E. (1998). Homocyseinemia due to cystatjionine beta synthase deficiency in Ireland: 25 years experience of a newborn screened and treated population with reference to a clinical outcome and biochemical control. *Journal of Inherited Metabolic Disease*, **21**, 738–47.

Chapter 17

Alcohol and coronary heart disease

M. Bobak and M. Marmot

17.1 Introduction

The cardioprotective effects of alcohol, and particularly of red wine, have been widely publicized. In fact, the notion that wine is protective against heart disease has become part of conventional wisdom. The relationship between alcohol and coronary heart disease (CHD), however, is more complex. The association is not linear, and high alcohol consumption can be associated with increased risk of CHD.

In this chapter, we will review the evidence on the consumption of alcohol and the risk of CHD and with mortality in general. The chapter has four general sections. We start with studies of 'average' volume of drinking and CHD. We will review the results of the studies, the potential biases in studies of alcohol, the biological mechanisms for the cardioprotective effects of alcohol, the possibility that the effect of alcohol is modified by background cardiovascular risk, and the public health implications of the results. The next section examines the role of drinking patterns, namely the effect of binge and heavy drinking on CHD. We then review the evidence linking different types of alcoholic beverages with CHD risk. Finally, we briefly summarize the effects of alcohol on all-cause mortality.

17.2 Overall drinking volume and CHD

Most studies to date have examined the risk of CHD in relation to overall volume or average volume of alcohol consumption; the average amount of alcohol consumed per day or per week is then used as the primary measure of alcohol consumption (Rehm 1998; Rehm and Gmel 2003). Analyses of drinking frequency largely assume similar alcohol intake per drinking occasion.

17.2.1 The U-shaped or L-shaped curve

Results of the numerous studies of alcohol and CHD are remarkably consistent (for reviews, see, e.g., Corrao *et al*. 2000; Doll 1997; Fagrell *et al*. 1999; Marmot 1984; Marmot and Brunner 1991; Rimm *et al*. 1996; Royal College of Physicians, Royal College of Psychiatrists and Royal College of General Practitioners 1995). The evidence suggests that the relation between alcohol and CHD, as well as stroke, follows a U-shaped or L-shaped curve. In nearly all studies, the lowest risk of cardiovascular and CHD was found among moderate drinkers. The risk is higher in non-drinkers and, in some but not all studies, also in heavier drinkers.

Figures 17.1 and 17.2 show mortality from CHD according to levels of alcohol intake in men and women included in the US Cancer Prevention Study (Thun *et al*. 1997). It examined drinking habits and other lifestyle factors in nearly half a million US adults, and recorded

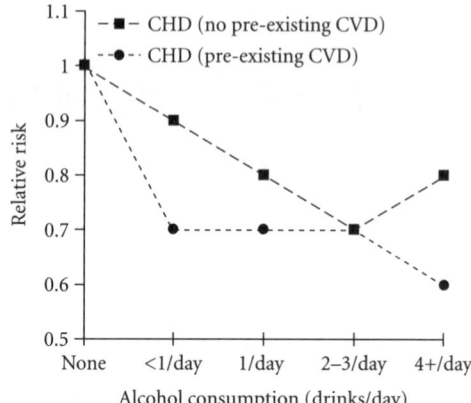

Fig. 17.1 Alcohol consumption and mortality from CHD in US men. (Based on Thun *et al.* 1997.)

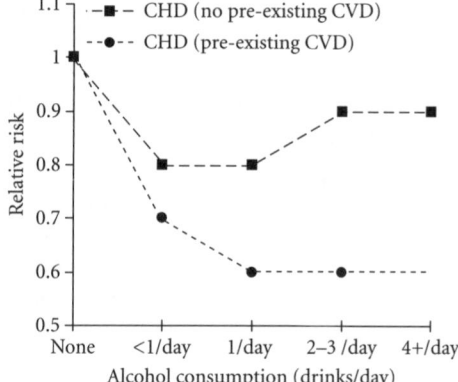

Fig. 17.2 Alcohol consumption and mortality from CHD in US women. (Based on Thun *et al.* 1997.)

deaths occurring in the subsequent 9 years. There was an L-shaped association with mortality from CHD in subjects with pre-existing cardiovascular disease (CVD), and an approximately U-shaped association in subjects without pre-existing disease, but the risk in the highest category did not exceed that of non-drinkers. The risk of all types of CVDs combined was lower in drinkers than in non-drinkers, and there was no apparent excess risk in the highest drinking category.

It is difficult to estimate the levels of alcohol intake associated with the maximum protection against CHD, because different studies used different measures and definitions, and because exact measurement of alcohol intake is difficult. A recent meta-analysis of 51 studies found that the risk of CHD was lowest (25% lower than among non-drinkers) at a consumption of 25 g of alcohol a day (Corrao *et al.* 2000). In a subset of 28 cohort studies judged as good quality, the maximum protection (20% lower risk) was seen at a daily consumption of 20 g of alcohol. It thus appears that consumption of 20–30 g of alcohol daily, corresponding to 2–3 drinks, is associated with maximum protection.

A U-shaped curve seems to exist for moderate alcohol intake and the risk of sudden cardiac death. Sudden cardiac deaths are a subgroup of deaths coded as CHDs; they account for about half of all cardiovascular deaths (Huikuri *et al.* 2001). The majority of sudden cardiac deaths are caused by arrhythmia, triggered by acute coronary events, such as myocardial infarction. The US Physicians Health Study found that, compared with non-drinkers, men drinking

2–4 drinks a week and 5–6 drinks a week had a relative risk of sudden cardiac death of 0.4 and 0.2, respectively; the risk was approaching unity at 2 drinks a day (Albert *et al.* 1999).

While the majority of studies produce consistent results, several issues remain unresolved. Some authors have suggested that all or part of the U-shaped curve may be due to a health selection bias. In addition, the biological mechanisms of the protective effect of alcohol, the possible interaction of alcohol with conventional risk factors or with cardiovascular risk score, and the effects of heavy drinking and of binge drinking should be clarified. These issues are briefly reviewed below.

17.2.2 Health selection bias and reverse causation

It has been argued that the protective effect is an artefact due to the fact that people with health problems caused by alcohol may have stopped drinking; this would lead to an artificially higher mortality among non-drinkers (Shaper *et al.* 1988). This explanation is not specific to CVDs; it would also apply to other causes of death and to all-cause mortality. However, available data do not support this hypothesis (Edwards *et al.* 1994; Klatsky 2001). Several groups have separated ex-drinkers and 'never drinkers', and have not confirmed the health selection hypothesis. Moreover, exclusion of deaths occurring in the first years of follow-up (which are more likely to result from pre-existing alcohol-related disease) does not change the results of the major studies (Gronbaek 2001). There is now a consensus that most of the protective effects of moderate drinking are genuine, not least because good evidence now exists of the biological mechanisms involved in the protective effect.

17.2.3 Biological mechanisms for the protective effect

One of the Bradford Hill criteria for accepting an association between an exposure and a disease as causal requires that biological mechanisms exist for the association (Bradford Hill 1965). This also applies to the case of the protective effects of moderate alcohol intake. There have been numerous experimental studies of the effect of alcohol on different physiological mechanisms. The pooled analysis of these studies (Rimm *et al.* 1999) is summarized in Table 17.1. Intake of alcohol is significantly associated with several biological risk factors of CHD. Using published associations between these risk factors and CHD, it has been estimated that the intake of 30 g of pure alcohol per day would reduce the risk of CHD by 25% (Rimm *et al.* 1999). This predicted reduction is consistent with the protective effect observed in prospective studies.

Table 17.1 Change of biological risk factors associated with an intake of 30 g of alcohol per day

Biological factor	Change (95% CI)
HDL cholesterol (mg/dl)	3.99 (3.25; 4.73)
Apolipoprotein A I (mg/dl)	8.82 (7.79; 9.86)
Triglycerides (mg/dl)	5.69 (2.49; 8.89)
Plasminogen (% of standard)	1.47% (−1.18; 4.42)
Fibrinogen (mg/dl)	−7.5 (−17.7; 32.7)
Lp(a) lipoprotein (mg/dl)	−0.70 (−3.38; 1.99)
Tissue type plasminogen activator antigen (ng/ml)	1.25 (20.31; 2.81)

Source: based on Rimm *et al.* 1999.

CI: confidence interval; HDL: high-density lipoprotein.

17.2.4 **Effect modification by coronary risk**

Available evidence suggests that the protective effect of alcohol is more pronounced among subjects at high risk of CHD. For example, the relation between alcohol and CHD is similar across different age groups (Mukamal *et al.* 2003), although for virtually all other coronary risk factors the relative risk reduces with increasing age. Fuchs *et al.* (1995) found that the effect of moderate alcohol intake was more pronounced among women with a higher prevalence of coronary risk factors than among women with more favourable risk factor profiles. The American Cancer Prevention cohort found similar results (Thun *et al.* 1997). The authors classified subjects into three categories by cardiovascular risk: 'low risk'(age less than 60, no history of heart disease or hypertension, and no medication for CHD, hypertension, stroke, or diabetes); 'medium risk' (younger than 60 but with presence of risk factors); and 'high risk' (aged 60 or more and with pre-existing disease). There was a J-shaped association between alcohol and all-cause mortality in the low risk group, a U-shaped association in the intermediate group, and an L-shaped association in the high risk group. Similar results were obtained where subjects were stratified by the presence of pre-existing CHD (Figs 17.1 and 17.2). However, the benefits of alcohol did not outweigh the large increase in mortality risk caused by smoking.

17.2.5 **Public health implications of the cardioprotective effect of alcohol**

Accepting the protective effect of alcohol against CVDs as genuine is an important issue. Because CVDs are the major cause of death worldwide, even a small protective effect has major implications for estimating the total burden of disease attributable to alcohol. The harmful effect on accidents or cancers could be counterbalanced by the positive effects on cardiovascular mortality. Calculations conducted for the World Bank/WHO Global Burden of Disease Project suggest that the impact of alcohol on mortality differs by age group. In younger age groups (below 44 years), the impact is clearly negative, mainly through deaths from injuries and accidents. Above the age of 70, alcohol seems to prevent more deaths (mainly from CVD) than it causes (Murray and Lopez 1996). Despite such calculations, however, alcohol poses a number of health hazards, and it is not to be recommended as a prevention strategy (Goldberg *et al.* 2001).

17.3 **Drinking patterns**

The vast majority of studies to date have relied on some indicator of 'average' consumption (mean intake or number of drinks per day or week, etc.). This is, however, a crude measure of drinking. Two persons consuming the same amount, say 140 g of alcohol per week, may drink very differently. One may drink 20 g of alcohol each day (regular or sustained drinking), while the second may consume the whole amount in one evening (episodic or binge drinking pattern). While this state of affairs has been recognized for a long time (Edwards *et al.* 1994), researchers have only recently addressed more systematically the question of whether regular and episodic drinking may have different health effects (Grant and Litvak 1998; Rehm *et al.* 2001). Other aspects of drinking patterns described in the literature include the social setting of drinking or drinking with meals, but most studies of drinking pattern focused on the amount of alcohol per occasion or the number of occasions (e.g. per year) with heavy drinking consumption.

17.3.1 **Heavy drinking and binge drinking**

While there is little doubt that regular moderate drinking has a protective effect against CVD, the issue of heavy drinking, either sustained or episodic, has not been resolved. This issue should not be underestimated. Despite the large number of studies of the effect of alcohol on CVDs, it is likely that heavy drinkers are under-represented in epidemiological studies. In the US Health Professionals Study, for example, only 3.5% of the men in the cohort drank 50 g of alcohol or more daily (Mukamal *et al.* 2003). Even in populations with high alcohol consumption, problem drinkers are particularly difficult to reach. It is therefore difficult to extrapolate the findings on 'heavy drinkers' included in epidemiological studies to heavy drinkers not included.

The effects of binge drinking on CHD have also not been systematically studied. It has been proposed that such drinkers have an elevated risk of sudden cardiac death (possibly resulting from ventricular arrhythmia) and cardiomyopathies (McKee and Britton 1998). Several studies reported increased CHD mortality in weekends or on Mondays, and binge drinking during weekends has been put forward to explain this observation (Chenet *et al.* 1998, 2001; Evans *et al.* 2000). Several individual-level studies suggested that binge drinking might increase the risk of myocardial infarction (Kauhanen *et al.* 1997; McElduff and Dobson 1997), as well as the risk of death after myocardial infarction (McElduff and Dobson 2001). This question may be important for explaining the high and fluctuating mortality rates in Russia and other parts of the former Soviet Union (Leon *et al.* 1997; Notzon *et al.* 1998). It has been proposed that the (suspected) predominant drinking pattern – binge drinking – may underlie the recent dramatic increase in cardiovascular mortality in the former Soviet Union (Britton and McKee 2000, see also Chapter 6 on Central and Eastern Europe).

Britton and colleagues subsequently conducted a systematic review of the literature on heavy alcohol consumption and CVDs (Britton and McKee 2000). This review confirmed the protective effect of moderate regular drinking described above, but highlighted the scarcity of studies on heavy or episodic drinking. For example, from 42 prospective studies which fulfilled the inclusion criteria, only 7 (in fact only 6, as one study was represented by two papers) examined drinking pattern or heavy drinking.

Results of these seven papers differed markedly from the remaining reports. Six reported a positive association between heavy alcohol consumption and CVDs, and one study found no association. The indices of heavy alcohol intake included: binge drinking (at least six bottles of beer in one session), frequency of hangovers or intoxication, being registered as a problem drinker (in Sweden), being admitted for alcohol treatment, and being unable to perform at work properly because of problems with alcohol. The relative risk of cardiac death among these heavy drinkers, compared with non-drinkers, ranged from 2 to 6, and seemed to be higher for sudden cardiac death than for myocardial infarction.

Two cohort studies published more recently provide some support for this view. A US-based investigation found that light drinkers who had episodes of heavy drinking (binges) had CHD mortality more than twice as high as light drinkers without heavy drinking episodes (Murray *et al.* 2002). A cohort study in Novosibirsk, Russia, found that the effect of drinking large amounts of alcohol depended on frequency: infrequent binge drinking was not related to CHD mortality, but frequent heavy drinkers had about a two-fold increase in CHD mortality risk compared to moderate drinkers (Fig. 17.3) (Malyutina *et al.* 2002).

The findings of the prospective studies are largely (but not entirely) supported by case-control studies and case series (Britton *et al.* 1998). In general, the risk of sudden cardiac death, myocardial infarction, atrial fibrillation, and supraventricular arrhythmia seemed to be

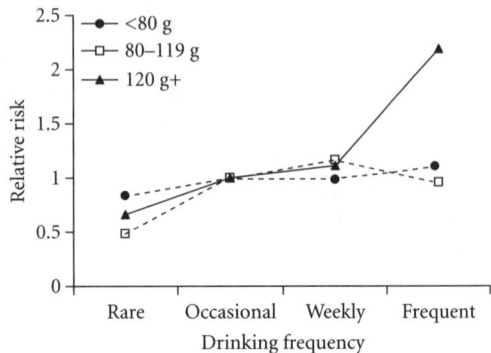

Fig. 17.3 Relative risk of CHD death by drinking frequency and mean dose per occasion in Novosibirsk, Russia. (From Malyutina *et al.* 2002.)

increased among heavy drinkers. There was some suggestion that people who died from sudden cardiac death were more likely to have consumed alcohol during the last hours before their death than persons who died from other cardiovascular causes. Analysis of the acute cardiac event register in New South Wales in Australia suggested that persons who consumed more than eight drinks at least twice a week had about twice the risk of both myocardial infarction and death following heart attack than non-drinkers (McElduff and Dobson 1997, 2001). The observation that frequent binge drinking increased the risk of myocardial infarction, but rare binge drinking did not (McElduff and Dobson 1997), is consistent with the Russian cohort study mentioned above (Malyutina *et al.* 2002).

In the meta-analysis by Corrao *et al.* (2000) mentioned above, it was estimated that daily consumption of 113 g alcohol and more was associated with risk of CHD significantly higher than among abstainers. In the subset of cohort studies, the risk of coronary mortality was significantly increased among those consuming 89 g or more daily. Although most studies included only a small number of subjects consuming high amounts of alcohol regularly, it appears that the protective effect is absent among such drinkers. Heavy drinkers may, in fact, have a higher risk of coronary death than abstainers.

The British Regional Heart Study has specifically addressed the question of whether the risk of sudden cardiac death is related to heavy drinking. The study found that the incidence of sudden cardiac death was about double among heavy drinkers (more than six drinks daily) compared with the rest (Wannamethee and Shaper 1992). The increased incidence of sudden death in heavy drinkers was similar in all social groups, more pronounced in older men, and strongest among men with no evidence of pre-existing CHD. Interestingly, however, there was an inverse relationship between non-sudden cardiac death and alcohol intake. As a result, the combined sudden and non-sudden deaths from heart disease showed an approximately U-shaped association with alcohol.

The elevated risk of coronary death among heavy drinkers may not be universal. Recently published results of a cohort of heavy drinkers in Italy did not find an increased risk of cardiovascular deaths, compared with the general population (Cipriani *et al.* 2002). However, there was also no protective effect on cardiovascular deaths, and there was a significantly increased risk of cardiac death from arrhythmia. In the meta-analysis by Corrao *et al.* (2000), the risk of CHD in heavy drinkers in non-Mediterranean countries was higher than that of abstainers, but it was slightly lower than in abstainers in Mediterranean populations. It is possible that the adverse cardiovascular effects of heavy drinking are contingent on the type of alcohol, drinking with meals, nutrition, or on the rates of heart disease in the population.

Biological mechanisms for the adverse effects of heavy/binge drinking

It has been proposed that sustained or episodic heavy drinking may have a different effect on biological risk factors compared with moderate regular drinking. The data, however, provide only weak support for this view. A review by McKee and Britton (1998) found that in animal models heavy alcohol intake did reduce the cardioprotective HDL cholesterol and increased LDL cholesterol concentrations, but this was not confirmed by research on humans. There are few data regarding the effect of heavy drinking on blood clotting, but withdrawal may lead to an increased risk of thrombosis (Hillbom *et al.* 1985; Renaud and Ruf 1996). In animal models, high doses of alcohol were found to disrupt the cardiac conducting system and damage heart muscle. Again, it is not known whether these effects are present at blood concentrations of alcohol which occur in humans. Blood pressure was found to be elevated in the intoxication phase during a binge and in sustained heavy drinkers (Seppa and Sillanaukee 1999; Seppa *et al.* 1994).

As yet, there is no general consensus on the cardiovascular effects of sustained heavy or episodic binge drinking. There is, however, sufficient evidence in the literature to raise this question and to issue a warning that heavy drinking may, in fact, involve increased risk of cardiovascular death, and to justify more research (Poikolainen 1998; Puddey *et al.* 1999).

17.4 **Beverage type and CHD**

The evidence summarized above demonstrates that light to moderate drinking is associated with lower risk of CHD, compared with non-drinkers, and that the protective effect appears to be genuine, independent of known biases and confounding factors. The evidence also suggests that heavy drinking does not provide protection against heart disease, and it may, in fact, be associated with higher risk, compared with non-drinkers. The question remains of whether among moderate drinkers wine is associated with a higher degree of protection against heart disease compared with other alcoholic beverages. This problem will be addressed in this section.

17.4.1 **The French paradox**

The hypothesis that wine protects against heart disease was originally proposed to explain the comparatively low mortality from CHD in France, despite relatively high levels of known coronary risk factors, such as smoking, blood pressure, cholesterol, fat intake, or obesity (the 'French paradox'). One proposed explanation was that the low rates of CHD are due to a high intake of wine (particularly red wine, which contains various substances with possible cardioprotective effects). Several studies based on international data on mortality rates and alcohol (wine) intake have supported this interpretation. Mortality from CHD was, in general, lower in countries with higher per capita intake of alcohol, and the link with alcohol appears stronger for wine intake than for alcohol (ethanol) in general or than for other beverages (Criqui and Ringel 1994; LaPorte *et al.* 1980; Leger *et al.* 2002).

The fact that, in France, mortality from heart disease is low and wine intake is high does not, of course, prove that wine reduces heart disease mortality. This is a purely ecological (geographical) association, based on comparing countries, rather than individuals. All sorts of biases and confounders cannot be controlled in such analyses. For example, identification and coding of different causes of death may vary by country; socio-economic characteristics must be taken into account; health behaviour patterns are different in different regions; dietary habits vary markedly; medical care also differs between countries, etc. There is, however, a more fundamental problem with this type of 'evidence': the so-called ecological fallacy

(Piantadosi *et al.* 1988). This bias is specific to ecological studies, and in principle it means that we cannot be sure that *individuals* who have a low risk of heart disease in countries with high wine intake are those who consume a lot of wine. In other words, these studies imply an extrapolation from populations (countries) to individuals, but since there are no data on individuals, this extrapolation is necessarily speculative. It needs to be confirmed by studies in individuals.

17.4.2 Studies in individuals

There have been very few studies directly comparing the effect of different types of alcoholic beverages on the risk of CHD. In the mid-1990s, Rimm and colleagues reviewed the literature and addressed this question (Rimm *et al.* 1996). They found clear evidence of a strong inverse relation between moderate total alcohol intake and CHD, but there was no consistent pattern of differential effects of different beverages. Out of 10 prospective studies, 4 found a significant protective effect of wine, 4 found this association with beer, and 4 found it for spirits. It appeared that the maximal protective effect was related to the beverage most frequently consumed in a given population, suggesting that it is the usual (not-excessive and regular) drinking that is protective, rather than a specific beverage. The authors concluded that if there were any extra cardioprotective effect of any specific beverage, it would be 'modest at best or possibly restricted to certain sub-populations'.

A more recent meta-analysis of studies of the relation between vascular risk (mainly including CHD outcomes) and consumption of wine and beer found that the effects of the two beverages were similar. Compared with non-drinkers, moderate wine intake was associated with relative risk of 0.68 (95% confidence interval: 0.59–0.77) and moderate beer intake was associated with relative risk of 0.78 (0.70–0.86); the small difference between the effects of wine and beer was not significant (Di Castelnuovo *et al.* 2002).

Two studies in particular provided some support for the wine hypothesis. In a prospective study of almost 130 000 US adults, Klatsky and Armstrong (1993) investigated whether different alcoholic beverages confer a varying risk of heart disease. The results suggested a tendency towards a lower risk of heart disease among those who preferred wine than among those who preferred beer or spirits. However, in later analyses of hospitalization for heart disease in the same cohort, the lowest risk was found among men preferring beer and (but not statistically significantly) women preferring wine (Klatsky *et al.* 1997). Red wine was no more protective than other types of wine.

The Copenhagen City Heart Study also examined directly the hypothesis that wine may be associated with a protective effect against heart disease that is greater than that provided by other alcoholic beverages (Gronbaek *et al.* 2000). In this study, more than 13 000 men and 11 500 women were followed for 10.5 years on average. The study found an L-shaped association between total alcohol intake and mortality from heart disease. However, when subjects were divided into wine drinkers and non-wine drinkers, light drinkers who avoided wine had 24% lower risk of death from heart disease than non-drinkers, while light drinkers who drank wine had 42% lower mortality. Compared to subjects who never drank wine, those who drank 3–5 glasses of wine per day had half of the risk of death from all causes (Gronbaek *et al.* 2000).

There is a potential measurement error here. Few people consume strictly one type of alcohol only. Most people drink several types of alcohol during a typical week (and often during one day). Classifying them into wine or non-wine drinkers is clearly a simplification.

It is even more difficult to exclude confounding by other risk factors. This will be discussed in the next subsection.

It is also possible to compare studies in different populations. If the protective effect were specific to wine only, studies in non-wine drinking populations should not find any protective effect of alcohol. This is clearly not the case. For example, studies in beer drinking populations found a clear U-shaped association between alcohol (beer) intake and heart disease (Bobak *et al.* 2000; Brenner *et al.* 2001; Keil *et al.* 1997). The magnitude of the effect was entirely consistent with studies in other populations, including wine drinking populations. A more detailed quantitative comparison of the size of the protective effects between studies in different populations (wine and non-wine drinking) would be problematic, for the reasons described for ecological studies, in addition to other important issues related to poor comparability between studies (study design; selection of subjects; alcohol measurement; measurement of other risk factors and other covariates; ascertainment of CHD; etc.).

Problems of studies in individuals

Studies in individuals – such as the Kaiser Permanente or the Copenhagen City Heart Study – are more reliable than ecological studies. Nevertheless, they are also prone to methodological problems that will be illustrated here.

One can start with a question about an ideal study to examine differential effects of different type of alcoholic beverages on heart disease. Such a study would be a randomized trial, where subjects would be randomly assigned to consumption of a standard dose of different types of alcohol. Unfortunately, such a trial is impossible, not only for ethical reasons, but also because people have different preferences for alcoholic beverages, and would probably not comply with the allocated 'intervention'. The second best design would be an observational study in a population where preferences for different types of alcohol (e.g. wine, beer, spirits) would be distributed randomly. And this illustrates the problem: preferences for alcoholic beverages are not distributed randomly in a given population, at least in most Western populations.

In the Whitehall II Study of British civil servants, for example, wine drinkers had higher social status, higher income, higher education, more favourable diet, and a more favourable risk profile than those who consumed predominantly beer or spirits (unpublished data). Analysis of the Copenhagen City Heart Study showed that wine drinkers were less likely to smoke, and had higher education and lower body mass index than beer and spirits drinkers (Gronbaek *et al.* 2000). Another large Danish population study found a similar pattern: wine drinkers had a more healthy diet (Tjonneland *et al.* 1999). In the cohort analysed by Klatsky *et al.*, those who preferred wine were more often non-smokers, college graduates, and had a more favourable coronary risk profile (Klatsky and Armstrong 1993). All these factors are also related to heart disease, and can confound the comparison between wine and other beverages (Klatsky 1999). For example, if wine drinkers are less likely to smoke than beer drinkers, one would expect a lower risk of heart disease among wine drinkers just because they smoke less.

It is possible to take such confounding factors into account and control, or adjust for them, usually in a statistical analysis. However, it is very difficult to remove all confounding, because it is virtually impossible to measure all potential confounding factors sufficiently precisely (Klatsky 1999). Thus it is plausible that the apparently greater protective effect of wine compared with other beverages, is due to residual confounding.

17.5 **Alcohol and all-cause mortality**

A brief review of the relation between alcohol and all-cause mortality may help to put the studies on CHD in a perspective. For all-cause mortality, virtually all prospective studies have found a U-shaped or J-shaped association with alcohol consumption (Royal College of Physicians, Royal College of Psychiatrists, and Royal College of General Practitioners 1995; Shaper *et al.* 1988). In general, moderate drinkers have lower mortality than non-drinkers; there seems to be little association between consumption and mortality within moderate intake levels. At higher intake levels, the mortality risk curve starts to rise again above that of non-drinkers. In most studies, the risk of death from all causes among heavier drinkers (above, say 50–60 g of alcohol per day) was some 20–50% higher than among non-drinkers (Royal College of Physicians, Royal College of Psychiatrists, and Royal College of General Practitioners 1995).

Most studies of alcohol mortality have focused on middle-aged and elderly subjects; consequently, little is known about younger people. The few studies including younger subjects suggest that the protective effect of moderate intake is not present among younger people (Andreasson *et al.* 1988; Gronbaek 2001). This is because the association between alcohol and all-cause mortality is an aggregate of the effects of alcohol on different causes of death.

Death from injury and accidents is more common among younger people, while cancers and CVD are more common in older age groups. Alcohol was found to be associated with increased mortality from several types of cancer, injuries and accidents, liver cirrhosis, and other health outcomes. The association with injury deaths among younger people is particularly strong. In addition, heavy drinking increases the risk of haemorrhagic stroke and may also increase that of ischaemic stroke and of CHD; on the other hand, moderate regular drinking seems protective against circulatory diseases, such as heart disease and ischaemic stroke. The sum of these effects is the familiar U-shaped or J-shaped curve.

17.6 **Conclusions**

There is clear evidence that mortality from CHD is some 20–30% lower among moderate regular drinkers, compared with non-drinkers. This reduction of coronary risk appears to be due to known biological effects of ethanol, largely on blood lipids and blood coagulation.

There is little evidence that wine provides a greater protection against heart disease than other alcoholic beverages. It is likely that the apparent beneficial effect of wine compared to spirits or beer found in a few studies is due to residual confounding by other factors. The much publicized beneficial biological effects of substances in red wine (polyphenols, antioxidants, etc.) found in cross-sectional studies and in animal or *in vitro* experiments do not provide definite evidence that wine is more beneficial than other types of alcohol. Existence of biological mechanisms (plausibility) is a weak criterion of causality. It has been proposed that beer also contains additional substances that can confer extra protection against heart disease (Ubbink *et al.* 1998; van der Gaag *et al.* 2000), but the researchers remain cautious and the media have not exaggerated these reports.

Finally, there is growing evidence that heavy drinking is not associated with lower rates of CHD; in fact, recent studies suggest that heavy drinking may increase the risk of cardiac death.

References

Albert, C. M., Manson, J. E., Cook, N. R., Ajani, U. A., Gaziano, J. M., and Hennekens, C. H. (1999). Moderate alcohol consumption and the risk of sudden cardiac death among US male physicians, *Circulation*, **100**, 944–50.

Andreasson, S., Allebeck, P., and Romelsjo, A. (1988). Alcohol and mortality among young men: longitudinal study of Swedish conscripts. *British Medical Journal*, **296**, 1021–5.

Bobak, M., Skodova, Z., and Marmot, M. (2000). Effect of beer drinking on risk of myocardial infarction: a population based case-control study. *British Medical Journal*, **320**, 1378–9.

Bradford Hill, A. (1965). The environment and disease: association or causation? *Proceedings of the Royal Society of Medicine*, **58**, 295–300.

Brenner, H., Rothenbacher, D., Bode, G., Marz, W., Hoffmeister, A., and Koenig, W. (2001). Coronary heart disease risk reduction in a predominantly beer-drinking population. *Epidemiology*, **12**, 390–5.

Britton, A. and McKee, M. (2000). The relation between alcohol and cardiovascular disease in Eastern Europe: explaining the paradox. *Journal of Epidemiology and Community Health*, **54**, 328–32.

Britton, A., McKee, M., and Leon, D. A. (1998). *Cardiovascular disease and heavy drinking: a systematic review. A report to the Health and Population Division of the United Kingdom Department of International Development*. London School of Hygiene and Tropical Medicine, London.

Chenet, L., McKee, M., Leon, D., Shkolnikov, V. M., and Vassin, S. (1998). Alcohol and cardiovascular mortality in Moscow: new evidence of a causal association. *Journal of Epidemiology and Community Health*, **52**, 772–4.

Chenet, L., Britton, A., Kalediene, R., and Petrauskiene, J. (2001). Daily variations in deaths in Lithuania: the possible contribution of binge drinking. *International Journal of Epidemiology*, **30**, 743–8.

Cipriani, F., Cucinelli, M. L., Dimauro, P. E., Angioli, D., Conte, M., Voller, F., and Buiatti, E. (2002). Mortality in a cohort of alcoholics from Arezzo in 1979–1997. *Epidemiologia e Prevenzione*, **25**, 63–70.

Corrao, G., Rubiatti, L., Bagnardi, V., Zambon, A., and Poikolainen, K. (2000). Alcohol and coronary heart disease: a meta-analysis, *Addiction*, **95**, 1505–23.

Criqui, M. H. and Ringel, B. L. (1994). Does diet or alcohol explain the French paradox? *Lancet*, **344**, 1719–23.

Di Castelnuovo, A., Rotondo, S., Iacoviello, L., Donati, M. B., and De Gaetano, G. (2002). Meta-analysis of wine and beer consumption in relation to vascular risk. *Circulation*, **105**, 2836–44.

Doll, R. (1997). One for the heart. *British Medical Journal*, **315**, 1664–8.

Edwards, G., Anderson, P., Babor, T. F., Casswell, S., Ferrence, R., Giesbrecht, C. *et al.* (1994). *Alcohol policy and the public good*. Oxford University Press.

Evans, C., Chalmers, J., Capewell, S., Redpath, A., Finlayson, A., Boyd, J. *et al.* (2000). 'I don't like Mondays' – day of the week of coronary heart disease deaths in Scotland: study of routinely collected data. *British Medical Journal*, **320**, 218–19.

Fagrell, B., de Faire, U., Bondy, S., Criqui, M., Gaziano, M., Gronbaek, M. *et al.* (1999). The effects of light to moderate drinking on cardiovascular diseases. *Journal of Internal Medicine*, **246**, 331–40.

Fuchs, C. S., Stampfer, M. J., Colditz, G. A., Giovannucci, E. L., Manson, J. E., Kawachi, I. *et al.* (1995). Alcohol consumption and mortality among women. *New England Journal of Medicine*, **332**, 1245–50.

Goldberg, I. J., Mosca, L., Piano, M. R., and Fisher, E. A. (2001). Wine and your heart: a science Advisory for Healthcare Professionals from the Nutrition Committee, Council on Epidemiology and Prevention, and Council on Cardiovascular Nursing of the American Heart Association. *Circulation*, **103**, 472–5.

Grant, M. and Litvak, J. (eds) (1998), *Drinking patterns and their consequences*. Taylor and Francis, Washington, DC.

Gronbaek, M. (2001). Factors influencing the relation between alcohol and mortality – with focus on wine. *Journal of Internal Medicine*, **250**, 291–308.

Gronbaek, M., Becker, U., Johansen, D., Gottschau, A., Schnohr, P., Hein, H. O. *et al.* (2000). Types of alcohol consumed and mortality from all causes, coronary heart disease and cancer. *Annals of Internal Medicine*, **133**, 411–19.

Hillbom, M., Kangasaho, M., Lowbeer, C., Kaste, M., Muuronen, A., and Numminen, H. (1985). Effect of ethanol on platelet function. *Alcohol*, **2**, 429–32.

Huikuri, H. V., Castellanos, A., and Myerburg, R. J. (2001). Sudden death due to cardiac arrhythmias. *New England Journal of Medicine*, **345**, 1473–82.

Kauhanen, J., Kaplan, G. A., Goldberg, D. E., and Salonen, J. T. (1997). Beer binging and mortality: results from the Kuopio ischaemic heart disease risk factors study, a prospective population based study. *British Medical Journal*, **315**, 846–51.

Keil, U., Chambless, L. E., Doering, A., Filipiak, B., and Stieber, J. (1997). The relation of alcohol intake to coronary heart disease and all-cause mortality in a beer-drinking population. *Epidemiology*, **8**, 150–6.

Klatsky, A. L. (1999). Is it the drink or the drinker? Circumstantial evidence only raises a probability. *American Journal of Clinical Nutrition*, **69**, 2–3.

Klatsky, A. L. (2001). Diet, alcohol, and health: a story of connections, confounders, and cofactors [Editorial]. *American Journal of Clinical Nutrition*, **74**, 279–80.

Klatsky, A. L. and Armstrong, M. A. (1993). Alcoholic beverage choice and risk of coronary artery disease mortality: do red wine drinkers fare best? *American Journal of Cardiology*, **71**, 467–9.

Klatsky, A. L., Armstrong, M. A., and Friedman, G. D. (1997). Red wine, white wine, liquor, beer, and risk of coronary artery disease hospitalization. *American Journal of Cardiology*, **80**, 416–20.

LaPorte, R. E., Cresanta, J. L., and Kuller, L. H. (1980). The relationship of alcohol consumption to atherosclerotic heart disease. *Preventive Medicine*, **9**, 22–40.

Leger, A. S., Cochrane, A. L., and Moore, F. (2002). Factors associated with cardiac mortality in developed countries, with particular reference to the consumption of wine. *Lancet*, **i**, 1017–20.

Leon, D. A., Chenet, L., Shkolnikov, V., Zakharov, S., Shapiro, J., Rakhmanova, G. *et al.* (1997). Huge variation in Russian mortality rates 1984–94: artefact, alcohol, or what? *Lancet*, **350**, 383–8.

Malyutina, S., Bobak, M., Kurilovitch, S., Gafarov, V., Simonova, G., Nikitin, Y., and Marmot, M. (2002). Relation between heavy and binge drinking and all-cause and cardiovascular mortality in Novosibirsk, Russia: a prospective cohort study. *Lancet*, **360**, 1448–54.

Marmot, M. G. (1984). Alcohol and coronary heart disease. *International Journal of Epidemiology*, **13**, 160–7.

Marmot, M. and Brunner, E. (1991). Alcohol and cardiovascular disease: the status of the U shaped curve. *British Medical Journal*, **303**, 565–8.

McElduff, P. and Dobson, A. J. (1997). How much alcohol and how often? Population based case-control study of alcohol consumption and risk of a major coronary event. *British Medical Journal*, **314**, 1159–64.

McElduff, P. and Dobson, A. J. (2001). Case fatality after an acute cardiac event: the effect of smoking and alcohol consumption. *Journal of Clinical Epidemiology*, **54**, 58–67.

McKee, M. and Britton, A. (1998). The positive relationship between alcohol and heart disease in eastern Europe: potential physiological mechanisms. *Journal of the Royal Society of Medicine*, **91**, 402–7.

Mukamal, K. J., Conigrave, K. M., Mittleman, M. A., Camargo, C. A., Jr., Stampfer, M. J., Willett, W. C., and Rimm, E. B. (2003). Roles of drinking pattern and type of alcohol consumed in coronary heart disease in men. *New England Journal of Medicine*, **348**, 109–18.

Murray, C. J. L. and Lopez, A. D. (1996). Quantifying the burden of disease and injury attributable to ten major risk factors. In *The global burden of disease* (ed. C. J. L. Murray and A. D. Lopez), pp. 295–324. World Health Organization, Geneva.

Murray, R. P., Connett, J. E., Tyas, S. L., Bond, R., Ekuma, O., Siversides, C. K., and Barnes, G. E. (2002). Alcohol volume, drinking pattern, and cardiovascular disease morbidity and mortality: is there a U-shaped function? *American Journal of Epidemiology*, **155**, 242–8.

Notzon, F. C., Komarov, Y. M., Ermakov, S. P., Sempos, C. T., Marks, J. S., and Sempos, E. V. (1998). Causes of declining life expectancy in Russia. *Journal of American Medical Association*, **279**, 793–800.

Piantadosi, S., Byar, D. P., and Green, S. B. (1988). The ecological fallacy. *American Journal of Epidemiology*, **127**, 893–904.

Poikolainen, K. (1998). It can be bad for the heart, too: drinking patterns and coronary heart disease [Editorial]. *Addiction*, **93**, 1757–9.

Puddey, I. B., Rakic, V., Dimmitt, S. B., and Beilin, L. J. (1999). Influence of pattern of drinking on cardiovascular disease and cardiovascular risk factors: a review. *Addiction*, **94**, 649–63.

Rehm, J. (1998). Measuring quantity, frequency, and volume of drinking. *Alcoholism: Clinical and Experimental Research*, **22** (Suppl.), 4S–14S.

Rehm, J. and Gmel, G. (2003). Alcohol consumption and total mortality/morbidity: definitions and methodological implications. *Best Practice and Research Clinical Gastroenterology*, **17**, 497–505.

Rehm, J., Greenfield, T. K., and Rogers, J. D. (2001). Average volume of alcohol consumption, patterns of drinking, and all-cause mortality: results from the US National Alcohol Study. *American Journal of Epidemiology*, **153**, 64–71.

Renaud, S. C. and Ruf, J. C. (1996). Effects of alcohol on platelet functions, *Clinica Chimica Acta*, **246**, 77–89.

Rimm, E. B., Klatsky, A., Grobbee, D., and Stampfer, M. J. (1996). Review of moderate alcohol consumption and reduced risk of coronary heart disease: is the effect due to beer, wine, or spirits? *British Medical Journal*, **312**, 731–6.

Rimm, E. B., Williams, P., Fosher, K., Criqui, M., and Stampfer, M. J. (1999). Moderate alcohol intake and lower risk of coronary heart disease: meta-analysis of effects on lipids and haemostatic factors. *British Medical Journal*, **319**, 1523–8.

Royal College of Physicians, Royal College of Psychiatrists, and Royal College of General Practitioners (1995). *Alcohol and the heart in perspective: sensible limits reaffirmed. Report of a working group*. Royal College of Physicians, London.

Seppa, K. and Sillanaukee, P. (1999). Binge drinking and ambulatory blood pressure. *Hypertension*, **33**, 79–82.

Seppa, K., Laippala, P., and Sillanaukee, P. (1994). Drinking pattern and blood pressure. *American Journal of Hypertension*, **7**, 249–54.

Shaper, A. G., Wannamethee, G., and Walker, M. (1988). Alcohol and mortality in British men: explaining the U-shaped curve. *Lancet*, **ii**, 1267–73.

Thun, M. J., Peto, R., Lopez, A. D., Monaco, J. H., Henley, J., Heath, C. W., and Doll, R. (1997). Alcohol consumption and mortality among middle-aged and elderly US adults. *New England Journal of Medicine*, **337**, 1705–14.

Tjonneland, A., Gronbaek, M., Stripp, C., and Overvad, K. (1999). Wine intake and diet in a random sample of 48763 Danish men and women. *American Journal of Clinical Nutrition*, **69**, 49–54.

Ubbink, J. B., Fehily, A. M., Pickering, J., Elwood, P. C., and Vermaak, W. J. (1998). Homocysteine and ischaemic heart disease in the Caerphilly cohort [see comments]. *Atherosclerosis*, **140**, 349–56.

van der Gaag, M. S., Ubbink, J. B., Sillanaukee, P., Nikkari, S., and Hendriks, H. F. (2000). Effect of consumption of red wine, spirits, and beer on serum homocysteine. *Lancet*, **355**, 1522.

Wannamethee, G. and Shaper, A. G. (1992). Alcohol and sudden cardiac death. *British Heart Journal*, **68**, 443–8.

Chapter 18

Fish consumption, n-3 fatty acids, and coronary heart disease

D. Kromhout

18.1 Introduction

The role of different fatty acids in the aetiology of coronary heart disease (CHD) is a subject that has been intensively investigated. By 1956 Sinclair had already noted the detrimental effects of saturated fatty acids and of unsaturated trans fatty acids produced by partial hydrogenation of polyunsaturated fatty acid-rich oils for margarine production (Sinclair 1956). He hypothesized that a high intake of saturated fatty acids and of unnatural trans fatty acids in combination with a chronic relative deficiency of essential fatty acids would promote coronary atherosclerosis and thrombosis. Essential fatty acids are polyunsaturated fatty acids from the n-6 family (i.e. linoleic acid and arachidonic acid) present in vegetable oils, and of the n-3 family (i.e. eicosapentaenoic acid and docosahexaenoic acid) present in seafood. These fatty acids may protect against coronary atherosclerosis and thrombosis.

It is hypothesized that a balanced intake of n-6 and n-3 fatty acids is of great importance in relation to prevention of CHD (Simopoulos 2001). During the Palaeolithic period the intake of n-6 and n-3 fatty acids was almost equal, and nowadays this ratio is about 15–20:1 in most Western diets. This is a result of a decrease in the consumption of seafood and an increased consumption of vegetable oils during the last century due to the development of modern agriculture and technology with an emphasis on grain feeds for domestic livestock. Because of this development, Western diets became 'deficient' in n-3 fatty acids.

Research on n-3 fatty acids, fish consumption, and CHD was stimulated by the pioneering studies of Bang, Dyerberg, and Sinclair among the Inuit (Eskimos) in Greenland (Bang *et al.* 1980). Therefore, in this chapter I begin by summarizing the results of the studies among the Inuit. Thereafter, the results on fish consumption and CHD mortality are reviewed at the population and individual levels. Evidence from experimental studies on fish and n-3 fatty acids and fatal CHD are also discussed. Finally, the importance of fish consumption in the prevention of CHD is discussed.

18.2 The Inuit studies

Dietary surveys were carried out among the Inuit from Greenland in the 1970s. In 1970 food specimens of seven people were collected during seven consecutive days using the duplicate portion technique (Bang *et al.* 1976). In 1976 a similar survey was carried out among 50 adult Inuit from Greenland (Bang *et al.* 1980). The results of these surveys are summarized in Table 18.1.

Table 18.1 Macronutrient content of the Inuit and Danish diet based on an energy intake of 3000 kcal/day

Macronutrient	Inuit		Danes	
	g	%E	g	%E
Protein	173	23	83	11
Carbohydrates	285	38	353	47
Total fat	130	39	140	42
Saturated fat	30	9	73	22
Monounsaturated fat	77	23	47	14
Polyunsaturated fat	23	7	17	5
n-3 PUFA	14	4.2	3	0.9
n-6 PUFA	5	1.5	10	3.0
Dietary cholesterol	0.79	0.26[a]	0.42	0.14[a]

Source: Bang et al. 1976, 1980.

%E = per cent of energy; PUFA = Polyunsaturated fatty acids.

[a] g/1000 kcal.

The consumption of whale and seal meat was very high and amounted to about 400 g/day (Bang and Dyerberg 1972). The average intake of n-3 and n-6 polyunsaturated fatty acids amounted to 14 and 5 g/day, respectively, assuming an energy intake of 3000 kcal/day (Dyerberg 1986). The total polyunsaturated fatty acid intake was 7% of total energy. The traditional diet of the Inuit can be characterized by a low amount of saturated fat (9% of energy) and a high P/S ratio (polyunsaturated/saturated fat ratio) of 0.84. The intake of dietary cholesterol was also high and amounted to 260 mg/1000 kcal.

The Inuit diet contained a large amount of fat (39% of energy). The Danish diet had a comparable amount of fat (42% of energy), but was much higher in saturated fat (22% of total energy) and contained 3 g of n-3 and 10 g of n-6 polyunsaturated fatty acids per day. The P/S ratio of the Danish diet was 0.24. These results suggest that the Inuit and the Danish diets do not differ in total fat. However, the amount of saturated and n-6 polyunsaturated fatty acids was substantially lower in the Inuit diet and the amount of n-3 polyunsaturated fatty acids was much higher in the Inuit compared to the Danish diet.

The difference in the intake of n-3 and n-6 polyunsaturated fatty acids between the Inuit and the Danes was reflected in the fatty acid composition of the platelets. The content of the n-6 polyunsaturated fatty acids, linoleic acid, and arachidonic acid was more than two times lower in the Inuit than the Danes (Dyerberg and Bang 1979). In contrast, much higher concentrations of n-3 polyunsaturated fatty acids eicosapentaenoic acid (EPA) and docosahexaenoic acid (DHA) were observed in the lipids of platelets of Inuit compared to Danes. These differences in polyunsaturated fatty acid intake were associated with a twice as long bleeding time in Inuit compared to Danes. Differences were also observed in blood lipid concentrations between the Inuit and the Danes (Bang et al. 1971). The most remarkable differences were 56% lower triglyceride levels and 45% higher high-density lipoprotein (HDL) cholesterol levels. Similar differences in blood lipids were reported in a more recent epidemiological study among Inuit carried out in 1993–94 (Bjerregaard et al. 1997). These differences were larger in Inuit who followed a more traditional diet.

The differences in diet and risk factors between Inuit and Danes were also associated with differences in cardiovascular disease patterns. A morbidity survey was carried out in the

Upernavik district in Northwest Greenland (Kromann and Green 1980). The study population of 1800 inhabitants was followed for 25 years between 1950 and 1974. The incidence of myocardial infarction was ~10 times lower among the Inuit compared to Danes. In contrast, the incidence of stroke was about twice as high among the Inuit compared to the Danes. Diabetes was very rare in the Inuit population. Between 1968 and 1983, mortality from CHD was also lower among Inuit compared to Danes (Bjerregaard and Dyerberg 1988). In accord with the results for morbidity, higher mortality rates from stroke were also observed among Inuit compared to Danes. These results suggest that the Inuit diet is associated with a substantially lower risk of CHD. On the other hand, the risk for stroke may be increased among the Inuit.

The pattern of cardiovascular diseases among the Inuit is probably due to the effect of their diet on haemostatic factors, illustrated by their increased bleeding time compared to the Danes (Dyerberg and Bang 1979). The low rates of CHD among the Inuit may also be attributed to less atherosclerosis in the coronary arteries. To test this hypothesis, the extent of atherosclerotic lesions in the coronary arteries and aortas from Alaskan natives (Inuit) and non-natives were compared (Newman *et al.* 1993). This comparative study showed that the prevalence of raised lesions in native specimens was consistently lower than in those from non-natives. I conclude from the results of these studies that the low rate of CHD among Inuit is the result of both less atherosclerosis and less thrombosis.

In order to prove causation in the relationships between the fatty acid composition of the diet, risk factors, and the occurrence of CHD in the Inuit, intervention studies are needed. Such intervention studies have not been carried out principally because ethical considerations ruled out a study in volunteers in view of the toxicity of the diet to those not adapted to it. Therefore Sinclair (1980) put himself on an Inuit diet for 100 days. This diet consisted solely of marine animal food (seal, fish, crustaceans, and molluscs) and water. His bleeding time rose from the normal value of 3–5 min to ~50 min, then declined to ~15 min. In addition, substantial decreases were observed in blood platelets, erythrocytes, packed cell volume, and haemoglobin. The triglyceride-rich very low-density lipoprotein (VLDL) fraction fell and the HDL fraction increased considerably. A substantial increase in the EPA concentration and a marked decrease in the linoleic acid concentration of the cholesteryl esters were noted.

The changes in fatty acid composition of cholesteryl esters, lipoproteins, bleeding time, and haemostatic factors in this human experiment were in accord with those observed in comparative studies between Inuit and Danes. Such an extreme diet is associated with a lower risk for CHD, but also with a possibly increased risk of stroke and an increased risk of accidents because of the prolonged bleeding time. Sinclair concluded from his experiment that it is necessary to have the right balance between n-3 and n-6 polyunsaturated fatty acids. A drastic alteration of n-6 to n-3 fatty acids greatly decreases platelet aggregation, to an undesirable extent. He concluded that the next step is to determine the amount of EPA which will cause optimum disaggregation of platelets and so prevent thrombotic disorders.

18.3 **Fish and CHD in the Seven Countries Study**

Besides Inuit, another population that is known for its high level of fish consumption is that of Japan. The average daily fish consumption in Japan is about 100 g/day and the Japanese are also known for their low mortality rate from CHD (Kagawa *et al.* 1982). Within Japan the lowest death rates from CHD are found on the island of Okinawa, where fish consumption is about twice as high as on the mainland of Japan. Comparisons between Inuit and Danes, and between different parts of Japan, do not answer the question of whether fish consumption levels of populations are related to CHD mortality rates in these populations. This question could be answered using data collected in large population studies.

In the Seven Countries Study, 12 763 men aged 40–59 were enrolled between 1958 and 1964 (Kromhout *et al.* 1996*a*). In these countries cohorts were established in rural areas in Finland, Italy, Greece, the former Yugoslavia, and Japan, two cohorts of railroad employees in the USA and Italy, one of workers in a large cooperative in Serbia, one of university professors in Belgrade, and one of inhabitants of a small commercial town in the Netherlands. Between 1959 and 1964 dietary information was collected in small random samples of 14 of the 16 cohorts (Kromhout *et al.* 1989). In the other two cohorts information was gathered around 1970. The weighed record method was used in all the dietary surveys. The average fish consumption was less than 20 g/day in cohorts from the USA, Western Finland, The Netherlands and Serbia, and between 20 and 60 g/day in cohorts from Eastern Finland, Italy, Slavonia, and Greece. An average consumption of ~100 g/day was observed in Dalmatia and in the Japanese cohort of Tanushimaru. Fishermen from the Japanese village of Ushibuka consumed on average ~200 g fish/day. The 25-year age-adjusted mortality rate from CHD in the 16 cohorts varied from 5% in Crete (Greece) and Tanushimaru (Japan) to 29% in Eastern Finland.

The logarithm of average fish consumption at baseline was inversely related to 25-year age-adjusted mortality rates from CHD in the 16 cohorts (Fig. 18.1). This relationship was no longer present after adjustment for the intake of saturated fat and flavonoids and the prevalence of cigarette smokers. At the population level fish consumption was positively associated with flavonoid intake and the prevalence of smokers, and inversely associated with the intake of saturated fat. Multivariate analysis of the Seven Countries Study data showed that the

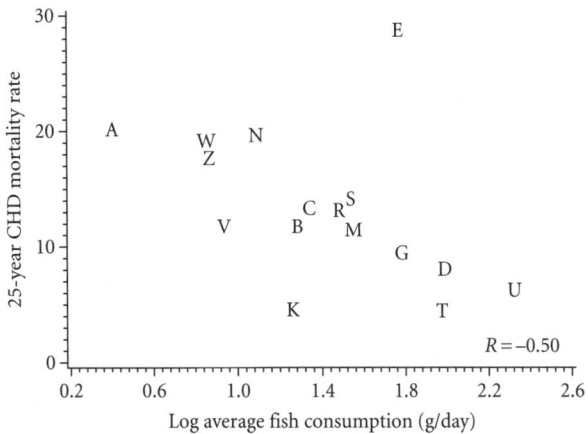

Fig. 18.1 Logarithm of average fish consumption in 1960 and 25-year age-adjusted mortality rates from CHD. Abbreviations: A: US Railroad; B: Belgrade, Serbia, former Yugoslavia; C: Crevalcore, Italy; D: Dalmatia, Croatia, former Yugoslavia; E: East Finland; G: Corfu; K: Crete; M: Montenegro, Italy; N: Zutphen, Netherlands; R: Rome; S: Slavonia, Croatia, former Yugoslavia; T: Tanushimaru, Japan; U: Ushibuka, Japan; V: Velika Krsna, Serbia, former Yugoslavia; W: West Finland; Z: Zrenjanin, Serbia, former Yugoslavia. (From Kromhout *et al.* 1996*a*.)

average population intake of saturated fat and flavonoids and the prevalence of cigarette smokers are the strongest determinants of population CHD mortality rates (Hertog *et al.* 1995; Kromhout *et al.* 1995*a*).

Other cross-cultural studies on fish consumption and CHD mortality used data from 21 and 36 countries, respectively (Crombie *et al.* 1987; Zhang *et al.* 1999). In these studies per capita fish consumption data and national CHD mortality rates were used. In the 21 countries study an inverse association was found which appeared stable over different periods of time (Crombie *et al.* 1987). This correlation was, however, very much dependent on the inclusion of Japan. Exclusion of Japan reduced the correlation between per capita fish consumption and CHD mortality rates. Multiple regression analyses including data from all 21 countries showed no relationship between per capita fish consumption and CHD mortality rates after inclusion of milk products and meat (a proxy for the intake of saturated fat) in the multivariate model.

The 36 countries study showed an inverse relation between the logarithm of per capita fish consumption and CHD mortality rates (Zhang *et al.* 1999). This relationship persisted whether the fish consumption data obtained were about 2, 12, or 30 years prior to the mortality examined, and also after multivariate analyses taking into account the confounding effects of animal fat, animal protein, and alcohol. The reason why the per capita fish consumption remained inversely related to CHD mortality in the 36 countries study may be the fact that in this study (in contrast to the Seven Countries Study) in the multivariate model flavonoid intake and the prevalence of cigarette smokers were not included as possible confounders of the relationship between average population fish consumption and CHD mortality rates.

I conclude that at the population level fish consumption is not a major determinant of CHD mortality rates. This does not mean that fish consumption is not important in the aetiology of CHD. The population level fish consumption was correlated with saturated fat, flavonoids, and cigarette smoking. The effects of these dietary and lifestyle variables on CHD mortality rates were stronger than that of fish consumption and overruled a possible protective effect of fish consumption.

18.4 Fish and CHD in individuals

In the first part of the 1980s information on the relationship between fish consumption and CHD mortality in individuals was not available.

The only information available was that populations with a high consumption of seafood, for example the Inuit and the Japanese, had low rates of CHD. We decided to test the hypothesis that at the individual level a low level of fish consumption protects against CHD mortality.

In the Zutphen cohort, the Dutch contribution to the Seven Countries Study, information on the habitual food consumption pattern was collected repeatedly since 1960 (Kromhout *et al.* 1985). The cross-check dietary history was used as the dietary survey method. This method provides information on the usual food consumption pattern of the participants in the 6–12 months before the interview. From this information fish consumption during a typical weekday was calculated. Other risk factors–serum cholesterol, blood pressure, smoking habits, anthropometric measures, physical activity, and occupation–were determined according to a standardized protocol. The vital status of 852 men aged 40–59 in 1960 and free from CHD was verified after 20 years of follow-up: 78 had died from CHD.

The average fish consumption of the Zutphen men was 20 g/day in 1960. About two-thirds consisted of lean fish (e.g. cod and plaice) and one-third consisted of fatty fish (e.g. herring

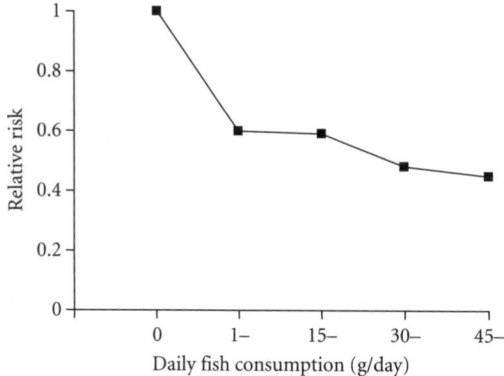

Fig. 18.2 Fish consumption in 1960 and 20-year mortality from CHD. (From Kromhout *et al.* 1985.)

and mackerel). About 19% of the men did not eat fish. The age-adjusted risk ratios for death from CHD decreased with increasing fish consumption (Fig. 18.2). This relationship persisted after multivariate analyses taking the confounding effects of different dietary and other risk factors into account. Compared to men who did not eat fish, the adjusted risk ratio was 36% lower in men who ate 1–14 g of fish per day. For men who consumed at least 30 g of fish per day the risk ratio was about 60% lower.

We also studied the relationship between fish consumption and CHD mortality among a small cohort of 272 persons aged 64 years and older in a general practitioner practice in Rotterdam (Kromhout *et al.* 1995*b*). In 1971 the dietary habits of these persons were investigated, also using the cross-check dietary history method. In 1971 60% of the cohort ate fish and 40% did not. The vital status was verified after 17 years of follow-up: 58 men had died from CHD. Multivariate analyses, taking into account the confounding effect of major risk factors, showed an inverse relationship between fish consumption and 17-year mortality from CHD. The risk ratio for fish eaters was 50% lower compared to that of no-fish eaters.

These two Dutch studies were too small to differentiate between the effect of lean and fatty fish in relation to CHD mortality. This was done in a combined analysis of the Dutch, Finnish, and Italian cohorts of the Seven Countries Study (Oomen *et al.* 2000). Around 1970, 553 Dutch, 1688 Finnish, and 1097 Italian men participated in a dietary survey. Fish consumption was again quantified using the cross-check dietary history method. The average daily fish consumption was 18 g in the Netherlands, 39 g in Finland, and 20 g in Italy. After 20 years of follow-up 105 men in the Netherlands, 242 men in Finland, and 116 men in Italy had died from CHD. Lean fish consumption was not associated with 20-year mortality from CHD in any country. Fatty fish compared to non-fatty fish consumption was associated with a lower CHD mortality rate. The adjusted pooled relative risk for fatty fish consumers was 34% lower compared to non-fatty fish consumers.

Several, but not all, cohort studies have found a protective effect of fish consumption on CHD mortality. Marckmann and Grønbaeck analysed 11 cohort studies and concluded that fish consumption at 40–60 g/day is associated with markedly reduced CHD mortality in high-risk populations (Marckmann and Grønbaeck 1999). However, fish consumption is not associated with CHD mortality in low-risk populations. Another reason for finding no relationship in populations with a relatively high level of fish consumption is probably the lack of a control group of no-fish eaters. An example of this is the Honolulu Heart Program, in which almost all men consumed fish (Curb and Reed 1985).

No effect, or even a harmful effect from fish consumption was observed in cohort studies from Finland (Oomen *et al.* 2000, Pietinen *et al.* 1997; Salonen *et al.* 1995). It has been hypothesized that the mercury content of fish may be responsible for the more harmful effect of fish observed in Finland. The Kuopio Study showed that lean fish, but not fatty fish, was associated with mercury intake and with excess risk from CHD (Salonen *et al.* 1995). This makes it likely that in the Finnish situation the association between fish consumption and CHD mortality is confounded by mercury. This was confirmed in another report from the Kuopio Study (Rissanen *et al.* 2000).

There is some evidence that the harder the CHD endpoint the stronger the association with fish consumption. The Physicians Health Study did not find a relationship between fish consumption and non-fatal CHD (Morris *et al.* 1995). Also, the recently reported results from the Nurses Health Study showed a stronger inverse relationship between fish consumption and 16-year mortality from CHD than with non-fatal myocardial infarction (Hu *et al.* 2002). In another analysis of the Physicians Health Study no association was found between fish consumption and 11-year mortality from CHD (Albert *et al.* 1998). However, at a level of fish consumption of less than one fish meal per week an inverse association was observed between fish consumption and sudden cardiac death. These results suggest that at a low level of fish consumption a protective effect can be shown for the hard endpoint sudden cardiac death.

In a case-control study carried out among 334 cases of primary cardiac arrest and 493 population-based controls, a dose–response relationship was observed between fish consumption and primary cardiac arrest (Siscovick *et al.* 1995). One fish meal per week was associated with a 50% reduction in the risk of primary cardiac arrest after adjustment for potential confounders. In this study both the intake of the n-3 polyunsaturated fatty acids EPA and DHA and the red blood cell level of these fatty acids were determined. For the intake of EPA and DHA the adjusted odds ratio for the fourth quartile of intake compared with no seafood consumption was 0.4 (95% CI: 0.2–0.7). The strongest association was, however, observed for the relationship between the EPA and DHA content of red blood cells and primary cardiac arrest. For the fourth quartile compared to the first quartile this risk ratio was 0.1 (95% CI: 0.1–0.4). The stronger association between the EPA and DHA content of red blood cells compared with dietary intake is due to less misclassification in using the red blood cell content of EPA and DHA as a marker for the intake of these fatty acids.

These results were confirmed in a recently reported nested-case control analysis carried out in the Physicians Health Study (Albert *et al.* 2002). Whole blood n-3 polyunsaturated fatty acids were determined by gas-liquid chromatography for 94 cases of sudden cardiac death and 184 controls originally free from cardiovascular diseases. Baseline levels of long-chain n-3 polyunsaturated fatty acids in whole blood were inversely related to the risk of sudden cardiac death. The adjusted relative risk of sudden cardiac death for men in the highest quartile of long-chain n-3 polyunsaturated fatty acids in blood compared with those in the first quartile was 0.19 (95% CI: 0.05–0.71).

In summary, the results of cohort studies suggest that, especially for hard endpoints such as CHD mortality and sudden cardiac death, inverse relationships are observed with fish consumption. These associations were even stronger in case-control comparisons of cardiac arrest and sudden cardiac death when blood levels of long-chain n-3 polyunsaturated fatty acids, instead of dietary intake data, were used as biomarkers for intake. There is, therefore, now firm evidence from observational studies that fish consumption is protective against hard endpoints of CHD.

18.5 **Experimental studies on fish consumption, n-3 polyunsaturated fatty acids, and CHD mortality**

For establishing cause and effect relationships, results of intervention trials are needed. The hypothesis that fatty fish prevents coronary death was tested in the DART trial (Burr *et al.* 1989). More than 2000 patients in Cardiff, Wales, who had recovered from a myocardial infarction were allocated to either an experimental group that was advised to eat fatty fish at least twice a week, or a control group, that did not receive such advice. The consumption of at least two dishes of fatty fish per week reduced cardiac death by 33% and all-cause mortality by 29%. No difference was observed in the occurrence of non-fatal myocardial infarction. The results of this trial are in accord with those of cohort studies showing a protective effect of fatty fish on fatal, but not on non-fatal, CHD.

The results of the DART trial suggest that long-chain n-3 polyunsaturated fatty acids present in fatty fish protect against fatal CHD. The hypothesis that a low-dose of long-chain n-3 polyunsaturated fatty acids protects against fatal and non-fatal cardiovascular diseases was tested in the GISSI-Prevenzione trial (GISSI-Prevenzione Investigators 1999). In this trial more than 11 000 patients surviving a recent myocardial infarction were randomized. The active treatment group received daily one gelatin capsule containing 850–882 mg EPA and DHA and the control group did not receive a supplement. These patients were followed for 3.5 years.

Treatment with a low-dose of n-3 polyunsaturated fatty acids lowered the risk for cardiovascular diseases by 11–20%. The benefit for cardiovascular death was 17–30%, for coronary death 20–35%, and for sudden death 26–45%. These results also suggest that the strongest effect is observed for the hardest endpoint, sudden death.

Compliance in this trial was about 70%. This means a daily intake of long-chain n-3 polyunsaturated fatty acids of about 600 mg/day. This corresponds to consumption of about 70 g of fatty fish per day or 3–4 fatty fish meals per week. This is a large amount of fatty fish, but a low amount of n-3 polyunsaturated fatty acids compared with the 'pharmacological' doses of more than 3 g/day used in experimental studies on mechanisms in relation to the aetiology of CHD.

Several mechanisms such as effects on blood lipids and lipoproteins, haemostatic factors, and electrical stability of the heart have been hypothesized as being the explanation for the protective effect of fatty fish and long-chain n-3 polyunsaturated fatty acids. However, it should be realized that in most research on mechanisms large doses of fish oil were used. This is not compatible with the results of observational and experimental studies showing a protective effect of fatty fish consumption and a low-dose of fish oil on CHD mortality.

We showed that a difference of one meal of fish per day during 26 years was associated with a 26% lower level of total triglycerides and a 38% lower level of the atherogenic intermediate-density lipoproteins (IDLs) (Kromhout *et al.* 1996b). This long-term difference of one fish meal per day was not associated with cutaneous bleeding time, platelet number, or collagen-induced platelet aggregation. However, the concentration of EPA in phospholipids was 100% higher and that of DHA 30% higher in fish consumers (Van Houwelingen *et al.* 1989). The higher content of these long-chain n-3 polyunsaturated fatty acids in phospholipids will increase membrane fluidity.

That a small amount of fish may have a large effect on pathology can be illustrated by two examples. Arterial compliance in non-fish eaters, as measured by Doppler ultrasonography, was significantly lower than that in persons who had one meal of fish per week (Wahlqvist *et al.*

1989). In patients who underwent percutaneous transluminal coronary angioplasty (PTCA) the reoccurrence of coronary stenosis was significantly lower in patients with an intake of at least 150 mg long-chain n-3 polyunsaturated fatty acids per day (Bairati *et al.* 1992). These results make clear that a small amount of fish has a profound effect on the pathology of CHD.

Both the DART and GISSI-Prevenzione trials had an open design. The interventions in both trials could not be blinded and placebos were not used. In order to get more definitive evidence on the association between a low-dose of long-chain n-3 polyunsaturated fatty acids and fatal CHD, results of double-blind placebo controlled trials are needed. Until recently this could not be done in dietary intervention trials. However, the appearance of functional foods on the market provides new opportunities for carrying out controlled dietary intervention trials.

We recently started a randomized controlled trial of 4000 cardiac patients aged 60–80. Over a period of 3 years these patients will receive four margarines: one placebo; one enriched with the long-chain n-3 polyunsaturated fatty acids, EPA, and DHA; one enriched with n-3 polyunsaturated fatty acid, α-linolenic acid; and one enriched with both EPA and DHA, and α-linolenic acid. The daily intake of EPA and DHA in this trial is estimated at about 400 mg/day. This trial will, therefore, test in a controlled fashion what the effect is of a low-dose of EPA and DHA on fatal CHD.

18.6 Conclusions

There are still unresolved questions on the metabolic effects of a low-dose of EPA and DHA and their association with fatal CHD. However, there is now some evidence from both observational epidemiology and experimental studies that a small amount of fish protects against fatal CHD and sudden cardiac death. It is, therefore, recommended to eat fish (preferably fatty fish) once or twice a week. Although fish is not a panacea, regular fish consumption is an important component of a healthy diet and lifestyle (Kromhout *et al.* 2002). It is, however, not enough to eat fish on a regular basis. This can be illustrated with the high mortality rate from CHD in the cohort from Eastern Finland of the Seven Countries Study. These men had a high consumption of fish (about 60 g/day), but also had a high intake of saturated fat and a low intake of flavonoids, and the cohort had a high prevalence of smokers. This example shows that a balanced diet and a healthy lifestyle are needed in order to achieve a low risk for CHD. Recently this was nicely illustrated by results from the Nurses Health Study (Stampfer *et al.* 2000; see also Chapter 38).

References

Albert, C. H., Hennekens, C. H., O'Donnell, J., Ajani, U. A., Carey, V. J., Willett, W. C. *et al.* (1998). Consumption of fish and risk of sudden cardiac death. *Journal of the American Medical Association*, **279**, 23–8.

Albert, C. M., Campos, H., Stampfer, M., Ridker, P., Manson, J. E., Willett, W. C., and Ma, J. (2002). Blood levels of long-chain n-3 fatty acids and the risk of sudden death. *New England Journal of Medicine*, **346**, 1113–18.

Bairati, I., Roy, L., and Meyer, F. (1992). Double-blind, randomized, controlled trial of fish oil supplements in prevention of recurrence of stenosis after coronary angioplasty. *Circulation*, **85**, 950–6.

Bang, H. O. and Dyerberg, J. (1972). Plasma lipids and lipoproteins in Greenlandic west coast Eskimos. *Acta Medica Scandinavica*, **192**, 85–94.

Bang, H. O., Dyerberg, J., and Nielsen, A. B. (1971). Plasma lipid and lipoprotein pattern in Greenlandic west-coast Eskimos. *Lancet*, **i**, 1143–6.

Bang, H. O., Dyerberg, J., and Hjorne, N. (1976). The composition of food consumed by Greenland Eskimos. *Acta Medica Scandinavica*, **200**, 69–73.

Bang, H. O., Dyerberg, J., and Sinclair, H. M. (1980). The composition of the Eskimo food in North Western Greenland. *American Journal of Clinical Nutrition*, **33**, 2657–61.

Bjerregaard, P. and Dyerberg, J. (1988). Mortality from ischaemic heart disease and cerebrovascular disease in Greenland. *International Journal of Epidemiology*, **17**, 514–19.

Bjerregaard, P., Mulvad, G., and Pedersen, H. S. (1997). Cardiovascular risk factors in Inuit of Greenland. *International Journal Epidemiology*, **26**, 1182–90

Burr, M. L., Fehily, A. M., Gilbert, J. F., Rogers, S., Holliday, R. M., Sweetnam, P. M. *et al.* (1989). Effects of changes in fat, fish and fibre intakes on death and myocardial re-infarction: diet and re-infarction trial (DART). *Lancet*, **ii**, 757–61.

Crombie, I. K., McLoone, P., Smith, W. S. C., and Tunstall-Pedoe, H. (1987). International differences in coronary heart disease mortality and consumption of fish and other foodstuffs. *European Heart Journal*, **8**, 560–3.

Curb, J. D. and Reed, D. M. (1985). Fish consumption and mortality from coronary heart disease [letter]. *New England Journal of Medicine*, **313**, 821.

Dyerberg, J. (1986). Linolenate-derived polyunsaturated fatty acids and prevention of atherosclerosis. *Nutrition Reviews*, **44**, 125–34.

Dyerberg, J. and Bang, H. O. (1979). Haemostatic function and platelet polyunsaturated fatty acids in Eskimos. *Lancet*, **2**, 433–5.

GISSI-Prevenzione Investigators (1999). Dietary supplementation with n-3 polyunsaturated fatty acids and vitamin E after myocardial infarction: results of the GISSI-Prevenzione trial. *Lancet*, **354**, 447–55.

Hertog, M. G. L., Kromhout, D., Aravanis, C., Blackburn, H., Buzina, R., Fidanza, F. *et al.* (1995). Flavonoid intake and long-term risk of coronary heart disease and cancer in the Seven Countries Study. *Archives of Internal Medicine*, **155**, 381–6.

Hu, F. B., Bronner, L., Willett, W. C., Rexrode, K. M., Albert, C. M., Hunter, D., and Manson, J. E. (2002). Fish and omega-3 fatty acid intake and risk of coronary heart disease in women. *Journal of the American Medical Association*, **287**, 1815–21.

Kagawa, Y., Nishizawa, M., Suzuki, M., Miyatake, T., Hamamoto, T. Goto, K. *et al.* (1982). Eicosapolyenoic acids of serum lipids of Japanese islanders with low incidence of cardiovascular diseases. *Journal of Nutritional Sciences and Vitaminology*, **28**, 441–53.

Kromann, N. and Green, A. (1980). Epidemiological studies in the Upernavik district, Greenland. *Acta Medica Scandinavica*, **208**, 401–6.

Kromhout, D., Bosschieter, E. B., and De Lezenne Coulander, C. (1985). The inverse relation between fish consumption and 20-year mortality from coronary heart disease. *New England Journal of Medicine*, **312**, 1205–9.

Kromhout, D., Keys, A., Aravanis, C., Buzina, R., Fidanza, F., Giampaoli, S. *et al.* (1989). Food consumption patterns in the nineteen sixties in Seven Countries. *American Journal of Clinical Nutrition*, **49**, 889–94.

Kromhout, D., Menotti, A., Bloemberg, B., Aravanis, C., Blackburn, H., Buzina, R. *et al.* (1995a). Dietary saturated and trans fatty acids, cholesterol and 25-year mortality from coronary heart disease: the Seven Countries Study. *Preventive Medicine*, **24**, 308–15.

Kromhout, D., Feskens, E. J. M., and Bowles, C. H. (1995b). The protective effect of a small amount of fish on coronary heart disease mortality in an elderly population. *International Journal of Epidemiology*, **24**, 340–5.

Kromhout, D., Bloemberg, B. P. M., Feskens, E. J. M., Hertog, M. G. L., Menotti, A., and Blackburn, H., for the Seven Countries Study Group (1996a). Alcohol, fish, fiber and antioxidant vitamins do not explain population differences in coronary heart disease mortality. *International Journal Epidemiology*, **25**, 753–9.

Kromhout, D., Katan, M. B., Havekes, L., Groener, A., Hornstra, G., and De Lezenne Coulander, C. (1996*b*). The effects of 26 years of habitual fish consumption on serum lipid and lipoprotein levels (The Zutphen Study). *Nutrition, Metabolism, and Cardiovascular Diseases*, **6**, 65–73.

Kromhout, D., Menotti, A., Kesteloot, H., and Sans, S. (2002). Prevention of coronary heart disease by diet and lifestyle: evidence from prospective cross-cultural, cohort, and intervention studies. *Circulation*, **105**, 893–8.

Marckmann, P. and Grønbaek, M. (1999). Fish consumption and coronary heart disease mortality: a systematic review of prospective cohort studies. *European Journal Clinical Nutrition*, **53**, 585–90.

Morris, M. C., Manson, J. E., Rosner, B., Buring, J. E., Willett, W. C., and Hennekens, C. H. (1995). Fish consumption and cardiovascular disease in the Physicians Health Study: a prospective study. *American Journal of Epidemiology*, **142**, 166–75.

Newman, W. P., Middaugh, J. P., Propst, M. T., and Rogers, D. R. (1993). Atheroscleroses in Alaska Natives and non-natives. *Lancet*, **341**, 1056–7.

Oomen, C. M., Feskens, E. J. M., Räsänen, L., Fidanza, F., Nissinen, A. M., Menotti, A. *et al.* (2000). Fish consumption and coronary heart disease mortality in Finland, Italy and the Netherlands. *American Journal of Epidemiology*, **151**, 999–1006.

Pietinen, P., Ascherio, A., Hartman, A. M., Willett, W. C., Albanes, D., and Virtamo, J. (1997). Intake of fatty acids and risk of coronary heart disease in a cohort of Finnish men: the Alpha-Tocopherol, Beta-Carotene Cancer Prevention Study. *American Journal of Epidemiology*, **145**, 876–87.

Rissanen, T., Voutelainen, S., Nyyssönen, K., Lakka, T. A., and Salonen, J. T. (2000). Fish oil derived fatty acids, docosahexaenoic acid and docosapentaenoic acid and the risk of acute coronary events: the Kuopio Ischaemic Heart Disease Risk Factor Study. *Circulation*, **102**, 2677–9.

Salonen, J. L., Seppänen, K. Nyyssönen, K., Korpela, H., Kaukanen, J. Kantola, M. *et al.* (1995). Intake of mercury from fish, lipid peroxidation, and the risk of myocardial infarction and coronary cardiovascular, and any death in Eastern Finnish men. *Circulation*, **91**, 645–55.

Simopoulos, A. P. (2001). Evolutionary aspects of diet, essential fatty acids and cardiovascular disease. *European Heart Journal*, **3** (Suppl. D), D8–D21.

Sinclair, H. M. (1956). Deficiency of essential fatty acids and atherosclerosis, etcetera. *Lancet*, **i**, 381–3.

Sinclair, H. (1980). Advantages and disadvantages of an Eskimo diet. In: *Drugs affecting lipid metabolism* (ed. D. Fumagalli, D. Kritchevsky, and R. Paoletti), pp. 363–70. Elsevier/North-Holland Biomedical Press, Amsterdam.

Siscovick, D. S., Raghunathan, T. E., King, I., Weinmann, S., Wicklund, K. G., Albright, J. *et al.* (1995). Dietary intake and cell membrane levels of long-chain n-3 polyunsaturated fatty acids and the risk of primary cardiac arrest. *Journal of the American Medical Association*, **274**, 1363–7.

Stampfer, M. J., Hu, F. B., Manson, J. E., Rimm, E. B., and Willett, W. C. (2000). Primary prevention of coronary heart disease in women through diet and lifestyle. *New England Journal of Medicine*, **343**, 16–22.

Van Houwelingen, A. C., Hornstra, G., Kromhout, D., and De Lezenne Coulander, C. (1989). Habitual fish consumption, fatty acids of serum phospholipids and platelet function. *Atherosclerosis*, **75**, 157–65.

Wahlqvist, M. L., Lo, C. S., and Myers K. A. (1989). Fish intake and arterial wall characteristics in healthy people and diabetic patients. *Lancet*, **ii**, 944–6.

Zhang, J., Sasaki, S., Amano, K., and Kesteloot, H. (1999). Fish consumption and mortality from all causes, ischemic heart disease and stroke: an ecological study. *Preventive Medicine*, **28**, 520–9.

Chapter 19

Exercise versus heart attack: history of a hypothesis

(reprinted from first edition)*

J. N. Morris

19.1 Introduction

The observation that physical activity can protect against heart attack was first made in studies of men in a variety of occupations. Conductors on London's double-decker buses (up and down stairs 11 days a fortnight, 50 weeks a year, often for decades) experienced half or less the incidence of acute myocardial infarction and 'sudden death' ascribed to coronary heart disease (CHD) in the sedentary bus drivers. Postmen (70% of their shift walking, cycling, and climbing stairs to deliver the mail) were similarly protected by comparison with postal clerks and miscellaneous other groups of sedentary government workers (Morris *et al*. 1953). The self-selection issue soon presented: conductors were manifestly more lightly built than drivers. Perhaps the conductors were generally healthier than the drivers (as manifest in their leanness) and so less likely to suffer heart attack – and also to choose more active jobs? However, prospective analysis of rates of sudden death in relation to uniform trouser-waist (central obesity?) in the bus population found that slim, average, or portly conductors suffered about half or less the incidence of the drivers (Heady *et al*. 1961). Subsequent occupational studies in the UK and elsewhere mostly confirmed the main observation and its 'independence' from a variety of other relevant, possibly confounding factors (Paffenbarger *et al*. 1970; Powell *et al*. 1987; Kristensen 1989).

By the 1960s it had already become evident that if physical activity was to contribute in the years ahead to prevention of CHD it would increasingly have to be the exercise taken off the job, in leisure time, by a population increasingly employed in physically undemanding work and otherwise physically inactive. Therefore a survey was mounted among a group of male sedentary/physically very light workers in the executive grade of the civil service to test the hypothesis drawn (not very perceptively) from these occupational studies that such men with high totals of physical activity in their leisure time would suffer less CHD than comparable men with low totals. There was no support for this in prospective study. Instead, it was found that only the men engaging in vigorous activity showed a reduced incidence of the disease (Fig. 19.1). Vigorous activity was defined as that liable to reach peaks of energy expenditure of 7.5 kcal/min (31.5 kJ/min), over six times basal oxygen uptake, say, and a gross oxygen uptake of 1.51/min or about 20 ml/kg/min. Furthermore, the men reporting dynamic vigorous aerobic exercise, in sports and getting about, showed much stronger and more consistent protection than those reporting heavy recreational 'work', the other form of vigorous activity (Morris *et al*. 1973, 1980).

....

* Copyright rests with the author, Professor J. N. Morris.

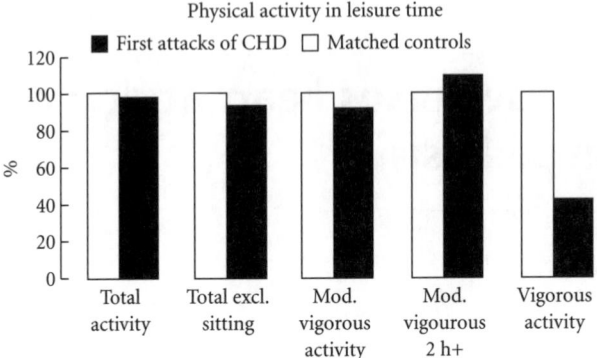

Fig.19.1 Prospective study (1968/70–78) of 16 882 British male executive grade civil servants, age 40–64 at entry. First 214 fatal and non-fatal clinical attacks of CHD and 428 controls. Activity logged, 5 min × 5 min, on sample Friday and Saturday. (Data from Morris et al. 1973.)

Table 19.1 CHD incidence (%)

	VE	No VE
Non-smokers		
Non-fatal first clinical attack	1.3	3.2
Fatal first clinical attack	0.85	1.7
Smokers		
Non-fatal	1.6	4.4
Fatal	3.3	5.2

VE: vigorous aerobic exercise.

Again, the benefits of such vigorous aerobic exercise were statistically independent of the other factors that were studied. For example, Table 19.1 shows the age-standardized percentage CHD incidence rates for men classified according to cigarette smoking and vigorous exercise at 8.5 years follow-up. The reductions were substantially greater in men aged 50–64 than in the younger entrants.

19.2 Variations of CHD

The advantage of men engaging in vigorous aerobic exercise was evident in the incidence of acute myocardial infarction (non-fatal and fatal), sudden death, angina pectoris, and coronary insufficiency.

In a cross-sectional approach a sample of 509 men was drawn from the cohort. Of these, 74 reported vigorous aerobic exercise. Their resting electrocardiograms (ECGs) were compared using the Minnesota Code (Rose and Blackburn 1968) with those of the 384 men reporting no vigorous exercise: 2.9% of the former (age-standardized) showed definite or possible ischaemia against 10.4% of the latter. Less expected were the differences in the frequency of ectopic beats (EBs). These were 2.9% in the 74 men reporting exercise versus 7.1% in the 384 others: 0 versus 10 instances of supraventricular EBs, 2 versus 17 instances of ventricular EBs, and 0 versus 14 instances of EBs comprising 10% or more of recorded cycles. Electrical instability?

Exclusion of men with evidence of clinical or subclinical cardiovascular disease did not affect this contrast. The 51 men reporting heavy recreational work showed no such immunity (Epstein *et al.* 1976).

19.3 **Next steps**

The indication that a threshold of intensity of exercise has to be reached for protection against CHD, and the further suggestion that vigorous *aerobic* exercise is distinctively effectual, raised questions for theory (Fentem *et al.* 1988; Pollock and Wilmore 1990) and for public health. Thus we could be identifying a level of activity in this homogeneous population of middle-aged, middle-class office workers whose health was average or above, sufficiently intense on average, that is, entailing over 50–60% of individual maximal aerobic power, and of sufficient quantity, to produce 'overload' and a training stimulus. And this could be improving cardiorespiratory fitness to moderately high levels. Plainly, health education messages would be affected if such a proposition superseded that of the benefits of high total physical activity levels (Morris 1975). Therefore a further survey was mounted in 1976 to test the new hypothesis directly.

19.3.1 **Fresh hypothesis**

The prospective survey of 1976–86, again in men of the executive grade in the civil service, was designed to test the following propositions.

1 Vigorous, habitual, frequent aerobic exercises in sports and in getting about would offer substantial protection against CHD.

2 More tentatively, heavy (vigorous) recreational work in jobs and hobbies in and about the house and garden and on the car (the other main form of physical activity in leisure time), which had shown an inconsistent and weaker association with incidence of CHD in the previous survey, would also confer some protection.

3 Other physical activity would not be protective.

4 High totals of energy expenditure per se would not be protective (Morris *et al.* 1990).

19.3.2 **Exercise and incidence**

Table 19.2 orders the data of this second survey in terms of the principal proposition 1. The total cohort consisted of 9375 men having no history or record of CHD. There were 474 first clinical events in a 9.3 year follow-up and 87 563 man-years' observation. Table 19.2 shows the data for men aged 55–64 at entry which relate to proposition 1.

Group 1 consists of the men (9% of the cohort) reporting vigorous sports (swimming, jogging, hill-climbing, rowing, soccer, and hockey (mostly refereeing), racket games, etc., at least twice a week), and/or rating the usual pace of their regular walking to and from work and in their leisure time as 'fast' (over 4 mph or 6.4 km/h), and/or recording considerable cycling. Group 2 comprises the next highest degree of such vigorous aerobic exercise, that is, vigorous sports at least once but less than twice a week, and/or 'fairly brisk' walking for over 30 min/day, and/or other cycling. Group 3 includes residual vigorous aerobic exercise, that is very little, occasional sports, and/or shorter 'fairly brisk' walks. Group 4, the largest, comprising just over half the men, is made up of those who reported no vigorous aerobic exercise. This category includes the very popular non-vigorous sports and games, the commoner regular walking at 'normal' pace or 'strolling', and a huge volume of recreational work in gardening and do-it-yourself, whether vigorous, moderate, or light.

Group 1 of the cohort had low CHD attack rates compared with the rest of the men ($p < 0.001$). This was evident in both non-fatal and fatal first clinical events. For younger men,

Table 19.2 Vigorous aerobic exercise, other CHD factors,[b] and the attack rate of CHD (1976–86) in male executive grade civil servants aged 55–64 at entry (rates per 1000 man-years)

	Group 1 (frequent vigorous aerobic exercise)	Group 2 (next lesser degree of this)	Group 3 (residual vigorous aerobic exercise)	Group 4 (no vigorous aerobic exercise)	p^a
Vigorous aerobic exercise	2.3	3.3	4.5	5.9	<0.001
Standardized for other factors	2.4	3.6	4.8	5.6	<0.005

Source: Morris *et al.* 1990.

Non-fatal first events, 55–59 years; fatal, 55–73 years.

[a] Tests for trend; tested for heterogeneity, the results are similar.

[b] Other factors, from data reported at entry, were premature parental mortality from CVD, stature, cigarette smoking, body mass index, history of high blood pressure, history of diabetes, positive/negative on LSHTM angina questionnaire (Rose and Blackburn 1968).

aged 45–54, there were no differences in attack rates among groups 2–4. However, the attack rate in entrants aged 55–64 was significantly lower in group 2 than in groups 3 and 4 ($p \approx 0.01$). Moreover, keep-fit exercises five or more times a week, and climbing 500 plus stairs each day – dynamic aerobic activities, plausibly vigorous items from the previous survey – which were not associated with incidence in the younger entrants did show significantly lower CHD rates in these older men. Therefore they have been included in group 2. This makes sense in terms of both the probable greater variability in intensity of these two activities on the one hand and the reduction with age of the oxygen utilization capacity of muscles on the other, so that less exercise is required for overload and a training stimulus (though of course it still has to be more intense than customary). The net result is that 30% of the older entrants showed such exercise-related reduction of heart disease.

In group 3 there is a non-significant continuation of the favourable trend in the older men. Thus there was some indication of dose – response of CHD with frequency/intensity in vigorous aerobic exercise. A threshold effect of such exercise alone is seen in the younger men, at the highest level of intensity that was identified (group 1). High coronary incidence at all ages was recorded in group 4.

Table 19.3 further illustrates the failure of popular non-vigorous sports and games (dancing was reported by 14% of the men and golf by 10%) to affect CHD rates. The outcome is similar with the quantity of regular walking if pace is disregarded. The negative findings with the detailed and more representative record in this survey of recreational work are clear; the results are the same for gardening. The situation chosen in Table 19.3 is that most likely to elicit association with coronary disease: first clinical events in men over 60 and the harder mortality data. At ages under 60 the results are the same for both non-fatal and fatal events. Because of the popularity and appeal of the non-vigorous sports and games, they were subjected to an intensive study, searching, for example, for possible associations with CHD in vulnerable groups such as cigarette smokers, the overweight, those with subclinical cardiovascular disease (CVD), and so on, which might be expected to show a response to such exercise of lower intensity. Again, none was found.

Table 19.3 Miscellaneous activities in leisure time and mortality from CHD in male executive grade civil servants (1976–86) aged 60–73 (rates per 1000 man-years)

Episodes in previous 4 weeks[a]	Ballroom dancing	Golf	Long walks[b]	Do-it-yourself		
				Heavy	Moderate	Light
0	4.2	4.2	4.4	4.3	4.2	4.0
1–3	4.3	4.0	3.8	3.9	3.9	3.6
4–7	5.5	5.1	4.1	4.7	5.4	5.1
≥8	(3.1)	6.2	4.2	6.5	3.4	4.6

Regular walking to and from work, and elsewhere, regardless of pace, per day: 0, 3.9 per 1000 man-years; ≤30 min, 4.2 per 1000 man-years; >30 min, 3.7 per 1000 man-years. (The 0 is an overstatement since episodes of activity <5 min were disregarded throughout.)

[a] Reported at entry in 1976. (Rates for less than five cases in brackets.)

[b] Walks of at least an hour, additional to 'regular' walking.

19.3.3 Multivariate analysis

The lower line of Table 19.2 controls for possible confounding by some CHD risk factors. The familiar dilemmas and limitations of such adjustment arise (Davey Smith and Phillips 1990), including circularity and double-counting of such factors as body mass, subclinical CVD (and blood cholesterol levels). These factors themselves are likely to be lowered by exercise, and may indeed be mechanisms of the effect of exercise on CHD. Therefore their introduction into the multivariate analysis may misleadingly reduce the value of the exercise factor itself in the outcome. This can be illustrated by data on 'personal control'.

In these men, there is a significant association between confidence in the possibility of personal control of future health and future coronary incidence. When the psychological variable is 'adjusted' for vigorous aerobic exercise, the association is considerably weakened, and if cigarette smoking is then introduced it disappears altogether. It is possible that this belief/attitude/knowledge is effectual through or mediated by these (and other health-directed) behaviours. This is attractive, but for understanding of aetiology – and for public health and its need to understand motives – how much is being lost by such computation and the summary dismissal of antecedent by later stages in the long natural history of CHD? (The difference in the precision of classification of exercise and smoking compared with that of the attitude, and how far this is responsible for the result, need not detain us now.)

Be all this as it may, the striking feature of Table 19.2 is the similarity of before and after profiles, again pointing to statistical independence of the exercise factor and some freedom from its confounding by the other factors studied. Of course, multivariate analyses are now ritual in epidemiological research, and in the relation between physical activity and CHD they have included all the standard risk factors and show the same general picture (Powell *et al.* 1987).

19.4 Overview

A few points can be made about some recent reports. First, a remarkable variety of populations have shown lower CHD rates with high physical activity. Thus the two most detailed studies are of elite affluent Harvard alumni (Paffenbarger *et al.* 1978) and our own British civil servants (social class II in the national scale) on modest incomes and generally without tertiary educational qualifications. The Finnish general population sample is from an area with a notably high prevalence of CHD (Salonen *et al.* 1988). The Honolulu Study follows a cohort of men of Japanese ancestry (Donahue *et al.* 1988). The Multiple Risk Factor Intervention Trial (MRFIT) is an experiment on American men selected for high risk of CHD by elevated lipid and blood pressure levels (Leon *et al.* 1987).

There are difficulties in interpreting discrepancies between the findings of these studies. Thus, in contrast with our findings, Paffenbarger *et al.* (1978) report substantial benefit from more than 2000 kcal per week of leisure time activity, however this is accomplished. On analysis, two-thirds of the men with such high totals engaged in vigorous sports, but those reporting other non-vigorous aerobic exercise also show some, albeit less, advantage. Could it be that the American cohort is basically less active and less fit than the British and thus capable of benefiting from less intense exercise? (The same point has previously been made on age.) Other obvious differences in the populations are that the British are subject to governmental medical recruitment and retirement policies, and that they are men actually in post and hence are a 'healthy worker' cohort. Comparative physiological studies on American and British men could be rewarding.

Another question arises with regard to the methods of assessment of physical activity that are being used and, in particular, on their probability of identifying training or conditioning exercise. Because of the frequency of do-it-yourself and gardening in our British study (90% of the men gardened and 80% reported moderate or heavy work), overall assessment of activity by totals of energy expenditure blur the picture: neither of these two classes of activity contain much of the sustained rhythmic contraction/relaxation of large muscle groups that is required for cardiorespiratory training. Again, as previously found, total physical activity estimates do not identify groups with different CHD risk in this population. Thus, in group 4, who reported no vigorous aerobic exercise, incidence rates per 1000 man-years by total physical activity in leisure time per week, summing all the forms previously considered, were as follows: <2000 kcal, 5.9; 2000–2999 kcal, 6.5; ≥3000 kcal, 7.0.

The other studies mentioned above are uniform and total in their assessments and do not seek to report predominantly aerobic exercise, vigorous or not, so that rival hypotheses can be tested. The fact that these studies produce positive results could mean that it is not training and fitness that matter but high total energy expenditure, thus refuting the British findings, or perhaps indicating that they apply only to a relatively healthy population. Alternatively, the overall profiles among those scoring high totals in these other studies may include enough vigorous aerobic exercise for benefit in their populations. It should be possible to disaggregate the data and extract such information. Highlighted by this discussion is the lack, exposed by the needs of epidemiological research, of physiological information on real-life everyday physical activities in leisure time (in people of disparate occupation): on caloric expenditures, dynamic/static, components, vascular reactions, metabolic responses, and short-, medium-, and long-term risk factor relationships. (The contrast with the richness of data on athletes and athleticism (Reilly *et al.* 1990) is striking.) Clinical and psychological data are frequently equally sparse.

19.5 Mechanisms of protection

With little qualification it can be said that exercise improves all physiological function, and of course there are also psychological and social benefits. In that sense exercise is a 'general cause' of good health (Morris 1975). Therefore, not surprisingly, major risk factors for CHD are liable to be diminished: lipid profiles, blood pressure, insulin sensitivity, glucose levels, and body mass (Powell *et al.* 1987; Fentem *et al.* 1988), At the same time, exercise both counteracts these risk factors and is some defence against them, as seen in the data previously given on smoking.

Table 19.4 History of exercise reported by male executive grade civil servants (1976–86)

	Cases 1976–86	Rate per 1000 man-years
Played no vigorous sports previously	128	5.7
Played up to 25 years of age	27	4.1
Played up to 30 years of age	54	6.4
Played up to 40 years of age	92	5.7
Played past 40 years of age	112	6.2

Thus it might be expected that coronary atherosclerosis will be retarded or reduced, but so far the evidence in humans is not impressive.

The more interesting suggestion in our study is that in such a different body of data it confirms and amplifies the observation by Paffenbarger *et al.* (1978) that, for benefit, the exercise has to be current. A history of exercise in the past, which has been abandoned, confers no protection. For example, Table 19.4 reports the experience among men who reported no vigorous sports in the 1976 survey. By the same token, men who reported taking part in vigorous sports in 1976 had the same low incidence over the period 1976–86 whether or not they had been 'athletic' when young (as attested by a record of the most vigorous sports such as squash, rugby, athletics, and wrestling). The future rates in men reporting vigorous sports at least once a week in 1976 were 3.2 and 3.0 per 1000 man-years, respectively, in those with and without such a record.

These observations point to the acute phases of the heart disease rather than the slow build-up of chronic coronary atherosclerosis as the main locus of protection by exercise: to acute ischaemia, thrombosis, occlusion, dysrhythmia and electrical instability. Evidence that exercise is related to improved haemostatic profile in particular is increasing (Davey Smith *et al.* 1989; Meade 1995). This is a field ripe for systematic study.

An alternative or complementary interpretation of the necessity for the exercise to be maintained is that the protection is related not so much to the exercise itself, for example the dynamic exercise that raises the level of high density lipoprotein cholesterol, as to the cardiorespiratory fitness and improved cardiac performance that is induced. It is well known that fitness cannot be stored; it depends on the maintenance of adequate aerobic exercise (Saltin *et al.* 1968). Studies of CHD incidence in relation to fitness are accumulating, mostly with positive results (Gyntelberg *et al.* 1980; Blair *et al.* 1989). A difficulty here is that endurance capacity or stamina, the manifestation of cardiorespiratory fitness likely to be most responsive to the exercise under consideration, cannot yet be readily measured in the field, and estimates of maximum aerobic power (VO_2 max) are not satisfactory substitutes. Interestingly, the association of cardiorespiratory fitness with CHD risk factors, as distinct from CHD incidence, is more controversial (Sedgwick *et al.* 1989, 1990; Bouchard *et al.* 1990*a*).

19.6 **Restatement of hypothesis**

The initial hypothesis has undergone several transformations in the course of its 40 years. It can now be stated as follows.

Adequate aerobic exercise in leisure time, which is habitual and ongoing, and the training and improved cardiorespiratory fitness and performance this produces, confer substantial protection against the occurrence of CHD in middle-aged and elderly men. The total death rate is also lowered. This is the case whatever the risk status of the men with respect to other factors. Protection by exercise is effectual mainly in the acute phases of the disease, in particular against thrombosis, though there is also some benefit from reducing and counteracting standard risk factors and the build-up of chronic coronary atherosclerosis.

In this statement 'adequate' refers to both vigour (intensity) and quantity (frequency/duration) of exercise. The hypothesis refers to ordinary relatively healthy men engaged in sedentary and physically light occupations, and not to athletes.

19.7 **From aetiology to public health**

There is now good reason to believe that the decline of physical activity in work, recreation, transport, and daily living is an integral part of the modern epidemic of CHD in developed industrial societies. This decline may well have been greatest in adequate aerobic exercise, and hence in cardiorespiratory fitness. Moreover, the increase in CHD has entailed an increase in coronary thrombosis – perhaps the main pathological change (Morris 1951) – and again a link with physical activity/inactivity can be postulated.

The UK is underachieving in several aspects of health, particularly in its persistent high rates of CHD, and the need to address major possible causes is now, at last, widely recognized. Exercise is today's best buy in public health, not only because of the need and potential, but because it is positive and acceptable, has insignificant side-effects, and can be inexpensive. Also, the opposition to be overcome is feeble in comparison with the tobacco barons and the Common Agricultural Policy, for instance.

In seminal papers, Rose (1981, 1985) has interpreted modern aetiological research for public health practice in the prevention of CHD. He describes two strategies: the individual high risk strategy involving case-finding and personal care, and the population strategy which, by attacking the causes of incidence, seeks to reduce the mean level of risk factors and 'to shift the whole distribution of exposure in a favourable direction'. Each has its advantages and its drawbacks, though there is no question about the importance of the population strategy for this mass scourge.

However, two points can be made in applying Rose's thesis to our present concern with exercise. Only a minority of the population takes anything worthy of the name of exercise, and only a small minority of the lower social classes that are most vulnerable to heart attack (*General Household Survey* 1989). Thus the majority, or the great majority, of the population is probably at high risk in these terms, and the approach to them and to the population at large must be much the same. Moreover, the 'prevention paradox' of the population strategy, that participating individuals will themselves derive little benefit from their contribution to the common good (for example by lowering their blood pressure), may not apply in the case of exercise. Altruistic participating individuals can be assured that by taking exercise, as encouraged, they will rapidly feel and function better as a result of the manifold benefits that exercise confers.

The evidence on CHD can be matched by that on the general benefits of exercise to physical capacity and mobility, mental and social function, and well-being, all perhaps most notably in the elderly; to the prevention of obesity, maturity onset diabetes, osteoporosis, and so on; and to the relief of anxiety and depression. Equally, benefits in the rehabilitation of chronic disease and in the life of people with disabilities could be included (Bouchard *et al.* 1990*b*). In the present chapter we have dealt with only one aspect.

19.7.1 **Practical application**

There are several practical messages for public health practice from the kind of positive and encouraging observations reported in the present chapter. The commitment to exercise manifestly has to be continuing and serious (Department of Health and Human Services 1980; American College of Sports Medicine 1986). Examples given here are vigorous aerobic exercise at least twice a week and the expenditure of more than 2000 kcal per week in leisure time activities. Therefore such a commitment has to be emphasized in health education. However, aetiological studies are urgently required in other social and occupational samples, particularly among the lower socio-economic groups, to aid the formulation of population strategy. Congruent with the physiology that, with adequate exercise, training is possible at all ages, there is encouragement for middle-aged men to start exercising and for the elderly to continue. Direct evidence on the former will soon be available (published by Paffenbarger 1993), and there is already some evidence of protection against CHD in the elderly (Donahue *et al.* 1988) and our own data for individuals up to 73 years of age.

19.7.2 **Individual and family, society and culture**

The appeal must be seen to apply to the whole population. At the same time exercise typifies the individual–social, personal–environmental, and private–public interactions and partnerships that health promotion and prevention of disease require today (Morris 1975). The individual takes exercise and can continue to do so. The individual alone can tell when he/she is taking enough exercise for 'overload' or too much for safety. We are slowly learning about individual and family motivations. However, culture and society have to reinforce motivation, help with education and research, and, above all, provide support with facilities. Among the civil servants in our study, swimming is the most popular and beneficial exercise: the provision of pools to generate and meet growing demand is under perennial threat from local government financial constraints. Similarly, both walking and cycling entail the partnership of individual and government; the latest British national plan to spend more than £12 billion on roads considers neither walking nor cycling.

The return of physical activity as the norm in everyone's everyday life – the 'restoration of biological normality' in Rose's words – will require cultural change on a scale similar to that which has occurred with smoking. Meanwhile, there is little advance among those who need it most. Hopefully, the findings of the National Fitness Survey (1990–91) may provide the impetus. The challenges to epidemiology are great: in a wide range of research, in information of the public, health service, and government, in teaching, in the example we set, and, as part of the wider public health movement, in our collective political message.

Acknowledgements

Readers of this account will know how much teamwork is required in these studies. I am deeply grateful to my colleagues for their contributions.

References

American College of Sports Medicine (1986). *Guidelines for exercise testing and prescription*, 3rd edn. Lea & Febiger, Philadelphia.

Blair, S. N., Kohl III, H. W., Paffenbarger, R. S., Jr, Clark, D. G., Cooper, K. H., and Gibbons, L. W. (1989). Physical fitness and all-cause mortality: a prospective study of healthy men and women. *Journal of the American Medical Association*, **262**, 2395–401.

Bouchard, C., Leon, A. S., Rao, D. C., Skinner, J. S., and Wilmore, J. H. (1990*a*). Cross-sectional and longitudinal relationships between physical fitness and risk factors for coronary heart disease in men and women: 'The Adelaide 1000'. *Journal of Clinical Epidemiology*, **43**, 1005–7.

Bouchard, C., Shephard, R. J., Stephens, T., Sutton, J. R., and McPherson, B. M. (eds) (1990*b*). *Exercise, fitness and health: a consensus of current knowledge*. Human Kinetics, Champaign, IL.

Davey Smith, G. and Phillips, A. (1990). Declaring independence: why we should be cautious. *Journal of Epidemiology Community Health*, **44**, 257–8.

Davey Smith, G., Marmot, M. G., Etherington, M., and O'Brien, J. (1989). A work stress-fibrinogen pathway as a potential mechanism for employment grade differences in coronary heart disease rates. [Abstracts.] 2nd International Conference on Preventive Cardiology, Washington, DC.

Department of Health and Human Services (1980). *Promoting health/preventing disease: objectives for the nation*. US Government Printing Office, Washington, DC.

Donahue, R. P., Abbott, R. D., Reed, D. M., and Yano, K. C. (1988). Physical activity and coronary heart disease in middle-aged and elderly men. *American Journal of Public Health*, **78**, 683–5.

Epstein, L., Miller, G. J., Stitt, F. W., and Morris, J. N. (1976). Vigorous exercise in leisure-time, coronary risk factors, and resting electrocardiogram in middle-aged male civil servants. *British Heart Journal*, **38**, 403–9.

Fentem, P. H., Bassey, E. J., and Turnbull, N. B. (1988). *The new case for exercise*. Health Education Authority and Sports Council, London.

General Household Survey 1986 (1989). HMSO, London.

Gyntelberg, F., Lauridsen, L., and Schubell, K. (1980). *Scandinavian Journal of Work and Environmental Health*, **6**, 170–8.

Heady, J. A., Morris, J. N., Kagan, A., and Raffle, P. A. B. (1961). Coronary heart disease in London busmen: a progress report with particular reference to physique. *British Journal of Preventive Social Medicine*, **15**, 143–53.

Kristensen, T. S. (1989). Cardiovascular diseases and the work environment. *Scandinavian Journal of Work and Environmental Health*, **15**, 165–79.

Leon, A. S., Connett, J., Jacobs, D. R., Jr, and Rauramaa, R. (1987). Leisure-time physical activity levels and risk of coronary heart disease and death. *Journal of the American Medical Association*, **258**, 2388–95.

Meade, T. W. (1995). Exercise and haemostatic function. *Journal of Cardiovascular Risk*, **2**, 323–9.

Morris, J. N. (1951). Recent history of coronary disease. *Lancet*, **i**, 1–7, 69–73.

Morris, J. N. (1975). *Uses of epidemiology*, 3rd edn. Churchill Livingstone, London (reprinted 1983).

Morris, J. N., Heady, J. A., Raffle, P. A. B., and Parks, J. W. (1953). Coronary heart disease and physical activity of work. *Lancet*, **ii**, 1053–7, 1111–20.

Morris, J. N., Chave, S. P. W., Adam, C., Sirey, C., and Epstein, L. (1973). Vigorous exercise in leisure-time and the incidence of coronary heart disease. *Lancet*, **i**, 333–9.

Morris, J. N., Everitt, M. G., Pollard, R., Chave, S. P. W., and Semmence, A. M. (1980). Vigorous exercise in leisure-time: protection against coronary heart disease. *Lancet*, **ii**, 1207–10.

Morris, J. N., Clayton, D. G., Everitt, M. G., Semmence, A. M., and Burgess, E. H. (1990). Exercise in leisure-time: coronary attack and death rate. *British Heart Journal*, **63**, 325–34.

Paffenbarger, R. S., Jr, Hyde, R. T., Wing, A. L., Lee, I. M., Jung, D. L., and Kampert, J. B. (1993). The association of changes in physical-activity level and other lifestyle characteristics with mortality among men. *New England Journal of Medicine*, **382**, 538–45.

Paffenbarger, R. S., Jr, Laughlin, M. E., Gima, A. S., and Black, R. A. (1970). Work activity of longshoremen as related to death from coronary heart disease and stroke. *New England Journal of Medicine*, **282**, 1109–13.

Paffenbarger, R. S., Jr, Wing, A. L., and Hyde, R. T. (1978). Physical activity as an index of heart attack risk in college alumni. *American Journal of Epidemiology*, **108**, 161–75.

Pollock, M. and Wilmore, J. H. (1990). *Exercise in health and disease*, 2nd edn. W. B. Saunders, Philadelphia.

Powell, K. E., Thompson, P. D., Caspersen, C. J., and Kendrick, J. S. (1987). Physical activity and the incidence of coronary heart disease. *Annual Review of Public Health*, **8**, 251–87.

Reilly, T., Secher, N., Snell, P., and Williams, C. (eds) (1990). *Physiology of sports*. Spon, London.

Rose, G. (1981). Strategy of prevention: lessons from cardiovascular disease. *British Medical Journal*, **282**, 1847–51.

Rose, G. (1985). Sick individuals and sick populations. *International Journal of Epidemiology*, **14**, 32–8.

Rose, G. and Blackburn, H. (1968). *Cardiovascular survey methods*. World Health Organization, Geneva.

Salonen, J. T., Slater, J. S., Tuomilehto, J., and Rauramaa, R. (1988). Leisure-time and occupational physical activity: risk of death from ischaemic heart disease. *American Journal of Epidemiology*, **127**, 87–94.

Saltin, B., Blomquist, G., Mitchell, J. H., Johnson, R. L., Wildenthal, K., and Chapman, C. B. (1968). Response to exercise after bed rest and after training. *Circulation*, **38** (Suppl. VII), 1–77.

Sedgwick, A. W., Thomas, D. W., Davies, M., Baghurst, K., and Rouse, I. (1989). Cross-sectional and longitudinal relationships between physical fitness and risk factors for coronary heart disease in men and women: 'The Adelaide 1000'. *Journal of Clinical Epidemiology*, **42**, 189–200.

Sedgwick, A. W., Thomas, D. W., Davies, M., Baghurst, K., and Rouse, I. (1990). Cross-sectional and longitudinal relationships between physical fitness and risk factors for coronary heart disease in men and women: 'The Adelaide 1000'. *Journal of Clinical Epidemiology*, **43**, 1007–12.

Addendum to Chapter 19

W. L. Haskell

19.1 Introduction

Slightly more than 50 years have passed since Professor Morris first proposed his 'heart attack protection through physical activity' hypothesis based on data collected from workers employed by the Transport Executive, Postal Service and other government offices in London (Morris *et al.* 1953). The author's interpretation of the data supporting this original hypothesis was that the total amount of occupational physical activity performed by healthy men in middle age was important in providing protection against CHD. However, based on data from a later survey of non-occupational physical activity in upper-grade civil servant workers (all with sedentary jobs), a revision in the hypothesis was made which focused on the need for ongoing vigorous aerobic exercise for protection against CHD (Morris *et al.* 1973). In this chapter by Morris, the major results from these landmark studies are summarized and their implication for public health action are well stated. Included in the chapter is a discussion that includes a great deal of what is now considered 'known' about the relation between habitual physical activity and CHD. This addendum will focus primarily on studies published over the past decade that shed additional light on the potential protective effects of physical activity for CHD, other selected chronic diseases and all-cause mortality.

19.2 Confirmation of the general hypothesis in middle-aged men

In addition to the continued research by Morris and colleagues, numerous other reports have been published since the early 1960s, with data confirming an inverse relationship between the amount of habitual activity performed (or estimated energy expenditure during activity) and CHD, cardiovascular disease (CVD) or all-cause mortality (Taylor *et al.* 1962; Paffenbarger and Hale 1975; Leon *et al.* 1987; Shaper and Wannamethee 1991). Several meta-analyses of prospective observational studies investigating physical activity and CHD, mainly in middle-aged men, have concluded that more active men experience significantly lower age-adjusted rates of CHD and all-cause mortality, with adjusted mortality rates for 'moderately' active men generally being 20–30% less than that experienced by the least active men (Powell *et al.* 1987; Berlin and Colditz 1990; Williams 2001). Some of the earlier studies classified men by occupation (longshoremen vs. clerks, postal carriers vs. postal clerks, railroad yardmen vs. clerks) while more recent studies (after1970) have primarily used questionnaires to obtain either 'leisure-time' (non-occupational) or total daily physical activity. In attempts to establish that physical activity causes a reduction in CHD, various analytical procedures have been used to eliminate people with disease at study entry, adjust for the effects of other risk factors, exclude early cases from the analysis, and attempt to relate a change in activity or fitness with CHD and all-cause mortality (Paffenbarger *et al.* 1993; Blair *et al.* 1995; Wannamethee and Shaper 1998).

19.3 **Expansion of the hypothesis to women and older men**

Up until the mid-1980s, studies investigating the relationship between habitual physical activity and CHD or all-cause mortality enrolled almost exclusively Caucasian men, with most being 65 years of age or younger at study entry. More recently, a number of published studies have included data on women and older men. Most studies have reported lower non-fatal and fatal CHD rates in the more active women (Kushi *et al.* 1997; Lee *et al.* 2001; Manson *et al.* 2002). In a majority of these studies involving women, physical activity has been assessed by questionnaires that evaluate non-occupational (leisure-time) physical activity. As with the earlier and concurrent studies of middle-aged men, the inverse associations between amount of physical activity and CHD incidence or all-cause mortality appear dose-dependent and largely independent of other personal characteristics or risk factors. For example, in the Women's Health Study Observational Cohort, the age-adjusted relative risk for non-fatal and fatal CHD by quintile of total activity expressed as MET hours (energy expenditure measured in metabolic equivalents) per week (low to high activity) were 1.0, 0.73 (95% CI: 0.53–0.99), 0.69 (0.53–0.99), 0.68 (0.50–0.96), and 0.47 (0.33–0.67) with the p value for trend <0.001 (Manson *et al.* 2002). Lee and colleagues observed similar results in a cohort of 39 372 healthy female health professionals aged 45 years and older living in the United States based on a questionnaire of non-occupational physical activity. Expressing activity as kilocalories per week, the risk ratios were 1.00 for <200; 0.59 (0.2–0.81) for 200–599; 0.42 (0.30–0.60) for 600–1499, and 0.51 (0.35–0.73) for ≥ 1500 kcal/week (p for trend <0.001) (Lee *et al.* 2001).

A number of studies have reported that the 'protective effect' of activity for CHD and all-cause mortality previously observed for middle-aged men also exists for men who were greater than 65 years old at study entry. For example, Dutch men aged 64–84 who reported spending more time performing physical activity had lower CHD, CVD, and all-cause mortality rates than those reporting less activity (Bijnen et al. 1998). CHD, CVD, stroke, and all-cause mortality were lower in the men in the middle and highest tirtiles of activity than those in the lowest tirtile (p for trend for these clinical outcomes ranged from 0.04 to <0.01).

19.4 **Use of cardiorespiratory fitness measures to support the hypothesis**

Habitual physical activity consists of a very complex set of behaviours that are difficult to accurately and reliably measure in large free-living populations. An alternative measurement is cardiorespiratory fitness, which can place people quite accurately and reliably into 'fitness' categories. It is well-established that such measures of fitness are determined in part by habitual level of activity (especially vigorous aerobic exercise), but also by heredity and other personal characteristics (age, gender, cigarette smoking, body composition). Standardized measurements of cardiorespiratory fitness have high subject and staff burden and thus have been performed in only a limited number of large population studies. The results of these studies have consistently supported the conclusion that men who have the lowest level of fitness have the highest rates of CHD and all-cause mortality. For example, in the first report on this relationship by Ekelund and colleagues the CHD, CVD, and all-cause mortality rates were significantly higher in unfit versus fit men, with adjusted relative risks somewhat higher for men with CVD diagnosed at baseline compared to healthy men (Ekelund *et al.* 1988). Blair and colleagues, using the Aerobics Center Longitudinal Study database, have repeatedly reported that healthy men and women who are least fit have higher rates of CHD, CVD, and all-cause mortality than even slightly more fit peers, with higher levels of fitness associated with even lower risk (Blair *et al.* 1989, 1996). That fitness level is predictive for future CHD clinical events in men with disease at study entry as well as for those with no evidence of disease has been demonstrated in several populations (Ekelund *et al.* 1988; Myers *et al.* 2002). While absolute clinic event rates are higher for patients with disease compared with those free of disease, the magnitude of the relationship between fitness level and clinical events appears similar between the two populations (Myers *et al.* 2002).

19.5 Possible mechanisms of action

Morris comments in the chapter on the value of knowing the biological mechanisms by which activity provides some protection against CHD, especially to help understand the characteristics of the activity that contribute to the benefit. He points out that there is good evidence that habitual activity of adequate amount and intensity improves a number of CHD risk factors that contribute to the progression of coronary atherosclerosis (e.g. obesity, blood pressure, high-density lipoprotein cholesterol (HDL-C), triglycerides, insulin action, fibrinolytic activity), but little direct evidence that activity decreases its development or progression. In fact, one of few studies to provide data on this issue was published by Morris and Crawford in 1958; when they reported on the autopsy results from the hearts of 3800 men who died suddenly but not from CVD (Morris and Crawford 1958). They observed that men who had jobs requiring heavy physical activity had significantly less 'ischaemic myocardial fibrosis' than men in jobs requiring light work, but that there was no significant relationship between activity of work and degree of coronary atherosclerosis. These results support the hypothesis that increased physical activity reduces CHD clinical events by processes other than, or in addition to, a decrease in the development of coronary atherosclerosis. Included here could be an increase in coronary artery size (angiogenesis), artery dilating capacity or myocardial efficiency (less oxygen required for the same total body work), and plaque stabilization. Any such change in response to an increase in activity could contribute to less myocardial damage and fewer CHD clinical events independent of a change in coronary atherosclerosis. Variable results have been obtained in different studies when adjustments were made for biological risk factors, frequently improved by an increase in activity and causally linked to the progression of atherosclerosis (body mass index, blood pressure, HDL-C, triglycerides). In some cases such adjustments have meaningfully reduced the relation between activity and CHD mortality, suggesting that activity might be working through these variables to reduce atherosclerosis, but in other studies such adjustments have had little or no effect on the relationship.

19.6 The issue of total amount of activity versus the need for intensity

An issue raised by Morris, as he continued to formulate his hypothesis, was that of the required intensity of the physical activity to achieve benefit. When initially evaluating occupational physical activity he hypothesized that total amount of activity (e.g. hours per week) was the important parameter, but later when evaluating non-occupational activity he concluded that 'vigorous' intensity was important. This issue has not yet been fully resolved, but it appears that both amount and intensity are important in providing protection against CHD. In a few recently published studies only activity classified as 'vigorous' appears to provide some protection against CHD (Yu *et al.* 2003), while others have demonstrated that brisk walking (considered moderate intensity at 4.8–6.4 km/hr) has a very similar inverse association with CHD or all-cause mortality as does vigorous or total activity (Lee *et al.* 2001; Manson *et al.* 2002). Several continuing problems complicating a comparative analysis across studies of the characteristics of activity needed for some CHD protection include non-standardization of activity classification by intensity, differences in the overall activity levels within each population, and the continued decline of habitual activity (occupational, leisure time, household, and transportation) in many populations. Also, other CHD risk factors that physical activity may interact with to provide some protection against CHD (obesity, lipoprotein profile, insulin resistance, etc.) vary from population to population and are changing over time.

19.7 **A new challenge: expanding the activity hypothesis to other chronic diseases**

While data will continue to be collected refining the Morris activity–CHD hypothesis, a major research challenge is to determine if low levels of habitual physical activity significantly contribute to other chronic diseases that inflict disability and premature mortality on large portions of many populations. For example, some prospective population studies have shown significant inverse associations between amount of activity and stroke (Lee *et al.* 2003), type II diabetes mellitus (Hu *et al.* 1999), and certain site-specific cancers (Thune and Furberg 2001). Many of these results are considered preliminary because of relatively few clinical events; they need verification in studies with more cases, where data on potentially confounding variables are collected and possible mechanisms of action investigated. Professor Morris and colleagues were successful in establishing and refining the physical activity–CHD hypothesis because of their use of sound epidemiological research methodology, persistence at addressing a number of issues raised by the hypothesis as it evolved, and their ability to collect, analyse, and interpret complex data. It will take similar approaches to determine if the activity–CHD hypothesis can appropriately be extended to these other chronic diseases.

References

Berlin, J. A. and Colditz, G. A. (1990). A meta-analysis of physical activity in the prevention of coronary heart disease. *American Journal of Epidemiology*, **132**, 612–28.

Bijnen, F. C. H., Casperson, C. J., Feshens, E. J. M., Saris, W. H. M., Mostera, W. L., and Kromhout, D. (1998). Physical activity and 10-year mortality from cardiovascular disease and all-causes: The Zutphen Elderly Study. *Archives of Internal Medicine*, **158**, 1499–1505.

Blair, S. N., Kohl, H. W., Paffenbarger, R. S., Clark, D. G., Cooper, K. H., and Gibbons, L. W. (1989). Physical fitness and all-cause mortality: a prospective study in healthy men and women. *Journal of the American Medical Association*, **262**, 2395–401.

Blair, S. N., Kohl, H. W., Barlow, C. E., Paffenbarger, R. S., Gibbons, L. W., and Macera, C. A. (1995). Changes in physical fitness and all-cause mortality. *Journal of the American Medical Association*, **273**, 1093–8.

Blair, S. N., Kampert, J. B., Kohl, H. W., Barlow, C. E., Macera, C. A., Paffenbarger, R. S., and Gibbons, L. W. (1996). Influences of cardiorespiratory fitness and other precursors on cardiovascular disease and all-cause mortality in men and women. *Journal of the American Medical Association*, **276**, 205–10.

Ekelund, L-G., Haskell, W. L., Johnson, J. L., Whaley, F. S., Criqui, M. H., and Sheps, D. S. (1988). Physical fitness as a predictor of cardiovascular mortality in asymptomatic North American men. *New England Journal of Medicine*, **319**, 1379–84.

Hu, F. B., Sigal, R. J., Rich-Edwards, J. W., Colidtz, G. A., Solomon, C. G., Willet, W. C. *et al.* (1999). Walking compared to vigorous physical activity and risk of type 2 diabetes in women: a prospective study. *Journal of the American Medical Association*, **282**, 1433–9.

Kushi, L. H., Fee, R. M., Folsom, A. R., Mink, P. J., Anderson, K. E., and Sellers, T. A. (1997). Physical activity and mortality in postmenopausal women. *Journal of the American Medical Association*, **277**, 1287–92.

Lee, C-D., Folsom, A. R., and Blair, S. N. (2003). Physical activity and stroke risk: a meta-analysis. *Stroke*, **34**, 2475–82.

Lee, I-M., Rexode, K. M., Cook, N. R., Manson, J. E., and Buring, J. F. (2001). Physical activity and coronary heart disease in women: is 'no pain, no gain', passé? *Journal of the American Medical Association*, **285**, 1447–54.

Leon, A. S., Connett, J., Jacobs, D. R., and Rauramaa, R. (1987). Leisure-time physical activity levels and risk of coronary heart disease and death: The Multiple Risk Factor Intervention Trial. *Journal of the American Medical Association*, **258**, 2388–95.

Manson, J. E., Greenland, P., LaCroix, A. Z., Stefanick, M. L., Mounton, C. P., Oberman, A. *et al.* (2002). Walking compared with vigorous exercise for the prevention of cardiovascular disease in women. *New England Journal of Medicine*, **347**, 716–25.

Morris, J. N. and Crawford, M. D. (1958). Coronary heart disease and physical activity of work: evidence of a national necropsy survey. *British Medical Journal*, **ii**, 1485–96.

Morris, J. N., Heady, J. A., Raffle, P. A. B., Roberts, C. G., and Parks, J. W. (1953). Coronary heart disease and physical activity of work. *Lancet*, **ii**, 1053–7, 1111–20.

Morris, J. N., Chave, S. P. W., Adam, C., Sirey, C., Epstein, L., and Sheehan, D. J. (1973). Vigorous exercise in leisure-time and the incidence of coronary heart disease. *Lancet*, **ii**, 333–9.

Myers, J., Prakash, M., Froelicher, V., Do, D., Partington, S., and Atwood, J. E. (2002). Exercise capacity and mortality among men referred for exercise testing. *New England Journal of Medicine*, **346**, 793–801.

Paffenbarger, R. S. and Hale, W. (1975). Work activity and coronary heart mortality. *New England Journal of Medicine*, **292**, 545–50.

Paffenbarger, R. S., Hyde, R. T., Wing, A. L., Lee, I-M., Jung, D. L., and Kampert, J. B. (1993). The association of changes in physical activity level and other lifestyle characteristics with mortality among men. *New England Journal of Medicine*, **328**, 538–45.

Powell, K. E., Thompson, P. D., Casperson, C. J., and Kendrick, J. S. (1987). Physical activity and the incidence of coronary heart disease. *Annual Review of Public Health*, **8**, 253–87.

Shaper, A. G. and Wannamethee, G. (1991). Physical activity and ischaemic heart disease in middle-aged British men. *British Heart Journal*, **66**, 384–94.

Taylor, H. L., Klepetar, E., Keys, A., Parlin, W., Blackburn, H., and Puchner, T. (1962). Death rates among physically active and sedentary employees of the railroad industry. *American Journal of Public Health*, **52**, 1697–707.

Thune, I. and Furberg, A-S. (2001). Physical activity and cancer risk: dose-response and cancer, all sites and site-specific. *Medicine and Science in Sports and Exercise*, **33** (Suppl.), S530–S550.

Wannamethee, S. G. and Shaper, A. G. (1998). Changes in physical activity, mortality and incidence of coronary heart disease in older men. *Lancet*, **351**, 1603–8.

Williams, P. T. (2001). Physical fitness and activity as separate heart disease risk factors: a meta-analysis. *Medicine and Science in Sports and Exercise*, **33**, 754–61.

Yu, Y., Yarnell, J. W., Sweetnam, P. M., and Murray, L. (2003). What level of physical activity protects against premature cardiovascular death? The Caerphilly study. *Heart*, **89**, 502–6.

Chapter 20

Obesity

A. R. Dyer, J. Stamler, and P. Greenland

20.1 Definitions of obesity and overweight

Obesity is a chronic disease defined as 'excess body fat relative to weight' (Foreyt and St Jeor 1997). The World Health Organization (WHO) (WHO 1997a) and the US National Institutes of Health (NHLBI Obesity Task Force 1998) define obesity based on the body mass index (BMI), a measure of weight corrected for height that is strongly correlated with body fat. The BMI is expressed as weight in kilograms divided by height in meters squared (kg/m^2). Overweight is defined as a BMI of 25–29.9 kg/m^2 and obesity as a BMI $\geq$ 30 kg/m^2. These categories are not mutually exclusive, however, since obese men and women are also overweight. A BMI of 30 is ~13.6 kg (30 lb) overweight and equivalent to 94.8 kg (209 lb) in a 1.78 m (5'10") man or to 79.4 kg (175 lb) in a 1.63 m (5'4") woman.

20.2 Trends in obesity

Obesity and overweight represent an escalating epidemic (WHO 1997b). In 1995, WHO estimated that there were 250 million obese adults worldwide, with the number increasing to more than 300 million in 2000 (WHO 2002a, b), including 115 million in developing countries. The increase to 300 million occurred 25 years sooner than projected, since in 1998 WHO had projected that the number of obese persons worldwide would not reach 300 million until 2025 (Visscher and Seidell 2001).

The prevalence of obesity varies widely among countries. In the WHO MONICA Project (Molarius *et al.* 2000), the prevalence of obesity in persons aged 35–64 ranged from 3–22% in men and from 10–43% in women at the first survey in 1979–89, and from 4–24% in men and from 8–43% in women at the second survey in 1989–96. It is estimated that the prevalence of obesity in Europe is ~10–20% in adult men and 15–25% in adult women (Seidell and Flegal 1997). The highest rates in the world are seen in Melanesians, Micronesians, and Polynesians (WHO 1997b). Up to 70% of women and 65% of men on the island of Nauru in Micronesia have a BMI between 30.0 and 34.9 kg/m^2. In a study of obesity among women aged 15–49 from developing countries (Martorell *et al.* 2000), the percentage of obese women was 0.1% in South Asia, 2.5% in sub-Saharan Africa, 9.6% in Latin America and the Caribbean, 15.4% in Central Eastern Europe, 17.2% in the Middle East and North Africa, and 20.7% in the US.

The prevalence of obesity is rising in most countries. Between the first and second surveys of the WHO MONICA Project (Molarius *et al.* 2000), prevalence increased in 21 of 26 population samples for men and 17 of 26 for women. In the US, data from national surveys indicate that the prevalence of obesity increased from 12.8 to 22.5% between 1960 and 1994 in adults aged 20–74 (NHLBI Obesity Task Force 1998). Data from the Behavioral Risk Factor Surveillance

System (Mokdad *et al.* 2001) indicate that the prevalence continued to rise throughout the 1990s, with an increase of 61% between 1991 and 2000.

Childhood obesity is also considered to be at epidemic proportions (Rocchini 2002; Strauss and Pollack 2001). Worldwide, approximately 22 million children under 5 years of age are overweight (Deckelbaum and Williams 2001). In the US, the number of overweight children has more than doubled in the last 30 years (Rocchini 2002). Between 1983 and 2000, the percentage of US preschool children categorized as overweight increased from 18.6 to 22.0% and the percentage categorized as obese increased from 8.5 to 10.0% (Deckelbaum and Williams 2001). Increases have been greater in African-Americans and Hispanic Americans than in whites (Strauss and Pollack 2001). The prevalence of overweight and obesity in children is also increasing in other countries. Between 1993 and 1997, the prevalence of overweight in Montreal children aged 10–12 increased at a rate of 1.3% per year, and the prevalence of obesity increased at a rate of 1.0% per year (O'Laughlin *et al.* 2000). In Australia (Margaray *et al.* 2001), the prevalence of overweight increased in boys from 9.3 to 15.0% between 1985 and 1995, and the prevalence in girls increased from 10.6 to 15.8%. Over the same period, the prevalence of obesity increased from 1.7 to 4.5% in boys and from 1.6 to 5.3% in girls.

20.3 Obesity and CHD risk

Both overweight and obesity are strongly associated with numerous cardiovascular disease (CVD) risk factors, including elevated levels of serum total cholesterol (TC), low-density lipoprotein cholesterol (LDL-C), triglycerides, blood pressure, fibrinogen, C-reactive protein, and insulin resistance or frank diabetes (NHLBI Obesity Task Force 1998; Stamler 1993; Stamler *et al.* 1998). Obesity and overweight are also associated with lower levels of the 'protective' CVD risk factor, high-density lipoprotein cholesterol (HDL-C) (NHLBI Obesity Task Force 1998). Thus, overweight and obesity would be expected to have important consequences on CVD morbidity and mortality.

Despite these strong and consistent associations of overweight and obesity with CVD risk factors, results of studies of the association of body weight, particularly as measured by BMI, with CVD and/or CHD mortality have not always been concordant with expectations (Barrett-Connor 1985; Manson *et al.* 1987). While many studies have shown significantly positive associations (Barrett-Connor *et al.* 1984; Cambien *et al.* 1985; Cochrane *et al.* 1980; Dorn *et al.* 1997; Dyer *et al.* 2004; Fitzgerald and Jarrett 1992; Garfinkel and Stellman 1988; Garn *et al.* 1983; Hubert *et al.* 1983; Jarrett *et al.* 1982; Johnson *et al.* 1986; Jousilahti *et al.* 1996; Lew and Garfinkel 1979; Manson *et al.* 1995; Prineas *et al.* 1993; Pyorala *et al.* 1979; Rabkin *et al.* 1977; Seidell *et al.* 1996; Selmer and Tverdal 1995; Semenciw *et al.* 1988; Shaper *et al.* 1997; Spataro *et al.* 1996; Stevens *et al.* 1992; Terry *et al.* 1992; Wilcosky *et al.* 1990; Yano *et al.* 1984), some of these same studies, as well as others, have also shown non-significant positive associations (Barrett-Connor *et al.* 1984; Dorn *et al.* 1997; Dyer *et al.* 2004; Hubert *et al.* 1983; Jarrett *et al.* 1982; Jousilahti *et al.* 1996; Prineas *et al.* 1993; Stevens *et al.* 1992; Terry *et al.* 1992; Wilcosky *et al.* 1990; Yao *et al.* 1991), no association (Cambien *et al.* 1985; Dorn *et al.* 1997; Dyer *et al.* 2004; Jarrett *et al.* 1982; Johnson *et al.* 1986; Jousilahti *et al.* 1996; Keys *et al.* 1984; Prineas *et al.* 1993; Rabkin *et al.* 1977; Rissanen *et al.* 1991; Semenciw *et al.* 1988), non-significant negative associations (Dorn *et al.* 1997; Dyer *et al.* 2004; Wilcosky *et al.* 1990; Yano *et al.* 1984), J-shaped associations (Dyer *et al.* 2004; Garfinkel and Stellman 1988; Jarrett *et al.* 1982; Jousilahti *et al.* 1996; Lew and Garfinkel 1979; Rissanen *et al.* 1989, 1991; Selmer and Tverdal 1995; Seidell *et al.* 1996; Semenciw *et al.* 1988; Shaper *et al.* 1997; Waaler 1984), U-shaped associations (Dyer *et al.* 1975, 2004; Fitzgerald and Jarrett 1992; Hanson *et al.* 1995; Harris *et al.* 1988; Lew and Garfinkel 1979; Rissanen *et al.* 1989; Rumpel *et al.* 1993; Seidell *et al.* 1996; Semenciw *et al.* 1988; Spataro *et al.* 1996), and in one instance a significant inverse association (Yao *et al.* 1991).

While some of the non-significant positive associations are likely due to low power, some investigators and review groups have suggested that the absence of a direct relation of body weight with mortality in many studies may be due to methodological problems (Manson *et al.* 1987; NHLBI Obesity Task Force 1998). The most frequently cited problems include: (a) failure to control for the confounding effect of cigarette smoking, which is generally associated with lower BMI; (b) 'inappropriate' control (or over-control) for biological effects of obesity, such as high blood pressure, elevated TC, and diabetes, all likely intermediates in the causal pathway; and (c) failure to eliminate early deaths (e.g. in the first 5 years) from the analysis, resulting in influences of disease on weight (i.e., weight loss) being evaluated in addition to effect of usual weight (Lee *et al.* 1993; Manson *et al.* 1987; NHLBI Obesity Task Force 1998). Other studies have also found weight to be related to CVD and/or CHD mortality only in the later years of long-term follow-up, for example, in years 15–22 in 22-year follow-up in the Western Electric Study (Spataro *et al.* 1996), and in the third decade of follow-up in a Finnish Study (Pekkanen *et al.* 1993). These studies suggest that the lack of long-term follow-up may also contribute to an underestimate of the impact of body weight on mortality.

We previously examined the importance of long-term follow-up (25 years) and the role of the three methodologicalal problems in associations of BMI with 25-year CVD mortality in men and women aged 18–39, 40–9, 50–9, and 60–74 from the Chicago Heart Association (CHA) Detection Project in Industry (Dyer *et al.* 2004). In 25-year follow-up with exclusion of deaths for 0–15 years, there was a positive association in all subcohorts, with seven significant, both with and without adjustment for smoking and obesity-related risk factors (systolic blood pressure (SBP), TC, diabetes). In contrast, with adjustment for obesity-related risk factors and no exclusion of early deaths in shorter-term (15-year) follow-up, there were two non-significant positive associations, three non-significant inverse associations, one significant positive association, and one significant quadratic association. These results clearly demonstrate that failure to address potential methodological problems and lack of long-term follow-up can substantially alter associations in BMI-mortality studies and may contribute to observed differences among studies.

We here examine the associations of BMI with 27-year CHD mortality in the same eight age–gender subcohorts from the CHA study to further illustrate how lack of long-term follow-up and failure to address the three methodological problems can impact findings on associations of BMI with CVD and CHD mortality.

20.4 The Chicago Heart Association Detection Project in Industry Study

Methods of the CHA study have been described (Stamler *et al.* 1975*a*, *b*, 1993). Briefly, 39 522 employed men and women aged 18 years and older at 84 companies and institutions in the Chicago area were surveyed between November 1967 and January 1973. Vital status was ascertained through 1997, with mean follow-up of 27 years. Underlying cause of death was coded using the Eighth Revision of the *International Classification of Diseases* (ICD-8), adapted for the United States (National Center for Health Statistics 1967), with CHD mortality defined as ICD-8 codes 410.0–414.9.

Two types of analyses on associations of BMI with CHD mortality are shown by sex for those ages 18–39, 40–9, 50–9, and 60–74 at baseline. First, BMI was divided into quintiles separately for each subcohort and three proportional hazards (Cox) regression models computed for two periods of follow-up: 0–15 years and 16–27 years. Model I included variables for BMI quintiles, age, ethnicity (black or non-black), and cigarettes/day. Model II removed cigarettes/day from Model I to assess impact of adjustment for smoking. Model III added SBP, serum TC, and clinical diagnosis of diabetes mellitus (yes/no) to Model II to assess impact of adjustment for variables pathogenetically related to obesity. Results for 16–27-year follow-up represent the impact of long-term follow-up, while Model III results for 0–15-year follow-up represent the impact of failure to address any of the methodological issues. In the second type of analysis, BMI was included as a continuous variable in each of the above models for each period of follow-up.

20.4.1 Associations of BMI with other risk factors

In CHA men and women, differences in mean BMI between the normal weight (BMI < 25 kg/m²) and obese (BMI ≥ 30 kg/m²) categories are 9–10 kg/m² for men and 1–13 kg/m² for women (Table 20.1). Mean SBP and diastolic blood pressure (DBP) increase progressively across the three categories, with differences between normal and obese categories of 11–16 mmHg for SBP and 6–10 mmHg for DBP. Mean serum TC is lowest in the normal category for all subcohorts, with differences between the normal and obese categories ranging from 0.2 mg/dl in women 60–74 to 20 mg/dl in men 18–39. Prevalence of diabetes is highest in the obese category for all subcohorts. Prevalence of smoking is highest in the normal category for seven subcohorts and lowest in the obese for all six subcohorts aged 40–74, with differences of 10–17% between the normal and obese categories in these six.

Observed differences in these risk factors by level of BMI clearly show that failure to adjust for cigarette smoking will result in underestimating associations between BMI and CHD mortality in these men and women, and that adjustment for SBP or DBP, serum TC, and diabetes can be expected to weaken associations.

20.4.2 BMI and CHD mortality

In 15-year follow-up, with adjustment for age, ethnicity, and smoking (Model I), BMI is positively and significantly related to CHD mortality in men 50–9 and 60–74, and in women 40–9, with hazard ratios of 1.16, 1.28, and 1.55 for BMI higher by one SD (Tables 20.2 and 20.3). In men 18–39 there is a non-significant positive association, and in women 50–9 and 60–74 there is a non-significant increase in risk in the fifth quintile, that is, hazard ratios of 1.69 and 1.79 relative to the first quintile.

With adjustment for age and ethnicity but not smoking (Model II), all hazard ratios are reduced relative to Model I. However, the hazard ratios for men 50–9 and 60–74 and women 40–9 for BMI higher by one SD are still significantly different from 1.0. Further, except for women 40–9, where mortality increases progressively from the first through fifth quintiles, all of the other subcohorts have one or more quintiles with hazard ratios less than 1.0, and for women 50–9 and 60–74 the second through fourth quintiles all show lower mortality relative to the first quintile.

As expected, addition of SBP, TC, and diabetes to Model II (Model III) for 15-year follow-up further weakens associations for all seven age–gender subcohorts. Compared to Model II, hazard ratios for the fifth quintile decrease from 1.48 to 0.57 (ages 18–39), 1.25 to 0.82

Table 20.1 Means or percentaged for study variables by age, gender, and BMI category: 38 379 men and women aged 18–74 at baseline in 1967–73, Chicago Heart Association Detection Project in Industry

Variable	BMI category[a]			All
	Normal	Overweight	Obese	
Men aged 18–39 (n = 11 106)				
BMI (kg/m^2)	22.8	27.1	32.7	26.0 ± 3.7
SBP (mmHg)	130.6	135.7	143.5	134.5 ± 15.4
DBP (mmHg)	75.3	79.1	84.4	78.1 ± 10.5
Serum TC (mg/dl)	180.3	195.9	200.1	189.9 ± 36.3
Diabetes (%)	1.2	0.7	1.9	1.1
Smoker (%)	50.2	45.3	46.3	47.5
Men aged 40–9 (n = 5154)				
BMI (kg/m^2)	23.1	27.3	32.6	27.1 ± 3.6
SBP (mmHg)	133.0	138.7	147.2	138.6 ± 18.3
DBP (mmHg)	79.1	83.3	88.7	83.1 ± 11.4
Serum TC (mg/dl)	203.3	213.2	214.8	210.7 ± 37.2
Diabetes (%)	2.6	2.0	3.4	2.4
Smoker (%)	48.9	42.0	39.0	43.4
Men aged 50–9 (n = 3944)				
BMI (kg/m^2)	23.1	27.4	32.7	27.3 ± 3.7
SBP (mmHg)	140.2	144.6	152.9	145.1 ± 21.2
DBP (mmHg)	81.7	85.4	90.8	85.5 ± 12.2
Serum TC (mg/dl)	207.7	216.7	215.0	214.0 ± 36.6
Diabetes (%)	4.2	4.8	5.8	4.9
Smoker (%)	48.3	36.2	34.4	39.0
Men aged 60–74 (n = 1528)				
BMI (kg/m^2)	23.2	27.4	32.5	27.2 ± 3.5
SBP (mmHg)	148.8	150.8	159.8	152.0 ± 21.9
DBP (mmHg)	84.5	86.2	90.8	86.6 ± 11.9
Serum TC (mg/dl)	207.7	211.2	212.3	210.4 ± 34.9
Diabetes (%)	6.1	6.6	9.1	6.9
Smoker (%)	39.4	26.2	24.5	29.5
Women aged 18–39 (n = 7729)				
BMI (kg/m^2)	21.1	26.9	34.1	22.8 ± 4.0
SBP (mmHg)	121.9	127.9	135.3	123.6 ± 13.8
DBP (mmHg)	71.8	75.7	80.3	72.9 ± 10.4
Serum TC (mg/dl)	178.8	187.9	190.9	180.9 ± 33.4
Diabetes (%)	0.9	0.8	1.4	0.9
Smoker (%)	44.8	43.8	46.6	44.7
Women aged 40–9 (n = 3852)				
BMI (kg/m^2)	22.1	27.0	34.0	24.8 ± 4.4
SBP (mmHg)	129.2	134.8	145.4	132.6 ± 18.8
DBP (mmHg)	77.2	80.2	87.0	79.1 ± 11.4
Serum TC (mg/dl)	206.7	209.2	210.6	207.8 ± 37.4
Diabetes (%)	1.5	2.1	4.8	2.0
Smoker (%)	42.8	35.1	30.7	39.3

Table 20.1 (continued)

Variable	BMI category[a]			All
	Normal	Overweight	Obese	
Women aged 50–9 (n = 3791)				
BMI (kg/m²)	22.3	27.1	33.6	25.5 ± 4.4
SBP (mmHg)	136.5	141.9	152.4	140.6 ± 20.9
DBP (mmHg)	79.7	82.4	88.0	81.8 ± 11.8
Serum TC (mg/dl)	228.4	231.3	232.2	229.9 ± 40.4
Diabetes (%)	2.1	2.9	4.1	2.7
Smoker (%)	38.8	28.7	23.7	33.3
Women aged 60–74 (n = 1275)				
BMI (kg/m²)	22.2	27.1	32.8	25.7 ± 4.2
SBP (mmHg)	145.4	149.7	157.9	149.0 ± 22.1
DBP (mmHg)	81.5	83.6	88.4	83.4 ± 11.8
Serum TC (mg/dl)	233.4	234.4	233.6	233.8 ± 40.2
Diabetes (%)	3.3	3.3	5.0	3.5
Smoker (%)	30.1	19.3	13.4	23.5

[a] Normal: BMI < 25.0 kg/m²; overweight: BMI 25.0–29.9 kg/m²; obese: BMI ⩾ 30 kg/m².

(ages 40–9), 1.47 to 1.08 (ages 50–9), and 2.26 to 2.07 (ages 60–74) in men, and from 4.28 to 2.89 (ages 40–9), 1.33 to 0.90 (ages 50–9), and 1.63 to 1.25 (ages 60–74) in women. With BMI as a continuous variable, while the association in women 40–9 is still positive with a hazard ratio of 1.25 for BMI higher by one SD, only the association in men 60–74 remains significant. However, this significant association is due primarily to increased risk in the fifth quintile. For men 40–9 and women 50–9 there are non-significant inverse associations, with quintiles 3–5 and quintiles 2–5, respectively, showing hazard ratios less than 1.0. For men 18–39 and 50–9 and women 60–74, hazard ratios from the continuous variable models are all close to 1.0.

If we based our conclusions on the associations of BMI with CHD mortality in CHA on the Model III results for 15-year follow-up, we would almost certainly conclude that there is little evidence that BMI is a risk factor for CHD mortality in these men and women.

In 16–27-year follow-up with adjustment for age, ethnicity, and smoking (Model I), BMI is now positively and significantly related to CHD mortality in seven of eight age–gender sub-cohorts (Tables 20.2 and 20.3); only in women 60–74 is there no association. Hazard ratios for BMI higher by one SD are 1.35, 1.24, 1.20, and 1.32 for men, 1.46, 1.75, 1.36, and 1.03 for women. These hazard ratios are larger than the corresponding hazard ratios for 0–15-year follow-up for all four groups of men, and for women 40–9 and 50–9. Risk is also significantly greater in the fifth quintile for all four groups of men, and in women 18–39, 40–9, and 50–9, with hazard ratios ranging from 1.79 to 4.13 in these seven subcohorts.

With adjustment for age and ethnicity, but not smoking (Model II), hazard ratios for BMI quintiles are generally somewhat smaller, with the largest differences occurring in women aged 40–9 and 50–9 in quintiles four and five. With BMI as a continuous variable, hazard ratios for men differ by no more than 0.01 between Models I and II. For women, differences range from −0.2 to 0.09.

With addition of SBP, TC, and diabetes to Model II (Model III) for 16–27-year follow-up, hazard ratios for BMI higher by one SD are smaller by 0.03–0.20 in men, and increase by 0.03

Table 20.2 Hazard ratios for CHD mortality by follow-up period by quintile of BMI: 21 732 men aged 18–74 at baseline, Chicago Heart Association Detection Project in Industry

Quintile mean	Years 0–15				Years 16–27			
	Deaths	HR-I[a]	HR-II	HR-III	Deaths	HR-I	HR-II	HR-III
Men aged 18–39								
21.4	8	1.00	1.00	1.00	19	1.00	1.00	1.00
24.0	14	1.45	1.40	1.29	23	1.04	1.02	0.88
25.7	11	1.04	1.00	0.84	37	1.57	1.53	1.23
27.5	11	1.01	0.96	0.69	38	1.61	1.54	1.12
31.4	17	1.49	1.48	0.87	60	2.51[b]	2.50[b]	1.55
Continuous[c]	61	1.21	1.21	1.01	177	1.35[b]	1.35[b]	1.15
Men aged 40–9								
22.5	28	1.00	1.00	1.00	44	1.00	1.00	1.00
25.2	36	1.36	1.28	1.11	56	1.36	1.27	1.25
26.8	28	1.07	0.99	0.82	46	1.14	1.05	0.97
28.6	38	1.38	1.33	0.99	59	1.40	1.34	1.11
32.3	35	1.33	1.25	0.82	72	1.88[b]	1.75[b]	1.45
Continuous	165	1.06	1.04	0.90	277	1.24[b]	1.23[b]	1.13
Men aged 50–9								
22.6	51	1.00	1.00	1.00	51	1.00	1.00	1.00
25.4	50	1.04	0.96	0.90	65	1.30	1.22	1.23
27.1	68	1.47[b]	1.35	1.21	64	1.37	1.30	1.28
28.8	47	0.99	0.89	0.70	80	1.68[b]	1.58[b]	1.50[b]
32.7	73	1.58[b]	1.47[b]	1.08	76	1.79[b]	1.70[b]	1.56[b]
Continuous	289	1.16[b]	1.13[b]	1.01	336	1.20[b]	1.19[b]	1.14[b]
Men aged 60–74								
22.7	31	1.00	1.00	1.00	31	1.00	1.00	1.00
25.2	43	1.33	1.30	1.33	28	0.87	0.86	0.88
27.0	35	1.09	1.04	1.06	39	1.19	1.17	1.19
28.8	32	1.02	0.97	0.97	48	1.60[b]	1.56	1.53
32.4	68	2.40[b]	2.26[b]	2.07[b]	47	1.98[b]	1.92[b]	1.83[b]
Continuous	209	1.28[b]	1.26[b]	1.21[b]	193	1.32[b]	1.32[b]	1.29[b]

[a] Model I includes age, ethnicity, and cigarettes/day; Model II removes cigarettes/day from Model I; and Model III adds SBP, serum TC, and diabetes (yes, no) to Model II.

[b] 95% confidence interval does not include 1.0.

[c] Hazard ratio for BMI higher by one SD.

in women 18–39 while decreasing by 0.08–0.26 in the other three groups of women. Nonetheless, the association remains non-significantly positive in men 18–39 and 40–9 and significantly positive in men 50–9 and 60–74, and in women 18–39, 40–9, and 50–9, with hazard ratios ranging from 1.13 to 1.49. (If smoking is added to this model, the association in men 40–9 is also significant, but not the association in men 18–39).

Thus, in contrast to our likely conclusions based on Model III results for 15-year follow-up of little association between BMI and CHD mortality, our conclusions based on Model I results for 16–27-year follow-up would be that the long-term consequence of an increased BMI is a direct independent association between body weight and CHD mortality.

Table 20.3 Hazard Ratios for CHD mortality by follow-up period by quintile of BMI: 16 647 women aged 18–74 at baseline, Chicago Heart Association Detection Project in Industry

Quintile mean	Years 0–15				Years 16–27			
	Deaths	HR-I[a]	HR-II	HR-III	Deaths	HR-I	HR-II	HR-III
Women aged 18–39								
19.5[b]					4	1.00	1.00	1.00
21.9					6	2.69	2.71	2.59
23.8					3	1.31	1.25	1.28
29.0					10	3.82[c]	3.77[c]	3.95[c]
Continuous[d]					23	1.46[c]	1.48[c]	1.49[c]
Women aged 40–9								
20.0	3	1.00	1.00	1.00	12	1.00	1.00	1.00
22.2	4	1.47	1.33	1.29	8	0.71	0.65	0.69
23.9	8	2.86	2.59	2.55	13	1.17	1.07	1.06
26.2	8	3.21	2.66	2.39	23	2.36[c]	1.99	2.08[c]
31.7	13	5.37[c]	4.28[c]	2.89	39	4.13[c]	3.39[c]	3.15[c]
Continuous	36	1.55[c]	1.47[c]	1.25	95	1.75[c]	1.66[c]	1.49[c]
Women aged 50–9								
20.4	18	1.00	1.00	1.00	41	1.00	1.00	1.00
22.9	15	0.90	0.80	0.73	38	0.94	0.87	0.90
24.8	17	1.08	0.95	0.83	51	1.42	1.30	1.32
27.1	12	0.76	0.64	0.52	47	1.24	1.10	1.11
32.3	24	1.69	1.33	0.90	69	2.10[c]	1.81[c]	1.72[c]
Continuous	86	1.12	1.05	0.90	246	1.36[c]	1.30[c]	1.21[c]
Women aged 60–74								
20.4	15	1.00	1.00	1.00	33	1.00	1.00	1.00
23.2	16	1.02	0.98	1.04	28	0.70	0.68	0.69
25.2	15	0.99	0.93	0.82	37	1.02	0.98	0.97
27.5	13	0.93	0.86	0.85	35	1.07	1.00	1.01
32.2	23	1.79	1.63	1.25	28	0.91	0.84	0.77
Continuous	82	1.22	1.19	1.07	161	1.03	1.00	0.95

[a] Model I includes age, ethnicity, and cigarettes/day; Model II removes cigarettes/day from Model I; and Model III adds SBP, serum TC, and diabetes (yes, no) to Model II.

[b] First two quintiles.

[c] 95% confidence interval does not include 1.0.

[d] Hazard ratio for BMI higher by one SD.

20.4.3 Findings in relation to other studies

The results presented here for BMI and 27-year CHD mortality and those previously reported for BMI and 25-year CVD mortality in this same cohort (Dyer *et al.* 2004) demonstrate that 'overadjustment' for obesity-related risk factors and failure to adjust for cigarette smoking represent important methodological problems that can hide or distort direct positive associations of BMI with CVD and CHD mortality. While some studies have found significant positive associations between weight and CVD and CHD mortality with adjustment for obesity-related risk factors (Barrett-Connor *et al.* 1984; Cambien *et al.* 1985; Dorn *et al.* 1997; Hubert *et al.* 1983; Johnson *et al.* 1986; Jousilahti *et al.* 1996; Lew and Garfinkel 1979; Pyorala *et al.* 1979;

Spataro *et al.* 1996; Wilcosky *et al.* 1990), associations in other studies have often become non-significant with such adjustment (Cambien *et al.* 1985; Jarrett *et al.* 1982; Jousilahti *et al.* 1996; Prineas *et al.* 1993; Stevens *et al.* 1992; Yano *et al.* 1984). In the CHA study, while associations of BMI with CVD and CHD mortality are significant only for men aged 60–74 in 15-year follow-up, in long-term follow-up, six of eight age–gender subcohorts for CHD (16–27 years) and seven of eight for CVD (16–25 years) (Dyer *et al.* 2004) show significant positive associations even with adjustment for obesity-related risk factors.

The results for BMI and CHD and CVD mortality in CHA also suggest that the lack of long-term follow-up and an inability to exclude early deaths for a period sufficient to remove effects of disease on weight have likely contributed importantly to lack of positive findings in some studies. In the Framingham Heart Study (Hubert *et al.* 1983), a strong and significant association between Metropolitan relative weight and CHD incidence did not emerge until 8-year follow-up, after which the strength of the association remained fairly constant through the 26-year follow-up period. Similarly, in the Manitoba Study (Rabkin *et al.* 1977) an association between BMI and CHD was not evident until 16 years of follow-up, with the strongest associations after 20 years of follow-up. In the Western Electric Study (Spataro *et al.* 1996), the association of BMI with CHD mortality was U-shaped through the first 14 years of follow-up, both with and without exclusion of deaths in the first 5 years. However, for years 15–22, BMI had a direct association, both with and without adjustment for obesity-related risk factors. In a Finnish study (Pekkanen *et al.* 1993), the highest tertile of BMI was related to CHD only in the third decade of follow-up.

20.5 Weight loss, weight gain, weight variability, and CHD mortality

Several studies have suggested that weigh fluctuation/variability is associated with increased risk for CVD and all-cause mortality (Blair *et al.* 1993; Hamm *et al.* 1989; Iribarren *et al.* 1995; Lissner *et al.* 1989, 1990, 1991; Stevens and Lissner 1990). Many studies have also found increased risk with weight loss or an inverse association with weight change (Avons *et al.* 1983; Blair *et al.* 1993; Deeg *et al.* 1990; Galanis *et al.* 1998; Hammond and Garfinkel 1969; Harris *et al.* 1988, 1993; Higgins *et al.* 1993; Iribarren *et al.* 1995; Lee and Paffenbarger 1992; Lissner *et al.* 1989, 1990, 1991; Paffenbarger *et al.* 1986; Pamuk *et al.* 1992, 1993; Rhoads and Kagan 1983; Rumpel *et al.* 1993; Sidney *et al.* 1987; Wannamethee and Shaper 1990; Wilcosky *et al.* 1990; Williamson *et al.* 1995), although several studies have also shown no increased risk with weight loss and/or increased risk associated with weight gain or weight change (Avons *et al.* 1983; Galanis *et al.* 1998; Hubert *et al.* 1983; Manson *et al.* 1990, 1995; Noppa 1980; Rexrode *et al.* 1997; Rhoads and Kagan 1983; Rimm *et al.* 1995; Schroll 1981; Sidney *et al.* 1987; Willett *et al.* 1995). Whether there is a causal association between weight loss or weight variability and increased mortality remains unclear, since underlying causes for weight loss or weight change are usually not determined. It is thus generally not known whether weight changes are an antecedent or a consequence of illness. These issues are of particular relevance to the prevention and treatment of obesity, given the current epidemic.

In a previous report from the Western Electric (WE) Study (Dyer *et al.* 2000), we examined associations of the variation and trend in BMI between 1958 and 1966 with subsequent 25-year CVD and all-cause mortality in men free of CHD and cancer between 1958 and 1966. In those analyses, we found that weight loss was significantly related to CVD and all-cause mortality in years 0–15 but not 16–25, and that weight gain was significantly related to all-cause mortality in years 0–15, while weight variability was not related to either CVD or all-cause mortality in either period. Here we report the associations of the variation and trend in BMI with 25-year CHD mortality in these men.

20.6 **Western Electric Study**

Methods of the WE Study have been described (Dyer *et al.* 2000; Paul *et al.* 1963). Participants were initially examined in 1957–58, with annual re-examinations through 1966. Data reported here are from the baseline exam and first seven or eight annual re-examinations. Of 2107 men aged 40–56 examined at baseline, 1281 aged 48–66 in 1965–66 met the inclusion criteria for these analyses (Dyer *et al.* 2000).

BMI was computed for each weight measurement. The slope of the regression line relating each man's BMI values to time from baseline was computed to assess his yearly rate of change. Two additional slope variables, representing weight loss and weight gain, respectively, were also computed to account for non-linear associations between slope and mortality. The weight loss slope was defined as the computed slope if it was less than or equal to zero, and zero otherwise. The weight gain slope was defined as the computed slope when it was greater than zero, and zero otherwise. The SD of BMI and the SD about the regression, which assess variation about the trend of BMI over the period, were computed as measures of weight fluctuation or variation. The average of all BMI measurements between 1958 and 1965–66 was used to assess overall level of BMI. Other variables included age at time of last weight measurement in 1965 or 1966, and average number of cigarettes smoked per day between baseline and 1965–66.

Death certificates were coded for underlying cause according to the Eighth Revision of the *International Classification of Diseases* (ICD-8), adapted for the United States (ICD-8) (National Center for Health Statistics 1967), with CHD mortality defined as ICD-8 codes 410.0–414.9. These analyses utilize mortality follow-up through 31 December 1990, which corresponds to an average of 25 years from the examination in 1965 or 1966.

Proportional hazards (Cox) regression was used to assess associations of BMI variability and trends with mortality. For one set of analyses, each variability measure was divided into quintiles. To categorize slope, non-positive slopes were divided at the median, and positive slopes were divided into tertiles, again creating five categories. Hazard ratios were then computed for each category or quintile, with adjustment for age and cigarettes/day.

In a second set of analyses, measures of variability and slope variables were entered as continuous variables. For these analyses, each variability measure was log transformed, since each had a highly skewed distribution. Models were fitted that included each measure of variability or the two slope variables, plus age and cigarettes/day. Subsequent multivariable models included the two slope variables, plus age, cigarettes/day, average BMI, and each variability measure in turn.

Because weight loss and weight variability could be a consequence of pre-existing disease, rather than an antecedent, associations were examined for 0–15 years of follow-up and years 16–25.

20.6.1 **Weight loss, weight gain, weight variability, and CHD mortality in WE men**

Between 1958 and 1965–66, the average BMI for these men was 25.8 kg/m^2, the average within-person SD was 0.75 kg/m^2, and the average within-person SD about the regression was

0.61 kg/m^2. Among 433 men who lost weight, the average decrease in BMI was 0.13 kg/m^2 per year, while among 848 men who gained weight, the average increase was 0.15 kg/m^2 per year.

The correlation between the slope and SD of BMI is 0.08 for all 1281 men, but -0.77 for the 433 men with negative slopes and 0.75 for the 848 men with positive slopes. These high correlations make it difficult to assess whether an observed association between the SD of BMI and mortality is a true association or rather reflects associations of weight loss and/or gain with mortality. Use of the SD about the regression does not entirely eliminate the problem of distinguishing between variability and the trend in weight over time, since correlations with the slope of -0.42 in men who lost weight and 0.24 in men who gained weight also indicate some overlap between this measure of variability and the trend in weight.

For the SD of BMI, the association with 15-year CHD mortality is J-shaped, with significantly increased risk in the fifth quintile relative to the first (Table 20.4). For the SD about the regression, risk generally increases progressively as the SD increases, also with significantly increased risk in the fifth quintile. In the continuous variable models, each variability measure is significantly related to 15-year mortality. In 16–25 year follow-up, associations are weaker

Table 20.4 Hazard ratios for CHD mortality by follow-up period by category of BMI variables: 1281 men from the Western Electric Study, aged 48–66 in 1965–66

Category mean	n	Years 0–15		Years 16–25	
		Deaths	HR[a]	Deaths	HR
SD of BMI					
0.35	256	23	1.00	24	1.00
0.51	256	20	0.87	27	1.11
0.66	257	20	0.96	21	0.85
0.86	256	31	1.52	26	1.16
1.36	256	36	1.84[b]	25	1.29
Continuous[c]			1.25[b]		1.11
SD about the regression					
0.28	256	21	1.00	22	1.00
0.42	256	21	0.99	26	1.11
0.54	257	26	1.27	26	1.15
0.68	256	26	1.32	24	1.05
1.13	257	36	1.91[b]	25	1.31
Continuous			1.22[b]		1.11
Slope of BMI					
-0.21	216	28	1.96[b]	23	1.00
-0.04	217	28	1.86[b]	21	0.91
0.04	282	21	1.00	33	1.00
0.13	284	14	0.74	21	0.62
0.29	282	39	2.16[b]	25	0.87
Negative slope			1.28[b]		1.09
Positive slope			1.17		1.03

[a] Hazard ratios adjusted for age and cigarettes/day.

[b] 95% confidence interval does not contain 1.0.

[c] Hazard ratios are computed for the log of the SD of BMI and the log of the SD about the regression higher by 0.05, for a 0.12 kg/m^2/year more negative slope, and for a 0.12 kg/m^2/year more positive slope.

than in 15-year follow-up, with no significant associations for the quintile models or the continuous variable models.

In analyses involving trends in weight between 1958 and 1965–66, men in each weight loss category and men in the highest tertile of weight gain all have significantly increased 15-year CHD mortality, relative to those in the lowest tertile of weight gain (Table 20.5). However, for 16–25-year follow-up, hazard ratios for all three of these categories are 1.0 or less. In the continuous variable models, the weight loss slope is significantly related to 15-year CHD mortality but not to 16–25-year mortality, and the weight gain slope is not significantly related to CHD mortality in either period. This latter result is due in part to the fact that for both periods of follow-up, men with the lowest mortality are those in the middle tertile of weight gain.

In the multivariable models, the weight loss slope is significantly related to 15-year CHD mortality with adjustment for the SD about the regression, but not with adjustment for the SD of BMI (Table 20.5). The weight loss slope is not related to 16–25-year mortality, and neither measure of variability is significantly related to mortality in either follow-up period. However, if slope is entered into the model as a single variable, instead of two variables representing weight loss and weight gain, the SD of BMI is significantly related to 15-year mortality with a relative risk of 1.21, but not to 16–25-year mortality, while the SD about the regression is not significantly related in either period of follow-up.

Associations were also examined in the multivariable models separately for smokers and non-smokers (Table 20.5). In these analyses, the weight loss slope is significantly related to

Table 20.5 Hazard ratios[a] for CHD mortality from multivariable models by follow-up period for all men, and smokers and non-smokers: 1281 men from the Western Electric Study aged 48–66 years in 1965–66

BMI variable	Regression SD models		SD of BMI models	
	0–15	16–25	0–15	16–25
All men (n = 1281)				
SD measure	1.11	0.97	1.07	0.95
Negative slope	1.21[b]	1.00	1.19	1.02
Positive slope	1.14	0.97	1.10	1.00
Non-smokers (n = 644)				
SD measure	1.20	0.99	1.26	0.94
Negative slope	0.99	1.09	0.90	1.15
Positive slope	0.91	0.84	0.81	0.87
Smokers (n = 637)				
SD measure	1.04	0.89	0.97	0.88
Negative slope	1.34[b]	0.90	1.37[b]	0.95
Positive slope	1.25[b]	1.11	1.28	1.20

[a] Hazard ratios are computed for the log of the SD about the regression and the log of the SD of BMI greater by 0.05, for a 0.12 kg/m^2/year more negative slope, and for a 0.12 kg/m^2/year more positive slope. Regression SD models included the regression SD, the two slope variables, plus average BMI, age, and cigarettes/day. SD of BMI models included the SD of BMI, the two slope variables, plus average BMI, age, and cigarettes/day.

[b] 95% confidence interval does not contain 1.0.

15-year CHD mortality in smokers with adjustment for each measure of variability, and the weight gain slope is significantly related to 15-year mortality with adjustment for the SD about the regression. While the 15-year regression coefficients for the weight loss and weight gain slopes in smokers do not differ significantly from those in non-smokers, the significant association for the weight loss slope for all 1281 men appears to be due to an association only in smokers, since the hazard ratio in non-smokers is near 1.0 for this period of follow-up.

20.6.2 Findings in relation to other studies

Several studies have found weight variability or weight fluctuation to be associated with increased risk for all-cause mortality and CVD morbidity or mortality (Blair *et al.* 1993; Hamm *et al.* 1989; Iribarren *et al.* 1995; Lissner *et al.* 1989, 1991). In an earlier report from the WE Study (Hamm *et al.* 1989), men who had large fluctuations in weight between ages 20 and 40 had twice the 25-year risk of CHD mortality compared to men who reported no substantial change in weight. In the Framingham Study (Lissner *et al.* 1991), the coefficient of variation of BMI was significantly related to 18-year all-cause and CHD mortality in both men and women. In the Multiple Risk Factor Intervention Trial (MRFIT) (Blair *et al.* 1993), the SD of weight, calculated from weights during the trial, was significantly related to subsequent 3.8-year all-cause and CVD mortality. In the Gothenburg studies (Lissner *et al.* 1989), the coefficient of variation of BMI was significantly related to 15-year all-cause and CHD mortality in men and 13-year all-cause mortality in women. In the Honolulu Heart Study (Iribarren *et al.* 1995), the SD about the regression of BMI was significantly related to 14.5-year all-cause and CVD mortality.

In contrast to these findings, in the Charleston Heart Study (Stevens and Lissner 1990) the coefficient of variation of BMI was not significantly related to 23-year all-cause mortality in men or women. In the Baltimore Longitudinal Study on Aging (Lissner *et al.* 1990), the SD about the regression of BMI was not significantly related to 16.5-year all-cause or CHD mortality in men.

The SD about the regression is a more appropriate measure of weight variability than the coefficient of variation or SD, since it does a better job of removing the portion of variability that is due to systematic gain or loss in weight. In the Honolulu Heart Study (Iribarren *et al.* 1995), the SD about the regression was related to all-cause and CVD mortality with adjustment for the trend in weight. In the Framingham Study (Lissner *et al.* 1991) and the Gothenburg studies (Lissner *et al.* 1989), but not MRFIT (Blair *et al.* 1993), associations were also adjusted for the slope of BMI using a single variable to represent the trend. In WE men, the SD of BMI is significantly related to 15-year all-cause, CVD, and CHD mortality, if the slope is included as a single continuous variable in the model (Dyer *et al.* 2000). However, with inclusion of slope variables that take into account the direction of the trend, neither measure of variability is significantly related to all-cause, CVD, or CHD mortality. Whether the results of these other studies would have been altered if the analytic models had included terms taking into account both positive and negative trends in weight is unclear. However, it is likely that the strength of the associations of BMI variability with mortality would have been reduced in such analyses.

Associations of weight change with mortality vary depending on how weight change is determined. Studies that define weight change as the difference in current weight and the highest lifetime weight have consistently shown weight loss to be associated with increased mortality (Harris *et al.* 1993; Pamuk *et al.* 1992, 1993; Rumpel *et al.* 1993; Sidney *et al.* 1987). In contrast, only a handful of the studies that define weight change as the difference between current weight and weight during young adulthood have shown increased risk with weight loss (Avons *et al.* 1983; Paffenbarger *et al.* 1986; Rhoads and Kagan 1983; Wilcosky *et al.* 1990). Most of these studies have shown no association between weight loss and mortality (Manson *et al.* 1995; Willett *et al.* 1995), or a positive association between weight gain or change and mortality (Galanis *et al.* 1998; Hubert *et al.* 1983; Manson *et al.* 1990, 1995; Rexrode *et al.* 1997; Rimm *et al.* 1995; Willett *et al.* 1995). Two studies that found increased risk with weight loss also found increased risk with weight gain (Avons *et al.* 1983; Rhoads and Kagan 1983). Studies that define weight change as the difference in weight between two exams are relatively consistent in showing an association between weight loss and increased risk (Blair *et al.* 1993; Deeg *et al.* 1990; Galanis *et al.* 1998; Hammond and Garfinkel 1969; Harris *et al.* 1988; Higgins *et al.* 1993; Iribarren *et al.* 1995; Lee and Paffenbarger 1992; Lissner *et al.* 1989; Wannamethee and Shaper 1990; Williamson *et al.* 1995). Only a few of these studies show an association between weight gain and increased risk (Galanis *et al.* 1998; Lee and Paffenbarger 1992; Noppa *et al.* 1980; Wannamethee *et al.* 1990).

These differences in results among weight change studies could be attributable to the influences of illness-related weight loss. Weight loss over a relatively short period of time, for example between two exams, is more likely to be influenced by illness than weight change from young adulthood. Similarly, decrease in weight from the highest lifetime weight appears more likely to be influenced by illness. Hence, it is perhaps not surprising that studies using weight change from young adulthood are the studies showing increased risk with weight gain and little or no increased risk with weight loss, whereas the other types of studies show an increased risk associated with weight loss.

Whether weight loss is causally related to increased mortality is unclear, since underlying reasons for weight loss or weight change are usually not determined. It is thus generally not known whether weight changes are intentional or unintentional, and thus whether changes in weight are an antecedent or a consequence of illness. In the WE men, associations between weight loss and CVD and CHD mortality are found only in smokers and only in the first 15 years of follow-up, suggesting that such associations are a consequence of illness rather than an antecedent.

Three studies were able to divide weight loss into intentional and unintentional loss (French *et al.* 1999; Williamson *et al.* 1995, 1999). Intentional weight loss among overweight women aged 40–64 with obesity-related conditions was generally associated with decreased mortality (Williamson *et al.* 1995). However, among women with no pre-existing illness, the association was equivocal. In the Iowa Women's Health Study of women aged 50–69 years (French *et al.* 1999), one or more intentional weight-loss episodes of 20 or more pounds ≥9.1 kg) was not significantly associated with higher total or CVD mortality risk compared to never losing 20 or more pounds. However, one or more unintentional weight loss episodes was associated with a 26–57% higher total mortality risk and a 51–114% higher CVD mortality risk, compared with never losing 20 or more pounds. In the third study (Williamson *et al.* 1999), neither intentional nor unintentional weight loss of 20 or more pounds in overweight men aged 40–64 was associated with total or CVD mortality in those with or without existing health problems.

20.7 Conclusions

The prevalence of obesity is rising at an alarming rate in both adults and children from both developed and developing countries. While both overweight and obesity are associated with numerous CVD risk factors, studies on associations of BMI with CVD and/or CHD morbidity and mortality have not always demonstrated the expected strong positive associations. The results presented here and previously from the CHA study demonstrate that the failure to find the expected results may be due in many studies to methodological problems, that is, failure to adjust for cigarette smoking, inappropriate adjustment for obesity-related risk factors (e.g. blood pressure, TC, and diabetes), and failure to exclude deaths for a sufficient period to eliminate the effects of illness-related weight loss. In the CHA study, in taking into account all three potential methodological problems by adjusting for smoking, but not obesity-related risk factors, and excluding deaths for the first 15 years of follow-up, BMI is significantly related to both CVD and CHD mortality in men aged 18–39, 40–9, 50–9, and 60–74, and in women aged 18–39, 40–9, and 50–9. In contrast, in 0–15-year follow-up with adjustment for obesity-related risk factors (SBP, TC, and diabetes), but not smoking, there are significant positive associations for both CVD and CHD only in men aged 60–74, with the other subcohorts showing each of the types of associations that have sometimes been reported, that is, non-significant positive associations, no association, non-significant inverse associations, and quadratic associations.

Based on review of all results from the CHA study and the many other studies on this topic, the *long-term* consequence of obesity is clear: a direct positive association, mediated in part by adverse effects of weight gain/obesity on other major risk factors, but persisting as an apparently independent additional adverse influence over and above these important and unfavourable influences.

The results of the WE study also indicate that any increased risk of CVD or CHD mortality associated with weight loss and/or weight fluctuation/variability is likely due to illness-related weight changes, since any increased risk with weight loss or weight variability did not persist beyond 15 years. Also, mortality associations with weight loss were present only in smokers, further supporting the judgement that the weight loss was a consequence of illness, rather than an antecedent.

Therefore, the long-term outlook for people with overweight and obesity is adverse. Overweight is soundly designated one of the major CHD/CVD risk factors. Concerted efforts are needed for its prevention and treatment.

References

Avons, P., Ducimetiere, P., and Rakotovo, R. (1983). Weight and mortality [letter]. *Lancet*, 1, 1104.

Barrett-Connor, E. L. (1985). Obesity, atherosclerosis, and coronary artery disease. *Annals of Internal Medicine*, 103, 1010–19.

Barrett-Connor, E., Suarez, L., Khaw, K-T., Criqui, M. H., and Wingard, D. L. (1984). Ischemic heart disease risk factors after age 50. *Journal of Chronic Diseases*, 37, 903–8.

Blair, S. N., Shaten, J., Brownell, K., Collins, G., and Lissner, L. (1993). Body weight change, all cause-mortality, and cause-specific mortality in the Multiple Risk Factor Intervention Trial. *Annals of Internal Medicine*, 119, 749–57.

Cambien, F., Chretien, J. M., Ducimetiere, P., Guize, L., and Richard, J. L. (1985). Is the relationship between blood pressure and cardiovascular risk dependent on body mass index? *American Journal of Epidemiology*, 122, 434–42.

Cochrane, A. L., Moore, F., Baker, I. A., and Haley, T. J. (1980). Mortality in two random samples of women aged 55–64 years followed up for 20 years. *British Medical Journal*, 280, 1131–3.

Deckelbaum, R. J. and Williams, C. L. (2001). Childhood obesity: the health issue. *Obesity Research*, 9(Suppl. 4), 239S–43S.

Deeg, D. J. H., Miles, T. P., Van Zonneveld, R. J., and Curb, J. D. (1990). Weight change, survival time and cause of death in Dutch elderly. *Archives of Gerontology and Geriatrics*, **10**, 97–111.

Dorn, J. M., Schisterman, E. F., Winkelstein, Jr., W., and Trevisan, M. (1997). Body mass index and mortality in a general population sample of men and women: The Buffalo Health Study. *American Journal of Epidemiology*, **146**, 919–31.

Dyer, A. R., Stamler, J., Berkson, D. M., and Lindberg, H. A. (1975). Relationship of relative and body mass index to 14-year mortality in the Chicago Peoples Gas Company Study. *Journal of Chronic Diseases*, **28**, 109–23.

Dyer, A. R., Stamler, J., and Greenland, P. (2000). Associations of weight change and weight variability with cardiovascular and all cause mortality in the Chicago Western Electric Company Study. *American Journal of Epidemiology*, **49**, 849–57.

Dyer, A. R., Stamler, J., Garside, D. B., and Greenland, P. (2004). Long-term consequences of body mass index for cardiovascular mortality: The Chicago Heart Association Detection Project in Industry Study. *Annals of Epidemiology*, **14**, 101–8.

Fitzgerald, A. P. and Jarrett, R. J. (1992). Body weight and coronary heart disease mortality: an analysis in relation to age and smoking habit. 15 years follow-up data from the Whitehall Study. *International Journal of Obesity*, **16**, 119–23.

Foreyt, J. P. and St Jeor S. T. (1997). Definitions of obesity and healthy weight. In *Obesity assessment: tools, methods, interpretations: a reference case: The RENO Diet-Heart Study* (ed. S. T. St Jeor), pp. 47–56. Chapman & Hall, New York.

French, S. A., Folsom, A. R., Jeffery, R. W., and Williamson, D. F. (1999). Prospective study of intentionality of weight loss and mortality in older women: the Iowa Women's Health Study. *American Journal of Epidemiology*, **149**, 504–14.

Galanis, D., Harris, T., Sharp, D. S., and Petrovitch, H. (1998). Relative weight, weight change, and risk of coronary heart disease in the Honolulu Heart Program. *American Journal of Epidemiology*, **147**, 379–86.

Garfinkel, L. and Stellman, S. D. (1988). Mortality by relative weight and exercise. *Cancer*, **62**, 1844–50.

Garn, S. M., Hawthorne, V. M., Pilkington, J. J., and Pesick, S. D. (1983). Fatness and mortality in the West of Scotland. *American Journal of Clinical Nutrition*, **38**, 313–19.

Hamm, P., Shekelle, R. B., and Stamler, J. (1989). Large fluctuations in body weight during young adulthood and twenty-five year risk of coronary death in men. *American Journal of Epidemiology*, **129**, 312–18.

Hammond, E. C. and Garfinkel, L. (1969). Coronary heart disease, stroke, and aortic aneurysm. *Archives of Environmental Health*, **19**, 167–82.

Hanson, R. L., McCance, D. R., Jacobson, L. T., Narayan, R. G., Pettitt, D. J., Bennett, P. H., and Knowler, W. C. (1995). The U-shaped association between body mass index and mortality: relationship with weight gain in a Native American population. *Journal of Clinical Epidemiology*, **48**, 903–16.

Harris, T., Cook, F., Garrison, R., Higgins, M., Kannel, W., and Goldman, L. (1988). Body mass index and mortality among nonsmoking older persons: The Framingham Heart Study. *Journal of the American Medical Association*, **259**, 1520–4.

Harris, T. B., Ballard-Barbasch, R., Madans, J., Makuc, D. M., and Feldman, J. J. (1993). Overweight, weight loss, and risk of coronary heart disease in older women: The NHANES I Epidemiologic Follow-up Study. *American Journal of Epidemiology*, **137**, 1318–27.

Higgins, M., D'Agostino, R., Kannel, W., and Cobb, J. (1993). Benefits and adverse effects of weight loss: observations from the Framingham Study. *Annals of Internal Medicine*, **119**, 758–63.

Hubert, H. H., Feinleib, M., McNamara, P. M., and Castelli, W. P. (1983). Obesity as an independent risk factor for cardiovascular disease: a 26-year follow-up of participants in the Framingham Heart Study. *Circulation*, **67**, 968–77.

Iribarren, C., Sharp, D. S., Burchfiel, C. M., and Petrovitch, H. (1995). Association of weight loss and weight fluctuation with mortality among Japanese American men. *New England Journal of Medicine*, **333**, 686–92.

Jarrett, R. J., Shipley, M. J., and Rose, G. (1982). Weight and mortality in the Whitehall Study. *British Medical Journal*, **285**, 535–7.

Johnson J. L., Heineman, E. F., Heiss, G., Hames, C. G., and Tyroler, H. A. (1986). Cardiovascular disease risk factors and mortality among black women and white women aged 40–64 years in Evans County, Georgia. *American Journal of Epidemiology*, **123**, 209–20.

Jousilahti, P., Tuomilehto, J., Vartiainen, E., Pekkanen, J., and Puska, P. (1996). Body weight, cardiovascular risk factors, and coronary mortality: 15-year follow-up of middle-aged men and women in Eastern Finland. *Circulation*, **93**, 1372–9.

Keys, A., Menotti, A., Aravanis, C., Blackburn, H., Djordevic, B. S., Buzina, R. *et al.* (1984). The Seven Countries Study: 2,289 deaths in 15 years. *Preventive Medicine*, **13**, 141–51.

Lee, I-M. and Paffenbarger, R. S., Jr. (1992). Change in body weight and longevity. *Journal of the American Medical Association*, **268**, 2045–9.

Lee, I. M., Manson, J. E., Hennekens, C. H., and Paffenbarger, R. S., Jr. (1993). Body weight and mortality: a 27-year follow-up of middle-aged men. *Journal of the American Medical Association*, **70**, 2823–8.

Lew, E. A. and Garfinkel, L. (1979). Variations in mortality by weight among 750,000 men and women. *Journal of Chronic Diseases*, **32**, 563–76.

Lissner, L., Bengtsson, C., Lapidus, L., Larsson, B., Bengtsson, B., and Brownell, K. (1989). Body weight variability and mortality in the Gothenburg prospective studies of men and women. In *Obesity in Europe 88: Proceedings of the First European Congress on Obesity* (ed. P. Bjorntorp and S. Rossner), pp. 55–60. John Libbey, London.

Lissner, L., Andres, R., Muller, D. C., and Shimokata, H. (1990). Body weight variability in men: metabolic rate, health and longevity. *International Journal of Obesity*, **14**, 373–83.

Lissner, L., Odell, P. M., D'Agostino, R. B., Stokes III, J., Kreger, B. E., Belanger, A. J., and Brownell, K. (1991). Variability of body weight and health outcomes in the Framingham population. *New England Journal of Medicine*, **324**, 1839–44.

Manson, J. E., Stampfer, M. J., Hennekens C. H., and Willett, W. C. (1987). Body weight and longevity: a reassessment. *Journal of the American Medical Association*, **257**, 353–8.

Manson, J. E., Colditz, G. A., Stampfer, M. J., Willett, W. C., Rosner, B., Monson, R. R. *et al.* (1990). A prospective study of obesity and risk of coronary heart disease in women. *New England Journal of Medicine*, **322**, 882–9.

Manson, J. E., Willett, W. C., Stampfer M. J., Colditz, G. A., Hunter, D. J., Hankinson, S. E. *et al.* (1995). Body weight and mortality in women. *New England Journal of Medicine*, **333**, 677–85.

Margarey, A. M., Daniels, L. A., and Boulton, T. J. (2001). Prevalence of overweight and obesity in Australian children and adolescents: reassessment of 1985 and 1995 data against new standard international definitions. *Medical Journal of Australia*, **174**, 561–4.

Martorell, R., Khan, L. K., Hughes, M. L., and Grummer-Strawn, L. M. (2000). Obesity in women from developing countries. *European Journal of Clinical Nutrition*, **54**, 247–52.

Mokdad, A. H., Bowman, B. A., Ford, E. S., Vinicor, F., Marks, J. S., and Koplan, J. P. (2001). The continuing epidemics of obesity in the United States. *Journal of the American Medical Association*, **286**, 1195–200.

Molarius, A., Seidell, J. C., Sans, S., Tuomilehto, J., and Kuulasmaa, K., for the WHO MONICA Project (2000). Educational level, relative body weight, and changes in their association over 10 years: an international perspective from the WHO Monica Project. *American Journal of Public Health*, **90**, 1260–8.

National Center for Health Statistics (1967). *International classification of diseases (adapted for use in the US), Eighth Revision.* US Government Printing Office, Washington, DC.

NHLBI Obesity Task Force (1998). Clinical guidelines on the identification, evaluation, and treatment of overweight and obesity in adults: the evidence report. *Obesity Research*, **6**(Suppl. 2), 51S–209S.

Noppa, H. (1980). Body weight change in relation to incidence of ischemic heart disease and change in risk factors for ischemic heart disease. *American Journal of Epidemiology*, **111**, 693–704.

O'Laughlin, J., Paradis, G., Meshefedjian, G., and Gray-Donald, K. (2000). A five-year trend of increasing obesity among elementary schoolchildren in multiethnic, low-income, inner-city neighborhoods in Montreal, Canada. *International Journal of Obesity and Related Metabolic Disorders*, **9**, 1176–82.

Paffenbarger, R. S., Jr., Hyde, R. T., Wing, A. L., and Hsieh, C. C. (1986). Physical activity, all-cause mortality, and longevity in college alumni. *New England Journal of Medicine*, **314**, 605–13.

Pamuk, E. R., Williamson, D. F., Madans, J., Serdula, M. K., Kleinman, J. C., and Byers, T. (1992). Weight loss and mortality in a national cohort of adults, 1971–1987. *American Journal of Epidemiology*, **136**, 686–97.

Pamuk, E. R., Williamson, D. F., Serdula, M. K., Madans, J., and Byers, T. E. (1993). Weight loss and subsequent death in a cohort of U.S. adults. *Annals of Internal Medicine*, **119**, 744–8.

Paul, O., Lepper, M. H., and Phelan, W. H. (1963). A longitudinal study of coronary heart disease. *Circulation*, **28**, 20–31.

Pekkanen, J., Tervahauta, M., Nissinen, A., and Karvonen, M. J. (1993). Does the predictive value of baseline coronary risk factors change over a 30-year follow-up? *Cardiology*, **82**, 181–90.

Prineas, R. J., Folsom, A. R., and Kaye, S. A. (1993). Central adiposity and increased risk of coronary artery disease mortality in older women. *Annals of Epidemiology*, **3**, 35–41.

Pyorala, K., Savolainen, E., Lehtovirta, E., Punsar, S., and Siltanen, P. (1979). Glucose tolerance and coronary heart disease: Helsinki Policemen Study. *Journal of Chronic Diseases*, **32**, 729–45.

Rabkin, S. W., Mathewsen, F. A. L, and Hsu, P. H. (1977). Relation of body weight to development of ischemic heart disease in a cohort of young North American men after 26-year observation period: the Manitoba Study. *American Journal of Cardiology*, **39**, 452–8.

Rexrode, K. M., Hennekens, C. H., Willett, W. C., Colditz, G. A., Stampfer, M. J., Rich-Edwards, J. W. *et al.* (1997). A prospective study of body mass index, weight change, and risk of stroke in women. *Journal of the American Medical Association*, **277**, 1539–45.

Rhoads, G. G. and Kagan, A. (1983). The relation of coronary disease, stroke, and mortality to weight in youth and in middle age. *Lancet*, **1**, 492–5.

Rimm, E. B., Stampfer, M. J., Giovannucci, E., Ascherio, A., Spiegelman, D., Colditz, G.A., and Willett, W. C. (1995). Body size and fat distribution as predictors of coronary heart disease among middle-aged and older US men. *American Journal of Epidemiology*, **141**, 1117–27.

Rissanen, A., Heliovaara, M., Knekt, P., Aromaa, A., Reunanen, A., and Maatela, J. (1989). Weight and mortality in Finnish men. *Journal of Clinical Epidemiology*, **42**, 781–9.

Rissanen, A., Knekt, P., Heliovaara, M., Aromaa, A., Reunanen, A., and Maatela, J. (1991). Weight and mortality in Finnish women. *Journal of Clinical Epidemiology*, **44**, 787–95.

Rocchini, A. P. (2002). Childhood obesity and a diabetes epidemic. *New England Journal of Medicine*, **346**, 854–5.

Rumpel, C., Harris, T. B., and Madans, J. (1993). Modification of the relationship between the Quetelet index and mortality by weight loss history among older women. *Annals of Epidemiology*, **3**, 343–50.

Schroll, M. (1981). A longitudinal epidemiological survey of relative weight at age 25, 50, and 60 in the Glostrup population of men and women born in 1914. *Danish Medical Bulletin*, **28**, 106–16.

Seidell, J. C., Verschuren, M., van Leer, E. M., and Kromhout, D. (1996). Overweight, underweight, and mortality: a prospective study of 48 287 men and women. *Archives of Internal Medicine*, **156**, 958–63.

Seidell, J. C. and Flegal, K. M. (1997). Assessing obesity: classification and epidemiology. *British Medical Bulletin*, **53**, 238–52.

Selmer, R. and Tverdal, A. (1995). Body mass index and cardiovascular mortality at different levels of blood pressure: a prospective study of Norwegian men and women. *Journal of Epidemiology and Community Health*, **49**, 265–70.

Semenciw, R. M., Morrison, H. I., Mao, Y., Johansen, H., Davies, J. W., and Wigle, D. T. (1988). Major risk factors for cardiovascular disease mortality in adults: results from the Nutrition Canada survey cohort. *International Journal of Epidemiology*, **17**, 317–23.

Shaper, A. G., Wannamethee, S. G., and Walker, M. (1997). Body weight: implications for the prevention of coronary heart disease, stroke, and diabetes mellitus in a cohort study of middle aged men. *British Medical Journal*, **314**, 1311–17.

Sidney, S., Friedman, G. D., and Siegelaub, A. B. (1987). Thinness and mortality. *American Journal of Public Health*, **77**, 317–22.

Spataro, J. A., Dyer, A. R., Stamler, J., Shekelle, R. B., Greenlund, K., and Garside, D. (1996). Measures of adiposity and coronary heart disease mortality in the Chicago Western Electric Company Study. *Journal of Clinical Epidemiology*, **49**, 849–57.

Stamler, J. (1993). Epidemic obesity in the United States [Editorial]. *Archives of Internal Medicine*, **153**, 1040–4.

Stamler, J., Rhomberg, P., Schoenberger, J. A., Shekelle, R. B., Dyer, A., Shekelle, S. *et al.* (1975a). Multivariate analysis of the relationship of seven variables to blood pressure: findings of the Chicago Heart Association Detection Project in Industry, 1967–1972. *Journal of Chronic Diseases*, **28**, 527–48.

Stamler, J., Stamler, R., Rhomberg, P., Dyer, A., Berkson, D. M., Reedus, W., and Wannamaker J. (1975b). Multivariate analysis of the relationship of six variables to blood pressure: findings from Chicago Community Surveys, 1965–1971. *Journal of Chronic Diseases*, **28**, 499–525.

Stamler, J., Dyer, A. R., Shekelle, R. B., Neaton, J., and Stamler, R. (1993). Relationship of baseline major risk factors to coronary and all-cause mortality, and to longevity: findings from long-term follow-up of Chicago cohorts. *Cardiology*, **82**, 191–222.

Stamler, J., Greenland, P., and Neaton, J. D. (1998). The established major risk factors underlying epidemic coronary and cardiovascular disease. *CVD Prevention*, **1**, 82–97.

Stevens, J. and Lissner, L. (1990). Body weight variability and mortality in the Charleston Heart Study [letter]. *International Journal of Obesity*, **14**, 385–6.

Stevens, J., Keil, J. E., Tyroler, H. A., Davis, C. E., and Gazes, P. C. (1992). Body mass index and body girths as predictors of mortality in black and white women. *Archives of Internal Medicine*, **152**, 1257–62.

Strauss, R. S. and Pollack, H. A. (2001). Epidemic increase in childhood overweight, 1986–1998. *Journal of the American Medical Association*, **286**, 2845–8.

Terry, R. B., Page, W. F., and Haskell, W. L. (1992). Waist/hip ratio, body mass index and premature cardiovascular disease mortality in US army veterans during a twenty-three follow-up study. *International Journal of Obesity*, **16**, 417–23.

Visscher, L. S. and Seidell J. C. (2001). The public health impact of obesity. *Annual Review of Public Health*, **22**, 355–75.

Waaler, H. T. (1984). Height, weight, and mortality: the Norwegian experience. *Acta Medica Scandinavia Supplement*, **679**, 1–56.

Wannamethee, G. and Shaper, A. G. (1990). Weight change, perceived health status and mortality in middle-aged British men. *Postgraduate Medical Journal*, **66**, 910–13.

Wilcosky, T., Hyde, J., Anderson, J. J. B., Bangdiwala, S., and Duncan, B. (1990). Obesity and mortality in the Lipid Research Clinics Program Follow-up Study. *Journal of Clinical Epidemiology*, **43**, 743–52.

Willett, W. C., Manson, J. E., Stampfer, M. J., Colditz, G. A., Rosner, B., Speizer, F. E., and Hennekens, C. H. (1995). Weight, weight change, and coronary heart disease in women. Risk within the 'normal' weight range. *Journal of the American Medical Association*, **273**, 461–5.

Williamson, D. F., Pamuk, E., Thun, M., Flanders, D., Byers, T., and Heath, C. (1995). Prospective study of intentional weight loss and mortality in never-smoking overweight US white women aged 40–64 years. *American Journal of Epidemiology*, **141**, 1128–41.

Williamson, D. F., Pamuk, E., Thun, M., Flanders, D., Byers, T., and Heath, C. (1999). Prospective study of intentional weight loss and mortality in overweight white men aged 40–64 years. *American Journal of Epidemiology*, **149**, 491–503.

WHO (World Health Organization) (1997a). Obesity: preventing and managing the global epidemic. Report of a WHO Consultation presented at the World Health Organization, 3–5 June 1997, Geneva. WHO/NUT/NCD/98.1, Geneva.

WHO (World Health Organization) (1997b). Obesity epidemic puts millions at risk from related diseases. Press release WHO/46, 12 June 1997; <http://www.who.int/archives/inf-pr-1997/en/pr97–46.html>.

WHO (World Health Organization) (2002a). Controlling the global obesity epidemic: the challenge; <http://www.who.int/nut/obs.htm>.

WHO (World Health Organization) (2002b). Global database on obesity and body mass index (BMI) in adults; <http://www.who.int/nut/db_bmi.htm>.

Yano, K., Reed, D. M., and McGee, D. L. (1984). Ten-year incidence of coronary heart disease in the Honolulu Heart program. *American Journal of Epidemiology*, **119**, 653–66.

Yao, C-H., Slattery, M. L., Jacobs, D. R., Jr., Folsom, A. R., and Nelson, E. T. (1991). Anthropometric predictors of coronary heart disease and total mortality: findings from the US Railroad Study. *American Journal of Epidemiology*, **134**, 1278–89.

Chapter 21

Metabolic syndrome, diabetes, and coronary heart disease

G. Hu, Q. Qiao, and J. Tuomilehto

21.1 Introduction

Diabetes is one of the fastest growing public health problems in both developing and developed countries due to increasing prevalence of obesity and sedentary behaviours (King *et al.* 1998; Zimmet *et al.* 2001). Cardiovascular disease (CVD) accounts for more than 70% of total mortality among patients with type 2 diabetes (Laakso 1999). Recent studies have shown that type 2 diabetes and CVD share many common risk factors such as obesity, hypertension, dyslipidaemia, and hyperglycaemia. These metabolic abnormalities were named as the 'metabolic syndrome' (WHO Consultation 1999). The pathogenesis of the metabolic syndrome is complex and so far incompletely understood, but obesity, sedentary lifestyle, dietary factors, and genetic factors are known to contribute and interact in its development (Reaven 1988; Liese *et al.* 1998). The most important dimension of the metabolic syndrome is its association with the risk of the development of atherosclerotic CVD. This chapter assesses the association of metabolic syndrome, diabetes, and coronary heart disease (CHD).

21.2 Definitions

21.2.1 Diagnostic criteria for diabetes mellitus

New diagnostic criteria for diabetes mellitus were approved by the American Diabetes Association (ADA) in 1997 and the World Health Organization (WHO) in 1999 (Expert Committee on the Diagnosis and Classification of Diabetes Mellitus 1997; WHO Consultation 1999). Subjects not previously diagnosed as diabetic are classified according to the following criteria: (1) 2-hour plasma glucose (2hPG) criteria alone: 2hPG $\geq$ 11.1 mmol/l for diabetes, 7.8–11.0 mmol/l for impaired glucose tolerance (IGT), and <7.8 mmol/l for normal glucose tolerance; and (2) fasting plasma glucose (FPG) criteria alone: FPG $\geq$ 7.0 mmol/l for diabetes, 6.1–6.9 mmol/l for impaired fasting glycaemia (IFG), and <6.1 mmol/l for normal fasting glucose. The major difference in the application of these diagnostic criteria for diabetes and glucose intolerance exists since ADA recommends the use of FPG alone, whereas the WHO consultation emphasizes the primary use of 2hPG together with FPG (see also Chapter 42). Multiple studies have shown that different people have high FPG than high 2hPG, and only one-third of asymptomatic diabetic subjects have both FPG and 2hPG simultaneously elevated (DECODE Study Group 1998, 2003*a*).

21.2.2 Definition of the metabolic syndrome

Subjects with diabetes or glucose intolerance are known as being associated with an adverse pattern of cardiovascular risk factors including obesity, hyperinsulinaemia, low high-density lipoprotein (HDL), high triglycerides, and hypertension compared to individuals with normal blood glucose. Since 1923 the clustering of some metabolic abnormalities has been recognized (Kylin 1923), but the mechanism of the clustering of these abnormalities is still poorly understood. The coining of the term 'syndrome X' in 1988 by Reaven (1988) renewed the impetus to conduct research concerning this syndrome. In his description of syndrome X, Reaven considered the following abnormalities: resistance to insulin-stimulated glucose uptake, glucose intolerance, hyperinsulinaemia, increased triglycerides, decreased high-density lipoprotein cholesterol (HDL-C), and hypertension. Since then, several additional components of the metabolic syndrome have been suggested, such as obesity, microalbuminuria, hyperuricaemia, abnormalities in haemostatic factors (DeFronzo and Ferrannini 1991; Kuusisto *et al.* 1995; Imperatore *et al.* 1998). Characterized by insulin resistance, this syndrome is also sometimes called the insulin resistance syndrome, or the metabolic syndrome (DeFronzo 1988; Reaven 1988; Liese *et al.* 1998). More recently, a term 'dysmetabolic syndrome', indicating the abnormality associated with this condition, has been launched in the United States with a specific ICD-code: 277.7. Despite the abundant research that has been published on the syndrome, definitions and cut-points for its components have varied widely (Reaven 1988; Liese *et al.* 1998). In 1999, the WHO (WHO Consultation 1999) named it as the metabolic syndrome and proposed the following working definition: IGT, or diabetes and/or insulin resistance together with two or more of the other components (hypertension, dyslipidaemia, central obesity, and microalbuminuria) (Fig. 21.1).

In 2001, the Third Report of the National Cholesterol Education Program (NCEP) Expert Panel on Detection, Evaluation, and Treatment of the High Blood Cholesterol in Adults (Adult Treatment Panel III) (ATP III) also provided a working definition of the metabolic syndrome

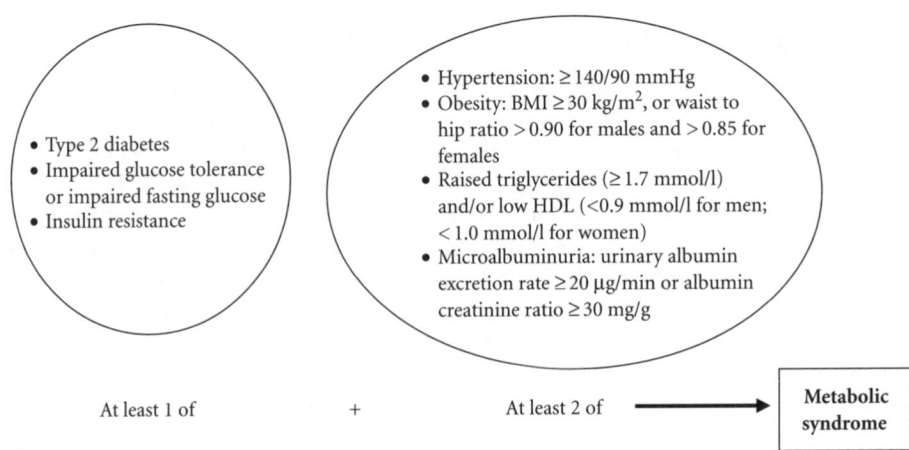

- Type 2 diabetes
- Impaired glucose tolerance or impaired fasting glucose
- Insulin resistance

- Hypertension: ≥ 140/90 mmHg
- Obesity: BMI ≥ 30 kg/m², or waist to hip ratio > 0.90 for males and > 0.85 for females
- Raised triglycerides (≥ 1.7 mmol/l) and/or low HDL (< 0.9 mmol/l for men; < 1.0 mmol/l for women)
- Microalbuminuria: urinary albumin excretion rate ≥ 20 μg/min or albumin creatinine ratio ≥ 30 mg/g

At least 1 of   +   At least 2 of ⟶ Metabolic syndrome

Fig. 21.1 Metabolic syndrome as defined by the WHO (WHO Consultation 1999). Insulin resistance is defined as being within the highest quartile for the relevant population.

(National Institute of Health 2001). People having three or more of the following criteria were defined as having the metabolic syndrome:

♦ Abdominal obesity: waist circumference >102 cm in men and >78 cm in women.

♦ Serum triglycerides ≥1.7 mmol/l.

♦ Serum HDL-C <1.04 mmol/l in men and <1.29 mmol/l in women.

♦ Blood pressure ≥130/85 mmHg.

♦ Fasting plasma glucose ≥6.1 mmol/l.

21.2.3 Global prevalence of diabetes and the metabolic syndrome

Diabetes is one of the fastest growing chronic diseases in the world. The global prevalence of diabetes was estimated to be 4.0% in 1995 and is projected to rise to 5.4% by the year 2025 (King *et al.* 1998). It is estimated that the number of adults with diabetes in the world will rise from 135 million in 1995 to 300 million in the year 2025. The major part of this numerical increase will occur in developing countries. There will be a 42% increase, from 51 to 72 million, in developed countries and a 170% increase, from 84 to 228 million, in developing countries. In developing countries the majority of people with diabetes are in the age range of 45–64 years, and in developed countries ≥65 years. This pattern will be accentuated by the year 2025.

The prevalence of the metabolic syndrome has varied markedly due to differences in definitions and populations studied (Meigs *et al.* 1997; Bonora *et al.* 1998; Hulthe *et al.* 2000; Isomaa *et al.* 2001; Ford *et al.* 2002). In the Botnia study, a follow-up study of family members of patients with type 2 diabetes in Finland, the metabolic syndrome (using the WHO definition) was found in 10% and 15% of subjects with normal glucose tolerance, in 42% and 64% of those with impaired glucose regulation, and in 78% and 84% of those with type 2 diabetes, in women and men, respectively (Isomaa *et al.* 2001). A recent study, using ATP III's new definition, estimated that 24% of US adults have the metabolic syndrome (Ford *et al.* 2002). Using the 2000 census data, ~47 million US residents have this syndrome. The prevalence of the metabolic syndrome in European and Asian populations, participating in the collaborative DECODE (Diabetes Epidemiology: collaborative analysis Of Diagnostic criteria in Europe) and the DECODA (Diabetes Epidemiology: collaborative analysis Of Diagnostic criteria in Asia) studies are shown in Tables 21.1 and 21.2.

21.3 Diabetes and CHD

The most common cause of death in adults with diabetes is CHD. Both type 1 diabetic and type 2 diabetic subjects present an excess risk of CHD compared with non-diabetic persons (Kannel and McGee 1979b; Stamler *et al.* 1993; Lee *et al.* 2000). There are wide differences in the prevalence of CHD in type 1 and type 2 patients between different populations. The follow-up study of 10 centres of the WHO Multinational Study of Vascular disease in diabetes (WHO MSVDD), including ~4700 patients with type 1 and 2 diabetes, showed that Japanese diabetic patients had a notably lower incidence of CHD than diabetic subjects from other parts of the world (Lee *et al.* 2001; Morrish *et al.* 2001). Furthermore, their CHD incidence rates were also lower than those of many non-diabetic Western populations. CVD was the most common cause of death, accounting for 44% of death from natural causes among patients with

Table 21.1 Age- and sex-specific prevalence of the metabolic syndrome and its components in European population, the DECODE Study

	NGT		IGR		Type 2 diabetes		Total	
	Male	Female	Male	Female	Male	Female	Male	Female
Metabolic syndrome[a]								
40–9 (years)	6.8	3.4	20.0	27.5	51.6	65.0	11.0	7.8
50–9	8.7	8.1	24.4	25.7	64.1	60.0	17.1	13.3
60–9	9.8	13.6	24.0	31.3	53.7	58.9	18.2	22.3
70+	6.9	11.7	24.2	26.7	38.8	64.8	17.2	25.0
Total	8.1	8.6	23.3	28.2	50.9	61.1	15.8	15.9
Obesity								
40–9	9.1	11.7	18.6	35.5	32.8	57.5	11.8	15.6
50–9	12.7	16.4	21.1	33.8	35.4	53.9	16.6	20.8
60–9	10.4	20.0	21.2	28.8	35.8	44.3	15.9	24.6
70 +	7.5	19.8	15.9	26.7	19.4	41.9	11.8	25.5
Total	10.3	16.4	19.5	31.1	29.3	47.4	14.3	21.1
Dyslipidaemia								
40–9	31.4	12.2	46.8	39.1	51.6	67.5	35.0	16.8
50–9	37.3	22.5	47.6	43.9	58.0	52.2	41.4	26.9
60–9	33.4	29.3	44.9	50.6	50.0	58.4	38.0	36.9
70+	23.7	24.6	39.5	41.2	43.0	54.3	31.3	33.9
Total	32.5	21.7	45.0	45.3	49.8	56.6	37.0	28.2
Hypertension								
40–9	32.9	17.5	52.5	37.0	62.5	45.0	37.6	20.4
50–9	42.3	37.0	61.7	48.3	71.8	60.0	49.2	39.8
60–9	48.1	48.2	58.8	65.0	69.1	69.2	53.0	54.0
70+	62.4	58.3	76.4	76.3	76.4	79.0	68.5	66.3
Total	44.1	36.4	62.4	57.1	71.9	67.0	51.0	42.1
Insulin resistance								
40–9	19.2	14.8	42.0	52.9	–	–	23.5	18.9
50–9	17.9	19.1	47.4	47.6	–	–	25.0	23.1
60–9	21.2	25.8	47.7	50.6	–	–	28.1	31.4
70 +	26.9	27.6	48.7	46.6	–	–	26.7	33.0
Total	18.8	20.4	46.6	49.4	–	–	25.6	25.3

NGT: normal glucose tolerance; IGR: impaired glucose regulation.

[a] The metabolic syndrome was defined using the WHO criteria. Insulin resistance was defined as the highest quartile of the $HOMA_{IR}$ index among subjects without diabetes; obesity: body mass index ≥ 30 kg/m^2; hypertension: blood pressure $\geq 140/90$ mmHg; dyslipidaemia: triglycerides ≥ 1.7 mmol/l and/or low HDL (<0.9 mmol/l in men, <1.0 mmol/l in women).

type 1 diabetes and 52% of the deaths in patients with type 2 diabetes (Morrish *et al.* 2001). In the EURODIAB IDDM Complication Study, involving 3250 type 1 diabetic patients from 16 European countries, the prevalence of CVD (a past history and electrocardiogram abnormality) was 9% in men and 10% in women. The prevalence increased with age (from 6% in patients 15–29 years old to 25% in patients 45–59 years old) and with duration of diabetes (Koivisto *et al.* 1996). In type 1 diabetic patients, the risk of CHD starts to increase dramatically after the onset of diabetic nephropathy. After 20 years' duration of diabetes up to 29% of childhood-onset type 1 diabetic patients with nephropathy will have CHD, while of

Table 21.2 Age- and sex-specific prevalence of the metabolic syndrome and its components in Asian populations, the DECODA Study[a]

	NGT		IGR		Type 2 diabetes		Total	
	Male	Female	Male	Female	Male	Female	Male	Female
Metabolic syndrome								
Indian (40–79 years)	–	–	21.8	31.9	32.4	45.0	10.4	15.4
Singaporean (40–69)	–	–	25.6	19.1	35.7	37.3	14.8	12.2
Japanese (60–79)	–	–	22.1	17.9	27.7	26.3	10.6	7.0
Chinese (40–89)	–	–	37.9	33.6	36.4	38.9	11.1	10.9
Obesity								
Indian	1.8	9.7	4.6	12.8	5.5	12.2	3.1	10.7
Singaporean	2.4	6.8	3.4	13.5	11.2	17.0	4.6	10.5
Japanese	0.6	1.6	1.7	2.5	2.0	6.9	1.1	2.4
Chinese	4.2	8.0	13.7	15.6	9.1	12.1	6.4	9.7
Dyslipidaemia								
Indian	46.0	40.4	54.0	52.1	63.7	71.1	51.2	49.7
Singaporean	39.3	18.9	55.7	33.7	55.9	60.8	47.4	31.0
Japanese	25.5	14.8	40.3	32.4	48.0	34.4	33.3	21.0
Chinese	34.7	24.7	60.0	39.8	45.5	51.7	40.3	31.1
Hypertension								
Indian	27.3	28.1	42.5	48.9	48.9	53.9	34.3	37.3
Singaporean	22.1	16.2	38.6	29.8	46.2	46.4	31.8	25.7
Japanese	33.6	23.4	48.3	42.7	50.5	51.9	40.4	31.0
Chinese	47.0	38.1	54.7	55.5	66.2	59.1	50.9	43.8

NGT: normal glucose tolerance; IGR: impaired glucose regulation.

[a] The metabolic syndrome was defined using the WHO criteria. Obesity: body mass index ≥ 30 kg/m^2; hypertension: blood pressure $\geq$ 140/90 mmHg; dyslipidaemia: triglycerides $\geq$ 1.7 mmol/l and/or low HDL (<0.9 mmol/l in men, <1.0 mmol/l in women).

non-nephropathic patients only 2–3% suffer from CHD (Tuomilehto *et al.* 1998). It seems that characteristics of the metabolic syndrome other than hyperglycaemia itself are the major contributing factors for CHD in type 1 diabetes (Orchard *et al.* 2003).

Several studies have compared the magnitude of CHD risk associated with a history of type 2 diabetes or previous CHD. Results from the 7-year follow-up of a Finnish Study (Haffner *et al.* 1998) and from 20-year follow-up of the Nurse's Health Study (Hu *et al.* 2001) found that patients with type 2 diabetes, but without any previous acute CHD event, have as high a risk of fatal CHD as non-diabetic patients who have suffered from a previous myocardial infarction (MI). The combination of type 2 diabetes and previous CHD identifies a particularly high risk of CHD death. The Nurse's Health Study also indicated a strong monotonic relation between duration of clinical diabetes and CHD mortality. Compared with non-diabetic persons, the multivariate relative risks of fatal CHD across categories of diabetes duration (≤ 5, 6–10, 11–15, 16–25, >25 years) were 2.75, 3.63, 5.51, 6.38, and 11.9 ($p < 0.001$ for trend), respectively.

The increased risk of CHD in subjects with diabetes is partly, but not fully, explained by abnormal levels of other cardiovascular risk factors such as high blood pressure, obesity, dyslipidaemia, and smoking. Thus, it has been hypothesized that the diabetic state itself or hyperglycaemia is responsible for the increased CHD risk. This question has been investigated during recent decades. In 1979, a series of papers from the International Collaborative Group (International Collaborative Group 1979) did not find consistent evidence for either a threshold or graded association between asymptomatic hyperglycaemia and CHD. The differences in glucose assay methods, glucose load and the time after loading, follow-up time, and the populations studied may have contributed to the inconsistent observations from the early studies. The National Diabetes Data Group (1979) and the WHO (WHO Expert Committee 1980) first advanced the diagnostic criteria for diabetes in 1979 and 1980, respectively, and this has created order out of the previous confusion in the diagnostic criteria for diabetes. Since then, several epidemiological studies in the past 20 years have shown an association between 2 hPG and the occurrence of CHD in the general population (Pyorala *et al.* 1979; Fuller *et al.* 1980; Fontbonne *et al.* 1989; Lowe *et al.* 1997; Barrett-Connor and Ferrara 1998; Barzilay *et al.* 1999; DECODE Study Group 1999, 2001; Rodriguez *et al.* 1999; Shaw *et al.* 1999; Tominaga *et al.* 1999; Saydah *et al.* 2001). In some studies the FPG was also associated with CHD (Scheidt-Nave *et al.* 1991; Shaten *et al.* 1991; Yarnell *et al.* 1994; Simons *et al.* 2000). A recent meta-analysis including 95 783 individuals from 20 epidemiological studies found a progressive relationship between glucose levels (both FPG and 2 hPG) and the incidence of cardiovascular events among non-diabetic people (Coutinho *et al.* 1999).

21.3.1 Impaired glucose tolerance, asymptomatic hyperglycaemia or diabetes, and CHD

The major disagreement between WHO and ADA criteria in the classification of individuals focuses on whether diabetes should be diagnosed using FPG or 2 hPG. While different people are identified as diabetic, and particularly as having impaired glucose regulation (IFG or IGT) when testing for FPG than 2 hPG, it is very interesting and clinically important to know how FPG and 2 hPG are related to mortality and CVD risk. Three early cohort studies, the Whitehall Study, the Paris Prospective Study, and the Helsinki Policemen Study, assessed the relationship between 2 hPG and CHD risk in European men (Pyorala *et al.* 1979; Fuller *et al.* 1980; Fontbonne *et al.* 1989). With known diabetes excluded, CHD mortality in those with high 2 hPG (>95th centile in the Whitehall Study and >80th centile in the Paris and Helsinki studies) was twice as high as in those with normal glucose levels. In the Japanese Funagata Diabetes Study, survival analysis concluded that IGT, but not IFG, was a risk factor for CVD (Tominaga *et al.* 1999). A recent Finnish study found that baseline IGT was an independent risk predictor for incidence of CHD and premature death from CVD and all-cause, which was not confounded by the development of clinically diagnosed diabetes during the follow-up (Qiao *et al.* 2003).

The 23-year follow-up of the Honolulu Heart Program suggested a dose–response relationship between 1 h glucose after 50 g load and CHD mortality (Rodriguez *et al.* 1999). The Chicago Heart Study of ~12 000 men without a history of diabetes showed that white men with asymptomatic hyperglycaemia (1 h glucose $\geq$ 11.1 mmol/l) had an increased risk of CVD mortality compared with men with low post-load glucose < 8.9 mmol/l (Lowe *et al.* 1997). The Rancho Bernardo Study indicated that older Californian women (but not men) with isolated post-challenge hyperglycaemia (2 hPG $\geq$ 11.1 mmol/l and FPG < 7.0 mmol/l) had a significantly increased risk of CVD (Barrett-Connor and Ferrara 1998). Several studies assessed the association of CHD with both FPG and 2 hPG. Based on longitudinal studies in Mauritius, Fiji, and Nauru, Shaw *et al.* also reported that people with isolated post-challenge hyperglycaemia doubled CVD mortality compared with non-diabetic persons, but no significant increase in mortality was associated with isolated fasting hyperglycaemia (FPG $\geq$ 7.0 mmol/l and 2 hPG < 11.1 mmol/l) (Shaw *et al.* 1999). In the Cardiovascular Health Study, including 4515 subjects aged >65 years, the relative risk for incident CHD was higher in individuals with abnormal glucose (including IGT, IFG, and newly diagnosed diabetes by both ADA and WHO criteria) than in those with normal glucose. However, ADA criteria based on FPG were less sensitive than the WHO criteria for predicting CHD among individuals with abnormal glucose (Barzilay *et al.* 1999). A recent analysis of the US Second National Health and Nutrition Survey data, including 3092 adults aged 30–74 years, found a graded mortality associated with abnormal glucose tolerance ranging from a 40% greater risk in adults with IGT to a 80% greater risk in adults with newly diagnosed diabetes (Saydah *et al.* 2001).

The most convincing evidence of increased CHD risk related to abnormal glucose tolerance was provided by the DECODE study. In this project, individual data from more than 10 prospective cohort studies including more than 22 000 subjects were analysed jointly (DECODE Study Group 1999, 2001). Death rates from all-causes, CVD, and CHD were higher in diabetic subjects diagnosed by 2 hPG criteria than in those not meeting these criteria. Significantly increased mortality was also observed in subjects with IGT, whereas there was no difference in mortality between subjects with IFG and those with normal fasting glucose. Multivariate Cox proportional hazard analyses showed that elevated 2 hPG was an independent predictor of mortality from all-causes, CVD, and CHD, but elevated FPG alone was not. A high 2 hPG was found to be associated with an increased risk of death, independent of the level of FPG, whereas increased mortality in people with elevated FPG was largely due to the simultaneous elevation of 2 hPG. On the other hand, FPG did not add any predictive information once 2 hPG was in the model. The largest absolute number of excess CVD deaths was observed in subjects with IGT, especially those with IGT but normal fasting glucose. The association between glucose and the incidence of CHD was assessed in five Finnish cohorts belonging to the DECODE study (Qiao *et al.* 2002). Multivariate Cox regression analyses showed that the hazards ratio for a one standard deviation increase in 2 hPG and FPG after logarithmic transformation was 1.17 (95% CI: 1.05–1.30) and 1.05 (0.94–1.17) for CHD incidence, respectively.

Thus, the DECODE study unequivocally confirmed that post-load hyperglycaemia independently increases cardiovascular morbidity and mortality and is a better predictor of events than high FPG. Next, however, it is necessary to demonstrate with controlled clinical trials that lowering of high 2 hPG will reduce the risk of CVD and the incidence of CHD. Such studies are underway.

So far, the largest trial in type 2 diabetic patients, the United Kingdom Prospective Diabetes Study (UKPDS) (UK Prospective Diabetes Study Group 1998*a*), did not find convincing evidence for the hypothesis that lowering blood glucose concentration by intensive antidiabetic treatment can reduce the risk of MI, although there was a 16% (almost significant) reduction in MI in the intensive treatment group compared with the conventional treatment group. In the UKPDS, however, post-load glucose excursion was not measured and over the 10 years the difference in HBA1c concentration between the intensive and conventional groups was only 0.9% (7.0 vs. 7.9%). Moreover, sulfonylureas, long-acting insulin, and metformin used for the intensive treatment in the UKPDS do not lower the post-prandial glucose excursions, but influence mainly fasting glucose levels.

The German Diabetes Intervention Study (DIS) is thus far the only intervention study that has demonstrated that controlling post-prandial hyperglycaemia (blood glucose measured 1 h after breakfast) had a greater impact on cardiovascular and all-cause mortality than controlling fasting blood glucose (Hanefeld *et al.* 1996). The DIS comprised newly diagnosed type 2 diabetic patients. During the 11-year follow-up the study showed that poor control of fasting glycaemia did not significantly increase the risk of MI or mortality, whereas poor control of prandial glucose was associated with a significantly higher mortality vs. good prandial glucose control. Mealtime glucose regulators or 'prandial' oral antidiabetic agents have now become available and offer possibilities to improve glycaemic control specifically during the postprandial state. These include α-glucosidase inhibitors, short-acting insulin secretagogues, and rapidly released insulin analogues. The first data evaluating the significance of post-prandial glucose control using acarbose in the prevention of diabetes in subjects with IGT have demonstrated its efficacy (Chiasson *et al.* 2002). Moreover, the early communications from secondary analyses of the STOP-NIDDM trial have revealed statistically significant reductions in cardiovascular event rates in patients receiving acarbose compared with placebo (Chiasson *et al.* 2003). This is the first demonstration that a treatment that specifically lowers post-prandial glucose will lead to a reduction in cardiovascular events.

21.3.2 Gender difference in CHD related to diabetes

Among middle-aged general populations, men have 2–5 times higher risk of CHD than women (Tuomilehto and Kuulasmaa 1989; Tunstall-Pedoe *et al.* 1994; Jousilahti *et al.* 1999). The Framingham Study was the first one to point out that women with diabetes seem to lose their relative protection against CHD compared with men (Kannel and McGee 1979*a*). The reason for the higher relative risk of CHD in diabetic women than diabetic men is still unclear. The 14-year follow-up of the Rancho Bernardo study showed that the multivariate-adjusted relative hazards of death from CHD in diabetic compared with non-diabetic subjects was 3.3 in women and 1.9 in men (Barrett-Connor *et al.* 1991). An 11.6-year follow-up study in Scotland found asymptomatic hyperglycaemia (casual blood glucose > 7.0 mmol/l) to be a significant risk factor for CVD in both genders, but stronger in women than in men (Janghorbani *et al.* 1994). A review about the impact of gender on the occurrence of atherosclerotic vascular disease in type 2 diabetes mellitus reported the overall relative risk for gender (men vs. women) in CHD mortality as 1.46 (95% CI: 1.21–1.95) in diabetic and 2.29 (2.05–2.55) in non-diabetic subjects (Orchard 1996). The results from the DECODE study, including 8172 men and 9407 women without known diabetes, showed that newly diagnosed diabetic women had a higher relative risk for CVD death than newly diagnosed diabetic men (DECODE Study Group 2003*b*). This association is statistically independent of age, body mass index, systolic blood pressure, total cholesterol, and smoking. The recent data related to hormone replacement therapy show that particularly in diabetic women the risk of CVD increases significantly (Kanaya *et al.* 2003).

21.3.3 The metabolic syndrome and CHD

Hyperinsulinaemia and CHD

Hyperinsulinaemia, or insulin resistance, has been shown to be associated with a cluster of CVD risk factors including hypertension, dyslipidaemia, obesity, and glucose intolerance. Any one or combination of them may increase the risk of CHD. However, the association of hyperinsulinaemia per se with CHD has been debated. In a review of 19 prospective epidemiological studies which had assessed the relationship between fasting plasma insulin and the risk of CHD, a positive association was observed in 10 studies, and in 8 of them the association was independent of other CVD risk factors (Pyorala *et al.* 1998). Nine studies found no association or even an inverse association. The differences in insulin assays, the populations studied, and statistical power may have contributed to the inconsistent observations. Therefore, at this moment it is still unclear whether hyperinsulinaemia is an independent risk factor for CHD or not. It is also important to note that during the progress to diabetes serum insulin levels rise in order to compensate peripheral insulin resistance, but in overt diabetes the production of insulin by pancreatic beta-cells will gradually fail and insulin production starts to fall. The duration of this process varies drastically between individuals. Thus, when fasting insulin is casually measured it may be difficult to determine the stage of this process and interpret fasting insulin concentration correctly.

The metabolic syndrome and CHD

The Framingham Offspring Study in subjects aged 19–74 years examined the clustering of metabolic factors and CHD risk (Wilson *et al.* 1999). The six metabolically linked risk factors considered were the lowest sex-specific quintile of HDL-C, and the highest quintiles of body mass index, systolic blood pressure, triglycerides, glucose, and serum total cholesterol. A cluster of three or more risk factors was associated with a 2.4 and 5.9 times increased risk of CHD in men and women, respectively. Cardiovascular morbidity and mortality was also assessed in 3606 subjects from the Botnia study in Western Finland, with a median follow-up of 6.9 years (Isomaa *et al.* 2001). The prevalence of CHD was increased three-fold in subjects with the metabolic syndrome, and cardiovascular mortality associated with the syndrome was markedly increased (12% in individuals with the syndrome versus 2.2% in those without; $p < 0.001$). Of the individual components of the metabolic syndrome, microalbuminuria conferred the strongest relative risk of cardiovascular death. Another Finnish study, the Kuopio Ischaemic Heart Disease Study, recently reported the results of an 11.4-year follow-up in middle-aged men, examining the predictive value of both the WHO and NCEP definitions of the metabolic syndrome and their modifications with regard to CHD, CVD, and all-cause mortality (Lakka *et al.* 2002). The prevalence of the metabolic syndrome ranged from 8.8 to 14.3%, depending on the definition. The metabolic syndrome as defined by the WHO was associated with 1.9 times higher all-cause mortality and 2.6 times higher CVD mortality, whereas the NCEP definition of the metabolic syndrome less consistently predicted all-cause and CVD mortality. The results from the DECODE study showed that multivariate-adjusted hazards ratios for CVD and CHD mortality, respectively, were 1.76 (95% CI: 1.43–2.17) and 1.51 (1.14–2.01) in men, and 2.34 (1.52–3.61) and 5.42 (2.47–11.91) in women with the metabolic syndrome compared to those without (Table 21.3).

Table 21.3 Multivariate-adjusted hazards ratios (95% confidence intervals) for mortality in subjects with the metabolic syndrome as compared with those without, in European populations, the DECODE study

	Men	**Women**
Cardiovascular diseases	1.76 (1.43–2.17)	2.34 (1.52–3.61)
Coronary heart disease	1.51 (1.14–2.01)	5.42 (2.47–11.91)

Hazards ratios adjusted for age, centre, and smoking.

21.4 Possible mechanisms linking metabolic factors to CHD

Type 2 diabetes and hyperglycaemia are consequences of impairments in insulin secretion and insulin action in peripheral tissues, and of an increase in the rate of endogenous hepatic glucose production (DeFronzo 1988; Ferrannini 1998; Pratley and Weyer 2001). The release of insulin in response to intravenous glucose is biphasic, with a rapid first phase lasting for 5–10 min, followed by a prolonged second phase, which continues for the duration of the stimulus (Ferrannini 1999; Pratley and Weyer 2001). During fasting, tissue insulin concentrations are low, lipolysis and circulating non-esterified fatty acids (NEFAs) are high, and the glucose requirements of the brain and other tissues are met through endogenous glucose production. The initial increase in plasma glucose upon ingestion of a meal stimulates a rapid increase in insulin secretion that optimally serves to increase interstitial insulin concentrations. The anti-lipolytic effect of insulin on adipocytes causes a rapid decrease in NEFAs and inhibition of endogenous glucose production. The early insulin response could also prime insulin-sensitive tissue to increase the efficiency of glucose disposal (Pratley and Weyer 2001). Thus, the loss of the early-phase insulin response after a meal due to the beta-cell dysfunction initially leads to post-prandial hyperglycaemia. The post-prandial state accounts for most of the hours of a day and has been considered to be an important contributing factor to the development of atherosclerosis (Ceriello 2000). Hyperglycaemia subsequently results in a high insulin output (hyperinsulinaemia) in order to restore blood glucose concentrations to normal (Ferrannini 1999; Pratley and Weyer 2001). Chronic hyperglycaemia, in turn, can also depress both beta-cell function and insulin sensitivity, so-called glucose toxicity (Unger and Grundy 1985; Leahy *et al.* 1986; Yki-Jarvinen 1992). In all these cycles of hypo- and hyperinsulinaemia, insulin's ability to suppress endogenous glucose production and to stimulate glucose uptake is compromised in the clinical abnormality of glucose intolerance and diabetes.

21.4.1 Mechanisms by which hyperglycaemia affects the atherogenic process

While clinical and epidemiological studies have convincingly demonstrated that cardiovascular morbidity and mortality increased in subjects with glucose intolerance and diabetes, the pathogenetic mechanisms involved are not yet fully understood, but currently under very intensive research. Studies have demonstrated that high serum triglycerides and an atherogenic lipoprotein profile in diabetes are related to hyperglycaemia (Howard 1987), and the control of post-prandial glucose excursions reduces the post-prandial increase in triglycerides (Hanefeld *et al.* 1991). Low-density lipoprotein (LDL) cholesterol oxidation in type 2 diabetic patients also increased after meals (Diwadkar *et al.* 1999), and the increase is directly related to the degree of hyperglycaemia (Ceriello *et al.* 1999). In both *in vitro* and *in vivo* studies high glucose concentrations could reduce the vasodilatory response to stimuli and result in a rise in blood pressure (Bohlen and Lash 1993; Marfella *et al.* 1995), and the rapid decrease in vasodilatation correlated inversely with the magnitude of post-prandial hyperglycaemia (Shige *et al.* 1999). Acute hyperglycaemia produces hypertension probably because it induces endothelial dysfunction (Giugliano *et al.* 1997; Kawano *et al.* 1999), which is likely to be linked to a reduction in the production/bioavailability of nitric oxide (NO) (Giugliano *et al.* 1997; Lash *et al.* 1999). It is, however, not yet clear whether hyperglycaemia actually reduces the production of NO (Lash *et al.* 1999) or whether it increases NO production together with an even greater increase in the production of its inhibitor, the superoxide anion (Cosentino *et al.* 1997) leading to an overall reduction in the bioavailability of NO (Bartels *et al.* 2000). Studies have also shown that acute glycaemic variations are accompanied by a series of alterations in the coagulation system that is likely to increase the risk of thrombosis in diabetic patients (Jones and Peterson 1979; Jones 1985; Ceriello *et al.* 1988, 1989, 1995, 1996; Sakamoto *et al.* 2000). The mechanisms by which acute hyperglycaemia may affect atherogenic process probably involves both non-enzymatic labile glycation (Ceriello *et al.* 1992) and the production of free radicals (Ceriello 1997). In labile glycation, glucose binds through a non-enzymatic bond with amino groups of circulating or vessel wall proteins, which subsequently rearrange to form the more stable Amadori-type early glycosylation products. These products continue to rearrange and will form advanced glycosylation end products (AGEs) (Brownlee 1995). Once formed, AGE protein adducts are virtually irreversible. AGEs promote atherosclerotic effects through various non-receptor mediating mechanisms (e.g. through extracellular matrix, functional alterations of regulatory proteins, lipoprotein modifications) and receptor-mediated mechanisms (e.g. inflammation promotion, induction of cellular proliferation, endothelial dysfunction).

Oxidative stress is a recognized pathogenetic process involved in complications of diabetes (Giugliano *et al.* 1996). Recently, Nishikawa *et al.* (2000) demonstrated that glucose can produce free radicals in a dose–response manner, providing further evidence to support the hypothesis that an acute increase in serum glucose levels can produce an equivalent increase in acute oxidative stress. A rapid production of free radicals from glucose can be obtained biochemically in three ways: during labile glycation (Mullarkey *et al.* 1990), directly from glucose through a process of auto-oxidation (Wolff and Dean 1987), and through intracellular activation of the sorbitol pathway (Williamson *et al.* 1993). Studies also suggested that antioxidant defences are diminished in diabetic patients (Ceriello *et al.* 1997) and that hyperglycaemia exacerbated the effects in the post-prandial state (Ceriello *et al.* 1999; Staprans *et al.* 1999).

21.4.2 The role of insulin resistance in atherosclerosis

Although clinical and epidemiological evidence showing that insulin resistance is probably a primary initiating defect behind the aberrations of the metabolic syndrome has accumulated, controversial opinions still exist. Lipolysis is highly insulin sensitive and insulin regulates the circulating NEFA concentration. The net systemic effect of insulin administration is a prompt, marked decline in circulating NEFA, indicating the switch of energy production from dominant fat oxidation to carbohydrate utilization (Ferrannini 1999). The action of insulin is impaired in subjects with insulin resistance, whether they are healthy individuals (Ferrannini *et al.* 1997), diabetic patients (Golay *et al.* 1987), or non-diabetic obese subjects (Frayn *et al.* 1996). This results in the liver being exposed to high NEFA concentrations, which stimulate both hepatic NEFA oxidation and hepatic glucose production. Triglyceride secretion is then stimulated, leading to reduction of HDL-C concentrations and enrichment of the LDL-cholesterol fraction with small, dense, strongly atherogenic particles (Ferrannini 1999). Chronically raised fatty acid levels antagonize insulin action on glucose uptake, and may further depress insulin secretion (Sako and Grill 1990; Zhou and Grill 1994). In the human body, increased levels of plasminogen activator inhibitor-1 (PAI-1) are associated with an increased risk of thrombosis. PAI-1 levels are elevated in subjects with hypertension (Cigolini *et al.* 1995), obesity (Vidal 2001) and dyslipidaemia (Hamsten *et al.* 1994; Festa *et al.* 1999). It was, thus, hypothesized that the role of PAI-1 in development of atherosclerosis may be associated with a mechanism whereby insulin resistance increases the risk of cardiovascular disease. Research has shown that glucose increases the gene expression of PAI-1, as dose proinsulin and split proinsulin, whereas insulin and insulin-like growth factor-1 increase the production of PAI-1 only by increasing the stability of the PAI-1 mRNA (Schneider *et al.* 1992). It was also reported that insulin resistance was associated with abnormal *in vivo* platelet calcium handling (Baldi *et al.* 1996).

21.5 Prevention of CHD in people with abnormal glucose regulation

While overall trends in CHD mortality have shown a significant downward trend in developed countries during recent decades, it has been suggested that in diabetic subjects the decline has been smaller, or even absent (Gu *et al.* 1999). On the other hand, accumulating evidence has shown that deterioration of IGT into type 2 diabetes can be effectively prevented by lifestyle intervention (Pan *et al.* 1997; Tuomilehto *et al.* 2001; Knowler *et al.* 2002). We need to demonstrate that the prevention and control of mealtime hyperglycaemia will lead to a reduction of mortality, CVD, and other late complications of type 2 diabetes. In addition, there is a need to reconsider the thresholds used to diagnose hyperglycaemia (DECODE Study Group 2003*c*). The majority of premature deaths due to hyperglycaemia occur in people with IGT (DECODE Study Group 1999, 2001); therefore, it is becoming important to pay more attention to people whose 2-hour post-challenge glucose level is within the IGT range. The first step is to detect such people through a systematic case finding among high-risk groups, for example, those with a family history of diabetes or subjects with hypertension, obesity, smoking, physical inactivity, and previous gestational diabetes. A systematic tool for this purpose has been recently developed and is now applied in some countries (Lindstrom and Tuomilehto 2003). The best way to prevent the negative health consequences of hyperglycaemia is to prevent the development of type 2 diabetes. In addition, it is clear from subgroup analyses of controlled trials that antihypertensive drug treatment in hypertensive patients with diabetes (Curb *et al.* 1996; UK Prospective Diabetes Study Group 1998b, Tuomilehto *et al.* 1999; The ALLHAT Officers and Coordinators for the Collaborative Research Group 2002) and statin therapy in those who have high serum cholesterol (Pyorala *et al.* 1997; Heart Protection Study Collaborative Group 2002) are efficient ways to prevent CHD in diabetic patients. In addition, it is currently recommended that patients with type 2 diabetes should receive acetosalicylic acid treatment if not contraindicated (American Diabetes Association 2002). The multifactorial, aggressive approach to influence the multiple risk factors for CHD in diabetic patients was recently well-demonstrated by the Steno-2 study (Gaede *et al.* 2003). Diabetes is one of the strongest factors leading to vascular complications through multiple pathways, not exclusively by hyperglycaemia, that may have a direct effect and also activate other pathophysiological processes (Heine and Dekker 2002). Thus, it is important that several, if not all, of these metabolic abnormalities are corrected, or preferably prevented in diabetic patients. Otherwise, it seems inevitable that they will continue to suffer from disproportionate rates of cardiovascular disease. Finally, one should not forget the importance of healthy lifestyle once a person has a severe disease such as diabetes – no smoking, sufficient physical activity and a healthy, balanced diet will do much to help.

Whether it is possible to prevent the development of CVD in people with asymptomatic hyperglycaemia is not known since we lack trial data on this question. What is known, however, is that the worsening of hyperglycaemia can be effectively halted by lifestyle intervention (Tuomilehto *et al.* 2001; Knowler *et al.* 2002) and certain antidiabetic drugs (Chiasson *et al.* 2002; Knowler *et al.* 2002). Whether this will then also result in a delay in the development of cardiovascular disease is still unclear. The communications from secondary analyses of the

STOP-NIDDM trial have revealed statistically significant reductions in cardiovascular event rates in patients receiving acarbose compared with placebo (Chiasson *et al.* 2003). Since acarbose specifically reduces post-prandial glucose excursions, this is the first demonstration that lowering post-prandial glucose may lead to a reduction in cardiovascular events. Such controlled clinical outcome trials among subjects with asymptomatic hyperglycaemia are now underway, but the results from these will only be available after several years. Meanwhile, the only way to make clinical treatment decisions in such subjects is to make inferences from the observational epidemiological data and pathophysiological studies.

References

American Diabetes Association (2002). Aspirin therapy in diabetes. *Diabetes Care*, **25**, S78–79.

Baldi, S., Natali, A., Buzzigoli, G., Galvan, A. Q., Sironi, A. M., and Ferrannini, E. (1996). In vivo effect of insulin on intracellular calcium concentrations: relation to insulin resistance. *Metabolism*, **45**, 1402–7.

Barrett-Connor, E. and Ferrara, A. (1998). Isolated postchallenge hyperglycemia and the risk of fatal cardiovascular disease in older women and men: The Rancho Bernardo Study. *Diabetes Care*, **21**, 1236–9.

Barrett-Connor, E. L., Cohn, B. A., Wingard, D. L., and Edelstein, S. L. (1991). Why is diabetes mellitus a stronger risk factor for fatal ischemic heart disease in women than in men? The Rancho Bernardo Study. *Journal of the American Medical Association*, **265**, 627–31.

Bartels, H., Berkels, R., Rosen, R., Kirmizigul, I., and Rosen, P. (2000). Short term high glucose stimulates the generation of reactive oxygen species, but eliminates free nitric oxide. *Diabetes*, **49**(Suppl. 1), 134A.

Barzilay, J. I., Spiekerman, C. F., Wahl, P. W., Kuller, L. H., Cushman, M., Furberg, C. D. *et al.* (1999). Cardiovascular disease in older adults with glucose disorders: comparison of American Diabetes Association criteria for diabetes mellitus with WHO criteria. *Lancet*, **354**, 622–5.

Bohlen, H. G. and Lash, J. M. (1993). Topical hyperglycemia rapidly suppresses EDRF-mediated vasodilation of normal rat arterioles. *American Journal of Physiology*, **265**, H219–25.

Bonora, E., Kiechl, S., Willeit, J., Oberhollenzer, F., Egger, G., Targher, G. *et al.* (1998). Prevalence of insulin resistance in metabolic disorders: the Bruneck Study. *Diabetes*, **47**, 1643–9.

Brownlee, M. (1995). The pathological implications of protien glycation. *Journal of Clinical Investigation*, **18**, 275–81.

Ceriello, A. (1997). Acute hyperglycaemia and oxidative stress generation. *Diabetic Medicine*, **14**, S45–9.

Ceriello, A. (2000). The post-prandial state and cardiovascular disease: relevance to diabetes mellitus. *Diabetes/Metabolism Research and Reviews*, **16**, 125–32.

Ceriello, A., Giugliano, D., Quatraro, A., Dello Russo, P., and Torella, R. (1988). Blood glucose may condition factor VII levels in diabetic and normal subjects. *Diabetologia*, **31**, 889–91.

Ceriello, A., Giugliano, D., Quatraro, A., Dello Russo, P., Marchi, E., and Torella, R. (1989). Hyperglycemia may determine fibrinopeptide A plasma level increase in humans. *Metabolism*, **38**, 1162–3.

Ceriello, A., Quatraro, A., and Giugliano, D. (1992). New insights on non-enzymatic glycosylation may lead to therapeutic approaches for the prevention of diabetic complications. *Diabetic Medicine*, **9**, 297–9.

Ceriello, A., Giacomello, R., Stel, G., Motz, E., Taboga, C., Tonutti, L. *et al.* (1995). Hyperglycemia-induced thrombin formation in diabetes: the possible role of oxidative stress. *Diabetes*, **44**, 924–8.

Ceriello, A., Taboga, C., Tonutti, L., Giacomello, R., Stel, L., Motz, E., and Pirisi, M. (1996). Post-meal coagulation activation in diabetes mellitus: the effect of acarbose. *Diabetologia*, **39**, 469–73.

Ceriello, A., Bortolotti, N., Falleti, E., Taboga, C., Tonutti, L., Crescentini, A. *et al.* (1997). Total radical-trapping antioxidant parameter in NIDDM patients. *Diabetes Care*, **20**, 194–7.

Ceriello, A., Bortolotti, N., Motz, E., Pieri, C., Marra, M., Tonutti, L. *et al.* (1999). Meal-induced oxidative stress and low-density lipoprotein oxidation in diabetes: the possible role of hyperglycemia. *Metabolism*, **48**, 1503–8.

Chiasson, J. L., Josse, R. G., Gomis, R., Hanefeld, M., Karasik, A., and Laakso, M. (2002). Acarbose for prevention of type 2 diabetes mellitus: the STOP-NIDDM randomised trial. *Lancet*, **359**, 2072–7.

Chiasson, J. L., Josse, R. G., Gomis, R., Hanefeld, M., Karasik, A., and Laakso, M. (2003). Acarbose treatment and the risk of cardiovascular disease and hypertension in patients with impaired glucose tolerance: the STOP-NIDDM trial. *Journal of the American Medical Association*, **290**, 486–94.

Cigolini, M., Targher, G., Seidell, J. C., Tonoli, M., Schiavon, R., Agostino, G., and De Sandre, G. (1995). Relationships of blood pressure to fibrinolysis: influence of anthropometry, metabolic profile and behavioural variables. *Journal of Hypertension*, **13**, 659–66.

Cosentino, F., Hishikawa, K., Katusic, Z. S., and Luscher, T. F. (1997). High glucose increases nitric oxide synthase expression and superoxide anion generation in human aortic endothelial cells. *Circulation*, **96**, 25–8.

Coutinho, M., Gerstein, H. C., Wang, Y., and Yusuf, S. (1999). The relationship between glucose and incident cardiovascular events: a metaregression analysis of published data from 20 studies of 95,783 individuals followed for 12.4 years. *Diabetes Care*, **22**, 233–40.

Curb, J. D., Pressel, S. L., Cutler, J. A., Savage, P. J., Applegate, W. B., Black, H. *et al.* (1996). Effect of diuretic-based antihypertensive treatment on cardiovascular disease risk in older diabetic patients with isolated systolic hypertension. Systolic Hypertension in the Elderly Program Cooperative Research Group. *Journal of the American Medical Association*, **276**, 1886–92.

DECODE Study Group (1998). Will new diagnostic criteria for diabetes mellitus change phenotype of patients with diabetes? Reanalysis of European epidemiological data. DECODE Study Group on behalf of the European Diabetes Epidemiology Study Group. *British Medical Journal*, **317**, 371–5.

DECODE Study Group (1999). Glucose tolerance and mortality: comparison of WHO and American Diabetes Association diagnostic criteria. The DECODE study group. European Diabetes Epidemiology Group. Diabetes Epidemiology: Collaborative analysis of Diagnostic criteria in Europe. *Lancet*, **354**, 617–21.

DECODE Study Group (2001). Glucose tolerance and cardiovascular mortality: comparison of fasting and 2-hour diagnostic criteria. *Archives of Internal Medicine*, **161**, 397–405.

DECODE Study Group (2003*a*). Age- and sex-specific prevalences of diabetes and impaired glucose regulation in 13 European cohorts. *Diabetes Care*, **26**, 61–9.

DECODE Study Group (2003*b*). Gender difference in all-cause and cardiovascular mortality related to hyperglycaemia and newly-diagnosed diabetes. *Diabetologia*, **46**, 608–17.

DECODE Study Group (2003*c*). Is the current definition for diabetes relevant to mortality risk from all-cause and cardiovascular and non-cardiovascular disease? *Diabetes Care*, **26**, 688–96.

DeFronzo, R. A. (1988). Lilly lecture 1987. The triumvirate: beta-cell, muscle, liver. A collusion responsible for NIDDM. *Diabetes*, **37**, 667–87.

DeFronzo, R. and Ferrannini, E. (1991). Insulin resistance: a multifaceted syndrome responsible for NIDDM, obesity, hypertension, dyslipidemia, and atherosclerotic cardiovascular disease. *Diabetes Care*, **14**, 173–94.

Diwadkar, V. A., Anderson, J. W., Bridges, S. R., Gowri, M. S., and Oelgten, P. R. (1999). Postprandial low-density lipoproteins in type 2 diabetes are oxidized more extensively than fasting diabetes and control samples. *Proceedings of the Society of Experimental Biological Medicine*, **222**, 178–84.

Expert Committee on the Diagnosis and Classification of Diabetes Mellitus (1997). Report of the Expert Committee on the Diagnosis and Classification of Diabetes Mellitus. *Diabetes Care*, **20**, 1183–97.

Ferrannini, E. (1998). Insulin resistance versus insulin deficiency in non-insulin-dependent diabetes mellitus: problems and prospects. *Endocrine Reviews*, **19**, 477–90.

Ferrannini, E. (1999). Insulin resistance and hyperinsulinemia: why are they important? *Current Opinion in Endocrinology & Diabetes*, **6**, S13–S16.

Ferrannini, E., Camastra, S., Coppack, S. W., Fliser, D., Golay, A., and Mitrakou, A. (1997). Insulin action and non-esterified fatty acids: the European Group for the Study of Insulin Resistance (EGIR). *Proceedings of the Nutrition Society*, **56**, 753–61.

Festa, A., D'Agostino, R., Jr., Mykkanen, L., Tracy, R., Howard, B. V., and Haffner, S. M. (1999). Low-density lipoprotein particle size is inversely related to plasminogen activator inhibitor-1 levels: the Insulin Resistance Atherosclerosis Study. *Arteriosclerosis, Thrombosis, and Vascular Biology*, **19**, 605–10.

Fontbonne, A., Eschwege, E., Cambien, F., Richard, J. L., Ducimetiere, P., Thibult, N. *et al.* (1989). Hypertriglyceridaemia as a risk factor of coronary heart disease mortality in subjects with impaired glucose tolerance or diabetes: results from the 11-year follow-up of the Paris Prospective Study. *Diabetologia*, **32**, 300–4.

Ford, E. S., Giles, W. H., and Dietz, W. H. (2002). Prevalence of the metabolic syndrome among US adults: findings from the third National Health and Nutrition Examination Survey. *Journal of the American Medical Association*, **287**, 356–9.

Frayn, K. N., Williams, C. M., and Arner, P. (1996). Are increased plasma non-esterified fatty acid concentrations a risk marker for coronary heart disease and other chronic diseases? *Clinical Science (London)*, **90**, 243–53.

Fuller, J. H., Shipley, M. J., Rose, G., Jarrett, R. J., and Keen, H. (1980). Coronary-heart-disease risk and impaired glucose tolerance. The Whitehall study. *Lancet*, **1**, 1373–1376.

Gaede, P., Vedel, P., Larsen, N., Jensen, G. V., Parving, H. H., and Pedersen, O. (2003). Multifactorial intervention and cardiovascular disease in patients with type 2 diabetes. *New England Journal of Medicine*, **348**, 383–93.

Giugliano, D., Ceriello, A., and Paolisso, G. (1996). Oxidative stress and diabetic vascular complications. *Diabetes Care*, **19**, 257–67.

Giugliano, D., Marfella, R., Coppola, L., Verrazzo, G., Acampora, R., Giunta, R. *et al.* (1997). Vascular effects of acute hyperglycemia in humans are reversed by L-arginine: evidence for reduced availability of nitric oxide during hyperglycemia. *Circulation*, **95**, 1783–90.

Golay, A., Swislocki, A. L., Chen, Y. D., and Reaven, G. M. (1987). Relationships between plasma-free fatty acid concentration, endogenous glucose production, and fasting hyperglycemia in normal and non-insulin-dependent diabetic individuals. *Metabolism*, **36**, 692–6.

Gu, K., Cowie, C. C., and Harris, M. I. (1999). Diabetes and decline in heart disease mortality in US adults. *Journal of the American Medical Association*, **281**, 1291–7.

Haffner, S. M., Lehto, S., Ronnemaa, T., Pyorala, K., and Laakso, M. (1998). Mortality from coronary heart disease in subjects with type 2 diabetes and in nondiabetic subjects with and without prior myocardial infarction. *New England Journal of Medicine*, **339**, 229–34.

Hamsten, A., Eriksson, P., Karpe, F., and Silveira, A. (1994). Relationships of thrombosis and fibrinolysis to atherosclerosis. *Current Opinions in Lipidology*, **5**, 382–9.

Hanefeld, M., Fischer, S., Schulze, J., Spengler, M., Wargenau, M., Schollberg, K., and Fucker, K. (1991). Therapeutic potentials of acarbose as first-line drug in NIDDM insufficiently treated with diet alone. *Diabetes Care*, **14**, 732–7.

Hanefeld, M., Fischer, S., Julius, U., Schulze, J., Schwanebeck, U., Schmechel, H. *et al.* (1996). Risk factors for myocardial infarction and death in newly detected NIDDM: the Diabetes Intervention Study, 11-year follow-up. *Diabetologia*, **39**, 1577–83.

Heart Protection Study Collaborative Group (2002). MRC/BHF Heart Protection Study of cholesterol lowering with simvastatin in 20,536 high-risk individuals: a randomised placebo-controlled trial. *Lancet*, **360**, 7–22.

Heine, R. J. and Dekker, J. M. (2002). Beyond postprandial hyperglycaemia: metabolic factors associated with cardiovascular disease. *Diabetologia*, **45**, 461–75.

Howard, B. V. (1987). Lipoprotein metabolism in diabetes mellitus. *Journal of Lipid Research*, **28**, 613–28.

Hu, F. B., Stampfer, M. J., Solomon, C. G., Liu, S., Willett, W. C., Speizer, F. E. *et al.* (2001). The impact of diabetes mellitus on mortality from all causes and coronary heart disease in women: 20 years of follow-up. *Archives of Internal Medicine*, **161**, 1717–23.

Hulthe, J., Bokemark, L., Wikstrand, J., and Fagerberg, B. (2000). The metabolic syndrome, LDL particle size, and atherosclerosis: the Atherosclerosis and Insulin Resistance (AIR) study. *Arteriosclerosis, Thrombosis, and Vascular Biology*, **20**, 2140–7.

Imperatore, G., Riccardi, G., Iovine, C., Rivellese, A. A., and Vaccaro, O. (1998). Plasma fibrinogen: a new factor of the metabolic syndrome. A population-based study. *Diabetes Care*, **21**, 649–54.

International Collaborative Group (1979). Asymptomatic hyperglycemia and coronary heart disease: a series of papers by the International Collaborative Group based on studies in fifteen populations. *Journal of Chronic Diseases*, **32**, 683–837.

Isomaa, B., Almgren, P., Tuomi, T., Forsen, B., Lahti, K., Nissen, M. *et al.* (2001). Cardiovascular morbidity and mortality associated with the metabolic syndrome. *Diabetes Care*, **24**, 683–9.

Janghorbani, M., Jones, R. B., Gilmour, W. H., Hedley, A. J., and Zhianpour, M. (1994). A prospective population based study of gender differential in mortality from cardiovascular disease and 'all causes' in asymptomatic hyperglycaemics. *Journal of Clinical Epidemiology*, **47**, 397–405.

Jones, R. L. (1985). Fibrinopeptide-A in diabetes mellitus: relation to levels of blood glucose, fibrinogen disappearance, and hemodynamic changes. *Diabetes*, **34**, 836–43.

Jones, R. L. and Peterson, C. M. (1979). Reduced fibrinogen survival in diabetes mellitus: a reversible phenomenon. *Journal of Clinical Investigation*, **63**, 485–93.

Jousilahti, P., Vartiainen, E., Tuomilehto, J., and Puska, P. (1999). Sex, age, cardiovascular risk factors, and coronary heart disease: a prospective follow-up study of 14 786 middle-aged men and women in Finland. *Circulation*, **99**, 1165–72.

Kanaya, A. M., Herrington, D., Vittinghoff, E., Lin, F., Grady, D., Bittner, V. *et al.* (2003). Glycemic effects of postmenopausal hormone therapy: the Heart and Estrogen/progestin Replacement Study. A randomized, double-blind, placebo-controlled trial. *Annals of Internal Medicine*, **138**, 1–9.

Kannel, W. B. and McGee, D. L. (1979*a*). Diabetes and cardiovascular disease: the Framingham study. *Journal of the American Medical Association*, **241**, 2035–8.

Kannel, W. B. and McGee, D. L. (1979*b*). Diabetes and glucose tolerance as risk factors for cardiovascular disease: the Framingham study. *Diabetes Care*, **2**, 120–6.

Kawano, H., Motoyama, T., Hirashima, O., Hirai, N., Miyao, Y., Sakamoto, T. *et al.* (1999). Hyperglycemia rapidly suppresses flow-mediated endothelium-dependent vasodilation of brachial artery. *Journal of the American College of Cardiology*, **34**, 146–54.

King, H., Aubert, R. E., and Herman, W. H. (1998). Global burden of diabetes, 1995–2025: prevalence, numerical estimates, and projections. *Diabetes Care*, **21**, 1414–31.

Knowler, W. C., Barrett-Connor, E., Fowler, S. E., Hamman, R. F., Lachin, J. M., Walker, E. A., and Nathan, D. M. (2002). Reduction in the incidence of type 2 diabetes with lifestyle intervention or metformin. *New England Journal of Medicine*, **346**, 393–403.

Koivisto, V. A., Stevens, L. K., Mattock, M., Ebeling, P., Muggeo, M., Stephenson, J., and Idzior-Walus, B. (1996). Cardiovascular disease and its risk factors in IDDM in Europe: EURODIAB IDDM Complications Study Group. *Diabetes Care*, **19**, 689–97.

Kuusisto, J., Mykkanen, L., Pyorala, K., and Laakso, M. (1995). Hyperinsulinemic microalbuminuria: a new risk indicator for coronary heart disease. *Circulation*, **91**, 831–7.

Kylin, E. (1923). Studien ueber das Hypertonie-Hyperglykämie-Hyperurikämiesyndrome. *Zentralblatt fuer Innere Medizin*, **44**, 105–27.

Laakso, M. (1999). Hyperglycemia and cardiovascular disease in type 2 diabetes. *Diabetes*, **48**, 937–42.

Lakka, H. M., Laaksonen, D. E., Lakka, T. A., Niskanen, L. K., Kumpusalo, E., Tuomilehto, J., and Salonen, J. T. (2002). The metabolic syndrome and total and cardiovascular disease mortality in middle-aged men. *Journal of the American Medical Association*, **288**, 2709–16.

Lash, J. M., Nase, G. P., and Bohlen, H. G. (1999). Acute hyperglycemia depresses arteriolar NO formation in skeletal muscle. *American Journal of Physiology*, **277**, H1513–1520.

Leahy, J. L., Cooper, H. E., Deal, D. A., and Weir, G. C. (1986). Chronic hyperglycemia is associated with impaired glucose influence on insulin secretion: a study in normal rats using chronic in vivo glucose infusions. *Journal of Clinical Investigation*, **77**, 908–15.

Lee, E. T., Keen, H., Bennett, P. H., Fuller, J. H., and Lu, M. (2001). Follow-up of the WHO Multinational Study of Vascular Disease in Diabetes: general description and morbidity. *Diabetologia*, **44**, S3–13.

Lee, W. L., Cheung, A. M., Cape, D., and Zinman, B. (2000). Impact of diabetes on coronary artery disease in women and men: a meta-analysis of prospective studies. *Diabetes Care*, **23**, 962–8.

Liese, A. D., Mayer-Davis, E. J., and Haffner, S. M. (1998). Development of the multiple metabolic syndrome: an epidemiologic perspective. *Epidemiologic Reviews*, **20**, 157–72.

Lindstrom, J. and Tuomilehto, J. (2003). The Diabetes Risk Score: a practical tool to predict type 2 diabetes risk. *Diabetes Care*, **26**, 725–31.

Lowe, L. P., Liu, K., Greenland, P., Metzger, B. E., Dyer, A. R., and Stamler, J. (1997). Diabetes, asymptomatic hyperglycemia, and 22-year mortality in black and white men: The Chicago Heart Association Detection Project in Industry Study. *Diabetes Care*, **20**, 163–9.

Marfella, R., Verrazzo, G., Acampora, R., La Marca, C., Giunta, R., Lucarelli, C. *et al.* (1995). Glutathione reverses systemic hemodynamic changes induced by acute hyperglycemia in healthy subjects. *American Journal of Physiology*, **268**, E1167–73.

Meigs, J. B., D'Agostino, R. B., Sr., Wilson, P. W., Cupples, L. A., Nathan, D. M., and Singer, D. E. (1997). Risk variable clustering in the insulin resistance syndrome: the Framingham Offspring Study. *Diabetes*, **46**, 1594–600.

Morrish, N. J., Wang, S. L., Stevens, L. K., Fuller, J. H., and Keen, H. (2001). Mortality and causes of death in the WHO Multinational Study of Vascular Disease in Diabetes. *Diabetologia*, **44**, S14–21.

Mullarkey, C. J., Edelstein, D., and Brownlee, M. (1990). Free radical generation by early glycation products: a mechanism for accelerated atherogenesis in diabetes. *Biochemical and Biophysical Research Communications*, **173**, 932–9.

National Diabetes Data Group (1979). Classification and diagnosis of diabetes mellitus and other categories of glucose intolerance. National Diabetes Data Group. *Diabetes*, **28**, 1039–57.

National Institute of Health (2001). Executive Summary of The Third Report of The National Cholesterol Education Program (NCEP) Expert Panel on Detection, Evaluation, and Treatment of High Blood Cholesterol in Adults (Adult Treatment Panel III). *Journal of the American Medical Association*, **285**, 2486–97.

Nishikawa, T., Edelstein, D., Du, X. L., Yamagishi, S., Matsumura, T., Kaneda, Y. *et al.* (2000). Normalizing mitochondrial superoxide production blocks three pathways of hyperglycaemic damage. *Nature*, **404**, 787–90.

Orchard, T. J. (1996). The impact of gender and general risk factors on the occurrence of atherosclerotic vascular disease in non-insulin-dependent diabetes mellitus. *Annals of Medicine*, **28**, 323–33.

Orchard, T. J., Olson, J. C., Erbey, J. R., Williams, K., Forrest, K. Y., Smithline Kinder, L. *et al.* (2003). Insulin resistance-related factors, but not glycemia, predict coronary artery disease in type 1 diabetes: 10-year follow-up data from the Pittsburgh Epidemiology of Diabetes Complications Study. *Diabetes Care*, **26**, 1374–9.

Pan, X., Li, G., Hu, Y., Wang, J., Yang, W., An, Z. *et al.* (1997). Effects of diet and exercise in preventing NIDDM in people with impaired glucose tolerance: the Da Qing IGT and Diabetes Study. *Diabetes Care*, **20**, 537–44.

Pratley, R. E. and Weyer, C. (2001). The role of impaired early insulin secretion in the pathogenesis of Type II diabetes mellitus. *Diabetologia*, **44**, 929–45.

Pyorala, K., Savolainen, E., Lehtovirta, E., Punsar, S., and Siltanen, P. (1979). Glucose tolerance and coronary heart disease: Helsinki policemen study. *Journal of Chronic Diseases*, **32**, 729–45.

Pyorala, K., Pedersen, T. R., Kjekshus, J., Faergeman, O., Olsson, A. G., and Thorgeirsson, G. (1997). Cholesterol lowering with simvastatin improves prognosis of diabetic patients with coronary heart disease: a subgroup analysis of the Scandinavian Simvastatin Survival Study (4S). *Diabetes Care*, **20**, 614–20.

Pyorala, M., Miettinen, H., Laakso, M., and Pyorala, K. (1998). Hyperinsulinemia predicts coronary heart disease risk in healthy middle-aged men: the 22-year follow-up results of the Helsinki Policemen Study. *Circulation*, **98**, 398–404.

Qiao, Q., Pyorala, K., Pyorala, M., Nissinen, A., Lindstrom, J., Tilvis, R., and Tuomilehto, J. (2002). Two-hour glucose is a better risk predictor for incident coronary heart disease and cardiovascular mortality than fasting glucose. *European Heart Journal*, **23**, 1267–75.

Qiao, Q., Jousilahti, P., Eriksson, J., and Tuomilehto, J. (2003). Predictive properties of impaired glucose tolerance for cardiovascular risk are not explained by the development of overt diabetes during follow-up. *Diabetes Care*, **26**, 2910–14.

Reaven, G. M. (1988). Banting lecture 1988. Role of insulin resistance in human disease. *Diabetes*, **37**, 1595–607.

Rodriguez, B. L., Lau, N., Burchfiel, C. M., Abbott, R. D., Sharp, D. S., Yano, K., and Curb, J. D. (1999). Glucose intolerance and 23-year risk of coronary heart disease and total mortality: the Honolulu Heart Program. *Diabetes Care*, **22**, 1262–5.

Sakamoto, T., Ogawa, H., Kawano, H., Hirai, N., Miyamoto, S., Takazoe, K. *et al.* (2000). Rapid change of platelet aggregability in acute hyperglycemia: detection by a novel laser-light scattering method. *Thrombosis and Haemostasis*, **83**, 475–9.

Sako, Y. and Grill, V. E. (1990). A 48-hour lipid infusion in the rat time-dependently inhibits glucose-induced insulin secretion and B cell oxidation through a process likely coupled to fatty acid oxidation. *Endocrinology*, **127**, 1580–9.

Saydah, S. H., Loria, C. M., Eberhardt, M. S., and Brancati, F. L. (2001). Subclinical states of glucose intolerance and risk of death in the U.S. *Diabetes Care*, **24**, 447–53.

Scheidt-Nave, C., Barrett-Connor, E., Wingard, D. L., Cohn, B. A., and Edelstein, S. L. (1991). Sex differences in fasting glycemia as a risk factor for ischemic heart disease death. *American Journal of Epidemiology*, **133**, 565–76.

Schneider, D. J., Nordt, T. K., and Sobel, B. E. (1992). Stimulation by proinsulin of expression of plasminogen activator inhibitor type-I in endothelial cells. *Diabetes*, **41**, 890–5.

Shaten, B. J., Kuller, L. H., and Neaton, J. D. (1991). Association between baseline risk factors, cigarette smoking, and CHD mortality after 10.5 years. MRFIT Research Group. *Preventive Medicine*, **20**, 655–9.

Shaw, J. E., Hodge, A. M., de Courten, M., Chitson, P., and Zimmet, P. Z. (1999). Isolated post-challenge hyperglycaemia confirmed as a risk factor for mortality. *Diabetologia*, **42**, 1050–4.

Shige, H., Ishikawa, T., Suzukawa, M., Ito, T., Nakajima, K., Higashi, K. *et al.* (1999). Endothelium-dependent flow-mediated vasodilation in the postprandial state in type 2 diabetes mellitus. *American Journal of Cardiology*, **84**, 1272–4, A9.

Simons, L. A., Friedlander, Y., McCallum, J., and Simons, J. (2000). Fasting plasma glucose in non-diabetic elderly women predicts increased all-causes mortality and coronary heart disease risk. *Australian and New Zealand Journal of Medicine*, **30**, 41–7.

Stamler, J., Vaccaro, O., Neaton, J. D., and Wentworth, D. (1993). Diabetes, other risk factors, and 12-yr cardiovascular mortality for men screened in the Multiple Risk Factor Intervention Trial. *Diabetes Care*, 16, 434–44.

Staprans, I., Hardman, D. A., Pan, X. M., and Feingold, K. R. (1999). Effect of oxidized lipids in the diet on oxidized lipid levels in postprandial serum chylomicrons of diabetic patients. *Diabetes Care*, 22, 300–6.

The ALLHAT Officers and Coordinators for the Collaborative Research Group (2002). Major outcomes in high-risk hypertensive patients randomized to angiotensin-converting enzyme inhibitor or calcium channel blocker vs diuretic: the Antihypertensive and Lipid-Lowering Treatment to Prevent Heart Attack Trial (ALLHAT). *Journal of the American Medical Association*, 288, 2981–97.

Tominaga, M., Eguchi, H., Manaka, H., Igarashi, K., Kato, T., and Sekikawa, A. (1999). Impaired glucose tolerance is a risk factor for cardiovascular disease, but not impaired fasting glucose: the Funagata Diabetes Study. *Diabetes Care*, 22, 920–4.

Tunstall-Pedoe, H., Kuulasmaa, K., Amouyel, P., Arveiler, D., Rajakangas, A. M., and Pajak, A. (1994). Myocardial infarction and coronary deaths in the World Health Organization MONICA Project: registration procedures, event rates, and case-fatality rates in 38 populations from 21 countries in four continents. *Circulation*, 90, 583–612.

Tuomilehto, J. and Kuulasmaa, K. (1989). WHO MONICA Project: assessing CHD mortality and morbidity. *International Journal of Epidemiology*, 18, S38–45.

Tuomilehto, J., Borch-Johnsen, K., Molarius, A., Forsen, T., Rastenyte, D., Sarti, C., and Reunanen, A. (1998). Incidence of cardiovascular disease in Type 1 (insulin-dependent) diabetic subjects with and without diabetic nephropathy in Finland. *Diabetologia*, 41, 784–90.

Tuomilehto, J., Rastenyte, D., Birkenhager, W. H., Thijs, L., Antikainen, R., Bulpitt, C. J. et al. (1999). Effects of calcium-channel blockade in older patients with diabetes and systolic hypertension: Systolic Hypertension in Europe Trial Investigators. *New England Journal of Medicine*, 340, 677–84.

Tuomilehto, J., Lindstrom, J., Eriksson, J. G., Valle, T. T., Hamalainen, H., Ilanne-Parikka, P. et al. (2001). Prevention of type 2 diabetes mellitus by changes in lifestyle among subjects with impaired glucose tolerance. *New England Journal of Medicine*, 344, 1343–50.

UK Prospective Diabetes Study Group (1998a). Intensive blood-glucose control with sulphonylureas or insulin compared with conventional treatment and risk of complications in patients with type 2 diabetes (UKPDS 33). UK Prospective Diabetes Study (UKPDS) Group. *Lancet*, 352, 837–53.

UK Prospective Diabetes Study Group (1998b). Tight blood pressure control and risk of macrovascular and microvascular complications in type 2 diabetes: UKPDS 38. UK Prospective Diabetes Study Group. *British Medical Journal*, 317, 703–13.

Unger, R. H. and Grundy, S. (1985). Hyperglycaemia as an inducer as well as a consequence of impaired islet cell function and insulin resistance: implications for the management of diabetes. *Diabetologia*, 28, 119–21.

Vidal, H. (2001). Gene expression in visceral and subcutaneous adipose tissues. *Annals of Medicine*, 33, 547–55.

WHO (World Health Organization) Consultation (1999). *Definition, diagnosis and classification of diabetes mellitus and its complications. Part 1: diagnosis and classification of diabetes mellitus*. World Health Organization, Geneva.

WHO (World Health Organization) Expert Committee (1980). WHO Expert Committee on Diabetes Mellitus: second report. *World Health Organization Technical Report Series*, 646, 1–80.

Williamson, J. R., Chang, K., Frangos, M., Hasan, K. S., Ido, Y., Kawamura, T. et al. (1993). Hyperglycemic pseudohypoxia and diabetic complications. *Diabetes*, 42, 801–13.

Wilson, P. W., Kannel, W. B., Silbershatz, H., and D'Agostino, R. B. (1999). Clustering of metabolic factors and coronary heart disease. *Archives of Internal Medicine*, 159, 1104–9.

Wolff, S. P. and Dean, R. T. (1987). Glucose autoxidation and protein modification: the potential role of 'autoxidative glycosylation' in diabetes. *Biochemistry Journal*, 245, 243–50.

Yarnell, J. W., Pickering, J. E., Elwood, P. C., Baker, I. A., Bainton, D., Dawkins, C., and Phillips, D. I. (1994). Does non-diabetic hyperglycemia predict future IHD? Evidence from the Caerphilly and Speedwell studies. *Journal of Clinical Epidemiology*, **47**, 383–8.

Yki-Jarvinen, H. (1992). Glucose toxicity. *Endocrine Reviews*, **13**, 415–31.

Zhou, Y. P. and Grill, V. E. (1994). Long-term exposure of rat pancreatic islets to fatty acids inhibits glucose-induced insulin secretion and biosynthesis through a glucose fatty acid cycle. *Journal of Clinical Investigation*, **93**, 870–6.

Zimmet, P., Alberti, K. G., and Shaw, J. (2001). Global and societal implications of the diabetes epidemic. *Nature*, **414**, 782–7.

Chapter 22

Women and cardiovascular heart disease

L. H. Kuller

22.1 **Introduction**

One of the most consistent findings in cardiovascular epidemiology is the substantially lower incidence and mortality due to coronary heart disease (CHD) for women as compared to men (Labarthe 1998; McGovern *et al.* 2001). This has been noted in practically every population that has been studied, including countries with very low, as well as those with very high death rates from CHD (Uemura and Pisa *et al.* 1988; Zhao *et al.* 1999). The higher prevalence of coronary atherosclerosis in men, as compared to women, is present even at young ages. In animal models the extent of experimental coronary atherosclerosis is greater in males than females. There are five important tenets (McGill *et al.* 2000*a, b, c*).

1 The sex differences are far greater for CHD incidence and death rates than for other manifestations of vascular disease such as stroke and peripheral vascular disease (NIH, NHLBI 1998).

2 The sex differences in the extent of atherosclerosis are also greater for the coronary arteries than the aorta or carotid arteries. There is little sex difference, for example, in the extent of atherosclerosis in the aorta. There is a high correlation in both men and women between the extent of atherosclerotic disease in the different vascular beds. The extent of atherosclerosis in vascular beds other than in the coronary arteries predicts the subsequent risk of CHD in both men and women. The extent of coronary atherosclerosis, that is, stenosis, predicts risk of clinical CHD for both men and women (Chambless *et al.* 1997; Kuller and Sutton-Tyrrell 1999; Newman *et al.* 1999; O'Leary *et al.* 1999; Solberg *et al.* 1980).

3 The incidence of CHD, especially myocardial infarction (MI), and sudden death remains much higher for men than women throughout the entire life span. The incidence of CHD for women does not catch up with that of men. There are no diseases that eliminate the differences in incidence of CHD between men and women (Psaty *et al.* 1999). For example, diabetes is associated with substantial increased risk of CHD in women. Diabetic men, however, have higher CHD incidence and mortality rates than women (Kuller *et al.* 2000*a*; Stamler *et al.* 1999; Stampfer *et al.* 2000).

4 The risk factors for incident CHD, elevated blood pressure (BP), cigarette smoking, diabetes, elevated low-density lipoprotein cholesterol (LDL-C) and decreased high-density lipoprotein cholesterol (HDL-C) are similar for men and women and are discussed elsewhere in this volume. These risk factors are the primary determinants of heart attack for both men and women. There is, furthermore, no evidence that any specific risk factor can account for the higher rates of CHD in men.

5 Treatments that reduce the risk of CHD have similar benefits for men and women. Sometimes the results of clinical trials may not be significant for women as compared to men primarily because of the smaller number of cases that occur in the studies among women, thus there is the loss of power. Reducing blood lipoprotein levels, treating hypertension, smoking cessation, and treatment of diabetes have similar effects in men as compared to women in reducing incidence and mortality due to CHD or stroke (Mosca et al. 1997; MRC/BHF Heart Protection Study Collaborative Group 1999).

Women respond similarly to men after exposures to lifestyle variables that increase the risk of heart attack, such as increased dietary saturated fat, cholesterol, etc. with a rise in LDL-C, and higher salt consumption with an increase in BP or increase in body weight and insulin resistance and diabetes (Ginsberg et al. 1998; Yu-Poth et al. 1999). Similarly, smoking is related to the risk of CHD for both men and women. There is some suggestion that there are small differences in the distribution of lipoprotein changes in relationship to diet in men and women.

Women with familial hypercholesterolemia have a substantially increased risk of coronary artery disease, especially at a younger age, but their absolute risk is much lower than that for men (Dreon et al. 1997; Herrington et al. 2002a, b; Jensen 1997).

There is a unique cardiovascular syndrome, primarily in women, of chest pain, consistent with the diagnosis of angina, with minimal or no coronary atherosclerosis or substantial elevated traditional risk factors for CHD. This syndrome, called cardiac syndrome X, is probably related to aberrant endothelial function in the coronary arteries and perhaps the release of nitric oxide, and may be related in some ways to estrogen metabolism. This syndrome often results in apparent increased incidence of angina pectoris in women and a higher ratio of angina to MI and sudden death among women. The syndrome is generally not associated with a major adverse outcome, that is, coronary disease deaths (Bairey et al. 1999).

Among 323 women enrolled in the Women's Ischemic Syndrome Evaluation (WISE Study), 34% had no detectable, 23% had measurable, but minimal, and 43% had significant (>75% diameter) stenosis of coronary arteries (Merz et al. 1999). Women with coronary artery disease usually had multi-vessel disease. The subsequent prognosis was better for those with as compared to without coronary stenosis. About half of the women with chest pain in the absence of coronary artery stenosis had microvascular dysfunction. It is possible that the microvascular disease is related to aberrant estrogen metabolism or to genetic polymorphisms of estrogen receptors and/or their protein products (Reis et al. 2001; Sharaf et al. 2001).

The use of the subclinical measurements of atherosclerosis has had a major impact on further testing of hypotheses related to the differences in atherosclerosis between men and women. Women have less coronary atherosclerosis, as measured by coronary calcium, than men even at very old ages (Newman et al. 2001). There are older women with almost no coronary calcium. Among both men and women the coronary calcium is a strong, independent predictor of the risk of clinical CHD. At any level of coronary calcium, however, the risk of a heart attack is higher in men than in women (Church et al. 2002).

The traditional cardiovascular risk factors are important determinants of the extent of subclinical disease among both men and women (Heiss et al. 1991; Kuller et al. 1999; Sutton-Tyrrell et al. 2002; Wong et al. 2002). There is a long incubation period between the initial levels or elevation of the risk factors and the development of high amounts of coronary calcium or other measures of subclinical atherosclerosis. The association of the risk factors measured concurrently among women and the amount of subclinical disease is, primarily, a function of the correlation of concurrent risk factors with risk factors years previously and the duration of exposure to such risk factors (Abbott *et al.* 2002; Edmundowicz *et al.* 2002; Wilsgaard *et al.* 2001).

22.2 Why do women have less heart disease?

Why do women have much less CHD than men, and less coronary atherosclerosis? Why is the sex difference so much greater for coronary atherosclerosis than for other vascular beds? There appear to be three major current hypotheses to explain these differences.

1 The lower risk among women is due to hormonal differences or tissue-specific hormone receptors (Kuller *et al.* 2000*a*; Reis *et al.* 1994).

2 Differences in the distribution of body fat and subsequent metabolic changes, including insulin resistance and distribution of lipoprotein particles, account for the differences in coronary atherosclerosis and clinical CHD among men and women (Bouchard 1990; Gallagher *et al.* 1996; Troiano *et al.* 1996; Wing *et al.* 1991).

3 Variations in immune response and inflammation are important determinants of differences in CHD between men and women.

These three hypotheses that may explain the lower rates of CHD among women are based on epidemiological, clinical, and animal experimental data (Tracy 1999).

22.2.1 Hormones

Premenopausal

Artificial menopause or premature natural menopause is associated with an increase in both coronary atherosclerosis and risk of heart attack (Novak and Williams 1966; Ritterband *et al.* 1963). An earlier age at menopause is an apparent risk factor for CHD. Similarly, animal models have demonstrated that progression of coronary atherosclerosis requires removal of the ovaries and an increase in dietary saturated fat and cholesterol to elevate the cholesterol levels (Adams *et al.* 1997; Wagner *et al.* 1997). There are, unfortunately, few good primate models of natural menopause and subsequent risk of atherosclerosis, and especially the development of CHD. The use of knock-out mouse models have provided a substantial amount of information about effects of specific lipoprotein receptors and metabolism, and relationship to atherosclerosis, but generally are not relevant to the study of the sex differences in CHD in humans.

There are a few diseases in women which are associated with an increase in premature CHD and may provide further evidence and interesting models for testing the reason for differences between men and women in CHD incidence. Premenopausal women with insulin-dependent diabetes are at increased risk of coronary atherosclerosis. They have very high prevalence of coronary calcium, a specific marker of atherosclerosis, as measured by electron beam computed tomography (EBCT) (Olson *et al.* 2000). The elevated levels of coronary calcium are related to the prevalence of heart disease. The higher risk of CHD is not primarily a function of the extent of the control of their diabetes, but rather with other risk factors, including renal disease, lipoprotein abnormalities, cigarette smoking, and hypertension (Olson *et al.* 2000). One possibility is that the risk of CHD among insulin-dependent diabetics is in part related to insulin resistance, as well as the relative hyperinsulinemia, secondary to insulin therapy.

The prevalence of systemic lupus is much higher among women than in men, and especially high among black women (Selzer *et al.* 2001; Thiagarajan 2001). Exposure to exogenous estrogen therapy may increase both morbidity and mortality in women with lupus, as well as an increase in the extent of disease during pregnancy. There is some suggestive evidence that abnormalities in estrogen metabolism are an important determinant of the risk of lupus. However, among women with lupus the risk of clinical CHD or measures of subclinical atherosclerosis is also strongly related to traditional risk factors for CHD (Manzi et al. 1997; Selzer et al. 2001).

Women with lupus have higher levels of acute phase proteins and inflammatory cytokines, both of which have been associated with an increased risk of CHD and also with the metabolic syndrome. Renal disease is often found among women with lupus, which also results in an increase in LDL-C and triglycerides, and especially an increase in small, dense, atherogenic lipoproteins that are also prevalent in the metabolic syndrome and are associated with an increased risk of CHD.

Polycystic ovary syndrome (PCO) is present in ~5% of premenopausal women and is a major cause of infertility (Talbott et al. 1999). The syndrome is associated with amenorrhea and anovulatory cycling, high levels of estrone and testosterone, lower peak levels of estradiol, and many of the components of the insulin-resistance syndrome (including elevated triglycerides, low HDL, central obesity, hyperinsulinemia and, often, elevated LDL-C levels). PCO can be diagnosed at a fairly early age, even among teenagers but, certainly, in the twenties. This syndrome can, therefore, provide an excellent test of the relationship of the metabolic syndrome among women to the risk of CHD (Talbott et al. 2002a).

Surprisingly, a longitudinal study in England suggested that there was little or no increased risk of CHD, only an increased risk of stroke and diabetes mellitus, among women with PCO (Pierpoint et al. 1998). The more recent studies from the Pittsburgh Polycystic Ovary study have reported an increase in CHD risk, especially among overweight women with polycystic ovary compared to overweight controls and also an increase in subclinical measures of atherosclerosis, including both increased prevalence of coronary calcium and greater intima-medial wall thickness (Talbott et al. 2000, 2002b). The amount of coronary calcium and intima-medial wall thickness is strongly related to measures related to the metabolic syndrome (Talbott et al. 2002b).

Postmenopausal

Androstenedione, a hormone produced by the adrenal gland, and subsequent aromatization in fat tissue is the primary source of postmenopausal estrogen (Simpson et al. 2001). The amount of body fat or obesity, and activity of aromatase enzyme, among postmenopausal women determines the production of estrone, the primary estrogen in postmenopausal women (Bjorntorp 1996).

The postmenopausal ovary may continue to produce some testosterone. The postmenopausal estradiol levels reflect primarily autocrine and paracrine activity in various tissues; they spill over into the blood and are a measure of the effects, that is, the local production of estradiol from estrone and possible effects on specific tissues, and are not necessarily a measure of overall estradiol production. This has substantially confounded the ability to study the relationship between sex steroid hormone levels and risk of CHD among postmenopausal women. Most studies suggest no relationship or a weak relationship between levels of sex steroid hormones and risk of CHD among women, or the extent of coronary atherosclerosis. This lack of an effect could, very simply, be a function of the inability to measure estradiol production from estrone in specific tissues, such as coronary arteries in postmenopausal women (Meilahn 1999).

Hormone therapy (HT)

Hormone therapy is reported in many observational studies, both case-control and longitudinal, to be associated with a substantial reduction in the risk of CHD (Kuller 2001). A secondary prevention trial, Hormone Estrogen Replacement Study (HERS), has cast substantial doubt on the benefits of HT (Herrington and Klein 2001; Hulley *et al.* 1998). It is important to note that most of the women in the HERS study, because they had already had a heart attack, have extensive coronary atherosclerosis; that is, HERS was a secondary prevention trial, and did not provide a test of whether HT prevents the development and progression of coronary athero-sclerosis. Studies which have measured the regression or progression of atherosclerosis either in the coronaries or in the carotids have primarily been limited to women who already have fairly extensive CHD. These studies have shown relatively little effect of HT on the progression of atherosclerosis. They do not provide a test of the hypothesis about whether continued long-term, high levels of hormones would prevent the development and early progression of atherosclerosis (Herrington and Klein 2001; Kuller 2003).

The Women's Health Initiative (WHI) tested the hypothesis that estrogens or estrogen plus progesterone (E + P) will reduce the risk of heart attack (Herrington and Klein 2001; Women's Health Initiative Study Group 1998). After 5.2 years of follow-up, the E + P arm of the trial, as compared to the placebo, was stopped because the global index of excess risk among the E + P users exceeded the predetermined statistical boundary and there was an excess of breast cancer for women on E + P (Writing Group for the Women's Health Initiative Investigators 2002). There was an excess also of CHD cases in the E + P arm, with a hazards ratio (HR) of 1.29 (1.02–1.63) based on 286 cases, and also for stroke with a HR of 1.41 (1.07–1.85). These results are not consistent with the 12.7% decrease in LDL-C and 7.3% increase in HDL-C in the E + P versus placebo arm. A 1% reduction in LDL-C has been estimated to result in about a 2% decrease in CHD, and for each 1% increase in HDL-C about a 3% decrease in CHD. We would have anticipated about a 30–5% decrease in CHD events based on these changes in lipopro-teins. E + P, however, also modifies the distributions of lipoproteins, primarily because of the increase in triglyceride levels associated with HT and a potential shift toward more dense LDL-C. Therefore, the levels of the lipoproteins after E + P therapy may not necessarily reflect changes in all classes of lipoprotein particle distribution and reduction of risk of CHD. It is likely that the clinical events in these trials over the 5, 6, or 7 years of follow-up primarily occurred in women who have fairly extensive atherosclerosis at entry to the study; that is, they will be at highest risk of CHD. The trial, therefore, has the potential of falsely concluding that HT is not beneficial in preventing the development and progression of coronary atherosclerosis.

We do not know the extent of coronary artery disease prior to the beginning of the trial. If HT primarily prevents the development of atherosclerosis, but is adverse for women who already have atherosclerosis, the lack of such information on the extent of atherosclerosis limits the interpretation of the results of the study to women with atherosclerosis.

Premenopausal lipoprotein levels prior to the onset of HT were not available and, therefore, there was no measure of the exposure (i.e., the incubation period) to the development of vascular disease prior to the HT. It may be possible that the prevention of the rise in LDL-C during the pre- to postmenopause is more a important factor in the benefit conferred from the use of HT than later in the postmenopausal years. For example, we have shown that the premenopausal lipoprotein levels of women are a strong predictor of the extent of coronary atherosclerosis as measured by coronary calcium 8–12 years later, in their middle 60 years of age. Postmenopausal HT does not reduce the average LDL-C level to that of the premenopausal levels. It is possible that drug therapy that fails to decrease the LDL-C premenopausal levels may be ineffective in reducing the risk of CHD, especially among women who already have some evidence of coronary atherosclerosis. Statin therapy, for example, has much greater lipid lowering effects than estrogens and does reduce the LDL-C level from the post- to below the premenopausal levels, and has been associated with a decrease in the risk of CHD among postmenopausal women (Wenger 2002).

A recent clinical trial report has suggested that raloxifene, a specialized estrogen receptor modulator, might be associated with a lower risk of CHD (Barrett-Connor *et al.* 2002). This was a secondary analysis based on a relatively small sample size and limited to higher risk women, and would need further replications. A larger study using tamoxifen, also a specialized estrogen receptor modulator, showed no effect on subsequent risk of CHD, and an increased risk of stroke among older women (Fisher *et al.* 1998).

Probably the only way to test the hypothesis that long-term HT prevents the development of coronary atherosclerosis in pre- to postmenopausal women would be a randomized trial that included women with minimal atherosclerosis in their forties and determined the rate of progression of atherosclerosis using non-invasive methods such as EBCT. The study might require a fairly large sample size, since the rate of progression of coronary atherosclerosis in women who have no or minimal coronary atherosclerosis at entry is small (Kuller *et al.* 2002*b*). Such a study would obviously be substantially confounded by changes of other risk factors, which would have to be carefully monitored in such a trial. At present, the evidence would suggest that for most postmenopausal women HT is unlikely to be beneficial, and could be hazardous for reasons which are still not determined but most likely relate to changes in risk of thrombosis and only moderate reduction of LDL-C, especially more atherogenic dense LDL (Kuller 2003).

HT, as well as specialized estrogen receptor modulators, has been associated with a substantial increased risk of venous thrombosis and pulmonary embolism. However, the factors related to clotting in the arterial and venous bed are different due to characteristics of blood flow. Markers associated with an increased risk of venous thrombosis have not necessarily been related to an increased risk of coronary atherosclerosis and thrombosis (Rosendaal *et al.* 2002).

22.3 Body fat distribution

The second hypothesis is based on the very high risk of CHD among both diabetics and women with metabolic syndrome X (Haffner *et al.* 1990, 1998; Kuller *et al.* 2000*b*). A higher waist circumference, an indirect measure of intra-abdominal fat, is an important risk factor for CHD among both men and women.

At any specific body weight, the percentage of body fat is higher in women than men. Men have greater muscle and bone mass than women. Men have a greater accumulation of central fat or obesity than women. The greater amount of peripheral and lower extremity body fat among women as compared to men is, in part, hormonally determined (Kuller 1995). Central obesity, especially intra-abdominal fat, is more strongly associated with lipoprotein changes, especially insulin resistance, elevated inflammatory markers, changes in clotting factors, and higher risk of heart attack (Kuller 1994). At increasing ages, the amount of central fat and intra-abdominal fat increases among women as measured by greater waist circumference. Women gain about one pound per year, during the peri- to the postmenopause (Wing *et al.* 1991), ~10–15 pounds between the ages of 45 and 55. This weight gain is associated with an increase in waist circumference, central obesity (Azziz 1989). The decline in estrogen production, may, in part contribute to the increase in central obesity. There is also some suggestion that decreasing resting metabolic rate and perhaps a reduction in leisure time physical activity may also be related to this increase in both body weight and central obesity (Poehlman 1993).

The distribution of body fat varies among women by race and ethnic group. Black women have a smaller percentage of central obesity, that is, intra-abdominal fat, at the same degree of obesity or total body fat as white women. Populations which have originally migrated from the Indian subcontinent or the South Pacific islands, including American Indians, have a high prevalence of obesity, insulin resistance, metabolic syndrome, and diabetes (Howard et al. 2000; McKeigue and Keen 1992). These populations often have an increased risk of CHD as the amount of saturated fat and cholesterol in their diet, the prevalence of cigarette smoking, and hypertension increase over time (Howard et al. 2000).

There is an association between measures of obesity or waist circumference and specific lipoprotein levels. Women with higher waist circumference, that is, possibly more intra-abdominal and visceral fat, will have greater levels of small, dense LDL, which may be the most atherogenic particle (Sniderman et al. 2001). Animal models (i.e., knock-out mouse) have further substantiated that the dense LDL (but not large LDL or very low-density lipoprotein (VLDL) particles) are associated with the development of atherosclerosis (Veniant et al. 2001).

Various techniques are now available to quantify the size distribution and the number of lipoprotein particles, LDL, HDL, and VLDL lipoproteins. Earlier studies using gradient gel electrophoresis, primarily case-control studies, noted that more dense LDL (so-called Pattern B) was more frequent among prevalent CHD patients as compared to controls. This was true in both men and women. Women had larger LDL size than men (Gardner et al. 1996; Lamarche et al. 1997; Stampfer et al. 1996).

The use of nuclear magnetic resonance imaging (NMR) has made it possible to quantify the specific LDL, HDL, and triglyceride particles, as well as the number of particles (Otvos et al. 1992). Recent data from the Women's Healthy Lifestyle Follow-up Study showed a strong association among the premenopausal cardiovascular risk factors (such as LDL-C, trigly-cerides, waist circumference, body mass index (BMI), HDL-C, and both internal carotid artery, intima-medial wall thickness and plaque, and the presence of coronary calcium) (Sutton-Tyrrell et al. 2002). A higher number of LDL particles and the presence of small LDL (L1 by NMR nomenclature) were strongly related to the presence of coronary calcium but the more common less dense (L3) was not related to coronary calcium. Large, but not small, HDL-C was also strongly associated with the presence of coronary calcium as were VLDL triglycerides. Small LDL was strongly correlated with waist circumference. The association of small LDL and extent of coronary calcium was independent of the HDL-C or total LDL-C measured by chemical methods (Kuller et al. 1999; Mackey et al. 2002).

In the Cardiovascular Health Study (CHS), the measure of the number of LDL particles and the small size or dense LDL were predictors of the risk of clinical CHD, MI, angina, and of CHD deaths among women, but not among men. These lipoproteins levels were also strongly related to the extent of subclinical cardiovascular disease among women without prevalent cardiovascular disease. There were very few men in this older age group who did not have subclinical or clinical coronary artery disease as compared to women. This probably accounted for the inability to show a relationship between the lipoproteins, size and distribution by NMR spectroscopy or LDL-C, triglycerides, etc. in men by traditional chemical methods and NMR spectroscopy (Kuller et al. 2001).

Estrogen or E + P therapy results in a decrease in total LDL-C and an increase in HDL-C. There is, however, an increase in triglyceride levels, especially associated with obesity or high waist circumference. The higher VLDL triglyceride levels are the precursors of smaller, more dense LDL and lower, large HDL-C levels through the activities of lipoprotein and hepatic lipase, and phospholipases and cholesterol ester transfer protein (Havel 2002). The phospholipase bilayer of the large VLDL triglyceride may also be associated with an increased risk of thrombosis (Martin *et al.* 1998).

An increase in free fatty acids to the liver results in greater production of triglycerides and secretion of VLDL triglycerides. Insulin suppresses the release of the free fatty acids. Insulin resistance is characterized by both reduced suppression of free fatty acid release (especially from visceral adipose tissue) as well as changes in glucose utilization in both the liver and muscle (Havel 2002). Increased intra-abdominal fat is associated with insulin resistance. Women have higher fasting free fatty acids levels but greater insulin sensitivity and suppression of free fatty acid release after stimulation by food than men (Laws *et al.* 1997). The gender effect on stimulated free fatty acid levels is primarily related to differences in visceral fat (Laws *et al.* 1997). Men have more central obesity or visceral fat than women. Two other protein hormones secreted by fat cells may also play an important role in energy metabolism and lipoprotein distribution. Levels of both leptin and adiponectin are higher in women than in men at, apparently, the same level of obesity (Havel 2002). Circulating levels of adiponectin are reduced in obese individuals and, apparently, may play an important role in atherosclerosis as well as the metabolic syndrome, especially in triglyceride and HDL metabolism. Both higher levels of leptin and adiponectin may also increase insulin sensitivity and suppress free fatty acid release to the liver.

HT decreases total LDL-C levels (Writing Group for the PEPI Trial 1995). However, the elevation in blood triglyceride levels with HT is associated with an increase in the dense LDL (L1). The levels of L1 have previously been reported to be higher in women on HT than women not on HT. In the Healthy Women Study (HWS) we showed that dense LDL (L1) was higher in women on HT while L3 (the more common LDL fraction) was lower in women on HT (Mackey *et al.* 2001). There was a strong, direct association between waist circumference and L1 among both hormone and non-hormone users. However, at every level of waist circumference, the L1 levels tended to be higher among hormone users. Therefore, if the level of dense LDL is an important atherogenic lipoprotein, the apparent reduction of LDL-C on HT would not necessarily be overly beneficial if limited primarily to less dense LDL-C, especially among overweight women.

There is also a striking inverse relationship between HDL (especially less dense HDL) and the levels of dense L1 (Kuller *et al.* 2002a). This is, again, consistent with the metabolism of lipoprotein particles. An important issue is whether it is the decrease in HDL or the increase in the dense LDL fraction that increases risk of atherosclerotic disease. There is strong epidemiological evidence in both women and in men that the levels of HDL are inversely related to the risk of CHD (Shah *et al.* 2001). Furthermore, several clinical trials have recently shown that increase of HDL-C reduces the risk of clinical coronary events (Rubins *et al.* 1999). In these studies, however, dense LDL-C also decreased and may be a potential explanation of efficacy of therapy. Animal experimental studies demonstrated that increasing ApoA-1 (the primary apoprotein in HDL) without an increase in LDL is not associated with increased risk of atherosclerosis. However, in the presence of higher LDL, or atherogenic high-fat diet, an increase in ApoA-1 or HDL is associated with protection against atherosclerosis in the animal model (Shah *et al.* 2001).

There are also several genetic disorders associated with low HDL in which the prevalence of atherosclerosis and clinical CHD is not very high. There are also several countries (especially in

Asia) where the rates of CHD are low in spite of low HDL-C. Such populations also have very low levels of LDL-C. The data, therefore, might be consistent with the hypothesis that denser LDL drives the development of atherosclerosis (Kuller 2002; St-Pierre et al. 2001; Walldius et al. 2001) but that the effects of HDL (both in terms of reverse cholesterol transport and other mechanisms such as antioxidant and anti-inflammatory effects) may be protective in the face of higher dense LDL (L1) (Shah et al. 2001).

A further issue is whether the difference in risk of CHD between men and women is a function of insulin resistance independent of related lipoprotein changes. Animal models have shown that the development of diabetes and substantial hyperglycaemia without concomitant hyperlipidemia is not associated with increased coronary atherosclerosis in a diabetic pig model (Gerrity et al. 2001). However, the combination of hyperlipidemia and diabetes is associated with much more severe atherosclerosis than hyperlipidemia alone. There is substantial variation in clinical CHD for both men and women among diabetics in different countries, which appears to be related to the lipoprotein levels (Morrish et al. 2001).

22.4 Vascular inflammation, immune-response

Sex differences in vascular response and, especially, inflammation and immunological changes have received increasing interest (Tracy 1999), centered on two areas: atherogenesis and plaque destabilization. Libby and his colleagues have identified T-lymphocytes in advanced atherosclerotic plaques and demonstrated their importance in the secretion of matrix metaloproteases (MMP) (Schonbeck et al. 1997).

T-cells have been implicated in the progression of atherosclerotic disease (Hansson 2001). Tracy and colleagues recently extended these studies in two ways (Huber et al. 1999, 2001). First, they used mouse models to explore the findings in human systems that chronic low level inflammation was associated with increased atherosclerosis and risk of cardiovascular events. They demonstrated that inflammation was in the causal pathway of atherosclerosis. During the course of their experiments they noted that IL-6 had an amplified effect on T helper (TH) cell production, which suggested to them that immune function may be a mechanism by which inflammatory mediators affect atherosclerosis. They then demonstrated that the TH-1 cell production, as compared to TH-2, was more important in the development of atherosclerosis and that the predominance of TH-2 cells was associated with a substantial reduction in atherosclerosis. It is interesting that women are more likely to have a predominant TH-2 response and men TH-1. The association of inflammatory markers such as c-reactive protein (CRP) and pro-inflammatory cytokine and risk of CHD is a major research direction. Central obesity, that is higher waist circumference, is associated with increased levels of CRP (Huber et al. 2001). Women on HT have higher levels of CRP (Huber et al. 2001) but not pro-inflammatory cytokines such as IL_6 (Cushman et al. 1999). The levels of CRP are directly related to risk of heart attacks among both men and women (Kuller et al. 1996; Ridker et al. 1998). There is also a strong association of levels of CRP and the metabolic syndrome (Yudkin et al. 1999) and direct correlation with levels of dense LDL (Kuller et al. 2001; Tracy 1999).

22.5 Discussion and summary

In summary, women have much less coronary atherosclerosis than men across the entire age spectrum. The sex difference for atherosclerosis in other vascular beds is much smaller and the reasons for these differences are still not determined. Women therefore have substantially lower incidence of CHD, especially MI and sudden CHD deaths than men. Traditional cardio-vascular risk factors such as elevated LDL-C, low HDL-C, smoking, hypertension, diabetes, and central obesity are major determinants of risk of coronary disease for men and women, but do not explain the differences in atherosclerosis or CHD rates between men and women. In animal models, exogenous estrogens are associated with reduced extent of atherosclerosis and oophorectomy will increase atherosclerosis in combination with an atherogenic diet. Oophorectomized women, or an early age natural menopause, increase the risk of CHD. Observational studies suggested that HT reduces the risk of clinical heart disease, but clinical trials do not show any significant reduction in CHD and possibly even an increased risk of CHD for women on HT. HT has not been shown to have any striking effect in slowing the progression of atherosclerosis among women who already have fairly significant coronary atherosclerosis or higher carotid intimal-medial wall thickness.

The distribution of lipoprotein particles is different between women and men. The athero-genic dense or small LDL particle is more prevalent in men than women, while less dense HDL is higher among women. Men have more central obesity and intra-abdominal fat than women, and the greater amount of intra-abdominal fat is strongly associated with more dense LDL-C, elevated VLDL, and triglycerides, and lower levels of less dense HDL. Women are more insulin sensitive than men. The distribution of body fat may be the important determinant of the sex differences in atherosclerosis and may be in part determined by hormonal factors. Genetic or lifestyle variations in estrogen metabolism and estrogen receptors on the vessel wall could also account for the sex differences in atherosclerosis specifically related to the coronary arteries (Iafrati *et al.* 1997).

There are several very important areas for future research. First, primary prevention of coron-ary atherosclerosis and heart attack among women should be feasible by preventing increased waist circumference, visceral fat, and resulting metabolic abnormalities of lipoprotein and glucose-insulin metabolism. Second, there is a paucity of information about determinants and prevention of CHD among older women, that is 75+, yet most of the heart attacks among women occur at older ages. Third, the reason why HT, and at least some of the selective estro-gen receptor modulators, failed to decrease CHD risk in spite of favorable lipoprotein changes needs to be clarified, especially determinants of thrombosis and possibly changes in VLDL triglyceride metabolism.

References

Abbott, R. D., Curb, J. D., Rodriguez, B. L., Masaki, K. H., Yano, K., Schatz, I. J. *et al.* (2002). Age-related changes in risk factor effects on the incidence of coronary heart disease. *Annals of Epidemiology*, **12**, 173–81.

Adams, M. R., Register, T. C., Golden, D. L., Wagner, J. D., and Williams, J. K. (1997). Medroxyprogesterone acetate antagonizes inhibitory effects of conjugated equine estrogen on coronary artery atherosclerosis. *Arteriosclerosis, Thrombosis, and Vascular Biology*, **17**, 217–21.

Azziz, R. (1989). Reproductive endocrinologic alterations in female asymptomatic obesity. *Fertility and Sterility*, **52**, 703–25.

Bairey, C. N., Kelsey, S. F., Pepine C. J., Reichek, N., Reis, S. E., Rogers, W. J. *et al.* for the WISE Study Group (1999). The Women's Ischemia Syndrome Evaluation (WISE) Study: Protocol Design, Methodology and Feasibility Report. *Journal of the American College of Cardiology*, **33**, 1453–61.

Barrett-Connor E., Grady, D., Sashegyi, A., Anderson, P. W., Hoszowski, K. *et al.* (2002). Raloxifene and cardiovascular events in osteoporotic postmenopausal women: four-year results from the MORE

(Multiple Outcomes of Raloxifene Evaluation) randomized trial. *Journal of the American Medical Association*, **287**, 847–57.

Bjorntorp, P. (1996). The regulation of adipose tissue distribution in humans. *International Journal of Obesity*, **20**, 291–302.

Bouchard, C., Bray, G. A., and Hubbard, V. S. (1990). Basic and clinical aspects of regional fat distribution. *American Journal of Clinical Nutrition*, **52**, 946–50.

Chambless, L. E., Heiss, G., Folsom, A. R., Rosamond, W., Szklo, M., Sharrett, A. R., and Clegg, L. X. (1997). Association of coronary heart disease incidence with carotid arterial wall thickness and major risk factors: the Atherosclerosis Risk in Communities (ARIC) Study, 1987–1993. *American Journal of Epidemiology*, **146**, 483–94.

Church, T. S., Blair, S., Nichaman, M., Cheng, Y.-L., Kimball, T., Gibbons, L. *et al.* (2002). Coronary artery calcium score and risk of CHD events [Poster presentation]. 42nd Annual Conference on Cardiovascular Disease Epidemiology and Prevention, American Heart Association. 23–26 April 2002, Honolulu, Hawaii.

Cushman, M., Legault, C., Barrett-Connor, E., Stefanick, M. L., Kessler, C., Judd, H. L. *et al.* (1999). Effect of postmenopausal hormones on inflammation-sensitive proteins: the Postmenopausal Estrogen/Progestin Interventions (PEPI) Study. *Circulation*, **100**, 717–22.

Dreon, D. M., Fernstrom, H. A., Williams, P. T., and Krauss, R. M. (1997). LDL subclass patterns and lipoprotein response to a low-fat, high-carbohydrate diet in women. *Arteriosclerosis, Thrombosis, and Vascular Biology*, **17**, 707–14.

Edmundowicz, D., Kuller, L., and Kriska, A. (2002). Lipoprotein levels at age 57 predict coronary calcium scores seventeen years later [Poster presentation]. 42nd Annual Conference on Cardiovascular Disease Epidemiology and Prevention, American Heart Association. 23–26 April 2002, Honolulu, Hawaii.

Fisher, B., Costantino, J. P., Wickerham, D. L., Redmond, C. K., Kavanah, M., Cronin, W. M. *et al.* (1998). Tamoxifen for prevention of breast cancer: report of the National Surgical Adjuvant Breast and Bowel Project P-1 Study. *Journal of the National Cancer Institute*, **90**, 1371–88.

Gallagher, D., Visser, M., Sepulveda, D., Pierson, R. N., Harris, T., and Heymsfield, S. B. (1996). How useful is body mass index for comparison of body fatness across age, sex, and ethnic groups? *American Journal of Epidemiology*, **143**, 228–39.

Gardner, C. D., Fortmann, S. P., and Krauss, R. M. (1996). Association of small low-density lipoprotein particles with the incidence of coronary artery disease in men and women. *Journal of the American Medical Association*, **276**, 875–81.

Gerrity, R. G., Natarajan, R., Nadler, J. L., and Kimsey, T. (2001). Diabetes-induced accelerated atherosclerosis in swine. *Diabetes*, **50**, 1654–65.

Ginsberg, H. N., Kris-Etherton, P., Dennis, B., Elmer, P. J., Ershow, A., Lefevre, M. *et al.* (1998). Effects of reducing dietary saturated fatty acids on plasma lipids and lipoproteins in healthy subjects: The DELTA Study, Protocol I. *Arteriosclerosis, Thrombosis, and Vascular Biology*, **18**, 441–9.

Haffner, S. M., Stern, M. P., Hazuda, H. P., Mitchell, B. D., and Patterson, J. K. (1990). Cardiovascular risk factors in confirmed prediabetic individuals: does the clock for coronary heart disease start ticking before the onset of clinical diabetes? *Journal of the American Medical Association*, **263**, 2893–8.

Haffner, S. M., Lehto, S., Ronnemaa, T., Pyorala, K., and Lakso, M. (1998). Mortality from coronary heart disease in subjects with type 2 diabetes and in nondiabetic subjects with and without prior myocardial infarction. *New England Journal of Medicine*, **339**, 229–34.

Hansson, G. K. (2001). Immune mechanisms in atherosclerosis. *Arteriosclerosis, Thrombosis, and Vascular Biology*, **21**, 1876–90.

Havel, P. J. (2002). Control of energy homeostasis and insulin action by adipocyte hormones: leptin, acylation stimulating protein, and adiponectin. *Current Opinion in Lipidology*, **13**, 51–9.

Heiss, G., Sharrett, A. R., Barnes, R., Chambless, L. E., Szklo, M., and Alzola, C. (1991). Carotid atherosclerosis measured by B-mode ultrasound in populations: associations with cardiovascular risk factors in the ARIC study. *American Journal of Epidemiology*, **134**, 250–6.

Herrington, D. M. and Klein, L. P. (2001). Cardiovascular trials of estrogen replacement therapy. *Annals of the New York Academy of Sciences*, **949**, 153–62.

Herrington, D. M., Howard, T. D., Brosnihan, B., McDonnell, D. P., Xiaolin, L., Hawkins, G. A. *et al.* (2002*a*). Common estrogen receptor polymorphism augments effects of hormone replacement therapy on E-selectin but not C-reactive protein. *Circulation*, **105**, 1879–82.

Herrington, D. M., Howard, T. D., Hawkins, G. A., Reboussin, D. M., Xu, J., Zheng, S. L. *et al.* (2002*b*). Estrogen receptor polymorphisms and effects of estrogen replacement on HDL cholesterol in women with coronary disease. *New England Journal of Medicine*, **346**, 967–75.

Howard, B. V., Robbins, D. C., Sievers, M. L., Lee, E. T., Rhoades, D., Devereux, R. B. *et al.* (2000). LDL cholesterol as a strong predictor of coronary heart disease in diabetic individuals with insulin resistance and low LDL: The Strong Heart Study. *Arteriosclerosis, Thrombosis, and Vascular Biology*, **20**, 830–5.

Huber, S. A., Sakkinen, P., Conze, D., Hardin, N., and Tracy, R. (1999). Interleukin-6 exacerbates early atherosclerosis in mice. *Arteriosclerosis, Thrombosis, and Vascular Biology*, **19**, 2364–7.

Huber, S. A., Sakkinen, P., David, C., Newell, M. K., and Tracy, R. P. (2001). T helper-cell phenotype regulates atherosclerosis in mice under conditions of mild hypercholesterolemia. *Circulation*, **103**, 2610–16.

Hulley, S., Grady, D., Bush, T., Furberg, C., Herrington, D., Riggs, B., and Vittinghoff, E., for the Heart and Estrogen/progestin Replacement Study (HERS) Research Group (1998). Randomized trial of estrogen plus progestin for secondary prevention of coronary heart disease in postmenopausal women. *Journal of the American Medical Association*, **288**, 605–13.

Iafrati, M. D., Karas, R. H., Aronovitz, M., Kim, S., Sullivan, T. R. Lubahn, D. B. *et al.* (1997). Estrogen inhibits the vascular injury response in estrogen receptor alpha-deficient mice. *Nature Medicine*, **3**, 545–8.

Jensen, E. V. (1997). History of the estrogen receptor concept and its relation to antiestrogens. In *Estrogens and antiestrogens: basic and clinical aspects* (ed. R. Lindsay, D. W. Dempster, and V. C. Jordan), pp. 3–8. Lippincott-Raven, Philadelphia.

Kuller, L. H. (1994). Eating fat or being fat and risk of cardiovascular disease and cancer among women. *Annals of Epidemiology*, **4**, 119–27.

Kuller, L. H. (1995). The etiology of breast cancer: from epidemiology to prevention. *Public Health Reviews*, **23**, 157–213.

Kuller, L. H. (2001). Hormone replacement therapy and coronary heart disease: a new debate. *Cardiology Clinics*, **19**, 327–41.

Kuller, L. H. (2002). Hyperlipidemia and cardiovascular disease. *Current Opinion in Lipidology*, **13**, 449–51.

Kuller, L. H. (2003). Hormone replacement therapy and risk of cardiovascular disease: implications of the results of the Women's Health Initiative. *Arteriosclerosis, Thrombosis, and Vascular Biology*, **23**, 11–16.

Kuller, L. H. and Sutton-Tyrrell, K. (1999). Aging and cardiovascular disease: use of subclinical measurements. *Cardiology Clinics*, **17**, 51–65.

Kuller, L. H., Tracy, R. P., Shaten, J., and Meilahn, E. N., for the MRFIT Research Group (1996). Relation of C-reactive protein and coronary heart disease in the MRFIT nested case-control study. *American Journal of Epidemiology*, **144**, 537–47.

Kuller, L. H., Matthews, K. A., Sutton-Tyrrell, K., Edmundowicz, D., and Bunker, C. H. (1999). Coronary and aortic calcification among women 8 years after menopause and their premenopausal risk factors: The Healthy Women Study. *Arteriosclerosis, Thrombosis, and Vascular Biology*, **19**, 2189–98.

Kuller, L. H., Matthews, K. A., and Meilahn, E. N. (2000*a*). Estrogens and women's health: interrelation of coronary heart disease, breast cancer and osteoporosis. *Journal of Steroid Biochemistry and Molecular Biology*, **74**, 297–309.

Kuller, L. H., Velentgas, P., Barzilay, J., Beauchamp, J. J., O'Leary, D. H., and Savage, P. J. (2000*b*). Diabetes mellitus: subclinical cardiovascular disease and risk of incident cardiovascular disease and all-cause mortality. *Arteriosclerosis, Thrombosis, and Vascular Biology*, **20**, 823–9.

Kuller, L. H., Tracy, R., Arnold, A., Otvos, J. D., Burke, G., Psaty, B. *et al.* (2001). Relationship between LDL size, number of particles and risk of coronary heart disease in the Cardiovascular Health Study [Abstract]. *Circulation*, **104** (Suppl. II), 826.

Kuller, L. H., Arnold, A., Tracy, R., Otvos, J., Burke, G., Psaty, B. *et al.* (2002*a*). NMR spectroscopy of lipoproteins and risk of CHD in the Cardiovascular Health Study. *Arteriosclerosis, Thrombosis, and Vascular Biology*, **22**, 1175–80.

Kuller, L. H., Edmundowicz, D., and Matthews, K. A. (2002*b*). Galloping atherosclerosis among postmenopausal women [Abstract]. *Circulation*, **105**, e86.

Labarthe, D. R. (1998). Age, sex, race, and heredity. In *Epidemiology and prevention of cardiovascular diseases: a global challenge* (ed. D. R. Labarthe), pp. 119–31. Aspen Publishers, Gaitherburg, MD.

Lamarche, B., Tchernof, A., Moorjani, S., Cantin, B., Dagenais, G. R., Lupien, P. J., and Despres, J. P. (1997). Small, dense low-density lipoprotein particles as a predictor of the risk of ischemic heart disease in men: prospective results from the Quebec Cardiovascular Study. *Circulation*, **95**, 69–75.

Laws, A., Hoen, H. M., Selby, J. V., Saad, M. F., Haffner, S. M., and Howard, B. V., for the Insulin Resistance Atherosclerosis Study (IRAS) Investigators (1997). Differences in insulin suppression of free fatty acid levels by gender and glucose tolerance status: relation to plasma triglyceride and apolipoprotein B concentrations. *Arteriosclerosis, Thrombosis, and Vascular Biology*, **17**, 64–71.

Mackey, R. H., Kuller, L. H., Sutton-Tyrrell, K., Matthews, K. A., Evans, R. W., and Holubkov, R. (2001). LDL subclass distribution is associated with coronary calcification in postmenopausal women [Abstract]. *Circulation*, **103**, 1349–50.

Mackey, R. H., Kuller, L. H., Sutton-Tyrrell, K., Evans, R. W., Holubkov, R., and Matthews, K. A. (2002). Lipoprotein subclasses and coronary artery calcium in postmenopausal women from the Healthy Women Study. *American Journal of Cardiology*, **90** (8A), 71I–76i.

Manzi, S., Meilahn, E. N., Rairie, J. E., Conte, C. G., Medsger, T. A. Jr., Jansen-Mcwilliams, L. *et al.* (1997). Age-specific incidence rates of myocardial infarction and angina in women with systemic lupus erythematosus: comparison with the Framingham study. *American Journal of Epidemiology*, **145**, 408–15.

Martin, P., Moyer, M. P., Tracy, R. P., Tracy, P. B., van't Veer, C., Sparks, C. E., and Mann, K. G. (1998). Plasma lipoproteins support prothrombinase and other procoagulant enzymatic complexes. *Arteriosclerosis, Thrombosis, and Vascular Biology*, **18**, 458–65.

McGill, H. C. Jr., McMahan, C. A., Herderick, E. E., Tracy, R. E., Malcom, G. T., Zieske, A. W., and Strong, J. P. (2000*a*). Effects of coronary heart disease risk factors on atherosclerosis of selected regions of the aorta and right coronary artery. The Pathobiological Determinants of Atherosclerosis in Youth (PDAY) Research Group. *Arteriosclerosis, Thrombosis, and Vascular Biology*, **20**, 836–45.

McGill, H. C. Jr., McMahan, C. A., Zieske, A. W., Sloop, G. D., Walcott, J. V., Troxclair, D. A. *et al.* (2000*b*). Associations of coronary heart disease risk factors with the intermediate lesion of atherosclerosis in youth. The Pathobiological Determinants of Atherosclerosis in Youth (PDAY) Research Group. *Arteriosclerosis, Thrombosis, and Vascular Biology*, **20**, 1998–2004.

McGill, H. C. Jr., McMahan, C. A., Zieske, A. W., Tracy, R. E., Malcom, G. T., Herderick, E. E., and Strong, J. P. (2000*c*). Association of coronary heart disease risk factors with microscopic qualities of coronary atherosclerosis in youth. *Circulation*, **102**, 374–9.

McGovern, P. G., Jacobs, D. R., Jr., Shahar, E., Arnett, D. K., Folsom, A. R., Blackburn, H., and Leupker, R. V. (2001). Trends in acute coronary heart disease mortality, morbidity, and medical care from 1985 through 1997: The Minnesota Heart Survey. *Circulation*, **104**, 19–24.

McKeigue, P. M. and Keen, H. (1992). Diabetes, insulin, ethnicity, and coronary heart disease. In *Coronary heart disease epidemiology: from aetiology to public health* (ed. M. Marmot and P. Elliott), pp. 217–32. Oxford University Press, New York.

Meilahn, E. (1999). Sex steroid hormonal influences on coronary artery disease. In *Health and disease among women: biological and environmental influences* (ed. R. B. Ness and L. H. Kuller), pp. 155–82. Oxford University Press, New York.

Merz, C. N. B., Kelsey, S. F., Pepine, C. J., Reichek, N., Reis, S. E., Rogers, W. J. *et al.* (1999). The Women's Ischemia Syndrome Evaluation (WISE) Study: protocol design, methodology and feasibility report. *Journal of the American College of Cardiology*, **33**, 1453–61.

Morrish, N. J., Wang, S. L., Stevens, L. K., Fuller, J. H., and Keen, H. (2001). Mortality and causes of death in the WHO multinational study of vascular disease in diabetes. *Diabetologia*, **44**, S14–21.

Mosca, L., Manson, J. E., Sutherland, S. E., Langer, R. D., Manolio, T., and Barrett-Connor, E. (1997). Cardiovascular disease in women: a statement for healthcare professionals from the American Heart Association. *Circulation*, **96**, 2468–82.

MRC/BHF Heart Protection Study Collaborative Group (1999). MRC/BHF Heart Protection Study of cholesterol-lowering therapy and of antioxidant vitamin supplementation in a wide range of patients at increased risk of coronary heart disease death: early safety and efficacy experience. *European Heart Journal*, **20**, 725–41.

Newman, A. B., Shemanski, L., Manolio, T. A., Cushman, M., Mittelmark, M., Polak, J. F. *et al.* (1999). Ankle-arm index as a predictor of cardiovascular disease and mortality in the Cardiovascular Health Study. *Arteriosclerosis, Thrombosis, and Vascular Biology*, **19**, 538–45.

Newman, A. B., Naydeck, B. L., Sutton-Tyrrell, K., Feldman, A., Edmundowicz, D., and Kuller, L. H. (2001). Coronary artery calcification in older adults to age 99: prevalence and risk factors. *Circulation*, **104**, 2679–84.

NIH, NHLBI (National Institutes of Health, National Heart, Lung, and Blood Institute) (1998). *Morbidity and mortality: 1998 chartbook on cardiovascular, lung, and blood diseases.* Washington DC: NIH.

Novak, E. R. and Williams, T. J. (1966). Autopsy comparison of cardiovascular changes in castrated and normal women. *American Journal of Obstetrics and Gynecology*, **80**, 863–72.

O'Leary, D. H., Polak, J. F., Kronman, R. A., Manolio T. A., Burke, G. L., and Wolfson, S. K., Jr. (1999). Carotid-artery intima and media thickness as a risk factor for myocardial infarction and stroke in older adults. *New England Journal of Medicine*, **340**, 14–22.

Olson, J. C., Edmundowicz, D., Becker, D. J., Kuller, L. H., and Orchard, T. J. (2000). Coronary calcium in adults with type 1 diabetes: a stronger correlate of clinical coronary artery disease in men than in women. *Diabetes*, **49**, 1571–8.

Otvos, J. D., Jeyarajah, E. J., Bennett, D. W., and Krauss, R. M. (1992). Development of a proton nuclear magnetic resonance spectroscopic method for determining plasma lipoprotein concentrations and subspecies distributions from a single, rapid measurement. *Clinical Chemistry*, **38**, 1632–8.

Pierpoint, T., McKeigue, P. M., Isaacs, A. J., Wild, S. H., and Jacobs, H. S. (1998). Mortality of women with polycystic ovary syndrome at long-term follow-up. *Journal of Clinical Epidemiology*, **51**, 581–6.

Poehlman, E. T. (1993). Regulation of energy expenditure in aging humans. *Journal of the American Geriatrics Society*, **41**, 552–9.

Psaty, B. M., Furberg, C. D., Kuller, L. H., Bild, D. E., Rautaharju, P. M., Polak, J. F. *et al.* (1999). Traditional risk factors and subclinical disease measures as predictors of first myocardial infarction in older adults: The Cardiovascular Health Study. *Archives of Internal Medicine*, **159**, 1339–47.

Reis, S. E., Gloth, S. T., Blumenthal, R. S., Resar, J. R., Zacur, H. A., Gerstenblith, G., and Brinker, J. A. (1994). Ethinyl estradiol acutely attenuates abnormal coronary vasomotor responses to acetylcholine in postmenopausal women. *Circulation*, **89**, 52–60.

Reis, S. E., Holubkov, R., Smith A. J. C., Kelsey, S. F., Sharaf, B. L., Reichek, N. *et al.* (2001). Coronary microvascular dysfunction is highly prevalent in women with chest pain in the absence of coronary artery disease: results from the NHLBI WISE study. *American Heart Journal*, **141**, 735–41.

Ridker, P., Buring, J., Shih, J., Matias, M., and Hennekens, C. H. (1998). Prospective study of C-reactive protein and the risk of future cardiovascular events among apparently healthy women. *Circulation*, **98**, 731–3.

Ritterband, A. B., Jaffe, I. A., Densen, P. M., Magagna, J. F., and Reed, E. (1963). Gonadal function and the development of coronary heart disease. *Circulation*, **26**, 237–51.

Rosendaal, F. R., Helmerhorst, F. M., and Vandenbroucke, J. P. (2002). Female hormones and thrombosis. *Arteriosclerosis, Thrombosis, and Vascular Biology*, **22**, 201–10.

Rubins, H. B., Robins, S. J., Collins, D., Anderson, C. L., Elam, J. W., Faas, M. B. *et al.* (1999). Gemfibrozil for the secondary prevention of coronary heart disease in men with low levels of high-density lipoprotein cholesterol. *New England Journal of Medicine*, **341**, 410–18.

Schonbeck, U., Mach, F., Sukhova, G., Murphy, C., Bonnefoy, J., Fabunmi, R., and Libby, P. (1997). Regulation of matrix metalloproteinase expression in human vascular smooth muscle cells by T lymphocytes: a role for CD40 signaling in plaque rupture? *Circulation Research*, **81**, 448–54.

Selzer, F., Sutton-Tyrrell, K., Fitzgerald, S., Tracy, R., Kuller, L., and Manzi, S. (2001). Vascular stiffness in women with systemic lupus erythematosus. *Hypertension*, **37**, 1075–82.

Shah, P. K., Kaul, S., Nilsson, J., and Cercek, B. (2001). Exploiting the vascular protective effects of high-density lipoprotein and its apolipoproteins: an idea whose time for testing is coming, Part I. *Circulation*, **104**, 2376–83.

Sharaf, B. L., Pepine, C. J., Kerensky, R. A., Reis, S. E., Reichek, N., Rogers, W. J. *et al.* (2001). Detailed angiographic analysis of women with suspected ischemic chest pain (pilot phase data from the NHLBI-sponsored Women's Ischemia Syndrome Evaluation [WISE] Study angiographic core laboratory). *American Journal of Cardiology*, **87**, 937–41.

Simpson, E. R., Clyne, C., Speed, C., Rubin, G., and Bulun, S. (2001). Tissue-specific estrogen biosynthesis and metabolism. *Annals of the New York Academy of Sciences*, **949**, 58–67.

Sniderman, A. D., Scantlebury, T., and Cianflone, K. (2001). Hypertriglyceridemic hyperapoB: the unappreciated atherogenic dyslipoproteinemia in type 2 diabetes mellitus. *Annals of Internal Medicine*, **135**, 447–59.

Solberg, L. A., Enger S. C., Hjermann, I. *et al.* (1980). Risk factors for coronary and cerebral atherosclerosis in the Oslo Study. In *Atherosclerosis V* (ed. A. M. Gotto and L. C. Smith), pp. 57–62. Springer-Verlag, New York.

Stamler, J., Stamler, R., Neaton, J. D., Wentworth, D., Daviglus, M. L., Garside, D. *et al.* (1999). Low risk-factor profile and long-term cardiovascular and noncardiovascular mortality and life expectancy: findings for 5 large cohorts of young adult and middle-aged men and women. *Journal of the American Medical Association*, **282**, 2012–18.

Stampfer, M. J., Krauss, R. M., Ma, J., Blanche, P. J., Holl, L. G., Sacks, F. M., and Hennekens, C. H. (1996). A prospective study of triglyceride level, low-density lipoprotein particle diameter, and risk of myocardial infarction. *Journal of the American Medical Association*, **276**, 882–8.

Stampfer, M. J., Hu, F. B., Manson, J. E., Rimm, E. B., and Willett, W. C. (2000). Primary prevention of coronary heart disease in women through diet and lifestyle. *New England Journal of Medicine*, **343**, 16–22.

St-Pierre, A. C., Ruel, I. L., Cantin, B., Dagenais, G. R., Bernard, P. M., Després, J. P., and Lamarche, B. (2001). Comparison of various electrophoretic characteristics of LDL particles and their relationship to the risk of ischemic heart disease. *Circulation*, **104**, 2295–9.

Sutton-Tyrrell, K., Kuller, L. H., Matthews, K. A., Holubkov, R., Patel, A., Edmundowicz, D., and Newman, A. (2002). Subclinical atherosclerosis in multiple vascular beds: an index of atherosclerotic burden evaluated in postmenopausal women. *Atherosclerosis*, **160**, 407–16.

Talbott, E. O., Wild, R. A., Remsberg, K. E., Gibson, L. B., and Casoglos, A. (1999). Epidemiology of polycystic ovary syndrome. In *Health and disease among women: biological and environmental influences* (ed. R. B. Ness and L. H. Kuller), pp. 225–46. Oxford University Press, New York.

Talbott, E. O., Guzick, D. S., Sutton-Tyrrell, K., McHugh-Pemu, K. P., Zborowski, J. V., Remsberg, K. E., and Kuller, L. H. (2000). Evidence for association between polycystic ovary syndrome and premature carotid atherosclerosis in middle-aged women. *Arteriosclerosis, Thrombosis, and Vascular Biology*, **20**, 2414–21.

Talbott, E., Mathur, T. M., Zborowski, J. V., and McHugh-Pemu, K. P. (2002*a*). Evidence for an increased prevalence of early-onset cardiovascular events among women with polycystic ovary syndrome [Poster presentation]. 42nd Annual Conference on Cardiovascular Disease Epidemiology and Prevention, American Heart Association. 23–26 April 2002, Honolulu, Hawaii.

Talbott, E. O., Zborowski, J. V., Guzick, D., Edmundowicz, D., McHugh-Pemu, K., and Kuller, L. H. (2002*b*). Excess coronary calcification in the Polycystic Ovary Syndrome (PCOS): association with metabolic cardiovascular syndrome (MCS) [Abstract]. *Circulation*, **105**, e86.

Thiagarajan, P. (2001). Atherosclerosis, autoimmunity, and systemic lupus erythematosus. *Circulation*, **104**, 1876–7.

Tracy, R. P. (1999). Inflammation markers and coronary heart disease. *Current Opinion in Lipidology*, **10**, 435–41.

Troiano, R. P., Frongillo, E. A., Jr., and Levitsky, D. A. (1996). The relationship between body weight and mortality: a quantitative analysis of combined information from existing studies. *International Journal of Obesity*, **20**, 63–75.

Uemura, K. and Pisa, Z. (1988). Trends in cardiovascular disease mortality in industrialized countries since 1950. *World Health Statistics Quarterly*, **41**, 155.

Veniant, M. M., Withycombe, S., and Young, S. G. (2001). Lipoprotein size and atherosclerosis susceptibility in Apoe and Ldlr mice. *Arteriosclerosis, Thrombosis, and Vascular Biology*, **21**, 1567–70.

Wagner, J. D., Cefalu, W. T., Anthony, M. S., Litwak, K. N., Zhang, L., and Clarkson, T. B. (1997). Dietary soy protein and estrogen replacement therapy improve cardiovascular risk factors and decrease aortic cholesteryl ester content in ovariectomized cynomolgus monkeys. *Metabolism*, **46**, 698–705.

Walldius, G., Jungner, I., Holme, I., Aastviet A. H., Kolar, W., and Steiner, E. (2001). High apolipoprotein B, low apolipoprotein A-I and improvement in the prediction of fatal myocardial infarction (AMORIS Study): a prospective study. *Lancet*, **358**, 2026–33.

Wenger, N. K. (2002). Clinical trial evidence for lipid lowering in women. *Clinical Journal of Women's Health*, **2**, 112–15.

Wilsgaard, T., Jacobsen, B. K., Schirmer, H., Thune, I., Lochen, M. L., Njolstad, I., and Arnesen, E. (2001). Tracking of cardiovascular risk factors: The Tromso Study, 1979–1995. *American Journal of Epidemiology*, **154**, 418–26.

Wing, R. R., Matthews, K. A., Kuller, L. H., Meilahn, E. N., and Plantinga, P. (1991). Waist to hip ratio in middle-aged women: associations with behavioral and psychosocial factors and with changes in cardiovascular risk factors. *Arteriosclerosis, Thrombosis, and Vascular Biology*, **11**, 1250–7.

Women's Health Initiative Study Group (1998). Design of the Women's Health Initiative clinical trial and observational study. *Controlled Clinical Trials*, **19**, 61–109.

Wong, N. D., Schreiner, P. J., Jacobs, D., Hilner, J., and Loria, C. M. (2002). Relation of baseline and longitudinal changes in lipids over 15 years with coronary artery calcium: the CARDIA study [Abstract]. *Circulation*, **105**, e86.

Writing Group for the PEPI Trial (1995). Effects of estrogen or estrogen/progestin regimens on heart disease risk factors in postmenopausal women. *Journal of the American Medical Association*, **273**, 199–208.

Writing Group for the Women's Health Initiative Investigators (2002). Risks and benefits of estrogen plus progestin in healthy postmenopausal women: principal results from the Women's Health Initiative randomized controlled trial. *Journal of the American Medical Association*, **288**, 321–33.

Yudkin, J. S., Stehouwer, C. D. A., Emeis, J. J., and Coppack, S. W. (1999). C-reactive protein in healthy subjects: associations with obesity, insulin resistance, and endothelial dysfunction: a potential role for cytokines originating from adipose tissue? *Arteriosclerosis, Thrombosis, and Vascular Biology*, **19**, 972–8.

Yu-Poth, S., Zhao, G., Etherton, T., Naglak, M., Jonnalagadda, S., and Kris-Etherton, P. M. (1999). Effects of the National Cholesterol Education Program's Step I and Step II dietary intervention programs on cardiovascular disease risk factors: a meta-analysis. *American Journal of Cardiology*, **69**, 632–46.

Zhao, D., Wu, Z., and Wang, W. (1999). Risk factors of cardiovascular diseases in China. *Cardiovascular Disease Prevention*, **2**, 252–6.

Chapter 23

Use of oral contraceptives

N. R. Poulter

23.1 History and background

Between the 1920s and 1950s the effects of various progestogens on the inhibition of ovulation were studied, with a view to developing an oral contraceptive (OC) pill. It appears that oestrogen became included in the first OC pills as a contaminant and hence the combined OC pill was developed by serendipity (Gillmer 1996)! Oral contraception entered clinical practice in May 1960 when the Federal Development Agency (FDA) in America approved evonid for the cyclical control of ovulation and shortly thereafter Searle launched the 'Pincus Pill', named after one of the earlier experimental investigators.

Because of their efficacy and convenience, the use of OCs increased rapidly thereafter such that, for example, by 1971–74, 21% of premenopausal women aged 15–44 years in the USA were using them (Russel-Brifel *et al.* 1985). This dramatic uptake of OCs was despite the fact that in the 3 years following the clinical introduction of OCs, cases of pulmonary embolus (Jordan 1961), stroke (Lorentz 1962), and myocardial infarction (Boyce *et al.* 1963) were reported in association with the use of OCs. Thereafter, further case reports and reviews of temporal changes in clinical experience (Masi and Dugdale 1970; Bickerstaff 1975), served to support the hypothesis that these cardiovascular (CV) events may be causally associated with OC use. More substantial support for these associations arose from case-control studies (Inman and Vessey 1968; Vessey and Doll 1969; Mann *et al.* 1975; Mann and Inman 1975; Jick *et al.* 1978; Shapiro *et al.* 1979; Krueger *et al.* 1980; Rosenberg *et al.* 1980; Adam *et al.* 1981; Slone *et al.* 1981; La Vecchia *et al.* 1987), and to a lesser extent, from the inevitably limited evidence available from cohort studies (Vessey *et al.* 1977; Petitti *et al.* 1979; Royal College of General Practitioners 1981) carried out during the 1960s and 1970s. Many of these studies were criticized for methodological defects (Realini and Goldzieher 1985) and certainly a large proportion of them, particularly the cohort studies, were too small to generate meaningful results. Nevertheless, by the 1980s it appeared to be established that, on the basis of the observational data available up to that time, the current use of combined OCs was associated with significantly increased risk in venous thromboembolic disease (VTE) – including deep vein thrombosis or pulmonary embolus, in ischaemic stroke and in acute myocardial infarction (Vessey 1980; Stadel 1981*a*, *b*).

The estimates of relative risk were variable from one study to another – in part dependent upon aspects of study design such as whether fatal or non-fatal events were included and whether current or ever users were compared with never or non-users. Several other issues regarding risks associated with OC use were much less well established. For example, OC-associated risks, if any, of haemorrhagic stroke were not clearly established, nor was it clear whether risk estimates were affected by duration of use and among past users. In addition, the role of oestrogen dose and progestogen type on risk estimates of any CV events was not established. This was particularly important since the studies hitherto related to OCs which contained higher doses of oestrogen and progestogen and different progestogen types than those increasingly used in standard practice by the late 1980s.

Presumably in response to concerns over CV health, not only had there been major changes in the formulation of OCs whereby oestrogen and progestogen doses were reduced, but there was also a change in prescribing practices of OCs towards their preferential use by younger women who did not have other risk factors for CV disease.

The impact of the presence or absence of other CV risk factors on risks of CV diseases associated with OC use was by no means clear, really reflecting the fact that studies up to the mid-1980s (and since) included too few cases to allow meaningful investigation.

Finally, given the extensive global use of combined OCs, no studies had attempted to evaluate risks of OC use in the majority of users worldwide – namely those arising from the developing world.

These missing pieces of information notwithstanding, the reports of adverse CV outcomes associated with the OC pill resulted in a decline in use, for example in the USA, from a high of 36.1% of married women using contraception in 1973 to 19.8% in 1982 (Pratt et al. 1984). This change in practice was not limited to women who intended no more pregnancies (and could opt for sterilization), since among married women who intended to become pregnant again, OC use dropped over the same time period from 61.1 to 44.6% of all methods used, with an increase in less effective contraceptive methods.

Hereafter, this chapter will focus on the association between OC use and risk of coronary heart disease (CHD).

23.2 OC use and CHD risk: summary of findings before 1990

Of three cohort studies started in 1968–69 (Vessey et al. 1977; Petitti et al. 1979; Royal College of General Practitioners 1981) only that of the Royal College of General Practitioners (1981) had found enough cases of myocardial infarction (MI) by 1981 to calculate a risk ratio, which turned out to be 4.1. This underlines the shortcomings of cohort studies in trying to evaluate the aetiology of rare disorders such as CHD in young women, and the consequent emphasis necessarily placed on data from case-control studies hereafter. Several case-control studies (Inman and Vessey 1968; Vessey and Doll 1969; Mann et al. 1975; Mann and Inman 1975; Jick et al. 1978; Shapiro et al. 1979; Krueger et al. 1980; Rosenberg et al. 1980; Adam et al. 1981; Slone et al. 1981; La Vecchia et al. 1987) estimated risks to be in the order of at least three for the development of a fatal or non-fatal MI in women without other risk factors or without a history of prior heart disease. The risk of smoking and OC use appeared to have a multiplicative effect on risk of MI, with one case-control study reporting a relative risk of 39 for heavy smoking OC users (Shapiro et al. 1979)! Possible interactions with other coexistent risk factors were not clearly evaluated, although in general risks were considered to be at least multiplicative (Stadel 1981b). Most studies had found no continuing risk of MI in women who stopped OC use, although one relatively large case-control study suggested a dose-related residual effect on risk after prolonged OC use (Slone et al. 1981). A brief survey of the case-control studies carried out and published by 1990 is shown in Table 23.1.

Table 23.1 Case-control studies of current[a] OC use and CHD events

Authors	Publication year	Years of CHD events	Setting	CHD end point	No of cases (OC users)	Adjusted OR (95% CI)
Inman and Vessey	1968	1966	England, Wales, and N. Ireland	Fatal	23	1.0 (NA)
Vessey and Doll	1969	1964–67	Northwest London	Non-fatal	2	1.0 (NA)
Mann et al.	1975	1968–72	3 regions in England	Non-fatal	17	4.0 (NA)
Mann and Inman	1975	1973	England and Wales	Fatal	31	2.3 (NA)
Jick et al.	1978	1975	USA	Non-fatal	20	14.0 (5.5–37)[b]
Shapiro et al.	1979	1976–78	USA	Non-fatal	29	4.0 (2.5–6.3)
Rosenberg et al.	1980	1964–76	USA	Non-fatal	23	1.6 (1.0–2.6)[c]
Krueger et al.	1980	1974–75	USA	Fatal	20	1.2 (0.6–2.3)
Slone et al.	1981	1976–79	USA	Non-fatal	41	3.5 (2.2–5.5)[c]
Adam et al.	1981	1978	England and Wales	Fatal	24	1.4 (0.8–2.4)[c]
La Vecchia et al.	1987	1983–85	Italy	Non-fatal	6	1.8 (0.3–11.5)[c]

NA = not available.

[a] Usually within 1 month of the index event.

[b] No other risk factors.

[c] Versus never users.

23.3 Mechanisms by which OCs might affect CHD risk

23.3.1 Coagulation

OCs produce endothelial proliferation, and an increase in various measures of coagulability (Bonnar 1987). Factors VIII and X are increased and antithrombin III is decreased in OC users (Meade 1982). These changes were considered largely secondary to the oestrogenic component of OCs, but there was some evidence of an effect of progestogen in low-dose OCs (i.e. <30 μg oestrogen) (Bonnar 1987). More recently, third generation progestogens (those containing desogestrel or gestodene) have been shown to have a more adverse clotting profile than second generation products (those containing levonorgestrel) (Rosing et al. 1999). When autopsy or arteriogram had allowed the visualization of the coronary vasculature in OC users suffering an MI, arteries reportedly showed relatively little atherosclerosis and instead showed obstruction by a solitary thrombus more often than in age-matched controls (Mann and Inman 1975). Nevertheless, it was and remains far from clear, if likely, that OCs have their effect on CV diseases through changes in coagulability. It was hypothesized that the decrease in antithrombin III associated with OC use leads to increased subclinical thrombosis, with subsequent fibrinolytic activity (Stadel 1981b). Those women with no reserve fibrinolytic activity would be expected to develop overt disease.

23.3.2 Lipid metabolism

Both oestrogens and progestogens were known to exert noticeable effects on lipid metabolism (Gaspard 1987; Crook 1996). In general, oestrogens have been found to produce a more favourable CV profile, and progestogens exert an adverse impact. Specifically, oestrogens increase the HDL-cholesterol, particularly the HDL2 subfraction, an increase in which has been found to be correlated with protection from CHD. The effect of oestrogens on LDL-cholesterol is not as well understood, but it appears that oestrogen slightly lowers this lipoprotein fraction. Although natural progesterone has no effect on lipoproteins, synthetic progestogens used in OCs, derived from 19-nortestosterone, have androgenic and anti-oestrogenic properties. These compounds produce an unfavourable CV profile, increasing the LDL-cholesterol and decreasing the HDL component, specifically the HDL2 subfraction. Combined OCs differ in their effects on lipoprotein metabolism depending on the relative amounts of the hormones present. OCs containing 50 μg oestrogen or more, combined with norethisterone, increased triglycerides and LDL-cholesterol and decreased HDL-cholesterol. Lower dose OCs (e.g. 35 μg oestrogen and less than 500 μg norethisterone) were found to have minimal effects on most lipoprotein fractions and to cause a slight increase in HDL-cholesterol. A more recent study of combined OCs showed that a lower dose of progestin and the newer third generation progestins (containing desogestrel) tended to reduce adverse metabolic effects (Godsland *et al.* 1991).

23.3.3 Carbohydrate metabolism

Oestrogens appear to have little effect on carbohydrate metabolism (Perlman *et al.* 1985; Godsland *et al.* 1991). Several studies show that progestogens adversely affect carbohydrate metabolism by producing hyperglycaemia with relative insulin deficiency. OCs affect glucose metabolism to varying degrees depending on the progestogen used, with norgestrel producing the greatest change in results of oral glucose tolerance tests. This effect increases with duration of use of OCs and one study found that 16% of OC users had abnormal oral glucose tolerance tests after 5 years of use (Perlman *et al.* 1985).

23.3.4 Blood pressure

A modest rise in blood pressure appears to be a relatively common occurrence in OC users (Poulter 1996), although it appears from one study (Nichols *et al.* 1993) that a return to baseline levels usually occurs after discontinuation of OCs. Few data exist to evaluate these effects accurately, or to compare the effect of OCs of different composition (Nichols *et al.* 1993). Since increasing blood pressure levels are an established risk factor for stroke and MI, it is possible that mild, OC-induced blood pressure elevation may contribute to increasing the incidence of these two conditions.

23.3.5 Summary

Alterations in coagulation, lipid metabolism, blood pressure, and carbohydrate metabolism are major risk factors for the development of CV diseases, as discussed in more detail in other chapters in this book. It is not known whether OCs exert their effects on CV disease by means of their adverse metabolic effects or if other mechanisms are involved. It is known, however, that some of the metabolic effects of OCs are affected by both oestrogen and progestogen dose and/or type.

23.4 Impact of low-dose OCs: early studies

Studies using reports of adverse drug reactions suggested that lower doses of oestrogen were linked with decreases in ischaemic heart disease risk (Bottiger *et al.* 1980; Meade *et al.* 1980) and that higher doses of levonorgestrel were associated with increased risk of stroke and CHD (Bottiger *et al.* 1980). In the light of these and the laboratory-based data described above, the composition of OCs had been changing. For example, in 1963 almost 50% of OC users in the UK were taking pills that contained 100 μg of oestrogen. By 1987, however, the majority of OC users in the UK were using pills containing up to 35 μg oestrogen (Thorogood and Vessey 1990) with a substantial increase in biphasic and triphasic OC usage (from 0 to 32.3% during the same 24-year period) and in progesterone-only OC usage (from 0 to 8.8%). The CV risks associated with progestogen-only contraceptives remain largely uninvestigated and hereafter results relate to risks associated with combined OCs (containing oestrogen and progestogen). Although the relative magnitude and distribution of these types of changes varied around the world, the trend was fairly consistent.

In 1975 one case-control study demonstrated that the relative risk of VTE was greater for users of OCs containing 100 μg of oestrogen or more when compared to users of OCs with less oestrogen (Stolley *et al.* 1975). However, a later case-control study (Mann 1982) found no difference in the risk of fatal MIs between users of OCs containing 50 μg oestrogen and users of OCs containing less oestrogen.

Thus, given the three major classes of progestogens, and the two types of oestrogen used in a multitude of possible combinations introduced during this period, no consistent data were available to assess the best dosage and composition of OCs in terms of minimizing associated CV morbidity or mortality.

The data on risk of MI in relation to duration of OC use were much less consistent than for VTE, which showed a plateau effect. One report suggested that duration of use may affect risk of stroke (Pettiti and Wingerd 1978), whereas the only study large enough to evaluate duration of use and MI risk with sufficient precision confirmed the results of smaller previous studies, which showed no relationship (Slone *et al.* 1981). More data from the same study, which was again the only one of sufficient size to adequately evaluate the question, showed that past OC use increased the risk of MI (Slone *et al.* 1981).

Clearly these data on duration and past use of OCs were inconsistent, and more data were required.

23.5 The WHO Collaborative Study of Cardiovascular Disease and Steroid Hormone Contraception

In the light of all the missing information regarding OC use and risk of CV diseases as of the late 1980s (Poulter *et al.* 1991), the World Health Organization Collaborative Study of Cardiovascular Disease and Steroid Hormone Contraception study was commissioned (WHO 1995). This was planned as – and turned out to be – the largest study of CV diseases and current OC use. It investigated VTE, stroke, and MI in association with OC use in four regions of the world. The objectives of the study in relation to CHD were:

Primary: to determine the association between current OC use and morbidity from acute MI in a combined group of European countries and a combined group of non-European ('developing') countries.

Subsidiary objectives included whether OC-associated risk of acute MI differed:

1 among subgroups of women (e.g. smokers);
2 by composition (i.e. oestrogen dose and progestogen type);
3 by duration of use;
4 among past OC users.

This study was a hospital-based, case-control study carried out in 21 countries subdivided between European countries and countries in Africa, Asia, and Latin America (including the Caribbean) combined ('developing'). The study recruited 368 women aged 20–44 years who had been admitted to one of the collaborating hospitals between February 1989 and January 1995 with a diagnosis of definite or possible MI based on standardized criteria (WHO Monica Project 1990). Women who died within 24 h of admission were excluded as were those with a past medical history of CHD, stroke, or VTE. A total of 941 age- and sex-matched hospital controls were recruited from the same hospitals as the cases. Further details of the methods used are published elsewhere (WHO 1995, 1997).

The odds ratios of an MI compared with never and past users combined (non-users) associated with current OC use in Europe and developing countries combined are shown in Table 23.2 before and after adjusting for confounding. Adjustment resulted in important increases in odds ratios, confirming that women with other risk factors (except smoking) were less likely to use OCs.

Table 23.3 shows similar data, but for past and current users separately compared with never users of OCs, and shows a non-significant increase in risk among past users of OCs. Age (<35 or ≥35 years) did not affect odds ratios significantly, in keeping with earlier reports (Stadel 1981a).

Table 23.2 Odds ratios for MI in relation to current use of combined OCs by region in the WHO/CVD/SHC study. Relative to non-user

Region and type of user	Cases	Controls	Odds ratio (95% CI)	
			Crude	Adjusted[a]
Europe				
Non-user	136	402	1.00	1.00
User	62	78	3.21 (1.94–5.32)	5.01 (2.54–9.90)
Developing countries				
Non-user	131	420	1.00	1.00
User	39	41	3.26 (1.94–5.49)	4.78 (2.52–9.07)

Source: WHO 1997.

[a] For confounding variables. Numbers included vary slightly in each group due to some missing data.

Table 23.3 Odds ratios for MI in relation to current and past use of combined OCs by region in the WHO/CVD/SHC study. Relative to never-users

Region and type of user	Cases	Controls	Odds ratio (95% CI)	
			Crude	Adjusted[a]
Europe				
Never	44	138	1.00	1.00
Past	92	264	1.16 (0.73–1.86)	1.23 (0.67–2.26)
Current	62	78	3.59 (1.95–6.60)	5.64 (2.49–12.8)
Developing countries				
Never	63	249	1.00	1.00
Past	68	171	1.56 (1.04–2.33)	1.48 (0.88–2.49)
Current	39	41	4.04 (2.30–7.09)	6.13 (2.99–12.6)

Source: WHO 1997.

[a] For confounding variables. Numbers included vary slightly in each group due to some missing data.

Higher oestrogen dose OCs ($\geq$50 μg) were associated with higher odds ratios for MI than lower dose OCs in developing countries, but not in Europe – the European data being more consistent with earlier findings (Shapiro *et al.* 1979; Adam *et al.* 1981).

The WHO study had no power to differentiate risk of MI associated with second or third generation progestogens. One consistent and obvious finding was that odds ratios for MI were higher among those who reported that their blood pressure had not been checked prior to the current episode of OC use, irrespective of age or oestrogen dose. Whether this effect (which has not been reported in earlier studies) was the result of the effect of screening out those women with higher blood pressures, or perhaps more likely, reflected other aspects of health care and/or health-seeking behaviour, is not known.

The coexistence of other risk factors such as history of high blood pressure (during or out-side pregnancy) or smoking appeared to produce an effect on OC-induced risk of MI which was at least multiplicative – particularly in the European countries (Table 23.4). For example, smoking (which showed a dose–response effect on risk) 10 or more cigarettes per day increased the OC-associated risk from an odds ratio of 3.96 to 87.0, albeit with confidence intervals (CIs) of 29.8–254!

Despite the size of the WHO study, the evaluation of the impact of duration of exposure lacked power. There was no significant effect among current users although, consistent with one earlier study (Slone *et al.* 1981), there was some suggestion of a possible duration-associated effect among past OC users.

Overall, the odds ratios for MIs associated with OC use were higher than shown in almost all studies reported up to 1990 (see Table 23.1) and thereafter, and the authors concluded that this finding may reflect the more frequent use of OCs by women with other CV risk factors and less screening than is currently carried out in, for example, the UK and USA. Hence it was hypo-thesized that the estimates of OC-associated risk had been inflated by an unknown proportion

Table 23.4 Odds ratios for MI in relation to current use of combined OCs according to other risk factors. European data from the WHO/CVD/SHC study

Factor	Non-users Cases/controls	Odds ratio[a] (95% CI)	OC users Cases/controls	Odds ratio[a] (95% CI)
History of hypertension other than in pregnancy (HBP)				
No	96/374	1.00	45/75	3.85 (1.88–7.89)
Yes	40/24	5.43 (2.39–12.4)	16/3	68.1 (6.18–751)
History of blood pressure problems in pregnancy (HIP)				
No	106/343	1.00	53/71	4.49 (2.19–9.20)
Yes	30/55	0.99 (0.45–2.19)	8/7	10.0 (2.40–42.0)
Current smoker				
No	29/261	1.00	15/49	3.96 (1.52–10.4)
<10 cigarettes/day	11/23	4.74 (1.65–13.6)	2/13	5.04 (0.78–32.4)
≥10 cigarettes/day	96/114	11.1 (5.68–21.8)	44/16	87.0 (29.8–254)
Reported risk factor status (HBP, rheumatic heart disease, diabetes, abnormal blood lipids, HIP, or smoking)				
No risk factor	16/205	1.00	10/41	3.07 (1.06–8.95)
At least one	120/193	8.18 (4.33–15.4)	51/37	37.3 (15.2–91.7)

Source: WHO 1997.

[a] For confounding variables. Numbers included vary slightly in each group due to some missing data.

Table 23.5 Estimated incidence rates and attributable risks per 10^6 woman-years associated with current OC use by age and smoking status among European women in the WHO/CVD/SHC study

	Incidence per 10^6 woman-years		Attributable risk
	Non-users of OCs	**Users of OCs**	
Women <35 years			
Non-smokers	0.83	3.56	2.73
Smokers	7.78	42.7	34.9
Women >35 years			
Non-smokers	9.45	40.4	31.0
Smokers	88.4	484.6	396.2

Source: WHO 1997.

of women who were inadequately screened and had undetected (and hence unrecorded) risk factors. Nevertheless, the odds ratio associated with current OC use among those with no other reported risk factors was still 3.1 (1.1–9.0) in the European part of the WHO study. Importantly, even with these apparently high odds ratios, the absolute risk of an MI associated with OC use was only importantly increased in women ≥ 35 years who smoked (see Table 23.5).

23.6 Other studies reported since 1990 (Table 23.6)

Whilst the WHO study was in progress, three other smaller case-control studies – one from the UK (Thorogood *et al.* 1991) and two from the USA (Rosenberg *et al.* 1990; Sidney *et al.* 1996) reported no significant increases in risk of an MI associated with current OC use. The UK study found odds ratios for a fatal MI of 1.9 (95% CI: 0.7–4.9) for current OC use and 1.9 (1.0–3.5) for past OC use, but the odds ratios were 4.2 (0.5–38.2) for current use of OCs containing 50 μg of oestrogen. The first of the two American studies was published in 1990 and, having included women aged 25–64 years, really focused on past use of OCs (Rosenberg *et al.* 1990). Those who had used OCs for at least 5 years in the past were found not to be at increased risk of MI (odds ratio (OR) = 1.1 (0.8–1.5)). This study only included six current OC users among the cases of MI and hence the risk estimate (OR = 1.1) for current use was of limited value. The second study from the USA (Sidney *et al.* 1996), published just before the WHO study, also found a non-significant increase in odds ratios for an MI associated with current OC use of 1.67 (0.48–5.85)), being a little higher in women over 35 years (OR = 1.98 (0.32–12.28)). This, too, was a small study, with only 29 MI cases who were current OC users. It is possible, limited study size notwithstanding, that due to effective pre-user screening, the prevalence of coexistent risk factors was lower in this group compared with those studied in the WHO study, and that odds ratios for MI were lower than those reported in the WHO study.

Prior to publication of the WHO study, two other case-control studies designed to evaluate whether the progestogen component of the OC used affected risk of MI were published (Jick *et al.* 1996; Lewis *et al.* 1996). The first of these two studies included only 11 cases (Jick *et al.* 1996). With the clear and inevitable serious limitations of size, it showed no difference in risk of an MI by progestogen type, but confirmed low absolute risk levels of MI in young women and the strong impact of smoking on these levels of risk. The second, somewhat larger study, included an undisclosed number of cases who were current OC users (Lewis *et al.* 1996). However, once again no significant difference between the impact of second and third generation progestogens on the risk of an MI was apparent, although there was some suggestion that third-generation products were associated with less risk. The full report of this second study (the Transnational Study) of OC use and risk of MI was reported (Lewis *et al.* 1997) shortly after the WHO study, and thereafter four others have since been published (Mant *et al.* 1998; Dunn *et al.* 1999; Rosenberg *et al.* 2001; Tanis *et al.* 2001).

The second report of the Transnational Study (Lewis *et al.* 1997) extended the database from the original report of the same study (Lewis *et al.* 1996) to include 57 OC-user cases of MI. In this analysis, current use of second generation OCs was associated with an increased risk of an MI (OR = 2.35 (1.42–3.89)) whereas third generation products were not, and the difference between pill types was significant. However, these findings were criticized for lack of adjustment for blood pressure screening – a variable which the WHO study had shown to be so important (WHO 1997).

In 1998 an update of data from the Oxford Family Planning Association Study was published (Mant *et al.* 1998). Despite the large cohort of 17 032 women originally recruited to the study between 1968 and 1974, this update only included eight cases of MI who had used an OC within the last year. Once again, this observation highlights the shortcomings of cohort studies for evaluating rare events such as CHD in young women, and the inability of this study design to contribute meaningfully to the database. Given these limitations, the reported odds ratios were 1.5 (0.6–3.2), but once again this study confirmed the important effect of smoking on risk estimates.

In 1999 the MICA case-control study from UK was published (Dunn *et al.* 1999). With 40 OC-user cases of MI they reported a non-significant increase in risk of MI (OR = 1.4 (0.78–2.52)) with no difference in risk between second and third generation products. In fact unlike the Transnational Study, the odds ratio for third generation products was higher than for second generation products. Because 87% of the MI cases included in this study of women aged under 45 were not current OC users and 88% of the cases had at least one known CV risk factor, the authors concluded that these other risk factors – and particularly smoking (80% smoked) – should be the focus of a preventive strategy.

Two case-control studies of MI risk and OC use were published in 2001 (Rosenberg *et al.* 2001; Tanis *et al.* 2001). The first was another small study from America (Rosenberg *et al.* 2001). Despite having recruited cases for over 14 years, this study included only 36 current OC users who had suffered an MI! The overall odds ratio for MI was 1.3 (0.8–2.2) compared with never users (as opposed to the usual comparator group of non-current users), but was also 1.3 for non-smokers. No variation in odds ratio was apparent by pill type or oestrogen dose, nor was past OC use associated with increased risk. However, given the restricted size of the study, these negative results are of uncertain value.

The most recent case-control study to address OC-associated risk of MI was a population-based study from the Netherlands (Tanis *et al.* 2001). This study included 99 MI cases aged 18–49 who currently used OCs and as such was the only study to approach the number of OC-user cases included in the WHO study (Table 23.6). This study reported an odds ratio of 2.0 (1.5–2.8) for MI risk associated with current OC use, and that second generation may produce higher risk than third generation products. The risk was independent of the presence or absence of a prothrombotic mutation (Factor V Leiden) but, in keeping with the European data from the WHO study, found no significant impact of oestrogen dose (<50 μg vs. ≥50 μg or 30 μg vs. 50 μg). Also in keeping with the WHO study, but contrary to

Table 23.6 WHO and other studies of current[a] OC use and CHD risk reported since 1990

Authors	Publication Year	Years of CHD events	Setting	CHD end point	No of cases (OC users)	Adjusted OR (95% CI)
WHO	1997	1989–95	Europe and developing countries	Non-fatal	101	5.0 (2.5–9.9)[b] 4.8 (2.5–9.0)[c]
Rosenberg et al.	1990	1985–88	New England	Non-fatal	6	1.1 (0.4–3.10)
Sidney et al.	1996	1991–94	North and south California	Non-fatal	10	1.65 (0.5–6.1)
Lewis et al.	1996	1993–96	5 European countries	Non-fatal	57	2.26 (1.3–3.9)[d]
Dunn et al.	1999	1993–95	England, Scotland, and Wales	Fatal and non-fatal	53	1.4 (0.8–2.5)
Rosenberg et al.	2001	1985–99	Boston/Philadelphia	Non-fatal	36[e]	1.3 (0.8–2.2)
Tanis et al.	2001	1990–95	Netherlands	Non-fatal	99[f]	2.0 (1.4–3.0)[g]
Thorogood et al.	1991	1986–88	England and Wales	Fatal	37	1.9 (0.7–4.9)

[a] Usually within 1 month of the index event.

[b] Europe.

[c] Developing countries.

[d] Matched analyses.

[e] Includes 1 × POP user.

[f] Includes 9 × POP users.

[g] Versus never user.

POP, progestogen only pill.

some earlier reports of small studies, was the finding that MI risk was significantly increased among non-smokers who currently used OCs. In addition, this study found, perhaps contrary to prior expectations, that among women with no known CV risk factors, OC use was associated with an odds ratio of 3.1 (1.0–9.2) for MI, a finding which almost exactly duplicated the findings of a similar analysis in the WHO study (Table 23.4). However, the possibly attenuating impact of BP screening on these risk estimates was not addressed in either analysis.

23.6.1 Summary

Risk of current OC use

- Prior to 1990, data from 11 relatively small case-control studies were largely consistent in showing a variable increase in risk of CHD events (see Table 23.1).

- Case-control studies published since then have been consistent in showing an increase in risk (see Tables 23.2, 23.3, and 23.6). However, most studies, particularly those from the USA, have been small and the largest studies, all of which were carried out in Europe (Lewis et al. 1997; WHO 1997; Tanis et al. 2001) do show an increase in risk of an MI even among non-smokers.

- The smaller estimates of risk from American studies (Rosenberg et al. 1990, 2001; Sidney et al. 1996) are more unstable than other studies seen in Table 23.6 due to limited size, but could possibly reflect (if true) the greater use of OCs among healthier women in America and/or different types of OCs.

- Even if the highest estimate of risk reported in any of the relatively recent large, well-conducted studies was correct (WHO 1997), the absolute risk for women is very small unless they are over age 35 and also smoke (Table 23.3).

Risk among past users of OCs

Good, robust evidence remains limited to a few studies, some of which do show some small residual risk, but overall best evidence suggests that any increase in risk, if it exists, is small (WHO 1997; Stampfer *et al.* 1988; Beral *et al.* 1999).

Risk and OC composition and oestrogen dose

◆ The data comparing second with third generation products are inconsistent although over-all most studies (Jick *et al.* 1996; Lewis *et al.* 1997; WHO 1997; Tanis *et al.* 2001), with one exception (Dunn *et al.* 1999), are compatible with the possibility that third generation products may be associated with a smaller increase in risk than second generation products. If true, any such benefits of third generation products need to be offset against the apparent (although still controversial) increase in risk of the far more frequently occurring VTE events associated with third generation products (Kemmeren *et al.* 2001; The European Agency for the Evaluation of Medicinal Products 2001).

◆ Somewhat surprisingly, and perhaps reflecting the small number of OC-using cases included in so many of the studies (Tables 23.1 and 23.2), the evidence that lower-dose oestrogen products are associated with lower risk is by no means clear. This lack of clarity may also reflect the effects of confounding, due to a prescription bias whereby lowest-dose products are supplied to higher-risk women. Nevertheless, it seems counter-intuitive not to recommend the use of lower-dose products (e.g. <50μg oestrogen (EE)) where they are well-tolerated and effective.

Impact of other risk factors on OC-associated risk

◆ Most studies have been underpowered to evaluate this question.

◆ Nevertheless it does seem that most cases of MI in young women who are OC users occur in those who also have at least one other CV risk factor. Where sample size has allowed investigation into the impact of coexistent risk factors on OC-associated risk, the effect appears multiplicative.

◆ Smoking is the commonest coexistent risk factor in OC-using women and most evidence suggests that the impact of smoking on OC-associated risk is at least multiplicative (WHO 1997). Targeted intervention to stop smoking would be far more effective in reducing the incidence of MI among young women than the withdrawal of combined OCs (Farley *et al.* 1998).

23.7 **Conclusions**

The small absolute excess risk of an MI due to the use of combined OCs should be balanced against the risks and benefits associated with the use of alternative forms of contraception and of the effect of OCs on other CV end points, on risk of, or protection against, certain forms of neoplasia, on quality of life, and ultimately on overall morbidity and mortality. The users of OCs are the only ones who can ultimately make this decision, but despite the small absolute risks involved, given the young age of OC users and the iatrogenic background to any complications induced, it is incumbent upon the medical research community to objectively evaluate the various pieces of information necessary to make such judgements. It is worrisome that, despite the large number of studies evaluating CV risk associated with OC use, definitive evidence regarding several issues – particularly whether risk varies with type of OC and oestrogen dosage – remains elusive. Such evidence cannot arise from cohort studies, nor will yet more underpowered case-control studies be helpful. Only a large-scale case-control study, or a huge randomized trial with a relatively short follow-up (e.g. 5 years), could provide the missing information. Whilst a trial is ideal, it is probably not a feasible project, and a very large case-control study probably remains the most realistic option for filling in the blanks. If the prospective multinational case-control study necessary were powered to evaluate MI risk effectively, it would also provide (with relatively limited add-on costs) more definitive evidence regarding the effects of OCs on other CV endpoints.

References

Adam, S. A., Thorogood, M., and Mann, J. I. (1981). Oral contraception and myocardial infarction revisited: the effects of new preparations and prescribing patterns. *British Journal of Obstetrics and Gynaecology*, **88**, 838–45.

Beral, V., Hermon, C., Kay, C., Hannaford, P., Darby, S., and Reeves, G. (1999). Mortality associated with oral contraceptive use: 25 year follow up cohort of 46 000 women from Royal College of General Practitioners' oral contraception study. *British Medical Journal*, **318**, 96–100.

Bickerstaff, E. R. (1975). *Neurological complications of oral contraceptives*. Clarendon Press, Oxford.

Bonnar, J. (1987). Coagulation effects of oral contraceptives. *American Journal of Obstetric Gynaecology*, **157**, 1042–8.

Bottiger, L. E., Boman, G., Eklund, G., and Westerholm, B. (1980). Oral contraceptives and thromboembolic disease: effects of lowering estrogen content. *Lancet*, **1**, 1097–101.

Boyce, J., Fawcett, J. W., and Noall, E. W. P. (1963). Coronary thrombosis and Conovid. *Lancet*, **ii**, 111.

Crook, D. (1996). Role of screening for vascular disease in pill users: lipids and lipoproteins. In *Evidence-guided prescribing of the pill* (ed. P. C. Hannaford and A. M. C. Webb), pp. 89–98. Parthenon, London.

Dunn, N., Thorogood, M., Faragher, B., de Caestecker, L., MacDonald, T. M., McCollum, C. *et al.* (1999). Oral contraceptives and myocardial infarction: results of the MICA case-control study. *British Medical Journal*, **318**, 1579–83.

Farley, T. M. M., Meirik, O., Chang, C. L., and Poulter, N. R. (1998). Combined oral contraceptives, smoking and cardiovascular risk. *Journal of Epidemiology and Community Health*, **52**, 775–85.

Gaspard, U. J. (1987). Metabolic effects of oral contraceptives. *American Journal of Obstetrics and Gynecology*, **157**, 1029–41.

Gillmer, M. D. G. (1996). The pill: an historical overview. In *Evidence-guided prescribing of the pill* (ed. P. C. Hannaford and A. M. C. Webb), pp. 15–26. Parthenon, London.

Godsland, I. F., Crook, D., and Wynn, V. (1991). Coronary heart disease risk markers in users of low-dose oral contraceptives. *Journal of Reproductive Medicine*, **36**(3S), 226–37.

Inman, W. H. W. and Vessey, M. P. (1968). Investigation of deaths from pulmonary, coronary and cerebral thrombosis and embolism in women of childbearing age. *British Medical Journal*, **ii**, 193–9.

Jick, H., Dinan, B., and Rothman, K. (1978). Oral contraceptives and non-fatal myocardial infarction. *Journal of the American Medical Association*, **239**, 1403–6.

Jick, H., Jick, S. S., Myers, M. W., and Vasilakis, C. (1996). Risk of acute myocardial infarction and low-dose combined oral contraceptives. *Lancet*, **347**, 627–8.

Jordan, W. M. (1961). Pulmonary embolism. *Lancet*, **ii**, 1146–7.

Kemmeren, J. M., Algra, A., and Grobbee, D. E. (2001). Third generation oral contraceptives and risk of venous thrombosis: meta-analysis. *British Medical Journal*, **323**, 131–4.

Krueger, D. E., Ellenberg, S. S., Bloom, S. *et al.* (1980). Fatal myocardial infarction and the role of oral contraceptives. *American Journal of Epidemiology*, 11, 655–74.

La Vecchia, C., Franceschi, S., Decarli, A., Pampalona, S., and Tognoni, G. (1987). Risk factors for myocardial infarction in young women. *American Journal of Epidemiology*, 125, 832–43.

Lewis, M. A., Heinemann, L. A. J., Spitzer, W. O., MacRae, D., and Bruppacher, R. for the Transnational Research Group on Oral Contraceptives and the Health of Young Women. (1997). The use of oral contraceptives and the occurrence of acute myocardial infarction in young women. *Contraception*, 56, 129–40.

Lewis, M. A., Spitzer, W. O., Heinemann, L. A. J. *et al.* (1996). Third generation oral contraceptives and risk of myocardial infarction: an international case-control study. *British Medical Journal*, 312, 88–90.

Lorentz, I. T. (1962). Parietal lesion and Enavid. *British Medical Journal*, ii, 1191.

Mann, J. I. (1982). Progestogens in cardiovascular disease: an introduction to the epidemiologic data. *American Journal of Obstetrics and Gynecology*, 142, 752–7.

Mann, J. I. and Inman, W. H. W. (1975). Oral contraceptives and death from myocardial infarction. *British Medical Journal*, ii, 245–8.

Mann, J. I., Vessey, M. P., Thorogood, M., and Doll, R. (1975). Myocardial infarction in young women with special reference to oral contraceptive practice. *British Medical Journal*, 2, 241–5.

Mant, J., Painter, R., and Vessey, M. (1998). Risk of myocardial infarction, angina and stroke in users of oral contraceptives: an updated analysis of a cohort study. *British Journal of Obstetrics and Gynecology*, 105, 890–6.

Masi, A. T. and Dugdale, M. (1970). Cerebrovascular diseases associated with the use of oral contraceptives. *Annals of Internal Medicine*, 72, 111–21.

Meade, T. W. (1982). Oral contraceptives, clotting factors and thrombosis. *American Journal of Obstetrics and Gynecology*, 142, 758–61.

Meade, T. W., Greenberg, G., and Thompson, S. G. (1980). Progestogens and cardiovascular reactions associated with oral contraceptives and a comparison of the safety of 50 and 30 μg estrogen preparations. *British Medical Journal*, 2, 1157–61.

Nichols, M., Robinson, G., Bounds, W., Newman, B., and Guillebaud, J. (1993). Effect of four combined oral contraceptives on blood pressure in the pill-free interval. *Contraception*, 47, 367–76.

Perlman, J. A., Russell-Briefel, R., Ezzati, T., and Liebnerknecht, G. (1985). Oral glucose tolerance and the potency of contraceptive progestins. *Journal of Chronic Diseases*, 38, 857–64.

Petitti, D. B. and Wingerd, J. (1978). Use of oral contraceptives, cigarette smoking and risk of subarachnoid hemorrhage. *Lancet*, 2, 234–7.

Petitti, D. B., Wingerd, J., Pellegrin, F., and Ramcharan, S. (1979). Risk of vascular disease in women. *Journal of the American Medical Association*, 242, 1150–4.

Poulter, N. R. 1996 Oral contraceptives and blood pressure. In *Evidence-guided prescribing of the pill* (ed. P. C. Hannaford and A. M. C. Webb), pp. 77–88. Parthenon, London.

Poulter, N. R., Chang, C. L., and Marmot, M. G. on behalf of The World Health Organization Collaborative Study of Cardiovascular Disease and Steroid Hormone Contraceptives (1991). Cardiovascular disease and oral contraception: what more can we learn from epidemiological studies? *Advances in Contraception*, 7(Suppl. 3), 6583.

Pratt, W. F., Mosher, W. D., Brachrack, C. A., and Horn, M. C. (1984). Understanding US fertility: findings from the National Survey of Family Growth, Cycle III. *Population Bulletin*, 39, 1042.

Realini, J. P. and Goldzieher, J. W. (1985). Oral contraceptives and cardiovascular disease: a critique of the epidemiologic studies. *American Journal of Obstetric Gynecology* 6, 729–98.

Rosenberg, L., Hennekens, C. H., Rosner, B., Belanger, C., Rothman, K. J., and Speizer, F. E. (1980). Oral contraceptive use in relation to non-fatal myocardial infarction. *American Journal of Epidemiology*, 111, 59–66.

Rosenberg, L., Palmer, J. R., Lesko, S. M., and Shapiro, S. (1990). Oral contraceptive use and the risk of myocardial infarction. *American Journal of Epidemiology*, **131**, 1009–16.

Rosenberg, L., Palmer, J. R., Rao, R. S., and Shapiro, S. (2001). Low-dose oral contraceptive use and the risk of myocardial infarction. *Archives of Internal Medicine*, **161**, 1065–70.

Rosing, J., Middlethorp, S., Curvers, J. *et al.* (1999). Low-dose oral contraceptives and acquired resistance to activated protein C: a randomised cross-over study. *Lancet*, **354**, 2036–40.

Royal College of General Practitioners (1981). Further analyses of mortality in oral contraceptive users. *Lancet*, **1**, 541–6.

Russel-Brifel, R., Ezzati, T., and Perlman, J. (1985). Prevalence and trends in oral contraceptive use in premenopausal females age 12–54 years, United States, 1971–80. *American Journal of Public Health*, **10**, 1173–5.

Shapiro, S., Slone, D., Rosenberg, L., Kaufman, D. W., Stoley, P. D., and Miettinen, O. S. (1979). Oral contraceptive use in relation to myocardial infarction. *Lancet*, **i**, 743–7.

Sidney, S., Petitti, D. B., Quesenberry, C. P., Klatsky, A. L., Ziel, H. K., and Wolf, S. (1996). Myocardial infarction in users of low dose oral contraceptives. *Obstetrics and Gynaecology*, **88**, 939–44.

Slone, D., Shapiro, S., Kaufman, D. W., Rosenberg, L., Miettinen, O. S., and Stolley, P. D. (1981). Risk of myocardial infarction in relation to current and discontinued use of oral contraceptives. *New England Journal of Medicine*, **305**, 420–4.

Stadel, B. V. (1981*a*). Oral contraceptives and cardiovascular disease, part 1. *New England Journal of Medicine*, **305**, 612–18.

Stadel, B. V. (1981*b*). Oral contraceptives and cardiovascular disease, part 2. *New England Journal of Medicine*, **305**, 672–7.

Stampfer, M. J., Willett, W. C., Colditz, G. A., Speizer, F. E., and Hennekens, C. H. (1988). A prospective study of past use of oral contraceptive agents and risk of cardiovascular diseases. *New England Journal of Medicine*, **319**, 1313–17.

Stolley, P. D., Tonascia, J. A., Tockman, M. S. *et al.* (1975). Thrombosis with low estrogen oral contraceptives. *American Journal of Epidemiology*, **102**, 197–208.

Tanis, B. C., Van den Bosch, M. A. A. J., Kemmeren, J. M., Cats, V. M., Helmerhorst, F. M., Algra A. *et al.* (2001). Oral contraceptives and the risk of myocardial infarction. *New England Journal of Medicine*, **345**, 1787–93.

The European Agency for the Evaluation of Medicinal Products (2001). Position Statement: CPMP concludes its assessment of 'third generation' combined oral contraceptives and the risk of venous thromboembolism. London, 28 September 2001. Document reference: EMEA/CPMP/2250/01/en/Final.

Thorogood, M. and Vessey, M. P. (1990). Trends in use of oral contraceptives in Britain. *British Journal of Family Planning*, **16**, 41–53.

Thorogood, M., Mann, J. I., Murphy, M., and Vessey, M. (1991). Is oral contraceptive use still associated with an increased risk of fatal myocardial infarction? Report of a case-control study. *British Journal of Obstetrics and Gynaecology*, **98**, 1245–53.

Vessey, M. P. (1980). Female hormones and vascular disease: an epidemiological overview. *British Journal of Family Planning*, **6S**, 1–12.

Vessey, M. P. and Doll, R. (1969). Investigation of relation between use of oral contraceptives and thromboembolic disease. *British Medical Journal*, **ii**, 651–7.

Vessey, M. P., McPherson, K., and Johnson, B. (1977). Mortality among women participating in the Oxford/Family Planning Association contraceptive study. *Lancet*, **2**, 731–2.

WHO (World Health Organization) Monica Project (1990). *MONICA manual*, part IV (a), 11–32. World Health Organization, Geneva.

WHO (World Health Organization) Collaborative Study of Cardiovascular Disease and Steroid Hormone Contraception (1995). A multinational study of cardiovascular disease and steroid hormone contraceptives: description and validation of methods. *Journal of Clinical Epidemiology*, **48**, 1513–47.

WHO (World Health Organization) Collaborative Study of Cardiovascular Disease and Steroid Hormone Contraception (1997). Acute myocardial infarction and combined oral contraceptives: results of an international multicentre case-control study. *Lancet*, **349**, 1202–9.

Chapter 24

Systematic review of prospective cohort studies of psychosocial factors in the aetiology and prognosis of coronary heart disease

H. Kuper, M. Marmot, and H. Hemingway

24.1 Introduction

There is widespread belief among the general public, fostered by the media, that psychological and social factors influence risk of disease. Over the last three decades the scientific community has picked up this interest in psychosocial factors, that is, those factors (such as work characteristics, depression, and social support) that link psychological phenomena to the social environment. Much of this research has focused on the effect of psychosocial factors on health, in particular coronary heart disease (CHD), in part because they may mediate the association between social class and health. Our previous systematic review of prospective studies published up until 1997 investigated the association between psychosocial factors and CHD aetiology and prognosis (Hemingway and Marmot 1999). Here, in updating this review to June 2001, we have used better search methods (and identified 71 new papers), improved summaries of the results, and discuss the results in an explicit framework of causality. Our objective for the review reported in this chapter is to assess the relative strength of the epidemiological evidence for causal links between psychosocial factors and CHD incidence among healthy populations and prognosis among CHD patients. The next two chapters explore aspects of mental illness and psychophysiology related to CHD.

24.1.1 Psychosocial factors as coronary risk factors

Over time there have been improvements in the measurement of psychosocial factors, moving away from the general idea of 'stress' to concepts based on theoretical models that can be tested. These psychosocial factors may relate to personality factors, such as type A behaviour, psychological disorders, for instance depression and anxiety, and to factors more explicitly involving the social environment, including work characteristics and social support. The validity and reliability of the questionnaire-based instruments used to measure the psychosocial factors have been improved through the use of psychometric techniques; increasingly studies use identical measurement scales. However, such standardization is more apparent for some factors, such as depression, than others, such as work characteristics.

Two aspects of the association between CHD and psychosocial factors have been researched intensively. The first aspect is the effect of psychosocial factors on CHD incidence, or newly diagnosed CHD. The second aspect is the impact of psychosocial factors on survival among people with CHD. Despite the large literature that has accumulated, the question of whether psychosocial factors are causally related to risk of, and survival from, CHD remains open for debate. Here we aim to highlight key issues in ascribing causal status to one or more psychosocial factor.

24.1.2 Are psychosocial–CHD associations causal?

An initial question to ask of an epidemiological association between psychosocial factors and CHD is: Can it be explained by bias? Most attention has been paid to bias intrinsic to study design as reported within a publication. One example is self-report bias that may arise if study participants tend to report adversely on both the psychosocial exposures and symptoms of heart disease. The review addresses this issue by emphasizing death and non-fatal myocardial infarction as outcomes rather than softer end points, such as angina, which may be more prone to reporting bias. However, for a systematic review a potentially more important set of biases lies extrinsic to individual published reports in the stages between hypothesis specification and communication to the scientific community. Of all the existing psychosocial–CHD data, an unknown amount remains unreported. Positive studies may be more likely to be published than negative studies; and, once published, positive studies may have greater impact than negative studies.

However, notwithstanding these potential biases, Bradford Hill (1965) outlined a set of interrelated criteria for judging an association to be causal. This is used as a framework for discussing the results of the studies.

Consistency

Finding the same association in different studies, in different populations, and under different circumstances, that is, consistency, strengthens the evidence for causation. As an example, depression is related to risk for CHD in Finland (Aromaa *et al.* 1994), the USA (Pratt *et al.* 1996), and the Netherlands (Penninx *et al.* 2001), as well as in both men and women (Cohen *et al.* 2001). However, as our review shows, studies are not unanimous for any psychosocial factor. These inconsistencies in the data may arise from, *inter alia*, differences in study designs or ways of measuring the psychosocial factors.

Temporal association

In order to address the requirement that exposure should precede the disease, we limited our review to prospective cohort studies. However, the presence of effects in shorter term follow-up studies, which are not found in longer term follow-up, raises the possibility that early manifestations of disease might have caused the psychosocial exposure.

Confounders, mediators, and biological mechanisms

Demonstration of biological pathways linking psychosocial factors and CHD might strengthen the evidence for a causal association. There are three plausible biological pathways by which psychosocial factors could be linked to the incidence of CHD. First, psychosocial factors may influence health-related behaviours, such as smoking, diet, alcohol consumption, and exercise, which in turn have pathophysiological consequences (Horsten *et al.* 1997; Brisson *et al.* 2000). If this is true, then studies that treat health behaviours as potential confounders in their analyses, arguing that preclinical disease and health behaviours are independently related to psychosocial factors, may be drawing incorrect conclusions. Nearly all studies do this in our review, therefore we are summarizing the independent effect of psychosocial factors on CHD events, net of lifestyle variables, and we are not assessing potential mediation of the association between psychosocial factors and CHD by health behaviours. Second, psychosocial factors, including social support or depression, may produce real or apparent hurdles to help-seeking behaviour and access to quality medical care, so that the progression of subclinical to clinical disease is more rapid in people with poor psychosocial characteristics. This possibility awaits adequate investigation. Third, psychosocial factors may produce direct or chronic physiological changes that increase the risk for CHD (Brunner 1997). Adverse psychosocial characteristics can induce biological arousal through neuroendocrine mechanisms affecting blood lipids, blood fibrinogen, and blood pressure, or neuroendocrine mechanisms that increase catecholamines and cortisol.

Strength

Stronger associations are more likely to be causal. This means that higher relative risks (RRs) give stronger evidence for causality than smaller RRs, so an RR of 2.86 (95% CI: 1.19–6.89) (Kawachi *et al.* 1998) is more indicative of an association between type A behaviour and CHD than an RR of 1.43 (0.63–3.26) (Everson *et al.* 1997).

Dose–response

The existence of a dose–response relationship between the exposure and disease also supports causation, and an example of this is the higher RRs for the association between major depression, than minor depression, and mortality in people with CHD (Ladwig *et al.* 1991; Barefoot *et al.* 1996).

24.2 Method of systematic review

The methods reported in this chapter, which updates our review of publications to 1997 (Hemingway and Marmot 1999), are similar to the first review in terms of qualitative data analysis, but use improved techniques for searching for papers and summarizing data.

24.2.1 Methodological quality filter

A methodological quality filter was used to determine inclusion of papers in the systematic review, so that the strength of evidence could be compared across psychosocial factors. For inclusion, papers had to meet four quality criteria relating to: design, size, psychosocial variable specification, and outcomes.

Study design

Since cross-sectional and retrospective case-control studies are subject to recall bias, we limited the review to prospective cohort studies. Nested case-control studies were not included in this review (Hearn *et al.* 1989), because our search methods may not distinguish nested and retrospective case-control studies.

Study size

This review was limited to studies that included at least 500 participants (aetiological studies in healthy populations) or 100 participants (prognostic studies in populations of patients with CHD). The number of participants included was taken as the total number reported after exclusion of ineligible subjects. Therefore, we do not report the restriction of the cohort for subgroup analyses, which was occasionally substantial.

Psychosocial variable specification

Psychosocial factors were included if they were used in at least two eligible study populations. Unspecified 'stress' was not considered a valid psychosocial factor, since it was too vague to be informative (Frasure-Smith 1991; Rosengren *et al.* 1991). Papers had to give details of precisely which measurement scale was used.

Outcomes

Valid outcomes were limited to fatal CHD, sudden cardiac death, incident non-fatal myocardial infarction (MI), incident angina, incident heart failure, and, for prognostic studies only, all-cause mortality.

24.2.2 Searching for eligible papers

The principal method of identifying new papers for updating the review was through the Science Citation Index (accessed on the web of science at www.webofscience.com[1]). The Science Citation Index is a database of bibliographic information gathered from scientific journals. The database is indexed so that a specific article can be searched for by subject, author, and journal. One of the pieces of information stored on the database is the article's cited reference list (that is, its bibliography), hence the database can also be searched for papers that cite a specific paper. This method was not available to us when the last review was carried out.

In June 2001 the Science Citation Index was used to identify papers that cited any of the 65 papers included in our original review. Abstracts of (the more than) 280 new papers identified with potentially relevant titles were extracted and those papers obviously not eligible were eliminated. This search strategy was compared to a search on PubMed, the database of scientific papers maintained by the National Library of Medicine, to ensure that no potentially eligible papers were missed. We found that all the eligible studies found using PubMed had already been identified using the Science Citation Index, but that many articles were retrieved through the Science Citation Index that were not identified using PubMed. Next, two independent researchers assessed full text versions of the more than 100 potentially relevant papers for inclusion criteria, as well as all the papers included in the first review. Finally, the bibliographies of all retrieved articles were manually searched to identify further studies, which lead to the inclusion of four more studies. Multiple papers from the same study were included if they met the eligibility criteria. Our search produced a total of 71 new papers for this review, of which 41 were published from 1998 to June 2001.

24.2.3 Summary of effect

We used RRs, where available, to summarize the association between the psychosocial factor and the outcome and this included incidence rate ratios, cumulative incidence ratios, hazard ratios, and odds ratios (occasionally these were calculated). Unless otherwise stated, we took RRs comparing the top (highest risk) versus bottom (lowest risk) category of exposure and statistical significance was inferred at p value <0.05; and, unlike the earlier review, we report confidence intervals. Where several effect estimates were reported, we took the most highly adjusted estimate, but avoided effect estimates that adjusted for other psychosocial factors, as this may reflect over-adjustment. Effect estimates were reported separately for men and women and for different outcomes, data permitting.

---

[1] Web address currently at ISI Web of Knowledge, isiknowledge.com.

Box 24.1 **Summary of effect**

The extent to which the paper supports the hypothesis that adverse psychosocial characteristics increase risk of, or mortality from, CHD is summarized in a single symbol ($-$, 0, +, or ++). The description of the summary symbols is as follows:

$-$ RR: <0.75
  'finding counter to hypothesis'
  Example: 1 standard deviation (SD) increase on the Bortner type A behaviour scale was protective for risk of mortality post-MI (RR = 0.70, 95% CI: 0.51–0.96) (Ahern *et al.* 1990).

0   RR: 0.75–1.50
  'lack of clear association'
  Example: Low social support was unrelated to risk of fatal CHD (RR = 1.42, 95% CI: 0.72–2.81) or risk of non-fatal MI (RR = 1.00, 95% CI: 0.58–1.71) (Kawachi *et al.* 1996).

+   RR $\geq$ 1.50 and <2.00
  'moderate association in line with hypothesis'
  Example: Depression increased risk for fatal and non-fatal MI (RR = 1.70, 95% CI = 1.23–2.34) (Barefoot *et al.* 1996).

++   Relative risk $\geq$ 2.00
  'strong association in line with hypothesis'
  Example: Job strain substantially increased the risk of fatal CHD and non-fatal CHD (RR = 4.95, *p* value = 0.03) (Haan 1988).

24.2.4 **Number of citations per paper**

In order to explore the extent to which the scientific influence of each study might relate to the degree of study positivity we recorded the number of times that each paper was cited as of September 2001 using the Science Citation Index. From this the mean number of citations across studies by the strength of the reported association was calculated separately for different years of publication.

24.3 **Results**

24.3.1 **Type A behaviour pattern and hostility (Table 24.1)**

The type A behaviour pattern (TABP) is a personality trait characterized by hard-driving and competitive behaviour, excessive job involvement, impatience, hostility, and vigorous speech stylistics and psychomotor activity. Early positive findings for the effect of TABP on CHD risk, reported by the Western Collaborative Group's Study and the Framingham Study, stimulated a great deal of interest in TABP and hostility as causes of CHD (Jenkins *et al.* 1974; Rosenman *et al.* 1976; Haynes *et al.* 1980). This interest ultimately led to the National Institutes of Health declaring type A to be an independent risk factor for CHD and to the implementation of a number of intervention trials, with moderately encouraging results, against TABP in an effort

Table 24.1 Studies of type A behaviour pattern and hostility and CHD

Author, year, country, study	Total sample (% women)	Age at entry	Exposure	Follow-up (years)	Type of events (n)	Adjustments	Relative risk	No. of citations (Sept 2001)	Summary
Aetiological studies									
Jenkins, 1974, USA, Western Collaborative Group Study	2750 (0)	39–59	Type A (JAS)	4 (max.)	NF MI, angina (120)	None	1.8 (ss)	N/A	+
Rosenman, 1976, USA, Western Collaborative Group Study	3154 (0)	39–59	Type A (SI)	8.5 (max.)	Fatal CHD, NF MI, angina (257)	Age, smoking, blood pressure, cholesterol, schooling (ages 39–49: corneal arcus, parental CHD, beta/alpha lipoprotein ratio) (ages 50–9: BMI, exercise)	Whole group aged 39–49:1.87 Men aged 50–9: 2.16	N/A	+
Haynes, 1980, USA, Framingham Heart Study	1674 (57)	45–77	Type A (Framingham)	8 (max.)	Fatal CHD, NF MI, coronary insufficiency, angina (170)	Age, smoking, blood pressure, cholesterol (men: number of promotions in past 10 years, anger-out) (women: glucose intolerance, anger-discuss)	*Standardized coefficient* Men: CHD = 0.380 ($p < 0.01$) MI = 0.544 ($p < 0.01$) Women: CHD = 0.453 ($p < 0.01$) Angina = 0.668 ($p < 0.01$)	N/A	+
Shekelle, 1983, USA, Western Electric Study	1877 (0)	40–55	Hostility (MMPI)	10 (max.) (incidence) 20 (max.) (mortality)	10-year fatal CHD, NF MI (139) 20-year coronary death (220)	Age, smoking, blood pressure, cholesterol, alcohol	10-year fatal CHD and NF MI: 1.47 ($p = 0.04$) 20-year CHD mortality: 1.27 ($p = $ ns)	344	0
Cohen, 1985, USA, Honolulu Heart Program	2187 (0)	57.8 (me)	Type A (JAS)	8 (max.)	Fatal CHD, NF MI, angina (190)	Smoking, blood pressure, cholesterol, BMI, alcohol, and other biological factors	1.43 (ns) Associated with prevalence, not incidence or post-mortem findings	43	0

Study	N (cases)	Age	Measure	Follow-up (years)	Outcome	Adjustment	Results	N	
Shekelle, 1985b, USA, MRFIT	12 772 (0)	35–57	Type A (JAS) and SI on subset (3110)	7.1 (me)	Fatal CHD, NF MI (554 in total group, 129 in subgroup)	Age, smoking, blood pressure, cholesterol, alcohol, education	Regression coefficient for point increase in TAB score: -0.006 (-0.015–0.003) In subgroup: 0.87 (0.59–1.28)	208	0
Appels, 1987, Netherlands, Kaunas-Rotterdam Intervention Study	3171 (0)	45–59	Type A (JAS)	9.5 (me)	Fatal CHD, NF MI (269), angina, coronary graft surgery without MI (75)	None	Fatal CHD/ NF MI: 0.90 (ns) Angina and CAGS: 1.11 (ns)	17	0
Johnston, 1987, UK, British Regional Heart Study	5936 (0)	40–59	Type A (Bortner)	6.2 (me)	Fatal CHD NF MI (254)	Age and social class	0.89 (ns)	25	0
Koskenvuo, 1988, Finland, Finnish Twin Cohort	3750 (0)	40–59	Hostility	3 (max.)	Fatal CHD, hospital discharge with CHD (29)	Age	0.77 (0.10–6.13)	91	0
Ragland, 1988a, USA, Western Collaborative Group Study	3154 (0)	39–59	Type A (SI)	22 (max.) (8.5 (max.) incidence)	Fatal CHD (214), incidence data: MI, SCD, angina pectoris (257)	Age, smoking, blood pressure, cholesterol	Mortality: 0.98 (0.85–1.12) Incidence: 1.38 (1.20–1.47)	69	0
Eaker, 1989, USA, Framingham Heart Study	1289 (56)	45–64	Type A (Framingham)	20 (max.)	Fatal CHD, NF MI (188); uncomplicated angina (125)	Age, smoking, blood pressure, cholesterol, BMI, diabetes, occupation, education	Men: Fatal CHD/NF MI: 1.0 (0.7–1.5) Angina: 2.2 (1.2–4.0) Women: Fatal CHD/NF MI: 1.0 (0.5–1.7) Angina: 2.6 (1.4–4.9)	16	Fatal CHD/ NF MI: 0 Angina: ++
Hollis, 1990, USA, MRFIT	12 772 (0)	35–57	Type A (JAS)	6 (max.)	Fatal CHD, NF MI (635); angina (not stated)	Age, smoking, blood pressure, cholesterol, life events, study group	Cox regression coefficients: Fatal CHD/NF MI: -0.04 (ns) Fatal CHD: -0.31 (ns) Angina: no association	20	0

Table 24.1 (continued)

Author, year, country, study	Total sample (% women)	Age at entry	Exposure	Follow-up (years)	Type of events (n)	Adjustments	Relative risk	No. of citations (Sept 2001)	Summary
Barefoot, 1995, Denmark, Glostrup	730 (44)	50	Hostility (Cook Medley)	27	NF MI (122)	Age, sex, smoking, blood pressure, triglycerides, sedentary work, sedentary leisure	Men: 1.26 (0.78–2.03) Women: 2.95 (1.37–6.35)	46	Men: 0 Women: ++
Bosma, 1995, Lithuania and Netherlands, Kaunas-Rotterdam Intervention Study	5817 (0)	45–60	Type A (JAS)	9.5 (me)	Fatal CHD, NF MI (394)	Age	No association	N/A	0
Everson, 1997, Finland, Kuopio Ischemic Heart Disease Risk Factor Study	1599 (0)	42–60	Cynical hostility (Cook Medley)	9 (max.)	MI (60)	Age, smoking, blood pressure, cholesterol, BMI, alcohol, exercise, prevalent disease, social support, income	1.43 (0.63–3.26)	34	0
Tunstall-Pedoe, 1997, Scotland, Scottish Heart Health Study	11629 (51)	40–59	Type A (Bortner)	7.6 (me)	Fatal CHD (206); NF MI, coronary artery surgery (581)	Age	HR for trend Men: Fatal CHD: 0.98 (0.87–1.10) CHD: 0.98 (0.91–1.05) Women: Fatal CHD: 0.77 (0.60–0.99) CHD: 0.82 (0.73–0.93)	68	Men: 0 Women: –
Whiteman, 1997, UK, Edinburgh Artery Study	1592 (49)	55–74	Hostility (Bedford-Foulds Personality Deviance Scales)	5 (max.)	Fatal CHD, NF MI (114); angina (89)	Age, smoking, blood pressure, cholesterol, triglycerides, BMI, alcohol, degree of baseline vascular disease, social class	1 SD increase in score Men: Total MI: 1.13 (0.89–1.41) Angina: 1.00 (0.74–1.35) Women: Total MI: 1.03 (0.70–1.39) Angina: 1.06 (0.74–1.53)	18	0
Kawachi, 1998, USA, Normative Aging Study	1305 (0)	40–90	Type A (MMPI-2)	7.0 (me)	Fatal CHD (20), MI (30), angina (60)	Age, smoking, blood pressure, cholesterol, BMI, alcohol, family history of CHD	Fatal CHD/ NF MI: 2.86 (1.19–6.89) Angina pectoris: 2.07 (1.00–4.27)	11	++

Prognostic studies

Study	Population	Age	Measure	Follow-up (years)	Outcome (n)	Adjustment	Results	n	Effect
Case, 1985, USA, Multicenter Post-Infarction Program	516 (18) patients <14 days post-MI	<70	Type A (JAS)	2 (me)	Fatal CHD (38)	Age, sex, hard-driving, job involvement, speed and impatience, education, rales, ejection fraction, New York Association functional class, ventricular premature beats	Type A continuous: 0.8 (0.5–1.5)	176	0
Shekelle, 1985a, USA, Aspirin Myocardial Infarction Study	2314 (11) patients post-MI	30–69	Type A (JAS)	3 (me)	Fatal CHD, NF MI (294)	Smoking, previous MI, angina, fasting glucose	*Partial regression coefficient* Men: −0.004 (se = 0.007) Women: −0.0216 (se = 0.0240)	122	0
Brackett, 1988, USA, Recurrent Coronary Prevention Project	1012 (8) patients 42 months (me) post-MI	53 (me)	Type A (SI)	4.5 (max.)	SCD (23), non-SCD (32), NF MI (87)	None	Mean type A score (*p* value for difference compared to no recurrence): No recurrence: 30 SCD: 36 (*p* = 0.02) Non-SCD: 28 (ns) NF MI: 30 (ns)	50	SCD: + Non-SCD and NF MI:0
Eaker, 1988, USA, Framingham Heart Study	204 (29) patients post-MI	45–77	Type A	5.5 (me)	All-cause mortality (67), fatal CHD (32), recurrent MI (31)	Age, smoking, blood pressure, cholesterol	Recurrent MI: Men: 0.6 (0.3–1.5) Women: 0.8 (0.1–5.0) CHD death: Men: 0.5 (0.2–1.3) Women: 0.9 (0.2–4.3) Total mortality: Men: 0.7 (0.3–1.3) Women: 0.8 (0.3–2.3)	7	Women: 0 Men: –
Koskenvuo, 1988, Finland, Finnish Twin Cohort	104 (0) with hypertension and/or previous IHD	40–59	Hostility	3 (max.)	Fatal CHD, hospital discharge with CHD (26)	Age and dyspnoea	21.10 (1.59–282)	91	++

Table 24.1 (continued)

Author, year, country, study	Total sample (% women)	Age at entry	Exposure	Follow-up (years)	Type of events (n)	Adjustments	Relative risk	No. of citations (Sept 2001)	Summary
Ragland, 1988b, USA, Western Collaborative Group Study	257 (0) with MI or angina	39–70	Type A (SI)	22 (max.)	Fatal CHD (91)	Age, smoking, blood pressure, cholesterol (long-term only: type of initial event)	Mortality within 24 h of follow-up: 0.96 (0.37–2.50) Mortality after 24 h of follow-up: 0.58 (0.35–0.96)	182	<24 h: 0 ≥24 h: –
Barefoot, 1989, USA, Duke Medical Center	1467 (18) patients with angiographic disease	52 (me)	Type A (SI) and hostility (Cook-Medley)	9.2 (max.)	Fatal CVD, NF MI (315)	Stratified on clinical prognostic factors	Type A: No association ($\chi^2 = 1.76$) No association between hostility and mortality	29	0
Ahern, 1990, USA, Cardiac Arrhythmia Pilot Study	353 patients 6–60 days post-MI	<75	Type A (Bortner)	1 (max.)	All-cause mortality, NF MI	Baseline ejection fraction, beta-blocker or digitalis use, presence of transmurality in qualifying MI, runs of ventricular premature complexes	0.70 (0.51–0.96) for 1 SD increase in measure of TABP	177	–
Palmer, 1992, Australia, Sydney	170 (25) patients 2–10 days after admission with MI	29–81	Type A (SI)	1 (max.)	Fatal CHD, NF MI (21)	Age	No significant multivariate association ($p = 0.85$)	4	0
Jenkinson, 1993, UK, Anglo-Scandinavian Study of Early Thrombolysis	1376 (22) within 7 days post-MI	25–84	Type A	3 (me)	All-cause mortality (247)	Age, sex, hypertension, previous MI, hospital complications, diabetes, car ownership	No significant multivariate association Survival at 3 years 83% in Type A and 82% in non-Type A group	17	0
Friedmann, 1995, USA, Cardiac Arrhythmia Suppression Trial ancillary study	369 (15) patients after acute MI with ventricular arrhythmias	63 (me)	Type A (JAS)	1 (max.)	All-cause mortality (20)	Diabetes, left ventricular ejection fraction, runs of ventricular premature beats, pet ownership, social support, anxiety, optimism	No significant multivariate association	17	0

Study	Sample (N)	Age	Measure	Follow-up	Outcome	Adjustments	Results		
Carinci, 1997, Italy, GISSI-2 Psychological Study	2449 (12) patients post-MI	3.7% > 70	Type A (JAS)	0.6 (me)	All-cause mortality (63)	Age, sex, hypertension, exercise test ineligibility, ventricular failure, recovery phase LF dysfunction, previous MI, exercise test positivity, electrical instability, extroversion	No significant multivariate association Unadjusted analyses: Type A: 1.4 (0.8–2.4)	7	0
Irvine, 1999, Canada, Canadian Amiodarone MI Arrhythmia Trial	671 (17) patients 6–45 days post-MI	32–89	Hostility (Cook-Medley)	2 (max.)	SCD (34)	Previous MI, previous CHF, depression, social network, social participation, dyspnoea/fatigue	No significant multivariate association	9	0
Kaufmann, 1999, USA, Pennsylvania	331 (34) patients 3–15 days post-MI	28–92	Hostility (Cook-Medley)	1 (max.)	All-cause mortality (33)	Left ejection fraction, history of chronic heart failure, previous stroke, diabetes	No significant multivariate association ($\chi^2 = 41.41$) Unadjusted analyses: Prevalence of hostility at 6 months 93.3% in non-survivors and 90.5% in survivors	8	0
Welin, 2000, Sweden, Gothenburg	275 (16) patients 3–6 days post first MI	30–65	Type A (JAS)	10 (max.)	All-cause mortality (67), fatal CHD (41), NF MI (55)	None	No association with fatal CHD ($p = 0.99$), all-cause mortality, or NF MI	1	0

BMI: body mass index;

CAGS: coronary artery graft surgery;

IHD: ischaemic heart disease;

JAS: Jenkins activity survey;

LF: low frequency;

me: mean or median;

MMPI: Minnesota Multiphasic Personality Inventory;

NF: non-fatal;

ns: non-significant;

se: standard error;

SI: structured interview;

ss: statistically significant;

TAB: Type A Behaviour.

to prevent CHD and improve prognosis in patients with CHD (Sebregts *et al.* 2000). As more data accumulated, however, the early positive findings were not confirmed and ideas shifted to the notion that hostility, rather than the more general TABP, was the aetiological agent.

In the current review 18 prognostic studies were included. As mentioned above, the three early studies provided moderate support for the hypothesis (Jenkins *et al.* 1974; Rosenman *et al.* 1976; Haynes *et al.* 1980), although two of these studies were published from the Western Collaborative Group Study and this association disappeared with extended follow-up (Ragland and Brand 1988*a*). Subsequently, 12 studies that did not show a clear effect were published, including two very large studies: MRFIT (Shekelle *et al.* 1985*b*) and the Scottish Heart Health Study (Tunstall-Pedoe *et al.* 1997), one of which showed evidence for a protective effect of TABP on CHD risk in women (Tunstall-Pedoe *et al.* 1997). Last, the three smallest studies strongly supported the hypothesis (Kawachi *et al.* 1998; Eaker *et al.* 1989; Barefoot *et al.* 1995), although for one the association was found only in women (Barefoot *et al.* 1995) and for the other only with respect to angina incidence (Eaker *et al.* 1989).

For the aetiological studies, 10 were not supportive of the underlying hypothesis that TABP worsened prognosis in patients with CHD. Three studies actually showed a significantly protective effect of TABP on prognosis after CHD, one of which was the Western Collaborative Group Study (Ragland and Brand 1988*b*), although for the Framingham Heart Study the effect was limited to men (Eaker and Castelli 1988). There was only one small study that showed a strong effect of hostility on prognosis, and one study that showed some increase in sudden cardiac death among patients post-MI with TABP. Therefore, there was little overall support for an association between TABP and CHD risk, nor was there evidence, as had been hypothesized, that hostility alone predicted CHD.

24.3.2 **Depression (Table 24.2)**

The association between depression and CHD has attracted a great deal of research interest in recent years, with 29 studies meeting our inclusion criteria published from 1998 to 2001. Depression and anxiety (Table 24.3) differ from the other psychosocial factors reported here, since they are defined psychiatric disorders and amenable to drug intervention. Furthermore, depression is a frequent result of CHD and, moreover, depression and CHD may share a common antecedent (e.g. social support or environmental stressors) so that elucidation of the cause and effect association becomes particularly difficult.

Table 24.2 shows the results from the 22 prospective studies that investigated the role of depression in the aetiology of CHD. Eight of these studies found a lack of clear association, five studies were moderately supportive, and four were strongly supportive of the hypothesis. The remaining five studies all reported strong effects of depression on CHD incidence limited to men (Penninx *et al.* 1998; Ferketich *et al.* 2000), angina incidence (Hallstrom *et al.* 1986; Sesso *et al.* 1998), or major depression (Ariyo *et al.* 2000). Interestingly, the three studies that separated angina from other outcomes reported stronger effects of depression on angina (Hallstrom *et al.* 1986; Sesso *et al.* 1998; Ariyo *et al.* 2000), suggesting the existence of reporting bias as angina is the CHD event least amenable to objective corroboration. There was no apparent difference in strengths of association reported between those studies that followed the participants for a longer period and those studies that had a shorter length of follow-up. This is important because studies with longer periods of follow-up are less likely to be confounded by the possibility of early disease causing depression. In certain studies there was over-adjustment for variables that either were potentially on the causal pathway between depression and CHD,

Table 24.2 Studies of depression and CHD

Author, year, country, study	Total sample (% women)	Age at entry	Exposure	Follow-up (years)	Type of events (n)	Adjustments	Relative risk	No. of citations (Sept 2001)	Summary
Aetiological studies									
Ostfeld, 1964, USA, Western Electric Company	1885 (0)	40–55	Depression (MMPI)	4.5 (max.)	MI (38), angina (50)	None	Mean (SD) depression score MI group: 57.4 (9.5) Angina group: 60.9 (11.4) Non-coronary group: 58.0 (10.7)	N/A	0
Hallstrom, 1986, Sweden, Gothenburg	795 (100)	38, 46, 50, and 54	Depression (DIS and Hamilton Rating Scale)	12 (max.)	MI (11), angina pectoris (25), ischaemic changes on ECG (39)	Age, social class, marital status, conventional risk factors	Angina significantly related, but other outcomes not Age adjusted only: Angina: 5.4 (ss)	27	Angina: ++ Other outcomes: 0
Haines, 1987, UK, Northwick Park Heart Study	1457 (0)	40–64	Depression (Crown–Crisp experiential index)	10 (me)	Fatal CHD (56), NF MI (57)	None	Mean depression score (lower quartile, upper quartile) Survivors: 2.2 (0.8–4.1) Fatal CHD: 3.3 (0.9–5.6) NF MI: 2.2 (0.8–5.6)	88	0
Anda, 1993, USA, National Health Examination Follow-Up Study	2832 (52)	45–77	Depressed affect (General Well-Being Schedule)	12.4 (me)	Fatal CHD (189), NF CHD (205)	Age, sex, smoking, blood pressure, cholesterol, BMI, alcohol, exercise, race, education, marital status	Fatal CHD: 1.5 (1.0–2.3) NF CHD: 1.6 (1.1–2.4)	145	+
Aromaa, 1994, Finland, Mini-Finland Health Survey	5355 (55)	40–64	Depression (GHQ-36 and PSE)	6.6 (me)	Fatal CHD (91)	Age	1.95 (ss) In those with no pre-existing CVD: 3.36 (ss)	5	++
Vogt, 1994, USA, Kaiser Permanente	2573 (54)	≥18	Depression (Langner Mental Health Index)	15 (max.)	Fatal and NF CHD (not stated)	Age, sex, smoking, self-reported health, social class, duration of health plan membership	0.94 (0.70–1.28)	40	0

Table 24.2 (continued)

Author, year, country, study	Total sample (% women)	Age at entry	Exposure	Follow-up (years)	Type of events (n)	Adjustments	Relative risk	No. of citations (Sept 2001)	Summary
Barefoot and Schroll 1996, Denmark, Glostrup	730 (44)	50 or 60	Depression (Obvious Depression Scale of MMPI)	27 (max.)	Fatal and NF MI (122)	Age, sex, smoking, blood pressure, triglycerides, exercise	1.70 (1.23–2.34)	146	+
Pratt, 1996, USA, Baltimore cohort of the Epidemiologic Catchment Area Study	1551 (62)	18–64	Major depressive episode (DIS), dysphoria (>2 weeks of sadness)	13 (max.)	NF MI (64)	Age, sex, hypertension, marital status, phobia, panic disorder, alcohol abuse/dependence, psychotropic medicine use, mutually	Compared to people with neither disorder: Major depression: 4.14 (1.48–11.62) Dysphoria: 2.06 (1.15–3.72)	103	++
Wassertheil-Smoller, 1996, USA, Systolic Hypertension in the Elderly Program	4367 (53)	≥60	Depression (CES-D)	4.5 (me)	Fatal and NF MI (126)	Age, sex, smoking, randomization group, history of MI, stroke and diabetes, ADL, race, education	No multivariate association Univariate RR = 0.99	68	0
Mendes de Leon, 1998, USA, Established Population for the Epidemiologic Study of the Elderly	2391 (66)	65–99	Depression (CES-D)	9 (max.)	Fatal CHD and NF MI (391)	Age, smoking, blood pressure, diabetes, exertional angina, physical functioning, education	Trend across five categories: Fatal CHD: Men: 0.98 (0.95–1.01) Women: 1.02 (0.99–1.05) Total CHD events: Men: 0.98 (0.95–1.01) Women: 1.01 (0.99–1.03)	12	0
Ford, 1998, USA, The Precursor Study	1190 (0)	26 (me)	Depression (DMMS)	37 (me)	All CHD (MI, sudden death, angina, chronic IHD, CAB surgery, PTCA) (163), MI (MI and sudden death) (103)	Age, smoking, cholesterol, exercise, hypertension, premature parental MI, diabetes	MI: 2.12 (1.11–4.06) CHD: 2.12 (1.24–3.63)	61	++

Study	N (%)	Age	Exposure measure	Follow-up	Outcome (n)	Adjustments	Results		Association
Penninx, 1998, USA, Established Population for the Epidemiologic Study of the Elderly	3701 (66)	70–103	Depression (CES-D)	4.0 (me)	CHD events (537)	Age, sex, smoking, blood pressure, BMI, alcohol, history of stroke, diabetes or cancer, physical disability, region	*Compared to never depressed:* Men: Newly depressed: 2.03 (1.28–3.24) Chronically depressed: 1.19 (0.58–2.46) Women: Newly depressed: 1.22 (0.83–1.80) Chronically depressed: 1.12 (0.76–1.65)	22	Men newly depressed: ++ Women newly depressed: 0 Chronically depressed: 0
Sesso, 1999, USA, Normative Aging Study	1305 (0)	21–80	Depression (MMPI-2D, MMPI-2DEP, SCL-90)	7.0 (me)	Fatal CHD, NF MI (50); angina (60)	Age, smoking, blood pressure, cholesterol, BMI, alcohol, family history	Fatal CHD and NF MI MMPI-2 D: 1.69 (0.70–4.05) MMPI-2 DEP: 1.88 (0.77–4.59) SCL-90: 0.67 (0.26–1.76) Angina: MMPI-2 D: 1.34 (0.63–2.82) MMPI-2 DEP: 2.30 (1.00–5.28) SCL-90: 3.33 (1.48–7.49)	13	Fatal CHD/NF MI: + Angina: ++
Chen, 1999, USA, Established Population for the Epidemiologic Study of the Elderly	1749 (59)	65–99	Depression (CES-D)	7.9 (me)	Heart failure (173)	Age, sex, blood pressure, BMI, diabetes, MI during follow-up	No significant multivariate association Unadjusted analysis: 1.10 (0.72–1.69)	6	0
Cole, 1999, USA, College Alumni Health Study	5053 (0)	65 (me)	Physician-diagnosed depression	12 (max.)	Fatal CHD (222)	Age, smoking, BMI, exercise, alcohol, hypertension, diabetes, hours of sleep, insomnia, use of sleeping pills or tranquillizers, mutually	1.20 (0.53–2.71)	1	0

Table 24.2 (continued)

Author, year, country, study	Total sample (% women)	Age at entry	Exposure	Follow-up (years)	Type of events (n)	Adjustments	Relative risk	No. of citations (Sept 2001)	Summary
Ariyo, 2000, USA, Cardiovascular Heart Study	4493 (61)	65–98	Depression (CES-D)	6 (me)	CHD (fatal CHD, MI, angioplasty, CABG, angina) (606); MI (270); angina without MI (298)	Age, sex, smoking, cholesterol, alcohol, exercise, triglycerides, hypertension, diabetes, angina, race, education, marital status	*5 unit increase in depression score:* MI: 1.12 (0.97–1.29) CHD: 1.11 (1.01–1.22) Angina: 1.13 (0.99–1.29)	4	+
Cohen, 2000, USA, 1199 National Benefit Fund Cohort	54997 (68)	43 (me)	Documented antidepressant medication use	3.6 (me)	Fatal or NF MI (207)	Age, sex, hypertension, hyperlipidaemia, diabetes, heart disease, anxiety, cancer	1.8 (1.1–3.1)	5	+
Ferketich, 2000, USA, First National Health and Nutrition Examination Study	7893 (63)	55 (me)	Depression (CES-D)	8.3 (me)	Fatal CHD (women: 129, men: 137); NF CHD (women: 187, men: 187)	Age, smoking, BMI, hypertension, diabetes, poverty (men: race also) Fatal: also adjust for NF CHD events	Men: Fatal CHD: 2.34 (1.54–3.56) NF CHD: 1.71 (1.14–2.56) Women: Fatal CHD: 0.74 (0.40–1.48) NF CHD: 1.73 (1.11–2.68)	8	Fatal CHD: Men: ++ Women: – NF CHD: +
Chang, 2001, USA, National Health and Nutrition Examination Study and Epidemiologic Follow-Up Study	10 766 (57)	35–74	Depression (General Well-Being Schedule)	21 (max.)	Fatal CHD (1401)	Age, smoking, cholesterol, BMI, exercise, hypertension, diabetes, replacement hormones, education	No significant association in multivariate analyses Unadjusted analyses: White men: 1.4 (1.0–2.0) Black men: 1.9 (0.9–4.0) White women: 1.3 (0.9–1.8) Black women: 0.8 (0.3–2.0)	0	0
Cohen, 2001, USA, New York	5564 (36)	53 (me)	History of treatment for depression	4.9 (me)	MI (112), cardiac events (138), IHD events (192)	Age, sex, smoking, blood pressure, cholesterol, BMI, alcohol, hypertension, diabetes, blood sugar, history of CVD, left ventricular hypertrophy, school, race, marital status	Men: MI: 2.03 (0.87–4.74) Cardiac event: 2.35 (1.13–4.91) IHD event: 1.86 (0.94–3.71) Women: MI: 2.42 (0.70–8.37) Cardiac event: 2.69 (0.90–8.05) IHD event: 2.66 (1.10–6.46)	1	++

Study	N (cases)	Age	Depression measure	Follow-up	Outcome (events)	Adjustment	Results	Deaths	Rating
Haines, 2001, UK, Northwick Park Heart Study	1408 (0)	40–64	Depression (Crown–Crisp experiential index)	20.9 (me)	Fatal CHD (127)	Age, smoking, blood pressure, cholesterol, BMI, fibrinogen, factor VIIc, social class	1 point increase: 1.07 (0.99–1.15)	0	+
Penninx, 2001, Netherlands, Longitudinal Aging Study Amsterdam	2397 (55)	55–85	Major depression (DIS) and minor depression (CES-D)	4.2 (me)	Cardiac mortality (91), CHD mortality (45)	Age, sex, smoking, BMI, alcohol, hypertension, diabetes, stroke, lung disease, cancer, education	Cardiac mortality Minor depression: 1.5 (0.9–2.6) Major depression: 3.9 (1.4–10.9) CHD mortality Minor depression: 1.3 (0.6–3.1) Major depression: 5.2 (1.5–17.7)	1	Minor depression:0 / major ++

Prognostic studies

Study	N (cases)	Age	Depression measure	Follow-up	Outcome (events)	Adjustment	Results	Deaths	Rating
Barefoot, 1989, USA, Duke Medical Center	1467 (18) patients with angiographic disease	52 (me)	Depression (MMPI)	9.2 (max.)	Fatal CVD, NF MI (315)	Stratified on clinical prognostic factors	No association between depression and mortality	29	0
Schleifer, 1989, USA, New York	283 (36) patients 8–10 days post-MI	64 (me)	Depression (Schedule for Affective Disorders and Schizophrenia, Hamilton Depression Rating Scale)	0.33 (max.)	All-cause mortality, reinfarction (25)	None	Minor depression: 0.83 (0.33–2.04) Major depression: 0.79 (0.28–2.29)	216	0
Ahern, 1990, USA, Cardiac Arrhythmia Pilot Study	353 patients 6–60 days post-MI	<75	Depression (BDI)	1 (max.)	All-cause mortality, NF MI	Baseline ejection fraction, beta-blocker or digitalis use, presence of transmurality in qualifying MI, runs of ventricular premature complexes	1 SD increase in measure of depression: 1.38 (0.99–1.93)	177	+

Table 24.2 (continued)

Author, year, country, study	Total sample (% women)	Age at entry	Exposure	Follow-up (years)	Type of events (n)	Adjustments	Relative risk	No. of citations (Sept 2001)	Summary
Ladwig, 1991, Germany, Post-Infarction Late Potential Study	560 (0) patients 3 weeks post-MI	29–65	Depression (PSYCHIS-Munchen)	0.5 (max.)	Fatal CHD (12)	Age, recurrent infarction, late potentials, dyspnoea, long-term ECG	Medium depressive disorder: 2.8 Major depressive disorder: 4.9 $p = 0.07$	105	++
Berkman, 1992, USA, Established Population for the Epidemiologic Study of the Elderly	194 (48) hospitalized with acute MI	≥65	Depression (CES-D)	0.5 (max.)	All-cause mortality (76)	None	1.08 (0.46–2.51)	157	0
Frasure-Smith, 1993, Canada, Montreal Heart Institute	222 (22) patients 5–15 days post-MI	24–88	Depression (DIS)	0.5 (max.)	All-cause mortality (12)	Warfarin, lack of close friends, Killip class, previous MI	3.44 (2.25–4.63)	460	++
Jenkinson, 1993, UK, Anglo-Scandinavian Study of Early Thrombolysis	1376 (22) within 7 days post-MI	25–84	Depression	3 (me)	All-cause mortality (247)	Age, sex, previous MI, hospital complications, diabetes, hypertension, car ownership	No association in multivariate analyses Survival at 3 years is 84% in depressed and 83% in non-depressed group	17	0
Ladwig, 1994, Germany Post-Infarction Late-Potential Study	377 (0) patients 17–21 days post-MI	29–65	Depression (interview)	0.5 (max.)	Angina (not stated)	Age, social class, recurrent infarction, rehabilitation, cardiac events, adherence to anti-anginal medication, pre-MI angina, helplessness	Severe depression: 2.31 (1.11–4.80)	78	++
Denollet, 1995, Belgium, Antwerp	105 (0) < 3–6 weeks post-MI	45–60	Depression (Zung)	3.8 (me)	All-cause mortality (15), fatal CHD (11)	Age, smoking, low exercise tolerance, previous or anterior MI	Depression not significantly related to total and cardiac mortality Unadjusted analyses: Total mortality: 4.57 (1.37–15.26) Fatal CHD: 5.38 (1.22–23.67)	21	0

Study	Sample	Age	Exposure	Follow-up (years)	Outcome (n)	Adjustments	Results	n	Rating
Frasure-Smith, 1995a, Canada, Montreal Heart Institute	222 (22) patients 5–15 days post-MI	24–88	Depressive symptoms (BDI) and major depression (DIS)	1.5 (max.)	Fatal CHD (19)	Age, previous MI, PVCs, Killip class	Depressive symptoms: 6.64 (1.76–25.09) Major depression: 2.68 (0.77–9.31)	278	++
Frasure-Smith, 1995b, Canada, Montreal Heart Institute	222 (22) patients 5–15 days post-MI	24–88	Depressive symptoms (BDI) and major depression (DIS)	1 (max.)	Recurrent cardiac events (arrhythmic death, fatal and NF MI, survived cardiac arrest and unstable angina) (48)	Previous MI, prescription of ACE inhibitors, anxiety	Depressive symptoms: 1.99 (0.92–4.31) Previous depression: 1.82 (0.85–3.90)	58	+
Friedmann, 1995, USA, Cardiac Arrhythmia Suppression Trial ancillary study	369 (15) patients after acute MI with ventricular arrhythmias	63 (me)	Depression (Zung)	1 (max.)	All-cause mortality (20)	Diabetes, LVEF, runs of ventricular premature beats, pet ownership, social support, optimism	No association	17	0
Hoffmann, 1995, Switzerland, Gais, Seewis and Le Noirmont	222 (0) patients 7 weeks (me) after first MI	30–60	Depression	1 (max.)	Poor medical outcome (death, reinfarction, New York Heart Association Class ≥ III, exercise capacity <100 W) (19)	Age, exercise, severity of MI, overprotection by friends, external locus of control	No association with poor medical outcome Associated with angina incidence ($p < 0.01$)	9	Poor medical outcome: 0 Angina: +
Oxman, 1995, USA, Dartmouth-Hitchcock Medical Center	232 (0) patients after elective open heart surgery	≥55	Depression (Hamilton Rating Scale for Depression)	0.5 (max.)	All-cause mortality (21)	Age, previous cardiac surgery, severe impairment, social support	No significant association Unadjusted 2.20 (0.94–5.11)	83	0

Table 24.2 (continued)

Author, year, country, study	Total sample (% women)	Age at entry	Exposure	Follow-up (years)	Type of events (n)	Adjustments	Relative risk	No. of citations (Sept 2001)	Summary
Barefoot et al. 1996, USA, Duke Medical Center	1250 (18) patients with angiographic disease	46–59	Depression (Zung)	15.2 (me)	All-cause mortality (604), fatal CHD (488)	Disease severity	Total mortality: Severe depression: 1.78 Mild depression: 1.57 Fatal CHD: Severe depression: 1.69 Mild depression: 1.38	93	+
Denollet, 1996, Belgium, Antwerp Cardiac Rehabilitation Programme	303 (12) patients with angiographic CHD	31–79	Depression (Millon behavioural health inventory)	7.9 (me)	All-cause mortality (38)	Left ventricular function, number of diseased vessels, low exercise tolerance, lack of thrombolytic therapy, type D personality	No significant multivariate association Unadjusted association: 2.38 (1.28–4.41)	59	0
Lesperance, 1996, Canada, Montreal Heart Institute	222 (22) patients 5–10 days post-MI	24–88	Depression (DIS and BDI)	1.5 (max.)	All-cause mortality(21)	None	3.96 (1.50–10.5)	73	++
Carinci, 1997, Italy, GISSI-2 Psychological Study	2449 (12) patients post-MI	3.7% >70	Depression (Cognitive Behavioural Assessment Hospital Form)	0.6 (me)	All-cause mortality (63)	Age, sex, hypertension, exercise test ineligibility, ventricular failure, recovery phase LF dysfunction, previous MI, exercise test positivity, electrical instability, extroversion	No significant association in multivariate Unadjusted analysis: 1.7 (0.9–3.1)	7	0
Krumholz, 1998, USA, Established Population for the Epidemiologic Study of the Elderly	292 (57) patients hospitalized with heart failure	80 (me)	Depression (CES-D)	1 (max.)	CVD death or readmission (142)	Age, sex, LVEF, physiology score, MI at current admission, hypertension, Rosow–Breslau or Nagi impairment, social support	No significant multivariate association Unadjusted analysis: 1.13 (0.87–1.48)	24	0

Study	Sample (%)	Age	Exposure	Follow-up	Outcome	Adjustment	Effect estimate		
Frasure-Smith, 1999, Canada, Montreal Heart Attack Readjustment Trial and Emotions and Prognosis Post-Infarct Study	896 (32) patients 7 days after MI	24–88	Depression (BDI)	1 (max.)	Fatal CHD (37)	Age, sex, smoking, Killip class, non-Q wave MI, LVEF	3.66 (1.68–7.99)	31	++
Irvine, 1999, Canada, Canadian Amiodarone Myocardial Infarction Arrhythmia Trial	671 (17) patients 6–45 days post-MI	32–89	Depression (BDI)	2 (max.)	SCD (34)	Previous MI, previous CHF, social participation, social network contacts, dyspnoea/fatigue	Amiodarone group: 0.47 (0.13–1.65) Placebo group: 1.73 (0.75–3.98)	9	0
Kaufmann, 1999, USA, Pennsylvania	331 (34) patients 3–15 days post-MI	28–92	Depression (DIS)	1 (max.)	All-cause mortality (33)	LVEF, history of chronic heart failure, previous stroke, diabetes	Depression not significant in multivariate analyses Unadjusted: 2.33 (1.16–4.65)	8	0
Murberg, 1999, Norway, Stavanger	119 (29) patients with congestive heart failure 61 months after diagnosis (me)	66 (me)	Depression (Zung)	2 (max.)	Fatal CHD (20)	Age, sex, disease severity (proANF)	Moderately depressed: 2.08 (ss)	5	++
Barefoot, 2000, USA, Duke Medical Center	1250 (18) patients with significant CAD	46–58	Depression (Zung)	15.2 (me)	Fatal CHD (488)	Age, sex, hazard scores, treatment status, income	2 SD increase in score: 1.37 ($p < 0.001$)	0	+
Denollet, 2000, Belgium, Antwerp	319 (8) patients in a cardiac rehabilitation program	35–70	Depression (Zung)	5 (max.)	Fatal CHD and NF MI (22)	Age, LVEF	Depression not significant in multivariate analyses Unadjusted analyses: Depression: 2.6 (1.1–6.3)	3	0

Table 24.2 (continued)

Author, year, country, study	Total sample (% women)	Age at entry	Exposure	Follow-up (years)	Type of events (n)	Adjustments	Relative risk	No. of citations (Sept 2001)	Summary
Herrmann, 2000, Germany, Gottingen	5057 (26) patients referred to cardiology department for exercise testing	54 (me)	Depression (Hospital Anxiety and Depression Scale)	5.7 (me)	All-cause mortality (457)	Age, sex, cardiac history, exercise performance, and mutually	1 SD increase in score: 1.16 (1.01–1.30)	1	+
Horsten, 2000, Sweden, Stockholm Female Coronary Risk Study	292 (100) 3–6 months post hospitalization for acute CHD	30–65	Depression (Pearlin)	4.8 (me)	CVD mortality, recurrent MI, revascularization (81)	Age, smoking, blood pressure, HDL, BMI, exercise, diagnosis at index event, heart failure, diabetes, hypertension, angina severity	1.8 (0.86–3.6)	4	+
Lane, 2000a, UK, West Midlands	288 (25) patients within 15 days post-MI	63 (me)	Depression (BDI)	0.33 (max.)	Fatal CHD (22)	None	1.31 (0.53–3.24)	1	0
Lane, 2000b, UK, West Midlands	288 (25) patients within 15 days post-MI	63 (me)	Depression (BDI)	1 (max.)	Recurrent CHD event (fatal and NF) requiring hospitalisation (82)	Peel index score, previous MI, hypertensive, angina, Killip class, thrombolysed, hypercholesterolaemia, diabetes, hospital stay	No multivariate association Unadjusted analyses: 0.97 (0.55–1.70)	1	0
Lesperance, 2000, Canada, Montreal Heart Institute	430 (29) patients mean 5 days after hospitalization with unstable angina	31–87	Depression (BDI)	1 (max.)	Fatal CHD and NF MI (28)	Electrocardiagraphic evidence of ischaemia, LVEF, number of diseased vessels	6.73 (2.43–18.64)	1	++

Welin, 2000, Sweden, Gothenburg	275 (16) patients 3–6 days post first MI	<65	Depression (Zung)	10 (max.)	All-cause mortality (67), fatal CHD (41), NF MI (55)	Sex, left ventricular failure, ventricular dysrhythmia, social support	Total mortality: 1.75 (1.02–2.99) Fatal CHD: 3.16 (1.38–7.25) Depression unrelated to NF MI	1	Total mortality: + Fatal CHD:++ NF MI:0
Baker, 2001, Australia, Adelaide	158 (26) patients undergoing CABG surgery	65 (me)	Depression (Depression Anxiety Stress Scale)	2.1 (me)	>30 day all-cause mortality (6)	None	6.24 (1.18–32.98)	0	++
Lane, 2001, UK, West Midlands	288 (25) patients within 15 days post-MI	31–89	Depression (BDI)	1 (max.)	Fatal CHD (27)	None	1.15 (0.49–2.67)	2	0
Penninx, 2001, Netherlands, Longitudinal Aging Study Amsterdam	450 (38) subjects with diagnosis of cardiac disease	55–85	Major depression (DIS) and minor depression (CES-D)	4.2 (me)	Cardiac mortality (93), CHD mortality (63)	Age, sex, smoking, BMI, alcohol, hypertension, diabetes, stroke, lung disease, cancer, education	Cardiac mortality Minor depression: 1.6 (1.0–2.7) Major depression: 3.0 (1.1–7.8) CHD mortality Minor depression: 2.1 (1.1–3.8) Major depression: 3.9 (1.3–11.8)	1	++

ADL: activities of daily living;
CAB: coronary artery bypass;
CABG: coronary artery bypass graft;
CVD: cardiovascular disease;
HDL: high-density lipoprotein;
LVEF: left ventricular ejection fraction;
PVC: premature ventricular contraction;
PTCA: percutaneous transluminal coronary angioplasty.

or else served as a proxy for CHD. One particular example of this is the study by Pratt *et al.* (1996) where psychotropic medicine use was adjusted for, although surprisingly a strong association between major depression and dysphoria with CHD was still detected. Both studies that focused on the degree of depression found that risk of CHD was higher among people seriously depressed than among those who were only moderately depressed (Pratt *et al.* 1996; Penninx *et al.* 2001), suggesting a dose–response association.

There were 34 studies looking at the effect of depression on prognosis for patients with CHD. Of these, 16 found a lack of clear association, 7 were moderately supportive, and 11 were strongly supportive studies. There was, therefore, no evidence that the association between depression and events differed between prognostic and aetiological studies, although where associations were observed, they were generally of greater magnitude for the prognostic studies. It is of note that for several prognostic studies depression is predictive of prognosis in the unadjusted analyses, but adjusting for traditional coronary risk factors and markers of disease severity explained much of the association, hence the association between depression and prognosis might be mediated by lifestyle factors, disease severity, and pharmacological interventions. This is in line with the scientific literature that shows that secondary prevention in patients with CHD is possible through changes in smoking and other health-related behaviours, as well as through medical interventions (Mehta and Eagle 1998; Sebregts *et al.* 2000). Five studies looked separately at the effect of moderate and severe depression on prognosis; one found a lack of clear association (Schleifer *et al.* 1989), three showed a higher risk among patients with major depression (Ladwig *et al.* 1991; Barefoot *et al.* 1996; Penninx *et al.* 2001), and the last found a lower risk of fatal CHD in patients with major depression compared to depressive symptoms (Frasure-Smith *et al.* 1995*a*).

24.3.3 **Anxiety and distress (Table 24.3)**

Anxiety, like depression, is a diagnosed psychiatric disorder that may be caused by CHD, and can be treated through drugs or counselling. Eight studies were published that explored the relationship between anxiety/distress and risk of CHD. Four studies showed little clear effect. Two papers, both published from the Israeli civil servant cohort, reported strong or moderate association between anxiety and incidence of angina (Medalie *et al.* 1973; Medalie and Goldbourt 1976). The remaining two studies gave evidence for an association between phobic anxiety and fatal CHD, but did not show a clear effect on non-fatal CHD or of free-floating anxiety (Haines *et al.* 1987; Kawachi *et al.* 1994). Furthermore, the studies with longer follow-up were less likely to find a positive association than the studies with less extended follow-up. This is exemplified by the Northwick Park Heart Study where the association between anxiety and fatal CHD found after 10 years of follow-up (Haines *et al.* 1987) disappeared when the follow-up was extended by another decade (Haines *et al.* 2001). Hence, anxiety may be a result of pre-clinical CHD rather than a cause of fatal CHD.

Eighteen studies were included that explored the association between anxiety and prognosis after a diagnosis of CHD. Half of these found a lack of clear association and one reported results significantly contrary to the hypothesis. Four studies showed a strong association between anxiety and prognosis and the remaining four studies showed some moderate support for an association, either in the entire group or in relation to a specific subgroup, exposure, or outcome. There was seemingly no effect of length of follow-up or measure of anxiety used on the chances of finding a positive result and there was no ability to test for a dose–response effect of anxiety on prognosis.

Table 24.3 Studies of anxiety and distress and CHD

Author, year, country, study	Total sample (% women)	Age at entry	Exposure	Follow-up (years)	Type of events (n)	Adjustments	Relative risk	No. of citations (Sept 2001)	Summary
Aetiological studies									
Medalie, 1973, Israel, Israeli Ischemic Heart Disease Study	8538 (0)	≥40	Anxiety (Anxiety Index)	5 (max.)	Angina (300)	Age and area	2.2	N/A	+ +
Medalie, 1976, Israel, Israeli Ischemic Heart Disease Study	8166 (0)	≥40	Anxiety (Anxiety Index)	5 (max.)	Angina (234)	Age, blood pressure, cholesterol, BMI, diabetes, ECG abnormalities, psychosocial problems	Beta coefficient: 0.29 ($p < 0.01$)	N/A	+
Haines, 1987, UK, Northwick Park Heart Study	1457 (0)	40–64	Free-floating anxiety and phobic anxiety (Crown–Crisp experiential index)	10 (me)	Fatal CHD (56), NF MI (57)	Age, smoking, blood pressure, cholesterol, factor VII activity, fibrinogen, social class, shift work	Fatal CHD: High phobic anxiety: 3.77 (1.64–8.64) NF MI: High phobic anxiety: 1.26 (0.62–2.54) Free-floating anxiety unrelated	88	*Phobic anxiety:* Fatal CHD: + + NF MI: 0 Free-floating anxiety: 0
Eaker, 1992, USA, Framingham Heart Study	749 (100)	45–64	Anxiety (Somatic Strain Scale)	20 (max.)	Fatal CHD, NF MI (69)	Age, smoking, blood pressure, cholesterol, HDL, BMI, diabetes	Unrelated for total women Homemakers (n =353): 7.8 (2–32.3)	67	0
Kawachi, 1994, USA, Health Professionals Follow-Up Study	33 999 (0)	42–77	Phobic anxiety (Crown–Crisp experiential index)	2 (max.)	Fatal CHD (40), NF MI (128)	Age, smoking, BMI, alcohol, exercise, hypertension, diabetes, hypercholesterolaemia, parental history of MI	Fatal CHD: 2.45 (1.00–5.96) NF MI: 0.89 (0.45–1.79)	114	Fatal CHD: + + NF MI: 0
Vogt, 1994, USA, Kaiser Permanente	2573 (54)	≥18	Worries (Bradburn Worries Index)	15 (max.)	Fatal CHD, NF CHD (not stated)	Age, sex, smoking, self-reported health, social class, duration of health plan membership	Worries: 1.18 (0.85–1.63)	40	0

Table 24.3 (continued)

Author, year, country, study	Total sample (% women)	Age at entry	Exposure	Follow-up (years)	Type of events (n)	Adjustments	Relative risk	No. of citations (Sept 2001)	Summary
Kubzansky, 1997, USA, Normative Aging Study	1759 (0)	21–80	Worry (Worries Scale)	13.7 (me)	Fatal CHD (86), NF MI (113), angina (124)	Age, smoking, blood pressure, cholesterol, BMI, alcohol, family history of CHD	Per point increase in scale of worry *Fatal CHD:* Social conditions: 0.94 (0.71–1.26) Health: 1.17 (0.82–1.66) Financial: 1.21 (0.86–1.70) Self-definition: 0.97 (0.74–1.29) Ageing: 1.05 (0.67–1.62) *NF MI:* Social conditions:1.49 (1.16–1.93) Health: 0.86 (0.63–1.17) Financial: 1.17 (0.87–1.56) Self-definition: 0.97 (0.74–1.26) Ageing: 1.06 (0.71–1.59) *Angina:* Social conditions: 1.17 (0.92–1.50) Health: 1.39 (1.04–1.87) Financial: 1.20 (0.91–1.58) Self-definition: 1.11 (0.86–1.42) Ageing: 1.28 (0.89–1.85)	36	*NF MI:* Worry about social conditions: + *Angina:* Worry about health: + Others: 0
Haines, 2001, UK, Northwick Park Heart Study	1408 (0)	40–64	Free-floating anxiety, phobic anxiety (Crown–Crisp experiential index)	20.9 (me)	Fatal CHD (127)	Age, smoking, blood pressure, cholesterol, BMI, fibrinogen, factor VIIc, social class	One point increase: Anxiety: 1.04 (0.99–1.10); Phobic anxiety: 1.07 (0.99–1.15)	0	0
Prognostic studies									
Ahern, 1990, USA, Cardiac Arrhythmia Pilot Study	353 patients 6–60 days post-MI	<75	Anxiety (STAI)	1 (max.)	All-cause mortality, NF MI	None	Mean (SD) trait anxiety: Survivors: 38.8 (8.0); Non-survivors: 39.5 (10.8); Mean (SD) state anxiety: Survivors: 35.7 (10.8); Non-survivors: 36.1 (11.2)	177	0

Study	Sample (n)	Age	Measure	Follow-up	Outcome	Adjustment		Results	Rating
Allison, 1995, USA, Mayo Clinic	381 (18) patients with CAD referred for cardiac rehabilitation	25–85	Psychologic distress (SCL-90-R)	0.5 (max.)	Cardiovascular rehospitalization (49) and recurrent cardiovascular event (fatal CHD, NF MI, cardiac arrest, cardiac operation, angiographic progression of CAD, CHF, embolic stroke, pulmonary embolus) (39)	Smoking, diabetes, ejection fraction, previous cardiac event, beta-blockers, bypass surgical procedure, or coronary angioplasty at index hospitalization	46	Cardiovascular rehospitalization: Distress: 3.05 ($p = 0.01$) Recurrent cardiovascular event: Distress: 4.39 ($p = 0.003$)	++
Denollet, 1995, Belgium, Antwerp	105 (0) patients 3–6 weeks post-MI	45–60	Distressed personality (STAI Heart Patients Psychological Questionnaire)	3.8 (me)	All-cause mortality (15), fatal CHD (11)	Age, smoking, low exercise tolerance, previous or anterior MI	21	Distressed personality significantly predicted total and fatal CHD Unadjusted analyses: Total mortality: 7.56 (2.62–21.82) Fatal CHD: 5.61 (1.80–17.55)	++
Frasure-Smith, 1995b, Canada, Montreal Heart Institute	222 (22) patients 5–15 days post-MI	24–88	Anxiety (STAI)	1 (max.)	Recurrent cardiac events (arrhythmic death, fatal and NF MI, survived cardiac arrest and unstable angina) (48)	Previous MI, prescription of ACE inhibitors, depression	58	2.52 (1.15–5.55)	++
Friedmann, 1995, USA, Arrhythmia Suppression Trial ancillary study	369 (15) patients after acute MI with ventricular arrhythmias	63 (me)	Anxiety (STAI)	1 (max.)	All-cause mortality (20)	Ejection fraction, diabetes, runs of ventricular premature beats, pet ownership, social support, optimism	17	Low state anxiety improved survival ($p = 0.09$)	0
Hoffmann, 1995, Switzerland, Gais, Seewis and Le Noirmont	222 (0) patients 7 weeks (me) after first MI	30–60	Anxiety (MAS)	1 (max.)	Poor medical outcome (death, reinfarction, New York Heart Association Class ≥ III, exercise capacity < 100 W)(19)	Age, severity of MI, exercise, overprotection by friends, external locus of control	9	No association with poor medical outcome Associated with angina incidence ($p < 0.01$)	Poor medical outcome: 0 Angina: +

Table 24.3 (continued)

Author, year, country, study	Total sample (% women)	Age at entry	Exposure	Follow-up (years)	Type of events (n)	Adjustments	Relative risk	No. of citations (Sept 2001)	Summary
Denollet, 1996, Belgium, Antwerp Cardiac Rehabilitation Programme	303 (12) patients with angiographic CHD	31–79	Type D personality (suppression of emotional distress) (STAI and HPPQ)	7.9 (me)	All-cause mortality (38)	Left ventricular function, number of diseased vessels, low exercise tolerance, lack of thrombolytic therapy	4.1 (1.9–8.8)	59	++
Carinci, 1997, Italy, GISSI-2 Psychological Study	2449 (12) patients post-MI	3.7% >70	Anxiety (Cognitive Behavioural Assessment Hospital Form)	0.6 (me)	All-cause mortality (63)	Age, sex, hypertension, exercise test ineligibility, ventricular failure, recovery phase LF dysfunction, previous MI, exercise test positivity, electrical instability, extroversion	No significant association in multivariate. Unadjusted analyses: Anxiety: 1.3 (0.8–2.1)	7	0
Perski, 1998, Sweden, Stockholm	171 (17) patients post-CABG surgery	43–80	Emotional distress (Nottingham Health Profile)	3 (max.)	Cardiac events (11) (fatal CHD, NF MI, revascularization, unstable angina)	Blood pressure, LDL/HDL ratio	1.89 (1.04–3.55)	3	+
Frasure-Smith, 1999, Canada, Montreal Heart Attack Readjustment Trial and Emotions and Prognosis Post-Infarct Study	896 (32) patients 7 days after MI	24–88	Anxiety (Spielberger's STAI)	1 (max.)	Fatal CHD (37)	Smoking, non-Q wave MI at baseline, LVEF	Men: 2.58 (1.06–6.30) Women: 0.63 (0.20–2.04)	31	Men: ++ Women: −
Irvine, 1999, Canada, Canadian Amiodarone Myocardial Infarction Arrhythmia Trial	671 (17) patients 6–45 days post-MI	32–89	Psychological distress (Symptom Check List)	2 (max.)	SCD (34)	Previous MI, previous CHF, social participation, social network contacts, dyspnoea/fatigue	Psychological distress not associated	9	0

Study	Sample (N)	Age	Measure	Length of follow-up	Outcome	Adjustments	Results	Quality	Type D / Anxiety
Denollet, 2000, Belgium, Antwerp	319 (8) patients in a cardiac rehabilitation program	35–70	Anxiety (State Anxiety Scale), Type D personality (DS16)	5 (max.)	Cardiac events (fatal CHD or NF MI), impaired QOL (22)	Age, LVEF	Type D: 8.9 (3.2–24.7) Anxiety not significant Unadjusted analyses: Type D: 7.6 (2.9–20.2) Anxiety: 2.0 (0.8–4.8)	3	Type D: ++ Anxiety: 0
Herrmann, 2000, Germany, Gottingen	5057 (26) patients referred to cardiology department for exercise testing	54 (me)	Anxiety (Hospital Anxiety and Depression Scale)	5.7 (me)	All-cause mortality (457)	Age, sex, cardiac history, exercise performance, and mutually	1 SD increase in score: survival: 1.19 (1.08–1.28)	1	–
Lane, 2000a, UK, West Midlands	288 (25) patients within 15 days post-MI	63 (me)	Anxiety (STAI)	0.33 (max.)	Fatal CHD (22)	None	1 unit increase in: State anxiety: 0.99 (0.96–1.03) Trait anxiety: 0.98 (0.93–1.02)	1	0
Lane, 2000b, UK, West Midlands	288 (25) patients within 15 days post-MI	63 (me)	Anxiety (STAI)	1 (max.)	Recurrent CHD event (fatal and NF) requiring hospitalization (82)	Peel index score, previous MI, hypertension, angina, Killip class, thrombolysed, hypercholesterolaemia, diabetes, hospital stay	No multivariate association Unadjusted 1 unit increase in: State anxiety: 1.00 (0.98–1.02) Trait anxiety: 0.98 (0.95–1.01)	1	0
Mayou, 2000, UK, Oxford Myocardial Infarction Incidence Study	344 (27) patients <3 days after hospitalization for suspected MI	30–79	Distress (HAD)	1.5 (max.)	All-cause mortality (28)	All significant unadjusted predictors of mortality (not stated which variables)	No association	5	0
Welin, 2000, Sweden, Gothenburg	275 (16) patients 3–6 days post first MI	<65	Anxiety (Trait anxiety inventory)	10 (max.)	All-cause mortality (67), fatal CHD (41), NF MI (55)	None	Total mortality: 0.91 (0.56–1.50) Fatal CHD: 1.08 (0.59–2.00) Anxiety unrelated to NF MI	1	0
Lane, 2001, UK, West Midlands	288 (25) patients within 15 days post-MI	31–89	Anxiety (STAI)	1 (max.)	Fatal CHD (27)	None	1 point increase State anxiety: 0.99 (0.96–1.03) Trait anxiety: 0.98 (0.94–1.02)	2	0

ACE: angiotensin-converting enzyme; CHF: congestive heart failure; LDL: low-density lipoprotein; N/A: not available; QOL: quality of life.

24.3.4 **Psychosocial work characteristics (Table 24.4)**

The belief that stress at work has a deleterious effect on health is common among the general public. To combat the lack of precision in defining job stress, various constructs have been made to explain how the interaction between a worker and the job environment causes stress, and how this affects health. The dominant model is the 'job strain' model proposed by Karasek and Theorell (Karasek 1979; Karasek and Theorell 1990). This model proposes that high demands at work (the need to work quickly and hard), in combination with low job control produces stress, as workers cannot moderate the pressure caused by high job demands by organizing their time, making new decisions, or learning new skills, and this stress has deleterious effects on health. Another model for psychosocial work characteristics is Siegrist's (Siegrist *et al.* 1990; Siegrist 1996) effort–reward imbalance model. Here the mismatch between high workload and low payback (in terms of money, esteem, promotion prospects, and job security) produces a condition of emotional distress, which increases risk for CHD.

Despite these models, work characteristics have been measured with a lesser degree of standardization than, for instance, depression and anxiety. Moreover, work characteristics can be measured either through self-report or ecological measurements (assigning a score on the basis of job title). Self-reports may be biased by early manifestations of disease, and ecological measurements may lack precision. The fact that so many different measures of the work environment have been reported is a challenge when evaluating this literature and for future researchers.

There were 13 aetiological studies investigating the effect of work characteristics on CHD that were included in this review. Of these, three found a lack of clear association between work characteristics and CHD, and five were either moderately supportive, or supportive only for a subset of the population, a particular outcome, or a particular exposure. The final five papers showed strong evidence for an effect of work stress on CHD incidence, although in three of these studies the effect was limited either to particular psychosocial work characteristics or to women. There is some evidence that CHD incidence was more closely related to individually, rather than ecologically, measured work characteristics. This could suggest either that there is more non-differential misclassification, and therefore bias towards the null, for ecological than individual measures, or that pre-clinical CHD influences subjective reporting of work characteristics. Of the four prognostic studies, two found a lack of clear association between work characteristics and prognosis, and two were moderately supportive of an association. Because of the lack of consistency in measuring psychosocial work characteristics it was difficult to compare the strength of evidence for the two theoretical models.

24.3.5 **Social support (Table 24.5)**

Social supports and networks relate to both the number and quality of a person's social contacts, and this includes emotional and confiding support. Social relationships may improve health through the emotional and instrumental support they provide; friends and family may encourage health-seeking behaviour and frown on unhealthy behaviour. Furthermore, isolation itself may induce an unfavourable mental state, and conversely the presence of social contacts could reduce physiological arousal and buffer the effect of environmental stressors. Reverse causation cannot be discounted: lack of social participation could be the result of subclinical coronary disease. Despite the interest in social support, there is little consensus on how it is measured, therefore variables ranging from 'high love and support from wife' to 'social network index' to 'social isolation' were included.

Table 24.4 Studies of psychosocial work characteristics and CHD

Author, year, country, study	Total sample (% women)	Age at entry	Exposure	Follow up (years)	Type of events (n)	Adjustments	Relative risk	No. of citations (Sept 2001)	Summary
Aetiological studies									
Theorell, 1977, Sweden, Building Construction Workers	5187 (0)	41–61	Workload index	2 (max.)	Fatal CHD, NF MI (31)	Age	1.98 (ss)	N/A	++
Lacroix, 1984, USA, Framingham Heart Study	876 (37)	45–64	Job control and demands (individual and ecological)	10 (max.)	Fatal CHD, NF MI, coronary insufficiency, angina (not stated)	Age, smoking, blood pressure, cholesterol	Women: 2.9 (ss) Men: no association Ecological exposure was associated with risk in men and women	20	*Individual:* Women:++ Men: 0 Ecological: +
Alfredsson, 1985, Sweden, 5 Swedish counties	958 096 (51)	20–64	Hectic work, few chances to learn new things, and monotonous work (ecological)	1 (max.)	NF MI hospitalizations (1201)	Age, smoking, 10 socio-demographic factors, heavy lifting	Men: Hectic work + non-learning: SMR = 128 (109–48) Hectic monotonous work: SMR = 118 (102–35) Women: Hectic monotonous work: SMR = 164 (112–233)	120	Men: 0 Women:+
Haan, 1988, Finland, Study of Metal Workers	902 (33)	17–65	Job strain (physical strain, variety, and control) (individual)	10 (max.)	Fatal CHD, NF CHD (60)	Age, sex, smoking, blood pressure, cholesterol, relative weight, alcohol	Strain (low control, low variety, high physical strain) 4.95 ($p = 0.03$)	26	++
Reed, 1989, USA, Honolulu Heart Program	4737 (0)	45–65	Strain (decision latitude and psychological demands) (ecological)	18 (max.)	Fatal CHD, NF MI (359)	Age, smoking, blood pressure, cholesterol, exercise, glucose	Job strain inversely associated with CHD incidence ($p = 0.07$) No significant effect of either job control or demand	73	0

Table 24.4 (continued)

Author, year, country, study	Total sample (% women)	Age at entry	Exposure	Follow up (years)	Type of events (n)	Adjustments	Relative risk	No. of citations (Sept 2001)	Summary
Netterstrom, 1993, Denmark, Urban Bus Drivers	2045 (0)	21–64	Job variety and satisfaction (individual)	10 (max.)	Fatal CHD (59)	Age	Choose same job: 2.2 (1.2–4.0) Not looking for new job: 6.5 (1.6–27.0) Job is special: 1.9 (1.1–3.1) Cannot use skills: 1.5 (0.9–2.5) High work pace: 0.9 (0.5–1.6) Passengers complain: 0.6 (0.4–1.2) Job varied: 1.6 (0.9–1.9) Job very varied: 2.5 (1.4–4.5)	22	Job satisfaction: ++ Job variety: + Others: 0
Suadicani, 1993, Denmark, Copenhagen Male Study	1638 (0)	59.7 (me)	Job influence, monotony, pace, satisfaction, ability to relax (individual)	4 (max.)	Fatal CHD, NF MI (46)	Age, smoking, blood pressure, cholesterol, HDL, triglycerides, BMI, alcohol, exercise, hypertension, selenium, social class	Only inability to relax after work associated with CHD 2.9 (1.3–6.1)	14	Inability to relax: ++ Others: 0
Alterman, 1994, USA, Western Electric Study	1683 (0)	38–56	Job strain (decision latitude and psychological demands) (ecological)	25 (max. mortality) 10 (max. incidence)	Fatal CHD (283) and NF CHD (115)	Age, smoking, blood pressure, cholesterol, alcohol, family history of CVD, education	Per tertile increase in exposure: Fatal CHD Job control: 0.76 (0.59–1.00) Job demands: 0.78 (0.48–1.26) Job strain: 1.40 (0.92–2.14) NF CHD Job control: 0.87 (0.57–1.31) Job demands: 1.07 (0.54–2.12) Job strain: 1.54 (0.85–2.80)	47	Control: + Demands: 0 Job strain: +
Bosma, 1997, UK, Whitehall II study	10 308 (33)	35–55	Job control, job demands, social support at work (individual and ecological)	5.3 (me)	Diagnosed CHD (166), angina (328)	Age, sex, smoking, blood pressure, cholesterol, BMI, drugs for hypertension	Low job control: CHD: 1.26 (0.67–2.39) Angina: 2.02 (1.22–3.34) Job demands and social support at work not related Ecological and individual measures similar	99	Control: Angina: ++ CHD: 0 Others: 0

Study	N (events)	Age	Exposure	Duration	Outcome (events)	Covariates	Results		
Lynch, 1997, Finland, Kuopio Ischemic Heart Disease Risk Factor Study	1727 (0)	42, 48, 54, or 60	Job demands, resources, income (individual)	10.8 (max.)	Fatal CHD, NF MI (89)	Age, behavioural, biological and psychosocial covariates	Demands/resources/income: (compared to low/high/high) High/low/low: 1.57 (0.78–3.18)	22	+
Steenland, 1997, USA, NHANES1	3575 (0)	25–74	Job strain (job control and job demand) (ecological)	16 (max.)	Fatal CHD and NF MI (519)	Age, smoking, blood pressure, cholesterol, BMI, diabetes, education	High control: 0.71 (0.54–0.93) High demands: 0.81 (0.61–1.09) Job strain: 1.08 (0.81–1.49)	15	0
Bosma, 1998, UK, Whitehall II study	10 308 (33)	35–55	Job control (also ecological), job demands, social support at work, effort–reward imbalance (individual)	5.3 (me)	Angina pectoris, doctor-diagnosed ischaemia (413)	Age, sex, smoking, cholesterol, BMI, hypertension, employment grade, negative affectivity, and mutually	Effort–reward imbalance: 2.15 (1.15–4.01) Low control (individual): 2.38 (1.32–4.29) Low job control (ecological): 1.56 (1.08–2.27) Job demands and social support at work unrelated	47	Effort–reward imbalance: ++ Job control: ++ Others: 0
Moore, 1999, Canada, Quebec	869 (0)	42–60	Occupational stress (individual)	10 (max.)	Fatal CHD, NF MI, angina (79)	None	Dissatisfied with: Work environment: 1.16 (0.62–1.15) Work schedule: 1.30 (0.73–2.29) Job context: 1.01 (0.52–1.97) Work responsibility: 0.89 (0.44–1.80) Support at work: 1.06 (0.61–1.86) Frequent stress at work: 1.19 (0.70–2.02)	3	0
Prognostic studies									
Hlatky, 1995, USA, Duke Medical Center	1489 (24) employed patients undergoing coronary angiography	41–59	Job strain, (decision latitude and psychological demands) (individual)	4 (me)	Fatal CHD (42), NF MI (70)	Ejection fraction, extent of coronary atherosclerosis, myocardial ischaemia	*Job strain* Fatal CHD: 1.01 (0.51–2.01) Total CHD: 0.96 (0.62–1.46)	40	0

Table 24.4 (continued)

Author, year, country, study	Total sample (% women)	Age at entry	Exposure	Follow up (years)	Type of events (n)	Adjustments	Relative risk	No. of citations (Sept 2001)	Summary
Hoffmann, 1995, Switzerland, Gais, Seewis and Le Noirmont	222 (0) patients 7 weeks (me) post first MI	30–60	Job workload	1 (max.)	Poor medical outcome (death, reinfarction, New York Heart Association Class ≥ III, exercise capacity < 100 W) (19)	Age, severity of MI, exercise, overprotection by friends, external class of control	High workload was positively associated with outcome ($p = 0.01$)	9	+
Orth-Gomer, 2000, Sweden, Stockholm Female Coronary Risk Study	292 (100) women post acute coronary event	30–65	Job strain (job demands, job control) (Karasek)	4.8 (me)	Fatal CHD, NF MI, revascularization procedure (81)	Age, smoking, blood pressure, HDL, triglycerides, oestrogen status, diabetes, diagnosis at index event, symptoms of heart failure, education	Severe work stress: 1.67 (0.64–4.32) Age adjusted only Low control: 1.62 (0.84–3.01) High demands: 1.21 (0.63–2.32)	2	+
Welin, 2000, Sweden, Gothenburg	275(16) patients 3–6 days post first MI	<65	Extra work, mental strain at work	10 (max.)	All-cause mortality (67), fatal CHD (41), NF MI (55)	None	No association between fatal CHD and extra work ($p = 0.26$), mental stress at work ($p = 0.99$) No association with total mortality or NF MI	1	0

SMR: standardized mortality ratio.

Table 24.5 Studies of social support and CHD

Author, year, country, study	Total sample (% women)	Age at entry	Exposure	Follow up (years)	Type of events (n)	Adjustments	Relative risk	No. of citations (Sept 2001)	Summary
Aetiological studies									
Medalie, 1976, Israel, Israeli Ischemic Heart Disease Study	8166 (0)	≥40	Perceived love and support from wife	5 (max.)	Angina (234)	None	High love and support from wife: 0.64 (0.43–0.96)	N/A	+
House, 1982, USA, Tecumseh Community Health Study	2754 (52)	35–69	Social relationships and activities (SI)	9–12	Fatal CHD	Age, baseline CHD, forced expiratory volume at 1 sec	Social relationships protective for fatal CHD, significantly so in women	N/A	+
Berkman, 1983, USA, Alameda County Residents	4725 (53)	30–69	Social network index	9 (max.)	Fatal CHD (120)	Age	2.13 (ss)	N/A	++
Reed, 1983, USA, Honolulu Heart Program	4653 (0)	52–71	Conceptual social networks score, factor-derived social networks score	8 (max.)	Fatal MI (76), NF MI (95), angina (47)	Age, smoking, blood pressure, cholesterol, BMI, alcohol, exercise, complex carbohydrate, glucose, uric acid, forced vital capacity, SES, and mutually	*Standardized logistic coefficients:* Conceptual social network: Fatal MI: −0.0505 (ns) NF MI: −0.0576 (ns) Angina: −0.1348 (ns) Factor-derived social network: Fatal MI: −0.0504 (ns) NF MI: −0.2146 (ns) Angina: −0.0851 (ns) Non-significant protective effect of social network	85	0
Kaplan, 1988, Finland, Kuopio and North Karelia	13 301	39–59	Social connections index	5 (max.)	Fatal CHD (223)	Age, smoking, blood pressure, cholesterol, BMI, family history of CHD, education, residence	Men only: 1.72 (0.77–3.84)	105	+
Vogt, 1992, USA, Northwest Kaiser Permanente	2603 (54)	≥18	Network scope, frequency, size (Household Interview Survey)	15 (max.)	Fatal CHD, NF CHD (not stated)	Age, sex, smoking, SES, baseline subjective health status	Network scope: 1.5 (1.0–2.3) Network frequency: 1.1 (0.8–1.5) Network size: 1.2 (0.9–1.6)	63	Network scope: + Others: 0

Table 24.5 (continued)

Author, year, country, study	Total sample (% women)	Age at entry	Exposure	Follow up (years)	Type of events (n)	Adjustments	Relative risk	No. of citations (Sept 2001)	Summary
Orth-Gomer, 1993, Sweden, Men Born in Gothenburg in 1933	736 (0)	50	Attachment, social integration	6 (max.)	Fatal CHD, NF MI (25)	Smoking, cholesterol, BMI, exercise, hypertension, diabetes	Low social integration: 3.8 (1.1–13.9) Low attachment: 3.1 (1.3–7.6)	77	++
Kawachi, 1996, USA, Health Professionals Follow-Up Study	32 624 (0)	42–77	Social Networks index (Berkman-Syme)	4 (max.)	Fatal CHD (128), NF MI (275)	Age, smoking, cholesterol, BMI, alcohol, exercise, hypertension, diabetes, angina, family history of MI, time period	Low social support: Fatal CHD: 1.42 (0.72–2.81) NF MI: 1.00 (0.58–1.71)	39	0
Chen, 1999, USA, Established Population for the Epidemiologic Study of the Elderly	1749 (59)	≥65	Emotional support	7.9 (me)	Heart failure (173)	Age, sex, blood pressure, BMI, diabetes, MI during follow-up	No significant multivariate association Unadjusted analysis: No emotional support: 1.48 (1.05–2.10)	6	0
Prognostic studies									
Ahern, 1990, USA, Cardiac Arrhythmia Pilot Study	353 patients 6–60 days post-MI	<75	Social Support	1 (max.)	All-cause mortality, NF MI	None	Mean (SD) social support Survivors: 22.8 (3.2) Non-survivors: 23.3 (2.6)	177	0
Berkman, 1992, USA, Established Population for the Epidemiologic Study of the Elderly	194 (48) hospitalized with acute MI	≥65	Emotional support from social, network, social network structure	0.5 (max.)	All-cause mortality (76)	Age, sex, Killip class, ejection fraction, reinfarction, comorbidity, functional disability, previous MI, ventricular tachycardia	No emotional support: 2.9 (1.2–6.9) Network support measure shows similar but less powerful or consistent trends (data not presented in paper)	157	++

Hedblad, 1992, Sweden, Men Born in 1914	98 (0) patients with ischaemic 24 h ECG	68	Social anchorage, contact frequency, social participation, emotional support, informational support, material support, social influence	4.5 (me)	Fatal CHD, NF MI (17)	Smoking, cholesterol, BMI, alcohol, exercise, triglycerides, previous CHD, hypertension, marital status, and mutually	Social anchorage: 1.8 (0.4–8.5) Contact frequency: 1.2 (0.3–4.9) Social participation: 0.5 (0.1–2.2) Emotional support: 4.1 (1.0–17.0) Informational support: 5.8 (1.4–24.5)	16	Support ++ Social anchorage: + Others 0
Williams, 1992, USA, Duke Medical Center	1368 (18) people with angiographic disease	52 (me)	Structural social support (marital status), functional social support	9 (me)	Cardiovascular mortality (237)	Age, sex, LVEF, non-invasive myocardial damage index, conduction disturbance on ECG, pain/ischaemia index, mitral regurgitation, no. of diseased vessels, % stenosis of left main stem and left anterior descending artery, year	Unmarried without a confidant compared to either married or with a confidant: 3.34 (1.84–6.20)	175	++
Gorkin, 1993, USA, Cardiac Arrhythmia Suppression Trial-1	1322 (17) with previous MI and ventricular premature complexes	61 (me)	Perceived social support, social functioning index, social integration index	0.8 (me)	All-cause mortality (not stated)	Sex, treatment, history of MI, ejection fraction, congestive heart failure, thrombolysis	No multivariate association for any social network score Unadjusted analyses: Social function: 0.82 (p = 0.02) Significant protective effect in placebo only group	16	0
Jenkinson, 1993, UK, Anglo-Scandinavian Study of Early Thrombolysis	1376 (22) within 7 days post-MI	25–84	Social isolation	3 (me)	All-cause mortality (247)	Age, sex, previous MI, hospital complications, diabetes, hypertension, car ownership	1.33 (0.89–1.98)	17	0

Table 24.5 (continued)

Author, year, country, study	Total sample (% women)	Age at entry	Exposure	Follow up (years)	Type of events (n)	Adjustments	Relative risk	No. of citations (Sept 2001)	Summary
Frasure-Smith, 1995b, Canada, Canadian Signal-Averaged ECG Trial	222 (22) patients 5–15 days post-MI	24–88	Social Support Scale (Blumenthal)	1 (max.)	Recurrent cardiac events (arrhythmic death, fatal and NF MI, survived cardiac arrest and unstable angina) (48)	Previous MI, prescription of ACE inhibitors, anxiety, depression	No association Unadjusted analyses: Low social support: 1.46 (0.70–3.07)	58	0
Friedmann, 1995, USA, Cardiac Arrhythmia Suppression Trial ancillary study	369 (15) patients after acute MI with ventricular arrhythmias	63 (me)	Social support (SSO6), social readjustment (social readjustment rating scale)	1 (max.)	All-cause mortality (20)	Diabetes, LVEF, runs of ventricular premature beats, pet ownership	Social support significantly increased survival $R = 0.06$, $p = 0.05$, Exp[β] = 0.94	17	+
Greenwood, 1995, UK, Anglo-Scandinavian Study of Early Thrombolysis	1283 (22) patients post-MI who survived 7 days	55–59 (me)	Social contact	5.6 (me)	All-cause mortality (302)	Age, sex, previous infarct, hospital complications, diabetes, beta-blockers, heart rate, hypertension, discharge diagnosis of MI, car owner	1.14 (0.78–1.67)	11	0
Oxman, 1995, USA, Dartmouth-Hitchcock Medical Center	232 (0) patients after elective open heart surgery	≥55	Social network (SNQ and ISSB), perceived social support (MSPSS), religion	0.5 (max.)	All-cause mortality (21)	Age, previous cardiac surgery, severe impairment, and mutually	No participation in: groups: 4.26 (1.15–15.73) No strength/comfort from religion: 3.25 (1.09–9.72)	83	++
Denollet, 1996, Belgium, Antwerp Cardiac Rehabilitation Programme	303 (12) patients with angiographic CHD	31–79	Social alienation (Millon behavioural health inventory)	7.9 (me)	All-cause mortality (38)	Left ventricular function, number of diseased vessels, low exercise tolerance, lack of thrombolytic therapy, type D personality	No significant multivariate association Unadjusted association: 2.33 (1.24–4.38)	59	0

Study	Sample	Age	Exposure	Follow-up	Outcome	Adjustment	Effect estimate		
Farmer, 1996, USA, Corpus Christi Heart Project	596 (35) patients 4–5 days post-MI	25–74	Social support (social support scale)	3.6 (me)	All-cause mortality > 28 days post-MI (115)	Age, sex, smoking, diabetes, hypertension, hypercholesterolaemia, ethnicity, education, employment	Low social support: 1.89 (1.20–2.97)	5	+
Woloshin, 1997, Canada, Manitoba	820 (35) patients 8–22months post-MI	67 (me)	Perceived adequacy of tangible support	1 (max.)	Total mortality (31)	Age, baseline PCS score, baseline MCS score, dyspnoea	Comparing those needing much more help to patients with no perceived need: 6.5 (2.0–21.6)	5	++
Herlitz, 1998, Sweden, Gothenburg	1290 (18) patients 3 months (mean) prior to CABG	32–86	Social isolation	5 (max.)	All-cause mortality (173)	Age, smoking, LVEF, CHF, diabetes, renal dysfunction, previous CVD, intermittent claudication	1.78 (1.17–2.71)	6	+
Krumholz, 1998, USA, Established Population for the Epidemiologic Study of the Elderly	292 (57) patients hospitalized with heart failure	≥65	Emotional support, instrumental support, social ties count	1 (max.)	CVD death or readmission (142)	Age, sex, LVEF, acute physiology score, MI at current admission, hypertension, Rosow–Breslau or Nagi impairment, and mutually	No social ties: 2.08 (0.95–4.54) No source of emotional support: 2.69 (1.22–5.94)	24	++
Frasure-Smith, 1999, Canada, Montreal Heart Attack Readjustment Trial and Emotions and Prognosis Post-Infarct Study	896 (32) patients 7 days post-MI	24–88	Social support (Perceived Social Support Scale)	1 (max.)	Fatal CHD (37)	None	Perceived social support: 1.25 (0.59–2.66)	31	0
Irvine, 1999, Canada, Canadian Amiodarone Myocardial Infarction Arrhythmia Trial	671 (17) patients 6–45 days post-MI	32–89	Social network contacts and social participation (Health and Daily Living Form)	2 (max.)	SCD (34)	Previous MI, previous CHF, depression, dyspnoea/fatigue, treatment group, and mutually	Point increase in score Social network contacts: 1.04 (1.01–1.07) Social participation: 0.98(0.96–1.01)	9	Network contacts:+ Participation: 0

Table 24.5 (continued)

Author, year, country, study	Total sample (% women)	Age at entry	Exposure	Follow up (years)	Type of events (n)	Adjustments	Relative risk	No. of citations (Sept 2001)	Summary
Horsten, 2000, Sweden, Stockholm Female Coronary Risk Study	292 (100) 3–6 months after hospitalization for acute coronary event	30–65	Attachment and social integration (ISSI)	4.8 (me)	Cardiovascular mortality, NF MI, revascularization procedure (81)	Age, smoking, blood pressure, HDL, BMI, exercise, diagnosis at index event, symptoms of heart failure, diabetes, hypertension, severity of angina symptoms	Low attachment: 1.4 (0.89 + 2.3) (age adjusted only) Low social integration: 2.3 (1.2–4.5)	4	Attachment: 0 Integration: ++
Orth-Gomer, 2000, Sweden, Stockholm Female Coronary Risk Study	292 (100) women post acute coronary event	30–65	Marital stress (Stockholm Marital Stress Scale)	4.8 (me)	Fatal CHD, NF MI, revascularization procedure (81)	Age, smoking, blood pressure, HDL, triglycerides, oestrogen status, diagnosis at index event, symptoms of heart failure, diabetes, education	Severe marital stress: 2.92 (1.30–6.54)	2	++
Welin, 2000, Sweden, Gothenburg	275 (16) patients 3–6 days post first MI	<65	Social relationships (ISSI, Broadhead questionnaire, social activities questionnaire)	10 (max.)	All-cause mortality (67), fatal CHD (41), NF MI (55)	Sex, left ventricular fatigue, ventricular dysrhythmia, depression	Social support: Total mortality: 1.67 (0.97–2.89) Fatal CHD: 2.75 (1.29–5.89) Unadjusted analyses for social activities: Total mortality: 2.07 (1.07–3.98) Fatal CHD: 1.89 (1.12–3.20) No association with NF MI	1	Fatal CHD: ++ Total mortality:+ NF MI: 0
Brummett, 2001, USA, Mediators of Social Support Study	430 (33) patients with angiographic disease	64 (me)	Network social support (Mannheim Social Support Interview)	4 (me)	Fatal CHD (120)	Age, number of diseased vessels, LVEF, CHF, comorbidity	≤3 network members: 2.43 (1.52–3.89)	1	++

MCS: mental component summary;

SES: socio-economic status;

PCS: physical component summary.

Nine studies were included that used social support as the proposed aetiological agent. Three studies showed no clear association, including the Health Professionals Follow-up Study (Kawachi *et al.* 1996). Four studies, using a range of different measures of social support, were moderately supportive of the hypothesis that social support is aetiologically linked to CHD. Finally, two studies were strongly supportive of an association between social support and risk of CHD.

Of the 21 prognostic studies, 10 were strongly supportive of the hypothesis, 4 were moderately supportive, and 7 showed no consistent effect. The strongly supportive studies included one of the largest studies (Williams *et al.* 1992) and two with extended follow-up (Williams *et al.* 1992; Welin *et al.* 2000), and they were generally highly adjusted for potential confounders, including lifestyle behaviours and indicators of disease severity. The stronger effect of social support on prognosis for people with CHD than on risk for CHD could potentially be explained if patients with CHD with high levels of social support are better taken care of or are more likely to seek medical care.

24.4 Discussion

24.4.1 Modification of psychosocial factors

Some primary prevention of CHD through modification of psychosocial factors may be possible, since depression and anxiety are amenable to intervention, but this may lie largely outside the remit of clinicians. This is because psychosocial factors themselves are determined largely by social, political, and economic factors and it is therefore policy makers who influence the structure and function of communities – in the public and private domains – who may have scope for primary prevention.

A meta-analysis of 23 randomized controlled trials found that psychosocial interventions are associated with improved survival after MI (Linden *et al.* 1996). However, two large randomized controlled trials of psychological rehabilitation after MI found no difference in anxiety and depression (Jones and West 1996; Frasure-Smith *et al.* 1997). Randomized controlled trials of modification of social supports after MI show a decrease in cardiac death or reinfarction rates (Bucher 1994). A multicentre trial of 3000 patients after MI (ENRICHD – enhancing recovery in coronary heart disease) is currently under way in the United States (Blumenthal *et al.* 1997). It is designed to target patients at high psychosocial risk (those who are depressed or socially isolated) and includes large numbers of women and ethnic minorities. The results, reported at the American Heart Association in November 2001, suggest no survival benefit of the intervention of cognitive behavioural therapy.

24.4.2 Challenges in improving this systematic review

Much of the literature used for this review was based on secondary analyses of data collected for other primary purposes; only a minority of studies were set up to investigate psychosocial factors in relation to CHD. A comparison with the systematic review of randomized trials is informative. Unlike trials, few, if any, studies reported in our review had published their hypotheses detailing primary exposure, confounder, and outcome relationships prior to reporting results. This is of concern given the possibility of multiple comparisons between numerous psychosocial variables and CHD outcomes within one study. Unlike the situation with randomized trials, there is no register of studies that are testing or could test psychosocial hypotheses. Such a register provides a 'denominator of hypotheses' which can then be tracked through the stages of analysis, manuscript preparation, submission, publication, and scientific impact, to determine the extent of any bias.

A number of psychosocial factors were examined in only a small number of studies, and these included anger, aggression, cynicism, dominance, hopelessness, neurosis, submissiveness, and vital exhaustion. It is apparent that these less commonly used psychosocial factors tended to report strong associations with the aetiology and prognosis of CHD. This is consistent with a role for publication bias.

In the absence of a true association, small studies are more likely to report results suggesting a relationship between a psychosocial factor and an outcome than larger, more powerful studies. However, should an effect truly exist, then the larger studies are more likely to show an association than are smaller studies. In this review, for social support null or negative studies were on average larger than the studies showing a role of social support in the aetiology or prognosis of CHD (Fig. 24.1a, b). This could suggest that a true causal association is absent. In contrast, for studies on depression, the studies that moderately supported the hypothesis were generally larger than the null or strongly supportive studies. This strengthens the claim of a role for depression in the aetiology and prognosis of CHD. For the other psychosocial factors, the trends were less apparent.

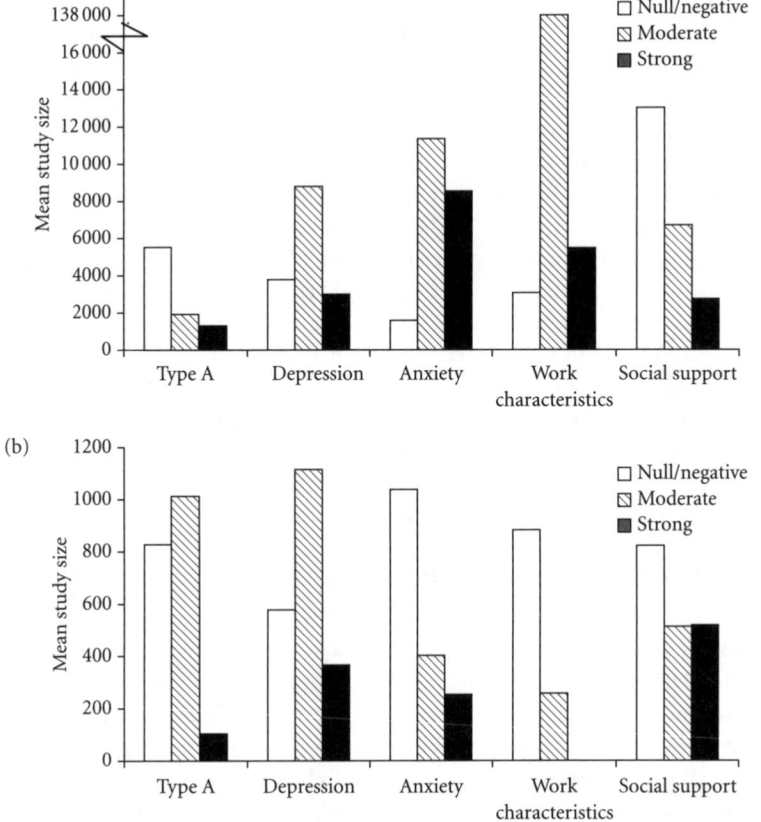

Fig. 24.1 (a) Association between support for the hypothesis and mean study size (aetiological studies). (b) Association between support for the hypothesis and mean study size (prognostic studies).

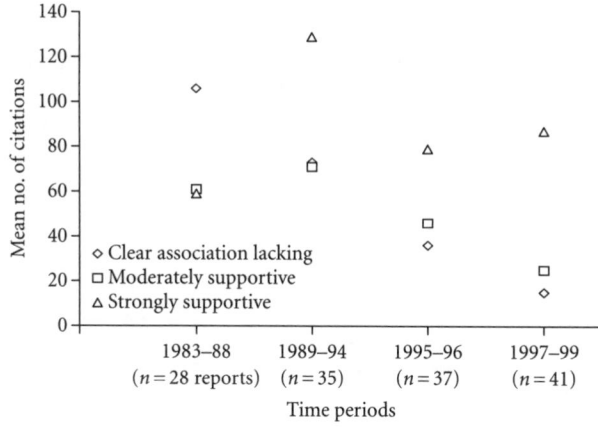

Fig. 24.2 The association between the size of the effect estimate and number of citations: an indicator of influence bias.

A further bias may occur after publication. Positive studies may be more influential than studies in which there is a lack of clear association. We attempted to evaluate the effect of such an influence bias, using the number of citations on the Science Citation Index. Figure 24.2 suggests that the frequency of citation was highest for strongly positive studies, intermediate for moderately positive studies, and lowest for those lacking a clear association. In the first period of assessment, studies not showing a clear association were cited most frequently, and this result is strongly influenced by the high frequency of citing the two major null studies on the TABP–CHD association (Shekelle *et al.* 1983, 1985*b*). This suggests that selective citing of positive studies, rather than using systematic reviews, may be used in specifying hypotheses. Moreover, it is clear from the tables that multiple reporting of results from the same study is an important issue, further increasing the opportunity for influence bias.

When summarizing whether the study was supportive overall of the hypothesis in question, although we did include confidence intervals, we did not consider the statistical significance of the effect estimate, for reasons of clarity. Although we are aware that this favours the reporting of large effect estimates by the less powerful study, this is to some extent mitigated by a restriction on study sample size. We also did not consider the influence of effect modification, although we did make an effort to report separate effect estimates by gender, where the data were available. We were unable to explore the effect of changes in, and cumulative exposure to, psychosocial factors on CHD events, even though several authors have looked at this association (Kaplan *et al.* 1988). We also did not explore the short- and long-term effects of psychosocial factors on CHD throughout the life course (Kuh and Ben-Shlomo 1997).

24.5 **Conclusions**

Our systematic review of prospective studies published up until 2001 identified 70 reports of aetiological effects and 92 reports of prognostic effects by psychosocial factors (Table 24.6). Based on prospective epidemiological data, there was indication for an association between depression, social support, and psychosocial work characteristics with CHD aetiology and prognosis. The randomized trials, to date, have been negative. Evidence for an effect of anxiety or type A behaviour was less consistent. We found some evidence that positive studies were more likely to be cited than negative studies.

Table 24.6 Summary of prospective studies investigating psychosocial factors and CHD

	Number of reports of aetiological studies (n = 70)				Number of reports of prognostic studies (n = 92)			
	−	0	+	++	+	0	+	++
Type A behaviour	1	11	5	1	3	10	1	1
Depression	0	8	5	9	0	16	7	11
Anxiety	0	4	1	3	1	9	4	4
Work characteristics	0	3	5	5	0	2	2	0
Social support	0	3	4	2	0	7	4	10

− = finding counter to hypothesis; 0 = lack of clear association; + = moderate association (relative risk ≥ 1.50 and < 2.00); ++ = strong association (relative risk ≥ 2.00).

This review suggests two challenges for future psychosocial research. The first challenge is obvious: more and better studies are needed. Further standardization of the scales used to measure psychosocial factors is crucial; proliferation of different scales used in small numbers of studies, sometimes with modification, will hamper progress. Further trials of modifying depression and social supports among CHD patients are awaited. The second challenge, while less obvious, is no less important. Given that much of the psychosocial literature is based on secondary analyses of data collected for other primary purposes, methods need to be developed to address the potential biases that occur between the stages of hypothesis specification and scientific influence. When this review is next updated the extent to which these challenges have been met can be assessed.

Information on any eligible studies we may have missed would be gratefully received.

Acknowledgements

Harry Hemingway is supported by a National Public Health Career Scientist Award from the Department of Health. Michael Marmot is supported by an MRC Research Professorship.

References

Ahern, D. K., Gorkin, L., Anderson, J. L., Tierney, C., Hallstrom, A., Ewart, C. *et al.* (1990). Biobehavioural variables and mortality/cardiac arrest in the cardiac arrhythmia pilot study. *American Journal of Cardiology*, **66**, 59–62.

Alfredsson, L., Spetz, C.-L., and Theorell, T. (1985). Type of occupation and near-future hospitalization for myocardial infarction and some other diagnoses. *International Journal of Epidemiology*, **14**, 378–88.

Allison, T. G., Williams, D. E., Miller, T. D., Patten, C. A., Bailey, K. R., Squires, R. W., and Gau, G. T. (1995). Medical and economic costs of psychologic distress in patients with coronary artery disease. *Mayo Clinical Proceedings*, **70**, 734–42.

Alterman, T., Shekelle, R. B., Vernon, S. W., and Burau, K. D. (1994). Decision latitude, psychologic demand, job strain, and coronary heart disease in the Western Electric study. *American Journal of Epidemiology*, **139**, 620–7.

Anda, R., Williamson, D., Jones, D., Macera, C., Eaker, E., Glassman, A., and Marks, J. (1993). Depressed affect, hopelessness, and the risk of ischaemic heart disease in a cohort of US adults. *Epidemiology*, **4**, 285–94.

Appels, A., Mulder, P., van, 't Hof, M., Jenkins, C. D., van Houtem, J., and Tan, F. (1987). A prospective study of the Jenkins Activity Survey as a risk indicator for coronary heart disease in the Netherlands. *Journal of Chronic Diseases*, **40**, 959–65.

Ariyo, A. A., Haan, M., Tangen, C. M., Rutledge, J. C., Cushman, M., Dobs, A., and Furberg, C. D. (2000). Depressive symptoms and risks of coronary heart disease and mortality in elderly Americans. Cardiovascular Health Study Collaborative Research Group. *Circulation*, **102**, 1773–9.

Aromaa, A., Raitasalo, R., Reunanen, A., Impivaara, O., Heliovaara, M., Knedt, P. *et al.* (1994). Depression and cardiovascular diseases. *Acta Psychiatrica Scandinavica Supplementum*, **377**, 77–82.

Baker, R. A., Andrew, M. J., Schrader, G., and Knight, J. L. (2001). Preoperative depression and mortality in coronary artery bypass surgery: preliminary findings. *Australian and New Zealand Journal of Surgery*, **71**, 139–42.

Barefoot, J. C. and Schroll, M. (1996). Symptoms of depression, acute myocardial infarction and total mortality in a community sample. *Circulation*, **93**, 1976–80.

Barefoot, J. C., Peterson, B. L., and Harrell, F. E. J. (1989). Type A behavior and survival: a follow-up study of 1,467 patients with coronary artery disease. *American Journal of Cardiology*, **64**, 427–32.

Barefoot, J. C., Larsen, S., von der Lieth, L., and Schroll, M. (1995). Hostility, incidence of acute myocardial infarction and mortality in a sample of older Danish men and women. *American Journal of Epidemiology*, **142**, 477–84.

Barefoot, J. C., Helms, M. J., Mark, D. B., Blumenthal, J. A., Califf, R. M., Haney, T. L. *et al.* (1996). Depression and long-term mortality risk in patients with coronary artery disease. *American Journal of Cardiology*, **78**, 613–17.

Barefoot, J. C., Brummett, B. H., Helms, M. J., Mark, D. B., Siegler, I. C., and Williams, R. B. (2000). Depressive symptoms and survival of patients with coronary artery disease. *Psychosomatic Medicine*, **62**, 790–5.

Berkman, L. F. and Breslow, L. (1983). *Health and ways of living*. Oxford University Press, New York.

Berkman, L. F., Leo-Summers, L., and Horwitz, R. I. (1992). Emotional support and survival after myocardial infarction: a prospective, population-based study of the elderly. *Annals of Internal Medicine*, **117**, 1003–9.

Blumenthal, J. A., O'Connor, C., Hinderliter, A., Fath, K., Hegde, S. B., Miller, G. *et al.* (1997). Psychosocial factors and coronary disease: a national multicenter clinical trial (ENRICHD). with a North Carolina focus. *North Carolina Medical Journal*, **58**, 440–4.

Bosma, H., Appels, A., and Sturmans, F. (1995). Psychosocial factors in the aetiology of coronary heart disease: follow-up to the Kaunas-Rotterdam intervention study (KRIS). *Cardiology*, **2**, 54–9.

Bosma, H., Marmot, M. G., Hemingway, H., Nicholson, A., Brunner, E. J., and Stansfeld, S. (1997). Low job control and risk of coronary heart disease in the Whitehall II (prospective cohort) study. *British Medical Journal*, **314**, 558–65.

Bosma, H., Peter, R., Siegrist, J., and Marmot, M. (1998). Two alternative job stress models and the risk of coronary heart disease. *American Journal of Public Health*, **88**, 68–74.

Brackett, C. D. and Powell, L. H. (1988). Psychosocial and physiological predictors of sudden cardiac death after healing of acute myocardial infarction. *American Journal of Cardiology*, **61**, 979–83.

Bradford Hill, A. (1965). The environment and disease: association or causation? *Proceedings of the Royal Society of Medicine*, **58**, 295–300.

Brisson, C., Larocque, B., Moisan, J., Vezina, M., and Dagenais, G. R. (2000). Psychosocial factors at work, smoking, sedentary behavior, and body mass index: a prevalence study among 6995 white collar workers. *Journal of Occupational and Environmental Medicine*, **42**, 40–6.

Brummett, B. H., Barefoot, J. C., Siegler, I. C., Clapp-Channing, N. E., Lytle, B. L., Bosworth, H. B. *et al.* (2001). Characteristics of socially isolated patients with coronary artery disease who are at elevated risk for mortality. *Psychosomatic Medicine*, **63**, 267–72.

Brunner, E. (1997). Stress and the biology of inequality. *British Medical Journal*, **314**, 1472–6.

Bucher, H. C. (1994). Social support and prognosis following first myocardial infarction. *Journal of General Internal Medicine*, **9**, 409–17.

Carinci, F., Nicolucci, A., Ciampi, A., Labbrozzi, D., Bettinardi, O., Zotti, A. M., and Tognoni, G. (1997). Role of interactions between psychological and clinical factors in determining 6-month mortality among patients with acute myocardial infarction: application of recursive partitioning techniques to the GISSI-2 database. Gruppo Italiano per lo Studio della Sopravvivenza nell' Infarto Miocardico. *European Heart Journal*, **18**, 835–45.

Case, R. B., Heller, S. S., Case, N. B., and Moss, A. J. (1985). Type A behavior and survival after acute myocardial infarction. *New England Journal of Medicine*, **312**, 737–41.

Chang, M., Hahn, R. A., Teutsch, S. M., and Hutwagner, L. C. (2001). Multiple risk factors and population attributable risk for ischemic heart disease mortality in the United States, 1971–1992. *Journal of Clinical Epidemiology*, **54**, 634–44.

Chen, Y. T., Vaccarino, V., Williams, C. S., Butler, J., Berkman, L. F., and Krumholz, H. M. (1999). Risk factors for heart failure in the elderly: a prospective community-based study. *American Journal of Medicine*, **106**, 605–12.

Cohen, J. B. and Reed, D. (1985). The type A pattern and coronary heart disease among Japanese men in Hawaii. *Journal of Behavoral Medicine*, **4**, 343–52.

Cohen, H. W., Gibson, G., and Alderman, M. H. (2000). Excess risk of myocardial infarction in patients treated with antidepressant medications: association with use of tricyclic agents. *American Journal of Medicine*, **108**, 2–8.

Cohen, H. W., Madhavan, S., and Alderman, M. H. (2001). History of treatment for depression: risk factor for myocardial infarction in hypertensive patients. *Psychosomatic Medicine*, **63**, 203–9.

Cole, S. R., Kawachi, I., Sesso, H. D., Paffenbarger, R. S., and Lee, I. M. (1999). Sense of exhaustion and coronary heart disease among college alumni. *American Journal of Cardiology*, **84**, 1401–5.

Denollet, J., Sys, S. U., and Brutsaert, D. L. (1995). Personality and mortality after myocardial infarction. *Psychosomatic Medicine*, **57**, 582–91.

Denollet, J., Sys, S. U., Stroobant, N., Rombouts, H., Gillebert, T. C., and Brutsaert, D. L. (1996). Personality as independent predictor of long term mortality in patients with coronary heart disease. *Lancet*, **347**, 417–21.

Denollet, J., Vaes, J., and Brutsaert, D. L. (2000). Inadequate response to treatment in coronary heart disease: adverse effects of type D personality and younger age on 5-year prognosis and quality of life. *Circulation*, **102**, 630–5.

Eaker, E. D. and Castelli, W. P. (1988). Type A behavior and mortality from coronary disease in the Framingham study. *New England Journal of Medicine*, **319**, 1480–1.

Eaker, E. D., Abbott, R. D., and Kannel, W. B. (1989). Frequency of uncomplicated angina pectoris in type A compared with type B persons (the Framingham Study). *American Journal of Cardiology*, **63**, 1042–5.

Eaker, E. D., Pinsky, J., and Castelli, W. P. (1992). Myocardial infarction and coronary death among women: psychosocial predictors from a 20-year follow-up of women in the Framingham Study. *American Journal of Epidemiology*, **135**, 854–64.

Everson, S. A., Kauhanen, J., Kaplan, G. A., Goldberg, D. E., Julkunen, J., Tuomilehto, J., and Salonen, J. T. (1997). Hostility and increased risk of mortality and acute myocardial infarction: the mediating role of behavioural risk factors. *American Journal of Epidemiology*, **146**, 142–52.

Farmer, I. P., Meyer, P. S., Ramsey, D. J., Goff, D. C., Wear, M. L., Labarthe, D. R., and Nichaman, M. Z. (1996). Higher levels of social support predict greater survival following acute myocardial infarction: the Corpus Christi Heart Project. *Behavoral Medicine*, **22**, 59–66.

Ferketich, A. K., Schwartzbaum, J. A., Frid, D. J., and Moeschberger, M. L. (2000). Depression as an antecedent to heart disease among women and men in the NHANES I study. National Health and Nutrition Examination Survey. *Archives of Internal Medicine*, **160**, 1261–8.

Ford, D. E., Mead, L. A., Chang, P. P., Cooper-Patrick, L., Wang, N. Y., and Klag, M. J. (1998). Depression is a risk factor for coronary artery disease in men: the precursors study. *Archives of Internal Medicine*, **158**, 1422–6.

Frasure-Smith, N. (1991). In-hospital symptoms of psychological stress as predictors of long-term outcome after acute myocardial infarction in men. *American Journal of Cardiology*, **67**, 121–7.

Frasure-Smith, N., Lesperance, F., and Talajic, M. (1993). Depression following myocardial infarction: impact on 6-month survival. *Journal of the American Medical Association*, **270**, 1819–25.

Frasure-Smith, N., Lesperance, F., and Talajic, M. (1995*a*). Depression and 18 month prognosis after myocardial infarction. *Circulation*, **91**, 999–1005.

Frasure-Smith, N., Lesperance, F., and Talajic, M. (1995*b*). The impact of negative emotions on prognosis following myocardial infarction: is it more than depression? *Health Psychology*, **14**, 388–98.

Frasure-Smith, N., Lesperance, F., Prince, R. H., Verrier, P., Garber, R. A., Juneau, M. *et al.* (1997). Randomised trial of home-based psychosocial nursing intervention for patients recovering from myocardial infarction. *Lancet*, **350**, 473–9.

Frasure-Smith, N., Lesperance, F., Juneau, M., Talajic, M., and Bourassa, M. G. (1999). Gender, depression, and one-year prognosis after myocardial infarction. *Psychosomatic Medicine*, **61**, 26–37.

Friedmann, E. and Thomas, S. A. (1995). Pet ownership, social support and one-year survival after acute myocardial infarction in the cardiac arrhythmia suppression trial (CAST). *American Journal of Cardiology*, **76**, 1213–17.

Gorkin, L., Schron, E. B., Brooks, M. M., Wiklund, I., Kellen, J., Verter, J. *et al.* (1993). Psychosocial predictors of mortality in the cardiac arrhythmia suppression trial-1 (CAST-1). *American Journal of Cardiology*, **71**, 263–7.

Greenwood, D., Packham, C., Muir, K., and Madeley, R. (1995). How do economic status and social support influence survival after initial recovery from acute myocardial infarction? *Social Science and Medicine*, **40**, 639–47.

Haan, M. N. (1988). Job strain and ischaemic heart disease: an epidemiologic study of metal workers. *Annals of Clinical Research*, **20**, 143–5.

Haines, A. P., Imeson, J. D., and Meade, T. W. (1987). Phobic anxiety and ischaemic heart disease. *British Medical Journal*, **295**, 297–9.

Haines, A., Cooper, J., and Meade, T. W. (2001). Psychological characteristics and fatal ischaemic heart disease. *Heart*, **85**, 385–9.

Hallstrom, T., Lapidus, L., Bengtsson, C., and Edstrom, K. (1986). Psychosocial factors and risk of ischaemic heart disease and death in women: a 12 year follow up of participants in the population study of women in Gothenburg, Sweden. *Journal of Psychosomatic Research*, **30**, 451–9.

Haynes, S. G., Feinleib, M., and Kannel, W. B. (1980). The relationship of psychosocial factors to coronary heart disease in the Framingham study: 3. Eight year incidence of coronary heart disease. *American Journal of Epidemiology*, **111**, 37–58.

Hearn, M. D., Murray, D. M., and Luepker, R. V. (1989). Hostility, coronary heart disease, and total mortality: a 33-year follow-up study of university students. *Journal of Behavioural Medicine*, **12** (2), 105–21.

Hedblad, B., Ostergren, P. O., Hanson, B. S., Janzon, L., Johansson, B. W., and Juul-Moller, S. (1992). Influence of social support on cardiac event rate in men with ischaemic type ST segment depression during ambulatory 24-h long-term ECG recording: the prospective population study 'Men born in 1914', Malmo, Sweden. *European Heart Journal*, **13**, 433–9.

Hemingway, H. and Marmot, M. (1999). Evidence based cardiology: psychosocial factors in the aetiology and prognosis of coronary heart disease. Systematic review of prospective cohort studies. *British Medical Journal*, **318**, 1460–7.

Herlitz, J., Wiklund, I., Caidahl, K., Hartford, M., Haglid, M., Karlsson, B. W. *et al.* (1998). The feeling of loneliness prior to coronary artery bypass grafting might be a predictor of short-and long-term postoperative mortality. *European Journal of Vascular and Endovascular Surgery*, **16**, 120–5.

Herrmann, C., Brand-Driehorst, S., Buss, U., and Ruger, U. (2000). Effects of anxiety and depression on 5-year mortality in 5,057 patients referred for exercise testing. *Journal of Psychosomatic Research*, **48**, 455–62.

Hlatky, M. A., Lam, L. C., Lee, K. L., Clapp-Channing, N. E., Williams, R. B., Pryor, D. B. *et al.* (1995). Job strain and the prevalence and outcome of coronary artery disease. *Circulation*, **92**, 327–33.

Hoffmann, A., Pfiffner, D., Hornung, R., and Niederhauser, H. (1995). Psychosocial factors predict medical outcome following a first myocardial infarction. Working Group on Cardiac Rehabilitation of the Swiss Society of Cardiology. *Coronary Artery Disease*, **6**, 147–52.

Hollis, J. F., Connett, J. E., Stevens, V. J., and Greenlick, M. R. (1990). Stressful life events, type A behavior, and the prediction of cardiovascular and total mortality over six years. MRFIT Group. *Journal of Behavoural Medicine*, **13**, 263–80.

Horsten, M., Wamala, S. P., Vingerhoets, A., and Orth-Gomer, K. (1997). Depressive symptoms, social support, and lipid profile in healthy middle-aged women. *Psychosomatic Medicine*, **59**, 521–8.

Horsten, M., Mittleman, M. A., Wamala, S. P., Schenck-Gustafsson, K., and Orth-Gomer, K. (2000). Depressive symptoms and lack of social integration in relation to prognosis of CHD in middle-aged women: the Stockholm Female Coronary Risk Study. *European Heart Journal*, **21**, 1072–80.

House, J. S., Robbins, C., and Metzner, H. L. (1982). The association of social relationships and activities with mortality: prospective evidence from the Tecumseh Community Health Study. *American Journal of Epidemiology*, **116**, 123–40.

Irvine, J., Basinski, A., Baker, B., Jandciu, S., Paquette, M., Cairns, J. *et al.* (1999). Depression and risk of sudden cardiac death after acute myocardial infarction: testing for the confounding effects of fatigue. *Psychosomatic Medicine*, **61**, 729–37.

Jenkins, C. D., Rosenman, R. H., and Zyzanski, S. J. (1974). Prediction of clinical coronary heart disease by a test of the coronary-prone behaviour pattern. *New England Journal of Medicine*, **290**, 1271–5.

Jenkinson, C. M., Madeley, R. J., Mitchell, J. R., and Turner, I. D. (1993). The influence of psychosocial factors on survival after myocardial infarction. *Public Health*, **107**, 305–17.

Johnston, D. W., Cook, D. G., and Shaper, A. G. (1987). Type A behaviour and ischaemic heart disease in middle-aged British men. *British Medical Journal*, **295**, 86–9.

Jones, D. A. and West, R. R. (1996). Psychological rehabilitation after myocardial infarction: multicentre randomised controlled trial. *British Medical Journal*, **313**, 1517–21.

Kaplan, G. A., Salonen, J. T., and Cohen, R. D. (1988). Social connections and mortality from all causes and from cardiovascular disease: prospective evidence from Eastern Finland. *American Journal of Epidemiology*, **128**, 370–80.

Karasek, R. A. (1979). Job demands, job decision latitude and mental strain: implications for job design. *Administrative Scientific Quarterly*, **24**, 285–308.

Karasek, R. A. and Theorell, T. (1990). *Healthy work: stress productivity and reconstruction of working life.* Basic Books, New York.

Kaufmann, M. W., Fitzgibbons, J. P., Sussman, E. J., Reed III, J. F., Einfalt, J. M., Rodgers, J. K., and Friccione, G. L. (1999). Relation between myocardial infarction, depression, hostility, and death. *American Heart Journal*, **138**, 549–54.

Kawachi, I., Colditz, G. A., Ascherio, A., Rimm, E. B., Giovannucci, E., Stampfer, M. J., and Willett, W. C. (1994). Prospective study of phobic anxiety and risk of coronary heart disease in men. *Circulation*, **89**, 1992–7.

Kawachi, I., Colditz, G. A., Ascherio, A., Rimm, E. B., Giovannucci, E., Stampfer, M. J., and Willett, W. C. (1996). A prospective study of social networks in relation to total mortality and cardiovascular disease in men in the USA. *Journal of Epidemiology and Community Health*, **50**, 245–51.

Kawachi, I., Sparrow, D., Kubzansky, L. D., Spiro III, A., Vokonas, P. S., and Weiss, S. T. (1998). Prospective study of a self-report type A scale and risk of coronary heart disease: test of the MMPI-2 type A scale. *Circulation*, **98**, 405–12.

Koskenvuo, M., Kaprio, J., Rose, R. J., Kesaniemi, A., Sarna, S., Heikkila, K., and Langinvainio, H. (1988). Hostility as a risk factor for mortality and ischemic heart disease in men. *Psychosomatic Medicine*, **50**, 330–40.

Krumholz, H. M., Butler, J., Miller, J., Vaccarino, V., Williams, C. S., Mendes de Leon, C. F. *et al.* (1998). Prognostic importance of emotional support for elderly patients hospitalized with heart failure. *Circulation*, **97**, 958–64.

Kubzansky, L. D., Kawachi, I., Spiro III, A., Weiss, S. T., Vokonas, P. S., and Sparrow, D. (1997). Is worrying bad for your heart? A prospective study of worry and coronary heart disease in the Normative Aging Study. *Circulation*, **95**, 818–24.

Kuh, D. and Ben-Shlomo, Y. (1997). *A life course approach to chronic disease epidemiology*. Oxford University Press, New York.

Lacroix, A. and Haynes, S. (1984). Occupational exposure to high demand/low control work and coronary heart disease incidence in the Framingham cohort. *American Journal of Epidemiology*, **120**, 481.

Ladwig, K. H., Kieser, M., Konig, J., Breithardt, G., and Borggrefe, M. (1991). Affective disorders and survival after acute myocardial infarction: results from the post-infarction late potential study. *European Heart Journal*, **12**, 959–64.

Ladwig, K. H., Roll, G., Breithardt, G., Budde, T., and Borggrefe, M. (1994). Post infarction depression and incomplete recovery 6 months after acute myocardial infarction. *Lancet*, **343**, 20–3.

Lane, D., Carroll, D., Ring, C., Beevers, D. G., and Lip, G. Y. (2000a). Effects of depression and anxiety on mortality and quality-of-life 4 months after myocardial infarction. *Journal of Psychosomatic Research*, **49**, 229–38.

Lane, D., Carroll, D., Ring, C., Beevers, D. G., and Lip, G. Y. (2000b). Do depression and anxiety predict recurrent coronary events 12 months after myocardial infarction? *Quarterly Journal of Medicine*, **93**, 739–44.

Lane, D., Carroll, D., Ring, C., Beevers, D. G., and Lip, G. Y. (2001). Mortality and quality of life 12 months after myocardial infarction: effects of depression and anxiety. *Psychosomatic Medicine*, **63**, 221–30.

Lesperance, F., Frasure-Smith, N., and Talajic, M. (1996). Major depression before and after myocardial infarction: its nature and consequences. *Psychosomatic Medicine*, **58**, 99–110.

Lesperance, F., Frasure-Smith, N., Juneau, M., and Theroux, P. (2000). Depression and 1-year prognosis in unstable angina. *Archives of Internal Medicine*, **160**, 1354–60.

Linden, W., Stossel, C., and Maurice, J. (1996). Psychosocial interventions in patients with coronary artery disease: a meta-analysis. *Archives of Internal Medicine*, **156**, 745–52.

Lynch, J., Krause, N., Kaplan, G. A., Tuomilehto, J., and Salonen, J. T. (1997). Workplace conditions, socioeconomic status, and the risk of mortality and acute myocardial infarction: the Kuopio ischaemic heart disease risk factor study. *American Journal of Public Health*, **87**, 617–22.

Mayou, R. A., Gill, D., Thompson, D. R., Day, A., Hicks, N., Volmink, J., and Neil, A. (2000). Depression and anxiety as predictors of outcome after myocardial infarction. *Psychosomatic Medicine*, **62**, 212–19.

Medalie, J. H. and Goldbourt, U. (1976). Angina pectoris among 10 000 men. II. Psychosocial and other risk factors as evidenced by a multivariate analysis of a five year incidence study. *American Journal of Medicine*, **60**, 910–21.

Medalie, J. H., Snyder, M., Groen, J. J., Neufeld, H. N., Goldbourt, U., and Riss, E. (1973). Angina pectoris among 10,000 men: 5 year incidence and univariate analysis. *American Journal of Medicine*, **55**, 583–94.

Mehta, R. H. and Eagle, K. A. (1998). Secondary prevention in acute myocardial infarction. *British Medical Journal*, **316**, 838–42.

Mendes de Leon, C. F., Krumholz, H. M., Seeman, T. S., Vaccarino, V., Willaims, C. S., Kasl, S. V., and Berkman, L. F. (1998). Depression and risk of coronary heart disease in elderly men and women: New

Haven EPESE, 1982–1991. Established Populations for the Epidemiologic Studies of the Elderly. *Archives of Internal Medicine*, **158**, 2341–8.

Moore, L., Meyer, F., Perusse, M., Cantin, B., Dagenais, G. R., Bairati, I., and Savard, J. (1999). Psychological stress and incidence of ischaemic heart disease. *International Journal of Epidemiology*, **28**, 652–8.

Murberg, T. A., Bru, E., Svebak, S., Tveteras, R., and Aarsland, T. (1999). Depressed mood and subjective health symptoms as predictors of mortality in patients with congestive heart failure: a two-years follow-up study. *International Journal of Psychiatry in Medicine*, **29**, 311–26.

Netterstrom, B. and Suadicani, P. (1993). Self-assessed job satisfaction and ischaemic heart disease mortality: a 10 year follow up of urban bus drivers. *International Journal of Epidemiology*, **22**, 51–6.

Orth-Gomer, K., Rosengren, A., and Wilhelmsen, L. (1993). Lack of social support and incidence of coronary heart disease in middle-aged Swedish men. *Psychosomatic Medicine*, **55**, 37–43.

Orth-Gomer, K., Wamala, S. P., Horsten, M., Schenck-Gustafsson, K., Schneiderman, N., and Mittleman, M. A. (2000). Marital stress worsens prognosis in women with coronary heart disease: the Stockholm Female Coronary Risk Study. *Journal of the American Medical Association*, **284**, 3008–14.

Ostfeld, A. M., Lebovits, B. Z., Shekelle, R. B., and Paul, O. (1964). A prospective study of the relationship between personality and coronary heart disease. *Journal of Chronic Diseases*, **17**, 265–76.

Oxman, T. E., Freeman, D. H. Jr, and Manheimer, E. D. (1995). Lack of social participation or religious strength and comfort as risk factors for death after cardiac surgery in the elderly. *Psychosomatic Medicine*, **57**, 5–15.

Palmer, K. J., Langeluddecke, P. M., and Jones, M. (1992). The relation of the type A behaviour pattern, factors of the structured interview, and anger to survival after myocardial infarction. *Australian Journal of Psychology*, **44**, 13–19.

Penninx, B. W., Guralnik, J. M., Mendes de Leon, C. F., Pahor, M., Visser, M., Corti, M. C., and Wallace, R. B. (1998). Cardiovascular events and mortality in newly and chronically depressed persons >70 years of age. *American Journal of Cardiology*, **81**, 988–94.

Penninx, B. W., Beekman, A. T., Honig, A., Deeg, D. J., Schoevers, R. A., van Eijk, J. T., and van Tilburg, W. (2001). Depression and cardiac mortality: results from a community-based longitudinal study. *Archives of General Psychiatry*, **58**, 221–7.

Perski, A., Feleke, E., Anderson, G., Samad, B. A., Westerlund, H., Ericsson, C. G., and Rehnqvist, N. (1998). Emotional distress before coronary bypass grafting limits the benefits of surgery. *American Heart Journal*, **136**, 510–17.

Pratt, L. A., Ford, D. E., Crum, R. M., Armenian, H. K., Gallo, J. J., and Eaton, W. W. (1996). Depression, psychotropic medication, and risk of myocardial infarction: prospective data from the Baltimore ECA follow-up. *Circulation*, **94**, 3123–9.

Ragland, D. R. and Brand, R. J. (1988a). Coronary heart disease mortality in the western collaborative group study: follow-up experience of 22 years. *American Journal of Epidemiology*, **127**, 462–75.

Ragland, D. R. and Brand, R. J. (1988b). Type A behaviour and mortality from coronary heart disease. *New England Journal of Medicine*, **318**, 65–9.

Reed, D., McGee, D., Yano, K., and Feinleib, M. (1983). Social networks and coronary heart disease among Japanese men in Hawaii. *American Journal of Epidemiology*, **117**, 384–96.

Reed, D. M., Lacroix, A. Z., Karasek, R. A., Miller, D., and MacLean, C. A. (1989). Occupational strain and the incidence of coronary heart disease. *American Journal of Epidemiology*, **129**, 495–502.

Rosengren, A., Tibblin, G., and Wilhelmsen, L. (1991). Self-perceived psychological stress and incidence of coronary artery disease in middle-aged men. *American Journal of Cardiology*, **68**, 1171–5.

Rosenman, R. H., Brand, R. J., Sholtz, R. I., and Friedman, M. (1976). Multivariate prediction of coronary heart disease during 8.5 year follow-up in western collaborative group study. *American Journal of Cardiology*, **37**, 903–9.

Schleifer, S. J., Macari-Hinson, M. M., Coyle, D. A., Slater, W. R., Kahn, M., Gorlin, R., and Zucker, H. D. (1989). The nature and course of depression following myocardial infarction. *Archives of Internal Medicine*, **149**, 1785–9.

Sebregts, E. H., Falger, P. R., and Bar, F. W. (2000). Risk factor modification through nonpharmacological interventions in patients with coronary heart disease. *Journal of Psychosometric Research*, **48**, 425–41.

Sesso, H. D., Kawachi, I., Vokonas, P. S., and Sparrow, D. (1998). Depression and the risk of coronary heart disease in the Normative Aging Study. *American Journal of Cardiology*, **82**, 851–6.

Shekelle, R. B., Gale, M., Ostfeld, A. M., and Paul, O. (1983). Hostility, risk of coronary heart disease and mortality. *Psychosomatic Medicine*, **45**, 109–14.

Shekelle, R. B., Gale, M., and Norusis, M. (1985*a*). Type A score (Jenkins activity survey), and risk of recurrent coronary heart disease in the aspirin myocardial infarction study. *American Journal of Cardiology*, **56**, 221–5.

Shekelle, R. B., Hulley, S. B., Neaton, J. D., Billings, J. H., Borhani, N. O., Gerace, T. A. *et al.* (1985*b*). The MRFIT behavior pattern study. II. Type A behavior and incidence of coronary heart disease. *American Journal of Epidemiology*, **122**, 559–70.

Siegrist, J. (1996). Adverse health effects of high-effort/low-reward conditions. *Journal of Occupational Health Psychology*, **1**, 27–41.

Siegrist, J., Peter, R., Junge, A., Cremer, P., and Seidel, D. (1990). Low status control, high effort at work and ischemic heart disease: prospective evidence from blue-collar men. *Social Science and Medicine*, **31**, 1127–34.

Steenland, K., Johnson, J., and Nowlin, S. (1997). A follow up study of job strain and heart disease among males in the NHANES1 population. *American Journal of Industrial Medicine*, **31**, 256–60.

Suadicani, P., Hein, H. O., and Gynetelberg, F. (1993). Are social inequalities as associated with the risk of ischaemic heart disease a result of psychosocial working conditions? *Atherosclerosis*, **101**, 165–75.

Theorell, T. and Floderus-Myrhed, B. (1977). 'Workload' and risk of myocardial infarction: a prospective psychosocial analysis. *International Journal of Epidemiology*, **6**, 17–21.

Tunstall-Pedoe, H., Woodward, M., Tavendale, R., Brook, R. A., and McCluskey, M. K. (1997). Comparison of the prediction by 27 different factors of coronary heart disease and death in men and women of the Scottish heart health study: cohort study. *British Medical Journal*, **315**, 722–9.

Vogt, T., Mullooly, J., Ernst, D., Pope, C., and Hollis, J. (1992). Social networks as predictors of ischemic heart disease, cancer, stroke and hypertension: incidence, survival and mortality. *Journal of Clinical Epidemiology*, **45**, 659–66.

Vogt, T., Pope, C., Mullooly, J., and Hollis, J. (1994). Mental health status as a predictor of morbidity and mortality: a 15-year follow-up of members of a health maintenance organization. *American Journal of Public Health*, **84**, 227–31.

Wassertheil-Smoller, S., Applegate, W. B., Berge, K., Chang, C. J., Davis, B. R., Grimm, R., Jr *et al.* (1996). Change in depression as a precursor of cardiovascular events: SHEP Cooperative Research Group (Systolic Hypertension in the elderly). *Archives of Internal Medicine*, **156**, 553–61.

Welin, C., Lappas, G., and Wilhelmsen, L. (2000). Independent importance of psychosocial factors for prognosis after myocardial infarction. *Journal of Internal Medicine*, **247**, 629–39.

Whiteman, M. C., Deary, I. J., Lee, A. J., and Fowkes, F. G. (1997). Submissiveness and protection from coronary heart disease in the general population: Edinburgh Artery Study. *Lancet*, **350**, 541–5.

Williams, R. B., Barefoot, J. C., Califf, R. M., Haney, T. L., Saunders, W. B., Pryor, D. B. *et al.* (1992). Prognostic importance of social and economic resources among medically treated patients with angiographically documented coronary artery disease. *Journal of the American Medical Association*, **267**, 520–4.

Woloshin, S., Schwartz, L. M., Tosteson, A. N., Chang, C. H., Wright, B., Plohman, J., and Fisher, E. S. (1997). Perceived adequacy of tangible social support and health outcomes in patients with coronary artery disease. *Journal of General Internal Medicine*, **12**, 613–18.

Chapter 25

Mental illness and coronary heart disease

S. Stansfeld and F. Rasul

25.1 Introduction

Mental illnesses, particularly severe illnesses such as psychosis, have long been associated with an increased risk of mortality (Schoevers *et al.* 2000). Besides mental illness-related causes of death such as suicide, it has been assumed that people with severe mental illness live less healthy lives, tending to have higher rates of smoking, and paying little attention to a healthy diet and to taking sufficient exercise. In addition, they may be further put at risk by alcohol and prescribed and non-prescribed drug use. However, in recent years there has also been evidence that less severe mental illness such as depressive and anxiety disorders may influence the aetiology and progression of CHD (CHD). At present it is helpful to distinguish the effects of these disorders on the aetiology and prognosis of CHD (Fig. 25.1).

Current evidence suggests that these effects are not specific to a single type of mental illness. Major depressive illness, minor depressive illness, and depressive symptoms have been associated with increased CHD risk (Barefoot and Schroll 1996; Ford *et al.* 1998), and phobic anxiety and even worrying have been associated with sudden death from cardiac causes (Kawachi *et al.* 1994*a*; Kubzansky *et al.* 1997). Also, non-specific psychological distress and less clear-cut conditions such as vital exhaustion have been associated with electrocardiographic evidence of CHD and increased mortality risk (Appels and Otten 1992). As yet it is not clear whether there is one underlying mechanism for these effects mediated through a single neurohormonal or biochemical pathway. The diversity of the effects suggests that even if affective disorder acts on CHD through a single mechanism it may act at different points in the pathogenic pathway.

This chapter describes the evidence linking mental illness and CHD, the associations between mental illness and risk factors for CHD, and the potential mechanisms through which mental illness may affect the heart.

25.2 Depression and CHD

Ideally, there should be studies in which structured interview measures of depressive illness are related prospectively to the incidence of CHD. In this way the link between precisely defined

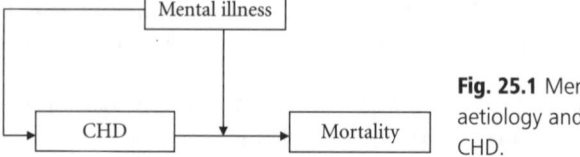

Fig. 25.1 Mental illness and the aetiology and prognosis of CHD.

types of mental illness and CHD could be tested. Until this has been achieved it is not certain the psychological measures used in current studies are indicative of primary mental illness. However, there have been prospective studies of depressive illness assessed by various proxy measures that have been linked to CHD (Table 25.1).

In the Johns Hopkins precursor's study (Ford *et al.* 1998) a cohort of medical students were followed up for 37 years. Depressive illness was measured by response to questions about depression and associated treatment rated by a panel of independent experts. The cohort was largely men in whom depressive illness was associated with an almost double risk of CHD measured as myocardial infarction, angina pectoris, chronic ischaemic heart disease, requirement for angioplasty, and bypass surgery.

One case control study that based a diagnosis of depression on Read-codes taken from British General Practice records found that men were three times more likely to develop CHD than control subjects (Hippisley-Cox *et al.* 1998). This risk was not found for CHD in women. The risk in men persisted after adjustment for smoking, diabetes mellitus, hypertension, and deprivation score. It is likely that depressive illness in this primary care sample was milder than that treated in secondary psychiatric care but, nevertheless, the diagnosis of depression does have some validity in this study.

25.3 Depressive symptoms and CHD morbidity and mortality

Whereas there have been few studies attempting to relate case-defined mental illness to CHD, there have now been several studies that have found longitudinal associations between questionnaire measures of depressive symptoms and both CHD morbidity (Anda *et al.* 1993; Barefoot and Schroll 1996; Sesso *et al.* 1998) and mortality (Ariyo *et al.* 2000) (Table 25.1). The questionnaires used have measured a range of overlapping constructs, including depressive thoughts, feelings of depression, pessimism, and hopelessness. Associations have particularly been found for depressive thoughts and hopelessness. In fact, moderate and severe hopelessness were related in a dose–response fashion with increasing risk of CHD (Anda *et al.* 1993).

It is not entirely clear what these depressive symptoms scales are measuring. It does not seem to be neuroticism or negative affectivity, as scales that measure this mood-dispositional dimension of negative emotionality, including nervousness, anger, and dissatisfaction, do not predict CHD mortality (Costa 1987). It may be that these symptomatic measures are identifying underlying severe depressive illness. In this case, respondents are checking questionnaire items relating to depression, scoring highly on scales that are designed to identify symptoms but not necessarily depressive illness. While people with depressive illness will score highly on scales of depressive symptoms, there are two reasons why depressive illness is unlikely to be the main construct measured by these scales. First, the prevalence of high scores on depressive symptom instruments is higher than the expected prevalence of depressive illness in the community. Second, repeated measures of depressive symptoms over a considerable time interval suggest that these measures are relatively stable over time, which would not be in keeping with the episodic nature of depressive illness.

A further possibility is that these measures of depressive symptoms are contaminated by the presence of physical ill health. Some of these scales contain non-specific symptoms such as sleep disturbance or fatigue which might equally be the result of a physical illness rather than depression. Most studies of depressive symptoms and CHD incidence have dealt with this either by excluding subjects with physical ill health at baseline (Anda *et al.* 1993; Ariyo *et al.* 2000; Sesso *et al.* 1998) or adjusting their analyses for physical ill health at baseline

Table 25.1 Prospective studies of the association between depression and CHD

Author and year	Total sample	Age at entry/sample	Depression measure	CHD measure	Follow-up (years)	Number of NF and F events	Adjustments	Relative risk	Summary
Anda 1993	2832	45–77 Community sample	General Well Being Scale	NF/F IHD	16	205 NF IHD, 189 F IHD	Age, sex, race, MS, SMK, CHOL, PASBP, BMI, ALC	NF 1.6 (1.10–2.40), F 1.5 (1.00–2.30)	Depressed affect and hopelessness predict F/NF IHD
Ariyo 2000	5888	65+ Community sample	CES-D	CHD, MI, angina, all-cause mortality	6	606 F/NF CHD, 270 F/NF MI, 298 NF angina, 614 deaths	Age, sex, race, ED, DIAB, HYP, SMK, CHOL, TGC, PA, HF	CHD 1.11 (1.01–1.22), MI 1.12 (0.97–1.29), angina 1.13 (0.99–1.29), death 1.13 (1.03–1.23)	Depressive symptoms an independent risk for CHD and mortality
Barefoot and Schroll 1996	730	60 Community sample	MMPI sub-scale (OBD)	Acute MI, all-cause mortality	10	122 NF, 290 F	Age, sex, SW, SL, SBP, TGC, SMK	MI 1.7 (1.23–2.34), death 1.6 (1.29–2.11)	Depressive symptoms predict MI and mortality
Ferketich 2000	7893	30–70+ Community sample	CES-D	F/NF CHD	11	Men: 187 NF, 137 F; women: 187 NF, 129 F	Age, race, SMK, HYP, PI, BMI, DIAB, NF-CHD	NF CHD men 1.7 (1.1–2.6), F 2.3 (1.5–3.6); NF CHD women 1.7 (1.1–2.7) F 0.74 (0.4–1.5)	Depression associated with increased risk of CHD in men and women, and CHD death in men
Ford 1998	1190	26 (average) Male medical students	Self-report of treatment of depression	CHD, MI	40	163 NF	SMK, COF, CHOL, HYP, DIAB, PA, PMI	CHD 2.1 (1.24–2.63), MI 2.1 (1.11–4.06)	Depression. Independent long-term predictor of MI and CHD
Mendes de Leon 1998	2391	65–99 Community sample	CES-D	NF MI, CHD mortality	9	208 NF, 255 F	Age, DIAB, EDUC, ANG, SMK, SBP, DBP	Men 0.99 (0.67–1.02), women 1.03 (1.01–1.05)	Depressive symptoms independent predictors of CHD only in women
Stansfeld 2002	10 308	35–55 Male and female occupational cohort	GHQ-30	CHD, abn. ECG	5	Men: 400 NF CHD, 163 abn. ECG; women: 252 NF CHD, 57 abn. ECG	Age, diet, SMK, ALC, BMI, EMP GRADE, FUP LENGTH	Men CHD 1.83 (1.5–2.3), ECG 1.54 (1.1–2.2); Women CHD 1.46 (1.1–2.0), ECG 0.66 (0.3–1.3)	Psychological distress increases risk of CHD in men but not women
Sesso 1998	1305	21–80 Community sample	MMPI-2-DEP, SCL-90	F/NF CHD	14	30 NF, 20 F	Age, BMI, SMK, ALC, SBP, DBP, FH	CHD 1.5 (0.82–2.58), MMPI 1.6 (0.93–2.64) SCL-90	Depressive symptoms possibly related to CHD

abn: abnormal; ALC: alcohol; ANG: angina; F: fatal; BMI: body mass index; CHOL: cholesterol; COF: coffee; DBP: diastolic blood pressure; DIAB: diabetes; EDUC: education; EMP GRADE: employment grade; FH: family history; FUP LENGTH: follow-up length; HF: heart failure; HYP: hypertension; MS: marital status; NF: non-fatal; PA: physical activity; PI: poverty index; PMI: parental myocardial infarction; SBP: systolic blood pressure; SL: sedentary leisure; SMK: smoking; SW: sedentary work.

(Barefoot and Schroll 1996; Ferketich *et al.* 2000). Often such adjustments have reduced the size of the effect, but not eliminated it. However, it is difficult to be certain that there is not some residual confounding from physical ill health. This may especially be the case because existing physical ill health may not always be identified at baseline in these studies, which employ the necessarily crude screening instruments used in large epidemiological studies. It is possible, as discussed below, that depression may have the largest effect in people who already have early CHD. Indeed, in Western populations it is difficult to find young adults who have not already developed a degree of atherosclerosis (Enos *et al.* 1953; McNamara *et al.* 1971). Therefore, ill health at baseline may be largely a matter of degree of ill health.

25.4 **Psychological distress, physical illness, and CHD**

While many studies suggest an independent association between psychological distress, usually depression, and CHD the origin of psychological distress is unclear. It is possible that either psychological distress reflects some underlying, undetected, chronic, physical ill health which influences CHD risk, or that psychological distress is indicative of depressive illness that still confers risk irrespective of any underlying chronic condition.

If it is accepted that psychological distress is a consequence of the pain, discomfort, and loss of functioning of some chronic condition of ill health, which also influences CHD risk, then the distress–CHD relationship can be explained by underlying physical ill health. Some studies have suggested that the association of psychological distress and CHD is explained by adjustment for physical ill health (Fredman *et al.* 1999).

Similarly, other studies have found that depressive symptoms are associated with mortality only among people in poor health (Black and Markides 1999; Fredman *et al.* 1999). Thus, mortality risk was greater in elderly Mexican men and women with chronic medical conditions and comorbid depression than those with a chronic medical condition but without depression, supporting a pathway explanation. Diabetic patients with depression had a three-fold greater mortality risk than diabetic patients without depression (Black and Markides 1999).

Is the risk of CHD morbidity and mortality associated with psychological distress confined only to people with physical ill health? The evidence seems to suggest it is not. In stratified analyses of women with, and without, baseline physical impairment of function there was a clear association between depression and CHD mortality in women without impairment of physical functioning (Mendes de Leon and Krumholz 1998). Similarly, other studies that have adjusted for pre-existing ill health such as cancer, stroke, diabetes, and past myocardial infarction (MI) still find an increased CHD risk associated with psychological distress (Everson *et al.* 1996; Ferketich *et al.* 2000; Penninx *et al.* 1998). It is plausible, however, that even after adjustment for ill health there remains some residual confounding. This may be the case particularly where self-report measures of ill health have been used in adjustment or the presence of undetected subclinical disease affects both psychological distress and CHD risk. An analytical strategy designed to deal with confounding effects of subclinical disease is to exclude the first 2 years of follow-up in the belief that this will eliminate participants with subclinical disease and therefore control the impact of subclinical disease on psychological distress and CHD. Adopting such a strategy, depression was still associated with non-fatal and fatal CHD in men and with non-fatal CHD in women (Ferketich *et al.* 2000). Therefore, these results strongly suggest that the association between psychological distress and CHD is not explained by subclinical disease.

One other strategy to control for the confounding effects of physical illness has been to develop measures of psychological distress, which specifically exclude symptoms scored positively by those with physical ill health. The 30-item general health questionnaire (GHQ), which measures depressive and anxiety disorders, was derived from the 60-item GHQ precisely to avoid contamination by physical illness. A study that used the GHQ-30 (Stansfeld *et al.* 2002) found that psychological distress was associated with an increased risk of self-reported CHD in men and women and ECG abnormalities only in men. However, the GHQ is a non-specific screening measure for psychological distress and it is still possible that it is identifying a decline in physical, as well as mental, functioning.

In summary, there is some evidence to indicate that the association between psychological distress and CHD morbidity and mortality is accounted for by pre-existing physical illness. In terms of causality, this would indicate that psychological distress is on the pathway between physical ill health and CHD risk. However, there is still sufficient and consistent evidence to suggest psychological distress is an aetiological agent that influences CHD risk independently of pre-existing physical ill health.

A useful classification of psychological risk factors for CHD based on duration of risk and proximity to cardiac events has been developed by Kop (1999). Chronic psychological factors such as hostility are distinguished from episodic psychological factors that have a duration ranging from several months to up to 2 years, and from other psychological risk factors such as anger or mental activity which may act as immediate triggers of cardiac events. Depression is included as an episodic risk factor, although it might also reasonably be considered as a chronic risk factor if dysthymia, recurrent episodic depression, and chronic pessimism are included. The elucidation of how the different manifestations of depression might fit in this model is an important future research goal.

25.5 Vital exhaustion and CHD

One episodic risk factor allied to depression is vital exhaustion made up of lack of energy, increased irritability, and demoralization. Most people who are depressed are also exhausted, but there is a subgroup who are exhausted but do not have the symptoms of sadness, guilt, and loss of self worth typical of depression (Kop 1999).

Exhaustion is a substantial predictor of MI within an 18-month period before the cardiac event (Appels and Mulder 1988; Appels and Schouten 1991). Because of its proximity to cardiac events, it has been supposed that it results from underlying cardiac insufficiency. However, the degree of exhaustion seems to be unrelated to exercise-induced ischaemia, electrocardiographic abnormalities, cardiac pump function, and the severity of CHD measured by angiography (Kop 1999; Kop *et al.* 1996). If fatigue is not a consequence of impaired cardiac function, it might be related to prolonged exposure to environmental stressors, or possibly to an inflammatory process.

Further precision in the definition of these psychological syndromes preceding CHD, and more specifically, cardiac events, would be helpful in elucidating the pathways between psychological states and cardiac pathophysiology.

25.6 Anxiety states and CHD

Overall, the evidence is established that depressive states are both aetiologically and prognostically associated with an increased CHD morbidity and mortality risk. However, an issue is whether other mental states/illnesses are also associated with CHD morbidity and mortality. Now, there is some evidence that less severe mental states such as anxiety are also associated with increased CHD morbidity and mortality (Table 25.2).

The evidence linking anxiety states to CHD mortality has come from studies of healthy subjects in the general population and also from subjects with established CHD. In one British prospective study of middle-aged men followed up for 6 years using the Crown–Crisp Index as a measure of phobic anxiety Haines et al. (1987) found that phobic anxiety was associated with an almost four-fold increased risk of fatal CHD. The association was present even after adjustment for CHD risk factors and was specific to fatal CHD. In another prospective follow-up study of over 33 000 male health professionals, again using the phobic anxiety scale of the Crown–Crisp Index, Kawachi et al. (1994a) found that men with an anxiety score of 4 or more had almost two and a half times greater risk of fatal CHD than men with a score of 0 or 1. Moreover, there was a dose–response relationship, such that risk of fatal CHD increased with levels of phobic anxiety. When fatal CHD was further categorized into sudden and non-sudden death the increased risk was confined to sudden death. Men with anxiety scores of 3 or more had a relative risk of 6.08 (95% confidence interval (CI): 2.35–15.73). These associations remained relatively unchanged after adjustment for CHD risk factors. However, phobic anxiety was not associated with risk of non-fatal MI or total CHD.

An explanation for the increased CHD mortality risk associated with phobic anxiety may be to do with drugs prescribed to treat phobic anxiety. Tricyclic antidepressants are known to promote arrhythmias (Roose and Glassman 1994) and are not recommended in patients with known ischaemic heart disease (Glassman 1998). However, their potential role in the aetiology of ischaemic heart disease is unclear. It may that their use is the underlying mechanism that contributes to the increased CHD risk. There is evidence linking psychotropic drugs, especially tricyclic antidepressants, with increased risk of MI (Penttinen and Valonen 1996; Thorogood et al. 1992), and ischaemic heart disease (Hippisley-Cox et al. 2001). It is not clear, however, whether the increased risk is associated with the adverse drug side effects or the underlying condition leading to their prescription. Further analysis by Kawachi et al. (1994a) provided evidence to support the view that it is in fact the underlying condition rather than adverse drug side effects that are associated with increased mortality risk. Analysis of a subgroup of men receiving no medication had similarly elevated risk of fatal CHD (Kawachi et al. 1994a).

The study by Kawachi et al. (1994a) specifically assessed the relationship between phobic anxiety and fatal CHD in male health professionals. Although the studies by Kawachi et al. demonstrated an increased risk of fatal CHD associated with phobic anxiety in male health professionals, it was not clear whether the risk would generalize to community samples and whether the risk was associated only with phobic anxiety or would be found with other anxiety disorders. These issues were examined in the Normative Aging Study (Kawachi et al. 1994b), a longitudinal community study of 2280 men in Greater Boston. In age-adjusted analysis anxiety was associated only with increased risk of fatal CHD (odds ratio (OR): 3.20, 95% CI: 1.27–8.09), but which became non-significant in multivariate analysis after adjustment for other factors related to anxiety (OR: 1.94, 95% CI: 0.70–5.41). Anxiety was not associated with other outcomes such as non-fatal CHD, MI, or total CHD in age adjusted or multivariate analysis. However, in further multivariate analyses, stratifying death as sudden or non-sudden, raised anxiety was associated with sudden death in men scoring 1 (OR: 2.96, 95% CI: 1.02–8.55) and also with men scoring 2 or more (OR: 4.46, 95% CI: 0.92–21.6) compared to men scoring 0 on the anxiety scale. Anxiety was not associated with non-sudden causes of death.

Table 25.2 Prospective studies of the association between anxiety and CHD

Author and year	Total sample	Age at entry/ sample	Anxiety measure	CHD measure	Follow-up (years)	Number of NF and F events	Adjustments	Relative risk	Summary
Haines 1987	3500	40–64 Occupational groups	Crown–Crisp Index	NF/F IHD	6	57 NF IHD, 56 F IHD		NF 1.26 (0.62–2.54), F 3.77 (1.64–8.64)	Phobic anxiety associated with CHD
Kawachi 1994a	51 529	40–75 Health professionals	Crown–Crisp Index	NF/F IHD	2	128 NF, 140 F	Age, SMK, CHOL, HYP, DIAB, FH, BMI, ALC, PA	NF 0.89 (0.45–1.79), F 2.45 (1.00–5.96)	An association between phobic anxiety and F CHD
Kawachi 1994b	2280	21–80 Community sample	5-item anxiety scale from Cornell Medical Index	NF/F IHD	32	137 NF, 131 F	Age, BMI, SBP, DBP, CHOL, ALC, SMK, FH	NF 0.71 (0.24–2.09), F 1.94 (0.70–5.41)	An association between anxiety and CHD
Kubzansky 1997	2280	21–80 Community sample	Worry scale	NF/F CHD	20	113 NF, 86 F	Age, DIAB, CHOL, BMI, FH, ALC, SMK, SBP, DBP	NF 2.41 (1.40–4.13), F 0.81 (0.45–1.44)	Worrying increases the risk of CHD

Anxiety is not a unitary concept and is made up of cognitive, behavioural, and biological components. Worry is related to the cognitive component of anxiety (Borkovec *et al.* 1983). Dysfunctionally high levels of worry are associated with anxiety disorders, so much so that extreme or chronic worriers fit the diagnostic and statistical manual of mental disorder (DSM-III-R) category of generalized anxiety disorder (Barlow 1988). Kubzansky *et al.* (1997) investigated the relationship between worry and CHD in the Normative Aging Study. Worry was assessed by a scale measuring five domains: social conditions, health, finances, self-definition, and ageing. Both moderate and high level worries about social conditions were associated with an increased risk of non-fatal MI adjusting for confounding factors in multivariate analysis. A one-unit increase in health worries was associated with a modest increase in risk of angina pectoris and with twice the risk of sudden cardiac death. Similarly, a one unit increase in financial worries was associated with a modest increase in risk of CHD, including angina, in age-adjusted analysis. Thus, not only anxiety but also worrying may be a risk factor for CHD in men.

25.7 Mental illness and CHD risk factors

As many epidemiological studies have suggested an independent association between depression and CHD morbidity and mortality, what plausible mechanisms may explain this association? Depression may be associated with changes in the balance between parasympathetic and sympathetic nerve activity, for example, either an increase in sympathetic nerve activity, a decrease in parasympathetic nerve activity, or both. Raised sympathetic activity may be associated with coronary vasospasm and increased allostatic load and the development of the metabolic syndrome predisposing to CHD (Julius and Nesbitt 1996).

One plausible pathway is that depression may lead to a poorer CHD risk factor profile, for example increased smoking, increased body weight, higher concentration of cholesterol, and high blood pressure. There is considerable evidence that depressed people have a poorer CHD risk factor profile (Lesperance *et al.* 1996). If these CHD risk factors are associated with depression might they be the link between depression and CHD?

What is the evidence that CHD risk factors are associated with depression? Studies linking depression to CHD risk factors may answer the question about whether or not the effects of depression on CHD morbidity and mortality are mediated through CHD risk factors, that is, increased smoking, raised cholesterol, hypertension, and increased body mass index (BMI).

Smoking is clearly associated with CHD morbidity and mortality, but to what extent is it associated with depression? A greater prevalence of psychological disorder has been found amongst smokers than non-smokers, even after taking into account various indicators of socio-economic circumstances (Anda *et al.* 1990; Jorm 1999; Rasul *et al.* 2001; Schoenborn and Horm 1993; Son *et al.* 1997). Psychological distress may make people more prone to take up smoking and less able to give up. Alternatively, smoking may give rise to psychological distress, perhaps related to repeated palliating of withdrawal symptoms (Jarvis 2002). It is plausible that the effects of psychological distress on CHD might be mediated through smoking. The effect of depression on CHD is more pronounced in smokers than non-smokers (Anda *et al.* 1993; Ford *et al.* 1998). However, differences in smoking status cannot entirely account for these findings, as the effect of depression on CHD morbidity and mortality was also found in non-smokers, and adjusting for the effects of smoking diminished the association between depression and CHD but did not remove it. Depression appears to increase risk of CHD morbidity and mortality independently of its association with cigarette smoking.

Hypertension, increased body weight, and raised cholesterol are conventionally associated with increased risk of CHD morbidity and mortality. It could be that the observed association between depression and increased CHD risk is mediated through the association of depression with these risk factors. Some studies have reported higher rates of depressive symptoms associated with hypertension (Coelho *et al.* 1999) raised cholesterol levels (Segers and Mertens 1976), and obesity (Carpenter *et al.* 2000; Haukkala and Uutela 2000; Istavan *et al.* 1992) while many others have not (Goldberg *et al.* 1980; Mann 1984; Monk 1980; Rasul *et al.* 2002; Roberts *et al.* 2000; Simonsick *et al.* 1995; Wardle 1994).

Generally, the evidence for the association between these CHD risk factors and depression is not strongly established. In a review of studies of the association between psychological well being and cholesterol the balance of evidence suggested a link between depression and low, rather than raised, levels of cholesterol (Wardle 1994). If raised cholesterol is not associated with depression, the effects of depression on CHD risk are unlikely to be mediated through raised cholesterol levels. Additionally, the evidence for a positive association between CHD risk factors and depression has come mainly from cross-sectional or correlational studies (Carpenter *et al.* 2000; Coelho *et al.* 1999; Haukkala and Uutela 2000; Istvan *et al.* 1992; Segers and Mertens 1976). The results from cross-sectional studies are less convincing than results from prospective studies, as they do not address whether CHD risk factors are related to onset of depression. Where depression has been examined prospectively as a precursor to hypertension (Simonsick *et al.* 1995), or obesity (Roberts *et al.* 2000), no association between these CHD risk factors and depression has been observed.

Possible mechanisms for the association of mental illness and CHD, morbidity, and mortality

One of the most plausible mechanisms, as discussed above, is that mental illness influences health behaviours such as smoking, eating an unhealthy diet, and taking little exercise (Bhui 2002). As has already been discussed, these may contribute only somewhat to the association between depression and CHD. If this is the case, what other possible pathways are there?

25.8 Early life and personality factors

There is increasing evidence that the seeds of future CHD are sown in infancy or even *in utero* (Barker and Osmond 1986). Might the same be true for psychosocial risk? Intriguing experiments in rats suggest that increased maternal attention to rat pups may lead to changes in adrenocortical receptors through increased expression of the gene, enabling the glucocorticoid receptor that establishes a lifelong predisposition to decreased adrenocortical responses to environmental stressors (Meaney *et al.* 1993). If this were paralleled in humans it could provide an explanation for physiological hyper-reactivity and damage to the cardiovascular system. Enduring negative emotional predispositions such as hostility, which may have roots in earlier life, have proved to be predictors of CHD (Barefoot *et al.* 1983; Shekelle *et al.* 1983; Williams *et al.* 1980). It is possible that depression or anxiety symptoms may be associated with hostility. This could arise either because hostility is a predictor of mental illness, or because people with high levels of hostility also score highly on mental illness screening instruments. Alternatively, depressive symptoms, hostility, hopelessness, and irritability in combination with vital exhaustion (Kop *et al.* 1996) all form part of a syndrome of pessimism and depressed mood that predicts CHD.

25.9 Adverse psychosocial circumstances

Exposure to acute life events, and to more chronic 'major difficulties' such as strained relationships with partners, financial problems, and poor housing are risk factors for depression (Brown and Harris 1978). Social isolation is a risk factor for both depression and CHD. Similarly, depression can be an outcome of a poor psychosocial work environment with high levels of demands, low social support at work, and low perceived control over work (Stansfeld et al. 1999). Low control at work has also been identified as a risk factor for CHD morbidity and mortality. Given these findings, could mental illness, especially depression, be an intervening variable between adverse psychosocial exposures both at work and at home and CHD? This hypothesis is not supported by findings from the Whitehall II study of British civil servants, in which the predictive power of low control on self-reported CHD was not diminished by adjustment for psychological distress (Bosma et al. 1998).

An alternative possibility is that depression is an outcome of adverse social circumstances but is not on the pathway to CHD. This would imply that the association between depression and CHD was an artefact of the association between adverse social circumstances, sometimes summarized as adverse social position, and CHD. It is difficult to entirely gainsay this explanation. However, many studies linking depression to CHD have adjusted for measures of social position or have examined relatively homogeneous social groups where social position has not been an issue and have still found associations between depression and CHD (Ford et al. 1998; Stansfeld et al. 2002). There is a further potential pathway, that mental illness leads to deterioration in working conditions or to reduced social support, which in turn predict CHD. Evidence from the Whitehall II study, linking psychological distress in men to increased risk of self-reported CHD and electrocardiographic abnormalities, and self-reported heart disease in women, suggest that the elevated coronary risk associated with psychological distress was not explained by health behaviours, social support, work characteristics, or hostility (Stansfeld et al. 2002).

25.10 Post-MI depression and mortality

Mental illness also has important effects in people who have already experienced a serious cardiac event. Traumatic life-threatening events like MI are often followed by depression. Major depression is present within 15–20% of patients following MI (Carney et al. 1987; Schleifer et al. 1989). Although major depressive episodes following MI are not uncommon, depressive symptoms are more prevalent. Schleifer et al. (1989) found prevalence rates of 18 and 27% for major and minor depression in MI patients. In another study moderate depression was more prevalent than severe depression, 22% compared to 14%, in men 3 weeks after MI (Ladwig et al. 1994).

Although the presence of post-MI depression is unrelated to severity of cardiac illness, it nevertheless has independent adverse effects on a patient's prognosis (Ladwig et al. 1994; Schleifer et al. 1989). For example, post-MI depression is associated with an increased mortality risk (Ahern et al. 1990; Frasure-Smith 1991; Frasure-Smith et al. 1993; Ladwig et al. 1991). Patients with high levels of post-MI depression are less likely to survive the first year than patients without, and also are more likely to die of cardiac causes over the subsequent 5 years than other patients (Ahern et al. 1990; Frasure-Smith 1991). The most convincing evidence comes from a prospective follow-up study of 222 patients from whom structured psychiatric examinations were obtained 5–15 days after they had suffered MI (Frasure-Smith et al. 1993).

During 6 months of follow-up 12 patients had died due to cardiac causes, 17% of the depressed and 3% of the non-depressed patients. Post-MI depression was associated with an almost six-fold increased risk in mortality in unadjusted analyses. After adjustment for other independent predictors of risk (previous MI, Killip class, left ventricular dysfunction, prescription of warfarin at discharge) the mortality risk for depressed patients was almost three and a half times greater than for non-depressed patients. This increased mortality risk was not due to more severe CHD amongst depressed patients at baseline 7 days after MI.

Is post-MI mortality risk associated only with major depression? Frasure-Smith *et al.* (1995) examined the relationship between major depression, depressive symptoms, and mortality using a modified version of the Diagnostic Interview Schedule (DIS) and the Beck Depression Inventory (BDI) (Beck *et al.* 1961). Multivariate analyses showed that both the DIS and the BDI were associated with an increased 18-month cardiac mortality risk. However, although the impact of major depression on cardiac mortality remained significant during the 18-month follow-up period, its impact occurred primarily in the first 6 months. Among patients who survived to 6 months major depression did not predict mortality. In contrast, the impact of BDI scores on mortality remained over time. After controlling for other significant predictors of mortality (previous MI, Killip class, premature ventricular contractions) BDI scores remained significantly associated with 18-month cardiac mortality (adjusted OR: 6.64, 95% CI: 1.76–25.09). However, the increased mortality risk associated with post-MI depression is not merely confined to the immediate hospitalization period or the initial months following hospitalization. Studies with longer follow-up times suggest that post-MI depression may be persistent or frequently recurrent in CHD patients and is associated with triggering cardiac events or progression of CHD or both (Barefoot *et al.* 1996). Compared with non-depressed coronary artery disease (CAD) patients, those with moderate to severe depression at baseline had an 84% greater mortality risk 5–10 years later and a 72% greater mortality risk after more than 10 years.

The distinction between major depression and depressive symptomatology may have little meaning in terms of prognosis in cardiac disease. Both may be presentations of the same chronic affective illness that is either persistent or recurrent over time, and independent of disease comorbidity (Ladwig *et al.* 1994). Further, the prognostic impact of depression is not limited to MI patients but has been demonstrated in patients with unstable angina (Lesperance *et al.* 2000). Using the BDI, depressed patients were more likely to experience cardiac death or non-fatal MI in the following year than non-depressed patients. The impact of depression remained after controlling for other significant prognostic factors, including baseline electrocardiographic evidence of ischaemia, left ventricular ejection fraction, and the number of diseased coronary vessels (adjusted OR: 6.73, 95% CI: 2.34–18.64). Thus, depression following an episode of unstable angina increased the risk of a cardiac event during the following year.

25.11 Mechanisms linking mental illness and CHD risk

There may be both common and individual mechanisms linking different types of mental illness with CHD. Elevated anxiety levels may promote ventricular arrhythmias and hence sudden death. Additionally, intense psychological states may affect neural input to the heart leading to fatal arrhythmias (Lown 1987). Furthermore, the lack of an association between phobic anxiety and non-fatal CHD, but a positive association with sudden cardiac death, suggests that different mechanisms may be involved to that in depression and CHD.

Low heart rate variability (HRV) has also been implicated as another pathophysiological mechanism. Chronically anxious patients have reduced HRV in response to stressors.

Men reporting higher levels of phobic anxiety had a higher heart resting rate and lower HRV even after adjusting for age, mean heart rate, and BMI (Kawachi *et al*. 1995). The effect of chronic exposure to adverse circumstances may be mediated through worrying, leading to chronic physiological arousal. Financial, social, and environmental conditions may impact on CHD through heightened arousal. Secondly, worrying implies a lack of control and lack of control, especially in the workplace, is known to contribute increased CHD risk (Bosma *et al*. 1997).

Mental illness, particularly depression, may induce biochemical and physiological changes, although these tend to be associated with more severe conditions. These include sympatho-adrenal hyperactivity, hypothalamic pituitary adrenal axis hyperactivity, diminished HRV, ventricular instability, and myocardial ischaemia in relation to mental stress and alterations in platelet receptors (King 1997). Sympatho-adrenal hyperactivity with raised plasma levels of noradrenaline represents a state marker of depression (Musselman *et al*. 1998), which may modify the function of circulating platelets and lipids. As with anxiety, HRV is decreased in depressed patients compared with non-depressed groups, predisposing to ventricular arrhythmias (Miyawaki and Salzman 1991).

Another mechanism that might be responsible for the association of depression and CHD is common vascular pathology affecting both the coronary arteries and arteries in the brain. In this case depression might be the outcome of cerebrovascular lesions (Stansfeld and Fuhrer 2002). A 'vascular depression' syndrome has been described in highly selected clinical samples. This is more likely to have an onset after 60 years, less likely to have a family history of depression, and more likely to be non-psychotic, also having more cognitive impairment, more retardation, less agitation, less guilt, and less insight (Alexopoulos *et al*. 1997; Krishnan *et al*. 1997). Vascular depression has been associated with lesions in the subcortical grey matter, deep white matter, and periventricular grey matter. In a community-based population study of elderly people, non-basal ganglia lesions identified on magnetic resonance imaging were associated with depressive symptoms adjusting for age, sex, history of stroke, and transient ischaemic attack. This association was abolished, however, after adjustment for cognitive and physical function. Thus either the brain lesion that creates the disability is also independently associated with depressive symptoms or the onset of depression is a reaction to the development of disability. Vascular depression might be an explanation for the association of depression and CHD in the elderly, but seems unlikely to explain how the experience of depression in early life leads to the much later development of CHD.

A number of potential behavioural and physiological mechanisms have been proposed to explain the relationship between post-MI depression and increased mortality risk. The direct effects of post-MI depression on CHD morbidity and mortality may involve at least two different pathophysiological mechanisms: ventricular arrhythmias and altered platelet function. It is conceivable that a combination of a vulnerable myocardium after an MI, acute ischaemia, and psychological distress may trigger fatal ventricular arrhythmias. Frasure-Smith *et al*. (1995) observed that the excess mortality amongst post-MI patients was due almost exclusively to sudden death. Frasure-Smith *et al*. investigated whether there was an interaction between depression and post-MI ventricular arrhythmias. They found a noticeable increase in mortality amongst post-MI patients who had both depression and even mild ventricular arrhythmias. In another study Jiang *et al*. (1996) found that mental stress-induced ischaemia in patients with CAD was associated with significantly higher rates of fatal and non-fatal cardiac events, independent of age, baseline left ventricular ejection fraction, and previous MI. The results were interpreted to suggest that the relationship between psychological stress and adverse cardiac events is mediated by myocardial ischaemia. This is likely as MI is the most significant factor in predisposition to ventricular instability (Musselman *et al.* 1998).

Altered platelet function, specifically platelet aggregability and heightened susceptibility to activation, have also been suggested as mechanisms linking post-MI depression and future coronary events, leading from plaque to coronary occlusion and then to a coronary event. A study by Musselman *et al.* (1996) found that, compared to a control group, depressed patients showed heightened susceptibility to platelet activation and changes in aggregation. The increased propensity for platelets to aggregate amongst depressed patients could be the reason for future coronary events.

There are also behavioural explanations linking depression with poor prognosis post-MI. Depression affects patients' abilities to cope with challenges and has a negative impact on compliance with medication and rehabilitation, including diet and exercise regimes. Severely depressed patients showed poorer adherence to prescribed medication (Ziegelstein *et al.* 1999). Frasure-Smith *et al.* (1995) found that depressed patients were more likely to continue smoking following MI. A number of studies have found consistent associations between increased CHD mortality risk and low levels of social support following MI (Farmer *et al.* 1996). It may be that the degree and quality of social support following MI influences subsequent mortality risk. Specifically, Berkman *et al.* (1992) suggested that lack of emotional support might be the mechanism by which social isolation exerts its effects to increase mortality risk following MI. They found that subjects with no emotional support were three times more likely to die 6 months after an MI than those who had one or more sources of support. Alternatively, it may be that social support exerts its effects through depression. However, studies that have examined the effects of social isolation and depression on mortality risk suggest that they have independent effects, and the effects of social isolation on increased mortality risk post-MI is not mediated through depression (Fuhrer *et al.* 1999; Horsten *et al.* 2000). The results of the ENRICHD randomized trial in 2481 post-MI patients demonstrated that a psychosocial intervention based on cognitive behaviour therapy and group therapy with selective serotonin reuptake inhibitor antidepressants did not improve event-free survival in intervention patients in comparison to a control group given usual care (Berkman *et al.* 2003). However, there was an improvement in depression and social isolation. It is possible the interventions were not sufficiently powerful to make changes that would affect the risk of new events within the follow-up period, but this study does not provide evidence for a causal role for depression in progression of CHD in post-MI patients.

25.12 Conclusions

In summary there is evidence that (a) depression is an independent predictor of CHD morbidity and mortality; (b) exhaustion is a predictor in the 18 months before cardiac events; (c) phobic anxiety predicts sudden cardiac death; and (d) depression post-MI predicts increased mortality rates. There is much that still needs to be understood about these associations, not least the pathophysiological pathways that underlie these associations.

In future research there is a need for better definition of the psychological variables, so that the risk factors are more specific and so that current depressive symptoms, depressive illness, vital exhaustion, and long-term pessimism/hopelessness can be distinguished in the same studies. Although smoking and lack of exercise may be partial mediators of the depression–CHD relationship, this does not seem to be the entire explanation. In fact, health behaviours may be more important in the association between depression and mortality in post-MI patients than in the aetiology of CHD.

It seems likely that pre-existing ill health or functional decline may precede depression in some instances which subsequently carry increased cardiovascular risk. In epidemiological studies more stringent investigation of baseline health and examination of the link between depression and early evidence of CHD is needed.

Kop's distinction between chronic and episodic risk factors and acute triggers of CHD is a useful one (Kop 1999). This provides a framework for future investigations and avoids the somewhat artificial distinction between aetiological and prognostic factors, given that atherosclerosis develops long before there is evidence of clinical CHD. Nevertheless, it is possible that risk factors such as depression have a different impact after a major cardiac trauma such as MI.

Ultimately this research can only be taken forward by gaining a better understanding of the biological mechanisms through which psychological states influence CHD (this is explored in the next chapter). This should help to refine the research questions and point the way to more suitable interventions to reduce CHD risk.

Acknowledgements

We would like to thank Lisa Kass for her help in preparing this chapter. Farhat Rasul was supported by the British Heart Foundation (Grant No PG/98170) during the first stage of writing this chapter.

References

Ahern, D. K., Gorkin, L., Anderson, J. L., Tierney, C., Hallstrom, A. Ewart, C. *et al.* (1990). Cardiac Arrhythmia Pilot Study (CAPS). Investigators: Biobehavioral variables and mortality or cardiac arrest in the Cardiac Arrhythmia Pilot Study (CAPS) study. *American Journal of Cardiology*, **66**, 59–62.

Alexopoulos, G. S., Meyers, B. S., Young, R. C., Kakuma, T., Silversweig, D., and Charlson, M. (1997). Clinically defined vascular depression. *American Journal of Psychiatry*, **154**, 562–5.

Anda, R. F., Williamson, D. F., Escobedo, L. G., Mast, E. E., Giovino, G. A., and Remington, P. L. (1990). Depression and the dynamics of smoking: a national perspective. *Journal of the American Medical Association*, **264**, 1541–5.

Anda, R., Williamson, D., Jones, D., Macera, C., Eaker, E., Glassman, A., and Marks, J. (1993). Depressed affect, hopelessness and the risk of ischaemic heart disease in a cohort of U. S. adults. *Epidemiology*, **4**, 285–94.

Appels, A. and Mulder, P. (1988). Excess fatigue as a precursor of myocardial infarction. *European Heart Journal*, **9**, 758–64.

Appels, A. and Otten, F. (1992). Exhaustion as precursor of cardiac death. *British Journal of Clinical Psychology*, **31**, 351–6.

Appels, A. and Schouten, E. (1991). Burnout as a risk factor for coronary heart disease. *Behavioural Medicine*, **17**, 53–9.

Ariyo, A. A., Haan, M., Tangen, C. M., Rutledge, J. C., Cushman, M., Dobs, A., and Furberg C. D. (2000). Depressive symptoms and risks of coronary heart disease and mortality in elderly Americans. *Circulation*, **102**, 1773–9.

Barefoot, J. C. and Schroll, M. (1996). Symptoms of depression, acute myocardial infarction, and total mortality in a community sample. *Circulation*, **93**, 1976–80.

Barefoot J. C., Dahlstrom, W. G., and Williams R. B. (1983). Hostility, CHD incidence, and total mortality: a 25-year follow-up study of 255 physicians. *Psychosomatic Medicine*, **45**, 59–63.

Barefoot, J. C., Helms, M. J., Mark, D. B., Blumenthal, J. A., Califf, R. M., Haney, T. L. *et al.* (1996). Depression and long-term mortality risk in patients with coronary artery disease. *American Journal of Cardiology*, **78**, 613–17.

Barker, D. J. P. and Osmond, C. (1986). Infant mortality, childhood nutrition and ischaemic heart disease in England and Wales. *Lancet*, **i**, 1077–81.

Barlow, D. H. (1988). *Anxiety and its Disorders*. Guilford Press, New York.

Beck, A. T., Ward, C. H., Mendelson, M., Mock, J., and Erbaugh, J. (1961). An inventory for measuring depression. *Archives of General Psychiatry*, **4**, 561–71.

Berkman, L. F., Leo-Summers, L., and Horwitz, R. I. (1992). Emotional support and survival after myocardial infarction: a prospective, population-based study of the elderly. *Annals of Internal Medicine*, **117**, 1003–9.

Berkman, L. F., Blumenthal, J., Burg, M., Carney, R. M., Catellier, D., Cowan, M. J. *et al.* (2003). Effects of treating depression and low perceived support on clinical events after myocardial infarction: the Enhancing Recovery in Coronary Heart Disease Patients (ENRICHD) Randomized Trial. *Journal of the American Medical Association*, **289**, 3106–16.

Bhui, K. S. (2002). Physical activity and stress. In *Stress and the heart* (ed. S. A. Stansfeld and M. G. Marmot), pp. 158–67. BMJ Books, London.

Black, S. A. and Markides, K. S. (1999). Depressive symptoms and mortality in older Mexican Americans. *Annals of Epidemiology*, **9** (1), 45–52.

Borkovec, T. D., Robinson, E., Pruzinsky, T., and Dupree, J. (1983). Preliminary explanation of worry: some characteristics and processes. *Behaviour Research and Therapy*, **21**, 9–16.

Bosma, H., Marmot, M. G., Hemingway, H., Nicholson, A., Brunner, E. J., and Stansfeld, S. A. (1997). Low job control and risk of coronary heart disease in the Whitehall II (prospective cohort) study. *British Medical Journal*, **314**, 558–65.

Bosma, H., Stansfeld, S. A., and Marmot, M. G. (1998). Job control, personal characteristics and heart disease. *Journal of Occupational Health Psychology*, **3**, 402–9.

Brown, G. W. and Harris, T. (1978). *Social origins of depression*. Tavistock, London.

Carney, R. M., Rich, M. W., Tevelde, A., Saini, J., Clarke, K., and Jaffe, A. S. (1987). Major depressive disorder in coronary artery disease. *American Journal of Cardiology*, **63**, 1273–5.

Carpenter, K. M., Hasin, D. S., Allison, D. B., and Faith, M. S. (2000). Relationships between obesity and DSM-IV major depressive disorder, suicide ideation, and suicide attempts: results from a general population study. *American Journal of Public Health*, **90**, 251–7.

Coelho, R., Santos, A., Ribeiro, L., Gama, G., Prata, J., Barros, H., and Polonia, J. (1999). Difference in behaviour profile between normotensive subjects and patients with white-coat and sustained hypertension. *Journal of Psychosomatic Research*, **46**, 15–27.

Costa, P. (1987). Influence of the normal personality dimension of neuroticism on chest pain symptoms and coronary artery disease. *American Journal of Cardiology*, **60**, 20–6.

Enos, W. F., Holmes, R. H., and Beyer, J. (1953). Coronary disease among United States soldiers killed in action in Korea. *Journal of the American Medical Association*, **152**, 1090–3.

Everson, S. A., Goldberg, D. E., Kaplan, G. A., Cohen, R. D., Pukkala, E., Tuomilehto, J., and Salonen, J. T. (1996). Hopelessness and risk of mortality and incidence of myocardial infarction and cancer. *Psychosomatic Medicine*, **58**, 113–21.

Farmer, I. P., Meyer, P. S., Ramsey, D. J., Goff, D. J., and Wear, M. L. (1996). Higher levels of social support predict survival following acute myocardial infarction: the Corpus Christi Heart Project. *Behavioural Medicine*, **22**, 59–66.

Ferketich, A. K., Schwartzbaum, J. A., Frid, D. J., and Moeschberger, M. L. (2000). Depression as an antecedent to heart disease among women and men in the NHANES I study. *Archives of Internal Medicine*, **160**, 1261–8.

Ford, D. E., Mead, L. A., Chang, P. P., Cooper-Patrick, L., Wang, N., and Klag, M. J. (1998). Depression is a risk factor for coronary artery disease in men: The Precursors Study. *Archives of Internal Medicine*, **158**, 1422–6.

Frasure-Smith, N. (1991). In-hospital symptoms of psychological stress as predictors of long term outcome after acute myocardial infarction in men. *American Journal of Cardiology*, **67**, 121–7.

Frasure-Smith, N., Lesperance, F., and Talajic, M. (1993). Depression following myocardial infarction: impact on 6-month survival. *Journal of the American Medical Association*, **270**, 1819–25.

Frasure-Smith, N., Lesperance, F., and Talajic, M. (1995). Depression and 18-month prognosis after myocardial infarction. *Circulation*, **91**, 999–1005.

Fredman, L. F., Magaziner, J., Hebel, R., Hawkes, W., and Zimmerman, S. I. (1999). Depressive symptoms and 6-year mortality among elderly community dwelling women. *Epidemiology*, **10**, 54–9.

Fuhrer, R., Dufouil, C., Antonucci, T. C., Shipley, M. J., Helmer, C., and Dartigues, J. F. (1999). Psychological disorder and mortality in French older adults: do social relations modify the association? *American Journal of Epidemiology*, **149**, 116–26.

Glassman, A. (1998). Cardiovascular effects of antidepressant drugs: updated. *Journal of Clinical Psychiatry*, **59** (15), 8–13.

Goldberg, E. L., Comstock, G. W., and Graves, C. G. (1980). Psychosocial factors and blood pressure. *Psychological Medicine*, **10**, 243–55.

Haines, A. P., Imeson, J. D., and Meade, T. W. (1987). Phobic anxiety and ischaemic heart disease. *British Medical Journal*, **295**, 297–9.

Haukkala, A. and Uutela, A. (2000). Cynical hostility, depression and obesity: the moderating role of education and gender. *International Journal of Eating Disorders*, **2**, 106–9.

Hippisley-Cox, J., Fielding, K., and Pringle, M. (1998). Depression as a risk factor for ischaemic heart disease in men: population based case-control study. *British Medical Journal*, **316**, 1714–18.

Hippisley-Cox, J., Pringle, M., Hammersley, V., Crown, N., Wynn, A., Meal, A., and Coupland, C. (2001). Antidepressants as risk factor for ischaemic heart disease: case-control study in primary care. *British Medical Journal*, **323**, 666–9.

Horsten, M., Mittleman, M. A., Wamala, S. P., Schenck-Gustaffson, K., and Orth-Gomer, K. (2000). Depressive symptoms and lack of social integration in relation to prognosis in middle-aged women: the Stockholm Female Coronary Risk Study. *European Heart Journal*, **21**, 1043–5.

Istavan, J., Zavelta, K., and Weidner, G. (1992). Body weight and psychological distress in NHANES I. *International Journal of Obesity*, **16**, 999–1003.

Jarvis, M. (2002). Smoking and stress. In *Stress and the heart* (ed. S. A. Stansfeld and M. G. Marmot), pp. 155–7. BMJ Books, London.

Jiang, W., Babyak, M., Krantz, D. S., Waugh, R. A., Coleman, R. E., Hanson, M. M. *et al.* (1996). Mental stress-induced myocardial ischemia and cardiac events. *Journal of the American Medical Association*, **275**, 1651–6.

Jorm, A. F. (1999). Association between smoking and mental disorders: results from an Australian National Prevalence Survey. *Australian and New Zealand Journal of Public Health*, **23**, 245–8.

Julius, S. and Nesbitt, S. (1996). Sympathetic overactivity in hypertension: a moving target. *American Journal of Hypertension*, **9**, 113S–120S.

Kawachi, I., Colditz, G. A., Ascherio, A., Rimm, E. B., Giovannucci, E., Stampfer, M. J., and Willett, W. C. (1994*a*). Prospective study of phobic anxiety and risk of coronary heart disease in men. *Circulation*, **89**, 1992–7.

Kawachi, I., Sparrow, D., Vokonas, P. S., and Weiss, S. T. (1994*b*). Symptoms of anxiety and risk of coronary heart disease: the Normative Aging Study. *Circulation*, **90**, 2225–9.

Kawachi, I., Sparrow, D., Vokonas, P. S., and Weiss, S. T. (1995). Decreased heart rate variability in men with phobic anxiety (data from the Normative Aging Study). *American Journal of Cardiology*, **75**, 882–5.

King, K. B. (1997). Psychologic and social aspects of cardiovascular disease. *Annals of Behavioral Medicine*, **19**, 264–70.

Kop, W. J. (1999). Chronic and acute psychological risk factors for clinical manifestations of coronary artery disease. *Psychosomatic Medicine*, **61**, 476–87.

Kop, W. J., Appels, A., Mendes de Leon, C. F., and Bar, F. W. (1996). The relationship between severity of coronary artery disease and vital exhaustion. *Journal of Psychosomatic Research*, **40**, 397–405.

Krishnan, K. R. R., Hays, J. C., and Blazer, D. G. (1997). MRI-defined vascular depression. *American Journal of Psychiatry*, **154**, 497–501.

Kubzansky, L. D., Kawachi, I., Spiro III, A., Weiss, S. T., Vokonas, P. S., and Sparrow, D. (1997). Is worrying bad for your heart? A prospective study of worry and coronary heart disease in the Normative Aging Study. *Circulation*, **95**, 818–24.

Ladwig, K. H., Kieser, M., Konig, J., Breithardt, G., and Borggrefe, M. (1991). Affective disorders and survival after acute myocardial infarction: results from the post-infarction late potential study. *European Heart Journal*, **12**, 959–64.

Ladwig, K. H., Roll, G., Breithardt, G., Budde, T., and Borggrefe, M. (1994). Post-infarction depression and incomplete recovery 6 months after acute myocardial infarction. *Lancet*, **343**, 20–3.

Lesperance, F., Frasure-Smith, N., and Talajic, M. (1996). Major depression before and after myocardial infarction: its nature and consequences. *Psychosomatic Medicine*, **58**, 99–110.

Lesperance, F., Frasure-Smith, N., and Juneau, M. (2000). Depression and 1-year prognosis in unstable angina. *Archives of Internal Medicine*, **160**, 1354–60.

Lown, B. (1987). Sudden cardiac death: biobehavioral perspective. *Circulation*, **76**, (1, Pt. 2), I186–I196.

Mann, A. H. (1984). Hypertension: psychological aspects and diagnostic impact in a clinical trial. *Psychological Medicine* (Monograph Supplement 5). Cambridge University Press.

McNamara, J. J., Molot, M. A., Stremple, J. F., and Cutting, R. T. (1971). Coronary artery disease in combat casualties in Vietnam. *Journal of the American Medical Association*, **216**, 1185–7.

Meaney, M. J., Bhatnagan, S., Dioria, J., Larocque, S., Francis, D., O'Donnell, D. *et al.* (1993). Molecular basis for the development of individual differences in the hypothalamic-pituitary-adrenal stress response. *Cell Molecular Neurobiology*, **12**, 321–47.

Mendes de Leon, C. F. and Krumholz, H. M. (1998). Depression and risk of coronary heart disease in elderly men and women: New Haven EPESE, 1982–1991. Established Populations for the Epidemiologic Studies of the Elderly. *Archives of Internal Medicine*, **158**, 2341–8.

Miyawaki, E. and Salzman, C. (1991). Autonomic nervous system tests in psychiatry: implications and uses of heart rate variability. *Integrated Psychiatry*, **7**, 21–8.

Monk, M. (1980). Psychological status and hypertension. *American Journal of Epidemiology*, **112**, 200–8.

Musselman, D. L., Tomer, A., Manatunga, A. K., Knight, B. T., Porter, M. R., Kasey, S. *et al.* (1996). Exaggerated platelet reactivity in major depression. *American Journal of Psychiatry*, **153**, 1313–17.

Musselman, D. L., Evans, D. L., and Nemeroff, C. D. (1998). The relationship of depression to cardiovascular disease: epidemiology, biology and treatment. *Archives of General Psychiatry*, **55**, 580–92.

Penninx, B. W. J. H., Guralnik, J. M., Mendes de Leon, C. F., Pahor, M., Visser, M., Corti, M. C., and Wallace, R. B. (1998). Cardiovascular events and mortality in newly and chronically depressed persons >70 years of age. *American Journal of Cardiology*, **81**, 988–94.

Penttinen, J. and Valonen, P. (1996). Use of psychotropic drugs and risk of myocardial infarction: a case-control study in Finnish farmers. *International Journal of Epidemiology*, **25**, 760–2.

Rasul, F., Stansfeld, S. A., Davey Smith, G., Hart, C. L., and Gillis, C. (2001). Socio-demographic factors, smoking and common mental disorder in the Renfrew and Paisley (MIDSPAN) study. *Journal of Health Psychology*, **6**, 149–58.

Rasul, F., Stansfeld, S. A., Davey Smith, G., Hart, C. L., and Gillis, C. (2002). Common mental disorder and physical illness in the Renfrew and Paisley (MIDSPAN) study. *Journal of Psychosomatic Research*, **53**, 1163–70.

Roberts, R. E., Kaplan, G. A., Shema, S. J., and Strawbridge, W. J. (2000). Are the obese at greater risk for depression? *American Journal of Epidemiology*, **152**, 163–70.

Roose, S. and Glassman, A. (1994). Antidepressant choice in the patient with cardiac disease: lessons from the cardiac arrhythmia suppression trial (CAST) studies. *Journal of Clinical Psychiatry*, **55**, (Suppl. A), 83–7.

Segers, M-J. and Mertens, C. (1976). Relationships between anxiety, depression self-ratings and CHD risk factors among obese, normal, and lean individuals. *Journal of Psychosomatic Research*, **20**, 25–35.

Shekelle, R. B., Gale, M., Ostfeld, A. M., and Paul, O. (1983). Hostility, risk of coronary disease and mortality. *Psychosomatic Medicine*, **45**, 219–28.

Sesso, H. D., Kawachi, I., and Vokonas, P. S. (1998). Depression and the risk of coronary heart disease in the Normative Aging Study. *American Journal of Cardiology*, **82**, 851–6.

Schleifer, S. J., Macari-Hinson, M. M., Coyle, D. A., Slater, W. R., Kahn, M., Gorlin, R., and Zucker, H. D. (1989). The nature and course of depression following myocardial infarction. *Archives of Internal Medicine*, **149**, 1785–9.

Schoenborn, C. A. and Horm, J. (1993). Negative moods as correlates of smoking and heavier drinking: implications for health promotion. *Advance Data from Vital and Health Statistics, No. 236*. Hyattsville Maryland, National Center for Health Statistics.

Schoevers, R. M., Geerlings, M. I., Beekman, A. T. F., Penninx, B. W. J. H., Deeg, D. J. H., Jonker, C., and Van Tilburg, W. (2000). Association of depression and gender with mortality in old age. *British Journal of Psychiatry*, **177**, 336–42.

Son, B. K., Markovitz, J. H., Winders, S., and Smith, D. (1997). Smoking, nicotine dependence and depressive symptoms in the CARDIA study: effects of educational status. *American Journal of Epidemiology*, **145**, 110–16.

Simonsick, E. M., Wallace, R. B., Blazer, D. G., and Berkman, L. F. (1995). Depressive symptomatology and hypertension associated morbidity and mortality in older adults. *Psychosomatic Medicine*, **57**, 427–35.

Stansfeld, S. A. and Fuhrer, R. (2002). Depression and coronary heart disease. In *Stress and the heart* (ed. S. A. Stansfeld and M. G. Marmot), pp. 101–23. BMJ Books, London.

Stansfeld, S. A., Fuhrer, R., Shipley, M. J., and Marmot, M. (1999). Work characteristics predict psychiatric disorder: prospective results from the Whitehall II study. *Occupational and Environmental Medicine*, **15**, 302–7.

Stansfeld, S. A., Fuhrer, R., Shipley, M. J., and Marmot, M. G. (2002). Psychological distress as a risk factor for coronary heart disease in the Whitehall II Study. *International Journal of Epidemiology*, **31**, 248–55.

Thorogood, M., Cowen, P., Mann, J., Murphy, M., and Vessey, M. (1992). Fatal myocardial infarction and use of psychotropic drugs in young women. *Lancet*, **340**, 1067–8.

Wardle, J. (1994). Cholesterol and psychological well being. *Journal of Psychosomatic Research*, **39**, 549–62.

Williams, R. B., Haney, T. L., Lee, K. L., Blumenthal, J. A., and Kong, Y. (1980). Type A behavior, hostility, and coronary atherosclerosis. *Psychosomatic Medicine*, **42**, 539–49.

Ziegelstein, R. C., Fauerbach, J. A., Stevens, S. S., Romanelli, J., and Richter, D. P. (1999). Patients with depression are less likely to follow recommendations to reduce cardiac risk during recovery from myocardial infarction. *Archives of Internal Medicine*, **160**, 1818–23.

Chapter 26

Psychophysiology

A. Steptoe

26.1 Introduction

Psychophysiology is concerned with dynamic associations between psychological factors and biological responses (Cacioppo *et al.* 2000). Psychophysiological processes can be defined as the pathways through which psychosocial factors such as emotional states and adverse life experiences influence physiological systems via central nervous system activation of autonomic, neuroendocrine, and immunological responses (Steptoe 1998). The principal psychophysiological methods used in health-related research are laboratory mental stress testing and naturalistic physiological monitoring. Mental stress testing involves the measurement of physiological reactions to, and recovery from, standardized acute emotional or behavioural tasks. Naturalistic monitoring takes the form of repeated measurement of variables such as blood pressure, the electrocardiogram, and cortisol in relation to activities and emotions in everyday life.

Until recently, these methods evolved relatively independently of cardiovascular epidemiological research. They have become important to epidemiology because of the growing acknowledgement of the role of psychosocial factors in coronary heart disease (CHD), reviewed in Chapters 24 and 25. Psychophysiological research contributes to our understanding of the pathways through which psychosocial factors increase risk of CHD prospectively, and trigger cardiac events in people with established CHD. This chapter will summarize applications of psychophysiological methods in CHD epidemiology. I hope to demonstrate that psychophysiological pathways are biologically plausible, and can be studied in ways that illuminate CHD aetiology. The contribution of psychophysiological processes within the multiple determinants of CHD risk will be presented in a schematic model at the end of the chapter.

26.1.1 Psychosocial risk factors and biological processes

There is substantial evidence that psychosocial factors are related both to cardiovascular risk factors and to CHD itself. For example, low socio-economic status is inversely associated with plasma fibrinogen, a pro-coagulant haemostatic profile, and with metabolic factors such as insulin resistance and unfavourable lipid levels (Brunner *et al.* 1996; Matthews *et al.* 1989; Wamala *et al.* 1999*b*). Social isolation and low levels of social support correlate with reduced heart rate variability, the metabolic syndrome, and other physiological variables (Horsten *et al.* 1999; Uchino *et al.* 1996). Adverse job characteristics such as high demands and low control at work are related to elevated rates of hypertension and other cardiovascular risks (Schnall *et al.* 1994). Depression is characterized by an inflammatory cytokine response (Maes 1999), and has also been linked to reduced parasympathetic cardiac tone, and with platelet activation (Hemingway *et al.* 2001; Nemeroff and Musselman 2000).

The question arises as to what causes these associations. Two sets of pathways are likely to be involved. The first is the behavioural pathway, whereby health behaviours such as smoking, food choice, physical activity, and alcohol consumption are influenced by psychosocial factors, and in turn modify CHD risk. For instance, depressed people are more likely to smoke and be physically sedentary than the non-depressed, while low socio-economic status is associated with smoking, patterns of alcohol consumption, dietary choice, and other behaviours (Stansfeld *et al.* 2002; Wardle *et al.* 1999). In the Air Traffic Controllers Health Change study, the accelerated rate of development of hypertension in controllers was found to be mediated by increased alcohol consumption (DeFrank *et al.* 1987).

The second route is the psychophysiological pathway, and involves more direct stimulation of biological dysfunction relevant to CHD. Some of the strongest evidence in favour of psychophysiological mechanisms comes from animal studies. A series of investigations carried out by Kaplan, Manuck, and colleagues have assessed the impact of the social stress caused by repeated disruption of social hierarchies in cynomolgus macaques. Manipulations of this kind lead to vascular endothelial dysfunction, abdominal fat deposition, and accelerated coronary atherosclerosis (Kaplan and Manuck 1999; Williams *et al.* 1993). Although species differences are present, other animal models have demonstrated more rapid progression of atherosclerosis in rabbits (McCabe *et al.* 2002), and hypertension in rodents (Henry *et al.* 1993) with social stress. Animal studies of this kind document an influence of social factors on the development of CHD that cannot be due to variations in diet, age, physical activity, or genetic factors. The complete sequence of disease development, from healthy individual to death, can be observed in a compressed time frame with random allocation of individuals to experimental conditions. However, the specific features in the social environments of animals that stimulate pathological responses are not necessarily the same as those operating in humans.

26.2 Stress responsivity and CHD

Laboratory mental stress testing involves the measurement of physiological responses to standardized stimuli such as problem-solving tasks or emotionally demanding social interactions. Early research often used mental arithmetic and the cold pressor test, but subsequently the array of stimuli has expanded to include speech tasks (involving impromptu public speaking), psychomotor tasks like mirror tracing, and colour/word interference tasks. In children, tasks based on computer games are frequently used. The crucial element is that conditions are perceived as stressful, challenging, and involving.

Two aspects of the physiological responses elicited by mental stress tests are important: reactivity (the magnitude of changes elicited), and recovery (the length of time taken before measures return to reference levels after the tasks are completed). For most physiological variables, high reactivity and delayed recovery are believed to be pathogenic, since they are indicative of dysfunction in physiological regulatory processes (Steptoe 1998). However, there are circumstances in which low physiological reactivity may be characteristic of people experiencing chronic life stress (McEwen 1998).

When applied carefully, mental stress testing induces consistent physiological responses with good test–retest reliability (Jain *et al.* 2001; Kamarck *et al.* 1994). Sophisticated measures of cardiovascular, metabolic, inflammatory, and haemostatic variables can be carried out repeatedly. Confounding factors can be monitored or eliminated, while the experimental manipulation of stimuli allows the causal factors responsible for the physiological responses to be determined. The disadvantages of mental stress testing are that studies are acute, so that only short-term responses are observed, and typically involve reactions to artificial stimuli that rarely occur in the real world. Generalizability across situations may also be an issue, and physiological responses adapt to repeat testing.

Two applications of mental stress testing are particularly relevant to CHD epidemiology. These are its use in the study of pathophysiology, and in the understanding of psychosocial processes.

26.2.1 Impact on pathophysiology

Research with mental stress testing began in the 1950s, when the principal physiological measures were heart rate, blood pressure, and corticosteroid metabolites. In the past decade, interest has focused on whether emotional stress has an impact on physiological parameters that are more directly implicated in atherogenesis.

The early stages of atherogenesis involve vascular endothelial dysfunction and inflammatory processes (Libby *et al.* 2002). Healthy endothelium maintains vascular tone and inhibits smooth muscle cell growth, the adhesion of white blood cells, and platelet aggregation through the production of nitric oxide. Cardiovascular risk factors induce endothelial dysfunction from an early age (Celermajer *et al.* 1992). It has now been shown that acute emotional stress also leads to transient endothelial dysfunction (Ghiadoni *et al.* 2000). In this study, we assessed endothelial dysfunction using the flow-mediated dilatation technique, involving high resolution ultrasound imaging of the brachial artery and its response to endothelial-dependent (reactive hyperaemia) and endothelial independent (glyceryl trinitrate) stimuli. Figure 26.1 illustrates the responses of a group of healthy middle-aged men before, and for up to 240 min after carrying out a stressful 3-min speech task. The saliva cortisol response is also illustrated, and this peaked at 20 min post-stress. It can be seen that stress induced a transient impairment of endothelial function which reached its maximum 90 min after the task, returning to baseline levels after 240 min. No changes were seen in the vascular response to glyceryl trinitrate, so endothelium-independent function was unchanged. There were also no changes in endothelial function in a control session without stress. It is interesting that the endothelial response evolved long after blood pressure and heart rate had returned to reference levels, indicating that a brief psychological stressor can elicit quite prolonged changes in vascular function. These findings have subsequently been replicated in a study that suggested that activation of endothelin-A receptors mediates the endothelial response to mental stress (Spieker *et al.* 2002).

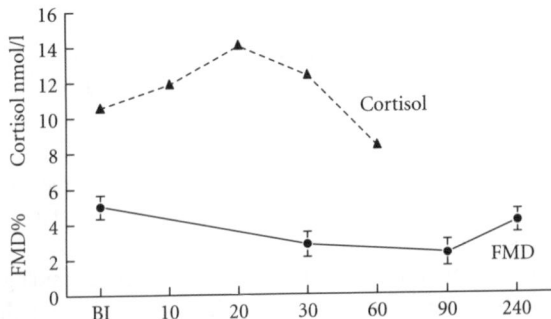

Fig. 26.1 Stress and endothelial dysfunction. Mean levels of flow-mediated dilatation (FMD, solid line), and salivary cortisol (dotted line) in healthy men before (B) and after a stressful speech task. The horizontal axis shows time in minutes after the stress test. Error bars are standard error of the mean. (Data based on Ghiadoni *et al.* 2000.)

Endothelial dysfunction in atherogenesis is associated with platelet activation and inflammatory cytokine release. Interleukin-6 (IL-6) induces endothelial dysfunction and the expression of adhesion molecules, and is also implicated in platelet activation. The cytokines tumour necrosis factor α (TNF-α) and interleukin-1 (IL-1) promote T-cell activation and foam cell formation, and induce macrophage colony stimulating factor. A number of investigators have shown that platelet activation is elevated by psychological stress, and we have shown that acute stress also stimulates increased levels of circulating IL-6 and TNF-α (Markovitz et al. 1996; Wallen et al. 1999). In one study, we found that the increase in IL-6 and TNF-α 2 h post-stress was positively correlated with blood pressure and heart rate during the stress tasks themselves (Steptoe et al. 2001). This suggests that individual differences in the magnitude of cardiovascular stress responses are important, and may partly determine which people are susceptible to psychosocial influences on atherogenic processes. Acute emotional stress affects other pathological processes as well, including low-density lipoproteins and haemostatic variables (Stoney et al. 1999; von Kanel et al. 2001).

Experimental studies also suggest that pathological processes involved in the early stages of atherogenesis are affected by chronic psychosocial factors as well as acute stress. For example, there is substantial evidence that clinical depression is associated with an inflammatory profile, including elevated levels of C-reactive protein, IL-6 and TNF-α (Maes 1999; Zorrilla et al. 2001). It has been demonstrated that endothelial function is impaired in depressed compared with non-depressed individuals (Rajagopalan et al. 2001). Heightened platelet activation has also been described in depression (Nemeroff and Musselman 2000).

At the other end of the cardiovascular disease spectrum, mental stress testing has been used to explore the myocardial responses of patients with advanced heart disease (Strike and Steptoe 2002). In one of the earlier studies, Deanfield et al. (1984) used positron emission tomography (PET) to image the hearts of 16 CHD patients while they performed mental arithmetic. Mental stress induced transient myocardial ischaemia in 75% of the sample, as indicated by abnormal regional myocardial perfusion. Since then, numerous studies have been carried out using echocardiography, radionuclide ventrilography, PET, and other techniques to evaluate myocardial function during mental stress (Goldberg et al. 1996; Rozanski et al. 1988). Rates of mental stress-induced myocardial ischaemia vary markedly between studies, depending on the clinical characteristics of the sample, the stressors used, and the imaging technique. These responses are rare in people without coronary artery disease, so ischaemia is most often induced by mental stress in people who already have diseased coronary vessels. Importantly, the large majority of episodes of stress-induced ischaemia are 'silent', and are not accompanied by chest pain. They also occur at a lower haemodynamic load (as indexed by rate–pressure product) than ischaemia induced by physical exercise. Quantitative angiography has shown that vasoconstriction occurs in diseased segments of coronary arteries during mental stress, in place of the dilatation that would be expected in healthy vessels (Yeung et al. 1991). Thus mental stress testing can be used to explore how emotional and behavioural factors affect pathophysiological processes at several stages of CHD aetiology.

26.2.2 Understanding psychosocial processes

The second use of mental stress testing in relation to CHD epidemiology is in understanding how psychosocial processes act on the cardiovascular system. Epidemiological studies have identified associations between CHD and socio-economic status, job control, and social isolation. These effects are accounted for in part by variations in health behaviours such as smoking, diet, alcohol consumption, and physical activity. However, the fact that associations persist in attenuated form when behaviours are taken into account suggests that other processes are involved as well (Lynch *et al.* 1996; Wamala *et al.* 1999*a*). Mental stress testing can illuminate the probable role of psychophysiological pathways. Work of this type has been carried out in relation to social support, job control, and hostility (Markovitz *et al.* 1996; Steptoe 2000; Uchino *et al.* 1996). However, I will illustrate the application of psychophysiological stress testing with research on socio-economic status.

It has been proposed that the social gradient in CHD is mediated in part through chronic stimulation of psychophysiological pathways, leading to low level sustained activation of pathophysiological processes (Steptoe and Marmot 2002). One way of assessing this possibility is to compare the physiological responses to acute mental stress of people of differing socio-economic status, testing the hypothesis that low status individuals are more stress responsive. Early research was inconclusive, with some studies showing heightened cardiovascular stress responsivity in people of lower socio-economic status, while others found the reverse (Carroll *et al.* 1997, 2000; Owens *et al.* 1993). We have argued that two factors are relevant. Firstly, psychophysiological responses need to be assessed in response to stimuli that are appraised similarly by people across the social spectrum. If one group feels more stressed and challenged by tasks than another, then their cardiovascular responses are likely to be greater. Secondly, the recovery as well as the reactivity arm of the psychophysiological stress response should be assessed, since differences in socio-economic status might be manifest through the failure of adaptation following challenge. This hypothesis is derived from the concept of chronic allostatic load developed by McEwen and colleagues (McEwen 1998; McEwen and Seeman 1999).

We carried out a study of psychophysiological reactivity and recovery in men and women from the Whitehall II cohort, recruited from higher, intermediate, and lower grades of employment (Steptoe *et al.* 2002). Ratings were obtained from participants after each task, and confirmed that the stimuli were perceived as equally stressful, challenging, involving, and uncontrollable by participants in different grades. As hypothesized, we found that the most striking differences between groups emerged in the post-stress recovery period, which lasted 45 min. We used the criterion that effective post-stress recovery implied a return to baseline levels. Compared with the higher grade of employment group, the odds of incomplete recovery in the lower grade group were 2.60 (95% confidence interval (CI): 1.20–5.6) for systolic blood pressure and 3.84 (CI: 1.48–10.0) for diastolic blood pressure, adjusting for sex, age, body mass, baseline blood pressure, and pressor reactions to tasks. It was also found that the lower grade of employment group was more likely to show incomplete post-stress recovery of heart rate variability (adjusted odds: 5.91, 95% CI: 1.88–18.6). The latter result is interesting in the light of the evidence that low heart rate variability is a marker of cardiac autonomic function, and predicts incident CHD and poor prognosis following myocardial infarction (Bigger *et al.* 1993; Liao *et al.* 1997). These results from mental stress testing are therefore consistent with the notion that disturbances of psychophysiological processes may partly mediate associations between low socio-economic status and CHD.

26.2.3 Stress reactivity and disease progression

From the clinical perspective, one of the most important questions about mental stress testing is whether it predicts disease, and provides useful information about the development and progression of CHD. This issue places the focus on individual differences in the magnitude of physiological responses, rather than on normative changes in physiological activity with stress. Animal studies indicate that heart rate responses to standard psychological stresses predict the development of coronary atherosclerosis (Manuck *et al.* 1983). An early report from the Seven Countries Study showed that blood pressure reactions to the cold pressor test predicted future CHD (Keys *et al.* 1971), but this has failed to be consistently replicated in later work (Carroll *et al.* 1998; Coresh *et al.* 1992). However, the cold pressor test (involving immersion of a hand or foot in iced water) is not simply a psychological stressor, but also a physiological stimulus involving reflex haemodynamic adjustments. Subsequent research has centred on whether responses to mental stress tests predict hypertension or increases in tonic blood pressure within the normal range. Again, the literature has been inconsistent, although a number of investigations have demonstrated that blood pressure or heart rate stress reactions make a significant contribution to the prediction of future blood pressure, independently of factors such as resting blood pressure and body weight (Steptoe 1997). In addition, stress-induced reactivity predicts left ventricular mass and the progression of carotid atherosclerosis (Georgiades *et al.* 1997; Jennings *et al.* 2004). Blood pressure stress reactivity (assessed as the anticipatory response to exercise) has also been found to predict 11-year incidence of stroke in middle-aged men independently of other risk factors (Everson *et al.* 2001).

Three factors need to be taken into account in considering the predictive role of stress responses. The first is that longitudinal studies have concentrated thus far on blood pressure and heart rate reactions, and not on stress responses in the more fundamental biological processes summarized earlier. Secondly, any influence of stress reactivity has to be set against the array of genetic, environmental, and behavioural factors that are known to affect CHD progression, and may indeed interact with these other factors in determining risk. Thirdly, mental stress testing assesses the propensity of the individual to respond to psychological challenges with large or small physiological adjustments. Whether this propensity is expressed depends on exposure to conditions that provoke stress responses in everyday life. Thus high stress reactivity per se may not predict future cardiovascular disease if people do not experience conditions in their lives that elicit responses (Steptoe and Cropley 2000). Interestingly, analyses of the Kuopio study have shown that cardiovascular stress reactivity predicts the progression of coronary atherosclerosis most strikingly in combination with high workplace demands and low socio-economic status (Everson *et al.* 1997; Lynch *et al.* 1998).

Evidence is also emerging that stress-induced myocardial ischaemia predicts the progression of CHD in patients with established coronary artery disease. At least four studies have been published to date that have followed patients for up to 5 years, and documented death, infarction, or other cardiac outcomes in relation to stress-induced ischaemia. These studies are summarized in Table 26.1. Different methods of assessing stress-induced ischaemia and adverse cardiac outcomes have been used across the studies; the number of adverse outcomes was smaller in the most recent investigation (Sheps *et al.* 2002), since the end point was death rather than non-fatal cardiac events. However, in each study, patients who demonstrated stress-induced myocardial ischaemia were more likely to have an adverse outcome than those who were stress-negative, and this effect was independent of severity of coronary artery disease and other clinical risk factors. An earlier study documented similar effects in a cohort of Italian patients (Specchia *et al.* 1991), but the end points were limited to revascularization and did not include major cardiac events. All these findings add weight to the evidence that mental stress testing is not only useful in understanding disease processes, but also provides important prognostic information.

Table 26.1 Mental stress-induced myocardial ischaemia (MSIMI) as a predictor of cardiac events in patients with CHD

Author	Patients	Mental stressor	Duration of follow-up (months)	Adverse cardiac outcomes	Adverse cardiac outcomes and MSIMI		Other factors
					MSIMI positive (%)	MSIMI negative (%)	
Jain et al. 1995	30 men, mean age 64	Mental arithmetic	12	Death, non-fatal MI, unstable angina requiring hospitalization	60	20	MSIMI defined as LVEF decrease ≥5%; positive and negative MSIMI groups do not differ demographically, on treadmill testing, or on myocardial perfusion imaging
Jiang et al. 1996	112 men, 14 women, mean age 59	Mental arithmetic, public speech, mirror tracing, interview	44	Death, non-fatal MI, revascularization	27.4	11.9	MSIMI defined as LVEF decrease ≥5%, new wall motion abnormality on radionuclide ventriculography, or ST segment depression; MSIMI effect significant after adjusting for age, history of MI, and baseline LVEF; no differences in risk factors
Krantz et al. 1999	76 men, 3 women, mean age 58	Mental arithmetic, public speech	42	Death, non-fatal MI, revascularization	44	23.5	MSIMI defined as wall motion abnormality on radionuclide ventriculography or echocardiography; positive and negative MSIMI groups do not differ demographically or on cardiovascular risk factors
Sheps et al. 2002	170 men, 26 women, mean age 63	Public speech, Stroop task	62	All-cause mortality	16.2	6.2	MSIMI defined as wall motion abnormality on radionuclide ventriculography; MSIMI effect significant after adjusting for age, history of MI, baseline LVEF, history of diabetes, hypertension, and duration of exercise tolerance test

References are the publications in which the MSIMI findings were originally presented.

LVEF: left ventricular ejection fraction;

MI: myocardial infarction.

26.3 **Naturalistic monitoring and CHD risk**

The second method used in psychophysiology is naturalistic monitoring in everyday life. Technical developments have lead to a substantial increase in the application of this method over the past two decades. In particular, ambulatory blood pressure monitoring allows relatively unobtrusive repeated measurement over the day and night in people going about their everyday lives. With Holter monitoring, heart rate, heart rate variability, and myocardial ischaemia can be assessed outside the clinic, while the measurement of hormones like cortisol and dehydroepiandrosterone (DHEA) sulfate from saliva has greatly expanded the opportunities for neuroendocrine assessment.

The great advantage of naturalistic monitoring is that it permits direct measurements of the impact of everyday experience on physiological functioning. The intricate social interactions and experiences that people have in their lives are impossible to replicate in the laboratory. By linking physiological measures with diary ratings of activities, moods, and social interaction, it is possible to come to a better understanding of how feelings and experiences covary with physiology in real-life situations. In addition, ambulatory measures of blood pressure and myocardial ischaemia themselves provide information of immediate clinical significance.

The limitations of naturalistic monitoring must also be recognized. The range of biological variables that can be measured is rather small compared with the laboratory. Physiological functions in everyday life are influenced by many factors, notably physical exercise, but also sleep patterns, posture, smoking, alcohol, and caffeine intake. Taking account of all these factors in order to demonstrate an independent effect of psychophysiological stimulation requires detailed measurement by paper or electronic diaries, together with advanced multilevel statistical techniques (Fahrenberg and Myrtek 2001). In addition, periods of naturalistic monitoring may not be entirely representative of normal life. People may restrict their activities, because they are embarrassed by the monitoring procedure, find it inconvenient in certain settings, or because they want to present a favourable cardiovascular risk profile. Using objective measures of energy expenditure, we have found that people are less active on a day of ambulatory blood pressure monitoring than on other days (Costa *et al.* 1999). Since cardiovascular activity is related to energy expenditure, this means that measures of blood pressure and heart rate are likely to be affected.

There are a number of applications of naturalistic monitoring in CHD epidemiology, and its potential will be illustrated here by studies of working life.

26.3.1 **Work, control, and psychophysiology**

There is an extensive epidemiological literature relating work characteristics to CHD, implicating factors such as low control, high demands coupled with low control (job strain), and effort–reward imbalance in disease risk (Steenland *et al.* 2000). One of the mechanisms that may mediate these effects is blood pressure elevation. Persistently raised blood pressure at work may either contribute directly to the development of hypertension, or else be a marker for the activation of other biological processes linked with atherogenesis. Ambulatory blood pressure monitoring has been crucial in establishing this link. Several studies have related blood pressure recorded at work to job characteristics, and have shown that blood pressure is raised in men in high demand/low control jobs. The association is more consistent for ambulatory blood pressure than for blood pressures measured casually or in clinic settings. For example, a French study of workers in a chemical company showed that diastolic blood pressure was on average 4.5 mmHg higher at work in high job-strain participants compared with the remainder, while there were no differences in casual measures or blood pressure monitored outside work (Fauvel *et al.* 2001). A 3-year reassessment of 195 men working in New York revealed that systolic pressure was on average 11.1 mmHg higher (and diastolic 9.1 mmHg higher) in the workplace in those experiencing persistent high job strain, compared with men who were not exposed at either time point (Schnall *et al.* 1998).

The pattern in women has been less consistent, with a number of studies failing to show clear effects of job strain or effort–reward imbalance (Light *et al.* 1992; Vrijkotte *et al.* 2000). One explanation is that family factors and non-work responsibilities may make a greater contribution to blood pressure in women, or that the obstacles faced by women at work change the nature of work stress, so that concepts such as high demand and low control are less relevant (Brisson *et al.* 1999; Light *et al.* 1995).

Blood pressure reductions in the evening after work are also associated with both job strain and family characteristics. In one study male and female schoolteachers were assessed, with ambulatory blood pressures recorded every 20 min over the working day, and every 30 min in the evening (Steptoe *et al.* 1999). Systolic blood pressure was typically lower after work than during the day, but this difference was smaller in the high job strain participants. People with high strain jobs may fail to unwind in the evening, a response that perhaps parallels the impairment in post-stress recovery observed in laboratory studies.

Attempts to relate cortisol recorded during the working day to factors such as job strain have generated mixed results, partly because the hormone has often been assessed from urine samples taken late in the day, when levels and variability are low (Pollard *et al.* 1996). Measurements from saliva allow cortisol to be monitored repeatedly over the day, so that a profile can be built up. Cortisol shows a marked circadian rhythm of output, with high levels early in the morning followed by gradual reductions over the day and evening. We have found that the high levels of cortisol early in the morning are more sensitive to work stress than are later values. In a study involving saliva sampling at 2-h intervals between 0800 h and 2200 h, it was found that levels were higher in people reporting job strain, but only in the first sample of the day; subsequently, the output of cortisol was identical in high and low job strain groups (Steptoe *et al.* 2000).

Naturalistic psychophysiological methods can be used not only to characterize responses to work, but also to investigate mediating processes. One reason why high job strain may increase CHD risk is because of the impact of low control on physiological responses. Animal studies indicate that low control stimulates neuroendocrine activation, immune suppression, and pathological outcomes (Steptoe 2000). In human laboratory studies, tasks over which an individual perceives little control elicit larger blood pressure and heart rate responses than more controllable conditions. It is possible, therefore, that the raised blood pressure at work of people in high strain jobs arises because they are exposed to conditions of low control during the working day.

This notion was tested in an analysis of blood pressures recorded over the day from schoolteachers, selected on the basis of high and low job strain ratings (Steptoe 2001). Blood pressure was measured every 20 min, and each recording was accompanied by a rating of how much control the person felt at the time, ranging from 1 = *no control* to 7 = *complete control*. A comparison was then made of the cardiovascular activity associated with relatively high perceived control (ratings of 6 or 7) and relatively low perceived control (ratings of 1–4). A within-person analysis was carried out, with all the blood pressure and heart rate values during episodes of high control being averaged for every individual, and compared with averages for episodes of low control.

Results are summarized in Fig. 26.2. It can be seen that low perceived control was associated with elevations in systolic pressure, diastolic pressure, and heart rate. Thus the perception

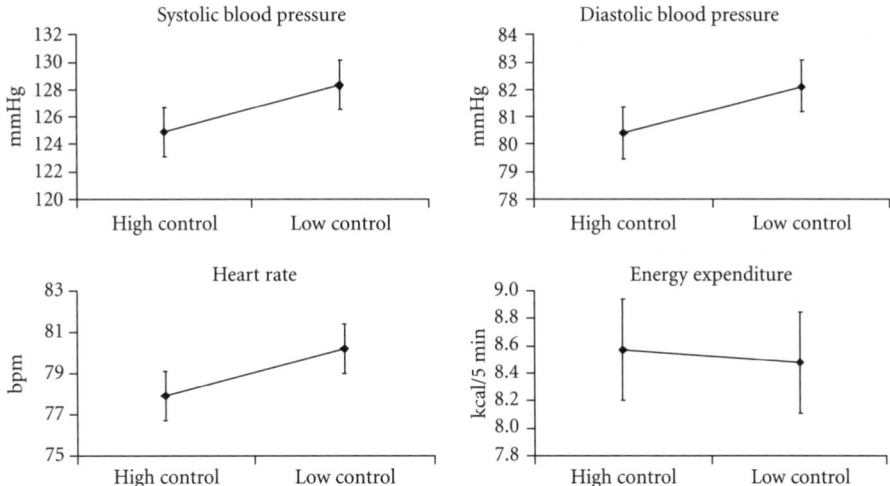

Fig. 26.2 Perceived control and cardiovascular activity at work. Mean levels of systolic pressure, diastolic pressure, heart rate, and energy expenditure during periods of high perceived control and low perceived control over the working day. Error bars are standard error of the mean. (Data based on Steptoe 2001.)

of having little control on a moment-to-moment basis at work stimulates small increases in cardiovascular activity. It is, of course, possible that people are simply more physically active when they feel that they have little control over situations in their lives. Since blood pressure and heart rate are partly dependent on physical activity (Kario *et al.* 1999), this might be an explanation of the pattern shown in Fig. 26.2. This possibility was assessed by measuring energy expenditure with accelerometers, and analysing activity at time points corresponding to blood pressure readings. The data in Fig. 26.2 indicates that there were no differences in energy expenditure between high and low perceived control conditions, so the cardiovascular effects of lack of control were not secondary to physical activity. It is more probable that the blood pressure and heart rate elevations during episodes of low control were stimulated by sympathetic nervous system activation.

Interestingly, there was no difference in the magnitude of the cardiovascular responses to lack of control in participants reporting high and low job strain. Thus, in this naturalistic setting, individuals experiencing high job strain were not more stress reactive to conditions of low perceived control. However, ratings of low perceived control were more frequent in the high job strain group. Thus individuals experiencing high job strain spent more of the day in situations over which they have little control than did the remaining participants. This suggests that the crucial distinction between groups lay not in differences in reactivity, but differences in exposure to adverse psychosocial conditions.

26.4 **Conclusions**

The main contribution that psychophysiology makes to CHD epidemiology at present is in understanding aetiological pathways. Figure 26.3 summarizes the hypothesized processes schematically. Individuals have a propensity to greater or lesser biological stress responsivity, based on a host of factors. These include genetic differences, such as polymorphisms of

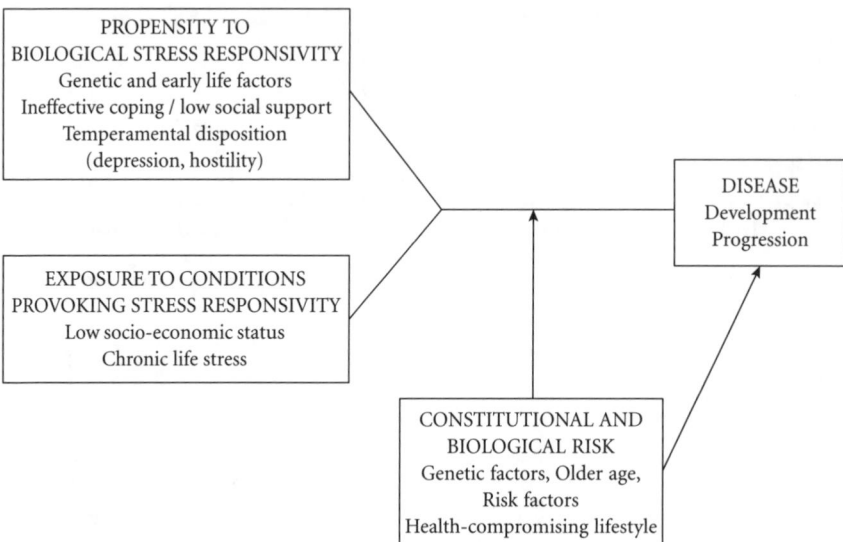

Fig. 26.3 Schematic summary of the contribution of psychophysiological processes to CHD.

beta-adrenergic receptor genes (McCaffery *et al.* 2002), early life factors that affect later responsivity (Heim and Nemeroff 2002), temperamental factors, ineffective coping responses, and lack of social support. The propensity to biological stress responsivity will vary in its expression with the degree of exposure to conditions that elicit responses. Low socio-economic status, for example, might increase the likelihood of expression, since lower status individuals experience greater chronic social stress than more privileged groups (Turner and Marino 1994). Exposure may also be high in racial minorities, due in part to low socio-economic status, and to racial discrimination (Williams and Neighbors 2001). In combination, these factors lead to a situation in which activation of psychophysiological processes occurs on a regular basis for months or years. Whether such responses lead to the development of CHD, or to the progression of disease in people with established CHD, depends on the interplay with constitutional and biological risk factors, and with health behaviours. Delineating these interactions in more detail, and quantifying the impact of psychophysiological processes, are among the main objectives of research over the next decade.

References

Bigger, J. T., Fleiss, J. L., Rolnitzky, L. M., and Steinman, R. C. (1993). The ability of several short-term measures of RR variability to predict mortality after myocardial infarction. *Circulation*, **88**, 927–34.

Brisson, C., Laflamme, N., Moisan, J., Milot, A., Masse, B., and Vezina, M. (1999). Effect of family responsibilities and job strain on ambulatory blood pressure among white-collar women. *Psychosomatic Medicine*, **61**, 205–13.

Brunner, E., Davey Smith, G., Marmot, M., Canner, R., Beksinska, M., and O'Brien, J. (1996). Childhood social circumstances and psychosocial and behavioural factors as determinants of plasma fibrinogen. *Lancet*, **347**, 1008–13.

Cacioppo, J. T., Tassinary, L. G., and Berntson, G. (eds) (2000). *Handbook of psychophysiology*, 2nd edn. Cambridge University Press, New York.

Carroll, D., Davey Smith, G., Sheffield, D., Shipley, M. J., and Marmot, M. G. (1997). The relationship between socioeconomic status, hostility, and blood pressure reactions to mental stress in men: data from the Whitehall II study. *Health Psychology*, **16**, 131–6.

Carroll, D., Davey Smith, G., Willemsen G., Sheffield, D., Sweetnam, P. M., Gallacher, J. E. J., and Elwood, P. C. (1998). Blood pressure reactions to the cold pressor test and the prediction of ischaemic heart disease: data from the Caerphilly Study. *Journal of Epidemiology and Community Health*, **52**, 528–9.

Carroll, D., Harrison, L. K., Johnston, D. W., Ford, G., Hunt, K., Der, G. *et al.* (2000). Cardiovascular reactions to psychological stress: the influence of demographic variables. *Journal of Epidemiology and Community Health*, **54**, 876–7.

Celermajer, D. S., Sorenson, K. E., Gooch, V. M., Spiegelhalter, D. J., Miller, O. I., Sullivan, I. *et al.* (1992). Non-invasive detection of endothelial dysfunction in children and adults at risk of atherosclerosis. *Lancet*, **340**, 1111–15.

Coresh, J., Klag, M. J., Mead, L. A., Liang, K.-Y., and Whelton, P. K. (1992). Vascular reactivity in young adults and cardiovascular disease: a prospective study. *Hypertension*, **19**, II-218–II-223.

Costa, M., Steptoe, A., Cropley, M., and Griffith, J. (1999). Ambulatory blood pressure monitoring is associated with reduced physical activity during everyday life. *Psychosomatic Medicine*, **61**, 806–11.

Deanfield, J. E., Shea, M., Kensett, M., Horlock, P., Wilson, R. A., De Landsheere, C. M. *et al.* (1984). Silent myocardial infarction due to mental stress. *Lancet*, **II**, 1001–4.

DeFrank, R. S., Jenkins, C. D., and Rose, R. M. (1987). A longitudinal investigation of the relationships among alcohol consumption, psychosocial factors, and blood pressure. *Psychosomatic Medicine*, **49**, 236–49.

Everson, S. A., Lynch, J. W., Chesney, M. A., Kaplan, G. A., Goldberg, D. E., Shade, S. B. *et al.* (1997). Interaction of workplace demands and cardiovascular reactivity in progression of carotid atherosclerosis: population based study. *British Medical Journal*, **314**, 553–8.

Everson, S. A., Lynch, J. W., Kaplan, G. A., Lakka, T. A., Sivenius, J., and Salonen, J. T. (2001). Stress-induced blood pressure reactivity and incident stroke in middle-aged men. *Stroke*, **32**, 1263–70.

Fahrenberg, J. and Myrtek, M. (eds) (2001). *Progress in ambulatory assessment*. Hogrefe & Huber, Gottingen.

Fauvel, J. P., Quelin, P., Ducher, M., Rakotomalala, H., and Laville, M. (2001). Perceived job stress but not individual cardiovascular reactivity to stress is related to higher blood pressure at work. *Hypertension*, **38**, 71–5.

Georgiades, A., Lemne, C., De Faire, U., Lindvall, K., and Fredrikson, M. (1997). Stress-induced blood pressure measurements predict left ventricular mass over three years among borderline hypertensive men. *European Journal of Clinical Investigation*, **27**, 733–9.

Ghiadoni, L., Donald, A., Cropley, M., Mullen, M. J., Oakley, G., Taylor, M. *et al.* (2000). Mental stress induces transient endothelial dysfunction in humans. *Circulation*, **102**, 2473–8.

Goldberg, A. D., Becker, L. C., Bonsall, R., Cohen, J. D., Ketterer, M. W., Kaufman, P. G. *et al.* (1996). Ischemic, hemodynamic, and neurohormonal responses to mental and exercise stress: experience from the Psychophysiological Investigations of Myocardial Ischemia Study (PIMI). *Circulation*, **94**, 2402–9.

Heim, C. and Nemeroff, C. B. (2002). Neurobiology of early life stress: clinical studies. *Seminars in Clinical Neuropsychiatry*, **7**, 147–59.

Hemingway, H., Malik, M., and Marmot, M. (2001). Social and psychosocial influences on sudden cardiac death, ventricular arrhythmia and cardiac autonomic function. *European Heart Journal*, **22**, 1082–101.

Henry, J. P., Liu, Y. Y., Nadra, W. E., Qian, C. G., Mormede, P., Lemaire, V. *et al.* (1993). Psychosocial stress can induce chronic hypertension in normotensive strains of rats. *Hypertension*, **21**, 714–23.

Horsten, M., Mittleman, M. A., Wamala, S. P., Schenck-Gustafsson, K., and Orth-Gomer, K. (1999). Social relations and the metabolic syndrome in middle-aged Swedish women. *Journal of Cardiovascular Risk*, **6**, 391–7.

Jain, D., Burg, M., Soufer, A., and Zaret, B. L. (1995). Prognostic implications of mental stress-induced silent left ventricular dysfunction in patients with stable angina pectoris. *American Journal of Cardiology*, **76**, 31–5.

Jain, D., Joska, T., Lee, F. A., Burg, M., Lampert, R., and Zaret, B. L. (2001). Day-to-day reproducibility of mental stress-induced abnormal left ventricular function response in patients with coronary artery disease and its relationship to autonomic activation. *Journal of Nuclear Cardiology*, **8**, 347–55.

Jennings, J. R., Kamarck, T. W., Everson-Rose, S. A., Kaplan, G. A., Manuck, S. B., and Salonen, R. (2004). Exaggerated blood pressure responses during mental stress are prospectively related to enhanced carotid atherosclerosis in middle-aged Finnish men. *Circulation*, **110**, 2198–203.

Jiang, W., Babyak, M., Krantz, D. S., Waugh, R. A., Coleman, R. E., Hanson, M. M. *et al.* (1996). Mental stress-induced myocardial ischemia and cardiac events. *Journal of the American Medical Association*, **275**, 1651–6.

Kamarck, T. W., Jennings, J. R., Pogue-Geile, M., and Manuck, S. B. (1994). A multidimensional measurement model for cardiovascular reactivity: stability and cross-validation in two adult samples. *Health Psychology*, **13**, 471–8.

Kaplan, J. R. and Manuck, S. B. (1999). Status, stress, and atherosclerosis: the role of environment and individual behavior. *Annals of the New York Academy of Sciences*, **896**, 145–61.

Kario, K., Schwartz, J. E., and Pickering, T. G. (1999). Ambulatory physical activity as a determinant of diurnal blood pressure variation. *Hypertension*, **34**, 685–91.

Keys, A., Longstreet, H., Blackburn, H., Brozek, J., Anderson, J. T., and Simonson, E. (1971). Mortality and coronary heart disease among men studied for 23 years. *Archives of Internal Medicine*, **128**, 201–24.

Krantz, D. S., Santiago, H. T., Kop, W. J., Merz, C. N. B., Rozanski, A., and Gottdiener, J. S. (1999). Prognostic value of mental stress testing in coronary artery disease. *American Journal of Cardiology*, **84**, 1292–7.

Liao, D., Cai, J., Rosamond, W. D., Barnes, R. W., Hutchinson, R. G., Whitsel, E. A. *et al.* (1997). Cardiac autonomic function and incident coronary heart disease: a population-based case-cohort study. The ARIC Study. Atherosclerosis Risk in Communities Study. *American Journal of Epidemiology*, **145**, 696–706.

Libby, P., Ridker, P. M., and Maseri, A. (2002). Inflammation and atherosclerosis. *Circulation*, **105**, 1135–43.

Light, K. C., Turner, J. R., and Hinderliter, A. L. (1992). Job strain and ambulatory work blood pressure in healthy young men and women. *Hypertension*, **20**, 214–18.

Light, K. C., Brownley, K. A., Turner, J. R., Hinderliter, A. L., Girdler, S. S., Sherwood, A. *et al.* (1995). Job status and high-effort coping influence work blood pressure in women and blacks. *Hypertension*, **25**, 554–9.

Lynch, J. W., Everson, S. A., Kaplan, G. A., Salonen, R., and Salonen, J. T. (1998). Does low socioeconomic status potentiate the effects of heightened cardiovascular responses to stress on the progression of carotid atherosclerosis? *American Journal of Public Health*, **88**, 389–94.

Lynch, J. W., Kaplan, G. A., Cohen, R. D., Tuomilehto, J., and Salonen, J. (1996). Do cardiovascular risk factors explain the relation between socio-economic status, risk of all-cause mortality, cardiovascular mortality, and acute myocardial infarction? *American Journal of Epidemiology*, **144**, 934–42.

Maes, M. (1999). Major depression and activation of the inflammatory response system. In *Cytokines, stress, and depression* (ed. R. Dantzer, E. E. Wollman, and R. Yirmiya), pp. 25–46. Kluwer, New York.

Manuck, S. B., Kaplan, J. R., and Clarkson, T. B. (1983). Behaviorally induced heart rate reactivity and atherosclerosis in cynomolgus monkeys. *Psychosomatic Medicine*, **45**, 95–102.

Markovitz, J. H., Matthews, K. A., Kriss, J., and Smitherman, T. C. (1996). Effects of hostility on platelet reactivity to psychological stress in coronary heart disease patients and in healthy controls. *Psychosomatic Medicine*, **58**, 143–9.

Matthews, K. A., Kelsey, S. F., Meilahn, E. N., Kuller, L. H., and Wing, R. R. (1989). Educational attainment and behavioral and biologic risk factors for coronary heart disease in middle-aged women. *American Journal of Epidemiology*, **129**, 1132–44.

McCabe, P. M., Gonzales, J. A., Zaias, J., Szeto, A., Kumar, M., Herron, A. J. *et al.* (2002). Social environment influences the progression of atherosclerosis in the Watanabe heritable hyperlipidemic rabbit. *Circulation*, **105**, 354–9.

McCaffery, J. M., Pogue-Geile, M. F., Ferrell, R. E., Petro, N., and Manuck, S. B. (2002). Variability within alpha- and beta-adrenoreceptor genes as a predictor of cardiovascular function at rest and in response to mental challenge. *Journal of Hypertension*, **20**, 1105–14.

McEwen, B. S. (1998). Protective and damaging effects of stress mediators. *New England Journal of Medicine*, **338**, 171–9.

McEwen, B. S. and Seeman, T. (1999). Protective and damaging effects of mediators of stress: elaborating and testing the concepts of allostasis and allostatic load. *Annals of the New York Academy of Sciences*, **896**, 30–47.

Nemeroff, C. B. and Musselman, D. L. (2000). Are platelets the link between depression and ischemic heart disease? *American Heart Journal*, **140**, 57–62.

Owens, J. F., Stoney, C. M., and Matthews, K. A. (1993). Menopausal status influences ambulatory blood pressure levels and blood pressure changes during mental stress. *Circulation*, **88**, 2794–802.

Pollard, T. M., Ungpakorn, G., Harrison, G. A., and Parkes, K. R. (1996). Epinephrine and cortisol responses to work: a test of the models of Frankenhaeuser and Karasek. *Annals of Behavioral Medicine*, **18**, 229–37.

Rajagopalan, S., Brook, R., Rubenfire, M., Pitt, E., Young, E., and Pitt, B. (2001). Abnormal brachial artery flow-mediated vasodilation in young adults with major depression. *American Journal of Cardiology*, **88**, 196–8, A7.

Rozanski, A., Bairey, C. N., Krantz, D. S., Friedman, J., Resser, K. J., Morell, M. *et al.* (1988). Mental stress and the induction of silent myocardial ischemia in patients with coronary artery disease. *New England Journal of Medicine*, **318**, 1005–11.

Schnall, P. L., Landsbergis, P. A., and Baker, D. (1994). Job strain and cardiovascular disease. *Annual Review of Public Health*, **15**, 381–411.

Schnall, P. L., Schwartz, J. E., Landsbergis, P. A., Warren, K., and Pickering, T. G. (1998). A longitudinal study of job strain and ambulatory blood pressure: results from a three-year follow-up. *Psychosomatic Medicine*, **60**, 697–706.

Sheps, D. S., McMahon, R. P., Becker, L., Carney, R. M., Freedland, K. E., Cohen, J. D. *et al.* (2002). Mental stress-induced ischemia and all-cause mortality in patients with coronary artery disease: results from the Psychophysiological Investigations of Myocardial Ischemia study. *Circulation*, **105**, 1780–4.

Specchia, G., Falcone, C., Traversi, E., La Rovere, M. T., Guasti, L., De Micheli, G. *et al.* (1991). Mental stress as a provocative test in patients with various clinical syndromes of coronary heart disease. *Circulation*, **83**, II108–14.

Spieker, L. E., Hurlimann, D., Ruschitzka, F., Corti, R., Enseleit, F., Shaw, S. *et al.* (2002). Mental stress induces prolonged endothelial dysfunction via endothelin-A receptors. *Circulation*, **105**, 2817–20.

Stansfeld, S. A., Fuhrer, R., Shipley, M. J., and Marmot, M. G. (2002). Psychological distress as a risk factor for coronary heart disease in the Whitehall II Study. *International Journal of Epidemiology*, **31**, 248–55.

Steenland, K., Fine, L., Belkic, K., Landsbergis, P., Schnall, P., Baker, D. *et al.* (2000). Research findings linking workplace factors to CVD outcomes. *Occupational Medicine*, **15**, 7–68.

Steptoe, A. (1997). Behavior and blood pressure: implications for hypertension. In *Handbook of hypertension: pathophysiology of hypertension* (ed. A. Zanchetti and G. Mancia), pp. 674–708. Elsevier Science, Amsterdam.

Steptoe, A. (1998). Psychophysiological bases of disease. In *Comprehensive clinical psychology*, Vol. 8, *Health psychology* (ed. M. Johnston and D. Johnston). Elsevier Science, New York.

Steptoe, A. (2000). Control and stress. In *Encyclopedia of stress*, Vol. 1 (ed. G. Fink), pp. 526–32. Academic Press, San Diego.

Steptoe, A. (2001). Perceptions of control and cardiovascular activity: an analysis of ambulatory measures collected over the working day. *Journal of Psychosomatic Research*, **50**, 57–63.

Steptoe, A. and Cropley, M. P. (2000). Persistent high job demands and reactivity to mental stress predict future ambulatory blood pressure. *Journal of Hypertension*, **18**, 581–6.

Steptoe, A. and Marmot, M. (2002). The role of psychobiological pathways in socio-economic inequalities in cardiovascular disease risk. *European Heart Journal*, **23**, 13–25.

Steptoe, A., Cropley, M., and Joekes, K. (1999). Job strain, blood pressure, and responsivity to uncontrollable stress. *Journal of Hypertension*, **17**, 193–200.

Steptoe, A., Cropley, M., Griffith, J., and Kirschbaum, C. (2000). Job strain and anger expression predict early morning elevations in salivary cortisol. *Psychosomatic Medicine*, **62**, 286–92.

Steptoe, A., Willemsen, G., Owen, N., Flower, L., and Mohamed-Ali, V. (2001). Acute mental stress elicits delayed increases in circulating inflammatory cytokine levels. *Clinical Science*, **101**, 185–92.

Steptoe, A., Feldman, P. J., Kunz, S., Owen, N., Willemsen, G., and Marmot, M. (2002). Stress responsivity and socioeconomic status: a mechanism for increased cardiovascular disease risk? *European Heart Journal*, **23**, 1757–63.

Stoney, C. M., Bausserman, L., Niaura, R., Marcus, B., and Flynn, M. (1999). Lipid reactivity to stress. II. Biological and behavioral influences. *Health Psychology*, **18**, 251–61.

Strike, P. C. and Steptoe, A. (2002). Systematic review of mental stress-induced myocardial ischaemia. *European Heart Journal*, **24**, 690–703.

Turner, R. J. and Marino, F. (1994). Social support and social structure: a descriptive epidemiology. *Journal of Health and Social Behavior*, **35**, 193–212.

Uchino, B. N., Cacioppo, J. T., and Kiecolt-Glaser, J. K. (1996). The relationship between social support and physiological processes: a review with emphasis on underlying mechanisms and implications for health. *Psychological Bulletin*, **119**, 488–531.

von Kanel, R., Mills, P. J., Fainman, C., and Dimsdale, J. E. (2001). Effects of psychological stress and psychiatric disorders on blood coagulation and fibrinolysis: a biobehavioral pathway to coronary artery disease? *Psychosomatic Medicine*, **63**, 531–44.

Vrijkotte, T. G., van Doornen, L. J., and de Geus, E. J. (2000). Effects of work stress on ambulatory blood pressure, heart rate, and heart rate variability. *Hypertension*, **35**, 880–6.

Wallen, N. H., Goodall, A. H., Li, N., and Hjemdahl, P. (1999). Activation of haemostasis by exercise, mental stress and adrenaline: effects on platelet sensitivity to thrombin and thrombin generation. *Clinical Science (London)*, **97**, 27–35.

Wamala, S. P., Mittleman, M. A., Schenck-Gustafsson, K., and Orth-Gomer, K. (1999a). Potential explanations for the educational gradient in coronary heart disease: a population-based case-control study of Swedish women. *American Journal of Public Health*, **89**, 315–21.

Wamala, S. P., Murray, M. A., Horsten, M., Eriksson, M., Schenck-Gustafsson, K., Hamsten, A. *et al.* (1999b). Socioeconomic status and determinants of hemostatic function in healthy women. *Arteriosclerosis, Thrombosis, and Vascular Biology*, **19**, 485–92.

Wardle, J., Farrell, M., Hillsdon, M., Jarivs, M., Sutton, S., and Thorogood, M. (1999). Smoking, drinking, physical activity and screening uptake and health inequalities. In *Inequalities in health* (ed. D. Gordon, M. Shaw, D. Dorling, and G. Davey Smith), pp. 213–39. Policy Press, Bristol.

Williams, D. R. and Neighbors, H. (2001). Racism, discrimination and hypertension: evidence and needed research. *Ethnicity and Disease*, 11, 800–16.

Williams, J. K., Kaplan, J. R., and Manuck, S. B. (1993). Effects of psychosocial stress on endothelium-mediated dilation of atherosclerotic arteries in cynomolgus monkeys. *Journal of Clinical Investigation*, 92, 1819–23.

Yeung, A. C., Vekshtein, V. I., Krantz, D. S., Vita, J. A., Ryan, T. J., Jr., Ganz, P. *et al.* (1991). The effect of atherosclerosis on the vasomotor response of coronary arteries to mental stress. *New England Journal of Medicine*, 325, 1551–6.

Zorrilla, E. P., Luborsky, L., McKay, J. R., Rosenthal, R., Houldin, A., Tax, A. *et al.* (2001). The relationship of depression and stressors to immunological assays: a meta-analytic review. *Brain, Behavior, and Immunity*, 15, 199–226.

Chapter 27

Chronic infection and circulating markers of inflammation

P. Whincup and J. Danesh

27.1 Introduction

The specific hypotheses under consideration in this chapter are that the presence of markers of chronic infective agents and of low-grade inflammation may increase the incidence of coronary atherosclerosis and its clinical complications. Although 'infective' and 'inflammatory' hypotheses are often described as 'novel' risk factors in coronary heart disease (CHD), each was originally proposed several decades ago (Frothingham 1911; Nieto 1998). The recent renewal of interest in them has been driven largely by advances in vascular pathology, in laboratory-based technology, and by the feasibility of measuring 'infective' and 'inflammatory' markers on a large scale in epidemiological study populations. Moreover, although it is often suggested that 'infective' and 'inflammatory' hypotheses are closely related to each other, there is little good epidemiological evidence to support this claim in the context of CHD, as larger and more rigorous studies in general populations (Danesh *et al.* 2000*a*) have not confirmed earlier suggestions that certain circulating markers of inflammation are associated with markers of specific chronic infections (Patel *et al.* 1995). The present discussion of these topics in one chapter is, however, appropriate because epidemiological studies of both issues have similar strengths and limitations and the relevance of each may be elucidated by more recent research strategies. The purpose of this chapter is, therefore, to provide a critical review of the available epidemiological and clinical evidence on CHD and markers of persistent infection and of inflammation, and to suggest ways in which further research can help to resolve existing uncertainties.

27.2 Methodological issues

Much of the epidemiological evidence on these topics derives from long-term prospective cohort studies of middle-aged individuals, with only a limited amount as yet from randomized intervention studies. In such observational studies, individuals who develop CHD after entry ('cases') are typically compared with an appropriate subset of those who remain disease-free ('controls'). The use of such 'nested' case-control studies in prospective cohorts with stored blood samples provides an efficient and rapid way to test many hypotheses. Moreover, in contrast with retrospective studies involving 'opportunistically' recruited groups of controls of uncertain validity, long-term prospective studies should reduce biases related to the selection of controls and should limit the influence of disease on the factors being investigated.

So far, however, individual observational studies have typically involved only a few hundred cases of CHD and only a few hundred controls. Due to their inherent statistical uncertainties, studies of such scale are prone to false-negative and false-positive results. The impact of random error can, moreover, be compounded by unduly data-dependent analyses and selective reporting. For example, spurious or exaggerated results may emerge when analytical cut-off values are chosen only after an exploration of the data has shown which seemed to be most strongly related to CHD (such as in studies of *Chlamydia pneumoniae*, where several different antibody titre values have been used in different studies to define 'seropositivity', often by the same group of investigators) (Danesh *et al.* 1997). Such biases can also arise when: (a) prominence is given to extreme findings in selected subgroups based on sparse data; (b) results are preferentially reported just for those few factors (out of the many measured) which show extreme associations; and (c) journals preferentially publish striking findings (Easterbrook *et al.* 1991).

To help minimize such potential biases, this chapter emphasizes evidence from systematic, quantitative reviews of available long-term prospective studies of chronic infective and of inflammatory hypotheses in CHD because such literature-based 'meta-analysis' should provide a better preliminary indication of the potential relevance of suspected risk factors than can individual studies involving just a few hundred cases and a few hundred controls. But, although such syntheses can help limit certain biases related to random error and selective publication, they may be less effective at reducing the impact of other potential biases found in individual observational studies: in particular, imprecise characterization of exposure, confounding, and reverse association.

In seroepidemiological studies of infective hypotheses, characterization of exposure to infection has generally been based on the presence of a high titre of specific antibodies. The presence of serum antibodies, however, does not necessarily indicate the persistence of active infection at any site, or persistent exposure of the coronary arteries to any type of insult. Moreover, although high titres of IgG antibody to *Helicobacter pylori* are generally stable markers of chronic gastric infection in the absence of specific antibiotic treatment, IgG antibodies to *C. pneumoniae* tend to fall after infection and those to cytomegalovirus (CMV) and other herpesviruses tend to fluctuate with repeated reactivation (Table 27.1). Such temporal variation in antibody titres means that any associations between CHD and antibody titres for *C. pneumoniae* and CMV measured at just one time will, due to regression dilution, be weaker than associations of CHD with long-term average antibody levels (Clarke *et al.* 1999).

Similar considerations apply to observational studies of CHD and circulating markers of inflammation, most of which have been based on measurements of inflammatory markers taken at a single baseline survey. Lack of serial assessment can lead to substantial underestimation of any association with CHD due to within-individual fluctuations of inflammatory factors over time (Table 27.2).

Whereas regression dilution generally leads to underestimation of any associations, 'confounding' by causative risk factors generally leads to exaggerated (or even spurious) associations between suspected risk factors and CHD (Greenland 1980). For example, only about half of the retrospective seroepidemiological studies of *C. pneumoniae* and CHD published before 1998 reported adjustment for cigarette smoking (Danesh *et al.* 2000b) – even though smoking appears to be an important determinant of *C. pneumoniae* seropositivity and is a known causal risk factor in CHD. But, even when observational studies attempt adjustment for potential confounding factors, the results may still be of uncertain validity. Residual biases are possible because baseline values of some confounders (for example, serum lipid concentrations) may be inaccurate measurements of their long-term 'usual' values or they may be only crude markers of a complex variable (for example, long-past exposures that are related to childhood socioeconomic status), thereby resulting in inadequate statistical adjustments.

Table 27.1 Characteristics of chronic infections possibly associated with vascular disease

Pathogen	H. pylori	C. pneumoniae	Cytomegalovirus	Periodontal disease
Type of organism	Gram-negative spiral bacterium	Gram-negative intracellular bacterium	Large herpesvirus	Various, especially certain Gram-negative anaerobes
Likely spread	Faecal–oral, oral–oral	Respiratory secretions	Faecal–oral, oral–oral, parenteral	?Oral–oral
Main site of persistence	Gastric mucus layer	?Alveolar macrophage	?Leucocyte	Periodontal pockets
Natural history	Persistent infection (usually from childhood)	?Moderately persistent, re-infections common	Persistent latent state, occasional re-activation	Persistent infection from early life
Antibody persistence	Persist until old age	Fluctuate with re-infection	Fluctuate with re-activation	?
UK prevalence, age 50	~40%	~50%	~50%	?
Correlates	Age (cohort effect), low socio-economic status	Age, periodic epidemics?, smoking	Age, low socio-economic status, immunosuppression	Age, low socio-economic status, smoking?, diet
Associated diseases	Chronic gastritis, peptic ulcer disease, some gastric cancers, non-ulcer dyspepsia?	Pneumonia, pharyngitis, sinusitis, bronchitis?, asthma	Protean manifestations (e.g. in adults: mononucleosis or pneumonitis)	Periodontitis, dental caries, gingivitis
Drug treatment	Two antibiotics (e.g. amoxycillin and clarithromycin) + omeprazole for 7 days)	Macrolide antibiotic (e.g. clarithromycin) for 7–14 days is effective in pneumonia	Ganciclovir (not curative; merely controls re-activation)	Broad-spectrum antibiotics (e.g. metronidazole and amoxycillin for 1 week)
Vaccine	Preventative and therapeutic vaccines in early trials	None available	Preventative vaccine of limited efficacy	None available

Table 27.2 Characteristics of fibrinogen, C-reactive protein, albumin, and leucocyte count

Characteristic	Fibrinogen	C-reactive protein	Albumin	Leucocyte count
Description	Large glycoprotein	Pentameric protein	Negatively charged protein	White blood cells
Effects in plasma	Haemostasis, increases viscosity, leucocyte adhesion	Opsonizes infections, activates complement, binds free DNA	Carriage of various ligands, maintains osmotic pressure (comprises 4% of plasma)	Various (e.g. antibody and cytokine synthesis, clearance of foreign host debris)
Main site of synthesis	Liver	Liver	Liver	Bone marrow
Main modulators	Various cytokines	Interleukins-1 and -6, TNF-α	Levels fall when cytokines switch liver to synthesis of acute phase proteins	Various cytokines
Main correlates	Age, smoking, LDL-C, physical inactivity, social class, alcohol abstinence	Age, smoking, possibly fibrinogen	Age, smoking, obesity, blood pressure, possibly social class	Age, smoking, obesity, blood pressure, possibly fibrinogen
Baseline mean (SD)	8.8 (2.4) μmol/l (0.30 (0.08) g/dl)	0.20 (0.33) $\log_{10}$ mg/l	40 (3.0) g/l	7.0 (1.8) × 10 g/l
Self-correlation (r)[a]	~0.6	~0.6	~0.7	~0.7
Usual values, top end and bottom thirds[b]	10.3 vs. 7.4 μmol/l (0.35 vs. 0.25 g/dl)	0.38 vs. 0.02 $\log_{10}$ mg/l	42 vs. 38 g/l	8.4 vs. 5.6 × 10⁹/l
Inflammatory response	~4-fold rise	~1000-fold rise	~20% fall	~3-fold rise

LDL-C: low-density lipoprotein cholesterol; SD: standard deviation; TNF: tumour necrosis factor α.

[a] Correlation coefficient (r) between two measurements of the same factors taken some years apart in the same individual.

[b] If a single baseline measurement is used to divide individuals into three equal-sized groups, the averages of the long-term 'usual' values in the top and bottom groups are estimated as baseline mean ±1.09 × SD.

In the context of infective hypotheses, reverse association is potentially relevant in pathology-based studies of atherosclerosis, where comparisons have been made of the frequency of various endovascular markers of infection in atherosclerotic specimens and in 'control' tissues. As discussed below, a difficulty in such studies is distinguishing between local infection predisposing to atheroma and the reverse sequence (Capron 1996). In the context of inflammatory hypotheses, an analogous difficulty is determining to what extent circulating markers of inflammation reflect the extent of pre-existing atherosclerosis and/or subclinical CHD at the 'baseline' survey rather than any direct impact on future CHD risk itself (Ross 1999).

As discussed later in this chapter, such methodological problems are being addressed by more recent research strategies that include randomized intervention studies of anti-infective strategies, collaborative re-analysis of individual participant data from long-term prospective studies, and large-scale observational studies of the genetic determinants of plasma markers of inflammation.

27.3 Chronic infection and CHD

The production of lesions in chickens resembling human atherosclerosis following experimental infection with avian herpesvirus in the 1970s revived interest in infective hypotheses in CHD (Fabricant *et al.* 1978). Since then, associations have been reported with a number of different infective agents, both acute and chronic. This chapter focuses on evidence related to a few common persistent infective agents (i.e., *H. pylori*, *C. pneumoniae*, and CMV) as well as on clinical markers of dental infection believed to be related to specific chronic infective agents (Mattila *et al.* 1989) (Table 27.1). *H. pylori*, identified in 1983, is a Gram-negative curved bacterium, usually acquired in childhood and implicated in the causation of peptic ulcer and, perhaps, gastric adenocarcinoma. *C. pneumoniae*, identified in 1986, is a Gram-negative intracellular bacterium that is responsible for infections of the lower respiratory tract. CMV, identified in 1956, is the largest of the herpesviruses, and is involved in a range of clinical illnesses.

27.3.1 *H. pylori*

Since the publication of the first report in 1994 (Mendall *et al.* 1994), a few dozen epidemiological studies have reported on associations between *H. pylori* antibody titres and CHD. A number of small retrospective studies with opportunistically selected controls have reported strongly positive associations (odds ratios >2), although the confidence intervals reported in these studies have generally been wide (Danesh *et al.* 1997). By about mid-2000, however, 10 long-term prospective studies of *H. pylori* IgG serology and CHD had been published, involving a total of 2916 cases of CHD death or non-fatal myocardial infarction (weighted mean age of cases: 67 years). In contrast with the generally smaller and less rigorous retrospective studies, these prospective studies yielded a combined odds ratio of just 1.15 (99% confidence interval: 0.96–1.37) in *H. pylori* seropositive individuals (Whincup *et al.* 2000; Ridker *et al.* 2001a), suggesting that the earlier studies were exaggerated by various potential biases. As *H. pylori* seropositivity is strongly correlated with markers of lower socio-economic status, two of the prospective studies (Wald *et al.* 1997; Ridker *et al.* 2001a), and one case-control study of sibling pairs (Danesh *et al.* 1999b), involved comparatively socially homogeneous populations that should minimize any residual biases related to social class. These three studies collectively involved a total of

1688 CHD cases, and again they yielded a weakly positive combined odds ratio that was not statistically significant (1.11, 95% confidence interval: 0.86–1.43).

As these prospective studies have suggested that any independent association between chronic *H. pylori* infection and CHD in late middle-age is likely to be null or only modest, studies have involved strategies to help detect any modest associations. Studies of early-onset CHD should provide more sensitive tests of the existence of any modest associations than do studies at older ages because established vascular risk factors (such as smoking, blood pressure, and blood cholesterol) tend be much stronger in younger individuals (Danesh *et al.* 1997). But, although a case-control study of 1122 comparatively young survivors of myocardial infarction (mean age: 44 years) and 1122 matched controls has reported an adjusted odds ratio of 1.87 (95% confidence interval: 1.42–2.47), it is not certain to what extent this result may have been influenced by residual confounding (Danesh *et al.* 1999*b*). Other studies have measured potentially more aggressive strains of *H. pylori* (such as strains positive for CagA, a cytotoxin-associated gene product A), since it may be that such putatively pro-inflammatory strains are more strongly related to CHD risk (Danesh *et al.* 1999*b*). But, although a small retrospective study involving a control group of uncertain validity reported a four-fold relative risk for CHD in individuals seropositive to CagA-positive strains of *H. pylori* (Pasceri *et al.* 1998), several larger and more rigorous studies have not observed strong associations (Gunn *et al.* 2000; Murray *et al.* 2000; Stone *et al.* 2001; Whincup *et al.* 2000). The lack of any good evidence that chronic *H. pylori* infection is related to established cardiovascular risk factors (Danesh and Peto 1998; Whincup *et al.* 2000), and the inability to detect *H. pylori* DNA consistently in atherosclerotic plaques in a few small pathology-based studies, have also weakened the plausibility of an important independent association with CHD (Blasi *et al.* 1996; Chiu *et al.* 1997; Danesh *et al.* 1999*a*; Farsak *et al.* 2000; Radke *et al.* 2001). It is not clear to what extent a few existing trials of *H. pylori* eradication treatment in the prevention of gastric cancer might help to resolve uncertainties about the reversibility of any modest association between *H. pylori* and CHD, as these studies may not record sufficient CHD events during scheduled follow-up to test the hypothesis reliably (Danesh 1999).

27.3.2 *C. pneumoniae*

The first reported association between seropositivity to *C. pneumoniae* and CHD appeared in 1988 (Saikku *et al.* 1988), and, a few years later, *C. pneumoniae* elementary bodies were directly observed by electron micrography in coronary plaques (Shor *et al.* 1992). Since then, dozens of seroepidemiological and pathology-based studies have reported on possible associations between *C. pneumoniae* and vascular disease (Danesh *et al.* 2000*b*), and several randomized trials of antibiotic treatments against the infection have already been reported (Danesh and Collins 2001).

As was the case for *H. pylori*, larger prospective studies of *C. pneumoniae* have not confirmed the suggestions of strong seroepidemiological associations originally reported in a number of smaller retrospective studies of uncertain validity. By about mid-2000, 15 long-term prospective studies of *C. pneumoniae* IgG serology and CHD had been published, involving a total of 3169 cases of CHD death or non-fatal myocardial infarction (weighted mean age of cases: 66 years). A combined analysis yielded an odds ratio of 1.15 (95% confidence interval: 0.97–1.36) in individuals with higher *C. pneumoniae* IgG titres (Danesh *et al.* 2000*b*), which is statistically compatible with a combined odds ratio of 1.25 (95% confidence interval: 1.03–1.53) observed in a synthesis of

10 prospective studies based on *C. pneumoniae* IgA serology, involving 2283 CHD cases (Danesh *et al.* 2002). Although these studies generally lacked correction for within-individual variation in *C. pneumoniae* antibody titres over time (Clarke *et al.* 1999), unpublished reproducibility data on 1065 adults in the UK with samples taken 3 years apart suggest that any underestimation due to regression dilution in *C. pneumoniae* serology was probably relatively modest (S. Clark, personal communication).

In contrast with the generally weak or null findings in seroepidemiological studies, a few dozen pathology-based studies, involving assessments of a total of about 1000 human arterial specimens for endovascular markers of *C. pneumoniae* (DNA, antigens, elementary bodies, or viable organisms), have reported a combined weighted odds ratio for atherosclerosis of about 20 (95% confidence interval: 15–32) (Danesh and Appleby 1998). What might account for this 20-fold discrepancy in different types of observational studies? Pathology-based studies have been retrospective (thereby creating uncertainty about whether local *C. pneumoniae* infection is a cause or consequence of atheroma), whereas the prospective serological studies assessed evidence of infection several years before the diagnosis of CHD. Most pathology-based studies have also been prone to selection biases and lacked any adjustment for possible confounders such as age, sex, and smoking, but this could not plausibly explain much of the 20-fold difference. It is also unclear to what extent the discrepancy can be accounted for by the different definitions of vascular disease (atheroma versus major coronary events) and the different markers of infection (endovascular markers such as DNA and antigens versus circulating antibody titres) used in these different sets of studies.

Such epidemiological uncertainties have prompted randomized intervention studies of antichlamydial antibiotic treatments. The results have been received (Fig. 27.1, Danesh 2005). Preliminary randomized placebo-controlled trials reported large cardioprotective effects in patients allocated antibiotic treatments (e.g. >30% reductions in CHD recurrences), but these studies were prone to chance fluctuations because each typically recorded only a few dozen CHD endpoints. These initial studies were also generally limited by brief treatment durations (e.g. lasting for a few weeks) and relatively brief durations of follow-up (e.g. lasting for several months) (Gurfinkel *et al.* 1997; Gupta *et al.* 1997; Gurfinkel *et al.* 1999; Sinisalo *et al.* 2002; Stone *et al.* 2002). By the end of 2004, data had been reported from a total of eleven such trials in the secondary prevention of CHD, involving a total of 19 221 patients recruited and 3 689 CHD endpoints recorded (Gurfinkel *et al.* 1997; Gupta *et al.* 1997; Gurfinkel *et al.* 1999; Muhlestein *et al.* 2000; Sinisalo *et al.* 2002; Stone *et al.* 2002; Cercek *et al.* 2003; O'Connor *et al.* 2003; Zahn *et al.* 2003; Cannon *et al.* 2004; Grayston *et al.* 2004). Several of the more recent trials involved much larger numbers of patients, much more prolonged antibiotic treatments, and more extended follow-up than did the earlier studies. In aggregate, the available trials have yielded a stratified risk of CHD with anti-chlamydial treatment of 0.96 (95% confidence interval: 0.90–1.01), which is not statistically significant and which does not vary materially by type of antibiotic treatment used (e.g. macrolide derivatives, such as azithromycin vs. other antibiotic treatments), by type of baseline CHD (stable disease vs acute coronary syndrome), and by baseline *C. pneumoniae* serostatus (Danesh 2005). Collectively, therefore, these trials have excluded the possibility of all but small benefits of these anti-chlamydial antibiotic regimens in the secondary prevention of CHD, although more extended follow-up should help address the possibility of any delayed benefits. These trials have not yet reported on any possible effects of these anti-chlamydial interventions against other chronic bacterial agents suspected in CHD, but, at least in the case of *H. pylori*, prolonged antibiotic monotherapy would be unlikely to achieve high bacterial kill rates.

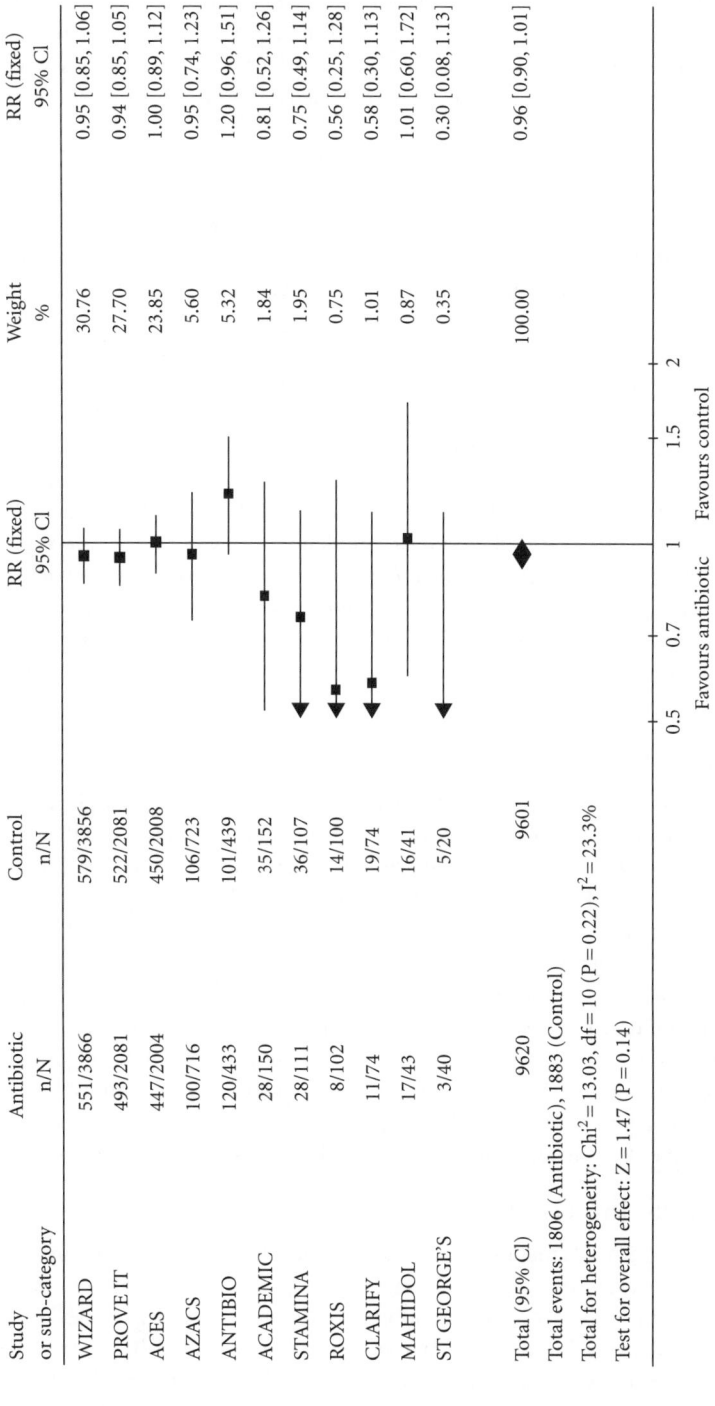

Study or sub-category	Antibiotic n/N	Control n/N	RR (fixed) 95% CI	Weight %	RR (fixed) 95% CI
WIZARD	551/3866	579/3856		30.76	0.95 [0.85, 1.06]
PROVE IT	493/2081	522/2081		27.70	0.94 [0.85, 1.05]
ACES	447/2004	450/2008		23.85	1.00 [0.89, 1.12]
AZACS	100/716	106/723		5.60	0.95 [0.74, 1.23]
ANTIBIO	120/433	101/439		5.32	1.20 [0.96, 1.51]
ACADEMIC	28/150	35/152		1.84	0.81 [0.52, 1.26]
STAMINA	28/111	36/107		1.95	0.75 [0.49, 1.14]
ROXIS	8/102	14/100		0.75	0.56 [0.25, 1.28]
CLARIFY	11/74	19/74		1.01	0.58 [0.30, 1.13]
MAHIDOL	17/43	16/41		0.87	1.01 [0.60, 1.72]
ST GEORGE'S	3/40	5/20		0.35	0.30 [0.08, 1.13]
Total (95% CI)	9620	9601		100.00	0.96 [0.90, 1.01]

Total events: 1806 (Antibiotic), 1883 (Control)
Total for heterogeneity: Chi² = 13.03, df = 10 (P = 0.22), I² = 23.3%
Test for overall effect: Z = 1.47 (P = 0.14)

0.5   0.7   1   1.5   2

Favours antibiotic   Favours control

Fig. 27.1 Randomized controlled trials of anti-chlamydial antibiotic treatments in the secondary prevention of CHD (Danesh 2005).

27.3.3 **CMV**

In 1983, an electron micrographic study reported the appearance of CMV antigen in human vascular tissue (Melnick *et al.* 1983), prompting further pathology-based studies as well as seroepidemiological studies of CMV and other herpesviruses in CHD. Although a number of retrospective seroepidemiological studies have reported strong associations between CMV IgG serology and vascular diseases, these studies have been limited by small sample sizes, the use of control groups of uncertain validity, and incomplete adjustment for potential confounders (Danesh *et al.* 1997). Furthermore, few of these studies were of classic CHD: by 1999, about 1400 of the 2100 available CHD cases in these studies were defined on the basis of coronary restenosis after atherectomy, or the development of lesions in transplanted hearts or in arteries outside the coronary circulation. So, even if CMV is causing such lesions, this may not be relevant to native coronary artery atherosclerosis. By 2002, six long-term prospective studies of CMV IgG serology and CHD had been published, involving a total of 1296 cases of CHD death or non-fatal myocardial infarction (weighted mean age of cases: 60.2 years) (Viik-Kajander *et al.* 1997; Ossewaarde *et al.* 1998; Ridker *et al.* 1998*a*, Strachan *et al.* 1999; Siscovick *et al.* 2000; Sorlie *et al.* 2000). They yielded a combined odds ratio of just 1.00 (95% confidence interval: 0.82–1.21) in CMV seropositive individuals. And, although about 20 pathology-based studies have reported on endovascular markers of CMV in human arterial lesions, with a combined weighted odds ratio of 1.6 (95% confidence interval: 1.5–1.7) for atherosclerosis (and a somewhat more extreme combined odds ratio of 2.6 (95% confidence interval: 2.3–2.9) in an analysis restricted to studies using the polymerase chain reaction, a potentially more sensitive assessment of low-level viral infection in arterial specimens) (Danesh and Appleby 1998), the causal relevance of local CMV infection to atherosclerosis is unknown since the sequence of infection and disease remains uncertain, as was the case for *C. pneumoniae*.

27.3.4 **Dental disease**

A number of studies have reported correlations of various markers of oral hygiene (for example, number of missing teeth, alveolar bone loss, the presence of periodontitis or other gum lesions) with risk of CHD (Danesh and Appleby 1998). By 1999, five long-term prospective studies of such markers of dental disease and CHD had been published, involving a total of 2369 cases of CHD death or non-fatal myocardial infarction (weighted mean age of cases at time of event: 67 years). Although these studies yielded a combined odds ratio of 1.24 (95% confidence interval: 1.10–1.38), it is possible that this association is largely or wholly an artefact of residual confounding due to differences in socio-economic status (a strong determinant of oral hygiene). For example, in one large study, there was a stronger correlation of gum disease with death from all causes than with CHD, which suggests that the associations were substantially confounded (DeStefano *et al.* 1993). Larger prospective studies reported since the previous meta-analysis have also generally failed to report positive associations (Howell *et al.* 2001).

27.3.5 **Multiple infection**

Despite the lack of good seroepidemiological evidence that any particular chronic infective agent is causally relevant to CHD, it has been suggested that co-infection by two or more of these agents (and possibly others) can substantially increase CHD risk (Nieto 1998). So far, however, available information on 'pathogen burden' and CHD has been restricted to a number of smaller retrospective studies (Zhu *et al.* 2001; Espinola-Klein *et al.* 2002) and a few prospective studies with limited statistical power (the latter have generally been unsupportive of the hypothesis, albeit with wide confidence intervals) (Ridker 2002). Reliably testing such detailed hypotheses is, however, even more demanding than investigating the relevance of a particular infective agent to CHD because larger sample sizes are required (since the hypotheses are essentially analyses of subgroups) and because confounding is likely to be compounded in studies that define relevant exposure as a composite of positive serological markers to a range of bacterial and viral infections.

27.4 Markers of systemic inflammation and CHD

Circulating concentrations of a variety of plasma components can fluctuate substantially during acute responses to tissue damage (Pepys 1995). Plasma concentrations of C-reactive protein and serum amyloid A can rise 10 000-fold; plasma concentrations of fibrinogen and von Willebrand factors (both of which also have important haemostatic activities) and the leucocyte count can each increase about three-fold; and the concentration of serum albumin can fall by about 20% (Danesh et al. 1998). These plasma alterations appear to reflect, at least in part, the impact of molecular cascades mediated by pro-inflammatory cytokines (such as interleukins-1 and -6 and tumour necrosis factor-α) on the liver and on other tissues (Libby et al. 2002). In recent years, such 'acute phase reactants' have been studied as potential markers of more subtle and persistent alterations that may be loosely called low-grade inflammation. Long-term circulating concentrations of these factors show a similar year-to-year consistency within individuals to levels of some classical vascular risk factors such as blood cholesterol and blood pressure (Table 27.3). Advances in laboratory assays have allowed detection of subtle variations of several 'inflammatory' factors (such as C-reactive protein and serum amyloid A protein) that would not previously have been noticed in general populations. Moreover, as several of these factors are stable in long-frozen blood, they can be measured fairly reliably in banked samples. These favourable biological characteristics have encouraged many blood-based epidemiological investigations of inflammatory factors and CHD.

Table 27.3 provides indirect comparisons of several of the most extensively studied inflammatory factors in CHD, by comparing the combined odds ratio of CHD (derived from literature-based meta-analyses of published prospective studies) in those with plasma concentrations in the top third with those in the bottom third of the distribution of these factors in the population (or, for serum albumin, bottom third versus top third). As shown by Table 27.3, the odds ratios for CHD of most of these factors appear to be less than two-fold, and are less extreme than the corresponding odds ratios for established risk factors such as cigarette smoking, blood pressure, and low-density lipoprotein cholesterol (MacMahon et al. 1990; Law et al. 1994; Parish et al. 1995; Lewington et al. 2002). Because these risk ratios are not very extreme, many of them might be largely or wholly accounted for by confounding. Rather than attempt to discuss the strengths and limitations of the epidemiological data on each of these dozen or so factors, this section focuses chiefly on plasma fibrinogen and C-reactive protein, two of the best studied of the inflammatory factors (fibrinogen is also of course a major haemostatic factor), since strategies that allow more detailed investigation of these two factors may be generally relevant to other factors.

27.4.1 Plasma fibrinogen

By 1998, 18 long-term prospective studies of plasma fibrinogen and CHD had been published, involving a total of 4018 cases of CHD death or non-fatal myocardial infarction (weighted mean age of cases: 64 years) (Danesh et al. 1998). A combined analysis of these studies has yielded an odds ratio of 1.8 (95% confidence interval: 1.6–2.0) in individuals in the top

Table 27.3 Literature-based meta-analyses of some 'inflammatory' factors studied in long-term prospective studies of general populations

Type of factor/examples	Reference source	No. of incident CHD cases	Risk ratio[a]
Acute-phase reactants			
Leucocyte count	Danesh *et al.* 1998	6000	1.4 (1.3–1.5)
Albumin	Danesh *et al.* 1998	3700	1.5 (1.3–1.7)[b]
C-reactive protein	Danesh *et al.* 2004	7000	1.5 (1.4–1.6)
Ferritin	Danesh and Appleby 1999	600	1.0 (0.8–1.3)
Serum amyloid A protein	Danesh *et al.* 2000a	600	1.6 (1.1–2.2)
Haemostatic			
Fibrinogen	Danesh *et al.* 1998	3000	1.8 (1.6–2.0)
von Willebrand factor	Whincup *et al.* 2002	1500	1.5 (1.1–2.0)
Cell adhesion molecules			
ICAM–1	Malik *et al.* 2001	1400	1.2 (1.0–1.6)
VCAM–1	Malik *et al.* 2001	1300	1.0 (0.8–1.3)
P-selectin	Malik *et al.* 2001	800	1.1 (0.7–1.4)
E-selectin	Malik *et al.* 2001	800	1.2 (0.9–1.6)

[a] Top third vs. bottom third.

[b] Bottom third vs. top third.

third compared with those in the bottom third of baseline values (corresponding to a long-term usual difference in plasma fibrinogen concentration of 1 g/l). The plasma fibrinogen concentration is, however, positively correlated with causative vascular risk factors such as cigarette smoking and low-density-lipoprotein cholesterol (Danesh *et al.* 1998). One important question, therefore, is whether the association of plasma fibrinogen with CHD would persist if full adjustment were made for smoking, lipids, and other potential confounders (as well as, of course, age and sex). Statistically reliable evidence about the effects of such adjustment is, however, possible only if large numbers of cases are available for analysis, and only if proper allowance is made for the effects of measurement errors in the factors for which adjustment is being made. As most published prospective studies have not fulfilled these conditions, other strategies are needed.

One approach involves detailed collaborative re-analysis of individual participant data from published long-term prospective studies of plasma fibrinogen and cardiovascular disease (Lewington *et al.* 2002). To help achieve this objective, the Fibrinogen Studies Collaboration was established in 1999. It involves almost 40 relevant studies (including several with repeated measurements which should help minimize biases due to regression dilution and residual confounding), involving about 150 000 individuals at baseline and >10 000 incident cardiovascular events (Fibrinogen Studies Collaboration 2004). In 2005, the Fibrinogen Studies Collaboration will report on its main findings, which should help quantify more precisely and reliably than previously possible any independent associations of plasma fibrinogen with CHD.

A complementary strategy involves investigation of the effects on CHD risk of genetic determinants of plasma fibrinogen (such as polymorphisms on the beta-fibrinogen gene that are associated with modest but definite differences in plasma fibrinogen concentrations). For, if plasma fibrinogen concentration directly affects the incidence of CHD, then sufficiently large case-control studies of these genotypes should reveal this. This is because in such comparisons any confounding should be eliminated, since individuals are effectively 'randomized' at conception, in a Mendelian fashion, to higher or lower long-term plasma fibrinogen concentrations (Youngman et al. 2000; Clayton and McKeigue 2001). A synthesis of 16 such studies reported by 2004, involving a total of 11 161 CHD cases and 18 068 controls, yielded a combined odds ratio of CHD per higher-fibrinogen allele of 1.00 (95% confidence interval: 0.96–1.05) (Keavney et al. submitted). This finding argues against causality as the main explanation for the odds ratio of 1.8 for CHD previously observed in those with 1 g/l higher usual plasma fibrinogen concentration. More generally, this approach suggests how observational epidemiological studies might be used to test the causal relevance of various plasma biomarkers, including inflammatory markers, by assessing the relevance to disease of genetic polymorphisms that influence the levels of these suspected risk factors.

27.4.2 C-reactive protein

By 2003, 22 long-term prospective studies of C-reactive protein and CHD in essentially general populations had been published, involving a total of about 7 000 cases of CHD death or non-fatal myocardial infarction (weighted mean age of cases: 69 years) (Danesh et al. 2004). A combined analysis of the larger of these studies yielded an odds ratio of 1.5 (95% confidence interval: 1.4–1.6) in individuals in the top third compared with those in the bottom third of baseline values (corresponding to a long-term usual difference in C-reactive protein concentration of about 1.5 mg/L). This result is less extreme than the combined odds ratio of 2.0 (95% confidence interval: 1.6–2.5) reported in a meta-analysis of 10 studies published in 2000, involving about 2 000 CHD cases, a difference which may be consistent with the selective publication of more striking findings in the earlier studies (Danesh et al. 2000a). C-reactive protein values are positively correlated with causative vascular risk factors, such as cigarette smoking and body mass index. By analogy with plasma fibrinogen, strategies that involve collaborative re-analysis of individual participant data from long-term prospective studies and/or of case-control studies of the genetic determinants of C-reactive protein may well be needed to help determine to what extent these associations are independent of classical risk factors.

Even if an independent association is established between plasma C-reactive protein concentrations and CHD, several questions would remain. Is C-reactive protein itself a direct mediator of vascular damage, or merely a marker of a more fundamental cause of disease – or both? There is no strong evidence so far for a direct role for C-reactive protein in vascular disease (Lagrand et al. 1999), but additional experimental research is clearly needed, as even the physiological role of C-reactive protein remains largely unknown. In apparently healthy people, there are close correlations between C-reactive protein values and other plasma acute-phase reactants associated with CHD in prospective studies (such as the factors listed in Table 27.3) (Danesh et al. 2000a). This suggests that it is the generally consistent pattern of some underlying processes related to inflammation, rather than plasma C-reactive protein per se, that may be relevant to CHD risk.

If so, what factors might be responsible for such inflammation? A number of suggestions have been made, ranging from factors within the arterial wall, such as oxidized low-density lipoprotein and local infection by agents such as *C. pneumoniae* or CMV (Danesh *et al.* 1997), to factors outside the circulation such as gastric infection with *H. pylori* or subclinical renal dysfunction (Baigent *et al.* 2000). In general, the evidence for these hypotheses is, as yet, both relatively sparse and weak, as there is uncertainty about whether any of these suspected risk factors are themselves associated with CHD (as described above for chronic infection). Some female sex hormones are produced in adipose tissue (a site of production of interleukin-6 and other cytokines), and the idea that oestrogens might promote low-grade inflammation has been suggested by a randomized trial that reported sustained increases in plasma C-reactive protein values in women treated with hormone therapy regimens (Cushman *et al.* 1999). However, high levels of oestrogens alone would not satisfactorily explain a role for low-grade inflammation in men with CHD. A partial genetic basis for low-grade inflammation is suggested by a study of several hundred apparently healthy twins in whom monozygotic pairs had closer correlations of circulating concentrations of C-reactive protein and serum amyloid A protein than did dizygotic pairs (MacGregor *et al.* 1999).

Despite incomplete knowledge about the factors responsible for persistent low-grade inflammation, several interventions have been proposed to prevent CHD by their presumed 'anti-inflammatory' actions. One report has suggested that the vascular protective effects of aspirin increase with increasing baseline C-reactive protein values (Ridker *et al.* 1997), but that claim is not statistically convincing and is not supported by large syntheses of randomized trials that have excluded much greater vascular benefits in patients taking higher ('anti-inflammatory') dosages of aspirin than in those taking lower dosages (Antithrombotic Trialists' Collaboration, 2002). The results of small trials of macrolides (antibiotics with anti-chlamydial and, perhaps, anti-inflammatory effects) suggested that these agents might reduce circulating levels of certain plasma markers of inflammation, including C-reactive protein. However, the results of subsequent trials have not provided consistent support for this possibility (Stone *et al.* 2002; Hillis *et al.* 2004). Long-term use of statins (3-hydroxy-3-methylglutaryl coenzyme A reductase inhibitors) appears to produce rapid and sustained reductions in plasma concentrations of C-reactive protein that are apparently unrelated to the degree of cholesterol lowering achieved (Ridker *et al.* 1998*b*, 1999, 2001*b, c*; Albert *et al.* 2001; Jialal 2001). Preliminary reports that cardioprotection with pravastatin or lovastatin may increase with increasing evidence of baseline inflammation (Ridker *et al.* 1998*b*, 2001*c*) require testing in much larger samples – as does a report claiming that lovastatin is not cardioprotective in individuals with lower than average plasma concentrations of low-density lipoprotein cholesterol and of C-reactive protein (as this analysis, based on a subgroup of 36 cases, was not statistically significant) (Ridker *et al.* 2001*c*).

27.5 **Conclusions**

Systematic quantitative reviews suggest that the epidemiological and clinical data on specific persistent infective agents and CHD is generally weak and inconclusive (in contrast with just a few years ago, when the available evidence was dominated by small retrospective studies of uncertain validity with strongly positive findings). Although larger and more rigorous studies now suggest that it is unlikely that chronic infection with *H. pylori*, *C. pneumoniae*, or CMV are strong determinants of CHD, available studies have been unable to confirm or exclude the existence of any modest associations. In aggregate, several randomized trails in the secondary prevention of CHD have excluded all but small effects of the anti-chlamydial antibiotic treatments tested.

Although meta-analyses of published long-term prospective studies suggest that there is reasonably consistent evidence of moderately strong associations between CHD and a number of plasma markers of inflammation (such as plasma C-reactive protein and serum amyloid A protein), it remains uncertain whether these markers are causes or consequences of CHD (or merely indicators of classical risk factors and/or early disease). Larger and more rigorous prospective studies of CHD (and more detailed syntheses of available studies) are needed to investigate these associations further, ideally, with serial measurements of inflammatory markers (and of potential confounding factors) to reduce residual biases. As has been the case for plasma fibrinogen, larger-scale observational studies are needed that can include complementary information on the genetic determinants of various inflammatory markers, thereby providing unconfounded tests of causality based on 'Mendelian randomization'. Such investigations should help to elucidate whether plasma inflammatory markers have any role in the prediction and prevention of CHD.

References

Albert, M. A., Danielson, E., Rifai, N., Ridker, P. M., and PRINCE Investigators (2001). Effect of statin therapy on C-reactive protein levels: the pravastatin inflammation/CRP evaluation (PRINCE): a randomized trial and cohort study. *Journal of the American Medical Association*, **286**, 64–70.

Anderson, J. L., Muhlestein, J. B., Carlquist, J., Allen, A., Trehan, S., Nielson, C. *et al.* (1999). Randomized secondary prevention trial of azithromycin in patients with coronary artery disease and serological evidence for Chlamydia pneumoniae infection: The Azithromycin in Coronary Artery Disease. Elimination of Myocardial Infection with Chlamydia (ACADEMIC) Study. *Circulation*, **99**, 1540–7.

Antithrombotic Trialists' Collaboration (2002). Collaborative meta-analysis of randomized trials of antiplatelet therapy for prevention of death, myocardial infarction and stroke in high-risk patients. *British Medical Journal*, **324**, 71–86.

Baigent, C., Burbury, K., and Wheeler, D. (2000). Premature cardiovascular disease in chronic renal failure. *Lancet*, **358**, 1356–60.

Blasi, F., Ranzi, M. L., Erba, M., Tarsia, P., Raccanelli, R., Fagetti, L., and Allegra, L. (1996). No evidence for the presence of Helicobacter pylori in atherosclerotic plaques in abdominal aortic aneurysm specimens. *Atherosclerosis*, **126**, 339–40.

Cannon, C. P., Braunwald, E., McCabe, C. H. *et al.* (2004). Provastatin or atorvastatin evaluation and infection therapy (TIMI 22). http://www.escardio.org/knowledge/congresses/hot/hot_2004.htm.

Capron, L. (1996). Chlamydia in coronary plaques: hidden culprit or harmless hobo? *Nature Medicine*, **2**, 856–7.

Cercek, B., Shah, P. K., Noc, M. *et al* (2003). Effect of short-term treatment with azithromycin on recurrent ischaemic events in patients with acute coronary syndrome in the Azithromycin in Acute Coronary Syndrome (AZACS) trial: a randomised controlled trial. *Lancet*, **361**, 809–13.

Chiu, B., Viira, E., Tucker, W., and Fong, I. W. (1997). Chlamydia pneumoniae, cytomegalovirus, and herpes simplex virus in atherosclerosis of the carotid artery. *Circulation*, **96**, 2144–8.

Clarke, R., Shipley, M., Lewington, S., Youngman, L., Collins, R., Marmot, M., and Peto R. (1999). Underestimation of risk associations due to regression dilution in long-term follow-up of prospective studies. *American Journal of Epidemiology*, **150**, 341–53.

Clayton, D. and McKeigue, P. M. (2001). Epidemiological methods for studying genes and environmental factors in complex diseases. *Lancet*, **358**, 1356–60.

Cushman, M., Legault, C., Barrett-Connor, E., Stefanick, M. L., Kessler, C., Judd, H. L. *et al.* (1999). Effect of postmenopausal hormones on inflammation-sensitive proteins: the Postmenopausal Estrogen/Progestin Interventions (PEPI) Study. *Circulation*, **100**, 717–22.

Danesh, J. (1999). Helicobacter pylori and gastric cancer: time for mega-trials? [Editorial.] *British Journal of Cancer*, **80**, 927–9.

Danesh, J. and Appleby, P. (1998). Persistent infection and vascular disease: a systematic review. *Expert Opinion on Investigational Drugs*, **7**, 691–713.

Danesh, J. and Appleby, P. (1999). Coronary heart disease and iron status: meta-analyses of prospective studies. *Circulation*, **99**, 852–4.

Danesh, J. and Collins, R. (2001). Antibiotics in the prevention of coronary heart disease: review of the randomized trials. In *Inflammatory and infectious basis of atherosclerosis* (ed. J. L. Mehta), pp. 237–42. Birkhauser Verlag, Basel, Switzerland.

Danesh, J. and Peto, R. (1998). Risk factors for coronary heart disease and infection with Helicobacter pylori: meta-analysis of 18 studies. *British Medical Journal*, **316**, 1130–2.

Danesh, J., Collins, R., and Peto, R. (1997). Chronic infections and coronary heart disease: is there a link? *Lancet*, **350**, 430–6.

Danesh, J., Collins, R., Appleby, P., and Peto, R. (1998). Association of fibrinogen, C-reactive protein, albumin, or leukocyte count with coronary heart disease: meta-analyses of prospective studies. *Journal of the American Medical Association*, **279**, 1477–82.

Danesh, J., Koreth, J., Youngman, L., Collins, R., Arnold, J. R., Balarajan, Y., McGee, J., and Roskell, D. (1999*a*). Is Helicobacter pylori a factor in coronary atherosclerosis? *Journal of Clinical Microbiology*, **37**, 1651.

Danesh, J., Youngman, L., Clark, S., Parish, S., Peto, R., and Collins, R. (1999*b*). Helicobacter pylori infection and early onset myocardial infarction: case-control and sibling pairs study. *British Medical Journal*, **319**, 1157–62.

Danesh, J., Whincup, P., Walker, M., Lennon, L., Thomson, A., Aleby, P. *et al.* (2000*a*). Low grade inflammation and coronary heart disease: prospective study and updated meta-analyses. *British Medical Journal*, **321**, 199–204.

Danesh, J., Whincup, P., Walker, M., Lennon, L., Thomson, A., Appleby, P. *et al.* (2000*b*). Chlamydia pneumoniae IgG titres and coronary heart disease: prospective study and meta-analysis. *British Medical Journal*, **321**, 208–13.

Danesh, J., Whincup, P., Lewington, S., Walker, M., Lennon, L., Thomson, A. *et al.* (2002). Chlamydia pneumoniae IgA titres and coronary heart disease. *European Heart Journal*, **23**, 371–5.

Danesh, J., Wheeler, J. G., Hirschfield, G. M., Eda, S., Eriksdottir, G., Rumley, A. *et al.* (2004). C-reactive protein and other circulating markers of inflammation in the prediction of coronary heart disease. *N Engl J Med*, **350**, 1387–97.

Danesh, J. (2005). Antibiotics in the prevention of coronary heart disease. *Lancet*, **365**, 365–7.

DeStefano, F., Anda, R. F., Kahn, H. S., Williamson, D. F., and Russell, C. M. (1993). Dental disease and risk of coronary heart disease and mortality. *British Medical Journal*, **306**, 688–91.

Easterbrook, P. J., Berlin, J. A., Gopalan, R., and Matthews, D. R. (1991). Publication bias in clinical research. *Lancet*, **337**, 867–72.

Espinola-Klein, C., Rurecht, H. J., Blankenberg, S., Bickel, C., Ko, H., Riin, G. *et al.* (2002). Impact of infectious burden on extent and long-term prognosis of atherosclerosis. *Circulation*, **105**, 15–21.

Fabricant, C. G., Fabricant, J., Litrenta, M. M., and Minick, C. R. (1978). Virus-induced atherosclerosis. *Journal of Experimental Medicine*, **148**, 335–40.

Farsak, B., Yildirir, A., Akyon, Y., Pinar, A., Oc, M., Boke, E. *et al.* (2000). Detection of Chlamydia pneumoniae and Helicobacter pylori DNA in human atherosclerotic plaques by PCR. *Journal of Clinical Microbiology*, **38**, 4408–11.

Fibrinogen Studies Collaboration (2004). Collaborative meta-analysis of prospective studies of plasma fibrinogen and cardiovascular disease. *Eur J Cardiovasc Prevention Rehab*, **11**, 9–17.

Frothingham, C. (1911). The relation between acute infectious diseases and arterial lesions. *Archives of Internal Medicine*, **8**, 153–62.

Grayston, J. T. (1999). Antibiotic treatment trials for secondary prevention of coronary artery disease events. *Circulation*, **99**, 1538–9.

Grayston, J. T., Kronmal, R., Jackson, L. A. *et al.* (2004). Antibiotic Treatment for Secondary Prevention of Coronary Events. http://www.escardio.org/knowledge/congresses/hot/hot_2004.htm.

Greenland, S. (1980). The effect of misclassification in the presence of covariates. *American Journal of Epidemiology*, **112**, 564–9.

Gunn, M., Stephens, J. C., Thompson, J. R., Rathbone, B. J., and Samani, N. J. (2000). Significant association of cagA positive Helicobacter pylori strains with risk of premature myocardial infarction. *Heart*, **84**, 267–71.

Gupta, S., Leatham, E. W., Carrington, D., Mendall, M. A., Kaski, J. C., and Camm, A. J. (1997). Elevated Chlamydia pneumoniae antibodies, cardiovascular events, and azithromycin in male survivors of myocardial infarction. *Circulation*, **96**, 404–7.

Gurfinkel, E., Bozovich, G., Daroca, A., Beck, E., and Mautner, B. (1997). Randomised trial of roxithromycin in non-Q-wave coronary syndromes: ROXIS Pilot Study. ROXIS Study Group. *Lancet*, **350**, 404–7.

Gurfinkel, E., Bozovich, G., Beck, E., Testa, E., Livellara, B., and Mautner, B. (1999). Treatment with the antibiotic roxithromycin in patients with acute non-Q-wave coronary syndromes: the final report of the ROXIS Study. *European Heart Journal*, **20**, 121–7.

Hillis, G. S., Pearson, C. V., Harding, S. A., Sutherland, S., Ludlam, C. A., Marion, J. C. *et al.* (2004). Effects of a brief course of azithromycin on soluble cell adhesion molecules and markers of inflammation in survivors of an acute coronary syndrome: a double-blind, randomized, placebo-controlled study. *Am Heart J*, **148**, 72–9.

Howell, T. H., Ridker, P. M., Ajani, U. A., Hennekens, C. H., and Christen, W. G. (2001). Periodontal disease and risk of subsequent cardiovascular disease in U. S. male physicians. *Journal of the American College of Cardiology*, **37**, 445–50.

Jialal, I., Stein, D., Halis, D., Grundy, S. M., Adams-Huet, B., and Devaraj, S. (2001). Effect of hydroxymethyl glutaryl coenzyme A reductase inhibitor therapy of highly sensitive C-reactive protein levels. *Circulation*, **103**, 1933–5.

Keavney, B., Danesh, J., Parish, S., Palmer, A., Clark, S., Delepine, M. *et al.* (submitted). Plasma fibrinogen and coronary heart disease in 4685 cases and 3460 controls: test of causality by 'Mendelian randomization'.

Lagrand, W. K., Visser, C. A., Hermens, W. T., Niessen, H. W., Verheugt, F. W., Wolbink, G. J., and Hack, C. E. (1999). C-reactive protein as a cardiovascular risk factor: more than an epiphenomenon? *Circulation*, **100**, 96–102.

Law, M. R., Wald, N. J., and Thompson, S. G. (1994). By how much and how quickly does reduction in serum cholesterol concentration lower risk of ischaemic heart disease? *British Medical Journal*, **308**, 367–72.

Lewington, S., Clarke, R., Qizilbash, N., Peto, R., Collins, R. Prospective Studies Collaboration. (2002). Age-specific relevance of usual blood pressure to vascular mortality: a meta-analysis of individual data for 1 million adults from 61 prospective studies. *Lancet*, **360**, 1903–13.

Libby, P., Ridker, P. M., and Maseri, A. (2002). Inflammation and atherosclerosis. *Circulation*, **105**, 1135–43.

MacGregor, A. J., Gallimore, J. R., Spector, T. D., and Pepys, M. B. (1999). Genetic factors determine baseline levels of C-reactive protein and serum amyloid A. *Annals of Rheumatic Disease*, **43**, 139.

MacMahon, S., Peto, R., Cutler, J., Collins, R., Sorlie, P., Neaton, J. *et al.* (1990). Blood pressure, stroke, and coronary heart disease. Part 1: Prolonged differences in blood pressure: prospective observational studies corrected for the regression dilution bias. *Lancet*, **335**, 765–74.

Malik, I., Danesh, J., Whincup, P., Bhatia, V., Papacosta, O., Walker, M. *et al.* (2001). Soluble adhesion molecules and prediction of coronary heart disease: a prospective study and meta-analysis. *Lancet*, **358**, 971–6.

Mattila, K. J., Nieminen, M. S., Valtonen, V. V., Rai, V. P., Kesaniemi, Y. A., Syrjala, S. L. *et al.* (1989). Association between dental health and acute myocardial infarction. *British Medical Journal*, **298**, 779–81.

Melnick, J. L., Petrie, B. L., Dreesman, G. R., Burek, J., McCollum, C. H., and DeBakey, M. E. (1983). Cytomegalovirus antigen within human arterial smooth muscle cells. *Lancet*, **2**, 644–7.

Mendall, M. A., Goggin, P. M., Molineaux, N., Levy, J., Toosy, T., Strachan, D. *et al.* (1994). Relation of Helicobacter pylori infection and coronary heart disease. *British Heart Journal*, **71**, 437–9.

Muhlestein, J. B., Anderson, J. L., Carlquist, J. F. *et al.* (2000). Randomized secondary prevention trial of azithromycin in patients with coronary artery disease: primary clinical results of the ACADEMIC Study. *Circulation*, **102**, 1755–60.

Murray, L. J., Bamford, K. B., Kee, F., McMaster, D., Cambien, F., Dallongeville J., and Evans, A. (2000). Infection with virulent strains of Helicobacter pylori is not associated with ischaemic heart disease: evidence from a population-based case-control study of myocardial infarction. *Atherosclerosis*, **149**, 379–85.

Nieto, F. J. (1998). Infections and atherosclerosis: new clues from an old hypothesis? *American Journal of Epidemiology*, **148**, 937–48.

O'Connor, C. M., Dunne, M. W., Pfeffer. M. A. *et al.* (2003). Azithromycin for the secondary prevention of coronary heart disease events. The WIZARD Study: a randomized controlled events. *JAMA*, **290**, 1459–66.

Ossewaarde, J. M., Feskens, E. J., De Vries, A., Vallinga, C. E., and Kromhout D. (1998). Chlamydia pneumoniae is a risk factor for coronary heart disease in symptom-free elderly men, but Helicobacter pylori and cytomegalovirus are not. *Epidemiology and Infection*, **120**, 93–9.

Parish, S., Collins, R., Peto, R., Youngman, L., Barton, J., Jayne, K. *et al.* (1995). Cigarette smoking, tar yields, and non-fatal myocardial infarction: 14,000 cases and 32,000 controls in the United Kingdom: The International Studies of Infarct Survival (ISIS) Collaborators. *British Medical Journal*, **311**, 471–7.

Pasceri, V., Cammarota, G., Patti, G., Cuoco, L., Gasbarrini, A., Grillo, R. L. *et al.* (1998). Association of virulent Helicobacter pylori strains with ischemic heart disease. *Circulation*, **97**, 1675–9.

Patel, P., Mendall, M. A., Carrington, D., Strachan, D. P., Leatham, E., Molineaux, N. *et al.* (1995). Association of Helicobacter pylori and Chlamydia pneumoniae infections with coronary heart disease and cardiovascular risk factors. *British Medical Journal*, **311**, 711–14.

Pepys, M. B. (1995). The acute phase response and C-reactive protein. In *Oxford textbook of medicine*, 3rd edn (ed. D. J. Weatherall, J. G. G. Ledingham, and D. A. Warrell), pp. 1527–33. Oxford University Press.

Radke, P. W., Merkelbach-Bruse, S., Messmer, B. J., vom Dahl, J., Dorge, H., Naami, A. *et al.* (2001). Infectious agents in coronary lesions obtained by endatherectomy: pattern of distribution, coinfection, and clinical findings. *Coronary Artery Disease*, **12**, 1–6.

Ridker, P. M. (2002). On evolutionary biology, inflammation, infection, and the causes of atherosclerosis. *Circulation*, **105**, 2.

Ridker, P. M., Cushman, M., Stampfer, M. J., Tracy, R. P., and Hennekens, C. H. (1997). Inflammation, aspirin, and the risk of cardiovascular disease in apparently healthy men. *New England Journal of Medicine*, **336**, 973–9.

Ridker, P. M., Hennekens, C. H., Stampfer, M. J., and Wang, F. (1998a). Prospective study of herpes simplex virus, cytomegalovirus, and the risk of future myocardial infarction and stroke. *Circulation*, **98**, 2796–9.

Ridker, P. M., Rifai, N., Pfeffer, M. A., Sacks, F. M., Moye, L. A., Goldman, S. *et al.* (1998b). Inflammation, pravastatin, and the risk of coronary events after myocardial infarction in patients with average cholesterol levels. Cholesterol and Recurrent Events (CARE) Investigators. *Circulation*, **98**, 839–44.

Ridker, P. M., Rifai, N., Pfeffer, M. A., Sacks, F., and Braunwald, E. (1999). Long-term effects of pravastatin on plasma concentration of C-reactive protein. The Cholesterol and Recurrent Events (CARE) Investigators. *Circulation*, **100**, 230–5.

Ridker, P. M., Danesh, J., Youngman, L., Collins, R., Stampfer, M. J., Peto, R., and Hennekens, C. H. (2001a). A prospective study of Helicobacter pylori seropositivity and the risk for future myocardial infarction among socioeconomically similar U. S. men. *Annals of Internal Medicine*, **135**, 184–8.

Ridker, P. M., Rifai, N., Clearfield, M., Downs, J. R., Weis, S. E., Miles, J. S., and Gotto, A. M. Jr (2001*b*). Measurement of C-reactive protein for the targeting of statin therapy in the primary prevention of acute coronary events. *New England Journal of Medicine*, **344**, 1959–65.

Ridker, P. M., Rifai, N., and Lowenthal, S. P. (2001*c*). Rapid reduction in C-reactive protein with cerivastatin among 785 patients with primary hypercholesterolaemia. *Circulation*, **103**, 1191–3.

Ross, R. (1999). Atherosclerosis is an inflammatory disease. *New England Journal of Medicine*, **340**, 115–26.

Saikku, P., Leinonen, M., Mattila, K., Ekman, M. R., Nieminen, M. S., Makela, P. H. *et al.* (1988). Serological evidence of an association of a novel Chlamydia, TWAR, with chronic coronary heart disease and acute myocardial infarction. *Lancet*, **2**, 983–6.

Shor, A., Kuo, C. C., and Patton, D. L. (1992). Detection of Chlamydia pneumoniae in coronary arterial fatty streaks and atheromatous plaques. *South African Medical Journal*, **82**, 158–61.

Sinisalo, J., Mattila, K., Valtonen, V. *et al.* (2002). Effect of 3 months of antimicrobial treatment with clarithromycin in acute non-Q-wave coronary syndrome. *Circulation*, **105**, 1555–60.

Siscovick, D. S., Schwartz, S. M., Corey, L., Grayston, J. T., Ashley, R., Wang, S. P. *et al.* (2000). Chlamydia pneumoniae, herpes simplex virus type 1, and cytomegalovirus and incident myocardial infarction and coronary heart disease death in older adults: the Cardiovascular Health Study. *Circulation*, **102**, 2335–40.

Sorlie, P. D., Nieto, F. J., Adam, E., Folsom, A. R., Shahar, E., and Massing, M. (2000). A prospective study of cytomegalovirus, herpes simplex virus 1, and coronary heart disease: the atherosclerosis risk in communities (ARIC) study. *Archives of Internal Medicine*, **160**, 2027–32.

Stone, A. F. M., Risley, P., Markus, H. S., Butland, B. K., Strachan, D. P., Elwood, P. C., and Mendall, M. A. (2001). Ischaemic heart disease and Cag A strains of Helicobacter pylori in the Caerphilly heart disease study. *Heart*, **86**, 506–9.

Stone, A. F. M., Mendall, M. A., Kaski, J. C. *et al.* (2002). Effect of treatment for *Chlamydia pneumoniae* and *Helicobacter pylori* on markers of inflammation and cardiac events in patients with acute coronary syndromes. *Circulation*, **106**, 1219–23.

Strachan, D. P., Carrington, D., Mendall, M. A., Butland, B. K., Sweetname, P. M., and Elwood, P. C. (1999). Cytomegalovirus seropositivity and incident ischaemic heart disease in the Caerphilly prospective heart disease study. *Heart*, **81**, 248–51.

Viik-Kajander, M., Roivainen, M., Manninen, V., Hovi, T., and Mantari, M. (1997). Herpes virus infections and the risk of myocardial infarction and coronary death. *Circulation*, **96** (Suppl. 1), 1–374.

Wald, N. J., Law, M. R., Morris, J. K., and Bagnall, A. M. (1997). Helicobacter pylori infection and mortality from ischaemic heart disease: negative result from a large, prospective study. *British Medical Journal*, **315**, 1199–201.

Whincup, P., Danesh, J., Walker, M., Lennon, L., Thomson, A., Appleby, P. *et al.* (2000). Prospective study of potentially virulent strains of Helicobacter pylori and coronary heart disease in middle-aged men. *Circulation*, **101**, 1647–52.

Whincup, P. H., Danesh, J., Walker, M., Lennon, L., Thomson, A., Appleby, P. *et al.* (2002). Von Willebrand factor and coronary heart disease: prospective study and meta-analysis. *European Heart Journal*, **23**, 1764–70.

Youngman, L. D., Keavney, B. D., Palmer, A., Parish, S., Clark, S., Danesh, J. *et al.* (2000). Plasma fibrinogen and fibrinogen genotypes in 4685 cases of myocardial infarction and in 6002 controls: test of causality by mendelian randomization. *Circulation*, **102** (Suppl. 1-II), 31–2.

Zahn, R., Schneider, S., Frilling, B. *et al.* (2003). Antibiotic therapy after acute myocardial infarction: a prospective randomized study. *Circulation*, **107**, 1253–59.

Zhu, J., Nieto, F. J., Horne, B. D., Anderson, J. L., Muhlestein, J. B., and Epstein, S. E. (2001). Prospective study of pathogen burden and risk of myocardial infarction or death. *Circulation*, **103**, 45–51.

Chapter 28

Coagulation, thrombosis, and coronary heart disease

T. W. Meade and P. K. MacCallum

28.1 Introduction

General recognition of the thrombotic component in arterial disease, particularly coronary heart disease (CHD), is comparatively recent. The term 'coronary thrombosis' appears to have been first used by Herrick (1912) early in the 1900s and it continued to be used until coronary or ischaemic heart disease became the preferred terminology after the Second World War, when the condition had reached epidemic proportions.

Epidemiological studies which started in the late 1940s – the work in the community of Framingham being the best known – began to establish the characteristics of those at particular risk of heart attacks. The main emphasis, however, was on the part played by lipid infiltration, which has tended to dominate thinking in North America ever since in comparison with a readier acceptance in Europe of a thrombotic component (as well as of atherogenesis). There was good reason for supposing that lipids play a major part: it was easy to demonstrate the presence of lipid-rich material, including cholesterol crystals, in the coronary arteries and it seemed logical to suggest that high-fat diets and blood cholesterol levels might contribute to atheroma. In 1951, however, Morris (1951) and Morris and Crawford (1958) in the MRC Social Medicine Unit at the (now Royal) London Hospital showed very clearly that while advanced atheroma obviously contributed, it could not explain the whole of the CHD epidemic. However, the implication that there must be another process involved – almost certainly thrombosis – was not fully recognized for at least another 20 years.

Interest in a thrombotic component to CHD started to re-emerge in the 1970s, but was initially characterized by a rather sterile debate as to whether thrombosis causes or is a consequence of myocardial infarction, settled in favour of causation by an unsatisfactory consensus method (Chandler *et al.* 1974). Evidence for the role of thrombosis in myocardial infarction was provided in convincing form when angiographic monitoring of the early use of thrombolytic therapy showed the development of occlusive thrombi preceding myocardial infarction (DeWood *et al.* 1980). One reason for doubting the involvement of thrombosis in sudden coronary death had been the failure to demonstrate thrombi at autopsy in many cases. In 1984, however, a particularly careful study (Davies and Thomas 1984) comparing the prevalence of thrombosis in sudden coronary death with sudden death from other causes gave the results summarized in Table 28.1, indicating that a degree of thrombosis is demonstrable in nearly all sudden coronary deaths. Other studies have generally confirmed this. It is now also recognized that the pathology of unstable angina pectoris is similar to that of myocardial infarction and of sudden coronary death in consisting of a significant thrombotic component (Falk 1987) and in responding to antithrombotic treatment.

Table 28.1 The presence of thrombus in 100 sudden coronary and 78 sudden non-coronary deaths

Thrombus type	Coronary (%)	Non-coronary (%)
Intraluminal	74	0
Intraluminal with plaque fissure	19	3.8
Intraintimal only	2	6
None	5	89.8

From Davies and Thomas 1984.

Further evidence for the role of thrombosis in CHD came with recognition of the effects of aspirin in modifying the aggregation of platelets and with the results of observational studies and early trials (Elwood *et al.* 1974) showing the reduction in CHD due to aspirin. However, no tests of platelet behaviour have convincingly been shown to be associated with the subsequent risk of first events of CHD (Meade *et al.* 1997) (although spontaneous platelet aggregation (Trip *et al.* 1990) and increased platelet volume (Martin *et al.* 1991) may help predict those at risk of recurrent episodes).

Until fairly recently, the contribution of the coagulation system to arterial thrombosis through fibrin formation was not considered to be of clinical significance. However, epidemiological studies of the coagulation system in thrombosis and CHD have now demonstrated its involvement and implications for its management and prevention.

28.2 **Epidemiological evidence**

Population-based studies started from the general proposition that high levels of procoagulatory clotting factors and low levels of anticoagulatory factors would predispose to CHD. Sceptics argued that (other than in obvious deficiency conditions such as haemophilia) clotting factors circulate well in excess of concentrations required for extravascular haemostasis and that no associations with CHD would therefore be demonstrable. However, requirements for haemostasis may not be a reliable guide to the influence of different levels of clotting factors on intravascular overactivity of the clotting system where a high level of a procoagulatory factor might facilitate thrombosis and a major coronary event.

Studies that demonstrate associations between different characteristics and the risk of CHD have two main purposes. One is to contribute to our understanding of the pathogenesis of the condition. The other is to identify characteristics with reasonably clear implications either for screening purposes and/or treatment and prevention. This distinction is important in the interpretation of the results of these studies. For screening, it is usually the additional, independent contribution of a risk factor that is required, largely regardless of other variables that determine its level or with which it is correlated. For studies concerned with mechanisms or pathways, however, multivariate techniques for analysing data should be used cautiously so that suggestive associations (say of the effect of smoking on the fibrinogen levels) are not overlooked by, in effect, removing possible determinants of a risk factor.

Figure 28.1 shows the main features of the coagulation system. Here and in the text the suffix 'a' signifies the activated form of the clotting factor. The coagulation process, resulting in the

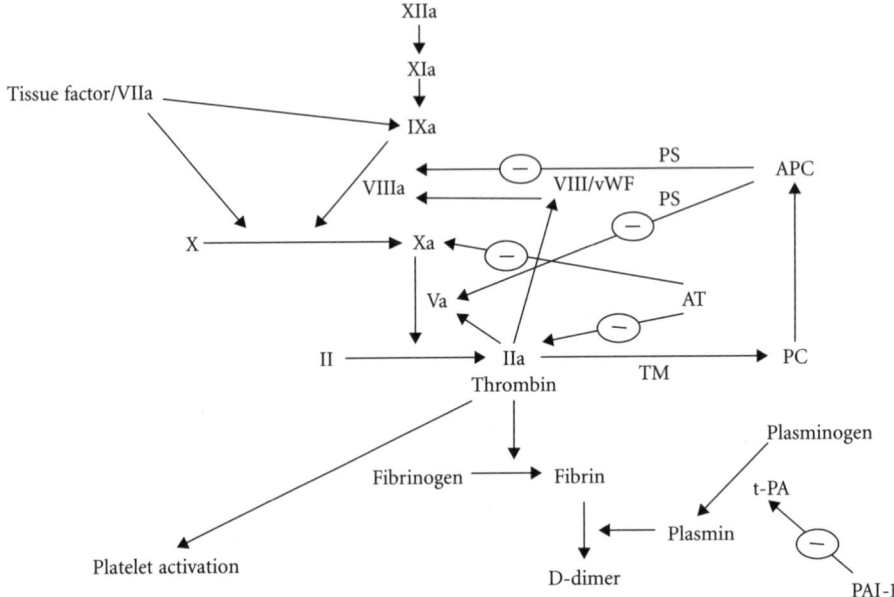

Fig. 28.1 Main features of the coagulation system. Activated forms of the clotting factors are denoted by the suffix 'a'. For simplicity, not all the precursor forms of activated factors are shown (e.g. XII for XIIa, etc.). (Abbreviations: vWF: von Willebrand factor; II: prothrombin; AT: antithrombin; PC: protein C; APC: activated protein C; TM: thrombomodulin; PS: protein S; t-PA: tissue-type plasminogen activator; PAI-1: plasminogen activator inhibitor type 1.) Arrows indicate direction of activation of one component by another, other than those shown [insert oval containing bar, as on diagram], which indicate inhibition.

generation of thrombin, can be initiated either through the extrinsic system, so called because it depends on the availability of tissue factor which has not generally been considered a component of the circulating blood, or through the intrinsic or contact system, which is not dependent on biochemical properties outside the circulating blood. It is generally considered that the extrinsic system is critical in the initiation of activation of coagulation. Tissue factor becomes available when atheromatous lesions leak or rupture. Besides its well-known function in converting soluble fibrinogen into insoluble fibrin, thrombin has numerous other properties. Among these is its action as a potent platelet-aggregating agent and it may exert this action at least as soon as (if not before) its action on fibrinogen, so that the coagulation system has a strong influence on platelet behaviour as well as on the deposition of fibrin. Other actions of thrombin include the activation of protein C, which together with protein S inhibits the coagulation process. Over the last few years the significance of a polymorphism in factor V, known as factor V Leiden, in leading to resistance to activated protein C, has become clear so far as venous thrombosis is concerned (Bertina *et al.* 1994), though what part it may play on the arterial side is much less obvious.

There have now been numerous cohort (prospective) and case-control or case-comparison studies of associations between different components of the coagulation system and the risk of CHD.

28.3 **Fibrinogen**

An overview of 18 cohort studies (Danesh *et al.* 1998) based on 4018 cases of CHD demonstrated that those in the top third of the fibrinogen distribution are at 1.8 times the risk of CHD compared with those in the bottom third, the findings being similar in the 12 studies concerned with first events and the other 6 with individuals known to have had previous episodes and followed for recurrences. The association of fibrinogen with the incidence of CHD is independent of other risk factors, is of a similar magnitude to the risk due to raised cholesterol, and is probably the same in women as in men. Besides first and recurrent events of CHD, high fibrinogen levels are also associated with the onset, recurrence, and progression of lower extremity arterial disease (Banerjee *et al.* 1992), with the incidence of graft occlusion following bypass surgery (Wiseman *et al.* 1989), and possibly with an increased risk of restenosis following coronary or lower limb angioplasty (Montalescot *et al.* 1995). Fibrinogen may also be associated with the occurrence of stroke (Wilhelmsen *et al.* 1984), but another and larger prospective study showed no association (Baker *et al.* 2002). There is much less evidence of this point than for CHD and it remains a largely unsettled but obviously important question.

28.4 **Factor VII**

The possible involvement of factor VII activity in CHD is of theoretical as well as practical interest, bearing in mind the importance of the extrinsic system in the initiation of blood coagulation, just referred to. When tissue factor is exposed to blood following the leakage or rupture of an atheromatous plaque, it binds with factor VII, so high levels of the latter might affect the amount of thrombin produced. However, the evidence is equivocal. Two cohort studies suggest that high levels increase risk (Junker *et al.* 1997; Meade *et al.* 1980, 1986), whilst others do not (Cooper *et al.* 2000; Folsom *et al.* 1997; Tracy *et al.* 1999). Case-control and cross-sectional studies have also given conflicting results. Several assay techniques have been used and it has been established that these may vary in their sensitivity to factor VII activity, which might partly account for the differing results (Miller *et al.* 1994).

28.5 **Factor VIII and von Willebrand factor**

Factor VIII circulates in a complex with von Willebrand factor (vWF). The two proteins serve different haemostatic functions and have different sites of production, but they are closely correlated in a statistical sense so that independent contributions of the two proteins cannot easily be demonstrated, if at all. The role of factor VIII in CHD has been reviewed by MacCallum and Meade (1999). Four cohort studies have shown high levels of factor VIII to confer an increased risk of CHD. Haemophiliac patients appear to have a lower than expected incidence of CHD (though a considerable excess of cerebrovascular disease because of bleeding) and carriers of haemophilia have a reduced standardized mortality rate from CHD. Autopsy data show that haemophilia does not prevent the development of atheroma, suggesting that the decreased risk of CHD in patients with haemophilia is due to the effect of low levels of factor VIII on thrombogenic potential and fibrin formation. Case-control data show that elevated levels of factor VIII are associated with an increased risk of venous thrombosis (Koster *et al.* 1995), where the potentially confounding effect of vessel wall disease on the factor VIII level is not as much of an issue as on the arterial side. The association of factor VIII with CHD therefore appears to be due to a direct contribution of the level of factor VIII in circulating blood and not to a chronic phase response to atheromatous vessel wall changes.

28.6 **Fibrinolytic activity**

Several cohort studies, whether concerned with first events or in patients with previous episodes of CHD, have led to the conclusion that impaired fibrinolytic activity is an independent risk factor for CHD or its recurrence. Different studies have used different methods. These have included global tests of fibrinolytic activity (Meade *et al.* 1993) such as the dilute clot lysis time, which takes account of both activators and inhibitors, and assays of specific components of the fibrinolytic system, principally tissue-type plasminogen activator (t-PA) plasminogen activator inhibitor type 1 (PAI-1), and of D-dimer, the main degradation product of fibrinolysis. The principal determinants of the dilute clot lysis time are PAI-1 and, in men, t-PA. High levels of t-PA antigen have been associated with CHD (Ridker *et al.* 1993), which seems counterintuitive since high levels of t-PA would be expected to confer protection. The explanation may be that t-PA antigen, which is what the studies in question have measured, complexes with PAI-1 that is present in higher concentration and for which t-PA antigen is a surrogate marker. Raised levels of D-dimer, indicating increased fibrin turnover, have been found to be predictive of future cardiovascular events (Danesh *et al.* 2001). The association of activity of PAI-1 with CHD is not seen after adjustment for the features of insulin resistance (body mass index, triglyceride, high-density lipoprotein cholesterol, blood pressure, and diabetes) so that the prognostic value of PAI-1 may be chiefly related to this syndrome (Juhan-Vague *et al.* 1996).

28.7 **Other factors**

Whereas inherited deficiencies of the naturally occurring inhibitors of coagulation such as antithrombin, protein C, and protein S clearly increase the risk of venous thromboembolism, the contribution that alterations in the levels of these proteins makes to arterial thrombosis is unclear. Anecdotally, case reports and case series have described deficiencies of these inhibitors in patients who have sustained arterial events. More formal studies have given conflicting and inconclusive results. What evidence there is suggests that low antithrombin levels may predispose to CHD (Meade *et al.* 1991; Thompson *et al.* 1995).

A high level of factor XIIa is associated with raised levels of a number of familiar risk factors for CHD, including plasma triglyceride and systolic blood pressure, and it is an independent predictor of CHD (Cooper *et al.* 2000).

Overall, the evidence shows that predisposition to thrombosis and CHD is associated with changes in several components of the coagulation system, as well as with platelet behaviour, and the question arises as to whether they represent causality. If so, what are the pathways involved and what are the implications for management and prevention through measures affecting the haemostatic system? There are three main ways in which these questions can be approached: (a) by detailed laboratory studies; (b) by the extent to which the associations of clotting factor with CHD are consistent with the effects of known risk factors such as smoking; and (c) by the ability of agents used in randomized controlled trials to affect particular pathways.

28.8 **Laboratory studies**

The effects of fibrinogen have been extensively studied and are summarized in Fig. 28.2. High fibrinogen levels make a substantial contribution to the viscosity of the whole blood and plasma and to the amount of fibrin deposited when coagulation is initiated: they increase platelet

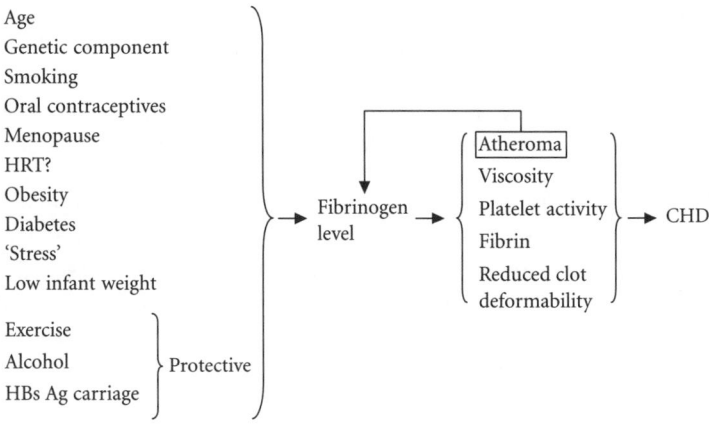

Age
Genetic component
Smoking
Oral contraceptives
Menopause
HRT?
Obesity
Diabetes
'Stress'
Low infant weight

Exercise
Alcohol } Protective
HBs Ag carriage

Fibrinogen level → { Atheroma
Viscosity
Platelet activity
Fibrin
Reduced clot deformability } → CHD

Fig. 28.2 Summary of determinants and thrombogenic pathways of fibrinogen in pathogenesis of CHD, showing possible fibrinogen-atheroma-fibrinogen sequence.

aggregability, enhance the binding of leucocytes to platelets and endothelial cells, decrease clot deformability, and contribute to the atheromatous process – all of which have been shown to, or are likely to, increase the risk of thrombosis and thus of clinical events.

A number of metabolic studies have shown associations of factor VII with dietary fat intake and with serum triglyceride concentrations. However, the inconsistent results of the epidemiological studies of factor VII, referred to earlier, need to be borne in mind. Factor VII assayed by conventional biological assay itself has little activity. Fully activated VII, VIIa, is associated with plasma levels of the activation peptide fragment 1 + 2, an indicator of thrombin generation that is released from prothrombin upon its conversion to thrombin. Dietary and other studies have shown a pivotal role for factor IXa on the level of blood coagulability (Miller *et al.* 1996). Factor VIII has been shown to increase the rate of activation of factor X by factor IXa in a dose-dependent manner.

28.9 **Consistency with known risk factors**

Very generally, associations of haemostatic variables with CHD are similar to the effects of more familiar risk factors. This is also best illustrated for fibrinogen in Fig. 28.2, in which many of the personal or lifestyle characteristics apparently influencing fibrinogen levels are known to be associated with the risk of CHD itself – for example the increased risk due to smoking and the protective effect of a moderate intake of alcohol. Indeed, the associations of smoking and of moderate alcohol consumption with fibrinogen are likely to explain, at least in part, how these aspects of lifestyle affect CHD itself. One feature absent from Fig. 28.2 is dietary intake, particularly of saturated fat. As an acute and chronic phase protein, fibrinogen levels also rise in response to inflammatory stimuli, of which underlying vessel wall pathology is likely to be an example. This has sometimes led to the view that fibrinogen is no more than a marker of the risk of CHD, whereas the likelihood seems to be that, whatever the original explanations for raised fibrinogen levels, these will increase risk. If so, fibrinogen may be considered to be both a marker and a causal feature as indicated in Fig. 28.2.

Obesity and the other features of the insulin resistance syndrome impair fibrinolytic activity, as does smoking.

The general conclusion is that the personal and lifestyle influences on the risk of CHD operate through effects on the haemostatic system and thrombotic tendency as well as through the more familiar lipid pathways. The implications for lifestyle modifications are therefore limited. However, to the extent that these operate on thrombogenicity, they may become effective over a shorter time period than on atherogenesis. The implications for pharmacological intervention are considerable (see below).

The original hypothesis that the haemostatic system contributes to CHD simply by a direct effect on thrombogenic potential, and thus through 'hypercoagulability', probably now requires modification. Account must be also taken of other processes involved in the pathogenesis of CHD, such as the inflammatory nature of the vessel wall damage in arterial disease to which changes in the coagulation system may be a secondary response (Miller 1999), although these changes may then still contribute to thrombotic potential.

28.10 Inflammatory markers and arterial disease

Recent years have seen widespread recognition that atheroma is an inflammatory process and the emergence of evidence that circulating markers of inflammation might be used to predict the risk of coronary events (Danesh *et al.* 1998; Ridker *et al.* 1997, 2000; see the previous chapter).

The most consistently observed association has been that of the acute-phase reactant, C-reactive protein (CRP) (Pearson *et al.* 2003), with coronary risk. In healthy, asymptomatic adults, a single CRP measurement (using a sensitive assay) in the high normal range is associated with increased risk of angina, acute myocardial infarction, and death. The association is independent of lipids and its strength is similar to that observed with other risk factors, including cholesterol and fibrinogen. CRP is also associated with the risk of recurrent events in those with established CHD.

Chronic respiratory infection (Danesh *et al.* 1997) or, in particular, recent more acute respiratory infection (Meier *et al.* 1998) may be important initiators of inflammatory stimuli in the onset of CHD.

28.11 Homocyst(e)ine

Although not itself a component of the haemostatic system, the sulphur-containing amino acid homocyst(e)ine has emerged in recent years as a potentially important risk factor for arterial disease and also for venous thromboembolism, with postulated mechanisms of effect that may be mediated in part through components of the haemostatic system.

It was first recognized in the 1960s that premature atherothrombosis was often seen in individuals with the rare inherited metabolic disorder homocystinuria, in which the plasma level of homocyst(e)ine is very high. Within the past decade, evidence has emerged from observational studies showing an association between homocyst(e)ine levels and the risk of vascular disease within the general population, although the causal nature of this association remains to be established (Homocyst(e)ine Studies Collaboration 2002; Wald *et al.* 2002) (see also Chapter 16). A number of possible explanations have been put forward but have often been based on *in vitro* studies that have used higher levels of homocyst(e)ine than those typically found clinically and should therefore be interpreted with some caution. They include effects on platelet adhesives or activation, activation of clotting factors V and X, and inhibition of fibrinolysis through enhanced binding of lipoprotein(a) to fibrin. Possible effects on the endothelium may result from oxidative damage and include increased tissue factor and decreased thrombomodulin expression, and inhibition of nitric oxide. Proliferation of smooth muscle may be enhanced.

Plasma homocyst(e)ine levels are influenced by a number of factors, both genetic and environmental (Hankey and Eikelboom 1999; Welch and Loscalzo 1998). Nutritional deficiency of folate is the most common cause of hyperhomocyst(e)inaemia and deficiencies of vitamin B_{12} and also B_6 also contribute. Other acquired causes of hyperhomocyst(e)inaemia include renal impairment, hypothyroidism, malignancy, severe psoriasis, and drugs that interfere with folate or B_6 metabolism. Levels rise with age and are higher in males than females and in smokers compared to non-smokers. The combined oral contraceptive pill and hormone replacement therapy appear to lower the concentration. Homocyst(e)ine should probably not be measured immediately after an occlusive vascular event as levels may be transiently depressed.

The epidemiological association between homocyst(e)ine and CHD may be of considerable public health significance. The magnitude of the reduction that is probably achievable with folic acid might result in a decrease of some 15% in CHD incidence and possibly more in stroke. However, this possibility must be confirmed by trials and a number (with folic acid alone or in combination with vitamin B_6 or B_{12}) are underway. Results should become available within the next few years. In the United States, meanwhile, flour has been fortified with folic acid since 1998 in order to reduce the risk of neural tube defect by ensuring improved folate status in women of child-bearing age. The level of fortification is likely to produce at least an extra 0.1 mg of folic acid per day in the diet and therefore lead to a partial lowering of homocyst(e)ine in the general population. Discussions are ongoing as to whether similar measures should be adopted in the UK. Concerns have been expressed that folic acid may mask subacute combined degeneration of the cord in patients with undiagnosed B_{12} deficiency. The extent of this theoretical risk is uncertain and probably extremely small, but no consensus has yet been reached on whether B_{12} deficiency should be excluded before starting higher doses of folic acid or whether vitamin B_{12} should be routinely administered in conjunction with folic acid.

28.12 Implications for clinical practice

Recent work on the haemostatic system has certainly led to improved understanding of the pathogenesis of CHD, but only some of the information gained so far has implications for clinical practice – in particular, attempting to identify those at increased risk of first or recurrent events. Measuring fibrinogen and assessing fibrinolytic activity are the two investigations that may be helpful. A high fibrinogen level is sometimes the only identifiable risk factor in a patient referred for investigation because of a strong family history of CHD, for example, or in some patients who have recovered from myocardial infarction and in whom there are no other risk factors. Although there is only limited evidence on the value of lowering fibrinogen levels (see below), information about this may be useful in deciding whether, for example, to recommend low-dose aspirin for primary prevention, even though aspirin does not lower fibrinogen. Measuring the euglobin lysis time and the activity of PAI-1 can also be helpful, though (see above) they are often to be explained by obesity and other features of the insulin resistance syndrome.

Fibrinogen and fibrinolytic activity should only be measured some time after an acute episode of CHD and in the absence of recent infection. As for other risk factors such as cholesterol and blood pressure, they should be measured more than once before an individual's habitual level can be established with any certainty. There is now a World Health Organization standard for fibrinogen, which means that ranges and values can be much more confidently compared between different centres than previously. Assays of factor VII activity are difficult to perform and (see above) the interpretation of results is uncertain. There are no established interventions for lowering levels of activity of factor VIII.

28.13 **Prevention**

Besides establishing the clinical value of antithrombotic therapy, randomized trials may (see above) help in confirming the causal nature of associations between the haemostatic variables and CHD that these agents alter. A limitation is that warfarin lowers the activity of all the vitamin K dependent factors, that is, factors II, VII, IX, and X, so that any benefit due to warfarin cannot be ascribed to any single one of them.

28.13.1 **Primary prevention**

In contrast to the value of aspirin in reducing recurrent major vascular events and mortality after a first attack (secondary prevention, see below), its main value in primary prevention seems on present evidence to be in reducing non-fatal myocardial infarction (Collaborative Group of the Primary Prevention Project 2001; Hansson et al. 1998; Medical Research Council's General Practice Research Framework 1998; Steering Committee of the Physicians' Health Study Research Group 1989). The risk of cerebral haemorrhage and other significant bleeding is increased, even at low doses (He et al. 1998). Considerably more thought than is commonly given to the use of aspirin in primary prevention is needed, especially as aspirin can be bought over the counter. Many middle-aged men take aspirin indiscriminately and not necessarily beneficially and safely, taking account simultaneously of benefits and hazards (Sanmuganathan et al. 2001).

One trial has evaluated low-dose aspirin (75 mg daily) and low-intensity oral anticoagulation with warfarin (aiming at an international normalized ratio of 1.5) either singly or in combination, in men at increased risk of CHD (Medical Research Council's General Practice Research Framework 1998). Both agents reduced the incidence of all major manifestations of CHD by ~20%. However, in common with the other evidence in primary prevention, aspirin achieved this as a result of reducing non-fatal events by just over 30% (and, if anything, slightly increasing the risk of fatal episodes). Warfarin reduced fatal episodes by 39%, perhaps by as much as 50% if the effect of full compliance is taken into account (Rudnicka et al. 2003), but had little effect on non-fatal events. The combination of both agents reduced events, whether fatal or non-fatal, by 34%. Warfarin may also have reduced the onset of angina pectoris slightly (Knottenbelt et al. 2002). There was no demonstrable difference in serious bleeding between the three active treatment groups (warfarin and aspirin together, warfarin alone, and aspirin alone) or between them and the placebo group (although minor bleeding was clearly more frequent in those on active treatment regimens). The assumption that warfarin is intrinsically more dangerous than aspirin was therefore not supported. The disadvantage of the need for dose monitoring when using warfarin is balanced by the possibility of a substantial reduction in fatal events, which needs to be considered alongside the inability to predict at all certainly which first major events of CHD will be fatal and the high proportion of those experiencing their first major event who die.

There is still only partial agreement about the optimal dose of aspirin: the evidence mostly points to the need for no more than 75 mg and certainly no more than 300 mg daily, both for antithrombotic effect and safety.

An important but still unresolved question is the value of lowering the plasma fibrinogen. Apart from ancrod, which is used only in emergencies and has to be given by infusion, there are at present no selective fibrinogen-lowering agents. Bezafibrate lowers fibrinogen by ~15% and also modifies the major components of the lipid profile in what would be expected to be a beneficial direction. A recent trial in men with lower extremity arterial disease suggested that bezafibrate may reduce the risk of CHD, especially non-fatal events (Meade *et al.* 2002). Four other trials, one using clofibrate (Report from the Committee of Principal Investigators 1978), two using bezafibrate (BIP 2000; Ericsson *et al.* 1996), and one using fenofibrate (Diabetes Atherosclerosis Intervention Study 2001) also suggest some benefit. However, the reduction in incidence or recurrence of major events has not been as much as would be expected from the fibrinogen-lowering and lipid-modifying effects of bezafibrate, which may be because it has now been shown to raise homocyst(e)ine levels. Another fibric acid derivative, gemfibrozil, clearly reduces events but is biochemically different from bezafibrate (Frick *et al.* 1987; Rubins *et al.* 1999).

28.13.2 Secondary prevention

Antithrombotic treatment in the early stages of myocardial infarction, in which a combination of aspirin and thrombolytic treatment is used and which reduces serious vascular events within the next month or so by some 50% (ISIS-2 1988), merges into the longer-term secondary prevention of further episodes. Here, aspirin reduces further major vascular events (myocardial infarction, stroke, or vascular death) by some 25% (Antiplatelet Trialists' Collaboration 1994; Antithrombotic Trialists' Collaboration 2002). The proportional benefits of aspirin are similar in older and younger patients, in men and women, in normotensive and hypertensive patients, and in non-diabetic and diabetic patients. Absolute reductions, however, are greater in the higher-risk groups (for example older, hypertensive, or diabetic patients) because of their higher event rates. There is little or no formal evidence on how long aspirin should be taken after an initial event, but since those who have already experienced episodes of arterial disease are likely to remain at high risk indefinitely, antithrombotic treatment should probably also be continued long term.

Despite the clear value of aspirin in secondary prevention, the benefits of oral anticoagulation should not be overlooked. First, it is possible that anticoagulation confers slightly greater protection against recurrence than aspirin, perhaps because of the effect of thrombin, which is reduced by warfarin, on platelets as well as fibrinogen. Despite the disadvantages of anticoagulation, this extra benefit (if real) may still be worthwhile for a common condition with a high risk of recurrence. It may be that warfarin also slightly reduces the incidence of malignant disease (Schulman and Lindmarker 2000). The potential value of combined antithrombotic regimens has been well illustrated in the postoperative treatment with aspirin and warfarin of patients undergoing heart valve surgery (Altman *et al.* 1976; Turpie *et al.* 1993). Aspirin with heparin followed by warfarin is also beneficial in the setting of acute coronary syndromes (Cairns *et al.* 2001). Some trials have cast doubt on the possible benefit of combined antithrombotic therapy for recurrent CHD, but they used fixed or capped low-dose warfarin, whereas it is almost certainly necessary to give warfarin in a dose-adjusted manner, that is, to achieve a specified target international normalized ratio. Combined regimens of agents modifying platelets and coagulation simultaneously (Hurlen *et al.* 2002) or different aspects of platelet function with aspirin and dipyridamole in the secondary prevention of stroke (Diener *et al.* 1996) further illustrate the potential value of considering more than one pathway at a time, provided the risk of serious bleeding is not unacceptably increased. An obvious question not so far tested in randomized trials is the potential value of the simultaneous use of antithrombotic and lipid-modifying agents.

References

Altman, R., Boullon, F., Rouvier, J. *et al.* (1976). Aspirin and prophylaxis of thromboembolic complications in patients with substitute heart valves. *Journal of Thoracic and Cardiovascular Surgery*, **72**, 127–9.

Antiplatelet Trialists' Collaboration (1994). Overview of randomized trials of antiplatelet therapy. I: Prevention of death, myocardial infarction, and stroke by prolonged platelet therapy in various categories of patients. III: Reduction in venous thrombosis and pulmonary embolism by antiplatelet prophylaxis among surgical and medical patients. *British Medical Journal*, **308**, 81–106, 235–46.

Antithrombotic Trialists' Collaboration (2002). Collaborative meta-analysis of randomised trials of antiplatelet therapy for prevention of death, myocardial infarction, and stroke in high risk patients. *British Medical Journal*, **324**, 71–86.

Baker, I. A., Pickering, J., Elwood, P. C. *et al.* (2002). Fibrinogen, viscosity and white blood cell count predict myocardial, but not cerebral infarction: evidence from the Caerphilly and Speedwell cohort. *Thrombosis and Haemostasis*, **87**, 421–5.

Banerjee, A. K., Pearson, J., Gilliland, E. L. *et al.* (1992). A six year prospective study of fibrinogen and other risk factors associated with mortality in stable claudicants. *Thrombosis and Haemostasis*, **68**, 261–3.

Bertina, R. M., Koelman, R. P. C., Koster, T. *et al.* (1994). Mutation in blood coagulation factor V associated with resistance to activated protein C. *Nature*, **369**, 64–7.

BIP (Bezafibrate Infarction Prevention) study (2000). Secondary prevention by raising HDL cholesterol and reducing triglycerides in patients with coronary artery disease. *Circulation*, **102**, 21–7.

Cairns, J. A., Theroux P., Lewis, H. D., Jr. *et al.* (2001). Antithrombotic agents in coronary artery disease. *Chest*, **119** (Suppl. 1), 228S–252S.

Chandler, A. B., Chapman, I., Erhardt, L. R. *et al.* (1974). Coronary thrombosis in myocardial infarction. *American Journal of Cardiology*, **34**, 823–33.

Collaborative Group of the Primary Prevention Project (PPP) (2001). Low dose aspirin and vitamin E in people at cardiovascular risk: a randomised trial in general practice. *Lancet*, **357**, 89–95.

Cooper, J. A., Miller, G. J., Bauer, K. A. *et al.* (2000). Comparison of novel hemostatic factors and conventional risk factors for prediction of coronary heart disease. *Circulation*, **102**, 2816–22.

Danesh, J., Collins, R., Peto, R. *et al.* (1997). Chronic infections and CHD: is there a link? *Lancet*, **350**, 430–6.

Danesh, J., Collins, R., Appleby, P. *et al.* (1998). Association of fibrinogen, C-reactive protein, albumin, or leukocyte count with CHD: meta-analyses of prospective studies. *Journal of the American Medical Association*, **279**, 1477–82.

Danesh, J., Whincup, P., Walker M. *et al.* (2001). Fibrin D-dimer and coronary heart disease: prospective study and meta-analysis. *Circulation*, **103**, 2323–7.

Davies, M. J. and Thomas A. (1984). Thrombosis and acute coronary-artery lesions in sudden cardiac ischemic death. *New England Journal of Medicine*, **310**, 1137–40.

DeWood, M. A., Spores, J., Notske, R. *et al.* (1980). Prevalence of total coronary occlusion during the early hours of transmural myocardial infarction. *New England Journal of Medicine*, **303**, 897–901.

Diabetes Atherosclerosis Intervention Study, a randomised study (2001). Effect of fenofibrate on progression of coronary-artery disease in type 2 diabetes. *Lancet*, **357**, 905–10.

Diener, H. C., Cunha, L., Forbes, C. *et al.* (1996). European Stroke Prevention Study. 2. Dipyridamole and acetylsalicylic acid in the secondary prevention of stroke. *Journal of the Neurological Sciences*, **143**, 1–13.

Elwood, P. C., Cochrane, A. L., Burr, M. L. *et al.* (1974). A randomized controlled trial of acetylsalicyclic acid in the secondary prevention of mortality from myocardial infarction. *British Medical Journal*, **i**, 436–40.

Ericsson, C. G., Hamsten, A., Nilsson, J. *et al.* (1996). Angiographic assessment of effects of bezafibrate on progression of coronary artery disease in young male postinfarction patients. *Lancet*, **347**, 849–53.

Falk, E. (1987). Thrombosis in unstable angina: pathologic aspects. In *Thrombosis and platelets in myocardial ischemia* (ed. J. L. Mehta, C. R. Conti, and A. N. Brest), pp. 137–49. F. A. Davis, Philadelphia.

Folsom, A. R., Wu, K. W., Rosamond, W. D. *et al.* (1997). Prospective study of hemostatic factors and incidence of coronary heart disease: the Atherosclerosis Risk in Communities (ARIC) study. *Circulation*, **96**, 1102–8.

Frick, M. H., Elo, O., Haapa, K. *et al.* (1987). Helsinki Heart Study: primary-prevention trial with gemfibrozil in middle-aged men with dyslipidemia. Safety of treatment, changes in risk factors, and incidence of coronary heart disease. *New England Journal of Medicine*, **317**, 1237–45.

Hankey, G. J. and Eikelboom, J. W. (1999). Homocysteine and vascular disease. *Lancet*, **354**, 407–13.

Hansson, L., Zanchetti, A., Carruthers, S. G. *et al.* (1998). Effects of intensive blood-pressure lowering and low-dose aspirin in patients with hypertension: principal results of the Hypertension Optimal Treatment (HOT) randomised trial. HOT Study Group. *Lancet*, **351**, 1755–62.

He, J., Whelton, P. K., Vu, B., Klag, M. J. (1998). Aspirin and risk of hemorrhagic stroke: a meta-analysis of randomized controlled trials. *Journal of the American Medical Association*, **280**, 1930–5.

Herrick, J. B. (1912). Clinical features of sudden obstruction of the coronary arteries. *Journal of the American Medical Association*, **59**, 2015–20.

Homocysteine Studies Collaboration (2002). Homocysteine and risk of ischaemic heart disease and stroke: a meta-analysis. *Journal of the American Medical Association*, **288**, 2015–22.

Hurlen, M., Abdelnoor, M., Smith, P. *et al.* (2002). Warfarin, aspirin, or both after myocardial infarction. *New England Journal of Medicine*, **347**, 969–74.

ISIS-2 (Second International Study of Infarct Survival) Collaborative Group (1988). Randomised trial of intravenous streptokinase, oral aspirin, both, or neither among 17 187 cases of suspected acute myocardial infarction: ISIS-2. *Lancet*, **2**, 349–60.

Juhan-Vague, I., Pyke, S. D. M., Alessi, M. C. *et al.*, on behalf of the ECAT Study Group (1996). Fibrinolytic factors and the risk of myocardial infarction or sudden death in patients with angina pectoris. *Circulation*, **94**, 2057–63.

Junker, R., Heinrich, J., Schulte, H. *et al.* (1997). Coagulation factor VII and the risk of coronary heart disease in healthy men. *Arteriosclerosis, Thrombosis, and Vascular Biology*, **17**, 1539–44.

Knottenbelt, C., Brennan, P. J., Meade, T. W. (2002). Antithrombotic treatment and the incidence of angina pectoris. *Archives of Internal Medicine*, **162**, 881–6.

Koster, T., Blann, A. D., Briet, E. *et al.* (1995). Role of clotting factor VIII in effect of von Willebrand factor on occurrence of deep-vein thrombosis. *Lancet*, **345**, 152–5.

MacCallum, P. K. and Meade, T. W. (1999). Haemostatic function, arterial disease and the prevention of arterial thrombosis. *Balliere's Clinical Haematology*, **12**, 577–99.

Martin, J. F., Bath, P. M., and Burr, M. L. (1991). Influence of platelet size on outcome after myocardial infarction. *Lancet*, **338**, 1409–11.

Meade, T. W., North, W. R. S., Chakrabarti, R. *et al.* (1980). Haemostatic function and cardiovascular death: early results of a prospective study. *Lancet*, **1**, 1050–4.

Meade, T. W., Mellows, S., Brozovic, M. *et al.* (1986). Haemostatic function and ischaemic heart disease: principal results of the Northwick Park Heart Study. *Lancet*, **ii**, 533–7.

Meade, T. W., Cooper, J. A., Miller, G. J. *et al.* (1991). Antithrombin III and arterial disease. *Lancet*, **338**, 850–1.

Meade, T. W., Ruddock, V., Stirling, Y. *et al.* (1993). Fibrinolytic activity, clotting factors, and long-term incidence of ischaemic heart disease in the Northwick Park Heart Study. *Lancet*, **342**, 1076–9.

Meade, T. W., Cooper, J. A., and Miller, G. J. (1997). Platelet counts and aggregation measures in the incidence of ischaemic heart disease (IHD). *Thrombosis and Haemostasis*, **78**, 926–9.

Meade, T., Zuhrie, R., Cook, C., and Cooper, J. (2002). Bezafibrate in men with lower extremity arterial disease: randomised controlled trial. *British Medical Journal*, **325**, 1139.

Medical Research Council's General Practice Research Framework (1998). Thrombosis prevention trial: randomized trial of low-intensity oral anticoagulation with warfarin and low-dose aspirin in the primary prevention of ischaemic heart disease in men at increased risk. *Lancet*, **351**, 233–41.

Meier, C. R., Jick, S. S., Derby, L. E. *et al.* (1998). Acute respiratory-tract infections and risk of first-time acute myocardial infarction. *Lancet*, **351**, 1467–71.

Miller, G. J., Stirling, Y., Esnouf, M. P. *et al.* (1994). Factor VII-deficient substrate plasmas depleted of protein C raise the sensitivity of the factor VII bio-assay to activated factor VII: an international study. *Thrombosis and Haemostasis*, **71**, 38–48.

Miller, G. J., Martin, J. C., Mitropoulos, K. A. *et al.* (1996). Activation of factor VII during alimentary lipemia occurs in healthy adults and patients with congenital factor XII or factor XI deficiency, but not in patients with factor IX deficiency. *Blood*, **87**, 4187–96.

Miller, G. J. (1999). Lipoproteins and the haemostatic system in atherothrombotic disorders. *Bailliere's Clinical Haematology*, **12**, 555–75.

Montalescot, G., Ankri, A., Vicaut, E. *et al.* (1995). Fibrinogen after coronary angioplasty as a risk factor for restenosis. *Circulation*, **92**, 31–8.

Morris, J. N. (1951). Recent history of coronary disease. *Lancet*, **1**, 1–7, 69–73.

Morris, J. N. and Crawford, M. D. (1958). Coronary heart disease and physical activity of work. *British Medical Journal*, **ii**, 1485–96.

Pearson, T. A., Mensah, G. A., Alexander, R. W. *et al.* (2003). Markers of inflammation and cardiovascular disease: application to clinical and public health practice. A statement for healthcare professionals from the Centers for Disease Control and Prevention and the American Heart Association. *Circulation*, **107**, 499–511.

Report from the Committee of Principal Investigators (1978). A co-operative trial in the primary prevention of ischaemic heart disease using clofibrate. *British Heart Journal*, **40**, 1069–118.

Ridker, P. M., Vaughan, D. E., Stampfer, M. J. *et al.* (1993). Endogenous tissue-type plasminogen activator and risk of myocardial infarction. *Lancet*, **341**, 1165–8.

Ridker, P. M., Cushman, M., Stampfer, M. J. *et al.* (1997). Inflammation, aspirin, and the risk of cardiovascular disease in apparently healthy men. *New England Journal of Medicine*, **336**, 973–9.

Ridker, P. M., Hennekens, C. H., Buring, J. E. *et al.* (2000). C-reactive protein and other markers of inflammation in the prediction of cardiovascular disease in women. *New England Journal of Medicine*, **342**, 836–43.

Rubins, H. B., Robins, S. J., Collins, D. *et al.* (1999). Gemfibrozil for the secondary prevention of coronary heart disease in men with low levels of high-density lipoprotein cholesterol: Veterans Affairs High-Density Lipoprotein Cholesterol Intervention Trial Study Group. *New England Journal of Medicine*, **341**, 410–18.

Rudnicka, A. R., Ashby, D., Brennan, P. J. *et al.* (2003). Thrombosis Prevention Trial: Compliance with warfarin treatment and investigation of a retained effect. *Archives of Internal Medicine*, 163, 1454–60.

Sanmuganathan, P. S., Ghahramani, P., Jackson, P. R. *et al.* (2001). Aspirin for primary prevention of coronary heart disease: safety and absolute benefit related to coronary risk derived from meta-analysis of randomised trials. *Heart*, 85, 265–71.

Schulman, S. and Lindmarker, P., for the Duration of Anticoagulation Trial (2000). Incidence of cancer after prophylaxis with warfarin against recurrent venous thromboembolism. *New England Journal of Medicine*, 342, 1953–8.

Steering Committee of the Physicians' Health Study Research Group (1989). Final report on the aspirin component of the ongoing Physicians' Health Study. *New England Journal of Medicine*, 321, 129–35.

Thompson, S. G., Kienast, J., Pyke, S. D. *et al.* (1995). Hemostatic factors and the risk of myocardial infarction or sudden death in patients with angina pectoris: European Concerted Action on Thrombosis and Disabilities Angina Pectoris Study Group. *New England Journal of Medicine*, 332, 635–41.

Tracy, R. P., Arnold, A. M., Ettinger, W. *et al.* (1999). The relationship of fibrinogen and factors VII and VIII to incident cardiovascular disease and death in the elderly: results from the Cardiovascular Health Study. *Arteriosclerosis, Thrombosis, and Vascular Biology*, 19, 1776–83.

Trip, M. D., Cats, V. M., van Capelle, F. J. L. *et al.* (1990). Platelet hyperactivity and prognosis and survivors of myocardial infarction. *New England Journal of Medicine*, 351, 233–41.

Turpie, A. G., Gent, M., Laupacis, A. *et al.* (1993). A comparison of aspirin with placebo in patients treated with warfarin after heart-valve replacement. *New England Journal of Medicine*, 329, 524–9.

Wald, D. S., Law, M., and Morris, J. K. (2002). Homocysteine and cardiovascular disease: evidence on causality from a meta-analysis. *British Medical Journal*, 325, 1202–8.

Welch, G. N. and Loscalzo, J. (1998). Homocysteine and atherothrombosis. *New England Journal of Medicine*, 338, 1042–50.

Wilhelmsen, L., Svardsudd, K., Korsan-Bengtsen, K. *et al.* (1984). Fibrinogen as a risk factor for stroke and myocardial infarction. *New England Journal of Medicine*, 311, 501–5.

Wiseman, S., Kenchington, G., Dain, R. *et al* (1989). Influence of smoking and plasma factors on patency of femoropopliteal vein grafts. *British Medical Journal*, 299, 643–6.

Chapter 29

Air pollution

C. A. Pope III

29.1 Introduction

It has long been suspected that elevated exposure to air pollution has adverse health effects (Brimblecombe 1987; Lipfert 1994). These suspicions were largely confirmed by several well-documented extreme air pollution episodes, including events that occurred in December 1930 in the Meuse Valley, Belgium (Firket 1931); in October 1948 in Donora, Pennsylvania (Ciocco and Thompson 1961); and in December 1952 in London (Logan 1953). In each of these episodes, stagnant air masses resulted in extremely elevated concentrations of combustion-related particulate and sulfur oxide air pollution which were associated with marked increases in cardiopulmonary morbidity and mortality. Early public policy efforts to improve air quality in the United States, Britain, and elsewhere were largely attempts to avoid or prevent these 'killer' episodes. Early studies of these episodes contributed to a prevailing opinion during the 1950s through much of the 1980s that appreciable health effects occurred only at very high concentrations (Holland *et al.* 1979).

During the relatively short time period of 1989–93, results of three loosely connected epidemiological research efforts from the US were reported, including:

1 The Harvard Six Cities prospective cohort study, which observed increased risk of respiratory illness in children (Dockery *et al.* 1989) and increased risk of cardiopulmonary mortality (Dockery *et al.* 1993).

2 A series of studies in Utah Valley that observed that particulate pollution was associated with respiratory and cardiovascular mortality (Pope *et al.* 1992) as well as various other respiratory health end points (Pope 1989, 1991; Pope and Dockery 1992; Pope and Kanner 1993; Pope *et al.* 1991; Ransom and Pope 1992).

3 A series of studies that linked daily changes in air pollution with both respiratory and cardiovascular daily mortality in several US cities (Dockery *et al.* 1992; Pope *et al.* 1992; Schwartz 1991, 1993; Schwartz and Dockery 1992a, b; Schwartz and Marcus 1990).

During this time period, results of other scattered studies from the US (Ostro 1990; Ostro *et al.* 1993; Thurston *et al.* 1992), Germany (Wichmann *et al.* 1989), Canada (Bates and Sizto 1989), Finland (Ponka 1991), and the Czech Republic (Bobak and Leon 1992) were published that also observed health effects at unexpectedly low concentrations of air pollution. The convergence of these findings resulted in a critical mass of evidence that prompted serious reconsideration of the contribution of particulate air pollution on human health and motivated abundant additional research. Several reviews of this research have been published (Bates 1996; Dockery 2001; Pope 2000a; Pope and Dockery 1999; Vedal 1997).

Although many of the epidemiological studies have focused on respiratory health end points, this review will focus on the growing epidemiological evidence of air pollution effects on cardiovascular disease. The plan of this chapter is as follows:

1 Review studies of day-to-day changes in acute exposure to air pollutants, including studies of early episodes of extremely elevated air pollution, more recent episodes with only moderately elevated concentrations of pollution, and results of numerous daily time-series studies of cardiovascular mortality and hospitalizations.

2 Review results of recent cohort-based studies that have evaluated mortality risk and chronic, long-term exposure to air pollution.

3 Discuss, in a selective way, the growing number of studies that attempt to look at specific physiological end points that may be part of the pathophysiological pathway linking cardiopulmonary mortality and particulate air pollution.

29.2 Acute exposure studies

Most epidemiological studies of health effects of particulate pollution have been designed to exploit two primary real-world dimensions of exposure variability. Acute exposure studies (often daily time-series studies) evaluate associations between various health end points with short-term (usually 1–5 day) temporal variability. Chronic exposure studies typically use average exposure for longer periods of time (usually 1 year or more) and spatial (or cross-sectional) differences as the source of exposure variability.

29.2.1 Simple episode studies

Some of the most compelling but methodologically simple studies of health effects of acute exposure to air pollution evaluated changes in mortality and/or morbidity before, during, and after pollution episodes that lasted a few days or weeks. The early studies of severe episodes, including the Meuse River valley in Belgium (Firket 1931), Donora, PA (Ciocco and Thompson 1961), and London (Logan 1953), suggested that elevated exposures to particulate and/or sulfur oxide air pollution over a period of several days exacerbate existing chronic cardiovascular and respiratory disease and increase the risk of becoming symptomatic, requiring medical care, or dying. In the notorious London episode of 5–8 December 1952 (Logan 1953), 80–90% of excess deaths associated with the air pollution episode were due to respiratory and cardiovascular disorders, often in combination (Ministry of Health 1954). Cause of death information obtained directly from death certificates or from analysis of coroners' records clearly indicated increases in cardiovascular as well as respiratory disease deaths during and for a week or two following the episode.

More recent studies of less severe episodes have been conducted. For example, Wichmann *et al.* (1989) studied a 5-day pollution episode that occurred in Germany in January 1985. They observed significant increases in cardiopulmonary deaths and hospitalizations. Interestingly, increases in cardiovascular diseases were greater than for respiratory diseases. Anderson *et al.* (1995) conducted a similar study of a December 1991 air pollution episode in London. Increases in cardiovascular and respiratory deaths and hospitalizations were observed, although these increases were generally not very statistically robust.

29.2.2 Daily time-series mortality studies

Formal daily time-series analysis has also been used to explore associations between short-term changes in mortality and air pollution. These studies have the advantage of using daily mortality and pollution data over long time periods and potentially provide more statistical power to evaluate effects of less extreme pollution exposure. Daily time-series mortality studies evaluate changes in daily death counts associated with short-term changes in air pollution using formal time-series regression modelling to estimate pollution effects while controlling for long-term time trends, seasonality, weather variables, and sometimes other time-dependent risk factors. These studies take advantage of available computerized mortality records to construct daily mortality counts, which can be combined with pollution, weather, and other daily co-risk factor data.

Many daily time-series mortality studies have now been conducted in many cities throughout the world (Levy *et al.* 2000; Pope 2000a; Pope and Dockery 1999; Samet *et al.* 2000) with over 150 published daily time-series mortality studies of air pollution. Daily mortality has been associated with various measures of air pollution, but the most consistent associations have been observed with respirable or fine particulate pollution. Various measurements of particulate pollution and various modelling strategies have been used, making precise comparisons of effect estimates across studies difficult. However, 0.5–1.5% changes in daily mortality associated with a 10 μg/m^3 increase in concentrations of inhalable particles (less than 10 μm in diameter) are commonly observed. In the large majority of these studies, the relative risk of mortality increased monotonically with particulate concentrations – usually in a near linear fashion (Daniels *et al.* 2000; Pope 2000b; Schwartz and Zanobetti 2000). Also, these studies often observed a lead–lag relationship between air pollution and mortality. The results suggested that the increased mortality occurred concurrently or within 1–5 days following an increase in air pollution.

Many of the daily time-series mortality studies also provided a breakdown of mortality by broad cause-of-death categories. A stylized summary of overall estimates of daily mortality effects of an increase in exposure to particulate air pollution by broad cause-of-death categories is provided in Table 29.1. These estimates are based on overall reviews of these studies reported elsewhere (Pope 2000a; Pope and Dockery 1999).

Measured in terms of cause-specific relative risk ratios for increases in exposure to particulate pollution, particulate pollution has a larger impact on respiratory disease mortality than on cardiovascular mortality. However, because cardiovascular deaths are much more common than respiratory deaths, cardiovascular disease deaths account for a much larger percentage of excess deaths attributable to particulate air pollution than respiratory disease deaths. Several studies have observed that pre-existing cardiovascular disease, including previous myocardial infarction, congestive heart failure, and coronary artery disease, in addition to diabetes, may predispose individuals to be more susceptible to dying due to short-term exposure to particulate air pollution (Bateson and Schwartz 2004; Goldberg *et al.* 2001; Kwon *et al.* 2001). In addition, one study that focused on stroke mortality reported that the risk of acute stroke mortality was significantly associated with exposures to particulate pollution in combination with various gaseous pollutants (Hong *et al.* 2002).

Table 29.1 Overall estimates of daily mortality effects of an increase in exposure to particulate air pollution by broad cause-of-death categories

Cause of death	Percentage of total deaths[a]	Cause-specific risk ratio (20 μg/m^3 increase in PM$_{2.5}$)[b]	Percentage of excess deaths due to PM exposure
All-cause[c]	100	1.032	100
Respiratory	8	1.111	28
Cardiovascular	45	1.050	69
Other disease	47	1.002	3

PM: particulate matter.

[a] Based on Vital Statistics of the United States; [b] Based on updated summary estimates from Pope and Dockery (1999) and Pope (2000); [c] Excluding accidents, suicide, homicide, etc. (ICD9 > 800).

29.2.3 **Daily time-series hospitalization studies**

Daily counts of hospital admissions can be analysed in the same way that daily counts of mortality have been assessed. Numerous time-series studies have reported associations between particulate air pollution and various respiratory hospitalization or related healthcare end points (Pope and Dockery 1999; Vedal 1997). Several studies that evaluated associations between particulate air pollution and hospitalizations for cardiovascular disease have also been conducted (Burnett *et al.* 1995; Poloniecki *et al.* 1997; Schwartz 1997, 1999; Schwartz and Morris 1995). Morris (2001) conducted a quantitative review of these studies from different cities. Positive associations between PM_{10} and cardiovascular disease hospitalizations were observed in all but one analysis and the positive associations were usually statistically significant. Several of the studies evaluated more specific cardiovascular outcomes. Associations between particulate air pollution and congestive heart failure and ischaemic heart disease were consistently positive and usually statistically significant. Associations between pollution and admissions for cerebrovascular accidents and dysrthymias were less consistent.

29.3 **Chronic exposure studies**

Several cohort-based mortality studies evaluated effects of longer term exposure. The first of these studies, reported by Dockery *et al.* (1993) and often referred to as the Harvard Six Cities study, involved a 14–16 year prospective follow-up of more than 8000 adults living in six US cities. It controlled for individual differences in age, sex, cigarette smoking, education levels, body mass index, and other risk factors. Cardiopulmonary mortality was significantly associated with mean sulfate and fine particulate concentrations over the years of the study period.

Two additional related studies (Pope *et al.* 1995, 2002) linked individual risk factor data from the American Cancer Society (ACS) Cancer Prevention Study II (CPS-II) with national ambient air pollution data. The analysis used data for more than 500 000 persons who lived in up to 151 different US metropolitan areas and who were followed prospectively from 1982 through 1998. The analysis controlled for individual differences in age, sex, race, cigarette smoking, and various other risk factors. Fine particle and sulfur oxide-related pollution were associated with all-cause mortality, cardiopulmonary mortality, and lung cancer mortality. Measures of coarse particles, total suspended particles, or most of the gaseous pollutants were not generally associated with mortality. In both the Harvard Six Cities study and the ACS study, the positive association between combustion-related air pollution and cardiopulmonary mortality was dominated by cardiovascular disease deaths.

Woodruff *et al.* (1997) conducted a study of post-neonatal infant mortality in the US. The National Center for Health Statistics birth and death records for infants born between 1989 and 1991 were linked with PM_{10} data from the Aerometric Database of the Environmental Protection Agency (EPA). The full data set included approximately 4 million infants in 86 US metropolitan areas. The analysis compared post-neonatal infant mortality across different levels of ambient PM_{10} concentrations during the first 2 months of life, controlling for individual differences in maternal race, maternal education, marital status, month of birth, maternal smoking during pregnancy, and temperature. Particulate pollution exposure was associated with post-neonatal infant mortality for all causes, respiratory causes, and sudden infant death syndrome (SIDS).

Comparisons of particulate pollution-related relative risks for mortality from the Six Cities study, both ACS studies, and the infant mortality study are presented in Table 29.2.

The estimated overall excess risk from the infant mortality study is similar to that estimated for adults in the Harvard Six Cities and ACS studies, even though the time frame of exposure

Table 29.2 Comparisons of mortality risk ratios (and 95% CI) for air pollution from the Harvard Six Cities, ACS-I, ACS-II, and post-neonatal infant mortality studies

Cause of death	Particulate air pollution (across observable range of particulate pollution)			
	Six Cities (18.6 μg/m³ PM$_{2.5}$)	ACS-I (24.5 μg/m³ PM$_{2.5}$)	ACS-II (20 μg/m³ PM$_{2.5}$)	Infant (56.9 μg/m³ PM$_{10}$)
All	1.26 (1.08–1.47)	1.17 (1.09–1.26)	1.13 (1.03–1.23)	1.25 (1.12–1.47)
Cardiopulmonary	1.37 (1.11–1.68)	1.31 (1.17–1.46)	1.19 (1.07–1.34)	—
SIDS, NBW[a]	—	—	—	1.91 (1.46–2.44)
Lung cancer	1.37 (0.81–2.31)	1.03 (0.80–1.33)	1.29 (1.09–1.52)	—
All others	1.01 (0.79–1.30)	1.07 (0.92–1.24)	1.01 (0.91–1.13)	1.00[a] (0.94–1.06)

Sources of data: Harvard Six Cities: Dockery *et al*. 1993; ACS-I: Pope *et al*. 1995; ACS-II: Pope *et al*. 2002; post-neonatal infant mortality study: Woodruff *et al*. 1997.

NBW: normal birth weight.

[a] Deaths due to causes other than SIDS or respiratory disease.

for the infants was clearly far shorter than for the adults. This observation suggests that the relevant time frame of exposure is short (a few months versus years), and/or that infants are at greater risk to exposure to air pollution. The majority of the excess mortality associated with air pollution in the adult studies was due to deaths that were recorded as cardiovascular deaths. For post-neonatal infant mortality, although respiratory deaths were associated with particulate pollution, SIDS deaths of normal birth weight children were the major contributor to excess mortality associated with air pollution. Parish (1997) notes that, although sudden cardiac death and SIDS are not generally regarded as the same disease, infants may be dying from stress-related causes similar to those associated with sudden cardiac death. The intriguing similarity of response of all-cause mortality to particulate air pollution in these studies makes it tempting to speculate on the role of exposure to particulate pollution and the risk of sudden cardiac death in children (included in the deaths recorded as SIDS) as well as adults.

Another cohort study has been conducted that related air pollution to 1977–92 mortality in 6338 non-smoking Seventh-Day Adventist adults living in California (Abbey *et al.* 1999). This study observed that all natural cause mortality, non-malignant respiratory mortality, and lung cancer mortality were significantly associated with ambient PM$_{10}$ concentrations in males, but not in females. Cardiopulmonary disease mortality was not statistically significantly associated with PM$_{10}$ in either males or females. Unfortunately this study did not have fine particulate (PM$_{2.5}$) data but relied on total suspended particulates (TSP) and PM$_{10}$ data. As noted above, in the Harvard Six Cities study (Dockery *et al.* 1993) and in the ACS studies (Pope *et al.* 1995, 2002), mortality was much more strongly associated with fine particles than with measures that included coarse particles.

A final cohort study from the Netherlands followed up 5000 adults aged 55–69 years over 8 years (Hoek *et al.* 2002). In this study Hoek and colleagues found the increased relative risk from a 10 μg/m³ increase in background black smoke exposure to be 1.34 (95% CI: 0.68–2.64). Although not statistically significant, this excess-risk estimate is roughly consistent with estimates from cohort studies in the USA. In addition, this study provides additional spatial resolution for estimated pollution exposure by using geographic information systems to determine whether individuals lived in areas with high traffic emissions. Living within 100 m of a highway or 50 m of a major roadway was associated with a relative risk of 1.95 (95% CI: 1.09–3.51). These results suggest that assessment of particulate exposure using only average background concentrations underestimates the health burden attributable to elevated concentrations in the vicinity of sources. In fact, the relative risk for a 10 μg/m³ increase in black smoke nearly doubled (1.71; 95% CI: 1.10–2.67) when local exposures in addition to background concentrations were modelled. This study provides important additional evidence that inhalable particulates or some closely related pollutant from road traffic is a risk factor for cardiopulmonary death.

29.4 Biological mechanisms

The epidemiological investigations briefly reviewed above provide reasonably compelling evidence of a link between particulate air pollution and cardiopulmonary morbidity and mortality. Although our understanding of the underlying biological mechanisms remains limited, some progress is being made. Seaton *et al.* (1995) hypothesized that particulate air pollution (especially ultrafine particles) may provoke a low-grade inflammatory response, resulting in the release of potentially harmful cytokines and increased blood coagulability. A related hypothesis suggested pollution induced lung damage (potentially including oxidative lung damage and inflammation), declines in lung function, respiratory distress, and potentially cardiovascular disease related to hypoxia (Pope *et al.* 1999a). It has also been suggested that the autonomic nervous system may play an important role in the pathophysiological pathway between particulate exposure and increased risk of cardiovascular disease death. Autonomic nervous system-activated changes in blood viscosity, as well as heart rate (HR) and heart rate variability (HRV), may increase the likelihood of cardiac death (Kennedy 1997; Stone and Godleski 1999). As has been appropriately emphasized by various researchers (Donaldson *et al.* 2001; Godleski *et al.* 2000; Pope *et al.* 2004a; Utell and Frampton 2000), it is likely that there are multiple mechanistic pathways with complex interdependencies. Nevertheless, there are a growing number of studies that attempt to look at specific physiological end points that may be part of the pathophysiological pathway linking cardiopulmonary mortality and particulate air pollution.

29.4.1 Pulmonary and systemic inflammation

Exposure to particulate pollution has been associated with various markers of pulmonary and systemic inflammation that suggests a low-grade inflammatory response to exposure to fine particulate pollution. For example, elevated levels of C-reactive protein (CRP) have been observed in people associated with exposure to air pollution episodes (Peters *et al.* 2001a; Pope *et al.* 2004b; Seaton *et al.* 1999). Recent studies have suggested that CRP, a marker of systemic inflammation, may be an important and independent predictor of cardiovascular disease in both men and women (Ridker *et al.* 1997, 2000). Evidence of inflammatory lung injury has been observed after bronchial instillation of air pollution particles largely from a steel mill (Ghio and Devlin 2001). Exposure to air pollution caused by forest fires was associated with bone marrow and blood cell responses, including elevated band cells as a percentage of polymorphonuclear leukocytes (Tan *et al.* 2000). Evidence of enhanced human alveolar macrophage production of proinflammatory cytokines has been observed associated with exposure to particles from various sources (Salvi *et al.* 2000; van Eeden *et al.* 2001). Two other related studies that evaluated effects of exposure to laboratory-generated ultrafine particles also observed evidence of effects on systemic markers of inflammation and leukocyte recruitment (Boscia *et al.* 2000; Frampton *et al.* 2001).

The proposition that particulate pollution-induced low-grade inflammation may increase the risk of adverse coronary events is bolstered by observations that elevated exposure to fine particulate air pollution, often in combination with other air pollutants, is also associated with the following: (a) increased risk of elevated blood plasma viscosity (Peters *et al.* 1997); (b) a small but statistically significant degree of brachial artery vasoconstriction (Brook *et al.* 2002); (c) a small increased risk of myocardial infarction within a few hours to one day following exposure (Peters *et al.* 2001*b*); and (d) evidence from a histopathological study in humans that observed the presence of inflammatory alterations in the lungs of individuals living in an area with higher levels of air pollution (Souza *et al.* 1998).

Several natural chronic animal experiments with inhalation of concentrated ambient particles have also observed evidence of fine particulate-induced inflammatory responses (Clarke *et al.* 1999, 2000*a, b*; Kodavanti *et al.* 2000). Studies using substantially larger doses by intratracheal instillation observed that repeated deposition of particulate matter from ambient air in the lungs of rabbits resulted in a systemic inflammatory response (Mukae *et al.* 2001). Repeated exposure to particles resulted in persistent increases in circulating band cells and a reduction in the transit time of polymorphonuclear leukocytes through the mitotic pool. The increases were related to the amount of particles phagocytosed by alveolar macrophages. Rabbits exposed repeatedly to cigarette smoke showed a similar bone marrow response (Terashima *et al.* 1997). The authors speculated that this inflammatory response to repeated low-level exposure to fine particles might accelerate atherosclerosis. In fact, a subsequent study did observe that repeated exposure of rabbits susceptible to atherosclerosis induced progression of atherosclerotic lesions (Suwa *et al.* 2002). They concluded that 'progression of atherosclerosis and increased vulnerability to plaque rupture may underlie the relationship between particulate air pollution and excess cardiovascular death.' In fact Kunzli *et al.* (2004) have reported associations between ambient concentrations of fine particulate air pollution across the Los Angeles region and carotid intima-media thickness (CIMT), a measure of sub-clinical atherosclerosis. Low-level exposure to fine particles from another source, second-hand tobacco smoke, has also been shown to promote atherosclerosis (Penn and Snyder 1993; Zhu *et al.* 1994) even at exposure to second-hand smoke of just one cigarette per day (Penn *et al.* 1994).

29.4.2 Cardiac autonomic response

The autonomic nervous system may play an important role in the pathophysiological pathway between particulate pollution exposure and cardiac risk. Recently a few epidemiological studies have evaluated such autonomic nervous system-related physiological measures and air pollution, although they have been limited and mostly only exploratory pilot studies. A daily time-series panel study of elderly subjects with repeated measures of blood oxygenation did not observe pollution-related hypoxia, but did observe that elevated particulate air pollution levels were associated with increased pulse rate (Pope *et al.* 1999*a*). Peters *et al.* (1999) also reported pollution-related increased heart rate. Using seven subjects from the previously discussed blood oxygenation and pulse rate study, repeated 24 h ambulatory ECG monitoring was conducted during episodes of high pollution and during periods of relatively low pollution (Pope *et al.* 1999*b*). HR was positively associated with particulate air pollution. Additionally, particulate air pollution was associated with reductions in various measures of HRV commonly used as markers of cardiac autonomic function. A subsequent analysis of 88 elderly subects also observed similar declines in cardiac autonomic function as measured by changes in HRV (Pope *et al.* 2004*b*).

Two other studies have also recently evaluated associations between particulate air pollution and HRV. One of these studies explored daily changes in HRV associated with daily changes in fine particulate air pollution with a panel of elderly subjects living in metropolitan Baltimore (Liao *et al.* 1999). Daily ECG monitoring was conducted with resting, supine, 6-min heart beat interval data being collected each day. The second study was conducted using 53–87-year-old subjects living in Boston (Gold *et al.* 2000). Weekly ECG monitoring was conducted using ambulatory (Holter) monitors continuously for 25 min, including 5 min of rest, 5 min of standing, 5 min of outdoor exercise, 5 min of recovery, and 20 cycles of slow breathing. Although the pollution levels were relatively low during the study periods in both of these studies, lower HRV was associated with elevated concentrations of fine particulate pollution and the association was strong for subjects with pre-existing cardiovascular conditions. In the currently available studies of particulate pollution exposure and HRV, a negative association with particulate exposure and overall HRV was observed. The results, however, are not entirely consistent, especially with measures of the short-term components of HRV. To what degree these inconsistencies across the studies can be explained by differences in ECG monitoring time frames, make-up of subjects, differences in pollution levels, or other differences needs to be explored.

Nevertheless, the proposition that exposure to particulate matter is associated with changes in cardiac autonomic function is further bolstered by:

1 A study of boilermakers that observed changes in HRV after occupational particulate matter exposure (Magari *et al.* 2001).

2 A study that observed HRV declines after just 2 h of second-hand cigarette smoke in an airport smoking lounge (Pope *et al.* 2001).

3 Two studies that observed an increase in systolic blood pressure during elevated exposure to particulate matter and other pollutants (Ibald-Mulli *et al.* 2001; Linn and Gong 2001).

4 Several studies of animals that observed changes in cardiac rhythm or function with ambient particles (Godleski *et al.* 1996, 2000; Nadziejko *et al.* 1997; Watkinson *et al.* 1998; Wellenius *et al.* 2002).

In addition, an interesting and novel pilot study of 100 cardiac patients who had received an implanted cardioverter defibrillator (ICD) has been conducted (Peters *et al.* 2000). These ICD devices continuously monitor cardiac rhythm for abnormalities and are able to initiate pacing or cardioverter shocks to restore proper electrical function. Associations between daily measures of air pollution and ICD therapeutic discharges were evaluated. Higher rates of ICD discharges indicating potentially life-threatening arrhythmias were associated with various measures of air pollution, especially black carbon particle mass and nitrogen dioxide.

29.4.3 **Biological plausibility**

Our knowledge about the underlying biological mechanisms remains limited and requires additional study. The results of the variety of epidemiological studies provide a pattern of effects that are biologically germane. Biological plausibility is enhanced by the observation of a coherent cascade of cardiopulmonary health effects and by the fact that non-cardiopulmonary health end points are not typically associated with the pollution. For example, a recent analysis of cardiovascular mortality and long-term exposure to particulate air pollution specifically evaluated the epidemiological evidence of various general pathophysiological pathways of disease (Pope *et al.* 2004*a*). Observed patterns of cause-specific pollution-mortality associations were consistent with fine particulate air pollution being a risk factor for cardiovascular disease mortality via mechanisms that likely include pulmonary and systemic inflammation, accelerated atherosclerosis, and altered cardiac autonomic function. Biological plausibility is further enhanced with the observation of a variety of specific physiological end points that may be part of the pathophysiological pathway linking cardiopulmonary mortality and particulate air pollution.

Table 29.3 Brief summary of observed associations between particulate air pollution and cardiovascular related effects

Acute exposure epidemiological studies

    ↑ Cardiovascular (and respiratory) mortality counts
    ↑ Cardiovascular (and respiratory) hospital admissions counts
    ↑ Onset of myocardial infarction

Chronic exposure epidemiological studies

    ↑ Risk of adult cardiopulmonary (and respiratory and lung cancer) mortality
    ↑ Risk of post-neonatal infant SIDS (and respiratory) mortality

Studies of various related cardiovascular physiology end points

    ↔ Hypoxaemia
    ↑ Markers of pulmonary and systemic inflammation
    ↑ Blood plasma viscosity
    ↑ Brachial artery vasoconstriction
    ↑ Atherosclerosis
    ↑ Pulse rate
    ↓ Heart rate variability
    ↑ Blood pressure
    ↑ Cardiac arrhythmias

Table 29.3 briefly summarizes the selected health effects that have been associated with elevated exposure to fine or respirable particulate air pollution. While these overall results are extremely intriguing, they are incomplete and difficult to interpret. They seem to suggest that interactions between pulmonary and systemic inflammation, abnormal haemostatic function, and altered cardiac autonomic function or cardiac rhythm may all play an important role in the pathogenesis of cardiopulmonary diseases related to fine particulate air pollution. As noted earlier, there are likely multiple mechanistic pathways with complex interdependencies. In an editorial dealing with air pollution as a cause of heart disease, Glantz (2002) pragmatically interprets the health effects evidence as follows: 'All these effects indicate that air pollution has an impact on heart disease. Some of these effects may occur over time, as with acceleration of the progression of atherosclerosis, or very quickly, as with an increase in the risk of an arrhythmia or MI by acute inflammatory responses, altering platelet function, or, perhaps, endothelial function. These effects may be independent of, or synergistic with, alteration in autonomic tone as reflected in increases in HR and reductions in HRV. In any event, it is clear that these risks are real and substantial.'

Biological plausibility is further enhanced by comparing the observed effect sizes with comparable particulate matter exposure from another common source, second-hand cigarette smoke. In the late 1970s and early 1980s annual average concentrations of ambient fine particles in US cities equalled ~10 μg/m^3 in the cleanest cities, rising to ~30 μg/m^3 for the most polluted cities (Pope *et al.* 2002), a difference in exposure equal to ~20 μg/m^3. Estimates of the relative risk of cardiopulmonary mortality associated with a 20 μg/m^3 increase in long-term exposure to fine particulate pollution range from 1.12 to 1.40, based on previously reviewed prospective cohort studies of air pollution (Dockery *et al.* 1993; Pope *et al.* 1995, 2002, 2004*a*). Similar estimates of excess risk are also observed for long-term average exposure to second-hand tobacco smoke. Particulate concentrations, on average, are ~20 μg/m^3 greater in homes with one smoker versus homes without smokers (Coultas *et al.* 1990; Spengler *et al.* 1981). A recent meta-analysis (Thun *et al.* 1999) estimated that the relative risk for fatal and non-fatal cardiovascular disease among never smokers married to smokers versus never smokers married to non-smokers was 1.25 (95% CI: 1.15–1.32). A similar relative risk of 1.21 (95% CI: 1.04–1.41) was estimated from a meta-analysis of studies evaluating relative risk of heart disease for workers occupationally exposed to second-hand tobacco smoke versus workers who were not (Steenland 1999).

29.5 Conclusions

There is substantial epidemiological evidence that air pollution, especially the fine particulate matter common to many urban and industrial environments, is an important risk factor for cardiovascular disease and mortality. This evidence comes from several types of epidemiological studies and includes:

1 Increases in both respiratory and cardiovascular disease deaths during and immediately following pollution episodes.

2 Associations between daily changes in particulate pollution and cardiovascular and respiratory disease deaths and hospitalizations.

3 Increased risk of adult cardiopulmonary disease mortality and increased risk of post-neonatal infant mortality associated with spatial differences in ambient fine particulate pollution concentrations.

In addition, particulate pollution has been associated with a variety of specific cardiovascular physiologic end points. The overall epidemiological results suggest that short-term exposures to fine particulate matter exacerbate existing cardiopulmonary disease and increase the number of persons in a population who become symptomatic, require medical attention, or die. Long term, repeated exposure may increase the risk of chronic cardiopulmonary disease. The overall evidence is somewhat consistent with the speculation that pollution-induced pulmonary and systemic inflammation, accelerated atherosclerosis, and altered cardiac autonomic function may be part of the pathophysiological mechanisms or pathways linking air pollution and cardiovascular mortality.

References

Abbey, D. E., Nishino, N., McDonnell, W. F., Burchette, R. J., Knutsen, S. F., Lawrence Beeson, W., and Yang, J. X. (1999). Long-term inhalable particles and other air pollutants related to mortality in nonsmokers. *American Journal of Respiratory and Critical Care Medicine*, **159**, 373–82.

Anderson, H. R., Limb, E. S., Bland, J. M., Ponce de Leon, A., Strachan, D. P., and Bower, J. S. (1995). Health effects of an air pollution episode in London, December 1991. *Thorax*, **50**, 1188–93.

Bates, D. V. (1996). Particulate air pollution. *Thorax*, **51** (Suppl. 2), S3.

Bates, D. V. and Sizto, R. (1989). The Ontario air pollution study: identification of the causative agent. *Environmental Health Perspectives*, **79**, 69–72.

Bateson, T. and Schwartz, J. (2002). Who is sensitive to the effects of particulate air pollution on mortality? A case-crossover analysis of effect modifiers. *Epidemiology*, **15**, 143–9.

Bobak, M. and Leon, D. A. (1992). Air pollution and infant mortality in the Czech Republic, 1986–1988. *Lancet*, **340**, 1010–14.

Boscia, J. A., Chalupa, D., Utell, M. J., Zareba, W., Konecki, J. A., Morrow, P. E. *et al.* (2000). Airway and cardiovascular effects of inhaled ultrafine carbon particles in resting, health, nonsmoking adults. *American Journal of Respiratory and Critical Care Medicine*, **161**, A239.

Brimblecombe, P. (1987). *The big smoke*. Methuen, London.

Brook, R. D., Brook, J. R., Urch, B., Vincent, R., Rajagopalan, S., and Silverman, F. (2002). Inhalation of fine particulate air pollution and ozone causes acute arterial vasoconstriction in healthy adults. *Circulation*, **105**, 1534–6.

Burnett, R. T., Dales, R. E., Krewski, D., Vincent, R., Dann, T., and Brook, J. R. (1995). Associations between ambient particulate sulfate and admissions to Ontario hospitals for cardiac and respiratory diseases. *American Journal of Epidemiology*, **142**, 15–22.

Ciocco, A. and Thompson, D. J. (1961). A follow-up on Donora ten years after: methodology and findings. *American Journal of Public Health*, **51**, 155–64.

Clarke, R. W., Catalano, P. J., Koutrakis, P., Krishna Murthy, G. G., Sioutas, C., Paulauskis, J. *et al.* (1999). Urban air particulate inhalation alters pulmonary function and induces pulmonary inflammation in a rodent model of chronic bronchitis. *Inhalation Toxicology*, **11**, 637–56.

Clarke, R. W., Catalano, P., Coull, B., Koutrakis, P., Krishna Murthy, G. G., Rice, T., and Godleski, J. J. (2000*a*). Age-related responses in rats to concentrated urban air particles (CAP's). *Inhalation Toxicology*, **12** (Suppl. 1), 73–84.

Clarke, R. W., Coull, B., Reinisch, U., Catalano, P., Killingsworth, C. R., Koutrakis, P. *et al.* (2000*b*). Inhaled concentrated ambient particles are associated with hematologic and bronchoalveolar lavage changes in canines. *Environmental Health Perspectives*, **108**, 1179–87.

Coultas, D. B., Samet, J. M., McCarthy, J. F., and Spengler, J. D. (1990). Variability of measures of exposure to environmental tobacco smoke in the home. *American Review of Respiratory Disease*, **142**, 602–6.

Daniels, M. J., Dominici, F., Samet, J. M., and Zeger, S. L. (2000). Estimating particulate matter-mortality dose-response curves and threshold levels: an analysis of daily time-series for the 20 largest U. S. cities. *American Journal of Epidemiology*, **152**, 397–406.

Dockery, D. W. (2001). Epidemiologic evidence of cardiovascular effects of particulate air pollution. *Environmental Health Perspectives*, **109** (Suppl. 4), 483–6.

Dockery, D. W., Speizer, F. E., Stram, D. O., Ware, J. H., Spengler, J. D., and Ferris, B. G. Jr. (1989). Effects of inhalable particles on respiratory health of children. *American Review of Respiratory Disease*, **139**, 587–94.

Dockery, D. W., Schwartz, J., and Spengler, J. D. (1992). Air pollution and daily mortality: associations with particulates and acid aerosols. *Environmental Research*, **59**, 362–73.

Dockery, D. W., Pope, C. A. III, Xu, X., Spengler, J. D., Ware, J. H., Fay, M. E. *et al.* (1993). An association between air pollution and mortality in six U. S. cities. *New England Journal of Medicine*, **329**, 1753–9.

Donaldson, K., Stone, V., Seaton, A., and MacNee, W. (2001). Ambient particle inhalation and the cardiovascular system: potential mechanisms. *Environmental Health Perspectives*, **109** (Suppl. 4), 523–7.

Firket, J. (1931). The cause of symptoms found in the Meuse Valley during the fog of December, 1930. *Bulletin De l'Academie Royale de Medecine de Belgique*, **11**, 683–741.

Frampton, M. W., Azadniv, M., Chalupa, D., Morrow, P. E., Gibb, F. R., Oberdorster, G. *et al.* (2001). Blood leukocyte expression of LFA-1 and ICAM-1 after inhalation of ultrafine carbon particles. *American Journal of Respiratory and Critical Care Medicine*, **163**, A264.

Ghio, A. J. and Devlin, R. B. (2001). Inflammatory lung injury after bronchial instillation of air pollution particles. *American Journal of Respiratory and Critical Care Medicine*, **164**, 704–8.

Glantz, S. A. (2002). Air pollution as a cause of heart disease: time for action [Editorial]. *Journal of the American College of Cardiology*, **39**, 943–5.

Gold, D. R., Litonjua, A., Schwartz, J., Lovett, E., Larson, A., Nearing, B. *et al.* (2000). Ambient pollution and heart rate variability. *Circulation*, **101**, 1267–73.

Goldberg, M. S., Burnett, R. T., Bailar, J. C. III, Tamblyn, R., Ernst, P., Flegel, K. *et al.* (2001). Identification of persons with cardiorespiratory conditions who are at risk of dying from the acute effects of ambient air particles. *Environmental Health Perspectives*, **109** (Suppl. 4), 487–94.

Godleski, J. J., Sioutas, C., Katler, M., and Koutrakis, P. (1996). Death from inhalation of concentrated air particles in animal models of pulmonary disease. *American Journal of Respiratory and Critical Care Medicine*, **153**, A15.

Godleski, J. J., Verrier, R. L., Koutrakis, P., and Catalano, P. (2000). Mechanisms of morbidity and mortality from exposure to ambient air particles. *Health Effects Institute*, **91**, 5–88.

Hoek, G., Brunkereef, B., Goldbohm, S., Fischer, P., and van den Brandt, P. A. (2002). Association between mortality and indicators of traffic-related air pollution in the Netherlands: a cohort study. *Lancet*, **360**, 1203–9.

Holland, W. W., Bennett, A. E., Cameron, I. R., Florey, C. V., Leeder, S. R., Schilling, R. S. *et al.* (1979). Health effects of particulate pollution: reappraising the evidence. *American Journal of Epidemiology*, **110**, 527–659.

Hong, Y. C., Lee, J. T., Kim, H., Kwon, H. J. (2002). Effects of air pollutants on acute stroke mortality. *Environmental Health Perspectives*, **110**, 187–91.

Ibald-Mulli, A., Stieber, J., Wichmann, H. E., Koenig, W., and Peters, A. (2001). Effects of air pollution on blood pressure: a population-based approach. *American Journal of Public Health*, **91**, 571–7.

Kennedy, H. L. (1997). Beta blockade, ventricular arrhythmias, and sudden cardiac death. *American Journal of Cardiology*, **80**, 29J–34J.

Kodavanti, U. P., Mebane, R., Ledbetter, A., Krantz, T., McGee, J., Jackson, M. *et al.* (2000). Variable pulmonary responses from exposure to concentrated ambient air particles in a rat model of bronchitis. *Toxicological Sciences*, **54**, 441–51.

Kunzli, N., Jarrett, M., Mack, W. J., Beckerman, B., LaBree, L., Gilliland, F. *et al.* (2004). Ambient air pollution and atherosclerosis in Los Angeles. *Environmental Health Perspectives* (http://dx.doi.org).

Kwon, H. J., Cho, S. H., Nyberg, F., and Pershagen, G. (2001). Effects of ambient air pollution on daily mortality in a cohort of patients with congestive heart failure. *Epidemiology*, **12**, 413–19.

Levy, J. I., Hammitt, J. K., and Spengler, J. D. (2000). Estimating the mortality impacts of particulate matter: what can be learned from between-study variability? *Environmental Health Perspectives*, **108**, 109–17.

Liao, D., Creason, J., Shy, C., Williams, R., Watts, R. Zweidinger, R. (1999). Daily variation of particulate air pollution and poor cardiac autonomic control in the elderly. *Environmental Health Perspectives*, **107**, 521–5.

Linn, W. S. and Gong, H. Jr. (2001). Air pollution, weather stress, and blood pressure. *American Journal of Public Health*, **91**, 1345–6.

Lipfert, F. W. (1994). *Air pollution and community health: a critical review and data sourcebook*. Van Nostrand Reinhold, New York.

Logan, W. P. D. (1953). Mortality in the London fog incident. *Lancet*, **1**, 336–8.

Magari, S. R., Hauser, R., Schwartz, J., Williams, P. L., Smith, T. J., and Christiani, D. C. (2001). Association of heart rate variability with occupational and environmental exposure to particulate air pollution. *Circulation*, **104**, 986–91.

Ministry of Health (1954). *Mortality and morbidity during the London fog of December 1952*. Reports on Public Health and Medical Subjects No. 95. Her Majesty's Stationery Office, London.

Morris, R. D. (2001). Airborne particulates and hospital admissions for cardiovascular disease: a quantitative review of the evidence. *Environmental Health Perspectives*, **109** (Suppl. 4), 495–500.

Mukae, H., Vincent, R., Quinlan, K., English, D., Hards, J., Hogg, J. C., and van Eeden, S. F. (2001). The effect of repeated exposure to particulate air pollution (PM_{10}) on the bone marrow. *American Journal of Respiratory and Critical Care Medicine*, **163**, 201–9.

Nadziejko, C., Chen, L. C., Zelikoff, I. T., and Gordon, T. (1997). Hematological and cardiovascular effects of acute exposure to ambient particulate matter (PM). *American Journal of Respiratory and Critical Care Medicine*, **155**, A247.

Ostro, B. D. (1990). Associations between morbidity and alternative measures of particulate matter. *Risk Analysis*, **10**, 421–7.

Ostro, B. D., Lipsett, M. J., Mann, J. K., Krupnick, A., and Harrington, W. (1993). Air pollution and respiratory morbidity among adults in southern California. *American Journal of Epidemiology*, **137**, 691–700.

Parish, A. R. (1997). Sudden infant death syndrome: a proposed discovery. *Medical Hypotheses*, **49**, 177–9.

Penn, A. and Snyder, C. A. (1993). Inhalation of sidestream cigarette smoke accelerates development of arteriosclerotic plaques. *Circulation*, **88**, 1820–5.

Penn, A., Chen, L. C., and Snyder, C. A. (1994). Inhalation of steady-state sidestream smoke from one cigarette promotes atherosclerotic plaque development. *Circulation*, **90**, 1363–7.

Peters, A., Doring, A., Wichmann, H. E., and Koenig, W. (1997). Increased plasma viscosity during the 1985 air pollution episode: a link to mortality? *Lancet*, **349**, 1582–7.

Peters, A., Perz, S., Doring, A., Stieber, J., Koenig, W., and Wichmann, H. E. (1999). Increases in heart rate during an air pollution episode. *American Journal of Epidemiology*, **150**, 1094–8.

Peters, A., Lui, E., Verrier, R. L., Schwartz, J., Gold, D. R., Mittleman, M. *et al.* (2000). Air pollution and incidence of cardiac arrhythmia. *Epidemiology*, **11**, 11–17.

Peters, A., Frohlich, M., Doring, A., Immervoll, T., Wichmann, H. E., Hutchingson, W. L. *et al.* (2001*a*). Particulate air pollution is associated with an acute phase response in men: results from the MONICA-Augsburg study. *European Heart Journal*, **22**, 1198–204.

Peters, A., Dockery, D. W., Muller, J. E., and Mittleman, M. A. (2001*b*). Increased particulate air pollution and the triggering of myocardial infarction. *Circulation*, **103**, 2810–15.

Poloniecki, J. D., Atkinson, R. W., de Leon, A. P., and Anderson, H. R. (1997). Daily time series for cardiovascular hospital admissions and previous day's air pollution in London, UK. *Occupational and Environmental Medicine*, **54**, 535–40.

Ponka, A. (1991). Asthma and low level air pollution in Helsinki. *Archives of Environmental Health*, **46**, 262–70.

Pope, C. A. III. (1989). Respiratory disease associated with community air pollution and a steel mill, Utah Valley. *American Journal of Public Health*, **79**, 623–8.

Pope, C. A. III. (1991). Respiratory hospital admissions associated with PM_{10} pollution in Utah, Salt Lake, and Cache Valleys. *Archives of Environmental Health*, **46**, 90–7.

Pope, C. A. III. (2000*a*). Epidemiology of fine particulate air pollution and human health: biologic mechanisms and who's at risk. *Environmental Health Perspectives*, **108** (Suppl. 4), 713–23.

Pope, C. A. III. (2000*b*). Invited commentary: particulate matter-mortality exposure-response relations and threshold. *American Journal of Epidemiology*, **152**, 407–12.

Pope, C. A. III and Dockery, D. W. (1992). Acute health effects of PM_{10} pollution on symptomatic and asymptomatic children. *American Review of Respiratory Disease*, **145**, 1123–8.

Pope, C. A. III and Dockery, D. W. (1999). Epidemiology of particle effects. In *Air pollution and health* (ed. S. T. Holgate *et al.*), pp. 673–705. Academic Press, London.

Pope, C. A. III and Kanner, R. E. (1993). Acute effects of PM_{10} pollution on pulmonary function of smokers with mild to moderate chronic obstructive pulmonary disease. *American Review of Respiratory Disease*, **147**, 1336–40.

Pope C. A. III, Dockery, D. W., Spengler, J. D., and Raizenne, M. E. (1991). Respiratory health and PM_{10} pollution: a daily time series analysis. *American Review of Respiratory Disease*, **144**, 668–74.

Pope, C. A. III, Schwartz, J., and Ransom, M. R. (1992). Daily mortality and PM_{10} pollution in Utah Valley. *Archives of Environmental Health*, **47**, 211–17.

Pope, C. A. III, Thun, M. J., Namboodiri, M. M., Dockery, D. W., Evans, J. S., Speizer, F. E., and Heath, C. W. Jr. (1995). Particulate air pollution as a predictor of mortality in a prospective study of U. S. adults. *American Journal of Respiratory and Critical Care Medicine*, **151**, 669–74.

Pope, C. A. III, Dockery, D. W., Kanner, R. E., Villegas, G. M., and Schwartz, J. (1999a). Oxygen saturation, pulse rate, and particulate air pollution: a daily time-series panel study. *American Journal of Respiratory and Critical Care Medicine*, **159**, 365–72.

Pope, C. A. III, Verrier, R. L., Lovett, E. G., Larson, A. C., Raizenne, M. E., Kanner, R. E. *et al.* (1999b). Heart rate variability associated with particulate air pollution. *American Heart Journal*, **138**, 890–9.

Pope, C. A. III, Eatough, D. J., Gold, D. R., Pang, Y., Nielsen, K. R., Nath, P. *et al.* (2001). Acute exposure to environmental tobacco smoke and heart rate variability. *Environmental Health Perspectives*, **109**, 711–16.

Pope, C. A. III, Burnett, R. T., Thun, M. J., Calle, E. E., Krewski, D., Ito, K., and Thurston, G. D. (2002). Lung cancer, cardiopulmonary mortality, and long-term exposure to fine particulate air pollution. *The Journal of the American Medical Association*, **287**, 1132–41.

Pope, C. A. III, Burnett, R. T., Thurston, G. D., Thun, M. J., Calle, E. E., Krewski, D. *et al.* (2004a). Cardiovascular mortality and long-term exposure to particulate air pollution: epidemiological evidence of general pathophysiological pathways of diesease. *Circulation*, **109**, 71–7.

Pope, C. A. III, Hansen, M. L., Long, R. W., Nielsen, K. R., Eatough, N. L., Wilson, W. E. *et al.* (2004b). Ambient particulate air pollution, heart rate variability, and blood markers of inflammation in a panel of elderly subjects. *Environmental Health Perspectives*, **112**, 339–45.

Ransom, M. R. and Pope, C. A. III. (1992). Elementary school absences and PM_{10} pollution in Utah Valley. *Environmental Research*, **58**, 204–19.

Ridker, P. M., Cushman, M., Stampfer, M. J., Tracy, R. P., and Hennekens, C. H. (1997). Inflammation, aspirin, and the risk of cardiovascular disease in apparently healthy men [published erratum appears in *New England Journal of Medicine*, 1997, **337**, 356]. *New England Journal of Medicine*, **336**, 973–9.

Ridker, P. M., Hennekens, C. H., Buring, J. E., and Rifai, N. (2000). C-reactive protein and other markers of inflammation in the prediction of cardiovascular disease in women. *New England Journal of Medicine*, **342**, 836–43.

Salvi, S. S., Nordenhall, C., Blomberg, A., Rudell, B., Pourazar, J., Kelly, F. J. *et al.* (2000). Acute exposure to diesel exhaust increases IL-8 and GRO-alpha production in healthy human airways. *American Journal of Respiratory and Critical Care Medicine*, **161**, 550–7.

Samet, J. M., Dominici, F., Curriero, F. C., Coursac, I., and Zeger, S. L. (2000). Fine particulate air pollution and mortality in 20 U. S. cities, 1987–1994. *New England Journal of Medicine*, **343**, 1742–9.

Seaton, A., MacNee, W., Donaldson, K., and Godden, D. (1995). Particulate air pollution and acute health effects. *Lancet*, **345**, 176–8.

Seaton, A., Soutar, A., Crawford, V., Elton, R., McNerlan, S., Cherrie, J. *et al.* (1999). Particulate air pollution and the blood. *Thorax*, **54**, 1027–32.

Schwartz, J. (1991). Particulate air pollution and daily mortality in Detroit. *Environmental Research*, **56**, 204–13.

Schwartz, J. (1993). Air pollution and daily mortality in Birmingham, Alabama. *American Journal of Epidemiology*, **137**, 1136–47.

Schwartz, J. (1997). Air pollution and hospital admissions for cardiovascular disease in Tucson. *Epidemiology*, **8**, 371–7.

Schwartz, J. (1999). Air pollution and hospital admissions for heart disease in eight U. S. counties. *Epidemiology*, **10**, 1–22.

Schwartz, J. and Dockery, D. W. (1992a). Increased mortality in Philadelphia associated with daily air pollution concentrations. *American Review of Respiratory Disease*, **145**, 600–4.

Schwartz, J. and Dockery, D. W. (1992b). Particulate air pollution and daily mortality in Steubenville, Ohio. *American Journal of Epidemiology*, **135**, 12–19.

Schwartz, J. and Marcus, A. (1990). Mortality and air pollution in London: a time series analysis. *American Journal of Epidemiology*, **131**, 185–94.

Schwartz. J. and Morris, R. (1995). Air pollution and hospital admissions for cardiovascular disease in Detroit, Michigan. *American Journal of Epidemiology*, **142**, 23–35.

Schwartz, J. and Zanobetti, A. (2000). Using meta-smoothing to estimate dose-response trends across multiple studies, with application to air pollution and daily death. *Epidemiology*, **11**, 666–72.

Souza, M. B., Saldiva, P. H. N., Pope, C. A. III, and Capelozzi, V. L. (1998). Respiratory changes due to long-term exposure to urban levels of air pollution: a histopathologic study in humans. *Chest*, **113**, 1312–18.

Spengler, J. D., Dockery, D. W., Turner, W. A., Wolfson, J. M., and Ferris, B. G. (1981). Long-term measurements of respirable sulfates and particles inside and outside homes. *Atmospheric Environment*, **15**, 23–30.

Steenland, K. (1999). Risk assessment for heart disease and workplace ETS exposure among non-smokers. *Environmental Health Perspectives*, **107** (Suppl. 6), 859–63.

Stone, P. H. and Godleski, J. J. (1999). First steps toward understanding the pathophysiologic link between air pollution and cardiac mortality. *American Heart Journal*, **138**, 804–7.

Suwa, T., Hogg, J. C., Quinlan, K. B., Ohgami, A., Vincent, R., and van Eeden, S. F. (2002). Particulate air pollution induces progression of atherosclerosis. *Journal of the American College of Cardiology*, **39**, 935–42.

Tan, W. C., Qiu, D., Liam, B. L., Ng, T. P., Lee, S. H., van Eeden, S. F. *et al.* (2000). The human bone marrow response to acute air pollution caused by forest fires. *American Journal of Respiratory and Critical Care Medicine*, **161**, 1213–17.

Terashima, T., Wiggs, B., English, D., Hogg, J. C., and van Eeden, S. F. (1997). Phagocytosis of small carbon particles (PM_{10}) by alveolar macrophages stimulates the release of polymorphonuclear leukocytes from the bone marrow. *American Journal of Respiratory and Critical Care Medicine*, **155**, 1441–7.

Thun, M., Henley, J., and Apicella, L. (1999). Epidemiologic studies of fatal and nonfatal cardiovascular disease and ETS exposure form spousal smoking. *Environmental Health Perspectives*, **107** (Suppl. 6), 841–6.

Thurston, G. D., Ito, K., Kinney, P. L., and Lippmann, M. (1992). A multi-year study of air pollution and respiratory hospital admissions in three New York State metropolitan areas: results for 1988 and 1989 summers. *Journal of Exposure Analysis and Environmental Epidemiology*, **2**, 429–50.

Utell, M. M. and Frampton, M. W. (2000). Acute health effects of ambient air pollution: the ultrafine particle hypothesis. *Journal of Aerosol Medicine*, **13**, 355–9.

van Eeden, S. F., Tan, W. C., Suwa, T., Mukae, H., Terashima, T., Fujii, T. *et al.* (2001). Cytokines involved in the systemic inflammatory response induced by exposure to particulate matter air pollutants (PM_{10}). *American Journal of Respiratory and Critical Care Medicine*, **164**, 826–30.

Vedal, S. (1997). Ambient particles and health: lines that divide. *Journal of the Air & Waste Management Association*, **47**, 551–81.

Watkinson, W. P., Campen, M. J., and Costa, D. L. (1998). Cardiac arrhythmia induction after exposure to residual oil fly ash particles in a rodent model of pulmonary hypertension. *Toxicological Sciences*, **41**, 209–16.

Wellenius, G. A., Saldiva, P. H., Batalha, J. R., Krishna Murthy, G. G., Coull, B. A., Verrier, R. L., and Godleski, J. J. (2002). Electrocardiographic changes during exposure to residual oil fly ash (ROFA) particles in a rat model of myocardial infarction. *Toxicological Sciences*, **66**, 327–35.

Wichmann, H. E., Mueller, W., Allhoff, P., Beckmann, M., Bocter, N., Csicsaky, M. J. *et al.* (1989). Health effects during a smog episode in West Germany in 1985. *Environmental Health Perspectives*, **79**, 89–99.

Woodruff, T. J., Grillo, J., and Schoendorf, K. C. (1997). The relationship between selected causes of postneonatal infant mortality and particulate air pollution in the United States. *Environmental Health Perspectives*, **105**, 608–12.

Zhu, B. Q., Sun, Y. P., Sievers, R. E., Glantz, S. A., Parmley, W. W., and Wolfe, C. L. (1994). Exposure to environmental tobacco smoke increases myocardial infarct size in rats. *Circulation*, **89**, 1282–90.

Chapter 30

Seasonal variations in all-cause and cardiovascular mortality and the role of temperature

M. B. Toledano, G. Shaddick, and P. Elliott

30.1 **Introduction**

Seasonal patterns in mortality have been recognized for well over a century. An increase in deaths during winter in England and Wales was reported by William Farr (GRO 1841) as early as 1841. More recently, seasonal variations in mortality, with consistent excess in winter, have been described in a number of countries across the world (Nayha 2002). The biggest single cause of excess deaths is cardiovascular disease (Keatinge and Donaldson 1995; Mackenbach et al. 1992).

Independent of season, both hot and cold temperatures are associated with increased mortality (Curriero et al. 2002; Huynen et al. 2001; Kunst et al. 1993). In the USA, while mortality associated with high ambient temperatures has been a widely acknowledged public health problem, the effects of cold temperatures have been largely unstudied (Taylor and McGwin 2000). In contrast, European researchers have mainly focused on cold-related deaths (Taylor and McGwin 2000), although recently there have been a number of reports of increased mortality associated with summer heatwaves across European cities (Bosch 2003b). Methods have varied considerably across studies (Pattenden et al. 2003), particularly with regard to the measures used; for example, season or daily, weekly, and monthly temperatures; allowance for potential lag effects; and degree of adjustment for potential confounders such as air pollution, wind, humidity, etc.

Previous reviews have mainly focused on either seasonal variation in death (Alderson 1985; Wyndham and Fellingham 1978) or the effects of cold weather on the risk of cardiovascular mortality (Keatinge 2002; Mercer 2003; Nayha 2002; Vuori 1987), and possible physiological mechanisms underlying this relationship (Keatinge and Donaldson 1995; Lloyd 1991). Recent interest in global warming has raised concerns over the effects that the predicted increased average global temperatures may have on the health of the world's population (Kalkstein 2000), but little attention has been given to reviewing the effects of heat on mortality (Basu and Samet 2002). This chapter aims to provide a current assessment of the relationship between ambient temperature and mortality or disease occurrence in adults, in particular from cardiovascular diseases. Studies investigating the possible association between temperature and infant mortality (see, for example, Hare et al. 1981; Murphy and Campbell 1987; Schluter et al. 1998) are not included here. Both studies of seasonal effects and time-series studies are considered.

30.2 **Studies of seasonal effects**

30.2.1 **Excess winter mortality**

Higher rates of mortality in the colder winter months have been described in many countries, including the USA (Bull and Morton 1978; Kloner *et al.* 1999; Lanska and Hoffmann 1999; Seto *et al.* 1998), Russia (McKee *et al.* 1998), China (Cheng 1993), Israel (Green *et al.* 1994), New Zealand (Douglas *et al.* 1990; Isaacs and Donn 1993; Marshall *et al.* 1988), Bangladesh (Becker and Weng 1998), Japan (Kagami 1983; Ornato *et al.* 1990), and throughout Europe (Cordioli *et al.* 2000; Douglas *et al.* 1995; Keatinge and Donaldson 1995; Kunst *et al.* 1993; Lerchl 1998; Mackenbach *et al.* 1992; Moran *et al.* 2000; Rose 1966). This phenomenon is referred to as 'excess winter mortality', and accounts for approximately 30 000–50 000 deaths per year in Britain alone (Aylin *et al.* 2001; Christophersen 1997; Curwen 1990/91; Curwen and Devis 1988; Keatinge 2002; Keatinge and Donaldson 1995; Laake and Sverre 1996); across Europe, there are approximately one-quarter of a million excess winter deaths each year (Mercer 2003). It is only partially explained by influenza epidemics (Curwen and Devis 1988; Donaldson and Keatinge 2002; Gemmell *et al.* 2000; Simonsen *et al.* 1997), estimated to account for less than 5% of the excess winter mortality in Britain over the last 10 years (Donaldson and Keatinge 2002; Keatinge 2002). Higher mortality rates in colder or more northern parts of a country have also been described within countries (Gyllerup 2000; Gyllerup *et al.* 1991; Law and Morris 1998; Nayha and Hassi 1995; Smith and Tunstall-Pedoe 1984).

Seasonal patterns of mortality are often described by comparing the number of deaths from December to March with those in the remaining months of the year (Aylin *et al.* 2001; Curwen 1990/91; Curwen and Devis 1988; Laake and Sverre 1996) or as the amplitude of a fitted cosine curve (Becker and Weng 1998; Douglas *et al.* 1990, 1991*b*), although other methods have also been used (Gemmell *et al.* 2000). The highest seasonal percentage increases in all-cause mortality from summer to winter are reported for the UK at ~30% (Douglas *et al.* 1991*a*; Gemmell *et al.* 2000; GRO 1987), with smaller summer to winter differences in other European countries of similar latitudes (Curwen 1990/91; McKee 1989).

Cardiovascular and respiratory causes of death are those most strongly and consistently linked to cold temperature (Aylin *et al.* 2001; Christophersen 1997; Douglas *et al.* 1995; Enquselassie *et al.* 1993; Haberman *et al.* 1981; Lanska and Hoffmann 1999; Mackenbach *et al.* 1992; Mannino and Washburn 1989; McKee 1990; McKee *et al.* 1998; van Rossum *et al.* 2001). Cardiovascular disease (CVD), including coronary heart disease (CHD) and cerebrovascular disease, accounts for approximately half of all the excess deaths (Curwen 1990/91; Huynen *et al.* 2001; Keatinge and Donaldson 1995) and up to 70% in some countries (Mackenbach *et al.* 1992; Mercer 2003). Respiratory disease generally accounts for up to half of the remaining excess cold-related mortality (Mackenbach *et al.* 1992; The Eurowinter Group 1997) and over three-quarters by some estimates (Christophersen 1997). Measured in terms of seasonal percentage increase, winter has a larger impact on mortality from respiratory disease than CVD (Aylin. 2001; Gemmell *et al.* 2000). However, as CVD is more common than respiratory disease mortality, CVD deaths account for a much larger percentage of the excess winter mortality.

There have been suggestions that excess winter deaths from all causes have been declining in a number of countries over the past few decades (Alderson 1985; Douglas *et al.* 1991*b*; Gemmell *et al.* 2000; Kunst *et al.* 1991; McDowell 1981; Nayha 2000), although weak, statistic-ally non-significant declines, or no change at all, have also been reported (Laake and Sverre 1996). Estimates for England and Wales suggest a drop of 500 excess deaths per year between

1949 and 1988 (Curwen and Devis 1988). Specifically, excess winter mortality from CHD is estimated to have fallen by 39.3% among old people in England and Wales during the period 1979–94, from cerebrovascular disease by 57.1%, and from respiratory disease by 36.9% (Donaldson and Keatinge 1997*a*).

Low temperatures have been implicated in explaining the amplitude of seasonal variation in mortality (Bull and Morton 1978; Elwood *et al.* 1993; Kunst *et al.* 1993; Lerchl 1998), though the steep increase in mortality in December/January is partly due to accumulation of frail individuals during the warmer season. Similarly, the low mortality in the summer is partly a consequence of survival of the fittest over the winter (Nayha 2000). Curwin and Devis (1988) used linear regression models to compare deaths in winters (December–March) to those in summer within England and Wales, and found that a drop of 1°C below the average temperature was associated with about 8000 excess winter deaths during the period 1976–85. A similar study by Aylin *et al.* (2001), using data for those aged 65 and older in Great Britain during 1986–96, also reported a significant association between all-cause and CHD mortality and temperature. There was 1.5% higher odds of dying in winter for every 1°C lower 24-h mean winter temperature.

Age and other risk factors

Since the majority of deaths from CVD occurs in the elderly, so does most of the excess winter mortality. Higher odds of dying in winter with increasing age have consistently been reported (Aylin *et al.* 2001; Christophersen 1997; Cordioli *et al.* 2000; Gemmell *et al.* 2000; Laake and Sverre 1996; Sheth *et al.* 1999; van Rossum *et al.* 2001). In the winter of 1996/97 in England and Wales, over three-quarters of the excess winter deaths were estimated to be among people aged 75 years and over, with women aged 85 and over accounting for nearly a third (Christophersen 1997).

In addition to age, other risk factors for cold-related mortality have been described (Table 30.1). While several studies support an association with indices of socio-economic deprivation (Donaldson and Keatinge 2003; Douglas *et al.* 1991*b*; Healy 2003; McKee 1989; O'Neill *et al.* 2003), others do not (Aylin *et al.* 2001; Gouveia *et al.* 2003; Lawlor 1999; Lawlor *et al.* 2000, 2002; Shah and Peacock 1999; van Rossum *et al.* 2001). This lack of consistency may reflect low sensitivity of the indices used to characterize living conditions or housing standards (Ballester *et al.* 2003) or the statistical 'removal' of socio-economic differentials by adjustment for other closely related variables, for example, air pollution (Keatinge 2003*a*).

30.2.2 Seasonal variations in CVD incidence

Excess winter mortality could reflect increased incidence (Anon 1970; Rose 1966) or decreased survival (Enquselassie *et al.* 1993; Pell *et al.* 1999) from higher case-fatality rates in winter or in low temperatures. Hospital-based studies are subject to referral and survival bias, as they only include patients who have survived long enough for admission (Danet *et al.* 1999; Rothwell *et al.* 1996).

The limited number of community-based studies on occurrence of CHD provides inconclusive evidence for an association with cold temperature. In New South Wales, Australia (part of the WHO MONICA project), coronary events, whether fatal or non-fatal, were 20–40% more likely to occur in winter and spring than summer, although low temperature was associated only with fatal coronary events, but not with non-fatal and incident cases of myocardial infarction (MI) (Enquselassie *et al.* 1993). A slight excess incidence of MI was found with below-zero temperatures in Helsinki (Sarna *et al.* 1977), while in Lille, France, a 10°C lower atmospheric

Table 30.1 Selected putative risk factors for temperature-related mortality

Cold	Heat
Demographic	*Demographic*
Elderly age	Elderly age
Socio-economic status	Socio-economic status
	Black
Social Behavioural	*Social Behavioural*
Poor housing quality/low levels of central heating	Lack of air conditioning
Less outdoor clothing	Social isolation
Greater time spent outdoors	Confinement to bed (unable to care for oneself)
Inactivity outdoors	Not leaving home daily
	Top floor of multi-storey buildings
	Excessive alcohol intake
	No access to transportation
	Excessive clothing
	Prolonged sun exposure
Clinical/Biological	*Clinical/Biological*
Seasonal variation in cardiovascular risk factors (e.g. cholesterol, fibrinogen, blood pressure)	Mental problem
Pre-existing medical illnesses (e.g. ischaemic heart disease, chronic bronchitis)	Pre-existing medical illnesses
	Tranquillizer or barbiturate use
	Medication use (e.g. anticholinergic drugs)
	Place of death (out-of-hospital mortality greater)

temperature was associated with 13% higher event rates for coronary deaths, and incident and recurrent MI, especially at older ages (Danet *et al.* 1999).

Spring and winter peaks in incident CHD were observed in a study of 47 281 admissions for CHD to all Scottish hospitals, 1962–66 (Dunnigan *et al.* 1970). In a further Scottish study over a similar time period, this bimodal pattern was observed only amongst males, whereas female hospital admissions showed a dominant winter/summer pattern (Douglas *et al.* 1995). In both studies, the spring peak declined with increasing age, while the winter peak became more prominent (Douglas *et al.* 1995; Dunnigan *et al.* 1970). Spring and winter peaks were also found in a study of hospital admissions from the National Registry of Myocardial Infarction in the USA (Ornato *et al.* 1996).

Concerning occurrence of strokes, population-based studies are inconsistent (Jakovljevic *et al.* 1996; Rothwell *et al.* 1996). Using data on 15 449 stroke events from the FINMONICA population-based stroke register in Finland, 1982–92, a significantly higher incidence of ischaemic strokes (12% (95% confidence interval (CI): 5–20%) in men and 11% (4–19%) in women) and intracerebral haemorrhages (28% (3–58%) in men and 33% (6–66%) in women) was observed in winter than summer, though subarachnoid haemorrhage did not vary significantly by season (Jakovljevic *et al.* 1996). Data from the SEPIVAC community-based stroke register in Umbria, Italy, also demonstrated a higher frequency of cerebral infarctions during winter and of primary intracerebral haemorrhages during late winter/autumn (Ricci *et al.* 1992).

In contrast, Rothwell *et al.* (1996) observed no significant seasonal variations in the incidence of all stroke subtypes from the Oxfordshire Community Stroke Project, UK, during the 1980s, although statistical power was limited due to small sample size. Neither was a significant winter excess in the incidence of stroke reported from the UK Medical Research Council trial of treatment for mild hypertension (Millar 1996), from a population-based register in the L'Aquila district of central Italy (Carolei *et al.* 1996) and from the Nijmegen morbidity register in the Netherlands (van Weel *et al.* 1996). Taken together, the limited number of studies to date are more suggestive of a possible seasonal influence on stroke fatality rate than on incidence (Rothwell *et al.* 1996).

30.2.3 Summer mortality and heatwaves

Numerous reports, predominantly from the USA, have shown that mortality increases during heatwaves (Allexenberg 1981; Anders *et al.* 1995; Applegate *et al.* 1981; Dardanoni *et al.* 1988; Donoghue *et al.* 1995; Ellis and Nelson 1978; Hawkins-Bell and Rankin 1994; Jones *et al.* 1982; MacFarlane 1978; MacFarlane and Waller 1976; Nashold *et al.* 1996; Ramlow and Kuller 1990; Rooney *et al.* 1998; Sartor *et al.* 1995; Semenza *et al.* 1996; Stewart *et al.* 1989; Voelker 1995). For example, in the summer of 1995, an estimated 460 and 619 extra deaths (relative to the expected number for that period) were recorded in Chicago (Anon 1995) and England and Wales (Rooney *et al.* 1998), respectively, as a result of extreme heatwaves when temperatures reached 40°C and 35.2°C, respectively. In the summer of 2003, average temperatures in Europe exceeded European summer temperatures over the last 100 years by around 2°C (Luterbacher *et al.* 2004), with excess mortality reported across European cities, for example in Spain, Portugal, Germany, France, and the UK (Bosch 2003*a, b*; Butler 2003; Hemon and Jougla 2003; McGregor 2003). Provisional estimates of mortality during the August heatwave, when temperatures soared above 35°C, suggest an excess of ~1700 deaths in England and Wales (McGregor 2003) and 14 800 deaths in France (Hemon and Jougla 2003).

Threshold temperatures, above which sharp rises in heat-related daily mortality have been observed in various countries across the world, commonly range between 36 and 38°C (Diaz *et al.* 2002*b*; Nakai *et al.* 1999; Whitman *et al.* 1997), although thresholds as low as 27.5°C and as high as 41°C have been reported (Diaz *et al.* 2002*a*; Sartor *et al.* 1995). In a study of seven warm and cold European regions, annual heat-related mortality averaged 217 per million population amongst those aged 65–74, significantly lower than the 2003 per million averaged annual cold-related deaths (Keatinge *et al.* 2000). In Britain, the number of heat-related deaths (the number of excess deaths on days hotter than 18°C) has averaged around 800 per year in recent years (Donaldson *et al.* 2001).

During heatwaves and with hot temperatures, cardiovascular (including cerebrovascular) and respiratory diseases are the leading causes of death (Ballester *et al.* 1997; Bull and Morton 1975; Ellis and Nelson 1978; Hemon and Jougla 2003; Kunst *et al.* 1993; MacFarlane 1978; Pan *et al.* 1995; Rooney *et al.* 1998; Saez *et al.* 1995; Wyndham and Fellingham 1978), with between 25 and 30% of heat-related deaths attributable to CVD (Huynen *et al.* 2001; Kunst *et al.* 1993) and nearly 25% to respiratory disease (Huynen *et al.* 2001). The proportion of heat- compared with cold-related mortality attributable to CVD is, therefore, smaller (26 vs. 57% according to Kunst *et al.* (1993)); most of the deaths attributed to these causes occur in persons with pre-existing cardiorespiratory illnesses, for example, CHD or stroke (Basu and Samet 2002).

Age and other risk factors

As with cold stress, the elderly (>60 years) are at highest risk of mortality from hot temperatures (Anon 1995; Applegate *et al.* 1981; Ballester *et al.* 1997; Ellis and Nelson 1978; Greenberg *et al.* 1983; MacFarlane 1978; Ramlow and Kuller 1990; Saez *et al.* 1995; Sartor *et al.* 1995; Schuman 1972; Smoyer-Tomic and Rainham 2001). Estimates from the heatwave of 2003 in

France suggest that excess mortality was 20% at ages 45–54 years, 40% at 55–74 years, 70% at 75–94 years, and 120% at ages 95 years and over (Hemon and Jougla 2003). In addition to age, most heat stress studies have identified a number of other demographic, social/behavioural and clinical/biological risk factors for mortality (see Table 30.1).

30.3 Time-series studies of temperature and mortality

Time-series studies have investigated the short-term relationship between temperature and mortality using data on daily death counts and daily temperatures. Long-term trends, for example, season, holiday periods, and influenza epidemics, need to be accounted for. A variety of approaches have been used to model this background variation, including both parametric and semi/non-parametric methods (smoothing). More recently, generalized additive models have become a common approach. These provide a flexible framework for modelling the underlying temporal patterns and the short-term changes in temperature and mortality (Schwartz 1994), which are non-linear when the full range of temperatures, that is, hot and cold extremes, are modelled simultaneously. Time-series studies require evaluation of the temporal scale of the temperature–mortality relationship; that is, whether effects are considered to be immediate, to occur after a lag, or are the sum of effects over a number of days. Different approaches to modelling the lag structure have been used, for example, multiple lags, simultaneously included in the same model (the effect of each day being identical) or distributed lag models that allow the influence of temperature to decline over time (Schwartz 2000; Zanobetti *et al.* 2000). In an attempt to reduce the problems associated with multicollinearity, temperature variables have often been constructed for groups of subsequent days (lag intervals) by averaging values for heat and cold over these periods (see, for example, Huynen *et al.* 2001; Kunst *et al.* 1993). Variables thought best to represent the effects of weather need to be selected, for example, mean, minimum, and maximum temperatures, with or without information on other time-varying meteorological variables such as humidity, or categories of synoptic weather patterns, and other potentially confounding factors such as air pollutants. Considerable variation in methods used in time-series studies to date attest to the uncertainty surrounding a number of key methodological issues, many of which are in common with the air pollution literature (Schwartz *et al.* 1996), complicating evaluation of the evidence from these studies. Distinguishing between true, artefactual, and spurious associations requires consideration of the following key questions:

◆ Have seasonal and longer-term trends been adequately adjusted for?

◆ Has multiple testing, for example, inclusion of multiple lag structures in a series of regression models, been adequately accounted for – is there spurious precision in effect estimates?

◆ Is the choice of lag periods appropriate, or has averaging temperatures over shorter or longer periods resulted in under/overestimation and/or reduced power to detect effects?

◆ Has the inherent multicollinearity of temperature and other variables in the fitted models given rise to biased estimates of effect?

◆ Could short-term 'mortality displacement' (i.e. the bringing forward of deaths by a few hours or days) account for any observed association?

◆ To what extent could another factor related to temperature, for example air pollution or humidity, confound or modify the effect of temperature on mortality?

Table 30.2 provides a summary of the findings of selected time-series studies to date. A variety of temperature exposure measurements, factors controlled for, and modelling methodologies have been used. Taken together, independent of season, these studies have mostly observed a U-, V-, or J-shaped relationship between temperature and mortality, that is, increased mortality associated with temperatures above and below some optimum temperature range (Alberdi *et al.* 1998; Huynen *et al.* 2001; Kunst *et al.* 1993; Saez *et al.* 1995) – usually in the range 15–20°C, but higher in regions with higher mean summer temperatures (Keatinge *et al.* 2000). Notable exceptions include Yekaterinburg, north-eastern Russia (mean winter temperature below −6°C), where mortality only increased at temperatures lower than 0°C (Donaldson *et al.* 1998*b*) and Yakutsk, eastern Siberia (mean winter temperature of −26.6°C), where mortality from CHD, cerebrovascular disease, and all causes did not rise as temperatures fell from 10.2 to −48.2°C (Donaldson *et al.* 1998*a*). Mortality is commonly estimated to increase by around 1 % for every 1°C fall in temperature below the optimal level.

Paradoxically, the cold temperature–mortality relation appears to be stronger in regions with milder climates, with higher incremental increases in mortality for the same drop in temperature for people living in warmer compared with colder climates (Eng and Mercer 1998; The Eurowinter group 1997, 2000). Similarly, regions with hot summers did not have higher annual heat-related mortality than cold regions (Curriero *et al.* 2002; Keatinge *et al.* 2000), and the effects of hot days on mortality were greater in cold cities, where hot days were less common than in hot cities (Braga *et al.* 2002). Explanations for these findings highlight differences in behavioural factors ascertained through surveys; for example, as temperatures fell from 10.2 to −48.2°C in Yakutsk, there was a tendency for people to wear more layers of clothing, to go outside less, and to sleep in heated bedrooms (Donaldson *et al.* 1998*a*). Similarly, as temperatures fell to 0°C in Yekaterinburg, Russia, people reported wearing progressively more clothing and spending less time stationary, and hence only 6.6% (95% CI: 2.6–9.6) reported shivering whilst outside (Donaldson *et al.* 1998*b*). Moreover, 94.2% of bedrooms were directly heated and living room temperatures averaged 19.8°C even when outside temperatures reached −25°C (Donaldson *et al.* 1998*b*). In the Eurowinter study of eight European regions (The Eurowinter Group 1997), significant associations were found between low living room temperatures, limited bedroom heating, low proportions of people wearing hats, gloves, and anoraks, inactivity, and shivering when outdoors and high indices of cold-related mortality from all causes and respiratory diseases (but not for deaths from CHD or stroke (The Eurowinter Group 1997)).

30.3.1 Lag periods

Most authors have described a time lag between a drop in ambient temperature and a change in all-cause mortality (Ballester *et al.* 1997; Bull and Morton 1978; Curriero *et al.* 2002; Donaldson and Keatinge 1997*b*; Huynen *et al.* 2001; Keatinge *et al.* 2000; Kunst *et al.* 1993). The lag that gives the highest regression coefficients for cold temperatures and all-cause mortality has been reported as 3 days in studies across Europe (Donaldson and Keatinge 1997*b*; Keatinge *et al.* 2000; The Eurowinter Group 1997), but the largest effect of temperature on daily deaths was seen at lag 0 in a number of US cities (Braga *et al.* 2001, 2002). Although Curriero *et al.* (2002) found only weak associations between mortality and temperature at lags greater than 4 days, most studies have reported cold effects lasting for at least 2 weeks (Ballester *et al.* 1997; Braga *et al.* 2001, 2002; Huynen *et al.* 2001; Kunst *et al.* 1993; Pattenden *et al.* 2003), and up to 40 days in a study in south-east England (Donaldson and Keatinge 1997*b*).

Table 30.2 Summary of selected time-series studies assessing the temperature–mortality relation

Author	Study population	Exposure	Outcome	Factors controlled for	Main findings
Studies of cold effects:					
Donaldson and Keatinge 1997b	50+ year-olds, south-east England, 1976–92	Daily mean temperatures	Daily mortality (digitally filtered together with mean daily temperatures for analysis) from: all-causes, ischaemic heart disease, cerebrovascular disease, respiratory disease	Daily mortality (digitally filtered together with mean daily temperatures for analysis) from: all-causes, ischaemic heart disease, cerebrovascular disease, respiratory disease	Cold-related mortality began to rise below 18°C, with linear increases below 15°C *For the temperature range 0–15°C, excess deaths per million population associated with short-term temperature displacements per 1 day fall of 1°C (% by which excess is greater than the overall seasonal increases in daily deaths per million per 1°C fall in temperature):* All causes: 24.68 (37%) IHD: 7.26 (52%) Respiratory disease: 5.81 (17%)
The Eurowinter Group 1997	50–59- and 65–74-year-olds in eight European regions: North and South Finland, Baden-Wurttemberg, Netherlands, London, North Italy, 1988–92, and Athens and Palermo, 1992	Daily mean temperatures below 18°C	Daily mortality (lagged on temperature by) from: all Causes (3 days), ischaemic heart disease (2 days), cerebrovascular disease (5 days), respiratory disease (12 days)	Deaths from Influenza averaged over 20 days, age and sex	*Mean (95% CI) % increase in all-cause mortality per 1°C fall from 18°C for coldest, medium, and hottest regions:* North Finland: 0.29 (0.10–0.48) London: 1.37 (1.20–1.54) Athens: 2.15 (1.20–3.10)

Reference	Population	Exposure	Outcome	Confounders	Results
Donaldson e al. 1998a	Residents aged 50–9 and 65–74 within 400 km of Yakutsk, eastern Siberia, 1989–95	Daily mean temperatures	Daily mortality (lagged on temperature by) from: all causes (3 days), ischaemic heart disease (2 days), cerebrovascular disease (5 days), respiratory disease (12 days)		**10.2 to −48.2°C:** *Mortality from:* All causes, ischaemic heart disease and cerebrovascular disease, no increase as temperatures fell to −48.2°C ($p > 0.05$) Respiratory disease, increased significantly from 4.69 (95% CI: 4.31–5.06) per million at 10.2°C to 5.07 (95% CI: 4.42–5.73) per million at −48.2°C
Donaldson et al. 1998b	Residents aged 50–9 and 65–74 within 140 km of Yekaterinburg, Russia, 1990–94	Daily mean temperatures	Daily mortality (lagged on temperature by) from: all causes (3 days), ischaemic heart disease (2 days), cerebrovascular disease (5 days), respiratory disease (12 days)	Deaths from Influenza averaged over 20 days, age and sex	**0 to −26.5°C:** No change in mortality from all causes and specific causes as temperatures fell to 0°C **0 to −29.6°C:** *Increase in mortality per 1°C decrease in temperature:* All causes: 1.15 (95% CI: 0.97–1.32) Relation between mortality and temperature for specific causes was not different to that for all Causes
Keatinge and Donaldson 2001a	Greater London, 1976–95, 50+ years of age	Daily mean temperatures	Daily mortality from: all causes	Daily relative humidity, rainfall, wind, and hours of sunshine; levels of SO_2, CO, smoke, and PM_{10}	V-shaped temperature–mortality relation, with point of minimum mortality 17°C *Excess deaths per million over a 24-day lag period following a 1°C fall in temperature for 1 day:* All causes: 2.77 (3.0% of the mean daily mortality of 92.4 per million)

Table 30.2 (continued)

Author	Study population	Exposure	Outcome	Factors controlled for	Main findings
Studies of heat effects					
Diaz et al. 2002a	Seville, Spain, 1986–97, 65+ years of age	Daily maximum temperatures	Daily mortality in summer months (June–September) from: all causes (except accidents), circulatory system disease, respiratory disease	Relative humidity, SO_2, TSP, NO_2, tropospheric ozone	Threshold of 41°C, above which temperature–mortality relation shown to increase abruptly. *% increase in daily mortality above the mean per 1°C increase above 41°C threshold:* All causes: 38 All causes (males): 29 All causes (females): 46 All causes (75+ years): 51 Circulatory: 49 Respiratory: 29 For pollutants: significant relationship between ozone and mortality only
Diaz et al. 2002b	Madrid, Spain, 1986–97, 65+ years of age	Daily maximum and minimum temperatures	Daily mortality in summer Months (June–September) from all causes (except accidents), circulatory System disease, respiratory disease	Relative humidity, influenza epidemic, periodicity, SO_2, TSP, nitric oxides, NO_2, tropospheric Ozone	Inflection point of rise in mortality observed at 36.5°C *(1) % increase in daily mortality above the mean per 1°C increase above 36.5°C threshold:* Circulatory (males, 65–74 years): 9.4 Circulatory (females, 65–74 years): 11.7 Circulatory (males, 75+ years): 9.3 Circulatory (females, 75+ years): 34.1 Respiratory (males, 65–74 years): 17.2 Respiratory (females, 65–74 years): 23.0 Respiratory (males, 75+ years): 26.1 Respiratory (females, 75+ years): 17.6 *(2) Persons increase in daily mortality per 1°C increase above 36.5°C threshold:* All causes (males, 65–74 years): 1.65 ($p < 0.001$) All causes (females, 65–74 years): 1.07 ($p < 0.01$) All causes (males, 75+ years): 2.51 ($p < 0.01$) All causes (females, 75+ years): 8.15 ($p < 0.001$)

Reference	Population/location	Exposure	Outcomes	Confounders	Results
Hajat et al. 2002	Greater London, UK, resident all-age deaths, January 1976 to December 1996	Daily mean temperatures	Daily mortality from: all causes (except accidents and violence), respiratory disease, CVD	Day of week, public holiday, relative humidity, SO_2, ozone, black smoke	Heat-related mortality began to rise at 19°C *% increase in mortality per 1°C average rise above 97th centile (21.5°C, excluding 1976 heatwave):* All causes: 3.34 (95% CI: 2.47–4.23) All causes (adjusted for air pollution): 3.18 (95% CI: 2.14–4.24) Respiratory: 5.46 (95% CI: 3.43–7.52) Cardiovascular: 3.01 (95% CI: 1.73–4.32)
Studies of cold and heat effects					
Kunst et al. 1993	Netherlands, 1979–87	Daily mean temperatures; effects also estimated by two groups: 'heat', where temperature >16.5°C and 'cold', where temperature was <16.5°C	Daily mortality from: all causes, neoplasms, CVDs, respiratory diseases, all other causes, external causes	Influenza incidence, lag periods, wind speed, relative humidity, season, SO_2	V-shaped temperature–mortality relation, with point of lowest mortality 16.5°C **Cold effects:** *(1) % increase in mortality per 1°C decrease in average temperature below 16.5°C over the preceding month:* All causes (unadjusted): 1.17 All causes (adjusted for influenza): 0.77 All causes (adjusted for SO_2): 1.34 *(2) Absolute no. of cold-related deaths per day per 1°C decrease in average temperature below 16.5°C over the preceding month (adjusted for influenza, season, SO_2):* All causes: 2.95 Cardiovascular diseases: 1.68 Respiratory diseases: 0.43

Table 30.2 (continued)

Author	Study population	Exposure	Outcome	Factors controlled for	Main findings
					Heat effects:
					(1) % increase in mortality per 1°C increase in average temperature above 16.5°C over the preceding month:
					All causes (unadjusted): 1.42
					All causes (adjusted for influenza): 1.10
					All causes (adjusted for SO$_2$): 1.75
					(2) Absolute no. of heat-related deaths per day per 1°C increase in average temperature above 16.5°C over the preceding month (adjusted for influenza, season, SO$_2$):
					All causes: 6.01
					Cardiovascular diseases: 1.54
					Respiratory diseases: 1.70
Pan et al. 1995	Taiwan, 1981–91, 25+ years of age	Daily mean temperatures	Daily mortality (residents only) from: CAD, CH, CIN	Year, area (surrounding each of the 14 weather monitoring stations)	U-shaped temperature–CIN and –CAD mortality relation, with MMR for CAD of 26–29°C and for CIN of 27–29°C.
					Cold effects:
					% increase in risk of mortality in >64 years per 1°C reduction from MMR:
					CAD: 2.8
					CIN: 3.0
					Heat effects:
					% increase in risk of mortality in >64 years at 32°C compared to MMR:
					CAD: 22 (95% CI: –2–51)
					CIN: 66 (95% CI: 33–108)
					Mortality from CH decreased with increasing temperature (range 9–32°C) at a rate of 3.3% per 1°C.

Reference	Location, years	Exposure measures	Outcome	Covariates	Results
Saez et al. 1995	Barcelona, Spain, 1985–89	Minimum and maximum temperatures, dew point temperature, relative humidity; effects estimated for unusual periods of weather increase (3 or more consecutive days where temperature exceeded 85th percentile)	Daily mortality from: all causes, CVD, respiratory disease	24 h average SO₂, black smoke, 1 h maximum SO₂, influenza epidemics	V-shaped temperature–mortality relation *% average increase in daily mortality following an unusual period of increased weather temperature:* All causes: 2 All causes >65 years of age: 2.6 Cardiovascular: 4.6 Respiratory: 21.6 Only unusual periods with an excess temperature and humidity were associated with mortality increases
Ballester et al. 1997	Valencia, Spain, 1991–93	Mean daily temperature and daily relative humidity; analysis stratified by cold (November–April) and hot (May–October) months.	Daily mortality (residents only) from: all causes, all causes (excluding external causes), CVD, respiratory disease, malignant tumours	Weekly influenza cases, day of week, holidays, heat, cold, lag periods, daily SO₂, and suspended particulates (black smoke).	V-shaped temperature–mortality relation with minimum mortality range of 22–25°C; lowest point of mortality 15°C and 24°C in colder and hotter months, respectively. **Cold effects** (in cold months with a 7–14 day lag): *Estimated relative risk of mortality per 1°C decrease in mean temperature below 15°C:* All causes: 1.032 (95% CI: 1.018–1.046) All causes (>70 years): 1.037 (95% CI: 1.021–1.054) CVD: 1.043 (95% CI: 1.021–1.064) Respiratory disease: 1.017 (95% CI: 0.976–1.060) **Heat effects** (in hot months with a 1–2 day lag): *Estimated relative risk of mortality per 1°C*

Table 30.2 (continued)

Author	Study population	Exposure	Outcome	Factors controlled for	Main findings
					increase in mean temperature above 24°C: All causes: 1.036 (95% CI: 1.012–1.060) All causes (>70 years): 1.050 (95% CI: (1.021–1.080) CVD: 1.023 (95% CI: 0.985–1.064) Respiratory disease: 1.057 (95% CI: 0.975–1.145)
Keatinge et al. 2000	65–74-year-olds in seven European regions: North and South Finland, Baden-Wurttemberg, Netherlands, London, North Italy, 1988–92 and Athens, 1992	Daily mean temperatures	Daily, all-cause mortality		**Cold effects** *Increase in daily mortality per million population per 1°C drop below minimum mortality band for coldest (14.3–17.3°C), medium (19.3–22.3°C) and hottest (22.7–25.7°C) regions:* North Finland: 0.58 (95% CI: 0.48–0.68) London: 1.25 (95% CI: 1.17–1.32) Athens: 1.60 (95% CI: 1.36–1.83) **Heat effects:** *Increase in daily mortality per million population per 1°C rise above minimum mortality band:* North Finland: 6.2 (95% CI: 4.0–8.4) London: 3.6 (95% CI: 1.5–5.8) Athens: 2.7 (95% CI: 0.9–4.6)
Saez et al. 2000	Barcelona, Spain, 1986–91, 45+ years of age	Daily mean temperatures, daily mean relative humidity	Daily mortality from: IHD	Influenza epidemics, annual seasonality, daily mean concentrations of black smoke SO_2, NO_2, and	V-shaped temperature–IHD mortality relation, with a downward gradient between 1.7–4.7°C and an upward gradient for temperatures above 21.06°C *Cold effects:* *(1) Relative risk of IHD mortality for each 1°C drop below 4.7°C:* 1.024 (95% CI: 1.001–1.048)

Reference	Population	Exposure	Outcomes	Covariates	Results
		daily 1 h maximum values of ozone			(2) *Relative risk of IHD mortality for each simultaneous (1°C and 1%) drop in temperature below 6.5°C and humidity below 70%:* 1.044 (95% CI: 1.001–1.089) **Heat effects:** (1) *Relative risks of IHD mortality for each 1°C rise above 21.06°C, by temperature bands:* 21.06–23.95°C: 1.013 (95% CI: 1.001–1.025) 23.96–24.95°C: 1.036 (95% CI: 0.991–1.083) ≥24.96°C: 1.041 (95% CI: 1.037–1.045) (2) *Relative risk of IHD mortality for each simultaneous (1°C and 1%) rise in temperature above 23°C and humidity above 85%:* 1.096 (95% CI: 1.005–1.194)
Huynen *et al.* 2001	Netherlands, 1979–97, 0–64 and 65+years of age	Daily mean temperatures, cold spells (at least 9 days of at least −5°C, including at least 6 days of −10°C) and heatwaves (at least 5 days of atleast 25°C, including at least 3 days of atleast 30°C)	Daily deaths from: all causes, malignant neoplasms, CVD, respiratory disease	Longer term trends, season, heat, cold, lag periods	V-shaped temperature–mortality relation with point of lowest mortality from all causes, respiratory, and CVDs among >65 years of age, 16.5°C **Cold effects:** (1) % increase in mortality per 1°C average drop below 16.5°C in the preceding month: All causes: 1.37 Malignant neoplasms: 0.22 CVD: 1.69 Respiratory disease: 5.15 (2) Average excess mortality during cold spells: All causes: 12.8% or 46.6 deaths/day **Heat effects:** (1) % increase in mortality per 1°C average rise above 16.5°C in the preceding month: All causes: 2.72 Malignant neoplasms: 0.47 CVD: 1.86 Respiratory disease: 12.82 (2) Average excess mortality during heatwaves: All causes: 12.1% or 39.8 deaths/day

Table 30.2 (continued)

Author	Study population	Exposure	Outcome	Factors controlled for	Main findings
Kassomenos et al. 2001	Athens, Greece, 1987–91	Meteorological data, including daily mean temperatures (same day and 2 day and 1–3 day lags), wind speed, relative humidity and cloudiness; analysis conducted using 8 categories of synoptic patterns and 11 categories of mesoscale weather types	Daily mortality, 1987–91, from: all causes	Long-term trends, season, day of the week, black smoke	Both synoptic and mesoscale classifications found to significantly explain daily variation in Mortality **Synoptic classification** (only categories with highest and lowest mortality shown): *% increase in daily deaths observed during days in cold period characterised by:* Southwesterly flow (humid and warm air): 10.4 (95% CI: 4.6–16.5) Northwesterly flow (cooler winds during summer, cold winters, low relative humidity): 1.5 (95% CI:-4.1–7.4) *% increase in daily deaths observed during days in cold period characterized by:* Southwesterly flow (humid and warm air): 9.6 (95% CI: 2.7–16.9) Northwesterly flow (cooler winds during summer, cold winters, low relative humidity): −0.7 (95% CI: −6.1–5.0) **Mesoscale classification** (only categories with highest mortality shown): *% increase in daily deaths observed during days in cold period characterized by:* Easterly flow (very low temperatures, weak winds, snow): 11.1 (95% CI: 2.6–20.3) *% increase in daily deaths observed during days in warm period characterized by:* Strong southerly flow (increased temperature, moist air masses): 9.4 (95% CI: 2.8–16.4)

Reference	Study	Methods	Outcome	Confounders	Results
Braga et al. 2002	12 US cities, 1986–93	Daily mean temperatures and humidity in distributed lag models; cities divided into two groups: hot and cold; effects estimated for cold days (24 h mean of –10°C) and hot days (24 h mean of 30°C)	Daily mortality from: pneumonia, COPD, CVD,MI	Season, long-term trend, day of the week, barometric pressure, demographic factors (e.g. college degree, % non-white)	No clear pattern for the effect of humidity *Cold cities* (low and high temperatures associated with increased CVD deaths): *% increase in daily deaths following 'cold days'* CVD: 5 (at lag zero) MI: 3 (at lag zero) *% increase in daily deaths following 'hot days'* CVD: 1 (at lag zero) MI: 6 (at lag zero) *Hot cities* (neither hot nor cold temperatures had much effect on CVD or pneumonia deaths): *% increase in daily deaths following 'hot days'* MI: 4 (4–6-day lags) COPD: 6 (3–4-day lags)
Curriero et al. 2002, 2003	11 cities of the Eastern US, 1973–94	Daily mean temperatures and daily mean dew point	Daily all-age mortality in study areas (residents only) from: all causes, CVD, respiratory disease, all other diseases	Season, latitude, census variables (e.g. poverty)	J-shaped temperature–mortality relation; inverse relation with latitude: minimum mortality temperature was 20.95°C in Boston (highest latitude), 21.42°C Washington (middle latitude), and 27.18°C in Miami (lowest latitude) *Cold effects* *% increase in relative risk of mortality per 10°F drop below the minimum mortality temperature:* Boston, Massachusetts: 3.20 Washington, DC: 1.93 Miami, Florida: 5.75 *Heat effects:* *% increase in relative risk of mortality per 10°F rise above the minimum mortality temperature:* Boston, Massachusetts:14.54 Washington, DC: 6.85 Miami, Florida: 11.54

Table 30.2 (continued)

Author	Study population	Exposure	Outcome	Factors controlled for	Main findings
Pattenden et al. 2003	44 701 all-age deaths, Sofia, 1996–99, and 256 464 all-age deaths, London, 1993–96	2 day and 2 week mean temperatures	Daily, all-cause mortality	Day of week, public holiday, particulate matter, relative humidity, heat, cold, season, and long-term trends	**Cold effects:** *(1) % increase in mortality per 1°C average drop below 10th centile over 2 weeks (5.25°C in London, −0.46°C in Sofia):* London: 4.24 (95% CI: 3.41–5.07) Sofia: 1.83 (95% CI: 0.59–3.90) *(2) % increase in mortality per 1°C average drop below V-shaped cut-off of 18°C:* London: 1.43 (95% CI: 1.28–1.58) Sofia: 0.70 (95% CI: 0.51–0.88) **Heat effects:** *(1) % increase in mortality per 1°C average rise above 90th centile over 2 days (21°C in London, 21.55°C in Sofia):* London: 1.86 (95% CI: 1.36–2.36) Sofia: 3.49 (95% CI: 2.23–4.76) *(2) % increase in mortality per 1°C average rise above V-shaped threshold of 18°C:* London: 1.30 (95% CI: 0.99–1.62) Sofia: 2.21 (95% CI: 1.55–2.87)

Goodman et al. 2004	Dublin, Eire, 1980–96, all ages	Daily minimum temperatures (using distributed lag functions to analyse simultaneous cumulative effects of temperature and air pollution)	Daily deaths (residents only) from: all causes (excluding trauma), CVD, respiratory disease, all other causes	Daily mean Black smoke, mean relative humidity on same and previous day, day of week, respiratory disease epidemics	**Cold effects:** *Cumulative 40-day % increase in mortality per 1°C decrease in mean temperature:* All causes: 2.6 (95% CI: 2.3–2.9) All causes (0–64 years): 1.4 (95% CI: 0.7–2.2) All causes (65–74 years): 2.8 (95% CI: 2.2–3.5) All causes (75+ years): 3.0 (95% CI: 2.6–3.5) CVD: 2.5 (95% CI: 2.0–3.0) Respiratory disease: 6.7 (95% CI: 5.8–7.6) **Heat effects:** *% increase in mortality per 1°C increase in same-day mean temperature:* All causes: 0.4 (95% CI: 0.1–0.6) All causes (0–64 years): −0.1 (95% CI: −0.7–0.5) All causes (65–74 years): 0.7 (95% CI: 0.2–1.3) All causes (75+ years): 0.3 (95% CI: −0.1–0.7) CVD: 0.0 (95% CI: −0.4–0.4) Respiratory disease: 0.8 (95% CI: 0.1–1.5)

CAD: coronary artery disease; CH: coronary haemorrhage; CI: confidence interval; CIN: cerebral infarction; COPD: chronic obstructive pulmonary diseases; IHD: ischaemic heart disease; MI: myocardial infarction; MMR: minimum mortality range; TSP: total suspended particulates.

Increases in mortality in Barcelona, Spain, were noted after at least 3 consecutive days of elevated temperature (Saez *et al.* 1995). Moreover, the greater the number of consecutive days of elevated mean temperatures, the higher the excess mortality (Bull and Morton 1978; Hemon and Jougla 2003). For example, in the Paris heatwave of 2003, excess mortality after 2–5 consecutive days of maximum temperatures above 35°C was approximately 52%, whereas after 6 consecutive days it was over 83% (Hemon and Jougla 2003). Isolated cold or hot days seem insufficient to cause an increase in mortality, though it is possible that studies of very short periods of high or low temperatures may lack the statistical power to show an effect.

There is limited evidence to suggest that lag intervals may differ by cause-specific mortality. In the Netherlands, cardiovascular causes of death were found to peak in January (when maximum temperature reaches its trough), whereas respiratory causes peak in March. This suggests possible different lag effects for cold weather, being almost instantaneous for the cardiovascular system, but delayed for respiratory illness (Goodman *et al.* 2004; Mackenbach *et al.* 1992). Donaldson and Keatinge (1997*b*) found that deaths from CHD and stroke peak ~3 and 4 days, respectively, after lowest cold temperatures, whereas respiratory deaths rise more slowly and only peak after ~12 days. Similarly, studies across Europe and Russia have lagged mortality on temperature by 2 days for CHD, 5 days for cerebrovascular disease, and 12 days for respiratory disease (Donaldson *et al.* 1998*a, b*; Keatinge *et al.* 2000; The Eurowinter Group 1997). Moreover, a recent study on the relationship between cold temperatures and general practice consultations amongst the elderly in London found that there was a delayed effect of a drop in temperature on consultations for respiratory disease; the strongest association was found with temperatures up to 15 days previously (Hajat and Haines 2002).

In contrast to cold effects that may persist for days, heat effects have consistently been observed to occur rapidly, ranging from the same day up to 1 or 2 days later (Braga *et al.* 2001, 2002; Diaz *et al.* 2002*a*; Goodman *et al.* 2004; Hajat *et al.* 2002; Huynen *et al.* 2001; Keatinge *et al.* 2000; Kunst *et al.* 1993; Oechsli and Buechley 1970; Pattenden *et al.* 2003). However, heat effects appear primarily to reflect mortality displacement (Braga *et al.* 2001), as a period of lower-than-average deaths is observed after the initial excess (Braga *et al.* 2001, 2002; Goodman *et al.* 2004; Huynen *et al.* 2001; Kunst *et al.* 1993; Pattenden *et al.* 2003; Sartor *et al.* 1995). For example, Braga *et al.* (2002) observed a 12% increase in MI deaths and a 3% increase in CVD deaths after 2 days from hot temperatures in cold US cities, which decreased to 4% and −0.6%, respectively, when looking at cumulative effects up to 7 days. In contrast, the effect of cold temperatures persisted for several days, with no evidence of a subsequent period of lower mortality.

30.3.2 Potential confounders of the temperature–mortality relationship

Cold and heat stress may not just be related to absolute temperature, but also to air movement and damp. Therefore, other time-varying meteorological phenomena, such as humidity and wind, have been considered as possible confounders/effect modifiers of the temperature–mortality relationship. These meteorological factors are usually included individually within models assessing the temperature–mortality relation, though the resultant interrelationships are inconsistent and inconclusive, possibly due to limited power to detect any interactions. There is limited evidence for an inverse relationship between relative humidity and mortality (Goodman *et al.* 2004; Saez *et al.* 2000), although this is not statistically significant in all studies (Ballester *et al.* 1997), and while some authors have shown a significant interaction between temperature and relative humidity (Diaz *et al.* 2002*a*; Kunst *et al.* 1993; Saez *et al.* 1995, 2000), others have not (Braga *et al.* 2002; Keatinge *et al.* 2000). A significant interaction between wind speed and cold temperatures has also been reported (Kunst *et al.* 1993), but not with hot temperatures (Keatinge *et al.* 2000; Kunst *et al.* 1993).

It has been argued that treating temperature and humidity as independent variables in multiple regression analyses ignores the natural correlation between them and the possibility of a combined effect (Kassomenos *et al.* 2001). More holistic approaches that group meteorological factors in order to create synoptic climatological classifications have, therefore, been proposed (Kalkstein 1991; Kalkstein *et al.* 1987; Kassomenos *et al.* 2001). Kassomenos *et al.* (2001) were the first to apply synoptic (large-scale systems that cover an area of at least 1 000 000 km^2) and mesoscale (medium-range systems that cover an area of, at most, 10 000 km^2) weather system classifications (based on atmospheric circulation schemes) to assess the effects of weather on daily mortality in Athens. Previously, Pope and Kalkstein (1996) and Samet *et al.* (1998) had applied the synoptic meteorological approach to time-series analysis of the association between air pollution and daily mortality in Utah Valley and Philadelphia, respectively. Pope and Kalkstein (1996) concluded that the synoptic climatological approach performed slightly better than traditional approaches to controlling for weather, whereas Samet *et al.* (1998) found this approach to be inferior to the traditional inclusion of either parametric or smoothed terms to control for weather. The most informative method for modelling weather remains unclear.

In recent years, much attention has been given to the short-term, or acute, effects of air pollution on both mortality and morbidity, particularly from cardiovascular and respiratory diseases (see Chapter 29). Concentrations of air pollutants may be driven by weather, with episodes of pollution associated with atypical patterns of prolonged cold weather (Keatinge and Donaldson 2001a). A notable example is the London smog episode of 1952, when a particularly cold spell and temperature inversion were accompanied by high concentrations of sulfur dioxide and black smoke that reached maximum daily levels of ~3800 and ~4500 $\mu g/m^3$, respectively, and a considerable excess of mortality was registered (Holland *et al.* 1979; Logan 1953). With the exception of ozone, winter levels of air pollutants are higher than summer ones (Saez *et al.* 2000). The question has arisen, therefore, as to whether observed air pollution–mortality associations could reflect inadequately controlled effects of weather on mortality (i.e., residual confounding), with both proponents of (Gamble and Lewis 1996) and detractors (Pope 1999) from this view. Most studies of air pollution have adjusted for weather in some form or another, whilst only a few studies of the temperature–mortality relation have adjusted for concentrations of air pollutants (Table 30.2).

A number of studies have assessed the interrelationships between temperature, air pollutants, and mortality (Biersteker and Evendijk 1976; Driscoll 1971; Goodman *et al.* 2004; Katsouyanni *et al.* 1993; Keatinge and Donaldson 2001a; Lippmann and Ito 1995; MacFarlane 1977; Mackenbach *et al.* 1993; Pope and Kalkstein 1996; Samet *et al.* 1998; Sartor *et al.* 1995; Shumway *et al.* 1988; Thurston and Ito 2001; Touloumi *et al.* 1996). Several have shown some evidence for air pollutants as confounders and/or effect modifiers of the temperature–mortality association (Kassomenos *et al.* 2001; Katsouyanni *et al.* 1993; MacFarlane 1977; Mackenbach *et al.* 1993; Pattenden *et al.* 2003; Sartor *et al.* 1995; Shumway *et al.* 1988; Touloumi *et al.* 1996), whilst others have not (Biersteker and Evendijk 1976; Driscoll 1971; Kalkstein 1991; Samet *et al.* 1998). Although there is general agreement that the adverse effects of air pollution on mortality are smaller than those from cold temperatures (Keatinge 2002), further studies examining the complex interrelations of temperature, air pollutants, and mortality are clearly warranted.

30.4 **Discussion**

Epidemiological investigation provides persuasive evidence for a relationship between ambient temperature and mortality, particularly from cardiovascular and respiratory causes. The association is consistent across different study designs and methodologies, countries worldwide, and varying time periods, despite the use of routine data and their inherent inaccuracies. Whilst both hot and cold temperatures are associated with increased deaths, the effects of hot temperatures appear to reflect mainly short-term mortality displacement, whilst cold temperatures appear to have prolonged effects on mortality. Elderly people, those with impaired health, or people from low social classes appear to be the most susceptible to the adverse impacts of weather. From the limited evidence to date, it remains unclear whether there is an excess in winter in the *incidence* of CVD. Further research is needed to clarify these possible effects on morbidity, the association with social class, and the role of other meteorological variables, to establish the size and importance of temperature effects on health.

The mechanisms by which exposure to hot or cold temperatures might increase the risk of death do not seem to be much clearer today than 20 years ago (Mercer and Sparr 2000). This is perhaps not surprising, given the multifactorial nature of CVD aetiology. Most of the cold-related cardiovascular deaths take place 2–3 days after exposure to cold. Several biologically plausible mechanisms for these deaths have been proposed, including the effects of changing temperature on haemostasis, blood viscosity, and vasoconstriction (Gordon *et al.* 1988; Neild *et al.* 1994; Woodhouse *et al.* 1994). Winter increases in plasma fibrinogen, plasma cholesterol, red and white blood cell counts, and blood pressure have been observed, all of which are indicators of CVD risk (Stout and Crawford 1991; Woodhouse *et al.* 1994). A strong inverse relation between blood pressure and temperature has been shown (Woodhouse *et al.* 1993), and changes in blood composition in people after exposure to mild cold include increased concentrations of red cells, plasma fibrinogen, plasma cholesterol, platelets, and blood viscosity (Kawahara *et al.* 1989; Keatinge 2002; Keatinge *et al.* 1984; Mercer *et al.* 1999; Qizibash *et al.* 1991; Stout and Crawford 1991). These changes appear to be initiated by cold-induced cutaneous vasoconstriction (Keatinge and Donaldson 1995). The protective protein C, a natural anticoagulant, however, does not increase in concentration (Neild *et al.* 1994). Short-term exposure to cold appears, therefore, to initiate a mild inflammatory reaction and an increased state of hypercoagulability. Moreover, these cold-induced haematological changes are more likely to lead to an increase in thrombosis in the elderly, often with atheromatous arteries, than the young (Keatinge 2002; Keatinge and Donaldson 1995). The question remains as to how much of the increased susceptibility among the elderly is due to age-related physiological changes in cold thermoregulation, and how much is due to other factors related to ageing (Smolander 2002). Whilst the elderly are less able to maintain core temperature, and have reduced thermal sensory perception and diminished vasoconstrictive response to cold (Smolander 2002), greater stress is imposed on their thermoregulatory system by, for example, immobility due to joint disorders, and decreased heart and lung capacity for exercise (Collins 1987).

Some cold-related deaths are directly respiratory deaths, others are cardiovascular deaths but occur in association with respiratory disease, and are delayed many days after the cold weather. Keatinge (2002) suggests that at least two factors help to explain why respiratory illnesses increase in winter: first, increased opportunities for cross-infection as a result of the tendency for people to congregate together in poorly ventilated spaces, and second, the reduced ability of the mucosa of the upper respiratory tract to protect against infection upon cooling. Respiratory infections are associated with increased plasma fibrinogen levels, which again lead to increased risk of CVD (Woodhouse et al. 1994).

Proposed mechanisms by which heat influences the pathogenesis of CVD focus on the loss of salt and water from sweating due to heat stress. The haemoconcentration that follows in turn causes increases in coronary and cerebral thrombosis (Keatinge et al. 1986). Those with pre-existing heart failure, and the elderly, with diminished thermoregulation (Kenney and Hodgson 1987) and elevated sweating thresholds (Foster et al. 1976), are unable to meet the need for increased cutaneous blood flow in the heat (Keatinge 2003b).

Seasonal variations in mortality, and cold- and hot-temperature related mortality, represent significant global public health challenges. Temperature-related deaths represent a larger problem than life lost in traffic accidents, yet much of this increase in mortality could be prevented by a combination of indoor and outdoor protective measures (Donaldson et al. 1998a, b; The Eurowinter Group 1997). The Eurowinter study (The Eurowinter Group 1997), with surveys of house temperatures and outdoor clothing, showed that cold-related mortality is more pronounced in European countries with milder winter climates relative to those with colder climates. They suggested that this finding could be explained by factors such as differences in home heating as well as individual thermoregulatory behaviour. Initially, this suggestion was met with some scepticism (MacKenzie 1997; Mather et al. 1997; Sperber and Weitzman 1997), but a growing body of evidence from different countries supports the notion that those living in colder climates do not experience the increases in cold-related mortality seen in regions with milder climates (Donaldson et al. 1998a, b; Eng and Mercer 1998). In addition, heat-related mortality is no higher in areas with hot climates than those with cold climates (Braga et al. 2001, 2002; Curriero et al. 2002; Keatinge et al. 2000). It does seem that populations acclimatize to their environments, and that individual and communal protective measures, as well as perceptions of risk and vulnerability, are important factors in understanding and tackling the effects of temperature on mortality.

Much debate remains as to where prevention efforts should best be concentrated. Some authors emphasize the relative importance of social measures, for example, housing standards and indoor temperature-stress (Clinch and Healey 2000; Mercer 2003) while others focus on outdoor exposures and clothing, that is, behavioural measures (Keatinge 1986; Keatinge and Donaldson 2001b). A campaign advising elderly people in Britain in the winter of 1986–87 to avoid outdoor exposures to cold was considered responsible for ~30 000 fewer winter deaths than expected that year (Keatinge and Donaldson 1995). In England and Wales, excess winter mortality from respiratory disease, but not CVD, was shown to decrease between 1964 and 1984 when the percentage of homes with central heating increased from 16 to 66% (Keatinge et al. 1989). According to Keatinge and Donaldson (1995) this suggests that cold indoor temperatures may play an important role in cold-related mortality from respiratory illnesses, whereas outdoor cold exposures may make a greater impact upon excess winter mortality from CVD. Aylin et al. (2001), however, in a small-area (ecological) study at electoral ward level, found that lack of central heating in Great Britain, 1986–96, was significantly associated with a higher risk of dying in winter from all causes, CHD, and stroke (odds ratio (OR) = 1.016, 95% CI: 1.009–1.022; OR = 1.017, 95% CI: 1.005–1.029; OR = 1.029, 95% CI: 1.011–1.048, respectively), but not with respiratory diseases (OR = 1.014, 95% CI: 0.998–1.031). Clearly, indoor and outdoor cold temperatures are related (Khaw 1995) and policies targeting the potential adverse impacts from both, at the individual and communal level, will provide the most effective prevention strategies.

An inverse association between mortality risk at 30°C and prevalence of air conditioning has been found in a study of 12 US cities (Braga *et al.* 2001); declines in heat-related mortality in the USA over the last few decades have been explained by increases in use of household air conditioning systems over the same time period (Davis *et al.* 2003; Keatinge 2003*b*). Recently, an initiative to develop heat- and health- watch warning systems in many large cities world-wide, for example Rome, Toronto, Shanghai, and various cities in the USA, has been under-taken (Kalkstein 2000). These warning systems are unique because they acknowledge the fact that the heat-related health burden will be city-specific, depending on the climate, social structure, and urban landscape. These holistic systems include media broadcasts suggesting simple protective measures such as staying in air-conditioned places and drinking plenty of fluids, as well as an emergency telephone 'heatline' service and a 'buddy system', whereby each street has a designated trained person to check on elderly and infirm people (Kalkstein 2000). Further studies are required to evaluate the effectiveness of these systems in reducing heat-related mortality.

The extent of the public health burden from temperature-related mortality in the future is complicated by predictions of global climate change. The Intergovernmental Panel on Climate Change (IPCC) predicts that average global surface temperatures will increase by 1.4–5.8°C by 2100 (Houghton *et al.* 2001). Changes in climate and rainfall patterns may have significant and wide-ranging impacts on human health, including those associated with extreme weather disasters; for example, an increased risk of communicable disease after floods, changes in the distribution and seasonality of vector-borne diseases, and changes in thermal stress (Greenough *et al.* 2001; Kovats *et al.* 1999; McMichael 1993). Predictions of global warming have left scientific opinion divided regarding the potential impact on temperature-related mortality. Some authors suggest that higher temperatures will result in fewer winter deaths each year (9000 fewer by one estimate, with the largest contribution being from CHD) (Langford and Bentham 1995; Martens 1998), whilst others predict large increases in mortality due to elevated ambient temperatures (Basu and Samet 2002; Kalkstein and Greene 1997). In addition, there have been suggestions that people may be able to acclimatize and adapt to warmer weather (Braga *et al.* 2001, 2002; Davis *et al.* 2003; Keatinge 2003*b*; Keatinge *et al.* 2000; McGeehin and Mirabelli 2001) with little sustained increase in heat-related mortality (Keatinge *et al.* 2000). Climate change may also affect levels of air pollutants, which, in turn, may impact upon the interrelations between weather, air pollutants, and mortality (Bernard *et al.* 2001).

A question remains, therefore, as to the net effect of global climate change on temperature-related mortality; that is, will the possible increases in heat-related mortality be offset by the potential decreases in cold-related mortality? An evaluation of possible impacts of global climate change on climate-mortality relationships in 44 large US cities estimated a sizeable net increase in weather-related mortality based on model predictions of a warmer climate (Kalkstein and Greene 1997). In contrast, in a study of 20 cities worldwide, Martens (1998) concluded that, as a result of decreasing winter mortality, most of the cities will experience a decline in overall temperature-related mortality due to global climate change. Global warming may, therefore, bring net health benefits to many regions (Keatinge 2002). Recent studies have shown the importance of taking into account regional weather differences in the assessment of climate change impact (Braga *et al.* 2001, 2002). However, there remains considerable uncer-tainty in forecasting specific regional and local changes in climate due to global warming (Houghton *et al.* 1996, 2001) and, consequently, any potential impacts on human health at the regional level. Whilst hot and cold weather patterns cannot be prevented, nor predicted with certainty, temperature-related morbidity and mortality can be reduced. Continued efforts are needed, therefore, to refine our understanding of the impacts of temperature on health and to further the formation of protective and preventive policies at the individual and societal levels, in order to minimize the adverse effects of temperature on human health on a global scale.

References

Alberdi JC, Diaz J, Montero JC, Miron IJ (1998). Daily mortality in Madrid community (Spain) 1986–1991: relationship with atmospheric variables. *European Journal of Epidemiology*, **14**, 571–8.

Alderson MR (1985). Season and mortality. *Health Trends*, **17**, 87–95.

Allexenberg RS (1981). Combating the heat wave of 1980: lessons for the future. *Urban Health*, **10**(7), 26–30.

Anders C, Jachimczyk JA, Green R *et al.* (1995). Heat-related illnesses and deaths: United States, 1994–1995. *Morbidity and Mortality Weekly Report*, **44**, 465–6.

Anon (1970). Winter and heart-disease. *Lancet*, **i**, 282–3.

Anon (1995). Heat-related mortality: Chicago, July 1995. *Morbidity and Mortality Weekly Report*, **44**, 577–9.

Applegate WB, Runyan JW Jr, Brasfield L, Williams ML, Konigsberg C, Fouche C (1981). Analysis of the 1980 heat wave in Memphis. *Journal of the American Geriatrics Society*, **XXIX**(8), 337–42.

Aylin P, Morris S, Wakefield J, Grossinho A, Jarup L, Elliott P (2001). Temperature, housing, deprivation and their relationship to excess winter mortality in Great Britain, 1986–1996. *International Journal of Epidemiology*, **30**, 1100–8.

Ballester F, Corella D, Perez-Hoyos S, Saez M, Hervas A (1997). Mortality as a function of temperature: a study in Valencia, Spain, 1991–1993. *International Journal of Epidemiology*, **26**, 551–61.

Ballester F, Michelozzi P, Iniguez C (2003). Weather, climate, and public health. *Journal of Epidemiology and Community Health*, **57**, 759–60.

Basu R and Samet JM (2002). Relation between elevated ambient temperature and mortality: a review of the epidemiologic evidence. *Epidemiologic Reviews*, **24**, 190–202.

Becker S and Weng S (1998). Seasonal patterns of deaths in Matlab, Bangladesh. *International Journal of Epidemiology*, **27**, 814–23.

Bernard SM, Samet JM, Grambsch A, Ebi KL, Romieu I (2001). The potential impacts of climate variability and change on air pollution-related health effects in the United States. *Environmental Health Perspectives*, **109**(Suppl. 2), 199–209.

Biersteker K and Evendijk JE (1976). Ozone, temperature, and mortality in Rotterdam in the summers of 1974 and 1975. *Environmental Research*, **12**, 214–17.

Bosch X (2003a). European heatwave causes misery and deaths. *Lancet*, **362**, 543.

Bosch X (2003b). France sets up action plan to tackle heat-related deaths. *Lancet*, **362**, 624.

Braga ALF, Zanobetti A, Schwartz J (2001). The time course of weather-related deaths. *Epidemiology*, **12**, 662–7.

Braga ALF, Zanobetti A, Schwartz J (2002). The effect of weather on respiratory and cardiovascular deaths in 12 U.S. cities. *Environmental Health Perspectives*, **110**(9), 859–63.

Bull GM and Morton J (1975). Relationships of temperature with death rates from all causes and from certain respiratory and other diseases in different age groups. *Age and Ageing*, **4**, 232–46.

Bull GM and Morton J (1978). Environment, temperature and death rates. *Age and Ageing*, **7**, 210–24.

Butler D (2003). Heatwave underlines climate-model failures. *Nature*, **424**, 867.

Carolei A, Marini C, De Matteis G, Di Napoli M, Baldassarre M (1996). Seasonal incidence of stroke (correspondence). *Lancet*, **347**, 1702–3.

Cheng G (1993). Investigation on the correlation between mortality of cerebrovascular diseases and the meteorological factors in Zhanjiang City. *Chinese Journal of Epidemiology* [*Chung-Hua Liu Hsing Ping Hsueh Tsa Chih*], **14**, 234–6.

Christophersen O (1997). Mortality during the 1996/7 winter. *Population Trends*, **90**, 11–17.

Clinch JP and Healy JD (2000). Housing standards and excess winter mortality. *Journal of Epidemiology and Community Health*, **54**, 719–20.

Collins KJ (1987). Effects of cold on old people. *British Journal of Hospital Medicine*, **December**, 506–14.

Cordioli E, Pizzi C, Martinelli M (2000). Winter mortality in Emilia-Romagna, Italy. *International Journal of Circumpolar Health*, **59**, 164–9.

Curriero FC, Heiner KS, Samet JM, Zeger SL, Strug L, Patz JA (2002). Temperature and mortality in 11 cities of the eastern United States. *American Journal of Epidemiology*, **155**, 80–7.

Curriero FC, Samet JM, Zeger SL (2003). On the use of generalized additive models in time-series studies of air pollution and health and temperature and mortality in 11 cities of the eastern United States [correspondence]. *American Journal of Epidemiology*, **158**, 93–4.

Curwen M (1990/91). Excess winter mortality: a British phenomenon? *Health Trends*, **22**(4), 169–75.

Curwen M and Devis T (1988). Winter mortality, temperature and influenza: has the relationship changed in recent years? *Population Trends*, **54**, 17–20.

Danet S, Richard F, Montaye M *et al.* (1999). Unhealthy effects of atmospheric temperature and pressure on the occurrence of myocardial infarction and coronary deaths. A 10-year survey: the Lille-World Health Organization MONICA project (monitoring trends and determinants in cardiovascular disease). *Circulation*, **100**, e1–e7.

Dardanoni G, Intonazzo V, La Rosa G, Lanzarone F (1988). Excess deaths related to hot weather in Palermo. *Bollettino Dell Istituto Sieroterapico Milanese*, **67**(3), 251–4.

Davis RE, Knappenberger PC, Michaels PJ, Novicoff WM (2003). Changing heat-related mortality in the United States. *Environmental Health Perspectives*, **111**(14), 1712–18.

Diaz J, Garcia R, Velazquez de Castro F *et al.* (2002*a*). Effects of extremely hot days on people older than 65 years in Seville (Spain) from 1986–1997. *International Journal of Biometeorology*, **46**, 145–9.

Diaz J, Jordan A, Garcia R *et al.* (2002*b*). Heat waves in Madrid 1986–1997: effects on the health of the elderly. *International Archives of Occupational and Environmental Health*, **75**, 163–70.

Donaldson GC and Keatinge WR (1997*a*). Mortality related to cold weather in elderly people in southeast England, 1979–94. *British Medical Journal*, **315**, 1055–6.

Donaldson GC and Keatinge WR (1997*b*). Early increases in ischaemic heart disease mortality dissociated from and later changes associated with respiratory mortality after cold weather in south east England. *Journal of Epidemiology and Community Health*, **51**, 643–8.

Donaldson GC and Keatinge WR (2002). Excess winter mortality: influenza or cold stress? Observational study. *British Medical Journal*, **324**, 89–90.

Donaldson GC and Keatinge WR (2003). Cold related mortality in England and Wales: influence of social class in working and retired age groups. *Journal of Epidemiology and Community Health*, **57**, 790–1.

Donaldson GC, Ermakov SP, Komarov YM, McDonald CP, Keatinge WR (1998*a*). Cold related mortalities and protection against cold in Yakutsk, eastern Siberia: observation and interview study. *British Medical Journal*, **317**, 978–82.

Donaldson GC, Tchernjavskii VE, Ermakov SP, Bucher K, Keatinge WR (1998*b*). Winter mortality and cold stress in Yekaterinburg, Russia: interview study. *British Medical Journal*, **316**, 514–18.

Donaldson GC, Kovats RS, Keatinge WR, McMichael AJ (2001). Heat- and cold-related mortality and morbidity and climate change. In *Health effects of climate change in the UK* (ed. RL Maynard), pp. 70–80. Department of Health, London.

Donoghue ER, Kalelkar MB, Boehmer MA *et al.* (1995). Heat-related mortality: Chicago, July 1995. *Morbidity and Mortality Weekly Report*, **44**(31), 577–8.

Douglas AS, Russell D, Allan TM (1990). Seasonal, regional and secular variations of cardiovascular and cerebrovascular mortality in New Zealand. *Australian and New Zealand Journal of Medicine*, **20**, 669–76.

Douglas AS, Allan TM, Rawles JM (1991*a*). Composition of seasonality of disease. *Scottish Medical Journal*, **36**, 76–82.

Douglas AS, Al-Sayer H, Rawles JM, Allan TM (1991*b*). Seasonality of disease in Kuwait. *Lancet*, **337**, 1393–7.

Douglas AS, Dunnigan MG, Allan TM, Rawles JM (1995). Seasonal variation in coronary heart disease in Scotland. *Journal of Epidemiology and Community Health*, **49**, 575–82.

Driscoll DM (1971). The relationship between weather and mortality in ten major metropolitan areas in the United States, 1962–1965. *International Journal of Biometeorology*, **15**, 23–39.

Dunnigan MG, Harland WA, Fyfe T (1970). Seasonal incidence and mortality of ischaemic heart disease. *Lancet*, **i**, 793–7.

Ellis FP and Nelson F (1978). Mortality in the elderly in a heat wave in New York City, August 1975. *Environmental Research*, **15**, 504–12.

Elwood PC, Beswick A, O'Brien JR *et al.* (1993). Temperature and risk factors for ischaemic heart disease in the Caerphilly prospective study. *British Heart Journal*, **70**, 520–3.

Eng H and Mercer JB (1998). Seasonal variations in mortality caused by cardiovascular diseases in Norway and Ireland. *Journal of Cardiovascular Risk*, **5**, 89–95.

Enquselassie F, Dobson AJ, Alexander HM, Steele PL (1993). Seasons, temperature and coronary disease. *International Journal of Epidemiology*, **22**(4), 632–6.

Foster KG, Ellis FP, Dore C *et al.* (1976). Sweat responses in the aged. *Age and Ageing*, **5**, 91–101.

Gamble JF and Lewis RJ (1996). Health and respirable particulate (PM_{10}) air pollution: a causal or statistical association? *Environmental Health Perspectives*, **104**(8), 838–50.

Gemmell I, McLoone P, Boddy FA, Dickinson GJ, Watt GCM (2000). Seasonal variation in mortality in Scotland. *International Journal of Epidemiology*, **29**, 274–9.

GRO (General Register Office) (1841). *Third annual report of births, deaths and marriages in England*, pp.102–9. HMSO, London.

GRO (General Register Office) (1987). *Quarterly variation in mortality in Scotland and 12 selected countries, since 1977*. HMSO, London.

Goodman PG, Dockery DW, Clancy L (2004). Cause-specific mortality and the extended effects of particulate pollution and temperature exposure. *Environmental Health Perspectives*, **112**(2), 179–85.

Gordon DJ, Hyde J, Trost DC *et al.* (1988). Cyclic seasonal variation in plasma lipid and lipoprotein levels: the Lipid Research Clinics Coronary Primary Prevention Trial placebo group. *Journal of Clinical Epidemiology*, **41**, 679–89.

Gouveia N, Hajat S, Armstrong B (2003). Socioeconomic differentials in the temperature-mortality relationship in Sao Paulo, Brazil. *International Journal of Epidemiology*, **32**, 390–7.

Green MS, Harari G, Kristal-Boneh E (1994). Excess winter mortality from ischaemic heart disease and stroke during colder and warmer years in Israel: an evaluation and review of the role of environmental temperature. *European Journal of Public Health*, **4**, 3–11.

Greenberg JH, Bromberg J, Reed CM, Gustafson TL, Beauchamp RA (1983). The epidemiology of heat-related deaths, Texas: 1950, 1970–79, and 1980. *American Journal of Public Health*, **73**, 805–7.

Greenough G, McGeehin M, Bernard SM, Trtanj J, Riad J, Engelberg D (2001). The potential impacts of climate variability and change on health impacts of extreme weather events in the United States. *Environmental Health Perspectives*, **109**(Suppl. 2), 191–8.

Gyllerup S (2000). Cold climate and coronary mortality in Sweden. *International Journal of Circumpolar Health*, **59**, 160–3.

Gyllerup S, Lanke J, Lindholm LH, Schersten B (1991). High coronary mortality in cold regions of Sweden. *Journal of Internal Medicine*, **230**, 479–85.

Haberman S, Capildeo R, Rose FC (1981). The seasonal variation in mortality from cerebrovascular disease. *Journal of the Neurological Sciences*, **52**, 25–36.

Hajat S and Haines A (2002). Associations of cold temperatures with GP consultations for respiratory and cardiovascular disease amongst the elderly in London. *International Journal of Epidemiology*, **31**, 825–30.

Hajat S, Kovats RS, Atkinson RW, Haines A (2002). Impact of hot temperatures on death in London: a time series approach. *Journal of Epidemiology and Community Health*, **56**, 367–72.

Hare EH, Moran PAP, MacFarlane A (1981). The changing seasonality of infant deaths in England and Wales, 1912–78 and its relation to seasonal temperature. *Journal of Epidemiology and Community Health*, **35**, 77–82.

Hawkins-Bell L and Rankin JT Jr (1994). Heat-related deaths: Philadelphia and United States, 1993–1994. *Morbidity and Mortality Weekly Report*, **43**(25), 453–5.

Healy JD (2003). Excess winter mortality in Europe: a cross country analysis identifying key risk factors. *Journal of Epidemiology and Community Health*, **57**, 784–9.

Hemon D and Jougla E (2003). Surmortalite liee a la canicule d'aout 2003 – rapport d'etape: Estimation de la surmortalite et principales caracteristiques epidemiologiques. Villejuif: Inserm.

Holland WW, Bennet AE, Cameron IR *et al.* (1979). Health effects of particulate pollution: reappraising the evidence. *American Journal of Epidemiology*, **110**, 527–659.

Houghton JT, Meiro Filho LG, Callander BA, Harris N, Kattenberg A, Maskell K (eds) (1996). Contribution of Working Group I to the Second Assessment of the Intergovernmental Panel on Climate Change. *Climate change 1995: the science of climate change*. Cambridge University Press, New York.

Houghton JT, Ding Y, Griggs DJ *et al.* (2001). Contribution of Working Group I to the Third Assessment Report of the Intergovernmental Panel on Climate Change. *Climate change 2001: the scientific basis*, pp. 583–638. Cambridge University Press, New York.

Huynen MMTE, Martens P, Schram D, Weijenberg MP, Kunst AE (2001). The impact of heat waves and cold spells on mortality rates in the Dutch population. *Environmental Health Perspectives*, **109**(5), 463–70.

Isaacs N and Donn M (1993). Health and housing: seasonality in New Zealand mortality. *Australian Journal of Public Health*, **17**, 68–70.

Jakovljevic D, Salomaa V, Sivenius J *et al.* (1996). Seasonal variation in the occurrence of stroke in a Finnish adult population: the FINMONICA stroke register. *Stroke*, **27**, 1774–9.

Jones TS, Liang AP, Kilbourne EM *et al.* (1982). Morbidity and mortality associated with the July 1980 heat wave in St Louis and Kansas City, Mo. *Journal of the American Medical Association*, **247**, 3327–31.

Kagami M (1983). Regional variance of cerebrovascular mortality in Japan. *Ecology of Disease*, **2**(4), 277–83.

Kalkstein LS (1991). A new approach to evaluate the impact of climate on human mortality. *Environmental Health Perspectives*, **96**, 145–50.

Kalkstein LS (2000). Saving lives during extreme weather in summer: interventions from local health agencies and doctors can reduce mortality. *British Medical Journal*, **321**, 650–1.

Kalkstein LS and Greene JS (1997). An evaluation of climate/mortality relationships in large U.S. cities and the possible impacts of a climate change. *Environmental Health Perspectives*, **105**(1), 84–93.

Kalkstein LS, Tan G, Skindlov J (1987). An evaluation of objective clustering procedures for use in synoptic climatological classification. *Journal of Climate and Applied Meteorology*, **26**, 717–30.

Kassomenos P, Gryparis A, Samoli E, Katsouyanni K, Lykoudis S, Flocas HA (2001). Atmospheric circulation types and daily mortality in Athens, Greece. *Environmental Health Perspectives*, 109(6), 591–6.

Katsouyanni K, Pantazopoulou A, Touloumi G *et al.* (1993). Evidence for interaction between air pollution and high temperature in the causation of excess mortality. *Archives of Environmental Health*, 48(4), 235–42.

Kawahara J, Sano H, Fukuzaki H, Saito K, Hirouchi H (1989). Acute effects of exposure to cold on blood pressure, platelet function and sympathetic nervous activity in humans. *American Journal of Hypertension*, 2, 724–6.

Keatinge WR (1986). Seasonal mortality among elderly people with unrestricted home heating. *British Medical Journal*, 293, 732–3.

Keatinge WR (2002). Winter mortality and its causes. *International Journal of Circumpolar Health*, 61, 292–9.

Keatinge WR (2003a). Commentary: mortality from environmental factors, but which ones? *International Journal of Epidemiology*, 32, 398–9.

Keatinge WR (2003b). Death in heat waves: simple preventive measures may help reduce mortality. *British Medical Journal*, 327, 512–13.

Keatinge WR and Donaldson GC (1995). Cardiovascular mortality in winter. *Arctic Medical Research*, 54 (Suppl. 2), 16–18.

Keatinge WR and Donaldson GC (2001a). Mortality related to cold and air pollution in London after allowance for effects of associated weather patterns. *Environmental Research Section A*, 86, 209–16.

Keatinge WR and Donaldson GC (2001b). Winter deaths: warm housing is not enough. *British Medical Journal*, 323, 166.

Keatinge WR, Coleshaw SRK, Corter F, Mattock K, Murphy M, Chelliah R (1984). Increases in platelets and red cell counts, blood viscosity, and arterial pressure during mild surface cooling: factors in mortality from coronary and cerebral thrombosis in winter. *British Medical Journal*, 289, 1405–8.

Keatinge WR, Coleshaw SRK, Easton JC, Cotter F, Mattock MB, Chelliah R (1986). Increased platelet and red cell count, blood viscosity, and plasma cholesterol levels during heat stress, and mortality from coronary and cerebral thrombosis. *American Journal of Medicine*, 81, 795–800.

Keatinge WR, Coleshaw SRK, Holmes J (1989). Changes in seasonal mortality with improvement in home heating in England and Wales 1964–1984. *International Journal of Biometeorology*, 33, 71–6.

Keatinge WR, Donaldson GC, Cordioli E *et al.* (2000). Heat related mortality in warm and cold regions of Europe: observational study. *British Medical Journal*, 321, 670–3.

Kenney WL and Hodgson JL (1987). Heat tolerance, thermoregulation and ageing. *Sports Medicine*, 4, 446–56.

Khaw KT (1995). Temperature and cardiovascular mortality. *Lancet*, 345, 337–8.

Kloner RA, Poole WK, Perritt RL (1999). When throughout the year is coronary death most likely to occur? A 12-year population-based analysis of over 220,000 cases. *Circulation*, 100, 1630–4.

Kovats RS, Haines A, Stanwell-Smith R, Martens P, Menne B, Bertollini R (1999). Climate change and human health in Europe. *British Medical Journal*, 318, 1682–5.

Kunst AE, Looman CWN, Mackenbach JP (1991). The decline in winter excess mortality in the Netherlands. *International Journal of Epidemiology*, 20, 971–7.

Kunst AE, Looman CWN, Mackenbach JP (1993). Outdoor air temperature and mortality in the Netherlands: a time-series analysis. *American Journal of Epidemiology*, 137, 331–41.

Laake K and Sverre JM (1996). Winter excess mortality: a comparison between Norway and England plus Wales. *Age and Ageing*, 25, 343–8.

Langford IH and Bentham G (1995). The potential effects of climate change on winter mortality in England and Wales. *International Journal of Biometeorology*, 38, 141–7.

Lanska DJ and Hoffmann RG (1999). Seasonal variation in stroke mortality rates. *Neurology*, **52**(5), 984–90.

Law MR and Morris KL (1998). Why is mortality higher in poorer areas and in more northern areas of England and Wales? *Journal of Epidemiology and Community Health*, **52**, 344–52.

Lawlor DA (1999). Deprivation and excess winter mortality [correspondence]. *Journal of Epidemiology and Community Health*, **53**, 807.

Lawlor DA, Harvey D, Dews HG (2000). Investigation of the association between excess winter mortality and socio-economic deprivation. *Journal of Public Health Medicine*, **22**(2), 176–81.

Lawlor DA, Maxwell R, Wheeler BW (2002). Rurality, deprivation, and excess winter mortality: an ecological study. *Journal of Epidemiology and Community Health*, **56**, 373–4.

Lerchl A (1998). Changes in the seasonality of mortality in Germany from 1946 to 1995: the role of temperature. *International Journal of Biometeorology*, **42**, 84–8.

Lippmann M and Ito K (1995). Separating the effects of temperature and season on daily mortality from those of air pollution in London: 1965–1972. *Inhalation Toxicology*, **7**, 85–97.

Lloyd EL (1991). The role of cold in ischaemic heart disease: a review. *Public Health*, **105**, 205–15.

Logan WPD (1953). Mortality in the London fog incident. *Lancet*, **i**, 336–8.

Luterbacher J, Dietrich D, Xoplaki E, Grosjean M, Wanner H (2004). European seasonal and annual temperature variability, trends, and extremes since 1500. *Science*, **303**, 1499–503.

MacFarlane A (1977). Daily mortality and environment in English conurbations. I: air pollution, low temperature, and influenza in Greater London. *British Journal of Preventive and Social Medicine*, **31**, 54–61.

MacFarlane A (1978). Daily mortality and environment in English conurbations. II: Deaths during summer hot spells in greater London. *Environmental Research*, **15**(3), 332–41.

MacFarlane A and Waller RE (1976). Short term increases in mortality during heatwaves. *Nature*, **264**, 434–6.

Mackenbach JP, Kunst AE, Looman CWN (1992). Seasonal variation in mortality in The Netherlands. *Journal of Epidemiology and Community Health*, **46**, 261–5.

Mackenbach JP, Looman CWN, Kunst AE (1993). Air pollution, lagged effects of temperature, and mortality: The Netherlands 1979–87. *Journal of Epidemiology and Community Health*, **47**, 121–6.

MacKenzie MA (1997). Cold exposure and winter mortality in Europe [correspondence]. *Lancet*, **350**, 590–1.

Mannino JA and Washburn RA (1989). Environmental temperature and mortality from acute myocardial infarction. *International Journal of Biometeorology*, **33**, 32–5.

Marshall RJ, Scragg R, Bourke P (1988). An analysis of the seasonal variation of coronary heart disease and respiratory disease mortality in New Zealand. *International Journal of Epidemiology*, **17**, 325–31.

Martens WJM (1998). Climate change, thermal stress and mortality changes. *Social Science and Medicine*, **46**(3), 331–44.

Mather K, Cooper D, Janson P, White M (1997). Cold exposure and winter mortality in Europe [correspondence]. *Lancet*, **350**, 591.

McDowell M (1981). Long term trends in seasonal mortality. *Population Trends*, **26**, 16–19.

McGeehin MA and Mirabelli M (2001). The potential impacts of climate variability and change on temperature-related morbidity and mortality in the United States. *Environmental Health Perspectives*, **109**(Suppl. 2), 185–9.

McGregor GR (2003). A preliminary synoptic climatological analysis of the summer heat waves and mortality in England and Wales. Available: <http://www.gees.bham.ac.uk/people/mcgregorresearch/heatmortality03.htm>.

McKee CM (1989). Deaths in winter: can Britain learn from Europe? *European Journal of Epidemiology*, **5**(2), 178–82.

McKee CM (1990). Deaths in winter in Northern Ireland: the role of low temperature. *Ulster Medical Journal*, **59**, 17–22.

McKee M, Sanderson C, Chenet L, Vassin S, Shkolnikov V (1998). Seasonal variation in mortality in Moscow. *Journal of Public Health Medicine*, **20**(3), 268–74.

McMichael AJ (1993). *Planetary overload: global environmental change and the health of the human species*. Cambridge University Press.

Mercer JB (2003). Cold: an underrated risk factor for health. *Environmental Research*, **92**, 8–13.

Mercer J and Sparr S (2000). Preface. In Proceedings from a seminar 'Old and cold: understanding excess winter mortality in the elderly' (ed. J Mercer J, S Sparr, J Leppaluoto). *International Journal of Circumpolar Health*, **59**, 152–3.

Mercer JB, Osterud B, Tveita T (1999). The effect of short term mild exposure on risk factors for cardiovascular disease. *Thrombosis Research*, **95**, 93–104.

Millar JA (1996). Seasonal incidence of stroke [correspondence]. *Lancet*, **347**, 1702.

Moran C, Johnson H, Johnson Z (2000). Seasonal patterns of morbidity and mortality in the elderly in Ireland. *International Journal of Circumpolar Health*, **59**, 170–5.

Murphy MF and Campbell MJ (1987). Sudden infant death syndrome and environmental temperature: an analysis using vital statistics. *Journal of Epidemiology and Community Health*, **41**, 63–71.

Nakai S, Itoh T, Morimoto T (1999). Deaths from heat-stroke in Japan: 1968–1994. *International Journal of Biometeorology*, **43**, 124–7.

Nashold RD, Jentzen JM, Peterson PL, Remington PL (1996). Heat-related deaths during the summer of 1995, Wisconsin. *Wisconsin Medical Journal*, **95**(6), 382–3.

Nayha S (2000). Seasonal variation of deaths in Finland: is it still diminishing? *International Journal of Circumpolar Health*, **59**, 182–7.

Nayha S (2002). Cold and the risk of cardiovascular diseases: a review. *International Journal of Circumpolar Health*, **61**(4), 373–80.

Nayha S and Hassi J (1995). Cold and mortality from ischaemic heart disease in northern Finland. *Arctic Medical Research*, **54**(Suppl. 2), 19–25.

Neild PJ, Syndercombe-Court D, Keatinge WR, Donaldson GC, Mattock M, Caunce M (1994). Cold-induced increases in erythrocyte count, plasma cholesterol and plasma fibrinogen of elderly people without comparable rise in protein C or factor X. *Clinical Science*, **86**, 43–8.

Oechsli FW and Buechley RW (1970). Excess mortality associated with three Los Angeles September hot spells. *Environmental Research*, **3**, 277–84.

O'Neill MS, Zanobetti A, Schwartz J (2003). Modifiers of the temperature and mortality association in seven US cities. *American Journal of Epidemiology*, **157**(12), 1074–82.

Ornato JP, Siegel L, Caren EJ, Nelson N (1990). Increased incidence of cardiac death attributed to acute myocardial infarction during winter. *Coronary Artery Disease*, **1**, 199–204.

Ornato JP, Peberdy MA, Chandra NC, Bush DE (1996). Seasonal pattern of acute myocardial infarction in the national registry of myocardial infarction. *Journal of the American College of Cardiology*, **28**, 1684–8.

Pan W-H, Li L-A, Tsai M-J (1995). Temperature extremes and mortality from coronary heart disease and cerebral infarction in elderly Chinese. *Lancet*, **345**, 353–5.

Pattenden S, Nikiforov B, Armstrong BG (2003). Mortality and temperature in Sofia and London. *Journal of Epidemiology and Community Health*, **57**, 628–33.

Pell JP, Sirel J, Marsden AK, Cobbe SM (1999). Seasonal variations in out of hospital cardiopulmonary arrest. *Heart*, **82**, 680–3.

Pope CA III (1999). Mortality and air pollution: associations persist with continued advances in research methodology. *Environmental Health Perspectives*, **107**(8), 613.

Pope CA III and Kalkstein LS (1996). Synoptic weather modelling and estimates of the exposure-response relationship between daily mortality and particulate air pollution. *Environmental Health Perspectives*, **104**(4), 414–20.

Qizibash N, Jones L, Warlow C, Mann J (1991). Fibrinogen and lipid concentration as risk factors for transient ischaemic attacks and minor ischaemic strokes. *British Medical Journal*, **303**, 605–9.

Ramlow JM and Kuller LH (1990). Effects of the summer heat wave of 1988 on daily mortality in Allegheny County, PA. *Public Health Reports*, **105**(3), 283–9.

Ricci S, Celani MG, Vitali R, La Rosa F, Righetti E, Duca E (1992). Diurnal and seasonal variations in the occurrence of stroke: community-based study. *Neuroepidemiology*, **11**(2), 59–64.

Rooney C, McMichael AJ, Kovats RS, Coleman MP (1998). Excess mortality in England and Wales, and in Greater London, during the 1995 heatwave. *Journal of Epidemiology and Community Health*, **52**, 482–6.

Rose G (1966). Cold weather and ischaemic heart disease. *British Journal of Preventive and Social Medicine*, **20**, 97–100.

Rothwell PM, Wroe SJ, Slattery J, Warlow CP (1996). Is stroke incidence related to season or temperature? *Lancet*, **347**, 934–6.

Saez M, Sunyer J, Castellsague J, Murillo C, Anto JM (1995). Relationship between weather temperature and mortality: a time series analysis approach in Barcelona. *International Journal of Epidemiology*, **24**, 576–82.

Saez M, Sunyer J, Tobias A, Ballester F, Anto JM (2000). Ischaemic heart disease mortality and weather temperature in Barcelona, Spain. *European Journal of Public Health*, **10**, 58–63.

Samet J, Zeger S, Kelsall J, Xu J, Kalkstein L (1998). Does weather confound or modify the association of particulate air pollution with mortality? *Environmental Research Section A*, **77**, 9–19.

Sarna S, Romo M, Siltanen P (1977). Myocardial infarction and weather. *Annals of Clinical Research*, **9**, 222–32.

Sartor F, Snacken R, Demuth C, Walckiers D (1995). Temperature, ambient ozone levels, and mortality during summer, 1994, in Belgium. *Environmental Research*, **70**, 105–13.

Schluter PJ, Ford RPK, Brown J, Ryan AP (1998). Weather temperatures and sudden infant death syndrome: a regional study over 22 years in New Zealand. *Journal of Epidemiology and Community Health*, **52**, 27–33.

Schuman SH (1972). Patterns of urban heat-wave deaths and implications for prevention: data from New York and St. Louis during July, 1966. *Environmental Research*, **5**, 59–75.

Schwartz J (1994). Non-parametric smoothing in the analysis of air pollution and respiratory illness. *Canadian Journal of Statistics*, **22**(4), 471–87.

Schwartz J (2000). The distributed lag between air pollution and daily deaths. *Epidemiology*, **11**(3), 320–6.

Schwartz J, Spix C, Touloumi G, et al. (1996). Methodological issues in studies of air pollution and daily counts of deaths or hospital admissions. *Journal of Epidemiology and Community Health*, **50**(Suppl. 1), S3–S11.

Semenza JC, Rubin CH, Falter KH et al. (1996). Heat-related deaths during the July 1995 heat wave in Chicago. *New England Journal of Medicine*, **335**(2), 84–90.

Seto T, Mittlemann M, Davis R, Taira D, Kawachi I (1998). Seasonal variation in coronary artery disease mortality in Hawaii: observational study. *British Medical Journal*, **316**, 1946–7.

Shah S and Peacock J (1999). Deprivation and excess winter mortality. *Journal of Epidemiology and Community Health*, **53**, 499–502.

Sheth T, Nair C, Muller J, Yusuf S (1999). Increased winter mortality from acute myocardial infarction and stroke: the effect of age. *Journal of the American College of Cardiology*, **33**(7), 1916–19.

Shumway RH, Azari AS, Pawitan Y (1988). Modeling mortality fluctuations in Los Angeles as functions of pollution and weather effects. *Environmental Research*, **45**, 224–41.

Simonsen L, Clarke MJ, Williamson G, Stroup DF, Arden NH, Schonberger LB (1997). The impact of influenza epidemics on mortality: introducing a severity index. *American Journal of Public Health*, **87**, 1944–50.

Smith WC and Tunstall-Pedoe H (1984). European regional variation in cardiovascular mortality. *British Medical Bulletin*, **40**(4), 374–9.

Smolander J (2002). Effect of cold exposure on older humans. *International Journal of Sports Medicine*, **23**, 86–92.

Smoyer-Tomic KE and Rainham DG (2001). Beating the heat: development and evaluation of a Canadian hot weather health-response plan. *Environmental Health Perspectives*, **109**, 1241–8.

Sperber AD and Weitzman S (1997). Mind over matter about keeping warm. *Lancet*, **349**, 1337–8.

Stewart SE, Gibson B, Land G, Rackers D, Donnell HD Jr, Graumann A (1989). Heat-related deaths: Missouri, 1979–1988. *Morbidity and Mortality Weekly Report*, **38**(25), 437–8.

Stout RW and Crawford V (1991). Seasonal variations in fibrinogen concentrations among elderly people. *Lancet*, **338**, 9–13.

Taylor AJ and McGwin G (2000). Temperature-related deaths in Alabama. *Southern Medical Journal*, **93**(8), 787–92.

The Eurowinter Group (1997). Cold exposure and winter mortality from ischaemic heart disease, cerebrovascular disease, respiratory disease, and all causes in warm and cold regions of Europe. *Lancet*, **349**, 1341–6.

The Eurowinter Group (2000). Winter mortality in relation to climate. *International Journal of Circumpolar Health*, **59**, 154–9.

Thurston GD and Ito K (2001). Epidemiological studies of acute ozone exposures and mortality. *Journal of Exposure Analysis and Environmental Epidemiology*, **11**, 286–94.

Touloumi G, Samoli E, Katsouyanni K (1996). Daily mortality and 'winter type' air pollution in Athens, Greece: a time series analysis within the APHEA project. *Journal of Epidemiology and Community Health*, **50** (Suppl. 1), S47–S51.

van Rossum CTM, Shipley MJ, Hemingway H, Grobbee DE, Mackenbach JP, Marmot MG (2001). Seasonal variation in cause-specific mortality: are there high-risk groups? 25-year follow-up of civil servants from the first Whitehall study. *International Journal of Epidemiology*, **30**, 1109–16.

van Weel C, van de Lisdonk E, van den Bosch W, van den Hoogen H, Bor H (1996). Seasonal incidence of stroke [correspondence]. *Lancet*, **347**, 1703.

Voelker R (1995). Probe of heat wave deaths under way. *Journal of the American Medical Association*, **274**, 595–6.

Vuori I (1987). The heart and the cold. *Annals of Clinical Research*, **19**, 156–62.

Whitman S, Good G, Donoghue ER, Benbow N, Shou W, Mou S (1997). Mortality in Chicago attributed to the July 1995 heat wave. *American Journal of Public Health*, **87**, 1515–18.

Woodhouse PR, Khaw KT, Plummer M (1993). Seasonal variation in blood pressure in relation to temperature in elderly men and women. *Journal of Hypertension*, **11**, 1267–74.

Woodhouse PR, Khaw KT, Plummer M, Foley A, Meade TW (1994). Seasonal variations of plasma fibrinogen and factor VII activity in the elderly: winter infections and death from cardiovascular disease. *Lancet*, **343**, 435–9.

Wyndham CH and Fellingham SA (1978). Climate and disease. *South African Medical Journal*, **53**, 1051–61.

Zanobetti A, Wand MP, Schwartz J, Ryan LM (2000). Generalized additive distributed lag models: quantifying mortality displacement. *Biostatistics*, **1**(3), 279–92.

Chapter 31

Gene–environment interaction in coronary artery disease: apolipoprotein E and smoking and the interleukin-6 gene and inflammation as examples

S. E. Humphries

31.1 Introduction

In common with all past genetic analyses of human disease, genetic research into coronary artery disease (CAD) has been based on two major premises. The first was that the identification of disease-causing mutations would lead to the development of DNA-based tests to identify those at risk. To date there has been little progress in developing such a 'battery' of tests. However, a detailed understanding of the way common genetic variations of modest effect interact with environmental factors suggests that this goal was always going to be difficult and technically challenging to achieve.

Since we would predict that the impact of single common mutations on CAD development will be modest (increasing relative risk (RR) by 20–40% at most), the main issue of clinical relevance is whether the conferred risk of such a mutation is very much higher in some population subgroups. To be clinically useful in any risk algorithm, we might require for any factor to have a RR of 2 or greater; this, for example, is the RR estimated to be associated with the smoking habit in middle-aged men (Doll and Hill 1966). Such subgroups might be those carrying a second important mutation in another gene (i.e. those with a gene–gene interaction), and such individuals might be identified using conventional genetic strategies. Alternatively, one might identify individuals exposed to a given environment, which amplifies the risk associated with that gene (i.e. gene–environment interaction). In the population, as shown in Fig. 31.1, there is a range of genetic risk profiles, with each individual occupying a position along the risk spectrum, from low to high genetic risk, depending on the number of CAD-risk variants each has inherited. Similarly, individuals adopt a different position on the environmental spectrum of risk by the lifestyle choices they make or the influences upon them. Increased risk of CAD occurs when a high genetic risk individual enters a high-risk environment. Either alone is unlikely to cause premature CAD. This chapter focuses on common genetic variants (at polymorphic frequency, i.e. >1% carrier frequency) which are associated with significant excess risk only when the individual is exposed to a 'high-risk' environment.

The second major goal of molecular genetic research has been to use molecular genetics to understand the pathological processes that are involved in determining CAD, and this aspect of the research has already made considerable contributions over the last 10 years. The detection of an association between a mutation in a particular enzyme and plasma levels of an 'intermediate

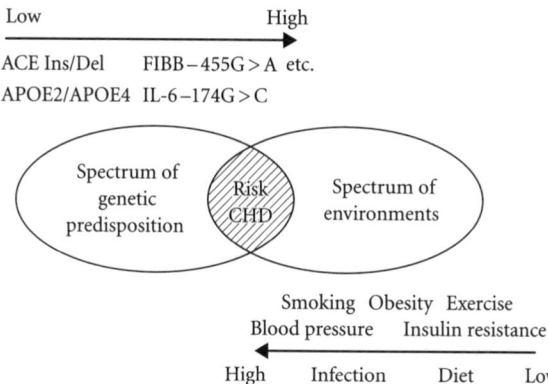

Low   High

ACE Ins/Del   FIBB − 455G > A etc.
APOE2/APOE4   IL-6 −174G > C

Spectrum of genetic predisposition   Risk CHD   Spectrum of environments

Smoking   Obesity   Exercise
Blood pressure   Insulin resistance

High   Infection   Diet   Low

Fig. 31.1 Model for gene–environment interaction.

phenotype' for CAD risk (e.g. plasma levels of lipids, clotting factors, or homocysteine) identifies the enzyme (and the pathway that the enzyme is involved in) as a pharmacological target. It highlights how understanding of the mechanisms by which these mutations interact with environmental factors sheds light on the pathological processes of disease, and may lead to novel therapeutic or interventional strategies to reduce an individual's risk of disease.

31.2 Risk factors for CAD

As a result of epidemiological and clinical studies over the last 20 years many CAD 'intermediate phenotypes' have been identified, with high risk being associated with elevated plasma levels of lipids (Castelli *et al.* 1986; Hokanson and Austin 1996), fibrinogen (Meade *et al.* 1986), and homocysteine (Ma *et al.* 1996), and with low levels of high-density lipoprotein-cholesterol (HDL-C) (Wilson *et al.* 1996). In addition, it is now recognized that the inflammatory system occupies a key role in the atherosclerotic process (Ross 1999), which may explain why elevated levels of markers of the acute phase response system such as C-reactive protein (CRP) (Ridker *et al.* 2000*a*), as well as cytokines such as interleukin-6 (IL-6), are also elevated in CAD subjects (Ridker *et al.* 2000*b*). Based on this understanding, it can similarly be predicted that what can be considered as an 'environmental challenge' which results in change in any of these phenotypes will be a 'risk-environment for CAD'. Such challenges include increasing age, male gender, dietary intake of fats or vitamins, use of cigarettes and alcohol, presence of hypertension, diabetes, and obesity, and as shown in Table 31.1 these have all been implicated in potential gene–environment interactions of clinical relevance, and are detailed in other chapters. Of these, smoking is particularly relevant, and will be examined further.

Smoking is known to roughly double life-time risk of CAD (Doll and Hill 1966), and is thought to increase cardiovascular risk by several different mechanisms. The products of tobacco combustion directly damage vascular endothelium, leading to increased secretion of adhesion molecules which enhance binding of platelets and monocytes to the vessel wall, thus promoting thrombosis and atherosclerosis (Allen *et al.* 1988; Blann 1992; Lowe 1993). Smoking disturbs lipoprotein metabolism by increasing insulin resistance and lipid intolerance, and is implicated in the production of small dense low-density lipoprotein (LDL). By stimulating catecholamines, smoking up-regulates hormone sensitive lipase, increasing circulating free fatty acid (FFA) levels (Eliasson *et al.* 1997), thus causing atherogenic dyslipidaemia. In addition, smoking-induced lung damage may lead to an IL-6-mediated inflammatory response, causing

Table 31.1 Examples of CAD itself or CAD risk traits which are affected by environment challenges, and reported examples of specific candidate gene–environment interaction in determining an individual's response

Plasma CAD risk trait	Environment stressor	Candidate genes	Reference
Cholesterol	Dietary fat	APOE/CETP/LPL	Ordovas and Schaefer 2000; Wallace et al. 2000
Triglyceride	Obesity/lack of exercise/smoking	LPL/APOC3	Fisher et al. 1995; Waterworth et al. 2000
HDL	Smoking/gender/alcohol	APOA1/CETP	Sigurdsson et al. 1992; Fumeron et al. 1995; Gudnason et al. 1997
Fibrinogen	Injury/infection/surgery/smoking	FIBB	Montgomery et al. 1996; Gardemann et al. 1997; Cotton et al. 2000
CRP/IL-6	Injury/infection/surgery/smoking	IL6	Fishman et al. 1998; Brull et al. 2001
Homocysteine	Low folate diet	MTHFR	Ma et al. 1996; Dekou et al. 2001
LV mass	Hypertension/exercise	ACE	Montgomery et al. 1997; Myerson et al. 2001
CAD	Smoking	LPL	Talmud et al. 2000
		APOE	Humphries et al. 2001a
		GST1[a]	Li et al. 2000, 2001

LV: left ventricular.

[a] Glutathione S-transferase.

hepatic up-regulation of fibrinogen expression (Dalmon *et al.* 1993) and increased risk of thrombosis (Meade *et al.* 1986). Smokers have lower levels of antioxidants such as ascorbate and tocopherol and thus smoking may favour the oxidation of LDL (Fickl *et al.* 1996).

31.3 Apolipoprotein E and effect on lipid levels and coronary heart disease risk

Of the candidate genes involved in the determination of lipid levels and coronary heart disease (CHD) risk, apolipoprotein E (apoE) is probably the most comprehensively studied, but it is only recently that the interaction of environmental factors with apoE variation has been examined. ApoE is synthesized both in the liver and intestine and is found in the plasma associated with triglyceride-rich lipoproteins. It is the ligand for removal of these particles and thus occupies a central role in determining the metabolic fate of these lipoproteins. There are three common isoforms of the protein, each differing from the other by one charged amino acid (reviewed in Davignon *et al.* 1988). The apoprotein designated apoE3 is the most common isoform in populations (frequency ~0.77) with apoE4 being present at a frequency of 0.15 and apoE2 at a frequency of 0.08 in Western Caucasian populations (Davignon *et al.* 1988). Carriers of apoE2, who represent ~12% of the population, have on average cholesterol levels 10% lower than E3E3 individuals, while apoE4 carriers represent ~25% of the population and have average cholesterol levels 5% higher than E3E3 individuals (Davignon *et al.* 1988). Based on this, and knowing the relationship between cholesterol levels and CAD risk, it can be predicted that variation at the *APOE* locus explains ~2–3% of the risk in myocardial infarction and this prediction is supported by several studies (e.g. Wilson *et al.* 1996). Compared to men homozygous for the common ε3 allele, subjects carrying the ε2 allele show protection from both coronary and carotid disease and stroke (Kessler *et al.* 1997), while those with the ε4 allele have higher risk. Recently, the ε4 allele has been reported to increase risk of coronary death in men in the Scandinavian Simvastatin Survival Study by 1.8-fold, but ε4 carriers also showed greatest benefit from statin treatment (Gerdes *et al.* 2000).

31.4 *APOE* genotype–smoking interaction

The interaction of *APOE* and smoking on CHD risk was examined in the UK-based Northwick Park Heart Study of more than 3000 men, followed prospectively for CHD events for over 6 years (Humphries *et al.* 2001*b*). The effect of smoking alone on CHD risk was 1.94 (95% CI: 1.25–3.01), in agreement with previous studies which found smoking to double CHD risk (Doll and Hill 1966). As expected, *APOE* genotype was associated with effects on cholesterol and apoB levels, with ε4 carriers having the highest and ε2 carriers the lowest levels, irrespective of smoking status. As presented in Fig. 31.2, compared to all genotype never smokers, where the hazard ratio was set at 1.00, in men who smoked, those with the genotype ε3/ε3 had a hazard ratio of 1.68 (95% CI: 1.01–2.83) compared to 1.18 (95% CI: 0.46–3.03) for ε2 carriers and 3.17 (95% CI: 1.82–5.51) in ε4 carriers. The effect of the interaction between smoking status and *APOE* genotype on CHD risk was significant ($p = 0.007$). In all genotype groups there was an increase in risk of CHD from never, to ex-smokers and in smokers the risk could be related to the number of cigarettes currently smoked per day, but the size of this effect was much greater in the ε4 carriers. Reassuringly, when apoε4 ex-smokers were examined it was found that their RR had fallen to 0.74 (0.34–0.1.55), suggesting that whatever the mechanism of higher risk, it is reversible upon smoking cessation.

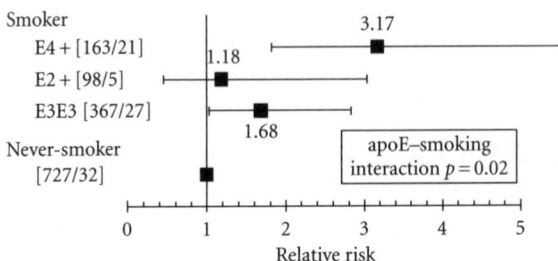

Fig. 31.2 ApoE–smoking interaction and CHD risk. For the non-smokers all genotype groups have been pooled and the hazard ratio (relative risk) set at 1. In this group there were 32 CHD events and 727 event-free men. In the smokers, divided on the basis of APOE genotype, there were 27 events and 367 event-free men in the $\varepsilon3\varepsilon3$ group, 21 events and 163 event-free men in the $\varepsilon4$ + group, and 5 events and 95 event-free men in the $\varepsilon2$ + group. Smoking increases risk in $\varepsilon3\varepsilon3$ by 68% but by >200% in the $\varepsilon4$ + group.

In these men the increased risk associated with smoking and carrying an $\varepsilon4$ allele was independent of body mass index (BMI), blood pressure, lipid levels, and markers of inflammation. Results from the PDAY study (Hixson 1991) also showed that *APOE* genotype had a significant effect on the extent of aortic lesions, again even after adjustment for cholesterol levels, suggesting that the *APOE* genotype effect on arterial wall lesions was over and above its effect on plasma cholesterol levels. Thus, although the mechanisms for these cholesterol-independent effects on arterial wall thickening are unclear, there is good evidence that *APOE* genotype influences lesion formation independently of its effects on fasting plasma lipid levels. The interaction of $\varepsilon4$ and smoking suggests that smoking exacerbates this.

The most likely mechanism to explain the $\varepsilon4$–smoking interaction on CHD risk appears to be through a direct effect on LDL oxidation. Several studies using recombinant apoE have demonstrated that the protection against oxidation *in vitro* is E2 > E3 > E4 (Smith *et al.* 1998). This effect may be due to the fact that E2 has two free SH-groups, E3 has one, and E4 none, or may be due to other effects of apoE isoforms on the physicochemical properties of lipoproteins that promote or protect from oxidation. *In vivo* studies have shown that *APOE* knock-out mice are highly susceptible to developing atherosclerosis (Plump *et al.* 1992), at least in part because their LDL is more susceptible to oxidation (Palinski *et al.* 1994), and this effect is reversible by vitamin E supplementation of their diet (Pratico *et al.* 1998). The differential oxidation of apoE isoforms has now been confirmed *in vitro* with, as expected, E4 being more susceptible than E3, which in turn is more susceptible to oxidation than E2 (Jolivalt *et al.* 2000).

31.5 Homeostasis and use of stressing the genotype to identify functional variants

In the context of a cell (or even an organ or organism), genes can be considered simply to code for the synthesis of proteins which allow the maintenance of intracellular homeostasis in the face of extracellular or environmental changes. At the basic level the cell requires oxygen, energy, and various chemicals, in order to reproduce and, in a Darwinian sense, to pass on its genes to the next generation. Naturally-occurring genetic variation means that some individuals are better able to maintain homeostasis than others in the face of the same environmental challenges. In the Western culture, people now experience many challenges to maintaining cardiovascular health, such as a high-fat diet, high levels of smoking and alcohol intake, and reduced physical exercise leading to obesity. Even in the face of these environmental 'insults', some individuals maintain cardiovascular health into old age, while others, with a different genetic make-up, fail to maintain homeostasis (e.g. plasma levels of cholesterol or fibrinogen within an optimal range), and thus develop atherosclerosis. Identifying the genes involved in maintaining cardiovascular homeostasis in the face of environmental challenge should thus lead to progress in understanding pathophysiology and aetiology, as well as in genetic risk prediction, since mutations in such genes are likely to be strongly predisposing to or protecting from CAD.

As an example of this, fibrinogen is a major acute phase reactant and levels rise rapidly after infection or injury. Since elevated fibrinogen levels are an independent risk factor for CAD (Meade *et al.* 1986), an individual who has a genetic predisposition to making particularly large responses may be at greater thrombotic risk than an individual with a genotype predis-posing to a modest response. For any individual, the measured level of fibrinogen in the blood is thus due to that individual's genetically determined ability to maintain homeostasis in response to the environment that has been, or is currently being, experienced. If genetic variation can be identified that distinguishes the 'plastic' from the 'stable' genotype, such informa-tion, in conjunction with information about current level, may add significantly to future risk prediction. Such genetic variation has been identified by us in the promoter region of the beta fibrinogen gene (*FIBB*), and is reviewed elsewhere (Humphries *et al.* 1997).

The impact of such variation can be examined in classical epidemiological studies by stratify-ing by the environmental factor of interest or can be examined by a 'genotype–stress' study, which has already been shown by us (e.g. Montgomery *et al.* 1996) and other groups to be an excellent way of magnifying modest genotype effects on traits. Other stress situations that have been used in CAD genetic research include a fatty meal (Gerdes *et al.* 1997) or a high-fat diet (Wallace *et al.* 2000), with some individuals having a modest response and others a very large response, determined in part by genotypes at the loci for apolipoproteins, *LPL*, and cholesterol ester transfer protein (CETP). Examples of where both approaches have identified gene–environment interactions are shown in Table 31.1.

31.6 Inflammation, IL-6 genotype, and coronary artery bypass surgery

Inflammatory processes are known to play a role in atherogenesis (Ross 1999), with the presence of chronic gastric, lung, and gum inflammation all being associated with the develop-ment of coronary disease (see Yudkin *et al.* 2000). The cytokine IL-6 is synthesized in response to diverse inflammatory stimuli and, as a key orchestrator of the inflammatory response, may play an important role in bridging the inflammatory and atherosclerotic processes. Elevated IL-6 levels are associated with the development (Ridker *et al.* 2000*a, b*) and severity of coronary disease (Gabriel *et al.* 2000), as well as with the transition to plaque instability (Crea *et al.* 1997; Biasucci *et al.* 1996) and subsequent poor outcome. As shown in Fig. 31.3, whilst such an effect might be mediated through the action of downstream acute phase proteins such as CRP and fibrinogen, IL-6 may itself be directly pathogenic. IL-6 stimulates endothelial activation, vascular smooth muscle cell proliferation, and leukocyte recruitment, effects that may lead to plaque growth or instability (see references in Yudkin *et al.* 2000).

However, despite such mechanistic data, the association of raised IL-6 levels with coronary disease is not proof of cause. Indeed, coronary lesions may be pro-inflammatory, causing

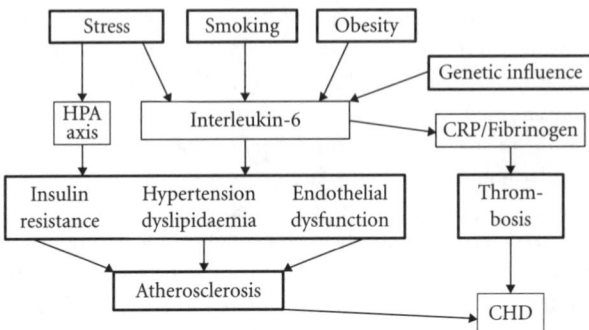

Fig. 31.3 The roles and regulation of IL-6 in CAD.

(rather than being caused by) rises in IL-6 levels. One way to clarify the issue of causation is to utilize a genetic approach. The association of a functional IL-6 polymorphism with CAD would suggest a causal, rather than passive, association of the cytokine and disease. It is thus of some importance to identify polymorphic variants of the IL-6 gene that are functional *in vivo* in humans. To date three common variants have been identified in the IL-6 gene promoter, of which −174G > C has been most widely studied (Fishman *et al.* 1998; Terry *et al.* 2000). The functionality *in vitro* has been examined using constructs of the 5' flanking region of the IL-6 gene in a luciferase reporter vector transiently transfected into HeLa cells. The −174C construct showed lower basal and stimulated (with LPS or IL-1) expression than the common allele −174G construct (Fishman *et al.* 1998).

However, *in vitro* studies using reporter gene constructs may be confounded by a number of factors. These include the type of cell line and culture conditions used, whether cells are at basal state or 'stimulated' by exogenous agents, the nature of the exogenous stimulation, and by the presence or absence of additional positive or negative regulatory elements contained within the sequences. Furthermore, varied lengths of DNA are used in the constructs, which are divorced from their normal chromatin context and the influence of distal enhancer or inhibitory regulatory elements that would further influence gene transcription. For all of these reasons, *in vitro* data must be extrapolated with care to the *in vivo* situation.

Further clarification of *in vivo* human functionality is thus required for the IL-6 polymorphisms and this can be best achieved by the utilization of a physiological stressor stimulus to increase gene expression (Montgomery *et al.* 1996; Myerson *et al.* 2001). We have applied this approach to the IL-6 gene polymorphisms (Brull *et al.* 2001) by investigating the genotype-dependence of the circulating IL-6 response to coronary artery bypass surgery (CABG). CABG is a well-characterized inflammatory stimulus that causes a substantial rise in circulating IL-6 levels that peak 6 h after patients are placed on cardiopulmonary bypass (CPB) (Corbi *et al.* 2000). Data for the IL-6 response to surgery are shown in Fig. 31.4. At baseline, there was no significant difference in IL-6 levels by genotype; however, 6 h after surgery mean IL-6 levels rose over 45-fold ($p < 0.001$, compared to baseline), and the magnitude of this rise was strongly genotype-dependent. Levels were 26% higher in those homozygous for the −174C allele, than amongst G allele carriers, and this difference was statistically significant even after adjustment for confounding variables ($p = 0.04$). Interestingly, subjects who were genotype −174GG reached peak IL-6 levels 24 h post-CPB and had higher IL-6 levels at this time point than carriers of one or more C allele (274.1 ± 23.7 vs. 214.4 ± 19, $p < 0.02$), perhaps reflecting a more damped response to the inflammatory stimulus.

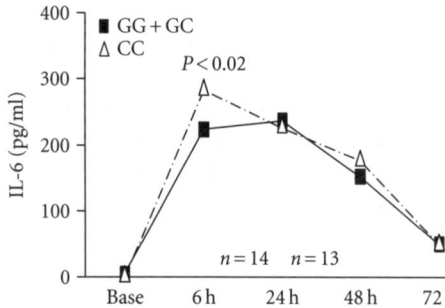

Fig. 31.4 The effect of IL-6 − 174C > C promoter genotype on IL-6 levels at baseline and 6 h post-CABG. Comparing the CC group to the GG + GC group combined.

These data suggest that this −174G > C variant is indeed functional *in vivo*. In contrast to *in vitro* data (Fishman *et al.* 1998), higher stimulated (6 h) IL-6 levels were observed amongst carriers of the −174C allele. This finding confirms the association between the −174C allele and increased IL-6 levels already reported in patients with aortic aneurysm – a disease known to be associated with an inflammatory response (Jones *et al.* 2001), and suggests important differences between *in vitro* and *in vivo* assessments of functionality.

The question remains as to what influence this higher IL-6 post-operation has on CHD risk. Whilst duration of intensive care or total in-hospital stay were independent of genotype, three of the five postoperative deaths occurred in −174CC homozygotes and the other two in −174G > C heterozygotes (−174GG vs. GC + CC, $p = 0.002$). It is tempting to speculate that the excess mortality seen in this group of patients for carriers of the IL-6 −174C allele might relate directly to the more exuberant acute inflammatory response they mount. However, this is based on five deaths overall and clearly requires much larger studies to obtain an accurate estimate of risk. However, as shown in Table 31.2, both case-control and prospective studies indicate that the −174C allele is associated with higher risk of CHD, with the risk effect magnified by smoking in at least one study (Humphries *et al.* 2001*a*).

The mechanism of the risk effect associated with the high IL-6 genotype is likely to be complex. IL-6 plays a pivotal role in generating the inflammatory response and regulating the hepatic synthesis of acute phase proteins such as CRP and fibrinogen, as well as having a wide range of effects relating to inflammation and tissue injury. IL-6 mRNA is found at high levels

Table 31.2 Relative risk CHD associated with IL-6 −174G > C genotype in reported studies

Study	Number Case/control	RR compared to GG (95% CI)	Reference
ECTIM (case/control)	640/719	GC 1.31 (1.05–1.73) CC 1.35 (0.95–1.84)	Georges *et al.* 2001
NPHS-II (prospective[a])	162/2589	GC 1.55 (1.06–2.22) CC 1.07 (0.65–1.77)	Humphries *et al.* 2001*b*
Aneurysms (prospective)	30/466	GC 2.83 (1.15–6.97) CC 3.41 (1.38–8.39)	Jones *et al.* 2001
WOSCOP (prospective) (Placebo group only)	259/579	GC 1.07 (0.77–1.48) GC 1.26 (0.83–1.91)	Basso *et al.* 2002

ECTIM: Etude Cas-Temoin de l'Infarctus du Myocarde; NPHS-II: Northwick Park Heart Study II.

[a] GC + CC in smokers vs. GG non-smokers, RR = 2.66 (1.64 – 4.32).

in atheromatous arteries (Rus *et al.* 1996) and colocalizes with macrophages in areas of plaque rupture. In addition, there is already a wealth of data supporting a role for IL-6 as a useful marker of cardiovascular risk. Elevated levels of IL-6 and CRP are predictive of future cardiovascular events in both healthy men (Ridker *et al.* 2000*b*) and women (Ridker *et al.* 2000*a*) and they are markers of poor prognosis in both chronic angina and following acute coronary syndromes. Despite this, it is still not known whether this association is causal or merely an epiphenomenon. The association between the genotype that results in high IL-6 in an inflammatory situation and high CHD risk adds weight to the argument that IL-6 is causal and not merely a marker of CAD.

31.7 Analytical problems for gene–environment interaction studies

A key factor in the identification and study of gene–environment interaction is that an individual carrying such a mutation will develop the phenotype, only if and when they enter the high-risk environment. Thus the mutation will only 'cause' high plasma cholesterol or high fibrinogen in the presence of this environmental challenge. This classical 'lack of penetrance' of a mutation will cause analytical problems and mis-phenotyping which will be particularly problematic with some sampling analytical designs. The problem that this 'context-dependency' of a mutation (i.e. gene x environment effect) creates, from an analytical point of view, has largely been overlooked in the field. The problem occurs when a second study fails to confirm a reported association between a candidate gene polymorphism and levels of intermediate traits or with risk of CAD. Although such a failure may cast doubt on the validity of the first report, it may also reflect the presence of a potentially interesting gene–environment interaction that requires further exploration. If, for example, smoking is the key environmental stress that amplifies or diminishes the genotype effect, then the different proportion of smokers in the samples being studied (and possibly the number of cigarettes being smoked) will have a major effect on the power of the sample to detect the association. However, simple power calculations can be carried out knowing the prevalence of the particular environmental factor in the sample under study, and the size of the sample to be studied can be increased accordingly. From a practical point of view this means that large samples are required for interactions to be statistically significant and that the characteristics of the sample being studied must be carefully recorded and compared between samples. As a minimum, it would be reasonable to propose that a statistically significant finding should be reproduced in three independent samples (preferably from different laboratories).

One area where environmental manipulation may be available to confirm gene–environment interaction observed in an association study would be to remove the environment (or the individual from the environment) and observe the decay of the induced phenotype effect over a period of time. Although this could not easily be done for the phenotype of atherosclerosis, requiring invasive serial coronary angiography, for example, it would be possible for some environments such as smoking, or dietary effects on plasma traits such as fibrinogen or cholesterol, or on the consequence of hypertension on left ventricular hypertrophy after antihypertensive therapy. The oxidative stress associated with smoking could be determined in subjects before and after quitting smoking, for example by measurement of F2-isoprostanes (see Pratico *et al.* 1998) and the relationship between levels and apoE genotype examined. The prediction would be that oxidative stress in $\varepsilon 4$ carriers should show a greater fall than in $\varepsilon 3\varepsilon 3$ subjects, and experiments to confirm this prediction could be an extremely powerful argument in support of causality. This is an area of research which has yet to be examined in detail.

31.8 When has a candidate gene won the election?

Before a mutation can be accepted as a proven CAD risk factor, it will be necessary to agree on the criteria that must be met. For this purpose the criteria proposed for causality of an infectious agent can be adapted.

The reproducibility of the effect in different laboratories and in different settings is one piece of evidence, but the problem of gene–environment interaction makes this less clear cut. As a minimum, it would be reasonable to propose that a statistically significant finding should be reproduced in three independent samples (preferably from different laboratories). If a particular mutation is associated with the same effect in different ethnic groups (even though its frequency may be quite different) this adds further weight to causality, as has been shown for the fibrinogen −455G > A in Caucasians and Japanese (Iso *et al.* 1995).

Biological plausibility of the effect of the mutation is important, and thus a mutation in the promoter of a gene that is having an *in vitro* demonstrated effect on transcription should affect the **levels** of a plasma risk factor, but not the **function** of the protein. Mutations that delete amino acids or that cause a premature stop codon are highly likely to affect function, as are non-conservative mis-sense mutations and those altering important cysteine disulfide bridges. Conservative amino acid changes and wobble position changes are less likely to be functional, but some have been reported to alter function dramatically. Sequence changes in introns may affect splicing efficiency or cause exon skipping, but many appear to be without effect. For every mutation it would be ideal to confirm effect in *in vitro* expression studies, but for some, the effects on function may be relatively mild (say, + 10% of activity), which would be difficult to prove using *in vitro* assays, but could still be of clinical importance in promoting atherosclerosis development over the lifetime of an individual. Improving the sensitivity and biological relevance of such *in vitro* assays is one of the aspects of the research into the genetic determinants of CAD risk that still needs considerable work.

A graded response of the mutation would be supportive evidence, such that carriers of a mutation would be expected to have levels (or activity) of a protein intermediate between non-carriers and homozygotes for the mutation. This is often the case for promoter mutations, for example, the fibrinogen promoter −445G > A (Tybjaerg Hansen *et al.* 1997). However, mutations in enzymes usually result in a 'recessive' pattern of inheritance when the product of the enzyme is the trait that is measured. A good example of this is one of the key enzymes of homocysteine metabolism, methylene tetrahydrofolate reductase (MTHFR), where a mis-sense mutation (A122V) causes a thermolabile variant of the enzyme which is associated with hyper-homocysteinaemia, and risk of CAD (Ma *et al.* 1996). Homozygotes for the rare allele thermolabile variant (~10% of the population) have significantly elevated levels of plasma homocysteine compared to non-carriers and carriers of the variant. Presumably this is because, in carriers, the slight reduction of MTHFR enzyme levels is sufficient to maintain homocysteine plasma homeostasis in the environment of adequate dietary folate levels, while in variant homozygotes, where MTHFR levels are considerably lower, the level of the enzyme is insufficient to cope even in the setting of an adequate folate intake and homocysteine levels are high.

Reversibility of effect is obviously not technically possible for a gene mutation in a patient, but where the strong effect of a mutation on an intermediate trait is the result of gene–environment interaction, removal of the high-risk environment should have a large effect on the trait. As an example of this, the triglyceride-raising effect associated with being a carrier of the LPL-N9 or −S291 mutations, is exacerbated by obesity (Fisher *et al.* 1997). This predicts that weight loss in carriers should be followed by a greater fall in triglyceride levels than following a similar weight loss in non-carriers, and experiments to confirm this prediction could be an extremely powerful argument in support of causality.

Expression in vitro and in vivo would be the 'gold standard' proof of causality. None of the criteria above rule out the possibility that the variation is not itself causal, but is rather a marker for another mutation elsewhere in the gene. Formally, this can only be proved by making a gene construct with the 'wild-type' and 'mutant' sequence and expressing it *in vivo*. If the phenotype of interest is myocardial infarction in a human subject, clearly this cannot be done because of ethical and logistic reasons. Such experiments can be carried out in knock-out and transgenic rabbits or mice, but the animal models do not result in myocardial infarction, and so at best can give information about effects of these mutations on intermediate traits. Even so, the findings from animals need to be extrapolated with care to humans because of the many differences in the metabolic pathways and particularly in the 'back-up' redundancy system in the different species.

31.9 Conclusions

So how should we expect the field to progress over the next 3–5 years? Concern has been raised about the apparent 'inconsistency' of genetic association studies, with genotypes being associated with large effects on CHD risk in the initial published report (often in high impact factor journals but on relatively small samples), but with subsequent (larger) studies failing to confirm this effect, or at best finding an effect of much more modest size. Luckily, this problem is amenable to meta-analysis and such an analysis of 36 associations in CHD, diabetes, hypertension, cancer, etc. was recently published (Ioannidis *et al.* 2001). Not surprisingly, the major discriminating factor in predicting whether an initial risk association was subsequently confirmed was the size of the original sample. With a sample size of less than 150 subjects the original observation was often refuted, while with more than 150 the majority showed no significant evidence for heterogeneity between the initial and subsequent studies. Even though the results of such a meta-analysis are confined to published studies, and the difficulty in publishing 'negative' studies raises concerns about publication bias, the overall message of this paper is extremely encouraging: namely that many of the reported associations between certain genotypes and CHD risk do stand up to the test of replication (e.g. for apoE), albeit with the estimated risk lower than that originally reported. Interestingly, while some initially exciting associations have not been replicated, others reported first of all to be not significantly associated with risk have subsequently turned out to have a significant effect (e.g. PAI-1 4G/5G and risk of myocardial infarction; Ioannidis *et al.* 2001).

The same sort of rules must be applied to the gene–environment interactions discussed in this chapter. It is obviously worth publishing such interactions providing they are carried out on a reasonable-sized sample, because they will stimulate workers in the field to try to replicate the observation. It should, however, be recognized that where a particular genotype is only associated with risk in the presence of a particular environment (e.g. cigarette smoking), the failure to observe an association between this genotype and risk in a second sample may be explained by the relatively lower prevalence of the important environmental factor. Clearly, we still have a lot of work to do to be able to tease out the genetic factors involved in CHD risk in the general population.

It should, in the near future, be possible to include genetic markers in risk algorithms to advise healthy subjects how best to avoid CAD (Khoury and Wagener 1995). If gene–environment interactions can also be confirmed, both by repeat studies and also by 'stress-experiments', it should be possible to agree on the necessary criteria for acceptability for a candidate gene common mutation to be deemed proven and useful for inclusion into a CAD-risk algorithm, such as has been prepared by Framingham (Wilson *et al.* 1998) using essentially non-genetic factors. This will give us the ability to be able to give genotype-specific lifestyle advice, or to tailor clinical and therapeutic decisions to an individual's genotype. It also reveals potential novel therapeutic possibilities, for example to prevent oxidative stress or inflammation, or the novel use of available drugs such as statins, to prevent disease in a molecularly rational manner.

Acknowledgements

The author is supported by grants from the British Heart Foundation (RG2000015), and thanks colleagues in the CVG group for intellectual input, particularly Philippa Talmud and Dave Brull.

References

Allen, D. R., Browse, N. L., Rutt, D. L., Butler, L., and Fletcher, C. (1988). The effect of cigarette smoke, nicotine, and carbon monoxide on the permeability of the arterial wall. *Journal of Vascular Surgery*, 7, 139–52.

Basso F, Lowe G. D. O., Rumley A., McMahon, A. D., and Humphries S. E. (2002). Interleukin-6 −174 G > C polymorphism and risk of coronary heart disease in West of Scotland Coronary Prevention Study (WOSCOPS). *Arteriosclerosis, Thrombosis, and Vascular Biology*, 22, 599–604.

Biasucci, L. M., Vitelli, A., Liuzzo, G., Altamura, S., Caligiuri, G., Monaco C. *et al.* (1996). Elevated levels of interleukin-6 in unstable angina. *Circulation*, 94 (5), 874–7.

Blann, A. D. (1992). The acute influence of smoking on the endothelium. *Atherosclerosis*, 96, 249–50.

Brull, D., Montgomery, H. E., Sanders, J., Dhamrait, S., Luong, L-A., Rumley, A. *et al.* (2001). Interleukin-6 gene −174G > C and −152G > C polymorphisms are strong predictors of plasma IL-6 levels after cardiopulmonary bypass. *Arteriosclerosis, Thrombosis, and Vascular Biology*, 21, 1458–63.

Castelli, S. P., Garrison, R. J., Wilson, P. W., Abbott, R. D., Kalousdian, S., and Kannel, W. B. (1986). Incidence of coronary heart disease and lipoprotein cholesterol levels: the Framingham Study. *Journal of the American Medical Association*, 256, 2835–8.

Corbi, P., Rahmati, M., Delwail, A., Potreau, D., Menu, P., Wijdenes, J. *et al.* (2000). Circulating soluble gp130, soluble IL-6R, and IL-6 in patients undergoing cardiac surgery, with or without extracorporeal circulation. *European Journal of Cardio-thoracic Surgery*, 18 (1), 98–103.

Cotton, J. M., Webb, K. E., Mathur, A., Martin, J. F., and Humphries, S. E. (2000). Impact of the −455G > A promoter polymorphism in the B fibrinogen gene on stimulated fibrinogen production following bypass surgery. *Thrombosis and Haemostasis*, 84, 926–7.

Crea, F., Biasucci, L. M., Buffon, A., Liuzzo, G., Monaco, C., Caligiuri, G. *et al.* (1997). Role of inflammation in the pathogenesis of unstable coronary artery disease. *American Journal of Cardiology*, 80 (5A), 10E–16E.

Dalmon, J., Laurent, M., and Courtois, G. (1993). The human β fibrinogen promoter contains a hepatocyte nuclear factor 1-dependent interleukin-6 responsive element. *Molecular and Cellular Biology*, 13, 1183–93.

Davignon, J., Gregg, R. E., and Sing, C. F. (1988). Apolipoprotein E polymorphism and atherosclerosis. *Arteriosclerosis*, 8, 1–21.

Dekou, V., Whincup, P., Papacosta, O., Lennon, L., Ebrahim, S., Humphries, S. E., and Gudnason, V. (2001). The effect of C677T and C1298A polymorphisms in methylenetetrahydrofolate reductase on plasma homocysteine levels in elderly men and women from the British Regional Heart Study. *Atherosclerosis*, **154**, 659–66.

Doll, R. and Hill, A. B. (1966). Mortality of British doctors in relation to smoking: observation on coronary thrombosis. *National Cancer Institute Monographs*, **99**, 205–68.

Eliasson, B., Mero, N., Taskinen, M. R., and Smith, U. (1997). The insulin resistance syndrome and postprandial lipid intolerance in smokers. *Atherosclerosis*, **129**, 79–88.

Fickle, H., Van Antwerpen, V. L., and Richards, G. A. *et al.* (1996). Increased levels of autoantibodies to cardiolipin and oxidised low density lipoprotein are inversely associated with plasma vitamin C status in cigarette smokers. *Atherosclerosis*, **124**, 75–81.

Fisher, R. M., Mailly, F., and Peacock, R. E., *et al.* (1995). Interaction of the lipoprotein lipase asparagine 291→serine mutation with body mass index determines elevated plasma triacylglycerol concentrations: a study in hyperlipidemic subjects, myocardial infarction survivors, and healthy adults. *Journal of Lipid Research*, **36**, 2104–12.

Fisher, R. M., Humphries, S. E., and Talmud, J. (1997). Common variation in the lipoprotein lipase gene: effects on plasma lipids and risk of atherosclerosis. *Atherosclerosis*, **13**, 145–59.

Fishman, D., Faulds, G., Jeffery, R., Mohamed-Ali, V., Yudkin, J. S., Humphries, S., and Woo, P. (1998). The effect of novel polymorphisms in the interleukin-6 (IL-6) gene on IL-6 transcription and plasma IL-6 levels, and an association with systemic onset juvenile chronic arthritis. *Journal of Clinical Investigation*, **102** (7), 1369–76.

Fumeron, F., Betoulle, D., Luc, G. *et al.* (1995). Alcohol intake modulates the effect of a polymorphism of the cholesteryl ester transfer protein gene on plasma high density lipoprotein and the risk of myocardial infarction. *Journal of Clinical Investigation*, **96** (3), 1664–71.

Gabriel, A. S., Ahnve, S., Wretlind, B., and Martinsson, A. (2000). IL-6 and IL-1 receptor antagonist in stable angina pectoris and relation of IL-6 to clinical findings in acute myocardial infarction. *Journal of Internal Medicine*, **248** (1), 61–6.

Gardemann, A., Schwartz, O., Haberbosch, W. *et al.* (1997). Positive association of the β fibrinogen H1/H2 gene variation to basal fibrinogen levels and to the increase in fibrinogen concentration during acute phase reaction but not to coronary artery disease and myocardial infarction. *Thrombosis and Haemostasis*, **77**, 1120–6.

Georges, J-L., Loukaci, V., Poirier, O., Evans, A., Luc, G., Arveiler, D. *et al.* (2001). Interleukin-6 gene polymorphisms and susceptibility to myocardial infarction: the ECTIM study. *Journal of Molecular Medicine*, **79**, 300–5.

Gerdes, C., Fisher, R. M., Nicaud, V., Boer, J., Humphries, S. E., Talmud, P. J., and Faergeman, O. on behalf of the EARS Group (1997). Lipoprotein lipase variants D9N and N291S are associated with increased plasma triglyceride and lower high-density lipoprotein cholesterol concentrations: studies in the fasting and post-prandial states; the European Atherosclerosis Research Studies. *Circulation*, **96** (3), 733–40.

Gerdes, L. U., Gerdes, C., Kervinen, K., Savolainen, M., Klausen, I. C., Hansen, P.S. *et al.* (2000). The apolipoprotein epsilon4 allele determines prognosis and the effect on prognosis of simvastatin in survivors of myocardial infarction: a substudy of the Scandinavian simvastatin survival study. *Circulation*, **101**, 1366–71.

Gudnason, V., Thormar, K., and Humphries, S. E. (1997). Interaction of the cholesterol ester transfer protein I405V polymorphism with alcohol consumption in smoking and non-smoking healthy men, and the effect on plasma HDL cholesterol and apoAI concentration. *Clinical Genetics*, **51**, 15–21.

Hixson, J. E. (1991). Apolipoprotein E polymorphisms affect atherosclerosis in young males. Pathobiological Determinants of Atherosclerosis in Youth (PDAY) Research Group. *Arteriosclerosis and Thrombosis*, **11**, 1237–44.

Hokanson, J. E. and Austin, M. A. (1996). Plasma triglyceride level is a risk factor for cardiovascular disease independent of high-density lipoprotein cholesterol level: a meta-analysis of population-based prospective studies. *Journal of Cardiovascular Risk*, **3**, 213–19.

Humphries, S. E., Thomas, A., Montgomery, H. E., Green, F., Winder, A., and Miller, G. (1997). Gene-environment interaction in the determination of plasma levels of fibrinogen. *Fibrinolysis & Proteolysis*, **11** (1), 3–7.

Humphries, S. E., Luong, L-A., Ogg, M. S., Hawe, E., and Miller, G. (2001*a*). The interleukin-6−174C > G promoter polymorphism is associated with risk of coronary artery disease and systolic blood pressure in healthy men. *European Heart Journal*, **22**, 2243–52.

Humphries, S. E., Talmud, P. J., Hawe, E., Bolla, M., Day, I. N., and Miller, G. J. (2001*b*). Apolipoprotein E4 and coronary heart disease in middle-aged men who smoke: a prospective study. *Lancet*, **358**, 115–19.

Ioannidis, J. P., Ntzani, E. E., Trikalinos, T. A., and Contopoulos-Ioannidis, D. G. (2001). Replication validity of genetic association studies. *Nature Genetics*, **29**, 306–9.

Iso, H., Folsom, A., Winklemann, J.C., Koike, K. *et al.* (1995). Polymorphisms of the beta fibrinogen gene and plasma fibrinogen concentration in Caucasian and Japanese population samples. *Thrombosis and Haemostasis*, **73**, 106–11.

Jolivalt, C., Leininger-Muller, B., Bertrand, P., Herber, R., Christen, Y., and Siest, G. (2000). Differential oxidation of apolipoprotein E isoforms and interaction with phospholipids. *Free Radical Biology and Medicine*, **28**, 129–40.

Jones, K. G., Brull, D. J., Brown, L. C., Sian, M., Greenhalgh, R. M., Humphries, S. E., and Powell, J. T. (2001). Interleukin-6 (IL-6) and the prognosis of abdominal aortic aneurysms. *Circulation*, **103**, 2260–5.

Kessler, C., Spitzer, C., Stauske, D., Mende, S., Stadlmuller, J., Walther, R., and Rettig, R. (1997). The apolipoprotein E and beta-fibrinogen G/A-455 gene polymorphisms are associated with ischemic stroke involving large-vessel disease. *Arteriosclerosis, Thrombosis, and Vascular Biology*, **17**, 2880–4.

Khoury, M. J. and Wagener, D. K. (1995). Epidemiological evaluation of the use of genetics to improve the predictive value of disease risk factors. *American Journal of Human Genetics*, **56** (4), 835–44.

Li, R., Boerwinkle, E., Olshan, A. F., Chambless, L. E., Pankow, J. S., Tyroler, H. A. *et al.* (2000). Glutathione S-transferase genotype as a susceptibility factor in smoking-related coronary heart disease. *Atherosclerosis*, **149**, 451–62.

Li, R., Folsom, A. R., Sharrett, A. R., Couper, D., Bray, M., and Tyroler, H. A. (2001). Interaction of the glutathione S-transferase genes and cigarette smoking on risk of lower extremity arterial disease: the Atherosclerosis Risk in Communities (ARIC) study. *Atherosclerosis*, **154**, 729–38.

Lowe, G. D. (1993). Blood viscosity and cardiovascular risk. *Current Opinion in Lipidology*, **4**, 283–7.

Ma, J., Stampfer, M.J., Hennekens, C. H. *et al.* (1996). Methylenetetrahydrofolate reductase polymorphism, plasma folate, homocysteine, and risk of myocardial infarction in US physicians. *Circulation*, **94**, 2410–16.

Meade, T. W., Mellows, S., Brozovic, M. *et al.* (1986). Haemostatic function and ischaemic heart disease: principal results of the Northwick Park Heart Study. *Lancet*, **ii**, 533–7.

Montgomery, H., Clarkson, P., Dollery, C. M. *et al.* (1997). Association of angiotensin-converting enzyme gene I/D polymorphism with change in left ventricular mass in response to physical training. *Circulation*, **96** (3), 741–7.

Montgomery, H. E., Clarkson, P., Nwose, O. M. *et al.* (1996). The acute rise in serum fibrinogen concentration with exercise is influenced by the G-453-A polymorphism of the beta-fibrinogen gene. *Arteriosclerosis, Thrombosis, and Vascular Biology*, **16**, 386–91.

Myerson, S. G., Montgomery, H. E., Whittingham, M., Jubb, M., World, M. J., Humphries, S. E., and Pennell, D. J. (2001). Left ventricular hypertrophy with exercise and the angiotensin converting enzyme gene I/D polymorphism: a randomised controlled trial with losartan. *Circulation*, **103**, 226–30.

Ordovas, J. M. and Schaefer, E. J. (2000). Genetic determinants of plasma lipid response to dietary intervention: the role of the APOA1/C3/A4 gene cluster and the APOE gene. *British Journal of Nutrition*, **83** (1), 127–36.

Palinski, W., Ord, V. A., Plump, A. S., Breslow, J. L., Steinberg, D., and Witztum, J. L. (1994). ApoE-deficient mice are a model of lipoprotein oxidation in atherogenesis: demonstration of oxidation-specific epitopes in lesions and high titers of autoantibodies to malondialdehyde-lysine in serum. *Arteriosclerosis, Thrombosis, and Vascular Biology*, **14**, 605–16.

Plump, A. S., Smith, J. D., Hayek, T., Aalto Setala, K., Walsh, A., Verstuyft, J. G. *et al.* (1992). Severe hypercholesterolemia and atherosclerosis in apolipoprotein E-deficient mice created by homologous recombination in ES cells. *Cell*, **71**, 343–53.

Pratico, D., Tangirala, R. K., Rader, D. J., Rokach, J., and FitzGerald, G. A. (1998). Vitamin E suppresses isoprostane generation in vivo and reduces atherosclerosis in ApoE-deficient mice. *Nature Medicine*, **4**, 1189–1192.

Ridker, P. M., Hennekens, C. H., Buring, J. E., Sc, D., and Rifai, N. (2000*a*). C-reactive protein and other markers of inflammation in the prediction of cardiovascular disease in women. *New England Journal of Medicine*, **342** (12), 836–43.

Ridker, P. M., Rifai, N., Stampfer, M. J., and Hennekens, C. H. (2000*b*). Plasma concentration of interleukin-6 and the risk of future myocardial infarction among apparently healthy men. *Circulation*, **101**, 1767–72.

Ross, R. (1999). Atherosclerosis: an inflammatory disease. *New England Journal of Medicine*, **340** (2), 115–26.

Rus, H. G., Vlaicu, R., and Niculescu, F. (1996). Interleukin-6 and interleukin-8 protein and gene expression in human arterial atherosclerotic wall. *Atherosclerosis*, **127** (2), 263–71.

Sigurdsson, G. Jr., Gudnason, V., Sigurdsson, G., and Humphries, S. E. (1992). Interaction between a polymorphisms of the apo A-I promoter region and smoking determines plasma levels of HDL and apo A-I. *Arteriosclerosis, Thrombosis, and Vascular Biology*, **12**, 1017–22.

Smith, J. D., Miyata, M., Poulin, S. E., Neveux, L. M., and Craig, W. Y. (1998). The relationship between apolipoprotein E and serum oxidation-related variables is apolipoprotein E phenotype dependent. *International Journal of Clinical and Laboratory Research*, **28**, 116–21.

Talmud, P., Bujac, S. R., Hall, S., Miller, G. J., and Humphries, S. E. (2000). Substitution of asparagine for aspartic acid at residue 9 (D9N) of lipoprotein lipase markedly augments risk of CAD in male smokers. *Atherosclerosis*, **149**, 75–81.

Terry, C. F., Loukaci, V., and Green, F. R. (2000). Cooperative influence of genetic polymorphisms on interleukin 6 transcriptional regulation. *Journal of Biological Chemistry*, **275** (24), 18138–44.

Tybjaerg Hansen, A., Agerholm Larsen, B., Humphries, S., Abildgaard, S., Schnohr, P., and Nordestgaard, B. G. (1997). A common mutation (G-455-A) in the beta-fibrinogen is an independent predictor of plasma fibrinogen, a risk factor for ischemic heart disease. *Journal of Clinical Investigation*, **99**, 3034–9.

Wallace, A. J., Mann, J. I., Sutherland, W. H. F., Williams, S., Chisholm, A., Skeaff, M. *et al.* (2000). Variants in the cholesterol ester transfer protein and lipoprotein lipase genes are predictors of plasma cholesterol response to dietary change. *Atherosclerosis*, **15**, 327–36.

Waterworth, D. M., Talmud, P. J., Bujac, S. R., Fisher, R. M., Miller, G. J., and Humphries, S. E. (2000). The contribution of apoCIII variants to the determination of triglyceride levels and interaction with smoking in middle-aged men. *Arteriosclerosis, Thrombosis, and Vascular Biology*, **20**, 2663–9.

Wilson, P. W., Abbott, R. D., Castelli, W. P. *et al.* (1996). High density lipoprotein cholesterol and mortality. *Arteriosclerosis*, **276**, 544–8.

Wilson, P. W., D'Agostino, R. B., Levy, D., Belanger, A. M., Silbershatz, H., and Kannel, W. B. (1998). Prediction of coronary heart disease using risk factor categories. *Circulation*, **97** (18), 1837–47.

Wilson, P. W., Schaefer, E. J., Larson, M. G., and Ordovas, J. M. (1996). Apolipoprotein E alleles and risk of coronary disease: a meta- analysis. *Arteriosclerosis, Thrombosis, and Vascular Biology*, **16**, 1250–5.

Yudkin, J. S., Kumari, M., Humphries, S. E., and Mohamed-Ali, V. (2000). Inflammation, obesity, stress and coronary heart disease: is interleukin-6 the link? *Atherosclerosis*, **148**, 209–14.

Section III

Aetiology

III.II Life course

Chapter 32

The developmental origins of coronary heart disease

D. J. P. Barker

32.1 Introduction

Until recently the search for the causes of coronary heart disease (CHD), and the way to prevent it, has been guided by a 'destructive' model. The principal causes to be identified are thought to act in adult life and to accelerate destructive processes, for example the formation of atheroma, rise in blood pressure, and loss of glucose tolerance. This model, however, has had limited success. Obesity, cigarette smoking, and psychosocial stress have been implicated, and evidence on dietary fat has accumulated to the point where a public health policy of reduced intake is prudent, if not proven. The effects of modifying adult lifestyle, when formally tested in randomized trials have, however, been disappointingly small (Ebrahim and Davey Smith 1997). The model has proved incapable of answering important questions. For example, in Western countries the steep increase in the disease has been associated with rising prosperity, so why do the poorest people in the poorest places now have the highest rates?

32.2 Developmental origins

The recent discovery that people who develop CHD grew differently to other people during fetal life and childhood has led to a new 'developmental' model for the disease (Barker *et al.* 1989). To explore the developmental origins of chronic disease required studies of a kind that had not hitherto been carried out. It was necessary to identify groups of men and women now in middle–late life, whose size at birth had been recorded at the time. Their birthweight could thereby be related to the later occurrence of CHD. In Hertfordshire, from 1911 onwards, when women had their babies they were attended by a midwife, who recorded the birthweight. A health visitor went to the baby's home at intervals throughout infancy, and the weight at 1 year was recorded. Table 32.1 shows the findings in 10 636 men born during the period 1911–30. Standardized mortality ratios for CHD fell with increasing birthweight. There were stronger trends with weight at 1 year.

A subsequent study confirmed a similar trend with birthweight among women, but no trend with weight at 1 year (Osmond *et al.* 1993). Table 32.2 shows findings for the first sample of men to have glucose tolerance tests (Hales *et al.* 1991). The percentage with impaired glucose tolerance or type 2 diabetes fell steeply with increasing birthweight, and with weight at 1 year. There were similar trends with birthweight among women.

The association between low birthweight and CHD has now been replicated among men and women in Europe, North America, and India (Forsén *et al.* 1997, 1999; Frankel *et al.* 1996; Leon *et al.* 1998; Rich-Edwards *et al.* 1997; Stein *et al.* 1996). The association between low weight

Table 32.1 Hazard ratios (95% CI) for death from CHD according to birthweight and weight at 1 year in 10 636 men in Hertfordshire

Weight (lb)	Death from CHD	
	Before 65 years	All ages
Birthweight		
≤5.5 (*n* = 486)	1.50 (0.98–2.31)	1.37 (1.00–1.86)
−6.5 (*n* = 1385)	1.27 (0.89–1.83)	1.29 (1.01–1.66)
−7.5 (*n* = 3162)	1.17 (0.84–1.63)	1.14 (0.91–1.44)
−8.5 (*n* = 3308)	1.07 (0.77–1.49)	1.12 (0.89–1.40)
−9.5 (*n* = 1564)	0.96 (0.66–1.39)	0.97 (0.75–1.25)
≥10 (*n* = 731)	1.00	1.00
p for trend	0.001	0.005
1 year old		
18 (*n* = 715)	2.22 (1.33–3.73)	1.89 (1.34–2.66)
−20 (*n* = 1806)	1.80 (1.11–2.93)	1.58 (1.15–2.16)
−22 (*n* = 3404)	1.96 (1.23–3.12)	1.66 (1.23–2.25)
−24 (*n* = 2824)	1.52 (0.95–2.45)	1.36 (1.00–1.85)
−26 (*n* = 1391)	1.36 (0.82–2.26)	1.29 (0.93–1.78)
>27 (*n* = 496)	1.00	1.00
p for trend	<0.001	<0.001

Table 32.2 Percentage of men aged 64 with impaired glucose tolerance or diabetes according to birthweight and weight at age 1 year in 370 men

	% (*n*) of men with 2-h glucose (mmol/l) of ≥7.8	Odds ratio (95% CI)[a]
Birthweight (lb)		
<5.5 (*n* = 20)	40	6.6 (1.5–28)
−6.5 (*n* = 47)	34	4.8 (1.3–17)
−7.5 (*n* = 104)	31	4.6 (1.4–16)
−8.5 (*n* = 117)	22	2.6 (0.8–8.9)
−9.5 (*n* = 54)	13	1.4 (0.3–5.6)
>9.5 (*n* = 28)	14	1.0
p for trend	<0.001	
Weight at age 1 year (lb)		
<18 (*n* = 23)	43	8.2 (1.8–38)
−20 (*n* = 63)	32	4.8 (1.2–19)
−22 (*n* = 107)	30	4.2 (1.1–16)
−24 (*n* = 105)	18	2.1 (0.5–7.9)
−26 (*n* = 48)	19	2.1 (0.5–9.0)
>27 (*n* = 24)	13	1.0
p for trend	<0.001	

[a] Adjusted for BMI.

gain in infancy and CHD in men has been confirmed in Helsinki (Eriksson *et al.* 2001). Low birthweight has been shown to predict altered glucose tolerance in studies around the world (Forsén *et al.* 2000; Lithell *et al.* 1996; McCance *et al.* 1994; Newsome *et al.* 2003; Rich-Edwards *et al.* 1999).

32.3 **Confounding variables**

These findings suggest that influences linked to early growth have an important effect on the risk of CHD and type 2 diabetes. It has been argued, however, that people whose growth was impaired *in utero* and during infancy may continue to be exposed to an adverse environment in childhood and adult life, and it is this later environment that produces the effects attributed to intrauterine influences. There is now strong evidence that this argument cannot be sustained.

In a number of studies, data on lifestyle, including smoking habits, employment, alcohol consumption, and exercise were collected. In the Nurses' Health Study in the USA allowance for these influences had little effect on the association between birthweight and CHD (Rich-Edwards *et al.* 1997). Similar results came from Sweden and the UK (Frankel *et al.* 1996; Leon *et al.* 1998). In studies of type 2 diabetes and blood pressure the associations with size at birth are again independent of social class, cigarette smoking, and alcohol consumption. Adult lifestyle, however, adds to the effects of early life: for example, the prevalence of impaired glucose tolerance is highest in people who had low birthweight but became obese as adults (Hales *et al.* 1991). As described later in this chapter, slow fetal growth may also alter the body's response to socio-economic influences in later life. Associations between low birthweight and altered glucose tolerance and raised blood pressure have been found in numerous studies of children, which is a further argument against these associations being the product of confounding variables in adult life.

32.4 **Biological basis**

Like other living creatures in their early life, human beings are 'plastic' and able to adapt to their environment. The development of the sweat glands provides a simple example of this. All humans have similar numbers of sweat glands at birth, but none of them function. In the first 3 years after birth a proportion of the glands become functional, depending on the temperature to which the child is exposed. The hotter the conditions, the greater the number of sweat glands that are programmed to function. After 3 years the process is complete and the number of sweat glands is fixed. Thereafter, the child who has experienced hot conditions will be better equipped to adapt to similar conditions in later life, because people with more functioning sweat glands cool down faster.

This brief description encapsulates the essence of developmental plasticity: a critical period when a system is plastic and sensitive to the environment, followed by loss of plasticity and a fixed functional capacity. For most organs and systems the critical period occurs *in utero*. There are good reasons why it may be advantageous, in evolutionary terms, for the body to remain plastic during development. It enables the production of phenotypes that are better matched to their environment than would be possible if the same phenotype was produced in all environments. Developmental plasticity is defined as the phenomenon by which one genotype can give rise to a range of different physiological or morphological states in response to different environmental conditions during development (West-Eberhard 1989). Plasticity during intrauterine life enables animals, and humans, to receive a 'weather forecast' from their mothers that prepares them for the type of world in which they will have to live (Bateson and Martin 1999). If the mother is poorly nourished she signals to her unborn baby that the environment it is about to enter is likely to be harsh. The baby responds to these signals by adaptations, such as reduced body size and altered metabolism, which help it to survive a shortage of food after birth. In this way plasticity gives a species the ability to make short-term adaptations, within one generation, in addition to the long-term genetic adaptations that come from natural selection. Since, as Mellanby (1933) noted long ago, the ability of a human mother to nourish her baby is partly determined when she herself is *in utero*, and by her childhood growth, the human fetus is receiving a 'weather forecast' based not only on conditions at the time of the pregnancy, but also on conditions a number of decades before. This may be advantageous in places which experience periodic food shortages.

Until recently we have overlooked a growing body of evidence that systems of the body which are closely related to adult disease, such as the regulation of blood pressure, are also plastic during early development. In animals it is surprisingly easy to produce lifelong changes in the blood pressure and metabolism of a fetus by minor modifications to the diet of the mother before and during pregnancy (Kwong *et al.* 2000; Widdowson and McCance 1963).

The different size of newborn human babies exemplifies plasticity. The growth of babies has to be constrained by the size of the mother, otherwise normal birth could not occur. Small women have small babies: in pregnancies after ovum donation they have small babies even if the woman donating the egg is large (Brooks *et al.* 1995). Babies may be small because their growth is constrained in this way or because they lack the nutrients for growth. As McCance (1962) wrote long ago, 'The size attained in utero depends on the services which the mother is able to supply. These are mainly food and accommodation.' Since mother's height or pelvic dimensions are generally not found to be important predictors of the baby's long-term health, research into the developmental origins of disease has focused on the nutrient supply to the baby, while recognizing that other influences such as hypoxia and stress also influence fetal growth. This focus on fetal nutrition was endorsed in a recent review (Harding 2001). In developing countries many babies are undernourished because their mothers are chronically malnourished. Despite current levels of nutrition in Western countries, the nutrition of many fetuses and infants remains suboptimal, because the nutrients available are unbalanced or because their delivery is constrained by the long and vulnerable fetal supply line. Around the world size at birth in relation to gestational age is a marker of fetal nutrition (Harding 2001).

32.5 Fetal origins hypothesis

The fetal origins hypothesis proposes that CHD, type 2 diabetes, stroke, and hypertension originate in developmental plasticity, in response to undernutrition during fetal life and infancy (Barker 1995; Barker *et al.* 2002a). Why should fetal responses to undernutrition lead to disease in later life? The general answer is clear. 'Life history theory', which embraces all living things, states that, during development, increased allocation of energy to one trait such as brain growth necessarily reduces allocation to one or more other traits, such as tissue repair processes. Smaller babies, who have had a lesser allocation of energy, must incur higher costs, and these it seems include disease in later life. A more specific answer to the question is that people who were small at birth are vulnerable to later disease through three kinds of process. First, they have fewer cells in key organs such as the kidney. One theory holds that hypertension is initiated by the reduced number of nephrons found in people who were small at birth (Brenner and

Chertow 1993). A reduced number necessarily leads to increased blood flow through each glomerulus. Over time this hyperfiltration is thought to lead to the development of glomerulosclerosis which, combined with the loss of nephrons that accompanies normal ageing, leads to accelerated age-related loss of glomeruli, and a self-perpetuating cycle of rising blood pressure and glomerular loss. Direct evidence in support of this hypothesis has come from a study of the kidneys of people killed in road accidents. Those being treated for hypertension had fewer but larger glomeruli (Keller *et al.* 2003).

Another process by which slow fetal growth may be linked to later disease is in the setting of hormones and metabolism. An undernourished baby may establish a 'thrifty' way of handling food. Insulin resistance, which is associated with low birthweight, may be viewed as persistence of a fetal response by which blood glucose concentrations were maintained for the benefit of the brain, but at the expense of glucose transport into the muscles and muscle growth (Phillips 1996).

A third link between low birthweight and later disease is that people who were small at birth are more vulnerable to adverse environmental influences in later life. Observations on animals show that the environment during development permanently changes not only the body's structure and function, but also its responses to environmental influences encountered in later life (Bateson and Martin 1999). Table 32.3 shows the effect of low income in adult life on CHD among men in Helsinki (Barker *et al.* 2001). As expected, men who had a low taxable income had higher rates of the disease. There is no agreed explanation for this, but the association between poverty and CHD is a major component of the social inequalities in health in many Western countries. Among the men in Helsinki the association was confined to those who had slow fetal growth and were thin at birth, defined by a ponderal index (birthweight/length^3) of less than 26 kg/m^3 (Table 32.3). Men who were not thin at birth were resilient to the effects of low income on CHD.

One explanation of these findings emphasizes the psychosocial consequences of a low position in the social hierarchy, as indicated by low income and social class, and suggests that perceptions of low social status and lack of success lead to changes in neuroendocrine pathways and hence to disease (Marmot and Wilkinson 2001). The findings in Helsinki seem consistent with this. People who are small at birth are known to have persisting alterations in responses to stress, including raised serum cortisol concentrations (Phillips *et al.* 2000). It is suggested that persisting small elevations of serum cortisol concentrations over many years may have effects

Table 32.3 Hazard ratios (95% CI) for CHD in 3629 men according to ponderal index at birth and taxable income in adult life

Household income (£/year)	Ponderal index (birthweight/length^3)	
	≤26.0 kg/m^3 (n = 1475)	>26.0 kg/m^3 (n = 2154)
>15 700	1.00	1.19 (0.65–2.19)
15 700	1.54 (0.83–2.87)	1.42 (0.78–2.57)
12 400	1.07 (0.51–2.22)	1.66 (0.90–3.07)
10 700	2.07 (1.13–3.79)	1.44 (0.79–2.62)
≤8 400	2.58 (1.45–4.60)	1.37 (0.75–2.51)
p for trend	<0.001	0.75

similar to those seen when tumours lead to more sudden, large increases in circulating glucocorticoid concentrations. People with Cushing's syndrome are insulin resistant and have raised blood pressure, both of which predispose to CHD.

32.6 **Childhood growth and CHD**

Figure 32.1 shows the growth of 357 men who were either admitted to hospital with CHD or died from it (Eriksson *et al.* 2001). They belong to a cohort of 4630 men who were born in Helsinki, and their growth is expressed as Z-scores. The Z-score for the cohort is set at zero, and a boy maintaining a steady position as large or small in relation to other boys would follow a horizontal path on the figure. Boys who later developed CHD, however, were small at birth, remained small in infancy, but had accelerated gain in weight and body mass index (BMI) thereafter. In contrast, their heights remained below average. Table 32.4 shows that, as in Hertfordshire, the hazard ratios for CHD fell with increasing weight at 1 year. Whereas in Hertfordshire measurements at 1 year were restricted to weight, in Helsinki length was also recorded. Table 32.4 shows that hazard ratios for CHD fell with increasing length and, more strongly, with BMI. Small size at this age predicted CHD independently of size at birth. There therefore appear to be at least two pathways of development that lead to CHD among men in this cohort. One begins with slow growth *in utero*, and low birthweight and thinness at birth, thought to be a consequence of fetal undernutrition. The other begins with poor weight gain during infancy, which is associated with two markers of poor living conditions, low parental socio-economic status and over-crowding in the home. The effect of rapid weight gain after infancy, shown in Fig. 32.1, is con-fined to men on the first pathway. Rapid weight gain has no effect on the risk of disease among men following the second pathway (Eriksson *et al.* 2001).

Among the 4130 girls in the same birth cohort, the 87 who later developed CHD showed a broadly similar pattern of growth to the boys (Forsén *et al.* 2004). They were, however, short at birth rather than thin. They had rapid height growth in infancy, but became thin. This persist-ed up to the age of 4 years, after which they gained weight rapidly. In both sexes disease risk was related to the tempo of weight gain rather than to body size at any particular age.

Table 32.5 shows hazard ratios for CHD according to birthweight and fourths of BMI at age 11 years among 13 517 men and women in Helsinki representing the combined older and younger birth cohorts, born during 1924–33 and 1934–44 (Barker *et al.* 2002a). The risks of

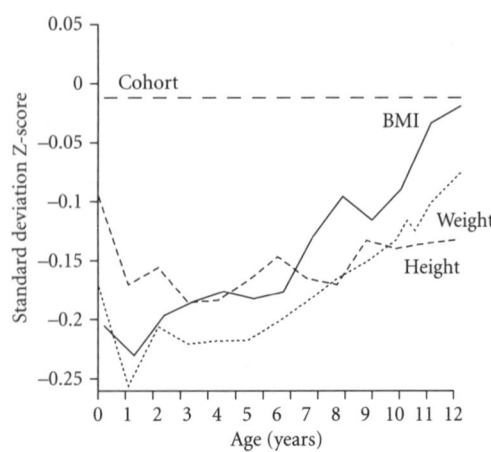

Fig. 32.1 Mean Z-scores for height, weight, and BMI during childhood in 357 boys who later developed CHD within a cohort of 4630 boys. At any age, the mean Z-score for the cohort is set at 0, while the standard deviation is set at 1.

Table 32.4 Hazard ratios for CHD according to body size at 1 year in 4630 men in Helsinki

	Hazard ratio (95% CI)	No. of cases/No. of men
Weight (kg)		
−9	1.82 (1.25–2.64)	96/781
−10	1.17 (0.80–1.71)	85/1126
−11	1.12 (0.77–1.64)	89/1243
−12	0.94 (0.62–1.44)	49/852
>12	1.00	38/619
p for trend	<0.0001	
Height (cm)		
−73	1.55 (1.11–2.18)	79/636
−75	0.90 (0.63–1.27)	68/962
−77	0.94 (0.68–1.31)	87/1210
−79	0.83 (0.58–1.18)	64/1011
>79	1.00	59/802
p for trend	0.007	
BMI (kg/m²)		
≤16	1.83 (1.28–2.60)	72/654
−17	1.61 (1.15–2.25)	89/936
−18	1.29 (0.91–1.81)	83/1136
−19	1.12 (0.77–1.62)	59/941
>19	1.00	54/954
p for trend	0.0004	

Table 32.5 Hazard ratios for CHD according to birthweight and BMI at 11 years among 13 517 men and women

Birthweight (kg)	BMI at 11 years (kg/m²)			
	−15.7	−16.6	−17.6	>17.6
No. of men and women				
−3.0	991	719	581	560
−3.5	1394	1422	1264	1246
−4.0	827	984	1122	1110
>4.0	167	254	413	463
Hospital admissions and deaths (1235 cases)				
−3.0	1.4	1.6	1.8	2.1
−3.5	1.3	1.5	1.5	1.6
−4.0	1.3	1.4	1.3	1.4
>4.0	1.0	1.2	1.1	1.0
Deaths (480 cases)				
−3.0	1.4	1.8	2.1	3.0
−3.5	1.4	1.9	2.2	2.7
−4.0	1.9	1.8	1.7	1.6
>4.0	1.0	1.4	1.6	1.3

disease fell with increasing birthweight and rose with increasing BMI. The pattern was similar in the two sexes.

32.7 Type 2 diabetes and hypertension

People who were small at birth remain biologically different from people who were larger, and these differences include an increased susceptibility to hypertension and type 2 diabetes. Table 32.6 is based on the same cohort of men and women shown in Table 32.5, and again shows odds ratios according to birthweight and fourths of BMI at age 11 years. The two disorders are associated with the same general pattern of growth as CHD (Barker *et al.* 2002*a*). Risk of disease falls with increasing birthweight and rises with increasing BMI.

Associations between low birthweight and type 2 diabetes, shown in Table 32.2, have been found in other studies (Forsén *et al.* 2000; Hales *et al.* 1991; Lithell *et al.* 1996; McCance *et al.* 1994; Newsome *et al.* 2003; Rich-Edwards *et al.* 1999). The association with hypertension has also been found elsewhere (Curhan *et al.* 1996). There is a substantial literature showing that birthweight is associated with differences in blood pressure and insulin sensitivity within the normal range (Hales *et al.* 1991; Huxley *et al.* 2000; Lithell *et al.* 1996; Newsome *et al.* 2003). These differences are found in children and adults, but they tend to be small. A 1 kg difference in birthweight is associated with ~3 mmHg difference in systolic pressure. The contrast between this small effect and the large effect on hypertension (Table 32.6) suggests that lesions that accompany poor fetal growth and tend to elevate blood pressure, which may include a reduced number of nephrons, have a small influence on blood pressure within the normal range because counter-regulatory mechanisms maintain normal blood pressure levels. As the lesions progress, however, these mechanisms are no longer able to maintain homeostasis and blood pressure rises. There may be a cycle of rise in blood pressure resulting in further progression of the lesions and further rise in blood pressure (Ingelfinger 2003). Evidence to support the development of self-perpetuating cycles comes from a study of elderly people in Helsinki among whom the effect of birthweight on blood pressure was confined to those being treated for hypertension (Ylihärsilä *et al.* 2003). Despite their treatment, the blood pressures of those

Table 32.6 Odds ratios (95% CI) for type 2 diabetes and hypertension according to birthweight and BMI at 11 years among 13 517 men and women

Birthweight (kg)	BMI at 11 years (kg/m²)			
	−15.7	−16.6	−17.6	>17.6
Type 2 diabetes (698 cases)				
−3.0	1.3 (0.6–2.8)	1.3 (0.6–2.8)	1.5 (0.7–3.4)	2.5 (1.2–5.5)
−3.5	1.0 (0.5–2.1)	1.0 (0.5–2.1)	1.5 (0.7–3.2)	1.7 (0.8–3.5)
−4.0	1.0 (0.5–2.2)	0.9 (0.4–1.9)	0.9 (0.4–2.0)	1.7 (0.8–3.6)
>4.0	1.0	1.1 (0.4–2.7)	0.7 (0.3–1.7)	1.2 (0.5–2.7)
Hypertension (2997 cases)				
−3.0	2.0 (1.3–3.2)	1.9 (1.2–3.1)	1.9 (1.2–3.0)	2.3 (1.5–3.8)
−3.5	1.7 (1.1–2.6)	1.9 (1.2–2.9)	1.9 (1.2–3.0)	2.2 (1.4–3.4)
−4.0	1.7 (1.0–2.6)	1.7 (1.1–2.6)	1.5 (1.0–2.4)	1.9 (1.2–2.9)
>4.0	1.0	1.9 (1.1–3.1)	1.0 (0.6–1.7)	1.7 (1.1–2.8)

Odds ratios adjusted for sex and year of birth.

who had low birthweight were markedly higher, whereas among the normotensive subjects birthweight was unrelated to blood pressure. Whether measured in the clinic or by ambulatory methods, there was a more than 20 mmHg difference in systolic pressure between those who weighed 2500 g (5.5 lb) or less at birth and those who weighed 4000 g (8.8 lb) or more. An inference is that by the time they reached old age most of the people with lesions acquired *in utero* had developed clinical hypertension. Studies in South Carolina bear on this issue. They showed that among 3236 hypertensive patients the blood pressures of those with low birth-weight tended to be more difficult to control (Lackland *et al.* 2002).

Figure 32.2 shows the growth of boys and girls who later developed type 2 diabetes, in the younger Helsinki cohort. They had below average body size at birth and at 1 year, after which their weights and body mass indices rose progressively to exceed the average (Eriksson *et al.* 2003).

Table 32.7 shows the relation between age at 'adiposity rebound' and later type 2 diabetes. After the age of 2 years the degree of obesity of young children, as measured by BMI, decreases to a minimum at ~6 years of age before increasing again – the so-called adiposity rebound.

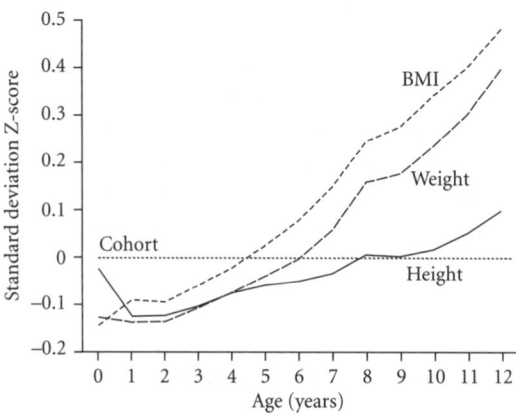

Fig. 32.2 Mean Z-scores for height, weight, and BMI during childhood in 290 boys and girls who later developed type 2 diabetes within a cohort of 8760 children. At any age, the mean Z-score for the cohort is set at 0 while the standard deviation is set at 1.

Table 32.7 BMI at 11 years of age and cumulative incidence of type 2 diabetes according to age at adiposity rebound in 8760 men and women

Age at adiposity rebound (years)	Mean BMI (kg/m²) at 11 years	Cumulative incidence of diabetes % (n)		
		Men	**Women**	**All**
≤4	19.7	8.1 (86)	8.9 (112)	8.6 (198)
5	17.6	6.2 (904)	2.5 (864)	4.4 (1768)
6	17.0	3.7 (1861)	2.5 (1456)	3.2 (3317)
7	16.8	2.4 (249)	2.1 (243)	2.2 (492)
≥8	16.7	3.0 (135)	0.7 (150)	1.8 (285)
p for trend	<0.001	<0.001	0.002	<0.001

Figures in parentheses are numbers of subjects.

The age at adiposity rebound ranges from around 3 years to 8 years or more. Table 32.7 shows that early adiposity rebound is strongly related to a high BMI in later childhood, as has previously been shown (Rolland-Cachera et al. 1987). It also predicts an increased incidence of type 2 diabetes in later life. This new observation has now been replicated in a longitudinal study in Delhi, India (Bhargava 2004). In both studies an early adiposity rebound was found to be associated with thinness at birth and at 1 year (Eriksson et al. 2003). It is not, therefore, the young child who is overweight who is at greatest risk of type 2 diabetes, but the one who is thin but subsequently gains weight rapidly.

32.8 Compensatory growth

When undernutrition during early development is followed by improved nutrition, many animals and plants stage accelerated or 'compensatory' growth (Barker et al. 2002a). Compensatory growth has costs, however, which in animals include reduced life-span (Metcalfe and Monaghan 2001). There are a number of processes by which, in humans, undernutrition and small size at birth followed by rapid childhood growth could lead to cardiovascular disease and type 2 diabetes in later life (Eriksson et al. 2001; Forsén et al. 2000). Rapid growth may be associated with persisting hormonal and metabolic changes. Larger body size may increase the functional demand on functional capacity that has been reduced by slow early growth – fewer nephrons, for example. Rapid weight gain may lead to an unfavourable body composition. Babies that are small and thin at birth lack muscle, a deficiency which will persist as the critical period for muscle growth occurs in utero and there is little cell replication after birth (Widdowson et al. 1972). If they develop a high body mass during later childhood they may have a disproportionately high fat mass in relation to lean body mass, which will lead to insulin resistance (Eriksson et al. 2002a).

32.9 Pathways to disease

New studies, especially the Helsinki studies with their detailed information on child growth and socio-economic circumstances, increasingly suggest that the pathogenesis of CHD and the disorders related to it depend on a series of interactions occurring at different stages of development. To begin with the effects of the genes acquired at conception may be conditioned by the early environment. Table 32.8 is based on a study of 476 elderly people in Helsinki (Eriksson et al. 2002b). It shows mean fasting plasma insulin concentrations according to which of two polymorphisms of the PPAR-γ (peroxisome proliferator-activated receptor) gene was present. The Pro12Pro polymorphism is known to be associated with insulin resistance, indicated by elevated fasting plasma insulin concentrations. Table 32.8 shows, however, that this effect occurs only among men and women who had low birthweight. Conversely, low birthweight has been consistently linked to later insulin resistance (Newsome et al. 2003), but Table 32.8 shows that this effect occurs only among people with the Pro12Pro polymorphism. As birthweight serves as a marker of fetal nutrition (Harding 2001), this gene–birthweight interaction may reflect a gene–nutrient interaction during development. Many such interactions are likely to be found in the future.

The effects of the intrauterine environment on later disease are conditioned not only by events at conception, but also by events after birth. Tables 32.5 and 32.6 showed how the effects are conditioned by childhood gain in BMI. Table 32.3 showed that the effects of low ponderal index at birth are conditioned by living conditions in adult life. Table 32.9 shows how the effects of low birthweight on later hypertension are conditioned by living conditions in childhood,

Table 32.8 Mean fasting insulin concentrations (*n*) in 476 elderly people according to PPAR-γ gene polymorphism and birthweight

	Birthweight (g)			*p* for difference
	−3000	−3500	>3500	
Fasting insulin (pmol/l)				
Pro12Pro (*n*)	84 (56)	71 (161)	65 (107)	0.003
Pro12Ala/Ala12Ala (*n*)	60 (37)	60 (67)	65 (48)	0.31
p for difference	0.008	0.02	0.99	

Table 32.9 Cumulative incidence (%) of hypertension according to birthweight and father's social class in 8760 men and women

Birthweight (g)	Father's social class			*p* for trend
	Labourer	Lower middle class	Upper middle class	
−3000	22.2	20.2	10.5	0.002
−3500	18.8	15.2	10.6	<0.001
−4000	14.5	12.5	10.3	0.04
>4000	11.1	15.6	15.7	0.11
p for trend	<0.001	0.05	0.79	

indicated by the occupational status of the father (Barker *et al.* 2002*b*). Among all the men and women low birthweight was associated with an increased incidence of hypertension, as has been shown before (Curhan *et al.* 1996). This association, however, was present only among those who were born into families where the father was a labourer or of lower middle-class.

It seems that the pathogenesis of cardiovascular disease and type 2 diabetes cannot be understood within a model in which risks associated with adverse influences at different stages of life add to each other (Kuh and Ben-Shlomo 1997). Rather disease is the product of branching paths of development. The branchings are triggered by the environment. The pathways determine vulnerability of each individual to what lies ahead. The pathway to CHD can originate either in slow fetal growth as a consequence of undernutrition, or in poor infant growth as a consequence of poor living conditions.

The effects of slow fetal growth and low birthweight, and the effects of postnatal development, depend on environmental influences and paths of development that precede and follow them. Low birthweight, or any other single influence, does not have 'an' effect that is best estimated by a pooled estimate from all published studies. A recent pooled estimate led to the conclusion that because the effects of birthweight on blood pressure within the normal range are small the effects on disease are small (Huxley *et al.* 2002). Such a conclusion is biologically fallacious for the reasons already described under 'developmental origins hypothesis'. It is also statistically fallacious because it discounts interactions of the kind described. As René Dubos wrote: 'the effects of the physical and social environments cannot be understood without knowledge of individual history' (*Mirage of health*, 1987). Unravelling disease causation, and hence the way to prevent it, will therefore require an understanding of heterogeneity.

32.10 **Strength of effects**

Low birthweight, though a convenient marker in epidemiological studies, is an inadequate description of the phenotypic characteristics of a baby that determine its long-term health. The wartime famine in Holland produced lifelong insulin resistance in babies who were *in utero* at the time, with little alteration in birthweight (Ravelli *et al.* 1998). In babies, as in children, slowing of growth is a response to a poor environment, especially undernutrition, but body size at birth does not adequately describe the long-term morphological and physiological consequences of undernutrition. The same birthweight can be attained by many different paths of fetal growth and each is likely to be accompanied by different gene–environment interactions (Harding 2001). Nevertheless, birthweight provides a basis for estimating the magnitude of the effects of the fetal phase of development on later disease, though it is likely to underestimate them.

Because the risk of cardiovascular disease is influenced both by small body size at birth and during infancy and by rapid weight gain in childhood, estimation of the risk of disease attributable to early development requires data on fetal, infant, and childhood growth. Currently the Helsinki studies are the main source of information (Barker *et al.* 2002a). Table 32.5 showed that men and women who had birthweights above 4 kg (8.8 lb) and whose prepubertal BMI was in the lowest fourth had around half the risk of CHD when compared with people who had birthweights below 3 kg (6.6 lb), but whose BMI was in the highest fourth. The hazard ratios for admissions and deaths were 0.80 (95% CI: 0.72–0.90) for each kilogram increase in birthweight and 1.06 (1.03–1.10) for each kg/m^2 increase in BMI at age 11 years. The hazard ratios for deaths alone were 0.83 (0.69–0.99) and 1.10 (1.04–1.16).

Table 32.10 is based on the younger Helsinki cohort, born 1934–44. Subjects are divided according to thirds of body size at birth and whether their standard deviation score for BMI decreased or increased between ages 3 and 11 years. Among men ponderal index at birth was more strongly related to CHD than birthweight; among women length at birth was stronger. If each man in the cohort had been in the highest third of ponderal index at birth, and each woman in the highest third of birth length, and if each man or woman had lowered their BMI score between ages 3 and 11 years, the incidence of CHD would have been reduced by 25% in men and 63% in women (Barker *et al.* 2002a).

Table 32.6 showed that men and women who had birthweights above 4 kg (8.8 lb) and whose prepubertal BMI was in the lowest fourth had around half the risk of type 2 diabetes and hypertension when compared with people who had birthweights below 3 kg (6.6 lb), but whose BMI was in the highest fourth. The odds ratio for type 2 diabetes was 0.67 (95% CI: 0.58–0.79) for each kilogram increase in birthweight and 1.18 (95% CI: 1.13–1.23) for each kg/m^2 increase in BMI at age 11 years. The corresponding figures for hypertension were 0.77 (95% CI: 0.71–0.84) and 1.07 (95% CI: 1.04–1.09).

In Table 32.11 subjects are again divided into six groups according to thirds of birthweight and whether their standard deviation score for BMI decreased or increased between ages 3 and 11 years. For both type 2 diabetes and hypertension there were independent effects of birthweight and change in BMI score. The patterns of odds ratios and incidence shown in Tables 32.6 and 32.11 were similar in the two sexes. Table 32.11 shows that the effect of increase in childhood BMI was greater for type 2 diabetes than for hypertension. If each individual in the cohort had been in the highest third of birthweight and had lowered their standard deviation score for BMI between 3 and 11 the incidence of type 2 diabetes would have been reduced by 52% and the incidence of hypertension by 25% (Barker *et al.* 2002a).

Table 32.10 Cumulative incidence, percent (no. of subjects), of CHD (hospital admissions and deaths) according to body size at birth and change in standard deviation score for BMI, 3–11 years of age, among 6345 men and women

Birth size	Change in standard deviation score for BMI, 3–11 years	
	Decrease	Increase
Men (279 cases)		
Birthweight (kg)		
−3.2	8.8 (512)	9.0 (476)
−3.6	6.9 (662)	11.3 (512)
>3.6	5.9 (740)	8.6 (521)
Ponderal index (kg/m³)		
−25	8.0 (411)	11.7 (394)
−27	7.6 (649)	10.8 (556)
>27	6.2 (838)	7.2 (539)
Women (66 cases)		
Birthweight (kg)		
−3.2	1.6 (563)	3.8 (604)
−3.6	1.5 (612)	2.5 (438)
>3.6	0.7 (450)	3.6 (334)
Birth length (cm)		
−49	1.5 (543)	4.2 (520)
−50	1.5 (452)	3.3 (338)
>50	0.8 (609)	2.6 (496)

Table 32.11 Cumulative incidence, percent (no. of subjects), of type 2 diabetes and hypertension according to birthweight and change in standard deviation score for BMI, 3–11 years of age, among 6424 men and women

Birthweight (kg)	Change in standard deviation score for BMI, 3–11 years	
	Decrease	Increase
Type 2 diabetes (227 cases)		
−3.2	3.1 (1075)	5.5 (1080)
−3.6	2.4 (1274)	4.3 (950)
>3.6	1.5 (1190)	5.4 (855)
Hypertension (1036 cases)		
−3.2	15.9 (1075)	21.3 (1080)
−3.6	14.8 (1274)	19.4 (950)
>3.6	12.0 (1190)	13.9 (855)

32.11 Maternal influences on fetal nutrition

Size at birth is the product of the fetus's trajectory of growth, which is set at an early stage in development, and the materno-placental capacity to supply sufficient nutrients to maintain that trajectory. In Western communities, randomized controlled trials of maternal macronutrient supplementation have had relatively small effects on birthweight (Kramer 1993). This has led to the view that regulatory mechanisms in the maternal and placental systems act to ensure that human fetal growth and development is little influenced by normal variations in maternal nutrient intake, and that there is a simple relationship between a woman's body composition and the growth of her fetus. Recent experimental studies in animals and observational data in humans challenge these concepts (Barker 1998). They suggest that a mother's own fetal growth and her dietary intakes and body composition can exert major effects on the balance between the fetal demand for nutrients and the materno-placental capacity to meet that demand. Specific issues that have not yet been adequately addressed include: (a) maternal effects on the trajectory of fetal growth; (b) intergenerational effects; (c) paradoxical effects on placental growth; (d) the importance of the mother's body composition and the balance of macronutrients in her diet.

32.11.1 The fetal growth trajectory

A rapid trajectory of growth increases the fetus's demand for nutrients. Though fetal demand for nutrients is greatest late in pregnancy, the magnitude of this demand is thought to be primarily determined by genetic and environmental effects on the trajectory of fetal growth, which is set at an early stage in development. Experimental studies of pregnant ewes have shown that, although a fast growth trajectory is generally associated with larger fetal size and improved neonatal survival, it renders the fetus more vulnerable to a reduced materno-placental supply of nutrients in late gestation. Thus, maternal undernutrition during the last trimester adversely affects the development of rapidly growing fetuses with high requirements, while having little effect on those growing more slowly (Harding *et al.* 1992). Rapidly growing fetuses were found to make a series of adaptations in order to survive, including fetal wasting and placental oxidation of fetal amino acids to maintain lactate output to the fetus (Barker 1998). Experiments in animals have shown that alterations in maternal diet around the time of conception can change the fetal growth trajectory. In a recent study, rats were fed a 9% casein low protein diet in the periconceptional period. This led to structural changes at the blastocyst stage of embryonic development, reduced fetal growth rates, small size at birth, and raised blood pressure in the offspring during adult life (Kwong *et al.* 2000). The sensitivity of the human embryo to its environment is being increasingly recognized with the development of assisted reproductive technology (Walker *et al.* 2000). The trajectory of fetal growth is thought to increase with improvements in periconceptional nutrition, and is faster in male fetuses. The consequent greater vulnerability of male fetuses to undernutrition may contribute to the higher death rates from CHD among men.

32.11.2 Intergenerational effects

Experimental studies in animals have shown that undernutrition can have effects on reproductive performance which may persist for several generations. Among rats fed a protein-deficient diet over 12 generations there was a progressive fall in fetal growth rates. When restored to a normal diet it took three generations before growth and development were normalized (Stewart *et al.* 1980).

Strong evidence for major intergenerational effects in humans has come from studies showing that a woman's birthweight influences the birthweight of her offspring (Emanuel *et al.* 1992). A study in the UK showed that whereas low birthweight mothers tended to have thin infants with a low ponderal index, the father's birthweight was unrelated to ponderal index at birth (Godfrey *et al.* 1997). The effect of maternal birthweight on thinness at birth is consistent with the hypothesis that in low birthweight mothers the fetal supply line is compromised and unable to meet fetal nutrient demand. Potential mechanisms underlying this effect include alterations in the uterine or systemic vasculature, changes in maternal metabolism, and impaired placentation.

32.11.3 Placental size and transfer capabilities

Though the size of the placenta gives only an indirect measure of its capacity to transfer nutrients to the fetus, it is nonetheless strongly associated with fetal size at birth. Experiments in sheep have shown that maternal nutrition in early pregnancy can exert major effects on the growth of the placenta, and thereby alter fetal development (Robinson *et al.* 1994). The effects produced depend on the nutritional status of the ewe in the periconceptional period. In ewes that were poorly nourished around the time of conception, low nutrient intakes in early pregnancy reduced the size of the placenta. Conversely, in ewes well nourished around the time of conception, low intakes in early pregnancy resulted in increased placental size (Robinson *et al.* 1994). Placental expansion may be an adaptation by the fetus to extract more nutrients from the mother; but seemingly it can only occur in previously well-nourished ewes. Although this suppression appears paradoxical, in sheep farming it is common practice for ewes to be put on rich pasture prior to mating and then on poor pasture for a period in early pregnancy.

There is evidence of a similar suppressive effect of high dietary intakes in early pregnancy on placental growth in humans (Godfrey *et al.* 1996). Among 538 women who delivered at term in Southampton, UK, those with high dietary intakes in early pregnancy, especially of carbohydrate, had smaller placentas, particularly if this was combined with low intakes of dairy protein in late pregnancy. These effects were independent of the mother's body size, social class, and smoking, and resulted in alterations in the ratio of placental weight to birthweight (placental ratio). Further evidence that maternal diet can alter placental growth has come from analyses of the Dutch famine, in which famine exposure in early pregnancy increased placental weight (Lumey 1998).

The U-shaped relation between the placental ratio and later CHD and raised blood pressure indicates that effects on placental growth may be of long-term importance (Barker *et al.* 1990; Martyn *et al.* 1996). Babies with a disproportionately small placenta may suffer as a consequence of an impaired placental supply capacity; those with a disproportionately large placenta may become catabolic and waste in order to supply amino acids for placental consumption (Robinson *et al.* 1995).

32.11.4 Maternal diet and body composition

Evidence supporting a long-term effect of levels of maternal nutrient intake during pregnancy has come from a follow-up study of children whose mothers took part in a randomized controlled trial of calcium supplementation in pregnancy in Argentina (Belizan *et al.* 1997). Supplementation was associated with lowering of the offspring's blood pressure in childhood, even though it was not associated with any change in birthweight. Follow-up studies following the Dutch famine of 1944–45 found that severe maternal caloric restriction at different stages of pregnancy was variously associated with obesity, dyslipidaemia, and insulin resistance in the offspring, and there is preliminary evidence of an increased risk of CHD (Ravelli *et al.* 1998; Roseboom *et al.* 2000*a, b*). Again, these effects were largely independent of size at birth.

In the Dutch studies, famine exposure per se was not associated with raised blood pressure in the offspring, but there was an effect of macronutrient balance. Maternal rations with a low protein density were associated with raised blood pressure in the adult offspring (Roseboom *et al.* 2001). This adds to the findings of studies in Aberdeen, UK, which showed that maternal diets with either a low or a high ratio of animal protein to carbohydrate were associated with raised blood pressure in the offspring during adult life (Campbell *et al.* 1996).

In the Aberdeen study maternal diets with a high protein density were not only associated with raised blood pressure in the offspring, but also with insulin deficiency and impaired glucose tolerance (Shiell *et al.* 2000). While it may seem counter-intuitive that a high protein diet should have adverse effects, these findings are consistent with the results of controlled trials of protein supplementation in pregnancy, which show that high protein intakes are associated with reduced birthweight (Rush 1989). The Aberdeen findings have recently been replicated in a follow-up study of men and women in Motherwell, UK, whose mothers were advised to eat a high meat protein, low carbohydrate diet during pregnancy (Shiell *et al.* 2001). Those whose mothers had high intakes of meat and fish in late pregnancy, but low intakes of carbohydrate, had raised blood pressure – particularly if the mother also had a low intake of green vegetables. Although raised blood pressure was also related to low birthweight, taking account of birthweight had little effect on the relation between maternal diet and offspring's blood pressure. One possibility is that the effect on blood pressure may be a consequence of the metabolic stress imposed on the mother by an unbalanced diet in which high intakes of essential amino acids are not accompanied by the micronutrients required to utilize them. Direct evidence for this comes from analysis of the offspring's fasting plasma cortisol concentrations (Herrick *et al.* 2003). Men and women whose mothers had high intakes of meat and fish and low intakes of green vegetables had raised cortisol concentrations.

The fetus does not live on the mother's diet alone: that would be too dangerous a strategy. It also lives off stored nutrients and the turnover of protein and fat in the mother's tissues (James 1997). Maternal size and body composition account for up to 20% of the variability in birthweight (Catalano *et al.* 1998). Gestational diabetes is known to be associated with adverse long-term outcomes in the offspring (Silverman *et al.* 1996). More recently, studies in Europe and India have shown that high maternal weight and adiposity are associated with insulin deficiency, type 2 diabetes, and CHD in the offspring (Fall *et al.* 1998; Forsén *et al.* 1997, 2000). Conversely, there is an increasing body of consistent evidence showing strong links between low maternal weight and BMI and insulin resistance and increased risk of type 2 diabetes in the adult offspring (Mi *et al.* 2000; Ravelli *et al.* 1998; Shiell *et al.* 2000). Table 32.12 shows plasma glucose and insulin concentrations in Chinese men and women aged around 45 years following a standard oral glucose challenge. Low maternal BMI at 38 weeks of pregnancy was associated with raised plasma glucose and insulin concentrations (Mi *et al.* 2000). Results for maternal BMI in early pregnancy, around 15 weeks, were stronger.

Table 32.12 Mean 2-h plasma glucose and insulin concentrations (*n*) according to maternal BMI in late pregnancy in 584 Chinese men and women

	Maternal BMI (kg/m²)				
	≤23	−24.5	−26	>26	*p* for trend
2-h glucose (mmol/l)	7.6 (137)	6.6 (119)	6.7 (121)	5.7 (103)	0.003
2-h insulin (pmol/l)	304	277	282	177	0.007

In contrast to these associations between maternal BMI and insulin resistance, thin maternal skinfold thicknesses and low pregnancy weight gain have been consistently associated with raised blood pressure in the offspring (Adair *et al.* 2001; Clark *et al.* 1998; Godfrey *et al.* 1994; Margetts *et al.* 1991). One of the metabolic links between maternal body composition and birth size is protein synthesis. Women with a greater lean body mass have higher rates of protein synthesis in pregnancy (Duggleby and Jackson 2001). Variation in rates of maternal protein synthesis explain around a quarter of the variability in birth length.

32.12 Conclusions

The demonstration that normal variations in fetal size and thinness at birth have implications for health throughout life has prompted a re-evaluation of the regulation of fetal development. Impetus has been added to this re-evaluation by recent findings showing that a woman's diet and body composition in pregnancy are related to levels of cardiovascular risk factors and the prevalence of CHD in her offspring in adult life. These observations challenge the view that the fetus is little affected by changes in maternal nutrition, except in circumstances of famine. There is an increasing body of evidence that a woman's own fetal growth, and her diet and body composition before pregnancy, play a major role in determining the future cardiovascular health of her children.

References

Adair, L. S., Kuzawa, C. W., and Borja, J. (2001). Maternal energy stores and diet composition during pregnancy program adolescent blood pressure. *Circulation* **104**, 1034–9.

Barker, D. J. P. (1995). Fetal origins of coronary heart disease. *British Medical Journal* **311**, 171–4.

Barker, D. J. P. (1998). *Mothers, babies and health in later life.* Churchill Livingstone, Edinburgh.

Barker, D. J. P., Osmond, C., Winter, P. D., Margetts, B., and Simmonds, S. J. (1989). Weight in infancy and death from ischaemic heart disease. *Lancet* **2**, 577–80.

Barker, D. J. P., Bull, A. R., Osmond, C., and Simmonds, S. J. (1990). Fetal and placental size and risk of hypertension in adult life. *British Medical Journal* **301**, 259–62.

Barker, D. J. P., Forsén, T., Uutela, A., Osmond, C., and Eriksson, J. G. (2001). Size at birth and resilience to the effects of poor living conditions in adult life: longitudinal study. *British Medical Journal* **323**, 1273–6.

Barker, D. J. P., Eriksson, J. G., Forsén, T., and Osmond, C. (2002a). Fetal origins of adult disease: strength of effects and biological basis. *International Journal of Epidemiology* **31**, 1235–9.

Barker, D. J. P., Forsén, T., Eriksson, J. G., and Osmond, C. (2002b). Growth and living conditions in childhood and hypertension in adult life: longitudinal study. *Journal of Hypertension* **20**, 1951–6.

Bateson, P. and Martin, P. (1999). *Design for a life: how behaviour develops.* Jonathan Cape, London.

Belizan, J. M., Villar, J., Bergel, E., del Pino, A., Di Fulvio, S., Galliano, S. V., and Kattan, C. (1997). Long term effect of calcium supplementation during pregnancy on the blood pressure of offspring: follow up of a randomised controlled trial. *British Medical Journal* **315**, 281–5.

Bhargava, S. K., Sachdev, H. S., Fall, C. H., Osmond, C., Lakshmy, R., Barker, D. J. *et al.* (2004). Relation of serial changes in childhood body-mass index to impaired glucose tolerance in young adulthood. *N Engl J Med*, **350**, 865–75.

Brenner, B. M. and Chertow, G. M. (1993). Congenital oligonephropathy: an inborn cause of adult hypertension and progressive renal injury? *Current Opinion in Nephrology and Hypertension* **2**, 691–5.

Brooks, A. A., Johnson, M. R., Steer, P. J., Pawson, M. E., and Abdalla, H. I. (1995). Birth weight: nature or nurture? *Early Human Development* **42**, 29–35.

Campbell, D. M., Hall, M. H., Barker, D. J. P., Cross, J., Shiell, A. W., and Godfrey, K. M. (1996). Diet in pregnancy and the offspring's blood pressure 40 years later. *British Journal of Obstetrics and Gynaecology* **103**, 273–80.

Catalano, P. M. Husten, L. P., Thomas, A. J., and Fung, C. M. (1998). Effect of maternal metabolism on fetal growth and body composition. *Diabetes Care* **21**, B85–B90.

Clark, P. M., Atton, C., Law, C. M., Shiell, A., Godfrey, K., and Barker, D. J. P. (1998). Weight gain in pregnancy, triceps skinfold thickness and blood pressure in the offspring. *Obstetrics and Gynecology* **91**, 103–107.

Curhan, G. C., Chertow, G. M., Willett, W. C. *et al.* (1996). Birth weight and adult hypertension and obesity in women. *Circulation* **94**, 1310–15.

Duggleby, S. L. and Jackson, A. A. (2001). Relationship of maternal protein turnover and lean body mass during pregnancy and birth length. *Clinical Science* **101**, 65–72.

Ebrahim, S. and Davey Smith, G. (1997). Systematic review of randomised controlled trials of multiple risk factor interventions for preventing coronary heart disease. *British Medical Journal* **314**, 1666–74.

Emanuel, I., Filakti, H., Alberman, E., and Evans, S. J. W. (1992). Intergenerational studies of human birthweight from the 1958 birth cohort. I. Evidence for a multigenerational effect. *British Journal of Obstetrics and Gynaecology* **99**, 67–74.

Eriksson, J. G., Forsen, T., Tuomilehto, J., Osmond, C., and Barker, D. J. P. (2001). Early growth and coronary heart disease in later life: longitudinal study. *British Medical Journal* **322**, 949–53.

Eriksson, J. G., Forsen, T., Jaddoe, V. W. V., Osmond, C., and Barker, D. J. P. (2002a). Effects of size at birth and childhood growth on the insulin resistance syndrome in elderly individuals. *Diabetologia* **45**, 342–8.

Eriksson, J. G., Lindi, V., Uusitupa, M. *et al.* (2002b). The effects of the Pro12Ala polymorphism of the peroxisome proliferator-activated receptor-γ2 gene on insulin sensitivity and insulin metabolism interact with size at birth. *Diabetes* **51**, 2321–4.

Eriksson, J. G., Forsen, T., Tuomilehto, J., Osmond, C., and Barker, D. J. P. (2003). Early adiposity rebound in childhood and risk of type 2 diabetes in adult life. *Diabetologia* **46**, 190–4.

Fall, C. H. D., Stein, C. E., Kumaran, K. *et al.* (1998). Size at birth, maternal weight, and type 2 diabetes in South India. *Diabetic Medicine* **15**, 220–7.

Forsén, T., Eriksson, J. G., Tuomilehto, J., Teramo, K., Osmond, C., and Barker, D. J. P. (1997). Mother's weight in pregnancy and coronary heart disease in a cohort of Finnish men: follow up study. *British Medical Journal* **315**, 837–40.

Forsen, T., Eriksson, J. G., Tuomilehto, J., Osmond, C., and Barker, D. J. P. (1999). Growth in utero and during childhood among women who develop coronary heart disease: longitudinal study. *British Medical Journal* **319**, 1403–7.

Forsén, T., Eriksson, J., Tuomilehto, J., Reunanen, A., Osmond, C., and Barker D. (2000). The fetal and childhood growth of persons who develop type 2 diabetes. *Annals of Internal Medicine* **133**, 176–82.

Forsén, T., Osmond, C., Eriksson, J. G., and Barker, D. J. P. (2004). The growth of girls who later develop coronary heart disease. *Heart*, **90**, 20–4.

Frankel, S., Elwood, P., Sweetnam, P., Yarnell, J., and Davey Smith, G. (1996). Birthweight, body mass index in middle age, and incident coronary heart disease. *Lancet* **348**, 1478–80.

Godfrey, K. M., Forrester, T., Barker, D. J. P., Jackson, A. A., Landman, J. P., Hall, J. St. E. *et al.* (1994). Maternal nutritional status in pregnancy and blood pressure in childhood. *British Journal of Obstetrics and Gynaecology* **101**, 398–403.

Godfrey, K., Robinson, S., Barker, D. J. P., Osmond, C., and Cox, V. (1996). Maternal nutrition in early and late pregnancy in relation to placental and fetal growth. *British Medical Journal* **312**, 410–14.

Godfrey, K. M., Barker, D. J. P., Robinson, S., and Osmond, C. (1997). Maternal birthweight and diet in pregnancy in relation to the infant's thinness at birth. *British Journal of Obstetrics and Gynaecology* **104**, 663–7.

Hales, C. N., Barker, D. J. P., Clark, P. M. S. *et al.* (1991). Fetal and infant growth and impaired glucose tolerance at age 64. *British Medical Journal* **303**, 1019–22.

Harding, J. (2001). The nutritional basis of the fetal origins of adult disease. *International Journal of Epidemiology* **30**, 15.

Harding, J. E., Liu, L., Evans, P., Oliver, M., and Gluckman, P. (1992). Intrauterine feeding of the growth-retarded fetus: can we help? *Early Human Development* **29**, 193–7.

Herrick, K., Phillips, D. I. W., Haselden, S., Shiell, A. W., Campbell-Brown, M., and Godfrey, K. M. (2003). Maternal consumption of a high-meat, low-carbohydrate diet in late pregnancy: relation to adult cortisol concentrations in the offspring. *Journal of Clinical Endocrinology and Metabolism,* **88**, 3554–60.

Huxley, R. R., Shiell, A. W., and Law, C. M. (2000). The role of size at birth and postnatal catch-up growth in determining systolic blood pressure: a systematic review of the literature. *Journal of Hypertension* **18**, 815–31.

Huxley, R., Neil, A., and Collins, R. (2002). Unravelling the fetal origins hypothesis. *Lancet* **360**, 2074–5.

Ingelfinger, J. R. (2003). Is microanatomy destiny? *New England Journal of Medicine* **348**, 99–100.

James, W. P. T. (1997). Long-term fetal programming of body composition and longevity. *Nutrition Reviews* **55**, S41–S43.

Keller, G., Zimmer, G., Mall, G., Ritz, E., and Amann, K. (2003). Nephron number in patients with primary hypertension. *New England Journal of Medicine* **348**, 101–8.

Kramer, M. S. (1993). Effects of energy and protein intakes on pregnancy outcome: an overview of the research evidence from controlled clinical trials. *American Journal of Clinical Nutrition* **58**, 627–35.

Kuh, D. and Ben-Shlomo, Y. (1997). *A life-course approach to chronic disease epidemiology.* Oxford University Press.

Kwong, W. Y., Wild, A., Roberts, P., Willis, A. C., and Fleming, T. P. (2000). Maternal undernutrition during the pre-implantation period of rat development causes blastocyst abnormalities and programming of postnatal hypertension. *Development* **127**, 4195–202.

Lackland, D. T., Egan, B. M., Syddall, H. E., and Barker, D. J. P. (2002). Associations between birthweight and antihypertensive medication in black and white Americans. *Hypertension* **39**, 179–83.

Leon, D. A., Lithell, H. O., Vagero, D. *et al.* (1998). Reduced fetal growth rate and increased risk of death from ischaemic heart disease: cohort study of 15 000 Swedish men and women born 1915–29. *British Medical Journal* **317**, 241–5.

Lithell, H. O., McKeigue, P. M., Berglund, L., Mohsen, R., Lithell, U. B., and Leon, D. A. (1996). Relation of size at birth to non-insulin dependent diabetes and insulin concentrations in men aged 50–60 years. *British Medical Journal* **312**, 406–10.

Lumey, L. H. (1998). Compensatory placental growth after restricted maternal nutrition in early pregnancy. *Placenta* **19**, 105–11.

Margetts, B. M., Rowland, M. G. M., Foord, F. A., Cruddas, A. M., Cole, T. J., and Barker, D. J. P. (1991). The relation of maternal weight to the blood pressures of Gambian children. *International Journal of Epidemiology* **20**, 938–43.

Marmot, M. and Wilkinson, R. G. (2001). Psychosocial and material pathways in the relation between income and health: a response to Lynch *et al. British Medical Journal* **322**, 1233–6.

Martyn, C. N., Barker, D. J. P., and Osmond, C. (1996). Mothers' pelvic size, fetal growth, and death from stroke and coronary heart disease in men in the UK. *Lancet* **348**, 1264–8.

McCance, D. R., Pettitt, D. J., Hanson, R. L., Jacobsson, L. T. H., Knowler, W. C., and Bennett, P. H. (1994). Birth weight and non-insulin dependent diabetes: thrifty genotype, thrifty phenotype, or surviving small baby genotype? *British Medical Journal* **308**, 942–5.

McCance, R. A. (1962). Food, growth and time. *Lancet* **2**, 621–6.

Mellanby, E. (1933). Nutrition and child-bearing. *Lancet* **2**, 1131–7.

Metcalfe, N. B. and Monaghan, P. (2001). Compensation for a bad start: grow now, pay later? *Trends in Ecological Evolution* **16**, 254–60.

Mi, J., Law, C., Zhang, K.-L., Osmond, C., Stein, C., and Barker, D. J. P. (2000). Effects of infant birthweight and maternal body mass index in pregnancy on components of the insulin resistance syndrome in China. *Annals of Internal Medicine* **132**, 253–60.

Newsome, C. A., Shiell, A. W., Fall, C. H. D., Phillips, D. I. W., Shier, R., and Law, C. M. (2003). Is birthweight related to later glucose and insulin metabolism: a systematic review. *Diabetic Medicine* **20**, 339–48.

Osmond, C., Barker, D. J. P., Winter, P. D., Fall, C. H. D., and Simmonds, S. J. (1993). Early growth and death from cardiovascular disease in women. *British Medical Journal* **307**, 1519–24.

Phillips, D. I. W. (1996). Insulin resistance as a programmed response to fetal undernutrition. *Diabetologia* **39**, 1119–22.

Phillips, D. I. W., Walker, B. R., Reynolds, R. M. *et al.* (2000). Low birth weight predicts elevated plasma cortisol concentrations in adults from 3 populations. *Hypertension* **35**, 1301–6.

Ravelli, A. C. J., van der Meulen, J. H. P., Michels, R. P. J. *et al.* (1998). Glucose tolerance in adults after prenatal exposure to famine. *Lancet* **351**, 173–7.

Rich-Edwards, J. W., Stampfer, M. J., Manson, J. E. *et al.* (1997). Birth weight and risk of cardiovascular disease in a cohort of women followed up since 1976. *British Medical Journal* **315**, 396–400.

Rich-Edwards, J. W., Colditz, G. A., Stampfer, M. J. *et al.* (1999). Birthweight and the risk for type 2 diabetes mellitus in adult women. *Annals of Internal Medicine* **130**, 278–84.

Robinson, J. S., Owens, J. A., de Barro, T. *et al.* (1994). Maternal nutrition and fetal growth. In *Early fetal growth and development* (ed. R. H. T. Ward, S. K. Smith, and D. Donnai), pp. 317–34. Royal College of Obstetricians and Gynaecologists, London.

Robinson, J. S., Chidzanja, S., Kind, K., Lok, F., Owens, P., and Owens, J. A. (1995). Placental control of fetal growth. *Reproduction, Fertility, and Development* **7**, 333–44.

Rolland-Cachera, M. F., Deheeger, M., Guilloud-Bataille, M., Avons, P., Patois, E., and Sempe, M. (1987). Tracking the development of adiposity from one month of age to adulthood. *Annals of Human Biology* **14**, 219–29.

Roseboom, T. J., van der Meulen, J. H., Osmond, C., Barker, D. J., Ravelli, A. C., and Bleker, O. P. (2000*a*). Plasma lipid profiles in adults after prenatal exposure to the Dutch famine. *American Journal of Clinical Nutrition* **72**, 1101–6.

Roseboom, T. J., van der Meulen, J. H., Osmond, C., Barker, D. J., Ravelli, A. C., Schroeder-Tanka, J. M. *et al.* (2000*b*). Coronary heart disease after prenatal exposure to the Dutch famine, 1944–45. *Heart* **84**, 595–8.

Roseboom, T. J., van der Meulen, J. H., van Montfrans, G. A., Ravelli, A. C., Osmond, C., Barker, D. J., and Bleker, O. P. (2001). Maternal nutrition during gestation and blood pressure in later life. *Journal of Hypertension* **19**, 29–34.

Rush, D. (1989). Effects of changes in maternal energy and protein intake during pregnancy, with special reference to fetal growth. In *Fetal growth* (ed. F. Sharp, R. B. Fraser, and R. D. G. Milner), pp. 203–33. Royal College of Obstetricians and Gynaecologists, London.

Shiell, A. W., Campbell, D. M., Hall, M. H., and Barker, D. J. (2000). Diet in late pregnancy and glucose-insulin metabolism of the offspring 40 years later. *British Journal of Obstetrics and Gynaecology* **107**, 890–5.

Shiell, A. W., Campbell-Brown, M., Haselden, S., Robinson, S., Godfrey, K. M., and Barker, D. J. P. (2001). A high meat, low carbohydrate diet in pregnancy: relation to adult blood pressure in the offspring. *Hypertension* **38**, 1282–8.

Silverman, B. L., Purdy, L. P., and Metzger, B. E. (1996). The intrauterine environment: implications for the offspring of diabetic mothers. *Diabetes Reviews* **4**, 21–35.

Stein, C. E., Fall, C. H. D., Kumaran, K., Osmond, C., Cox, V., and Barker, D. J. P. (1996). Fetal growth and coronary heart disease in South India. *Lancet* **348**, 1269–73.

Stewart, R. J. C., Sheppard, H., Preece, R., and Waterlow, J. C. (1980). The effect of rehabilitation at different stages of development of rats marginally malnourished for ten to twelve generations. *British Journal of Nutrition* **43**, 403–12.

Walker, S. K., Hartwick, K. M., and Robinson, J. S. (2000). Long-term effects on offspring of exposure of oocytes and embryos to chemical and physical agents. *Human Reproduction Update* **6**, 564–7.

West-Eberhard, M. J. (1989). Phenotypic plasticity and the origins of diversity. *Annual Review of Ecology and Systematics* **20**, 249.

Widdowson, E. M., and McCance, R. A. (1963). The effect of finite periods of undernutrition at different ages on the composition and subsequent development of the rat. *Proceedings of the Royal Society of London Series B* **158**, 329–42.

Widdowson, E. M., Crabb, D. E., and Milner R. D. G. (1972). Cellular development of some human organs before birth. *Archives of Diseases of Childhood* **47**, 652–5.

Ylihärsilä, H., Eriksson, J. G., Forsén, T., Kajantie, E., Osmond, C., and Barker, D. J. P. (2003). Self-perpetuating effects of birth size on blood pressure levels in elderly people. *Hypertension* **41**, 446–50.

Chapter 33

Life course influences on coronary heart disease

G. Davey Smith and J. Lynch

33.1 Introduction

Until relatively recently most of the focus of coronary heart disease (CHD) epidemiology has been on understanding how behavioural, physiological, and social factors measured in middle age influence disease risk. The possibility that factors acting earlier in life could influence the risk of CHD had been considered at various times from the 1930s to the 1970s (Kuh and Davey Smith 1997), but interest in this issue was particularly stimulated by the work of Anders Forsdahl beginning in the early 1970s (Forsdahl 1973; 1977). Forsdahl suspected that adverse environmental conditions in infancy and early childhood could increase the risk of CHD in late adult life. Forsdahl studied the high mortality in the Norwegian county of Finnmark and drew attention to a possible cause 'which has not been discussed earlier, namely that the considerably high mortality today is a late consequence of the adverse circumstances to which a large part of the population was exposed during their childhood and adolescence' (Forsdahl 1973). He showed that the main contributor to this high mortality was CHD and that the current pattern of conventional risk factors – such as smoking and diet in adulthood – did not seem to account for this (Forsdahl *et al.* 1974). He then analysed data across the whole of Norway and demonstrated that infant mortality rates early in the twentieth century correlated strongly with CHD mortality rates 70 years later (Forsdahl 1977) (Fig. 33.1). Forsdahl speculated that permanent damage may be caused by nutritional deficits in early life that rendered individuals less able to tolerate particular forms of fat in their adult diet – a hypothesis he went on to test (Forsdahl 1978).

Forsdahl's finding of an ecological association between past infant mortality and present CHD mortality was replicated in different countries by several authors with somewhat differing

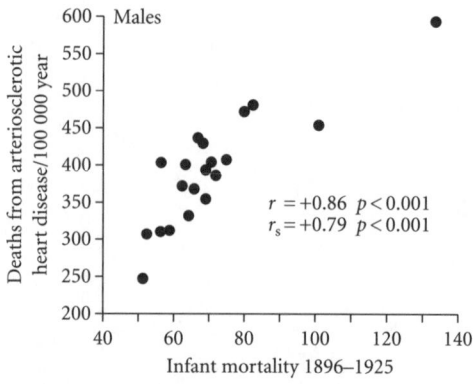

Fig. 33.1 Correlation between mortality from arteriosclerotic heart disease, 1964–67, in men aged 40–69 years (standardized rates/100 000 population) and infant mortality rates, 1896–1925. (From Forsdahl 1977.)

interpretations of the meaning of the observed associations. However, by far the most influential replication and development of this work was by David Barker and Clive Osmond in 1986 (Barker and Osmond 1986). In their early studies Barker and colleagues interpreted their findings as indicating an influence of childhood nutrition, but the focus of their investigations quickly came to rest on exposures in the prenatal environment (Barker *et al.* 1989). From these initial observations, the now well-known 'Barker' or 'Fetal Origins Hypothesis' was developed, which focused on the long-term effects of *in utero* biological programming associated with maternal and fetal undernutrition. Only after a decade of almost exclusive concentration on the prenatal period have these studies again embraced the potentially modifying influence of experiences acting in later life (Barker *et al.* 2001; Forsen *et al.* 2000). To some epidemiologists working on the aetiology of CHD, the 'fetal origins of adult disease' hypothesis stimulated broader thinking about a range of influences acting from before birth and then right through the life course. In 1997 a book edited by Diana Kuh and Yoav Ben-Shlomo, *A life course approach to chronic disease epidemiology* (Kuh and Ben-Shlomo 1997), collected together contributions from across the disciplinary and disease spectrum, and for many researchers helped establish life course thinking as central to the epidemiological endeavour.

A key problem with the initial studies in the early life or fetal origins field was that when relating early life exposures to health outcomes many decades later the intervening anthropometric, biological, behavioural, psychological, and social trajectories of individuals might be correlated with a particular indicator of early life exposure. Thus, because birthweight may influence subsequent weight in childhood, at puberty, and in adulthood, it was not clear whether early life exposures were linked to adult disease only through their links with later life distributions of exposures. For instance, in regard to early life social deprivation, those born into poor circumstances would tend to have less favourable social trajectories (in regard to their subsequent education, occupation, and income) than those individuals who entered the world as members of more comfortably off families. Ben-Shlomo and Davey Smith demonstrated this potential problem with respect to the studies that have correlated past infant mortality rates with present day mortality rates (Ben-Shlomo and Davey Smith 1991). The findings of Forsdahl and Barker, showing that areas with high levels of infant mortality in the early part of the twentieth century had high CHD mortality among elderly adults in the 1980s, were replicated (Fig. 33.2), but then statistical adjustment for an area-based measure of current

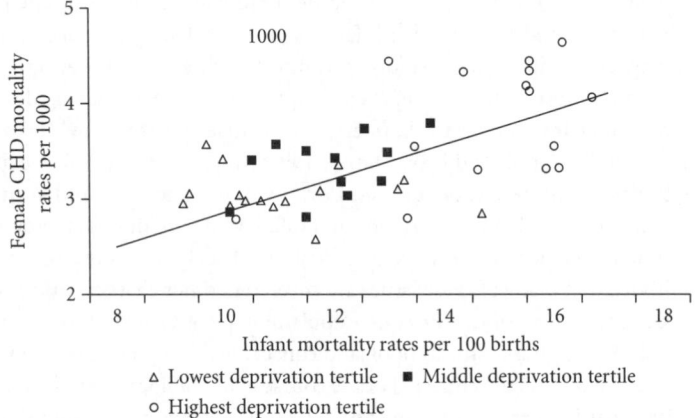

Fig. 33.2 Infant mortality rate, 1905–08, and CHD mortality of females aged 65–74 in 1969–73.

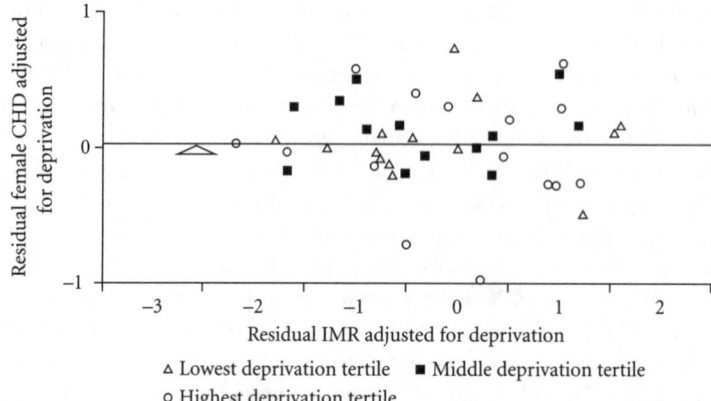

Fig. 33.3 Infant mortality rates (IMR), 1905–08, and CHD mortality of females aged 65–74 in 1969–73 after control for measures of adult deprivation. (From Ben-Shlomo and Davey Smith 1991.)

socio-economic disadvantage abolished this association (Fig. 33.3). However, the authors did not dismiss the importance of early life factors, but rather concluded that it 'is unhelpful to consider an either/or model, which would exclude the possible interaction and cumulative effect of factors acting early and later in life. These ecological associations, however, do clearly point out the importance of considering a life course approach to disease aetiology' (Ben-Shlomo and Davey Smith 1991). The implications of these findings for CHD epidemiology were that detailed data for periods covering the entire life course were required to identify the contribution of exposures acting at particular time periods.

Research on early life factors appeared against the background of the huge amount of epidemiological work that was carried out during the second half of the twentieth century on adulthood behaviours (smoking, diet, exercise), physiological parameters (blood pressure, cholesterol and other lipid-related elements, haemostatic factors), socio-economic position (social class, education) and psychosocial factors (psychological dispositions, social networks, and stress in its various guises). Some of these areas are covered in detail in this volume (see the other chapters in this section). The flurry of reports on the fetal origins of CHD produced somewhat polarized opinions, with many epidemiologists emphasizing the primacy of the already well-characterized adulthood risk factors (as indicated by the success of intervention studies – in particular with regard to blood pressure and cholesterol lowering), while a minority began to focus almost exclusively on events happening very early during development. The partial synthesis that arose under the banner of 'life course epidemiology' (Davey Smith 2003; Davey Smith et al. 1997; Kuh and Davey Smith 1997; Kuh and Hardy 2002), explicitly investigated how timing of discrete exposures and/or how the sequencing and accumulation of a variety of exposures from before birth, through infancy and childhood, to adulthood and old age might be of aetiological importance. A partial list of such factors is given in Box 33.1. It is clear from this list that many of these issues are covered in other chapters of this volume and so a comprehensive treatment of the life course epidemiology of CHD in this chapter would both be repetitive of much material in this book and constitute a complete treatise on the disease.

Therefore we will outline the concepts of life course epidemiology as applied to CHD, discuss evidence with regard to early life factors and CHD (with an emphasis on infancy and childhood, given the discussion of fetal origins in Chapter 32), consider the recently debated issue as

Box 33.1 Putative life course risk factors for CHD

- Parental history of CHD.
- Maternal health before and during pregnancy.
- Maternal diet and behaviour before and during pregnancy.
- Maternal psychosocial stress before and during pregnancy.
- Low birthweight/growth retardation.
- Infant feeding.
- Poor maternal attachment.
- Socio-economic deprivation from childhood onwards.
- Stress from childhood onwards.
- Poor growth in childhood.
- Short leg length in childhood.
- Obesity in childhood.
- Certain infections acquired in childhood.
- Diet from childhood onwards.
- Blood pressure in late adolescence.
- Serum cholesterol level in late adolescence.
- Smoking from late adolescence onwards.
- Little physical activity from late adolescence onwards.
- Number of children borne (for women).
- Blood pressure in adulthood.
- Serum cholesterol level in adulthood.
- Obesity in adulthood.
- Quitting smoking in adulthood.
- Job insecurity and unemployment in adulthood.
- Short stature in adulthood.
- Binge alcohol drinking in adulthood.
- Diabetes and components of syndrome X in adulthood.
- Elevated levels of fibrinogen and other acute phase reactants in adulthood.
- Certain infections acquired in adulthood.

Source: Davey Smith *et al.* 2002

to whether there is any need to continue searching for additional CHD risk factors above the well-established adulthood factors, examine how well CHD trends fit with life course approaches (given the importance of time and historical context to life course thinking), and conclude by reviewing some of the remaining important issues in CHD epidemiology from a life course perspective.

33.2 **Theoretical models of life course influences on adult disease**

Many studies of how socially patterned exposures acting at different stages of the life course affect health outcomes use general measures such as all-cause mortality or overall subjective health ratings. These composite outcomes will be influenced by a wide range of exposures – for example, there are multiple aetiological pathways that could generate a self-report of poor health. Similarly, all the aetiological factors relating to the component causes of death will relate to all-cause mortality. Detailed models of how exposures acting at different stages of life come together to influence the final health outcome cannot be clearly specified with respect to such summary measures. The development of life course epidemiology within particular health domains shows that different processes come into play with respect to different health outcomes. This is also likely to be important for gaining greater insights into the contributions of different types of exposures over the life course to CHD – itself a relatively diverse pathological entity with both acute and chronic components.

Ben-Shlomo and Kuh have developed a helpful typology of models for life course epidemiology (Ben-Shlomo and Kuh 2002) (see Box 33.2), some of which are illustrated by considerations of CHD aetiology.

A simple model of life course influences is that **accumulation of risk** occurs, such that an adverse exposure early in life that increases disease risk has an additive effect with later life adverse influences. Cumulative effects are certainly seen with respect to CHD mortality when combining early and later life socio-economic and behavioural factors (smoking and excess drinking), as shown in Table 33.1 (Davey Smith and Hart 2002; Davey Smith *et al.* 2000a). In these cases the adverse exposures could either be uncorrelated – for example, high alcohol consumption is not strongly related to childhood or adulthood social class – or they could cluster. Clustering could occur either because poor social circumstances predispose individuals to a variety of other exposures, such as smoking and diet, or they could reflect more direct causal links – as when poor childhood educational attainment leads to an unfavourable adulthood occupation. Such clustering of risk across the life course may be one reason why adult indicators of socio-economic disadvantage are strongly linked to CHD risk. Indicators of adult deprivation can be effective summaries of negative social, behavioural, anthropometric, and physiological trajectories over time.

An alternative set of models sees the time window of exposure as key. This is well understood in a variety of situations, such as with prenatal infections or drug exposure, where during a

---

Box 33.2 **Conceptual life course models**

Critical period model

With or with out later life risk factors.
With later life effect modifiers.

Accumulation of risk

With independent and uncorrelated insults.
With correlated insults.
  'Risk clustering'.
  'Chains of risk' with additive or trigger effects.

(Source: Ben-Shlomo and Kuh 2002)

Table 33.1 Age-adjusted relative rates of CHD mortality by father's social class and later life risk factors: the Collaborative Study

Risk factor	Father's social class	
	Non-manual	Manual
Smoking		
Other	1	1.56 (1.18–2.07)
Current cigarette	2.01 (1.46–2.77)	2.78 (2.12–3.63)
Alcohol		
<15 units/week	1	1.44 (1.18–1.75)
≥15 units/week	1.17 (0.80–1.70)	1.86 (1.50–2.31)
Screening social class		
Non-manual	1	1.46 (1.18–1.82)
Manual	1.53 (1.06–2.21)	1.78 (1.45–2.17)

Sources: Davey Smith and Hart 2002; Davey Smith *et al.* 2000*a*.

particular period of fetal development these can lead to devastating permanent developmental changes, whereas if they were experienced just a few days earlier or later they would have no long-term impact. Such **critical period** effects can also extend from before conception right through the growing period and beyond. The fetal origins hypothesis is, of course, one example of a hypothesized critical periods model of adult disease. Other examples include how the exact age of acquisition of *Helicobacter pylori* may be related to the particular disease outcome that results (gastric cancer, peptic ulcer, stomach cancer). As with other infections, such as hepatitis B, very early infection (which mainly occurs in developing countries) appears to increase the risk many decades later of developing cancer. The age of acquisition of human papillomavirus through unprotected sexual intercourse may also influence the risk of subsequently developing cervical cancer, just as the particular age at which lead exposure occurs will influence its neuro-developmental consequences. It is reasonable to say that there are, as yet, no well-established and broadly accepted examples of strictly defined critical periods for CHD. However, a less restrictive conceptualization of critical period could include the idea that the ultimate outcome of exposures experienced at such critical periods can depend upon later life influences. A simple illustration of this is that antibiotic treatment to eradicate *H. pylori* dramatically reduces risk of developing stomach cancer (Uemura *et al.* 2001). For CHD, poor *in utero* growth appears to have greater detrimental consequences if followed by rapid catch-up growth and obesity in later life (Frankel *et al.* 1996).

Thus, CHD appears to be an exemplary condition in which factors acting right across the life course are of importance – either at particular critical periods or in particular time-dependent interactions, or through simple accumulation of influence with other exposures.

33.3 Evidence of early life influences on CHD risk

33.3.1 Biological and behavioural factors

As recently documented in an extensive review (McCarron and Davey Smith 2003), blood pressure, blood cholesterol, and body mass index (BMI) measurements taken in adolescence or early adulthood predict CHD risk up to 50 years later. Table 33.2, for example, documents the

Table 33.2 Cumulative incidence of CHD among 1017 men in the Johns Hopkins Precursors Study after 40 years of follow-up according to baseline serum cholesterol level

Variable	No. of events	Quartile of cholesterol level (mmol/l)				p for trend
		3.05–4.46	4.47–4.90	4.91–5.39	5.40–8.15	
CHD	97	6.9	11.5	17.5	35.2	<0.001
MI	62	3.4	5.1	7.2	29.2	<0.001
Angina	49	5.7	4.2	13.4	9.2	<0.001

Source: Klag *et al.* 1993.

MI: myocardial infarction.

incidence of CHD over a 40-year follow-up of men in the Johns Hopkins Precursor study (Klag *et al.* 1993), with a remarkable gradient between blood cholesterol level and later incidence of CHD being seen. Similar results are seen with cholesterol measured slightly later in the life course in the Chicago Heart Association Detection Project in Industry, where measures among 18–39-year-olds were considerably more strongly associated with CHD than measures taken among 40–59-year-olds (relative risks per 1.04 mmol/l higher cholesterol 1.92 (95% CI: 1.64–2.24) for the former and 1.18 (1.12–1.25) for the latter, *p* value for interaction <0.001) (Navas-Nacher *et al.* 2001). Studies that measured cholesterol in childhood demonstrate that this predicts markers of atherosclerosis – carotid artery intima-media thickness – as strongly, or more strongly, than cholesterol measured in adulthood, and that the childhood measures remain predictors after adulthood measures are taken into account (Li *et al.* 2003; Raitakari *et al.* 2003). Long-term exposure to circulating cholesterol is a stronger risk factor than single measures in either childhood or adulthood (Li *et al.* 2003). This is in accord with data from three other sources. First, Geoffrey Rose demonstrated that ecological correlations between cholesterol levels and CHD mortality were stronger for cholesterol measured many years before CHD mortality was assessed, than if contemporaneous cholesterol measures were correlated with contemporaneous CHD mortality (Rose 1982). Second, data from randomized controlled trials find relative reduction in CHD risk amongst those allocated to statins that increases with duration of treatment (Heart Protection Study Collaborative Group 2002*a*). Third, evidence from 'Mendelian randomization' approaches demonstrates that the lifetime differences in cholesterol levels generated by genetic variants such as familial defective apolipoprotein B are consistent with considerably greater effects of lifetime cholesterol levels than are seen with single cholesterol measures (Davey Smith and Ebrahim 2003, 2004).

For blood pressure, the situation is somewhat different. While blood pressure measured in early adulthood predicts future CHD risk, as demonstrated in the association between blood pressure in early adulthood and CHD mortality up to 50 years later in the Glasgow University students cohort (McCarron *et al.* 2000) (Table 33.3), the effects are certainly no greater than those seen for adulthood measures (Li *et al.* 2003; Miura *et al.* 2001; Navas-Nacher *et al.* 2001; Raitakari *et al.* 2003).

Cholesterol measurements taken during adolescence or early adulthood reflect long-term exposure to such factors and are uninfluenced by early stages of the disease that can lead to declines in such physiological measures and thus underestimation of the causal associations with CHD. Thus, cholesterol measured in early life generally produces greater prediction than do such measurements taken in later life. This may reflect long-term accumulative atherosclerotic process. Blood pressure levels in early life, while influencing later disease, do not show the

Table 33.3 Baseline JNC-VI blood pressure classification, blood pressure category, and CHD mortality hazard ratios for former male Glasgow University students, CHADPI men, and MRFIT men

JNC-VI classification	Blood pressure mmHg	Glasgow HR (95% CI)	Chicago HR (95% CI)	MRFIT HR
Optimal	<120/80	1.00	1.39 (0.67–2.86)	1.00
Normal	120–9/80–4	1.19 (0.62–2.32)	1.00	1.30
High normal	130–9/85–9	1.65 (0.88–3.12)	1.37 (0.81–2.30)	1.67
Stage 1 HT	140–59/90–9	1.66 (0.88–3.13)	1.62 (1.00–2.61)	2.56
Stage 2 HT	160–79/100–9	2.73 (1.26–5.92)	2.51 (1.44–4.37)	4.57[a]
Stage 3 HT	180/110 or above	2.91 (0.80–10.55)	3.60 (1.71–7.59)	
Trend across categories		0.002	–	<0.001

Sources: McCarron et al. 2000; Miura et al. 2001; Stamler et al. 1993; The Sixth Report of the Joint National Committee on prevention, detection, evaluation, and treatment of blood pressure 1997.

CHADPI: Chicago Heart Association Detection Project in Industry; HR: hazard ratio; HT: hypertension; MRFIT: Multiple Risk Factors Intervention Trial.

[a] HR for stage 2 and stage 3 HT combined.

enhanced association seen for cholesterol. However, the basic point that influencing conventional risk factors in adolescence or early adulthood should reduce risk of CHD many decades hence appears to apply. This is also seen with respect to where smoking amongst adolescents or young adults is strongly related to later disease risk (McCarron et al. 2001a). The biological and behavioural factors that serve as causal factors for CHD in middle-age also serve this purpose in earlier life.

A well-established finding is that greater height is associated with lower risk of CHD (Davey Smith et al. 2000b; McCarron et al. 2002). Height in early adulthood is as strongly associated with later CHD risk as is height measured in middle age; thus influences on growth in early life, rather than on height loss from middle age onwards, seem to be key (Davey Smith et al. 2000b). The association between height and CHD risk appears to be independent of birthweight (Rich-Edwards et al. 1995; Yarnell et al. 1992) and recent evidence suggests that a particular component of total stature – leg length – is key (Davey Smith et al. 2001a; Lawlor et al. 2004). Leg length appears to be particularly influenced by nutrition and possibly infection in infancy and prepubertal childhood. Leg length is inversely related to measures of insulin resistance in adulthood (Lawlor et al. 2002b) and while, statistically, this fails to account for the association between leg length and CHD in existing studies, this may be due to poor characterization of insulin resistance with the single measurements usually available.

33.3.2 Socio-economic disadvantage

There have been several studies investigating early and later socio-economic disadvantage and heart disease (many studies used the combined category of cardiovascular disease (CVD), but this grouping is dominated by CHD). We recently systematically reviewed (Galobardes et al. 2004) studies that investigated associations between childhood socio-economic position (SEP) and adult CVD (Barker et al. 2001; Beebe-Dimmer et al. 2004; Bobák et al. 2000; Brasche et al. 2001; Burr and Sweetnam 1980; Claussen et al. 2003; Coggon et al. 1990; Davey Smith et al. 1998, 2001b; Dedman et al. 2001; Donnan et al. 1994; Eriksson et al. 2000; Forsen et al. 1999;

Frankel *et al.* 1999; Gliksman *et al.* 1995; Hasle 1990; Heslop *et al.* 2001; Kaplan and Salonen 1990; Lynch *et al.* 1994; Marmot *et al.* 2001; Notkola 1985; Notkola *et al.* 1985; Pensola and Valkonen 2002; Vågerö and Leon 1994; Wannamethee *et al.* 1996). There were 7 case-control, 15 prospective, and 2 cross-sectional/cumulative prevalence studies. A variety of measures of childhood SEP were used including father's and sometimes mother's occupation and/or education, and housing conditions. Many of the studies adjusted for one or more measures of adulthood social position and/or adult risk factors. Of the 24 studies, 14 used information on childhood socio-economic circumstances recalled during adulthood, while 10 prospective studies collected data either in childhood or early life (before age 20). Presumably, the data collected in early life should be more reliable than that recalled in adulthood. Overall these studies show stronger effects of childhood SEP on CVD than studies that collected the early life SEP data in adulthood. Moreover, all these studies with SEP data collected in early life used objectively defined CVD outcomes and controlled for indicators of adulthood SEP. After adjustment for later life SEP, with only a few exceptions, poorer socio-economic conditions in childhood showed increased CVD risk of between 50 and 250%, depending on the study population.

Some persuasive evidence comes from a follow-up of students who attended Glasgow University between 1948 and 1968 (Davey Smith *et al.* 2001*b*). This study showed more than two-fold increased CVD mortality risk for men with fathers from social classes IV and V after adjustment for age, systolic blood pressure, and smoking. This is strong evidence for the importance of early life socio-economic effects because external data suggest that the adult social circumstances of the large majority of these graduates of Glasgow University (over 75%) (OPCS 1978) was affluent, and so reduces the likelihood of severe residual confounding by adult SEP. Indeed, in a recent follow-up survey just under 95% of the students were in social class I or social class II occupations in middle age. Also worth noting is that in the Glasgow students study, as in several other studies, the relative effects of childhood socio-economic disadvantage are stronger for CVD than other causes of death (Davey Smith *et al.* 1998). For instance, Beebe-Dimmer *et al.* (2004) found that among a population-based sample of 3087 women in California, USA lower childhood SEP was more strongly associated with CVD (relative hazard (RH) = 1.31, 95% CI: 1.11–1.56) than with all-cause mortality (RH = 1.13; 95% CI: 1.00–1.28) after adjustment for education, income, and occupation. This study (along with others) (Davey Smith *et al.* 1998) highlights that there may be unique contributions of socio-economic disadvantage from several life course stages to heart disease risk, and suggests that there may be different pathways that mediate the effects of lower SEP during childhood (effects of early life diet and exercise habits), lower education (less cognitive integration of health information into behaviours), poorer working conditions (less likely to encounter conditions conducive to quitting smoking), and lower income (less capacity to purchase good diet and engage in exercise) on increased risk of heart disease.

While not measuring childhood socio-economic environment directly, some early studies of links between childhood SEP and CHD investigated the 'social incongruity' and apparent stress associated with moving from a disadvantaged background into the hypothesized stressful environment of the professional and managerial world (Marks 1967). While this general hypothesis was influential in directing thinking about how social processes affected CHD risk (Cassell 1995), there is in fact little evidence that upward mobility from poor childhood background to advantaged adult social position increases the risk of CHD through generating the stress of status incongruity. In fact, some evidence would suggest the opposite – that upward social mobility is protective relative to the socio-economic group of origin (Lynch *et al.* 1994) – although those who are upwardly mobile seem not to attain the same levels of health as those who were advantaged over the whole life course (Hart *et al.* 1998). Downward intergenerational social mobility – from a non-manual occupational background of father to a manual occupation in middle age – has rarely been directly studied in the context of adult CHD. Data from Finland showed that intergenerationally downwardly mobile men had the highest cardiovascular risk of any social group (Lynch *et al.* 1994), but without detailed information on the precise timing of downward mobility it is hard to know which particular life course processes might be implicated in generating these adult health differences. Early life critical period exposures, followed by later effect modifiers, and accumulation models, are all possible explanations for the downward mobility effects on adult heart disease (Hallqvist *et al.* 2004; Kuh *et al.* 2004).

How could socio-economic disadvantage at different stages of the life course be linked to risk of CHD? The suggestion by Forsdahl that the effects of early life deprivation are mediated through high blood cholesterol concentrations in adulthood has received little support (Davey Smith *et al.* 2002; Notkola *et al.* 1985). In the West of Scotland cohort, CVD risk factors were analysed in relation to childhood and adult social class (Blane *et al.* 1996). Men with manual social class fathers had lower, rather than higher, total serum cholesterol concentrations compared to men with non-manual fathers. Behavioural risk factors, such as smoking and exercise, were more dependent on adult than parental social class, supporting the notion that in some circumstances behaviours like smoking were powerfully affected by the social environment experienced during adult life, and that modifying such behaviours is dependent upon the presence of the social circumstances required for maintaining favourable health-related behaviours. Blood pressure and lung function were associated with both current and parental social class, but more strongly with the former. This suggests that smoking and occupational exposures for lung function, or alcohol and other dietary factors for blood pressure are, in this male cohort, more dependent upon adult than childhood social circumstances. However, BMI and triglyceride levels were dependent on childhood social class rather than current social class. Men with manual fathers had higher body mass indices and higher triglyceride levels than men with non-manual fathers, and once father's social class was taken into account there was no association of current social class with BMI and a reverse association for triglycerides. High BMI and elevated triglycerides are components of the insulin resistance syndrome. This is compatible with evidence that the concomitants of adverse childhood socio-economic circumstances are associated with an elevated risk of diabetes and impaired glucose tolerance in adulthood (Lawlor *et al.* 2002a). The components of insulin resistance syndrome may cluster in childhood (Bao *et al.* 1994; Raitakari *et al.* 1994) and, as described above, this clustering tracks into adulthood (Berenson *et al.* 1998a) suggesting that a common factor, already active in young childhood, may underlie the risk of insulin resistance syndrome.

The relatively few studies that have examined the influence of early and later life socio-economic factors on risk factors have consistently found associations, but the patterning of links between socio-economic factors in early life and particular heart disease risk factors is somewhat inconsistent across studies (Brunner *et al.* 1996; Davey Smith *et al.* 2002; Forsdahl 1978; Hardy *et al.* 2000; Kuh *et al.* 2002; Lynch *et al.* 1997; Notkola *et al.* 1985; Power and Matthews 1997; van de Mheen *et al.* 1998). See Davey Smith and Lynch (2004) for a more complete description. Interpretation of these mixed findings is complicated by the fact that the studies are in different countries with cohorts of different ages and there is no need to assume that the influence of SEP at different life course stages on risk factors should necessarily show the same patterns in different contexts or times. Life course socio-economic patterning of behaviours like smoking, diet, and exercise may show complicated period and cohort effects that will be reflected in their biological sequelae and thus be specific to particular cohorts, countries, regions and subgroups of the population.

For example, in Britain there is evidence that early life social circumstances have a stronger influence on smoking among women than among men (Graham and Der 1999), although this is not necessarily the case in other countries or in other time periods. These potential gender and cohort differences are evident in the educational patterning of smoking initiation in Switzerland, where higher education was a risk factor for early smoking initiation, but over time eventually became protective, and this effect was lagged by 20 years in women compared to men (Curtin *et al.* 1997). In the US there are different education by sex by race/ethnic group patterns for smoking uptake by different birth cohorts (Escobedo and Peddicord 1996). These studies show how socio-economic factors can leave very different imprints on patterns of smoking initiation and cessation according to gender, race/ethnicity, and birth cohort, which in turn may correspond to the timing of subgroup-specific experiences of the overall trends in smoking and subsequent CHD at the population level.

Such patterns could not be revealed without socio-economic data from across the life course and may provide useful information on heterogeneity of risk among adult socio-economic groups, even under social conditions where powerful period changes occur in the link between adult SEP and a risk factor such as smoking. Similar period by socio-economic group differences may also be present for other life course CHD risk factors such as the period rise (in the early twentieth century) and social distribution of high fat diets in the US, followed by the socially patterned shifts to greater consumption of fruit and vegetables by the more affluent. Tastes for certain foods may be 'programmed' early in life, but are also then subject to later modification based on adult socio-economic influences (Lynch *et al.* 1997).

33.3.3 Psychosocial exposures

Early life socio-economic disadvantage could also be linked to increased risk of CHD in adulthood via psychosocial mechanisms. There is some evidence that adult psychosocial risk factors such as depression, hostility, and hopelessness may also partly have their roots earlier in life. A study of Finnish men showed that those whose parents both had less than a primary school education were more likely to report higher levels of cynical hostility and hopelessness, regardless of their own education and adult occupation and income (Harper *et al.* 2002). On the other hand, patterns of adult depressive symptoms were much more sensitive to current socio-economic circumstances than to early life socio-economic indicators, although in a US study there was evidence for an early life component to adult depression (Gilman *et al.* 2002).

In addition, there is evidence that childhood experiences of abuse and neglect may predispose to poorer adult health behaviours (Kendall-Tacket 2002). For example, smoking, poorer diet, and obesity in adulthood is related to a group of childhood experiences including emotional, physical, and sexual abuse, parental neglect, separation or divorce, and growing-up with a substance-abusing, mentally ill, or incarcerated household member (Anda *et al.* 1999; Diaz *et al.* 2002; Felitti *et al.* 1998; Lissau and Sorenson 1994). There is also evidence that such factors influence later health status (Taylor *et al.* 1997), including the health of future generations through adverse influences on birth outcomes among women. A life course approach to chronic disease in adulthood must consider the full range of material and psychosocial factors acting across the life course, which may be precursors of disease onset.

33.4 CHD risk factors: enough already?

It has frequently been suggested that the established CHD risk factors – smoking, blood pressure, blood cholesterol, obesity, and insulin resistance/diabetes – account for relatively little of the population distribution of CHD. A recent polemical version of this suggested that while the conventional risk factors have received the lion's share of attention 'they account for peanuts' (Evans 2002). Recently, however, a strong case has been made that the conventional risk factors can, indeed, account for most of the population distribution of CHD (Beaglehole and Magnus 2002; Canto and Iskandrian 2003; Greenland *et al.* 2002). This proposition is based on the fact that single measures of risk factors underestimate their potential explanatory power, particularly when it is recognized that lifetime exposure is the key factor and that this would not be adequately indexed by single measurements taken in middle age.

Acceptance of the notion that conventional risk factors are key does not, of course, mean that understanding the aetiology of CHD is solved. It merely suggests that if exposures such as poor intrauterine growth or psychosocial factors are advanced as being important causal factors for CHD their influence must, at a proximal level, be mediated through the established behavioural or physiological risk factors. The important issue then becomes one of explaining the distribution of these conventional risk factors in a population. For behavioural risk factors such as smoking, diet, and exercise the determinants are, of course, political, economic, and social. For physiological risk factors the processes influencing these – such as diet with its effect on serum cholesterol and insulin resistance, or alcohol and salt consumption and their influence on blood pressure – have the same ultimate determinants. There is also evidence that other processes, some of them acting in early life – such as genetic make-up determined at conception, growth during the intrauterine period, or infant and child growth – influence the distribution of the established physiological risk factors.

Consideration of time-trends in established physiological risk factors can point to important periods in the life course for their determination. It is well known that blood pressure levels in many countries, including the UK and US, have been declining for many decades. However, recent evidence from cross-sectional surveys suggests that this stepwise decline by birth year was already evident among adolescents and young adults 50 years ago (McCarron *et al.* 2001*b*). Similarly, in the US formal analysis has suggested strong birth cohort influences in the downward shift of blood pressure there (Goff *et al.* 2001). This evidence suggests that the factors that are influencing secular declines in blood pressure – declines that were seen before the widespread introduction of effective antihypertensive medication – are set in train in early life. Changes in birthweight are not of a magnitude that can explain the blood pressure declines, given the known strength of association between birthweight and blood pressure. Diet (especially increased access to fruits and vegetables) and growth in infancy and childhood may be of importance, and in this respect evidence from a randomized controlled trial that lower sodium intake during infancy results in lower blood pressure in adolescence (Geleijnse *et al.* 1997) provides intriguing provisional evidence regarding one potential dietary influence that requires replication in future studies.

33.4.1 Life course approaches and the twentieth century epidemic of CHD

Trend data on smoking provide some support for the contention that the established risk factors explain the bulk of the CHD epidemic. Figure 33.4 shows male and female heart disease mortality and sex ratio in the US from 1900 to 1998. This demonstrates the twentieth century epidemic of heart disease that was dominated by male heart disease mortality. It is important to note that the category of 'heart disease' used here is comprised of a diverse set of pathological entities with potentially disparate causal mechanisms. The generic term of heart disease includes

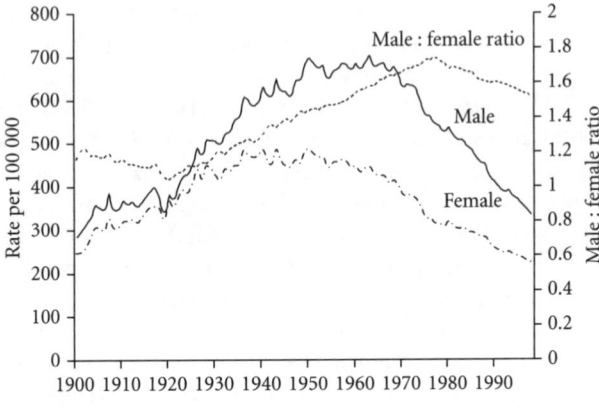

Fig. 33.4 Age-adjusted mortality rates from heart disease by sex, and male:female ratio for heart disease mortality, USA, 1900–98.

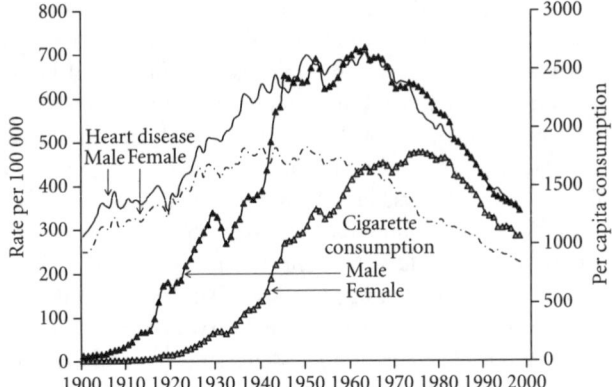

Fig. 33.5 Age-adjusted mortality rates from heart disease by sex, and estimated annual adult per capita cigarette consumption, USA, 1900–98.

not only CHD, but also congestive heart failure, rheumatic heart disease, arrhythmia, hypertensive heart disease, and others. In addition, the relative contributions of these sub-components of the generic category of heart disease has changed over time. Nevertheless, it is reasonable to propose that the largest contributor to the rise and subsequent fall in the twentieth century epidemic of heart disease was CHD.

From individual-level data on sex-specific smoking prevalences by birth cohort (Burns *et al.* 1997; Escobedo and Peddicord 1996) and historical data on cigarette consumption (Centers for Disease Control and Prevention 2002), we have estimated sex-specific cigarette consumption trends over the century and show them in relation to sex-specific heart disease trends in Fig. 33.5. For males, these patterns suggest that at the population level the effect of smoking on heart disease is rather immediate, in that there seems little or no time lag between the rapid rise of smoking in the population and the equally steep increase and decline in smoking and heart disease. This is not the case for women, where the peak in heart disease occurs 25–30 years before the zenith of smoking. This may reflect secular trends in other CHD risk factors such as lipids and blood pressure. There is a need to examine sex-specific links between smoking, the other major risk factors, and CHD rates in more detail, including the age of initiation of smoking in various birth cohorts (Glied 2003), their total exposure to smoking, and age at quitting.

There are three main processes implicated in heart disease: the development of atheroma, thrombo-embolic processes, and arrhythmia. Smoking may not only affect development of atheroma, but also operate through the thrombo-embolic and/or arrhythmic pathways, thus plausibly being able to almost instantaneously influence heart disease, given underlying susceptibility due to the development of vulnerable atherosclerotic plaque – itself associated with diet, blood lipids, and blood pressure. The point of these graphs is to show how long-term trends in smoking are reasonably compatible (at least for men) with CHD trends. However, it is difficult to make definitive judgements on the contribution of single risk factors to population trends in disease, given the wide range of plausible time lags between exposure and outcome.

Data on blood pressure trends in the US shows strong birth cohort shifts in the whole distribution of blood pressure from the 1950s onwards (Goff *et al.* 2001). This suggests that each successive generation born after the last decades of the nineteenth century carried with it a more favourable distribution of blood pressure. The US epidemic of heart disease peaked in the 1960s for men – among cohorts born around the turn of the century. The rapid declines in heart disease after the 1960s are thus compatible with both period declines in smoking and cohort declines in blood pressure in the population, and suggest different influences across different birth cohorts in both early and later life experiences of the conditions predisposing to adverse risks for adopting (and maintaining) smoking and developing hypertension.

With this mixture of cohort effects in the increases (and decreases) for some risk factors, but period effects in others, combined with the generally multiplicative nature of combined influence of CHD risk factors (and thus influences on CHD risk that are extra-additive), it is difficult to predict whether cohort or period effects in CHD should be seen. A re-analysis of UK data suggested that both were evident, but period effects were stronger (Charlton *et al.* 1997). If we could obtain integrated measures of the main CHD risk factors over the life course of the successive generations who contributed to these patterns of heart disease, then explaining the causes of epidemic CHD might not be so complicated. From a life course perspective, even if we can explain the bulk of the epidemic of CHD during the twentieth century with the traditional risk factors, we still do not understand the determinants of the changing distributions of these risk factors in different birth cohorts over time. Exercise, for example, is a determinant of insulin resistance and perhaps blood pressure. Early life social circumstances seem to be important for insulin resistance in a way we do not understand fully. One important implication, from a life course perspective, would be that apparently novel life course CHD risk factors – whether these are deprivation in childhood, poor *in utero* growth, psychosocial factors in adulthood, or income inequality (Lynch *et al.* 2004) – are likely to increase CHD risk through the conventional risk factors, both at the individual and population levels.

An important exception to this general pattern is illustrated in the case of sudden cardiac death, where contemporaneous exposure may be particularly important in triggering acute events and in understanding population trends. The example of the mortality crisis in Russia after the fall of the Soviet Union shows that massive social upheaval can be almost simultaneously translated into large increases in CHD (Shkolnikov *et al.* 2001). Figure 33.6 shows trends in CHD, violence and accidents, breast cancer, rheumatic heart disease, and stomach cancer from 1965 to 1999. The rapid rise of deaths from CHD and accidents/violence has been attributed largely to arrhythmia and cardiomyopathy resulting from binge consumption of alcohol (Leon *et al.* 1997). Thus, a contemporaneous exposure in the population such as increases in binge alcohol consumption can generate large increases in sudden cardiac death (see Chapter 17). So rather than cohort differences in the acquisition of risk from across the life course, as may be the case of CHD trends in the US, the Russian example highlights the importance of examining acute period exposures on a specific component of CHD – arrhythmia. CHD is a grouped phenomenon, with chronic atheromatous disease and acute electrical instability having somewhat

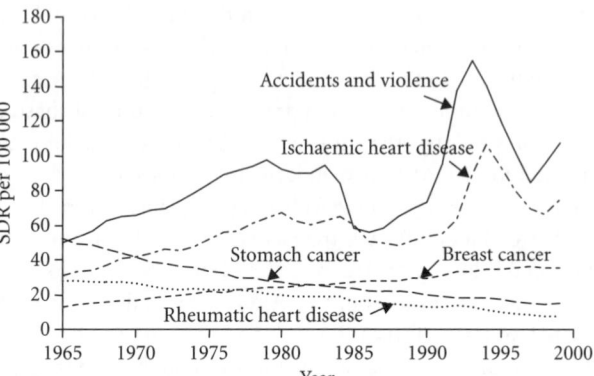

Fig. 33.6 Trends in selected causes of death for women aged 30–59 in Russia, 1965–99. (SDR: standardized death rate) (Adapted from Shkolnikov *et al.* 2001.)

different determinants acting at different life course stages. Having said this, the idea that chronic atheromatous CHD and sudden cardiac death from arrhythmia can have different aetiological time lags and therefore different determinants understates the complex interactions of social conditions and risk factors over the life course. Thus while binge alcohol consumption may contribute to sudden cardiac death, there are social determinants of who is more likely to engage in this pattern of behaviour. Thus, the susceptibility to engage in binge drinking is itself influenced by social and economic circumstances from across the life course. A recent study of Finnish men has shown that patterns of binge alcohol consumption in adulthood are influenced by socio-economic and family influences in childhood net of adult socio-economic conditions. It is also interesting to note that Fig. 33.6 shows the lack of effect of rapid economic change on mortality from rheumatic heart disease and breast and stomach cancer – these continue their historical trends unaffected by the massive social changes experienced in Russia. These are all conditions with important early life determinants (Davey Smith 2003), so this finding is expected. It does, however, highlight the value of examining specific outcomes in regard to their particular determinants.

33.5 Epidemiological implications of life course approaches

There has been considerable recent debate regarding the individualistic focus of much epidemiology on the lifestyles or physiological profiles of people abstracted from their social context (Diez-Roux 1998; Koopman and Lynch 1999; Krieger 1994). These authors point out that there are broader social determinants of the risks to health that people suffer, and that attempts to reduce these risks should recognize this fundamental social determination. Others have strongly taken issue with this view (Rothman *et al.* 1998).

The weaknesses of epidemiological approaches which fail to locate exposure–disease associations within their historical, political, and social contexts have been convincingly elaborated on (Diez-Roux 1998; Koopman and Lynch 1999; Krieger 1994; Schwartz and Carpenter 1999). Perhaps less widely acknowledged is that the abstraction of such associations from their particular context can lead to misleading conclusions about disease aetiology. Take, for example, the extensive research on vitamin C consumption and the risk of CVD. A strong observational inverse association between plasma vitamin C levels and CHD mortality (Khaw *et al.* 2001) was rendered implausible by a subsequent large randomized controlled trial of a vitamin supplement that raised plasma vitamin C levels substantially, but left 5-year CHD mortality unchanged. In this case the range of plasma vitamin C levels in the observational study and the

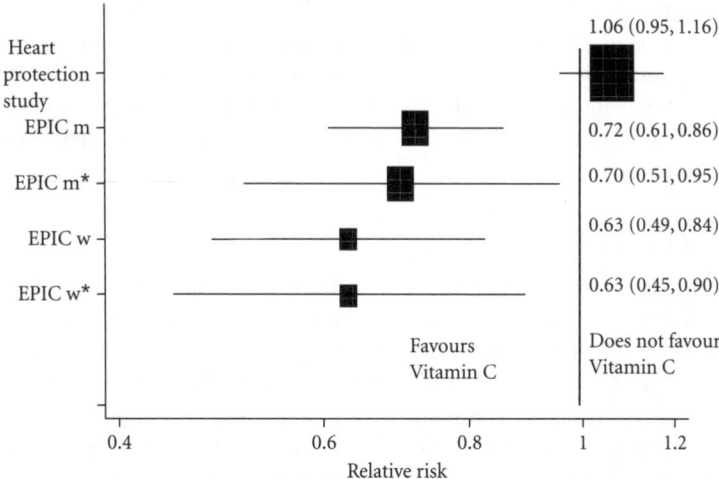

Fig. 33.7 Estimates of the effects of an increase of 15.7 mmol/l plasma vitamin C on CHD 5-year mortality estimated from observational epidemiological EPIC study and randomized controlled Heart Protection Study. (EPIC m = men, age-adjusted; EPIC m* = men, adjusted for systolic blood pressure, cholesterol, BMI, smoking, diabetes, and vitamin supplement use; EPIC w = women, age-adjusted; EPIC w* = women, adjusted for systolic blood pressure, cholesterol, BMI, smoking, diabetes, and vitamin supplement use).

change introduced by supplementation were similar, yet the outcomes of observation and experiment were very different (see Fig. 33.7) (Heart Protection Study Collaborative Group 2002*b*). There are now a series of similar examples: hormone replacement therapy (Chapter 22), vitamin E, and beta carotene intake in relation to CVD among them (Chapter 15). What these examples have in common is that the groups of people who were apparently receiving protection from these substances in the observational studies were very different from the groups not using them, on a whole host of characteristics of their lives. In a cross-sectional study of late middle-aged women, blood vitamin C levels were measured and it was found that women with higher vitamin C levels were less likely to have had a father in a manual social class job, less likely to have had no bathroom in their homes as a child, less likely to have had no hot water in their homes as a child, less likely to have come from a family with no car, less likely to have only completed minimal education, less likely to be in a manual social class adulthood, less likely to have no car as an adult, less likely to be a smoker, more likely to have moderate daily alcohol intake, more likely to exercise in their leisure time, more likely to eat a low fat diet, less likely to be obese, more likely to be tall, more likely to have longer legs (Lawlor *et al.* 2003). It is clear that a large range of confounding factors from right across the life course would generate an apparent protective effect of vitamin C levels on CHD, even when no causal association exists. As mentioned earlier, indicators of adult SEP can be effective (but not exhaustive) summaries of different life course trajectories. Similarly, levels of Vitamin C can be thought of as an embodied biological crystallization of people's entire life course experiences.

Believing that the full range of differences – accumulated over the life course – between people with different vitamin C intakes could be summed up in measures of a few 'potential confounders' and adequately adjusted for in statistical analyses fails to recognize the complexity of the reasons why people differ with regard to particular and general characteristics of their lives, and reinforces the view that the causes of CHD need to be sought with data from across the life course and considered within the historically contextualized conditions of successive generations. To advance understanding of the specific role of factors such as vitamin C in CHD aetiology approaches other than the purely observational – such as Mendelian randomization (Davey Smith and Ebrahim 2004; Davey Smith and Ebrahim 2003), or randomized controlled trials, need to be deployed.

33.6 Conclusions

CHD is clearly influenced by factors acting across the life course. CHD is a heterogeneous category, however, and in different places and at different times its composition (and therefore the balance of aetiological factors) may differ. Ultimately it appears that a limited range of established risk factors mediate between processes acting at different stages of the life course and CHD. Therefore the (non-comprehensive, but extensive) list of putative life course risk factors for CHD, given in Box 33.1, will ultimately be channelled through a limited range of proximal processes. The social, economic, political, and cultural influences on the broad range of life course factors in Box 33.1 will all influence population CHD rates. Further, the factors driving trends and levels of CHD in different countries, and at different times within the same country, may differ.

A life course perspective may simultaneously simplify considerations of CHD aetiology – by suggesting that as far as proximal processes are concerned, the hunt for novel risk factors for epidemic CHD is not necessary – while at the same time adding the complexity of having to consider the changing broader contexts of the times through which different cohorts of people have lived and the implications for acquiring CHD risk factor profiles.

References

Anda, R. F., Croft, J. B., Felitti, V. J., Nordenberg, D., Giles, W. H., Williamson, D. F., and Giovino, G. A. (1999). Adverse childhood experiences and smoking during adolescence and adulthood. *Journal of the American Medical Association* **282**, 1652–8.

Bao, W., Srinivasan, S. R., Wattigney, W. A., and Berenson, G. S. (1994). Persistence of multiple cardiovascular risk clustering related to syndrome X from childhood to young adulthood. *Archives of Internal Medicine* **154**(16), 1842–7.

Barker, D. J. P. and Osmond, C. (1986). Infant mortality, childhood nutrition and ischaemic heart disease in England and Wales. *Lancet* **i**, 1077–81.

Barker, D. J. P., Osmond, C., Winter, P. D., Margetts, B., and Simmonds, S. J. (1989). Weight in infancy and death from ischaemic heart disease. *Lancet* **ii**, 577–80.

Barker, D. J. P., Forsén, T., Uutela, A., Osmond, C., and Eriksson, J. G. (2001). Size at birth and resilience to the effects of poor living conditions in adult life: longitudinal study. *British Medical Journal* **323**, 1273–6.

Beaglehole, R. and Magnus, P. (2002). Coronary heart disease prevention: act now, research at leisure. *International Journal of Epidemiology* **31**, 1134–5.

Beebe-Dimmer, J., Lynch, J. W., Turell, G., Lustgarten, S., Raghunathan, T., and Kaplan, G. A. (2004). Childhood and adult socioeconomic conditions and 31-year mortality risk in women. *American Journal of Epidemiology* **159**, 481–90.

Ben-Shlomo, Y. and Davey Smith, G. (1991). Deprivation in infancy or in adult life: which is more important for mortality risk? *Lancet* **337**, 530–4.

Ben-Shlomo, Y. and Kuh, D. (2002). A lifecourse approach to chronic disease epidemiology: conceptual models, empirical challenges and interdisciplinary perspectives. *International Journal of Epidemiology* **31**, 285–93.

Berenson, G. S., Srinivasan, S. R., Bao, W., Newman, W. P., Tracy, R. E., and Wattigney, W. A. (1998a). Association between multiple cardiovascular risk factors and atherosclerosis in children and young adults. *New England Journal of Medicine* **338**, 1650–6.

Blane, D., Hart, C. L., Davey Smith, G., Gillis, C. R., Hole, D. J., and Hawthorne, V. M. (1996). Association of cardiovascular disease risk factors with socioeconomic position during childhood and during adulthood. *British Medical Journal* **313** (7070), 1434–8.

Bobák, M., Hertzman, C., Skodová, Z., and Marmot, M. (2000). Own education, current conditions, parental material circumstances, and risk of myocardial infarction in a former communist country. *Journal of Epidemiology and Community Health* **54**, 91–6.

Brasche, S., Galbas, C., and Störl, B. (2001). Kindheit und Herzinfarkt: sozioökonmische und psychosoziale Kindheitseinflüsse auf das Herzinfarktrisiko. *Sozial Und Präventivmedizin* **46**, 311–19.

Brunner, E., Davey Smith, G., Marmot, M., Canner, R., Beksinska, M., and O'Brien, J. (1996). Childhood social circumstances and psychosocial and behavioural factors as determinants of plasma fibrinogen. *Lancet* **347**(9007), 1008–13.

Burns, D. M., Lee, L., Shen, L. Z., Gilpin, E., Tolley, H. D., Vaughn, J., and Shanks, T. G. (1997). Cigarette smoking behavior in the United States. In *Smoking and tobacco control*, Monograph 8: *Changes in cigarette-related disease risks and their implications for prevention and control* (ed. D. M. Burns, L. Garfinkel, and J. M. Samet), pp. 13–42. US Dept. of Health and Human Services, National Cancer Institute, Bethesda, MD.

Burr, M. L. and Sweetnam, P. M. (1980). Family size and paternal unemployment in relation to myocardial infarction. *Journal of Epidemiology and Community Health* **34**(2), 93–5.

Canto, J. G. and Iskandrian, A. E. (2003). Major risk factors for cardiovascular disease: debunking the 'only 50%' myth. *Journal of the American Medical Association* **290**, 947–9.

Cassell, J. (1995). The contribution of the social environment to host resistance. [Originally published 1976.] *American Journal of Epidemiology* **141**, 798–814.

Centers for Disease Control and Prevention, Tobacco Information and Prevention Source. Consumption Data. Available at: <http://www.cdc.gov/tobacco/research_data/economics/consump1.htm> (accessed 11 September 2002).

Charlton, J., Murphy, M., Khaw, K., Ebrahim, S., and Davey Smith, G. (1997). Cardiovascular diseases. In *The health of adult Britain 1841–1994*, Vol. 2 (ed. J. Charlton, M. Murphy, K. Khaw, S. Ebrahim, and G. Davey Smith), pp. 60–80. The Stationery Office, London.

Claussen, B., Davey Smith, G., and Thelle, D. (2003). The impact of childhood and adulthood socioeconomic position on cause-specific mortality: The Oslo Mortality Study. *Journal of Epidemiology and Community Health* **57**, 40–5.

Coggon, D., Margetts, B., Barker, D. J. *et al.* (1990). Childhood risk factors for ischaemic heart disease and stroke. *Paediatric and Perinatal Epidemiology* **4**(4), 464–9.

Curtin, F., Morabia, A., and Bernstein, M. (1997). Smoking behaviour in a Swiss urban population: the role of gender and education. *Preventive Medicine* **26**(5 Part 1), 658–63.

Davey Smith, G. (2003). *Health inequalities: lifecourse approaches*. Policy Press, Bristol.

Davey Smith, G. and Ebrahim, S. (2003). 'Mendelian randomization': can genetic epidemiology contribute to understanding environmental determinants of disease? *International Journal of Epidemiology* **32**, 1–22.

Davey Smith, G. and Ebrahim, S. (2004). Mendelian randomization: prospects, potentials, and limitations. *International Journal of Epidemiology* **33**, 30–42.

Davey Smith, G. and Hart, C. (2002). Lifecourse socioeconomic and behavioural influences on cardiovascular disease mortality: the Collaborative study. *American Journal of Public Health* **92**, 1295–8.

Davey Smith, G. and Lynch, J. W. (2004). Socioeconomic differentials. In *Lifecourse approach to chronic disease epidemiology*, 2nd edn (ed. D. Kuh D and Y. A. Ben-Shlomo), pp. 77–115. Oxford University Press.

Davey Smith, G., Hart, C. L., Blane, D., Gillis, C., and Hawthorne, V. (1997). Lifetime socioeconomic position and mortality: prospective observational study. *British Medical Journal* **314**, 547–52.

Davey Smith, G., Hart, C., Blane, D., and Hole, D. (1998). Adverse socioeconomic conditions in childhood and cause specific adult mortality: prospective observational study. *British Medical Journal* **316** (7145), 1631–5.

Davey Smith, G., Gunnell, D., and Ben-Shlomo, Y. (2000*a*). Life-course approaches to socio-economic differentials in cause-specific adult mortality. In *Poverty, inequality and health* (ed. D. and G. Walt), pp. 88–124. Oxford University Press.

Davey Smith, G., Hart, C., Upton, M., Hole, D., Gillis, C., Watt, G., and Hawthorne, V. (2000*b*). Height and risk of death among men and women: aetiological implications of associations with cardiorespiratory disease and cancer mortality. *Journal of Epidemiology and Community Health* **54**, 97–103.

Davey Smith, G., Greenwood, R., Gunnell, D., Sweetnam, P., and Elwood, P. (2001*a*). Leg length, insulin resistance, and coronary heart disease risk: The Caerphilly Study. *Journal of Epidemiology and Community Health* **55**, 867–72.

Davey Smith, G., McCarron, P., Okasha, M., and McEwen, J. (2001*b*). Social circumstances in childhood and cardiovascular disease mortality: prospective observational study of Glasgow university students. *Journal of Epidemiology and Community Health* **55**, 340–1.

Davey Smith, G., Ben-Shlomo, Y., and Lynch, J. (2002). Life course approaches to inequalities in coronary heart disease risk. In *Stress and the heart* (ed. S. A. Stansfeld and M. G. Marmot), pp. 20–49. BMJ Books, London.

Dedman, D. J., Gunnell, D., Davey Smith, G., and Frankel, S. (2001). Childhood housing conditions and later mortality in the Boyd Orr cohort. *Journal of Epidemiology and Community Health* **55**(1), 10–15.

Diaz, A., Simantov, E., and Rickert, V. I. (2002). Effect of abuse on health: results of a national survey. *Archives of Pediatrics and Adolescent Medicine* **156**, 811–17.

Diez-Roux, A. V. (1998). Bringing context back into epidemiology: variables and fallacies in multilevel analysis. *American Journal of Public Health* **88**, 216–22.

Donnan, S. P. B., Ho, S. C., Woo, J. *et al.* (1994). Risk factors for acute myocardial infarction in a Southern Chinese population. *Annals of Epidemiology* **4**, 46–58.

Eriksson, J. G., Forsén, T., Tuomilehto, J., Osmond, C., and Barker, D. J. P. (2000). Early growth, adult income, and risk of stroke. *Stroke* **31**(4), 869–74.

Escobedo, L. and Peddicord, J. (1996). Smoking prevalence in US birth cohorts: the influence of gender and education. *American Journal of Public Health* **86**(2), 231–6.

Evans, R. (2002). *Interpreting and addressing inequalities in health: from Black to Acheson to Blair to . . . .* Office of Health Economics, London.

Felitti, V. J., Anda, R. F., Nordenberg, D., Williamson, D. F., Spitz, A. M., Edwards, V. *et al.* (1998). Relationship of childhood abuse and household dysfunction to many leading causes of death in adults: The Adverse Childhood Experiences (ACE) Study. *American Journal of Preventive Medicine* **14**, 245–58.

Forsdahl, A. (1973). Momenter til belysning ar den høye dødelighet; Finnmark Fylke. *Tidsskr Nor Lægeforen* **93**, 661–7. [Translated and reprinted as Forsdahl A. (2002). Observations throwing light on the high mortality in the county of Finnmark: is the high mortality today a late effect of very poor living conditions in childhood and adolescence? *International Journal of Epidemiology* **31**, 302–8.]

Forsdahl, A. (1977). Are poor living conditions in childhood and adolescence an important risk factor for arteriosclerotic heart disease? *British Journal of Preventive & Social Medicine* **31**, 91–5.

Forsdahl, A. (1978). Living conditions in childhood and subsequent development of risk factors for arteriosclerotic heart disease. *Journal of Epidemiology and Community Health* **32**, 34–7.

Forsdahl, A., Salmi, H., and Forsdahl, F. (1974). Finskættede i Sør-Varanger kommune II. *Tidsskrift for den Norske Lægeforening* **94**, 1565–72.

Forsen, T., Eriksson, J., Tuomilehto, J., Reunanen, A., Osmond, C., and Barker, D. (2000). The fetal and childhood growth of persons who develop type 2 diabetes. *Annals of Internal Medicine* **133**, 176–82.

Forsen, T., Eriksson, J. G., Tuomilehto, J., Osmond, C., and Barker, D. J. (1999). Growth in utero and during childhood among women who develop coronary heart disease: longitudinal study. *British Medical Journal* **319**, 1403–7.

Frankel, S., Davey Smith, G., and Gunnell, D. (1999). Childhood socioeconomic position and adult cardiovascular mortality: the Boyd Orr cohort. *American Journal of Epidemiology* **150**, 1081–4.

Frankel, S., Elwood, P., Sweetnam, P., Yarnell, J., and Davey Smith, G. (1996). Birthweight, body-mass index in middle age, and incident coronary heart disease. *Lancet* **348**, 1478–80.

Galobardes, B., Davey Smith, G., and Lynch, J. W. (2004). Childhood socioeconomic position and adult CVD. *Epidemiological Reviews* **26**, 7–21.

Geleijnse, J. M., Hofman, A., Witteman, J. C., Hazebroek, A. A., Valkenburg, H. A., and Grobbee, D. E. (1997). Long-term effects of neonatal sodium restriction on blood pressure. *Hypertension* **29**, 913–17.

Gilman, S. E., Kawachi, I., Fitzmaurice, G. M., and Buka, S. L. (2002). Socioeconomic status in childhood and the lifetime risk of major depression. *International Journal of Epidemiology* **31**, 359–67.

Glied, S. (2003). Is smoking delayed smoking averted? *American Journal of Public Health* **93**, 412–16.

Gliksman, M. D., Kawachi, I., Hunter, D. *et al.* (1995). Childhood socioeconomic status and risk of cardiovascular disease in middle aged US women: a prospective study. *Journal of Epidemiology and Community Health* **49**(1), 10–15.

Goff, D. C., Howard, G., Russell, G. B., and Labarthe, D. R. (2001). Birth cohort evidence of population influences on blood pressure in the United States, 1887–1994. *Annals of Epidemiology* **111**, 271–9.

Graham, H. and Der, G. (1999). Influences on women's smoking status: the contribution of socioeconomic status in adolescence and adulthood. *European Journal of Public Health* **9**, 137–41.

Greenland, P., Gidding, S. S., and Tracy, R. P. (2002). Lifelong prevention of atherosclerosis: the critical importance of major risk factor exposures. *International Journal of Epidemiology* **31**, 1129–34.

Hallqvist, J., Lynch, J. W., Blane, D., Bartley, M., and Lange, T. (2004). Critical period, accumulation and social trajectory: can we empirically distinguish lifecourse processes? *Social Science and Medicine* **58**, 1555–62.

Hardy, R., Wadsworth, M., and Kuh, D. (2000). The influence of childhood weight and socioeconomic status on change in adult body mass index in a British national birth cohort. *International Journal of Obesity Related Metabolic Disorders* **24**(6), 725–34.

Harper, S., Lynch, J. W., Everson, S. A., Hsu, W.-L., Raghunathan, T., and Kaplan, G. A. (2002). Lifecourse socioeconomic position and depression, cynical hostility and hopelessness in adulthood. *International Journal of Epidemiology* **31**, 395–403.

Hart, C. L., Davey Smith, G., and Blane, D. (1998). Social mobility and 21 year mortality in a cohort of Scottish men. *Social Science & Medicine* **47**(8), 1121–30.

Hasle, H. (1990). Association between living conditions in childhood and myocardial infarction. *British Medical Journal* **300**(6723), 512–13.

Heart Protection Study Collaborative Group (2002a). MRC/BHF Heart Protection Study of cholesterol lowering with simvastatin in 20,536 high-risk individuals: a randomised placebo-controlled trial. *Lancet* **360**, 7–22.

Heart Protection Study Collaborative Group (2002b). MRC/BHF Heart Protection Study of antioxidant vitamin supplementation in 20536 high-risk individuals: a randomised placebo-controlled trial. *Lancet* **360**, 23–33.

Heslop, P., Davey Smith, G., Macleod, J., and Hart, C. (2001). The socioeconomic position of employed women, risk factors and mortality. *Social Science & Medicine* **53**, 477–85.

Kaplan, G. A. and Salonen, J. T. (1990). Socioeconomic conditions in childhood and ischaemic heart disease during middle age. *British Medical Journal* **301**, 1121–3.

Kendall-Tacket, K. (2002). The health effects of childhood abuse: four pathways by which abuse can influence health. *Child Abuse and Neglect* **26**, 715–29.

Khaw, K.-T., Bingham, S., Welch, A., Luben, R., Wareham, N., Oakes, S., and Day, N. (2001). Relation between plasma ascorbic acid and mortality in men and women in EPIC-Norfolk prospective study: a prospective population study. *Lancet* **357**, 657–63.

Klag, M. J., Ford, D. E., Mead, L. A., He, J., Whelton, P. K., Liang, K. Y. *et al.* (1993). Serum cholesterol in young men and subsequent cardiovascular disease. *New England Journal of Medicine* **328**, 313–18.

Koopman, J. S. and Lynch, J. W. (1999). Individual causal models and population system models in epidemiology. *American Journal of Public Health* **89**, 1170–4.

Krieger, N. (1994). Epidemiology and the web of causation: has anyone seen the spider? *Social Science & Medicine* **39**, 887–903.

Kuh, D. and Ben-Shlomo, Y. (eds) (1997). *A life course approach to chronic disease epidemiology.* Oxford University Press.

Kuh, D. and Davey Smith, G. (1997). The life course and adult chronic disease: an historical perspective with particular reference to coronary heart disease. In *A life course approach to chronic disease epidemiology* (ed. D. Kuh and S. Ben-Shlomo), pp. 15–41. Oxford University Press.

Kuh, D. and Hardy, R. (eds) (2002). *A lifecourse approach to women's health.* Oxford University Press.

Kuh, D., Hardy, R., Chaturvedi, N., and Wadsworth, M. E. (2002). Birth weight, childhood growth and abdominal obesity in adult life. *International Journal of Obesity and Related Metabolic Disorders* **26**(1), 40–7.

Kuh, D., Ben-Shlomo, Y., Lynch, J., Hallqvist, J., and Power, C. (2003). A glossary for lifecourse epidemiology. *Journal of Epidemiology and Community Health* **57**, 774–83.

Lawlor, D. A., Ebrahim, S., and Davey Smith, G. (2002*a*). Socioeconomic position in childhood and adulthood and insulin resistance: cross sectional survey using data from British women's heart and health study. *British Medical Journal* **325**(7368), 805.

Lawlor, D. A., Ebrahim, S., and Davey Smith, G. (2002*b*). The association between components of adult height and Type II diabetes and insulin resistance: British Women's Heart and Health Study. *Diabetologia* **45**, 1097–106.

Lawlor, D. A., Davey Smith, G., *et al.* (2003). Those confounded vitamins: what can we learn from the difference between observational versus randomised trial evidence? *Lancet* **363**, 1724–7.

Lawlor, D. A., Taylor, M., Davey Smith, G., Gunnell, D., and Ebrahim, S. (2004). The associations of components of adult height with coronary heart disease in postmenopausal women: the British Women's Heart and Health Study. *Heart* **90**, 745–9.

Leon, D., Chenet, L., Shkolnikov, V. M., Zakharov, S., Shapiro, J., Rakhmanova, G. *et al.* (1997). Huge variation in Russian mortality rates, 1984–1994: artefact, alcohol, or what? *Lancet* **350**, 383–8.

Li, S., Chen, W., Srinivasan, S. R., Bond, M. G., Tang, R., Urbina, E. M., and Berenson, G. S. (2003). Childhood cardiovascular risk factors and carotid vascular changes in adulthood: The Bogalusa Heart Study. *Journal of the American Medical Association* **290**, 2271–6.

Lissau, I. and Sorenson, T. (1994). Parental neglect during childhood and risk of obesity in young adulthood. *Lancet* **343**, 324–7.

Lynch, J. W., Kaplan, G. A., Cohen, R. D. *et al.* (1994). Childhood and adult socioeconomic status as predictors of mortality in Finland. *Lancet* **343**, 524–7.

Lynch, J. W., Kaplan, G. A., and Salonen, J. T. (1997). Why do poor people behave poorly? Variation in adult health behaviours and psychosocial characteristics by stages of the socioeconomic lifecourse. *Social Science & Medicine* **44**(6), 809–19.

Lynch, J. W., Davey Smith, G., Harper, S., and Hillemeier, M. (2004). Is income inequality a determinant of population health? Part 2. US National and Regional Trends in Income Inequality and Age- and Cause-specific Mortality. *Milbank Memorial Fund Quarterly* **82**, 355–400.

Marks, R. U. (1967). Social stress and cardiovascular disease: factors involving social and demographic characteristics. A review of empirical findings. *Milbank Memorial Fund Quarterly* **45**(Part 2): Suppl., 51–108.

Marmot, M., Shipley, M., Brunner, E., and Hemingway, H. (2001). Relative contribution of early life and adult socioeconomic factors to adult morbidity in the Whitehall II study. *Journal of Epidemiology and Community Health* **55**, 301–7.

McCarron, P. and Davey Smith, G. (2003). Physiological measurements in children in young people and risk of coronary heart disease in adults in: National Heart Forum *Young@heart*. National Heart Forum, London.

McCarron, P., Davey Smith, G., Okasha, M., and McEwen, J. (2000). Blood pressure in young adulthood and mortality from cardiovascular disease. *Lancet* **355**, 1430–1.

McCarron, P., Davey Smith, G., Okasha, M., and McEwen, J. (2001*a*). Smoking in adolescence and young adulthood and mortality in later life: prospective observational study. *Journal of Epidemiology and Community Health* **55**, 334–5.

McCarron, P., Okasha, M., McEwen, J., and Davey Smith, G. (2001*b*). Changes in blood pressure among students attending Glasgow University between 1948 and 1968: analyses of cross sectional surveys. *British Medical Journal* **322**, 885–9.

McCarron, P., Okasha, M., McEwen, J., and Davey Smith, G. (2002). Height in young adulthood and risk of death from cardiorespiratory disease: a prospective study of male former students of Glasgow University, Scotland. *American Journal of Epidemiology* **155**, 683–7.

Miura, K., Daviglus, M. L., Dyer, A. R., Liu, K., Garside, D. B., Stamler, J. *et al.* (2001). Relationship of blood pressure to 25-year mortality due to coronary heart disease, cardiovascular diseases, and all causes in young adult men: the Chicago Heart Association Detection Project in industry. *Archives of Internal Medicine* **161**, 1501–8.

Navas-Nacher, E. L., Colangelo, L., Beam, C., and Greenland, P. (2001). Risk factors for coronary heart disease in men 18 to 39 years of age. *Annals of Internal Medicine* **134**, 433–9.

Notkola, V. (1985). Living conditions in childhood and coronary heart disease in adulthood. *Commentationes Scientiarum Socialium* **29**, 15–119.

Notkola, V., Punsar, S., Karvonen, M. J., and Haapakoski, J. (1985). Socioeconomic conditions in childhood and mortality and morbidity caused by coronary heart disease in adulthood in rural Finland. *Social Science & Medicine* **21**(5), 517–23.

OPCS (Office of Population Censuses and Surveys) (1978). *The General Household Survey 1975.* HMSO, London.

Pensola, T. H. and Valkonen T. (2002). Effect of parental social class, own education and social class on mortality among young men. *European Journal of Public Health* **12**, 29–36.

Power, C. and Matthews, S. (1997). Origins of health inequalities in a national population sample. *Lancet* **350**(9091), 1584–9.

Raitakari, O. T., Porkka, K. V., Rasanen, L., Ronnemaa, T., and Viikari, J. S. (1994). Clustering and six year cluster-tracking of serum total cholesterol, HDL-cholesterol and diastolic blood pressure in children and young adults. *Journal of Clinical Epidemiology* **47**(10), 1085–93.

Raitakari, O. T., Juonala, M., Kähönen, M., Taittonen, L., Laitinen, T., Mäki-Tokko, N. *et al.* (2003). Cardiovascular risk factors in childhood and carotid artery intima-media thickness in adulthood: The Cardiovascular Risk in Young Finns Study. *Journal of the American Medical Association* **290**, 2277–83.

Rich-Edwards, J. W., Stampfer, M. J., Colditz, G. A. *et al.* (1995). Height and the risk of cardiovascular disease in women. *American Journal of Epidemiology* **142**, 1909–17.

Rose, G. (1982). Incubation period of coronary heart disease. *British Medical Journal* **284**, 1600–1.

Rothman, K. J., Adami, H. O., and Trichopoulos, D. (1998). Should the mission of epidemiology include the eradication of poverty? *Lancet* **352**, 810–13.

Schwartz, S. and Carpenter, K. M. (1999). The right answer for the wrong question: consequences of type III error for public health research. *American Journal of Public Health* **89**, 1175–80.

Shkolnikov, V., McKee, M., and Leon, D. A. (2001). Changes in life expectancy in Russia in the mid-1990s. *Lancet* **357**, 917–21.

Stamler, J., Stamler, R., and Neaton, J. D. (1993). Blood pressure, systolic and diastolic, and cardiovascular risks: US population data. *Archives of Internal Medicine* **153**, 598–615.

Taylor, S. E. and Repetti, R. L. (1997). Health psychology: what is an unhealthy environment and how does it get under the skin? *Annual Review of Psychology* **48**, 411–47.

The sixth report of the Joint National Committee on prevention, detection, evaluation, and treatment of high blood pressure (1997). *Archives of Internal Medicine* **157**, 2413–46.

Uemura, N., Okamoto, S., Yamamoto, S., Matsumura, N., Yamaguchi, S., Yamakido, M. *et al.* (2001). Helicobacter pylori infection and the development of gastric cancer. *New England Journal of Medicine* **345**, 784–9.

Vågerö, D. and Leon, D. (1994). Effect of social class in childhood and adulthood on adult mortality. *Lancet* **343**, 1224–5.

van de Mheen, H., Stronks, K., Looman, C. W. N., and Mackenbach, J. P. (1998). Does childhood socioeconomic status influence adult health through behavioural factors? *International Journal of Epidemiology* **27**, 431–7.

Wannamethee, S. G., Whincup, P. H., Shaper, G., and Walker, M. (1996). Influence of fathers' social class on cardiovascular disease in middle-aged men. [See comments.] *Lancet* **348**, 1259–63.

Yarnell, J. G. W., Limb, E. S., Layzell, J. M. *et al.* (1992). Height: a risk marker for ischaemic heart disease. *European Heart Journal* **13**, 1602–5.

Chapter 34

Emergence of risk factors in children

D. R. Labarthe

34.1 **Importance**

In 1990, the Cardiovascular Disease (CVD) Unit of the World Health Organization (WHO) published its Expert Committee Report *Prevention in childhood and youth of adult cardio-vascular diseases: time for action* (WHO 1990). Reflecting the deliberations of an international panel of experts convened in the late 1980s, this report urged that:

> countries develop and pursue a comprehensive population strategy for the primary prevention of [atherosclerotic and hypertensive] diseases as part of their long-term national health development plan. This strategy should emphasize primary prevention beginning in early childhood and continuing throughout childhood and youth, in order to avoid the emergence of the established major risk factors for adult CVD and prevent their persistence on a mass scale in the community.

The three pillars of the recommended programs were:

- improvements in eating patterns that will prevent hyperlipidaemia, obesity, hypertension, and diabetes while assuring an adequate intake of all the nutrients essential for optimal growth and development;
- the elimination of smoking and other forms of tobacco use;
- improvements in exercise habits that will enhance cardiopulmonary fitness and help prevent obesity, hyperlipidaemia, hypertension, and diabetes.

These excerpts from deliberations well over a decade ago accord with our current under-standing of the major risk factors for atherosclerotic and hypertensive diseases, their main immediate determinants, and the potential for preventing or reversing the epidemic of the risk factors themselves. The subtitle, *Time for Action*, was a deliberate addition by the Committee, which judged that the recommended actions were already long overdue. Strasser had expressed a decade earlier, in 1978, the urgency of mounting worldwide efforts for 'primordial preven-tion,' or prevention of risk factor epidemics (Strasser 1978). There was a sense in the Expert Committee's discussion and report that this recommendation had received insufficient notice and little if any practical implementation.

This WHO report has equal or greater force today, as the global pandemic of atherosclerotic and hypertensive diseases and their risk factors continues to expand. Its importance is heightened by the perception of an abrupt increase in the prevalence of obesity in some parts of the world, often including children and adolescents, with serious implications for further progression of the pandemic.

The focus of this chapter on the 'emergence' of the risk factors emphasizes the progressive development of the risk factors within the individual person, from all relevant antecedent conditions – genetic endowment, social and environmental conditions (perhaps including the intrauterine environment), and behavioural patterns – to the expression of these as manifest risk factors such as obesity, dyslipidaemia, high blood pressure, and diabetes. This emphasis is distinct from the emergence of population-wide epidemics of the risk factors anticipated by Strasser, which would entail a different approach that characterizes long-term trends in risk factor distributions in populations. That approach, although worthy of attention, is beyond the scope of the present review. Because the earliest and latest aspects of the progressive development noted above – possibly beginning in fetal life and extending into advanced age – are addressed in the other chapters in this section, the focus of this discussion is the period of childhood and adolescence.

34.2 **Risk factors**

This section addresses the risk factors for atherosclerosis and hypertension singly and in combination. Because each risk factor is reviewed in other chapters, only those aspects of particular importance in childhood and adolescence are discussed here. Such aspects are mainly issues of definition, classification, and measurement, and of patterns of development within this period of life (essentially the school years, ages 6–18), including specific influences on this development.

34.2.1 **Obesity**

Definition, classification, and measurement

'Obesity' may refer to any of several characteristics related to absolute or relative body size, body composition, or body fat distribution. Each of these characteristics is measured as a continuous trait. However, the term obesity implies, respectively, the upper extreme of body size, a relatively high proportion of body mass that is adipose tissue, or a relatively high concentration of adipose tissue in the abdomen (abdominal, central, or truncal adiposity/obesity). Several methods of measurement are available for each of these characteristics. Surprisingly, reports addressing obesity often fail to specify either the characteristic under discussion or the underlying methods and criteria. Probably the most widely used measure for children and adolescents as well as other age groups is the body mass index (BMI), calculated as total weight in kilograms divided by the square of height in metres. Unlike adults, children and adolescents are typically classified by relative rather than absolute values of BMI, for example, values above the sex- and age-specific 85th or 95th percentile value of a reference distribution (Troiano *et al.* 1995).

Development with age

After a transient decrease in the first years of life, BMI increases continuously throughout childhood and adolescence in both males and females. This increase reflects general growth of body mass relative to growth in height. The proportionate contributions of lean and fat mass differ by sex, females having a greater and nearly constant proportion of fat mass, males experiencing a greater proportionate increase in lean mass relative to fat mass from the beginning of adolescence. Thus, the interpretation of BMI as an index of adiposity requires qualification as to age and sex. For this reason, the terms 'overweight' and 'at risk for overweight' have sometimes been used to refer to BMI at or above the 95th percentile and between the 85th and 95th percentiles of a reference population, respectively, in preference to 'obese' (Troiano *et al.* 1995). Prevalence estimates of overweight and at risk for overweight in a national probability sample of US children and adolescents in 1988–91 were, overall, 22.0 and 10.9% among survey participants at ages 6–17 years. Marked variation by age, sex, and race or ethnicity was found, with generally higher prevalence in both categories for two minority populations, non-Hispanic blacks, and Mexican Americans.

Other measures may either resemble or differ strikingly from BMI in their patterns of development with age, as shown in longitudinal data (Dai *et al.* 2002*a*). Abdominal circumference, a measure of central adiposity, closely resembles BMI in this respect. By contrast, percentage of body fat, which is estimated from selected skinfold measurements and bioelectrical impedance, and multiple skinfolds (whether two or six measurements in combination) differ from BMI and abdominal circumference by being greater in females (especially in black females) than in males at all ages and in decreasing sharply in males after a peak at age 10 (percentage of body fat) or 12 (skinfolds).

Other aspects

Major influences on development of overweight and obesity in children and adolescents are thought to be those bearing on energy imbalance – that is, dietary imbalance and physical inactivity, with their multiple underlying determinants. Contributions of genetics, socio-economic status, and psychosocial factors have also been studied. A particular focus of attention is television watching, a modern habit of children and adolescents (as well as adults) that combines physical inactivity with both simultaneous consumption of nutritionally undesirable foods and beverages and extensive exposure to advertising of similar food products. More detailed discussion of this aspect of obesity and its relationships to risk factors is presented in an extensive recent review (Obarzanek 1999).

34.2.2 **Blood lipids**

Definition, classification, and measurement

The US National Cholesterol Education Program (NCEP) has provided an example of the classification of total and low-density lipoprotein cholesterol (LDL-C) concentrations in children and adolescents, in this case relying on the study population of the Lipid Research Clinics (NCEP 1991). The NCEP adopted as screening criteria for ages 2–19 years values said to approximate the 95th and 75th percentile values of this population, expressed in mg/dl, without regard to variation by age or sex. Per the NCEP, high total cholesterol is a concentration of ≥200 mg/dl (5.2 mmol/l; high LDL-C, ≥130 mg/dl (3.4 mmol/l). 'Borderline' concentrations are, in turn, 170–199 mg/dl (4.4 to <5.2 mmol/l) and 110–129 mg/dl (2.8 to <3.4 mmol/l). Detailed algorithms for evaluating and managing elevated cholesterol concentrations are presented in the NCEP's 'Report of the Expert Panel on Blood Cholesterol Levels in Children and Adolescents'.

Well-standardized methods for determining blood lipids are widely available, most notably the National Reference System for Cholesterol Measurements operated by the Centers for Disease Control and Prevention and the National Bureau of Standards in the US. Issues of the reliability of desktop analysers for rapid screening of total cholesterol concentrations have been examined and require consideration in use of these devices (US General Accounting Office 1994). Increasing attention to other components of the blood lipid profile (most frequently LDL-C, as well as HDL-C and triglycerides) further requires attention to the fasting state, as the LDL-C concentration is calculated in a manner sensitive to the concentration of triglycerides, which may change rapidly after food intake.

Development with age

Numerous cross-sectional surveys have established that blood lipids change with age, and longitudinal studies have confirmed and refined the patterns of change suggested by the surveys. Among the earliest of these population surveys was the multicentre study of the Lipid Research Clinics Program, noted above (NCEP 1991). The age-specific values of the mean, 5th, 10th, 25th, 50th, 75th, 90th, and 95th percentiles of total cholesterol distribution for each of four age categories, 0–4, 5–9, 10–14, and 15–19 years, were presented for both males and females. In this representation, only seemingly minor variation in mean values with age was apparent from birth to 19 years.

When survey data on blood lipids are presented by single year of age, rather than by 5-year age categories, a pattern becomes clearly evident that is obscured by the cruder age classification. This result of more detailed observation might be expected, because in childhood and adolescence the pace or tempo of change in such fundamental characteristics as body size and composition and sexual development is so rapid. In the case of blood lipids, changes are in part fluctuations that are simply overlooked unless year-to-year or even shorter-term variation is captured. This necessitates observation in much narrower age categories, or with much greater frequency, in this period than in adulthood if the unfolding processes are to be demonstrated. Surveys designed to address a wide range of ages, by single years or finer categories of age, are especially revealing. First, they show a sharp increase from the newborn period to age 3–5 years. Second, values appear to be somewhat lower at ages around 14–16 years than at either 10–12 years or 17 and older. Finally, values after age 16 are somewhat higher than at any earlier age.

Longitudinal data, like cross-sectional data, are more informative when they permit finer resolution by age at observation. For this reason Project HeartBeat!, a longitudinal study of development of CVD risk factors from ages 8–18 years, used examinations every 4 months for up to 4 years, in successive cohorts aged 8, 11, or 14 years at first observation (Labarthe *et al.* 1997a, b). In this study, 678 Texas children and adolescents provided more than 5400 observations for analysis of change in blood lipids with age in a mixed longitudinal, or synthetic cohort, design. The true longitudinal patterns of change in total, LDL-C, and high-density lipoprotein cholesterol (HDL-C) and triglycerides can be examined on the basis of these data, by multilevel modelling with MLwiN software (Rabash *et al.* 2000).

Using Project HeartBeat! data, the trajectories of change from ages 8–18 years can be described for each blood lipid component (Fig. 34.1a–d). Total cholesterol concentration varies sharply with age for both males and females, with notable differences by sex. In both sexes, however, total and LDL-C decline sharply from ages 10 or 11 to about age 14. The peak and nadir are somewhat later for males, who also show a greater decrease over time in total cholesterol than do females. LDL-C declines more among males than females and among blacks than whites. Through about age 14, the decline in LDL-C accounts quantitatively for the decline in total cholesterol. HDL-C differs much more than total or LDL-C between males and females and between blacks and whites, and does not decrease at any point for females. In all four sex–race groups, HDL-C increases after ages 14 or 15, largely accounting for the increase in total cholesterol in the later teenage years. The concentration of triglycerides increases continuously from age 8 in males, but reaches a plateau at about age 13 in females.

Population differences

Surveys in adult populations, whether conducted independently or under a standard protocol, have suggested substantial between-population differences in lipids in the thirties or even

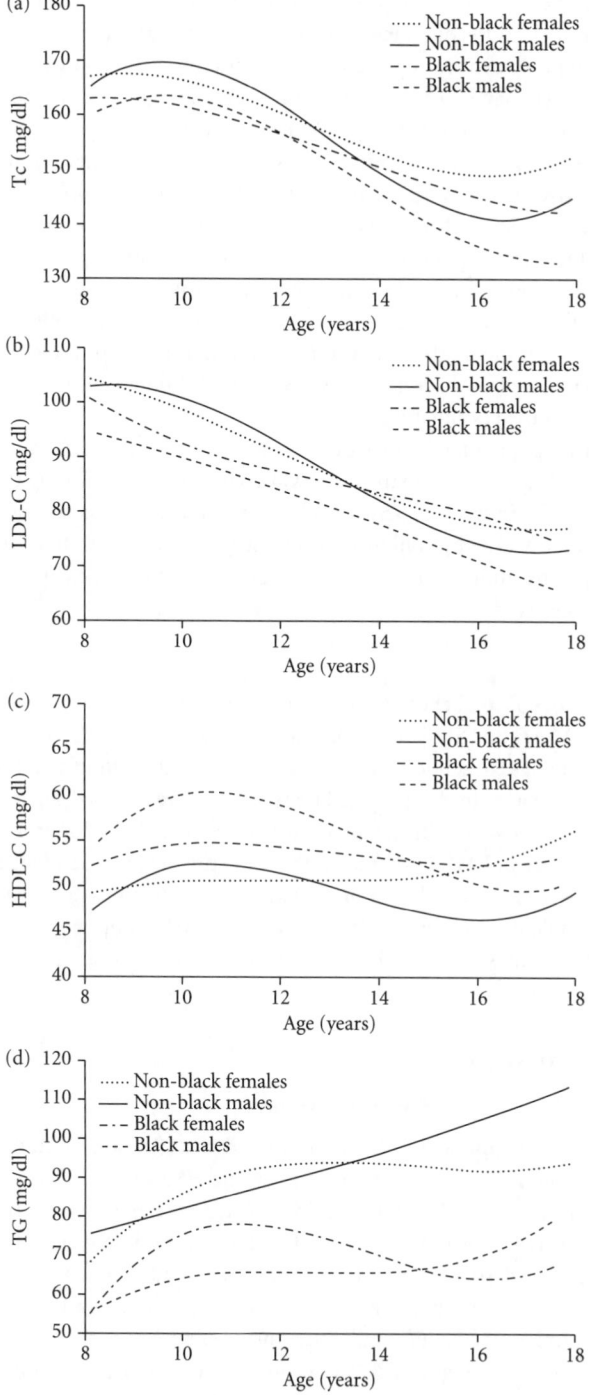

Fig. 34.1 Trajectories of change in concentrations of blood lipid components by sex and race, Project HeartBeat!, 1991–95. (a) Total cholesterol. (b) LDL-C. (c) HDL-C. (d) Triglycerides.

twenties. It would be interesting to know how early such differences arise, if they are real. Differences in total cholesterol concentration by year of age from newborn to as much as 19 years have been presented from population surveys in several countries, including the US, Finland, and Japan (Labarthe *et al.* 1991); differences in age-specific mean values as great as 40–50 mg/dl (1.0–1.3 mmol/l) were apparent over much of the age range of these three surveys. In another array of surveys within the US alone, much smaller population differences were found (15 mg/dl (0.4 mmol/l) or less), possibly related to improved reliability through the studies' use of the Center for Disease Control (CDC)'s Lipid Standardization Program or to a true greater homogeneity of the populations. Equally apparent in the two groups of surveys was the general similarity in age pattern of total cholesterol concentration, with definitely lower values generally around ages 13–15 than at immediately prior or later years. Thus, while the magnitude of absolute population differences cannot yet be described with confidence, the pattern of lower total cholesterol in early adolescence appears to be a general occurrence among studied populations.

The most extensive population comparison through a coordinated set of surveys was reported by Knuiman and colleagues (Knuiman *et al.* 1980), who studied total and HDL-C in boys aged 13 years in 16 countries in Europe, Africa, and South Asia and used a central laboratory for all lipid determinations. Marked population differences were found in both lipid components, but differences by population in growth tempos could not be excluded as a partial explanation of the differences observed.

Other aspects

Insight into predictors of total cholesterol concentration from school age into early adulthood is provided by the Muscatine Study (Mahoney *et al.* 1991). Contributions to variability in total cholesterol at various ages in school and high values (above the 90th percentile for age and sex) on re-measurement at ages in the early or late twenties were assessed separately in males and females. For males, the two significant predictors of later high cholesterol were the previous value itself and increase in BMI. For females, the same predictors were identified, as was use of oral contraceptives. More recently, we have examined for females in Project HeartBeat! the relation between apolipoprotein E genotypes and blood lipid components (Fulton *et al.* 1999). Presence of the E2 allele is associated with significantly lower total cholesterol, attributable entirely to lower LDL-C.

34.2.3 **Blood pressure**

Definition, classification, and measurement

An example of evolving approaches to definition and classification of blood pressure in children and adolescents is the series of reports from the US National Heart, Lung, and Blood Institute that culminated in the 1996 version (National High Blood Pressure Education Working Group on Hypertension Control in Children and Adolescents 1996). Similar to the system for blood lipids, classification of blood pressure in children and adolescents is based on percentile values in a reference population distribution of systolic and (currently) fifth-phase diastolic pressure. Unlike the NCEP guidelines, these reference values are derived from a pool of population surveys with geographical variation nationally and are specific by sex and year of age. Furthermore, in the current approach, the percentile values are specific for age- and sex-specific percentile values of height, from 1 to 17 years, derived from the same surveys.

Hypertension is defined as values ≥95th percentile, while 'high-normal' blood pressure refers to values ≥90th percentile but <95th. Because of the intra-individual variability of blood pressure, this classification is to be based on average values of systolic or diastolic pressure recorded on at least two occasions.

Measurement of blood pressure is addressed in detail in these reports, which emphasize the importance of standardization of measurement conditions, apparatus, and observers. Use of automated devices is discussed with reference to their uncertain reliability, and a preference is expressed for standard auscultation. (Recent environmental policies in the US intended to eliminate potential exposures to mercury, and hence use of mercury sphygmomanometers, may seriously affect the standardization of blood pressure measurement.)

Development with age

Cross-sectional surveys of blood pressure are abundant in the literature. To gain an impression of the general pattern of change in blood pressure with age, we identified some 80 published reports with sex-specific mean values reported by single year of age over at least three levels of age (Brotons et al. 1989). Because the population-specific patterns appeared quite similar, we evaluated the general picture by pooling the data from all contributing surveys. Doing so provided some 250 000 observations for systolic pressure and ~125 000 observations each for fourth- and fifth-phase diastolic pressure.

Mean systolic blood pressure appears to rise year to year over almost the entire range from 6 to 18 years. Males and females diverge at age 14, with males increasing up to age 17, then staying the same at age 18. Females have modest increases from ages 14–16 and then appear to have lower values at 17 and 18. The pattern for fourth-phase diastolic pressure is similar but less pronounced. For fifth-phase diastolic pressure, in contrast, patterns for males and females are virtually identical, with higher values for each successive age level from 6 to 18 years in both sexes.

Longitudinal data, again from Project HeartBeat!, in which systolic, fourth- and fifth-phase diastolic pressures were recorded, mainly confirm and amplify these impressions from cross-sectional surveys (Labarthe et al. 1998) (Fig. 34.2a–c). The trajectory for systolic pressure is best fitted to a cubic function of age and shows a late separation of curves for males and females, confirming the actual decrease in systolic pressure for older teenage females. The trajectory for fourth-phase diastolic pressure is best fitted with a quadratic function of age, with the rate of increase declining toward the upper limit of the age range. For fourth-phase diastolic pressure, in contrast to systolic pressure, in Project HeartBeat! significantly higher mean values were found for blacks than whites. For fifth-phase diastolic pressure, a linear model by age is the best fit; no difference was observed by sex, but the black–white difference seen in fourth-phase diastolic pressure was present here as well.

These longitudinal data confirm the differences in patterns between the three blood pressure measures (systolic, diastolic fourth and fifth phase) suggested by survey data. Furthermore, they reinforce the impression that these three measures of haemodynamic function convey different information and represent distinct physiological phenomena. These differences may be important in evaluating predictive relationships – whether blood pressure is the predictor or the outcome variable – and in understanding the effects of interventions on blood pressure, because the three blood pressure indices are clearly not equivalent.

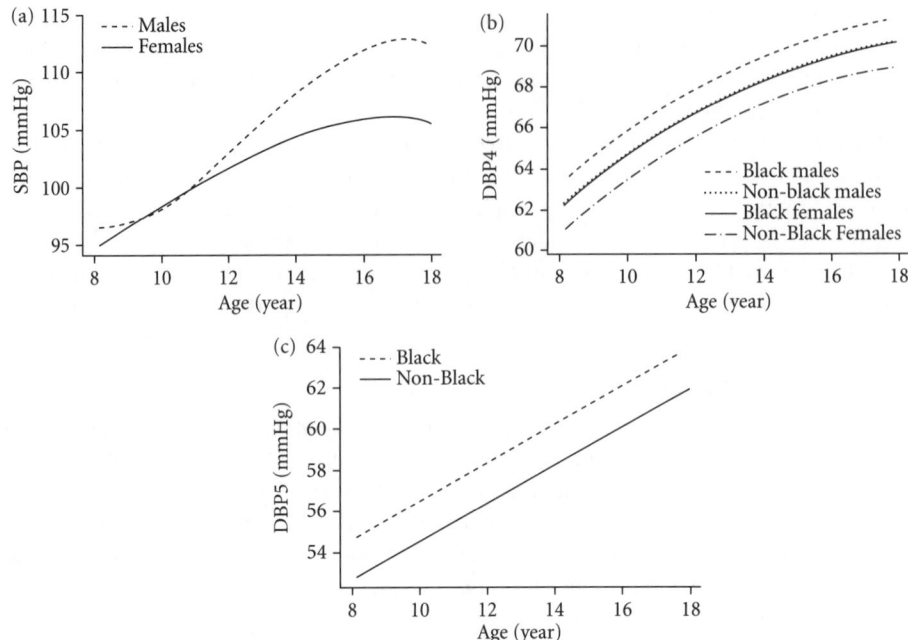

Fig. 34.2 Trajectories of change in blood pressure, Project HeartBeat!, 1991–95. Sex and race trajetories are shown when differences are statistically significant. (a) Systolic blood pressure. (b) Diastolic blood pressure phase 4. (c) Diastolic blood pressure phase 5.

Population comparisons

Population comparisons of blood pressure levels can be made from the collected survey reports described above (Brotons *et al.* 1989). For this purpose, those surveys with the widest age representation were selected as being most informative. For systolic blood pressure, surveys in six populations were compared: China, Greece, India, the Netherlands, Yugoslavia (two surveys), and the US. At any age, for both males and females, differences of as much as 10 mmHg were found across populations. Whether these were true differences or reflected measurement differences alone is unknown. Regardless, the general patterns of increments in blood pressure with age were consistent across populations. Unfortunately, unlike the case for population studies of blood lipids, the degree of standardization provided by a central laboratory is unavailable, and even strict implementation of a common measurement protocol has rarely, if ever, been used in comparative population surveys of blood pressure in children and adolescents.

Other aspects

For blood pressure, as for cholesterol, the Muscatine Study offered an opportunity to identify potential predictors of high levels (>90th percentile) at re-examination at ages in the twenties (Mahoney *et al.* 1991). For both males and females, the predictors of high systolic blood pressure were the previous mean level, the maximum level recorded over the course of follow-up in the study, and the calculated left ventricular mass. For diastolic pressure only the previous measurement was a significant predictor, and here the relation was much weaker than for systolic pressure.

34.2.4 **Diabetes**

Definition, classification, and measurement

Diabetes in childhood and adolescence has in the past been represented almost entirely by juvenile, or type 1, diabetes. Recently, however, both adult-onset, or type 2, diabetes and the cluster of characteristics that constitute the 'metabolic syndrome' have appeared frequently in young people, causing great concern among public health authorities (see Chapter 21). In the Proceedings of the Prevention Conference VI: Diabetes and Cardiovascular Disease, convened in January 2001, current issues of definition, classification, and measurement in this increasingly important area are reviewed (Grundy *et al.* 2002). Briefly, based on fasting plasma glucose determination, values of $\geq$126 mg/dl (7 mmol/l) define diabetes, and values in the range of 110–125 mg/dl (6.1 to <7 mmol/l) define impaired fasting glucose, which is linked with the metabolic syndrome. Also termed the 'insulin resistance syndrome', this set of conditions has been described as comprising hyperinsulinaemia, hypertension, dyslipidaemia, and obesity (Sinaiko 2000). Assessment of hyperinsulinaemia in population studies of children and adolescents has been based primarily on determination of fasting insulin concentrations. Only a few such studies have used the 'insulin clamp' method, which indicates cellular glucose uptake and is considered a much more precise indicator of glucose metabolism.

Development with age

Study of fasting blood glucose concentrations in the Bogalusa Heart Study has provided an illustrative cross-sectional view of changes with age in children and adolescents aged 5–17 years (Radhakrishnamurthy *et al.* 1985). In this study ($n = 3555$) median glucose values in males rose gradually with age to a peak of ~95 mg/dl (5.3 mmol/l) at 13 years and were slightly lower at older ages. In females, mean values below those for males were found in a generally parallel pattern with age. A more definite decrease in mean values was observed in females older than 13, where the peak concentration was ~90 mg/dl (5.0 mmol/l). Insulin concentrations measured in 400 participants increased steeply with age in both males and females. Studies in Finland and Belgium yielded similar findings (Ronnemaa *et al.* 1991; Guillaume *et al.* 1996). Few longitudinal data are available to indicate change in insulin concentrations, but associations between baseline insulin values and later measures of other risk factors suggest potentially important links (Sinaiko 2000). Further studies are needed to characterize the age- and sex-related patterns of change in insulin levels in childhood and adolescence and their relation to change in other risk factors.

Other aspects

The Prevention VI Conference report summarized changes in frequency of diabetes in children and adolescents and indicated increasing frequencies of type 1, especially in Europe, and type 2, particularly in the US (Grundy *et al.* 2002). Evidence in the US is limited mainly to clinical reports, but is supported by population studies in some racial and ethnic groups.

34.2.5 **Smoking**

Definition, classification, and measurement

Assessment of tobacco use in children and adolescents requires consideration not only of cigarette smoking but also of other forms of tobacco use, especially plug, dipping, or chewing tobacco, or snuff, as well as exposure to environmental tobacco smoke. Quantitation of past and current tobacco use and ages at points of change in use are needed to classify smoking behaviour in accordance with the succession from 'preparatory stage,' 'trying stage', 'experimental stage', and 'regular use', to 'addiction/dependent smoker' that characterizes the progressive adoption of the smoking habit (US Department of Health and Human Services 1994). Various strictures on using tobacco contribute to unreliability of self-reported use and make direct measurement of metabolic products of nicotine such as cotinine or thiocyanate in blood or saliva desirable.

Development with age

Smoking often begins in childhood and is considered unlikely to become a habit if not started before adulthood. Accordingly, a particularly strong public health emphasis is placed on youth, both to evaluate preventive strategies and to monitor influences of advertising and other factors on smoking behaviour (Chapter 45). Reported prevalence of smoking in youth varies widely among populations, reflecting in part both the extent of social controls and methods of assessment. The US Youth Risk Behavior Surveillance study of 1999 reported cigarette smoking and smokeless tobacco use among six categories of high school students – males and females who were non-Hispanic whites, non-Hispanic blacks, or Hispanics (American Heart Association 2002). Smoking was most common among whites (38–39%) and least common among blacks (18–22%), while smokeless tobacco use was practised (per the self-reports) by nearly 19% of white males and 6% of Hispanic males, but by fewer than 3% of the other groups.

34.3 Combined factors

Numerous reports indicate the coexistence of multiple risk factors among individual youth within childhood and adolescence, especially in association with abdominal obesity (Gillum 1987; Gidding 1993; Daniels *et al.* 1999; Chen *et al.* 2000). In the most recent of these examples, from the Bogalusa Heart Study, clustering of four factors – the insulin resistance index, BMI, the triglycerides/HDL-C ratio, and mean arterial pressure – was studied among black and white participants at ages from 5 to 37 years (Chen *et al.* 2000). The intraclass correlations among these four characteristics by age group and race were generally stronger among whites than blacks. In both races the correlations decreased in strength from ages 8–10 (~0.37–0.40) to 14–17 years (~0.14–0.25) and then increased to reach the same magnitude as at ages 8–10 by ages 31–37. This age pattern was largely absent after adjustment for BMI. The authors' interpretation suggested that the observed clustering was an effect of insulin resistance, mediated by obesity as measured by BMI.

34.4 Tracking

'Tracking' in connection with CVD risk factors in children and adolescents typically refers to persistently high values of cholesterol, blood pressure, or other continuously distributed traits on repeated measurement, often on only two occasions some years apart. Measurements might be taken within childhood or adolescence alone or include one taken in early adulthood. Two ways to assess the degree of tracking are to examine the strength of correlations between paired absolute values, or to see whether there is a persistence of high rank order, such as the uppermost decile or highest quintile. If conventional statistical tests show the correlation coefficients to be strong or the proportions of participants in a decile or quintile to exceed expectation, tracking is said to be present.

Examples of the tracking of CVD risk factors include the Muscatine Study (Clarke *et al.* 1978), the Bogalusa Heart Study (Webber *et al.* 1991), the Cardiovascular Risk in Young Finns Study (Porkka *et al.* 1994), and the Amsterdam Growth and Health Study (Twisk *et al.* 1996). These and other studies have established that some degree of consistency of values or ranks over time is observable for most of the risk factors, and consistency tends to be greater for traits with less measurement error and shorter intervals between measurements. There is little disagreement that tracking occurs for blood pressure, blood lipids, BMI, and other studied traits, although the strength of the tracking is sometimes debated. Usual study designs rely on only one observation at each of two time points, often years apart, and fail to take measurement variability into account (Porkka *et al.* 1994; Dai, personal communication, 2002). Therefore, the strength of measures of tracking is clearly underestimated. Better insights into determinants of tracking will depend on wider use of improved designs.

34.5 Links with vascular pathology

Perhaps the strongest evidence of the importance of risk factors for atherosclerosis and hypertension during childhood and adolescence is the repeated demonstration of their links with vascular pathology. Following early population studies of the pathology of coronary atherosclerosis in young adults, two approaches were adopted to extend these observations back to the adolescent ages or even earlier. In one approach, the Bogalusa Heart Study conducted postmortem examinations of aortic and coronary artery samples from participants who had died some time after having risk factor measurements in the original study (Newman *et al.* 1986, 1991). The 66 deaths under study (Newman *et al.* 1991) occurred at ages from 7 to 26 years, and risk factors had last been measured at ages 3–18 years. In the second approach, persons dying at ages from 15 to 34 years who were free of known coronary heart disease were identified in one of eight collaborating centres (PDAY 1990; Strong *et al.* 1999). Their records and examination at autopsy were used to assess risk factor levels at the time of death, and sections of abdominal and thoracic aorta and right coronary artery were studied in detail under a standard protocol. The 1999 report represented 2876 decedents, including both black and white men and women.

The Bogalusa Heart Study demonstrated associations between prior measurements of systolic and diastolic blood pressure, LDL-C, and HDL/LDL + VLDL-cholesterol concentrations and the presence or absence of fibrous plaques in the coronary artery (Newman *et al.* 1991). Other findings implicated total, LDL-, and VLDL cholesterol in the extent of fatty streak involvement of the coronary arteries. The PDAY Study first investigated the relation of blood lipids and smoking (as indicated by serum thiocyanate concentration at the time of death) to the percentage involvement of the thoracic and abdominal aorta and right coronary artery with atherosclerotic lesions. Positive associations for LDL- + VLDL-cholesterol and thiocyanate concentrations and an inverse association for HDL-C were found in the initial phase of the study (PDAY 1990). Based on the full study sample, later analysis extended the description of pathological findings, and, with larger numbers, included separate analysis for females. Detailed computer mapping of observed lesions, by type, grade, and location in the vessel wall demonstrated the early occurrence of fatty streaks and raised lesions, even within the 15–19-year age group, and progressively greater involvement across the age range to 34 years. Furthermore, it was clearly demonstrated that areas of greatest involvement with fatty streaks at one 5-year age level were the areas with greatest concentration of raised lesions in the next 5-year age group. These studies contribute importantly to understanding the role of the risk factors in producing atherosclerotic lesions well before adulthood and to the direct link between fatty streaks and more advanced lesions. Future studies in clinical settings may take advantage of intravascular ultrasound examination of the coronary arteries, a non-invasive technique permitting assessment of atherosclerosis in living study subjects (Tuzcu *et al.* 2001). In addition, computed tomography of the coronary arteries has been used in the Muscatine Study to assess predictive relations between risk factors measured at school age and detectable calcified lesions in early adulthood (Mahoney 2000).

34.6 Changing coronary risk in children

An adverse change in risk factor distributions in children and adolescents can be inferred in populations where obesity as defined earlier is increasing in prevalence, an issue addressed in several recent reports. Little direct evidence is available on the other risk factors themselves, however, because of insufficient monitoring of population trends in blood pressure, blood lipid profiles, or blood insulin concentrations in children and adolescents.

34.7 Implications for theory, research, and practice

The emergence of cardiovascular risk factors in childhood and adolescence has been shown to be characterized in general by (a) a progressive shift in risk factor distributions with increasing age toward undesirable levels; (b) a tendency for clustering of multiple factors within individual persons; (c) tracking of risk factor values at the higher-risk extreme; and (d) an association with the extent and severity of atherosclerotic lesions observed well before adulthood. Variation in the trajectories of change in mean values of specific risk factors – such as distinct components of blood lipids, blood pressure, or blood glucose and insulin concentrations – indicates some complexity in these patterns and suggests that they may differ in some important aspects of causation and prevention.

What are the implications of this knowledge for theory, practice, and further research? For theory, the main conclusion is that early development of the risk factors is not simply a matter of normal growth and development, but also underlies a progressive increase in CVD risk and the pathogenesis of atherosclerosis. For practice, the immediate implication is that risk factors in childhood and adolescence should be recognized as a significant public health challenge in their own right, receiving at least the level of attention urged one to two decades ago by WHO and by Strasser (Strasser 1978; WHO Expert Committee 1990), as well as by others more recently (NCEP 1991; National High Blood Pressure Education Working Group on Hypertension Control in Children and Adolescents 1996). For research priorities, a task force reporting to the US National Heart, Lung and Blood Institute nearly a decade ago urged that research on prevention of CVD risk in the first place was the single greatest opportunity for progress in CVD prevention (National Heart, Lung and Blood Institute 1994). Clearly, the implications of the findings of more than three decades of research highlighted here direct greatly increased attention to the period of childhood and adolescence in the continuing effort to reverse or to stem the rising tide of CVD and its risk factors as a global health challenge.

References

American Heart Association (2002). *Heart and stroke statistical update 2002.* American Heart Association, Dallas.

Brotons, C., Singh, P., Nishio, T., and Labarthe, D. R. (1989). Blood pressure by age in childhood and adolescence: a review of 129 studies worldwide. *International Journal of Epidemiology*, **18**, 824–29.

Chen, W., Bao, W., Begum, S., Elkasabany, A., Srinivasan, S. R., and Berenson, G. S. (2000). Age-related patterns of the clustering of cardiovascular risk variables of syndrome X from childhood to young adulthood in a population made up of black and white subjects: The Bogalusa Heart Study. *Diabetes*, **49**, 1042–8.

Clarke, W. R., Schrott, H. G., Leaverton, P. E., Connor, W.E ., and Lauer, R. M. (1978). Tracking of blood lipids and blood pressure in school age children: The Muscatine Study. *Circulation*, **58**, 626–34.

Dai, S., Labarthe, D. R., Grunbaum, J. A., Harrist, R. B., and Mueller, W. H. (2002*a*). Longitudinal analysis of changes in indices of obesity from age 8 years to age 18 years: Project HeartBeat! *American Journal of Epidemiology*, **156**, 720–9.

Daniels, S. R., Morrison, J. A., Sprecher, D. L., Khoury, P., and Kimball, T. R. (1999). Association of body fat distribution and cardiovascular risk factors in children and adolescents. *Circulation*, **99**, 541–5.

Fulton, J. E., Dai, S., Grunbaum, J. A., Boerwinkle, E., and Labarthe, D. R. (1999). Apolipoprotein E affects serial changes in total and low-density lipoprotein cholesterol in adolescent girls: Project HeartBeat! *Metabolism*, **48**, 285–90.

Gidding, S. S. (1993). Relationships between blood pressure and blood lipids in childhood. *Pediatric Clinics of North America*, **40**, 41–9.

Gillum, R. F. (1987). The association of the ratio of waist to hip girth with blood pressure, serum cholesterol and serum uric acid in children and youths aged 6–17 years. *Journal of Chronic Diseases*, **40**, 413–20.

Grundy, S. M., Howard, B., Smith, Jr. S., Eckel, R., Redberg, R., and Bonow, R. O. (2002). Prevention Conference VI: Diabetes and Cardiovascular Disease. Executive summary: conference proceeding for healthcare professionals from a special writing group of the American Heart Association. *Circulation*, **105**, 2231–9.

Guillaume, M., Lapidus, L., Beckers, F., Lambert, A., and Bjorntorp, P. (1996). Cardiovascular risk factors in children from the Belgian province of Luxembourg: The Belgian Luxembourg Child Study. *American Journal of Epidemiology*, **144**, 867–80.

Knuiman, J. T., Hermus, R. J., and Hautvast, J. G. (1980). Serum total and high density lipoprotein (HDL) cholesterol concentrations in rural and urban boys from 16 countries. *Atherosclerosis*, **36**(4), 529–37.

Labarthe, D. R., O'Brien, B., and Dunn, K. (1991). International comparisons of plasma cholesterol and lipoproteins. *Annals of the New York Academy of Sciences*, **623**, 108–19.

Labarthe, D. R., Nichaman, M. Z., Harrist, R. B., Grunbaum, J. A., and Dai, S. (1997*a*). Change in blood lipid components during adolescence differs importantly by sex and is not consistently related to change in body fat: Project HeartBeat! [Abstract.] *Canadian Journal of Cardiology*, **13**(Suppl. B), 162B.

Labarthe, D. R., Nichaman, M. Z., Harrist, R. B., Grunbaum, J. A., and Dai, S. (1997*b*). Development of cardiovascular risk factors from age 8 to 18 in Project HeartBeat! Study design and patterns of change in plasma total cholesterol concentration. *Circulation*, **95**, 2636–42.

Labarthe, D. R., Dai, S., and Harrist, R. B. (1998). True longitudinal change in blood pressure in childhood and adolescence demonstrates marked differences in patterns among blood pressure components: Project Heartbeat! [Abstract.] *Circulation*, **98**(Suppl.), I-858.

Mahoney, L. T. (2000). Noninvasive identification of youth with cardiovascular disease. *CVD Prevention*, **3**, 155–8.

Mahoney, L. T., Lauer, R. M., Lee, J., and Clarke, W. R. (1991). Factors affecting tracking of coronary heart disease risk factors in children: The Muscatine Study. *Annals of the New York Academy of Sciences*, **623**, 120–32.

NCEP (National Cholesterol Education Program) (1991). Check date Report of the Expert Panel on Blood Cholesterol Levels in Children and Adolescents. NIH Publication No. 91-2732. National Cholesterol Education Program, National Heart, Lung and Blood Institute, National Institutes of Health, Public Health Service, US Dept. of Health and Human Services, Bethesda, Maryland.

National Heart, Lung and Blood Institute (1994). *Report of the Task Force on Research in Epidemiology and Prevention of Cardiovascular Diseases*. US Department of Health and Human Services, Public Health Service, National Institutes of Health, Bethesda, Maryland.

National High Blood Pressure Education Working Group on Hypertension Control in Children and Adolescents (1996). Update on the 1987 Task Force report on high blood pressure in children and adolescents: a working group report from the National High Blood Pressure Education Program. *Pediatrics*, **98**, 649–58.

Newman, W. P. III, Freedman, D. S., Voors, A. W., Gard, P. D., Srinivasan, S. R., Cresanta, J. L. *et al.* (1986). Relation of serum lipoprotein levels and systolic blood pressure to early atherosclerosis. *New England Journal of Medicine*, **314**, 138–44.

Newman, W. P. III, Wattigney, W., and Berenson, G. S. (1991). Autopsy studies in United States children and adolescents: relationship of risk factors to atherosclerotic lesions. *Annals of the New York Academy of Sciences*, **623**, 16–25.

Obarzanek, E. (1999). Obesity in children, adolescents, and families. In *Obesity: impact on cardiovascular disease* (ed. G. F. Fletcher, S. M. Grundy, and L. L. Hayman), pp. 31–53. Futura Publishing, Armonk, NY.

PDAY (Pathobiological Determinants of Atherosclerosis in Youth) Research Group (1990). Relationship of atherosclerosis in young men to serum lipoprotein cholesterol concentrations and smoking: a preliminary report from the Pathobiological Determinants of Atherosclerosis in Youth (PDAY) Research Group. *Journal of the American Medical Association*, **264**, 3018–24.

Porkka, K. V. K., Viikari, J. S. A., Taimela, S., Dahl, M., and Ckerblom, H. K. (1994). Tracking and predictiveness of serum lipid and lipoprotein measurements in childhood: a 12-year follow-up. The Cardiovascular Risk in Young Finns Study. *American Journal of Epidemiology*, **140**, 1096–110.

Rabash, J., Browne, W., Goldstein, H., Yang, M., Plewis, I., Healy, M. *et al.* (2000). *A user's guide to MLwiN, Version 2.1*. Multilevel Models Project, Institute of Education, University of London.

Radhakrishnamurthy, B., Srinivasan, S. R., Webber, L. S., Dalferes, Jr., E. R., and Berenson, G. S. (1985). Relationship of carbohydrate intolerance to serum lipoprotein profiles in childhood: The Bogalusa Heart Study. *Metabolism: Clinical and Experimental*, **34**, 850–60.

Ronnemaa, T., Knip, M., Lautala, P., Viikari, J., Uhari, M., Leino, A. *et al.* (1991). Serum insulin and other cardiovascular risk indicators in children, adolescents and young adults. *Annals of Medicine*, **23**, 67–72.

Sinaiko, A. R. (2000). Insulin resistance syndrome in children. *CVD Prevention*, **3**, 153–4.

Strasser, T. (1978). Reflections on cardiovascular diseases. *Interdisciplinary Science Reviews*, **3**, 225–30.

Strong, J. P., Malcom, G. T., McMahan, C. A., Tracy, R. E., Newman, W. P. III, Herderick, E. E., and Cornhill, J. F. (1999). Prevalence and extent of atherosclerosis in adolescents and young adults: implications for prevention from the Pathobiological Determinants of Atherosclerosis in Youth Study. *Journal of the American Medical Association*, **281**, 727–35.

Troiano, R. P., Flegal, K. M., Kuczmarski, R. J., Campbell, S. M., and Johnson, C. L. (1995). Overweight prevalence and trends for children and adolescents: The National Health and Nutrition Examination Surveys, 1963 to 1991. *Archives of Pediatrics and Adolescent Medicine*, **149**, 1085–91.

Tuzcu, E. M., Kapadia, S. R., Tutar, E., Ziada, K. M., Hobbs, R. E., McCarthy, P. M. *et al.* (2001). High prevalence of coronary atherosclerosis in asymptomatic teenagers and young adults: evidence from intravascular ultrasound. *Circulation*, **103**, 2705–10.

Twisk, J. W., Kemper, H. C., Mellenbergh, D. J., and van Mechelen, W. (1996). Factors influencing tracking of cholesterol and high-density lipoprotein: The Amsterdam Growth and Health Study. *Preventive Medicine*, **25**, 355–64.

US Department of Health and Human Services (1994). *Preventing tobacco use among young people: a report of the Surgeon General*. US Department of Health and Human Services, Public Health Service, Centers for Disease Control and Prevention, National Center for Chronic Disease Prevention and Health Promotion, Office on Smoking and Health, Atlanta.

US General Accounting Office (1994).

Webber, L. S., Srinivasan, S. R., Wattigney, W. A., and Berenson, G. S. (1991) Tracking of serum lipids and lipoproteins from childhood to adulthood: The Bogalusa Heart Study. *American Journal of Epidemiology*, **133** (9), 884–99.

WHO (World Health Organization) Expert Committee (1990). *Prevention in childhood and youth of adult cardiovascular diseases: time for action*. Technical Report Series 792. World Health Organization, Geneva.

Chapter 35

Risk factors in the elderly

J. G. van der Bom and D. E. Grobbee

35.1 Size of the problem

The proportion of older subjects in Westernized societies is gradually increasing. This trend has now been present for a number of decades and will continue well into the present century. It is estimated that by the year 2035 nearly one in four individuals living in the industrialized countries will be 65 years of age or older (http://www.census.gov/ipc/www/idbagg.html). In addition, life expectancy has increased since the beginning of the last century. As a consequence, the survival curve for men as well as for women has rectangularized, indicating a compression of mortality towards a likely maximum life span of around 80 or 90 years (Fries 1980) (Fig. 35.1). While more people will live longer, similar compression of morbidity has, however, not taken place. This is well illustrated by mortality trends from atherosclerotic cardiovascular diseases (Tunstall-Pedoe *et al.* 1999). In many countries rates of fatal coronary heart disease (CHD) and stroke have shown a steady decline since the late sixties or early seventies. This decline is likely to reflect both a reduced incidence of myocardial infarction (MI) and stroke, and a lower case-fatality rate. The latter is probably a result of a combination of improved acute medical care and a change towards the occurrence of milder forms of disease.

Not all age groups have benefited to the same extent. The largest reductions of mortality have occurred in middle-aged men, so called 'premature' mortality, while women, and particularly the elderly, have not shown such substantial decreases in fatal cardiovascular diseases (Fig. 35.2). Rather, the burden of chronic disease has dramatically increased in older age groups. Rates for stable and unstable angina pectoris, heart failure, and other forms of chronic cardiovascular diseases have all shown a steady increase in elderly subjects and the

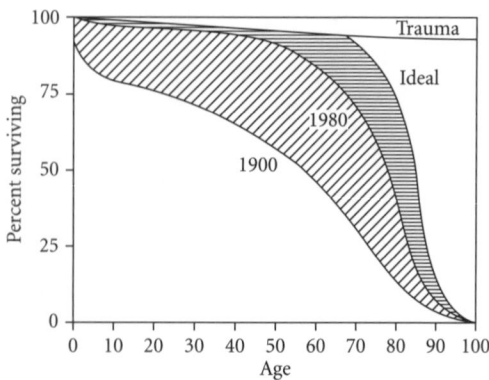

Fig. 35.1 Survival curve changes over the last century. (Reproduced with permission from Fries *et al.* 1980.)

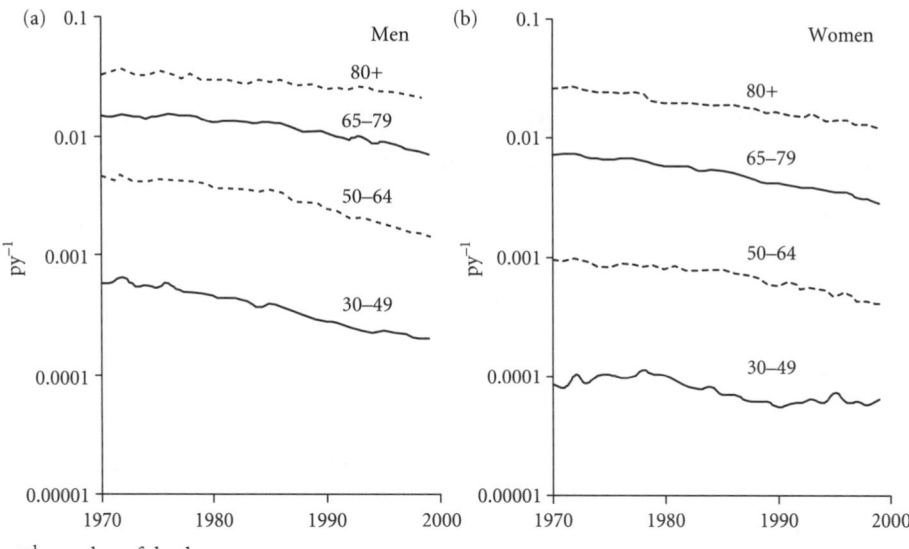

py^{-1}: number of deaths per person year.

Fig. 35.2 Trends in mortality from CHD according to age of dying for (a) men and (b) women. (Based on vital statistics of Statistics Netherlands <http://www.cbs.nl/default.asp>, accessed June 2001; with thanks to Luc G. A. Bonneux.)

number of coronary revascularization procedures has boomed (Cowie *et al.* 1997; Kalache and Aboderin 1995).

35.2 Age-associated cardiovascular changes

Over 80% of all cardiovascular deaths occur in those aged 65 years and above. Thus, age per se is the most important risk factor for cardiovascular diseases. One way to conceptualize why the effect of risk factors on cardiovascular diseases, the clinical manifestations and the prognosis of cardiovascular diseases, change with age is that in older individuals the specific pathophysiological mechanisms that cause clinical disorders are superimposed on heart and vessels that are modified by the ageing process. Ageing is associated with vascular alterations that may lead to an increased susceptibility to cardiovascular diseases (Weinsaft and Edelberg 2001). Clinical and experimental studies have demonstrated that ageing is associated with systemic and cardiac differential regulation of the three basic vascular functions: rheology (Egashira *et al.* 1993; Taddei *et al.* 1995), haemostasis (Hager *et al.* 1989), and vascular repair/angiogenesis (Marinho *et al.* 1997; Pili *et al.* 1994). Endothelial cells play a central role in modulating each of these functions (Reed *et al.* 2000; Vanhoutte 2002).

The age-associated changes in cardiac and vascular properties alter the manifestations of cardiovascular diseases in several ways (Lakatta 2002). First, they lower the extent of disease severity required to cross the threshold that results in clinically significant signs and symptoms. For example, a mild degree of ischaemia-induced cardiac relaxation abnormalities that may be asymptomatic in a younger individual may cause dyspnoea in an older one, who, by virtue of age alone, has a slowed and delayed early diastolic relaxation. Age may also alter the manifestations and presentation of cardiovascular diseases. In older patients with acute infarction, the diagnosis may be delayed because atypical symptoms may result in increased time to onset of therapy (de Bruyne *et al.* 1997). Age-associated changes also influence the response to, and therefore the selection of, different therapeutic interventions in older individuals.

35.3 Atherosclerosis and other risk factors for cardiovascular diseases in the different phases of life

It is becoming ever more clear that atherosclerosis is not the only process involved in symptomatic cardiovascular diseases; several other mechanisms may determine whether an individual, in the presence of atherosclerosis, will eventually experience a MI or another manifestation of ischaemic vascular diseases. As early as the 1950s it was demonstrated from autopsy studies of soldiers killed in action that early atherosclerotic lesions are present in a significant proportion of young healthy individuals (Enos *et al.* 1953). Subsequent findings in studies such as the Bogalusa Heart Study and the PDAY study have shown that lesions in coronary arteries and the aorta may be present in teenagers and younger children (Newman *et al.* 1986; PDAY 1990). Rupture of the atherosclerotic plaque has gained increased recognition as the proximate causes of disability and death due to related syndromes such as acute MI. Plaque composition and vulnerability have emerged as more critical determinants of plaque rupture than the degree of luminal stenosis (Robbie and Libby 2001).

Atherosclerosis, from early slight wall alterations to full calcified and complicated lesions, may take almost a lifetime to develop. By the age of 60 or 70 a sizeable proportion of the population in Westernized societies have some degree of atherosclerosis in the major arteries. In contrast, the sequence of events leading to symptomatic angina, infarction, or sudden death takes hours or seconds. It does not take too much imagination to conclude that certain phenomena, in addition to atherosclerosis, must be involved to explain why some suffer from their atherosclerosis and others do not. Alternatively, it seems likely that these other factors only start to play a role in the presence of atherosclerosis. Therefore, their importance may increase in old age.

A lucid view of the major determinants of cardiovascular events, given the presence of atherosclerosis, was given by Oliver (1986). According to the scheme in Fig. 35.3, symptoms of CHD

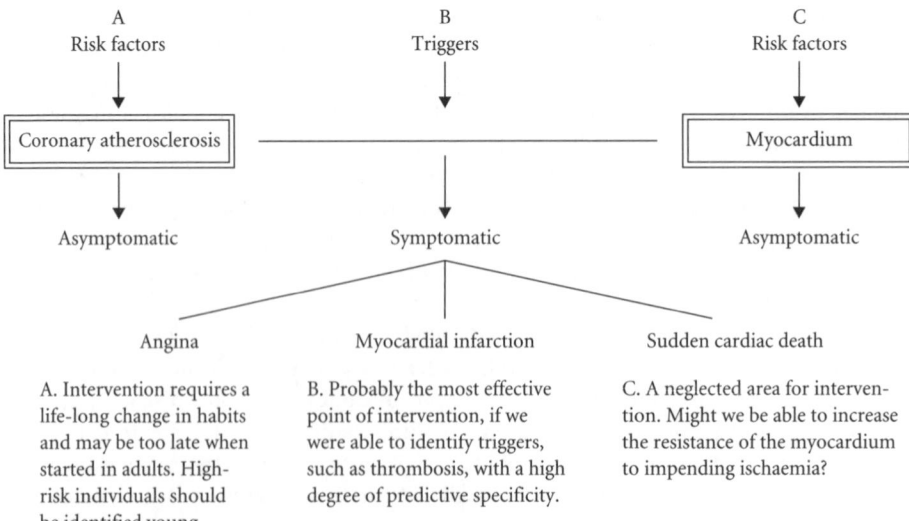

Fig. 35.3 Scheme for the development of symptomatic cardiovascular disease and points for intervention. Where is it best to intervene? (Reproduced with permission from Oliver 1986.)

are particularly likely to manifest themselves in subjects that have a myocardium that is vulnerable to reduced coronary flow and ischaemia. In addition, sudden reductions of coronary flow and ischaemia may be triggered by factors that promote rapid occlusion of vessels already compromised by atherosclerosis. While particularly clear for CHD, the scheme is also likely to apply to ischaemic symptoms in other vascular beds. The concept of trigger factors is of vital importance in understanding the final phase of atherosclerotic cardiovascular diseases. The observation that important sporting events were associated with increased mortality from CHD suggests that such events may provoke a sufficient level of stress to trigger symptomatic cardiovascular disease (Witte *et al.* 2000). Other convincing data to support this concept come from studies demonstrating circadian variation in the occurrence of ischaemic symptoms, MI, and sudden cardiac death (Mulcahy *et al.* 1991). It seems likely that trigger factors particularly promote arterial thrombosis. The importance of thrombosis in the acute phase of MI, and probably in angina pectoris, is beyond debate. Moreover, circadian variation has been shown, for example, for platelet activity and fibrinolytic capacity. In the Physicians' Health Study (Ridker *et al.* 1990), the use of aspirin diluted the circadian pattern in the occurrence of MI compared to placebo (Fig. 35.4).

There is a growing body of evidence pointing at disturbances in haemostatic function and fibrinolysis at multiple levels, leading to an increased tendency of thrombosis, in patients at increased risk for cardiovascular diseases (see Chapter 28). Previous studies have demonstrated that ageing is associated with increased coagulation activity (Van Der Bom *et al.* 2001) and decreased endothelial fibrinolytic potential, which may explain the increased predisposition of older individuals to the risk of cardiovascular events. Large-scale population-based studies have demonstrated an association between advanced age and increased levels of d-dimer and plasma coagulation factors (Mari *et al.* 1995; Pieper *et al.* 2000; Van Der Bom *et al.* 1999). The expression of plasminogen activator inhibitor-1, a fibrinolytic enzyme inhibitor associated with coronary thrombosis and MI, is upregulated in senescent human endothelial cells (Comi *et al.* 1995; Fay *et al.* 1996; Wiman *et al.* 2000). In addition, thrombotic tendency increases with age (Mari *et al.* 1995) and the production of coagulation inhibitors as antithrombin decreases with increasing age (Van Der Bom *et al.* 1996). These observations provide evidence of a potential age-associated increase in systemic vascular thrombotic potential. In addition to thrombogenic factors, there are other candidates to act as 'triggers', although they may eventually also affect thrombogenesis: sympathetic nervous system activity, vasoactive hormones, and smoking, to name a few.

Similarly important is the third part of the equation, illustrated in Fig. 35.3: myocardial vulnerability to ischaemic burden. Despite the fact that it is the source of pain, arrhythmias, failure,

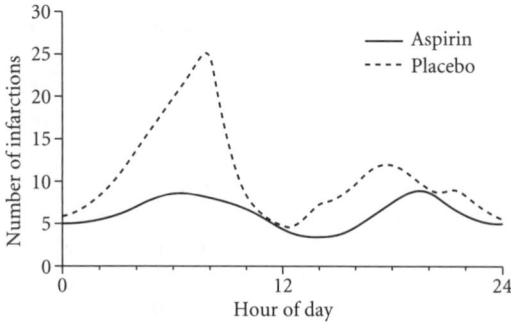

Fig. 35.4 Circadian variation of the incidence of coronary events according to the use of aspirin. (Reproduced with permission from Ridker *et al.* 1990.)

and death, the role of the myocardium in the development of cardiovascular disease has received much less attention than that of atherosclerosis and the 'classic' risk factors. Yet, one of the most likely ways whereby physical activity protects against cardiovascular disease is by improving myocardial perfusion. The ability to develop collateral arterial circulation may constitute an important response to vascular occlusive disease and determines, in part, the severity of residual tissue ischaemia (Sasayama and Fujita 1992). Conditions such as left ventricular hypertrophy, heart failure, rhythm disturbances, and scars from previous MI are common in older individuals (Mosterd *et al.* 1999a, 2001). Smoking also compromises the condition of the myocardium in subjects suffering from coronary atherosclerosis. Metabolic abnormalities, including diabetes and hyperinsulinemia, and neurohumoral effects may be important too.

Although atherosclerosis can be viewed as a systemic disorder, the expression of the disease in specific preferred locations is striking. Haemodynamic factors may play an important role in this context, but there is no adequate explanation for the fact that in some people atheros-clerotic changes mainly occur in leg arteries, in some in coronary arteries, and in others mainly in cerebral arteries. Similarly, there is no explanation for the observation that the effect of risk factors differs for the various manifestations of cardiovascular diseases. It is obvious that numerous factors including genetic constitution have an impact on the processes mentioned above.

Figure 35.2 illustrates that the decline in mortality from cardiovascular diseases applies especially to middle-aged men, and that it is less clear among the elderly. This may indicate that a change has mainly occurred in the early stages of the development of atherosclerosis and less in the factors that exacerbate the process and provoke the occurrence of ischaemic symptoms. The understanding of trigger factors and determinants of vulnerability, in concert with (risk factors of) atherosclerosis offers new potential for prevention and intervention, particularly in the older age groups.

35.4 Effects of the established risk factors in the elderly

The importance of preventing cardiovascular disease events in older people has led in recent years to a re-examination of the role of the conventional risk factors in large-scale studies focusing on older subjects. We will discuss findings from studies on serum cholesterol, blood pressure, smoking, and type 2 diabetes mellitus. Additionally, we will discuss some of the risk factors that are an expression of damage already present in the heart and arteries: electrocardiogram (ECG) deviations, left ventricular hypertrophy, and changes in the wall of the (carotid) arteries.

35.4.1 Cholesterol and the incidence of cardiovascular diseases in older people

Hypercholesterolaemia is a major risk factor for *coronary heart disease* in the general population according to many observational and intervention studies. However, in older people, the association between high serum total cholesterol levels and CHD is still disputed (Faergeman 2002). The results of some studies, in particular those among the very old (Weverling-Rijnsburger *et al.* 1997) suggest that there is no association between serum cholesterol levels and the incidence of CHD (Casiglia *et al.* 2002; Krumholz *et al.* 1994; Simons *et al.* 1995; Zimetbaum *et al.* 1992). However, the results of several other studies demonstrate a positive association between serum total cholesterol and the risk for CHD in men aged 65 years and older (Corti *et al.* 1997; Houterman *et al.* 1999, 2000, 2002; Rubin *et al.* 1990). The Framingham study showed a reduction of the CHD risk ratio between the highest and the lowest quartiles for serum total cholesterol for men aged 50 years and older, compared to younger men (Kronmal *et al.* 1993). Similarly, among older women, results are conflicting. A positive association was found among elderly women in some studies (Corti *et al.* 1995; Houterman *et al.* 1999; Zimetbaum *et al.* 1992), but it was absent in other studies (Casiglia *et al.* 2002; Simons *et al.* 1995; Weverling-Rijnsburger *et al.* 1997).

Low levels of high-density lipoprotein cholesterol (HDL-C) are another risk factor for CHD in the general population. In the elderly, findings on the association between low levels of HDL and the incidence of CHD are again less consistent. Some studies showed that low HDL-C was associated with an increased risk for CHD in older men and women (Corti *et al.* 1995; Houterman *et al.* 1999); others did not confirm the presence of this association (Krumholz *et al.* 1994). The Dubbo and the Bronx Ageing studies found it to be a risk factor in men only (Simons *et al.* 1995; Zimetbaum *et al.* 1992). The FINE Study, which included men from three countries, found low HDL-C to be related to CHD mortality in Finnish men, as well as in lean Italian men who drank more than 40 g of alcohol daily (Houterman *et al.* 2000).

One of the major differences between middle-aged and older populations is an increased prevalence in the older population of poorer health status, which is often the result of co-occurring disease or comorbidity. Older 'frail' persons with a high burden of disease and resultant acquired low cholesterol levels are more likely to have decreased survival than are those with little or no disease and chronically low cholesterol levels. The report by Corti *et al.* showed that in the EPESE study only after adjustment for markers of poor health, such as low serum iron and albumin levels, and exclusion of deaths that occurred within the first year, were elevated total cholesterol levels associated with an increased risk of death from CHD (Corti *et al.* 1997). This confirms that in the older population, the burden of multiple concomitant conditions can markedly alter observed associations between risk factors and outcomes that are well established in middle-aged populations. Thus, the heavy burden of chronic disease and frailty may simply hide the effect of lifelong elevated cholesterol levels when cholesterol levels are lowered near the end of life. Additionally, a direct pathophysiological effect of chronic disease on CHD may explain the absence of an association between cholesterol and cardiovascular disease in the older population. For example, in chronically ill persons, production of procoagulant and pro-inflammatory molecules could lead to increased risk for CHD (Esmon 2000).

While the level of risk appears to be smaller and less consistent in studies among the elderly than among the middle aged, the general consensus seems to be that lipid levels are a risk factor for coronary artery disease in the elderly. The relationship of hypercholesterolaemia with *stroke* incidence, however, is controversial not only for the elderly but also for middle-aged subjects. Some have reported a positive association between levels of serum total cholesterol and the risk of total stroke (Harmsen *et al.* 1990) and cerebral infarction (Benfante *et al.* 1994; Lindenstrom *et al.* 1994; Salonen *et al.* 1982); others showed little or no association with total stroke (Prospective Studies Collaboration 1995) or cerebral infarction (Haheim *et al.* 1993; Wolf *et al.* 1991). Some demonstrated an inverse relation between total cholesterol and death from haemorrhagic stroke (Gatchev *et al.* 1993; Iso *et al.* 1989). Few prospective studies have examined the association between HDL-C and stroke. Three prospective population-based studies on the association between serum HDL-C and risk of stroke showed a tendency towards a higher risk of cerebral infarction with lower HDL levels (Gordon *et al.* 1981; Tanne *et al.* 1997). A fourth study showed similar results for men, but increased HDL levels were significantly associated with an increased risk for non-fatal stroke and cerebral infarction in women (Bots *et al.* 2002).

One of the major limitations in analysing the possible relationship between cholesterol and stroke is the heterogeneous nature of the disease, which includes haemorrhagic and non-haemorrhagic stroke. About 80% of first strokes are non-haemorrhagic, and can be further divided into atherothrombotic, cardioembolic, lacunar, etc. The results from the Kaiser Permanente Medical Care program showed that, in men aged 65 or older, low serum cholesterol levels compared with high levels were associated with a higher risk of intracerebral haemorrhage (relative risk of 2.7 (95% CI: 1.4–5.0)) (Iribarren *et al.* 1996). Therefore meta-analyses such as the Prospective Studies Collaboration (1995) which included studies with no reference to stroke subtype are difficult to interpret. The heterogeneous nature of non-haemorrhagic stroke may also obscure the possible association with cholesterol, as strokes caused by atherothrombotic process involving extracranial vessels may be more likely to be associated with high cholesterol levels than cardioembolic or lacunar strokes. Determining precisely the aetiology of stroke is technically difficult and not carried out routinely, and therefore data from most existing studies are incomplete. The absence of an association between cholesterol and stroke may also be explained by competing CHD. Stroke typically occurs later in life than CHD, probably because of the time-related development of atherosclerotic lesions first in the aorta, then in the coronary arteries, and finally in the cerebral arteries (Strong 1992). When in populations the incidence of CHD early in life is relatively higher than that of stroke, the association with stroke may be attenuated. Many people with increased cholesterol may die from CHD before a stroke can occur. This leaves subjects at risk of stroke whose cardiovascular system for some reason is relatively resistant to the effects of cholesterol. Finally, it should be noted that the importance of one risk factor is relative to the presence of other potential factors contributing to the disease of interest. In industrial societies smoking, increased blood pressure, and diabetes mellitus may reduce the relative importance of increased cholesterol as a risk factor for stroke.

35.4.2 Effect of cholesterol lowering on the occurrence of cardiovascular diseases in the older population

Most of the evidence on the effects of cholesterol lowering on CHD and total mortality in the older population are derived from secondary prevention trials such as the Scandinavian Simvastatin Survival Study (4S) (Miettinen *et al.* 1997; Scandinavian Simvastatin Survival Study Group 1995), Cholesterol and Recurrent Events (CARE) study, and the Long-Term Intervention with Pravastatin in Ischemic Disease (LIPID) study that included men and women aged 65 years and older. A marked reduction in coronary events in the older age group was found, similar to the reduction observed in patients aged less than 65 years. The major limitation of these studies is that they included 'young' elderly subjects up to age 75 years. However, as the effects of cholesterol lowering with these hydroxy-methylglutaryl-coenzyme A reductase inhibitors (HMG-CoA) do not show a tendency to decrease with advancing age, it is reasonable to extrapolate these results to the 'older' elderly, as long as the patient is in relatively general good health. Only one primary-prevention trial with an HMG-CoA reductase inhibitor included a large number of older people: the Air Force/Texas Coronary Atherosclerosis Prevention Study (AFCAPS/TEXCAPS) (Downs *et al.* 1998). The 6605 participants in the trial included 1416 men and women aged over 65 years. The results showed a marked reduction of 37% in major coronary events in the whole group, and similar results were observed in the older age group. No significant adverse events were reported related to drug therapy in this study. The study suggests that primary prevention with HMG-CoA reductase inhibitors is beneficial in the elderly, at least in the 'young' elderly, without significant adverse effect.

An early overview of results of trials on the efficacy of cholesterol lowering suggested that there was no significant reduction in *fatal or non-fatal stroke* incidence with lipid lowering regimens compared to placebo treatment (Hebert *et al.* 1995). A more recent trial among 6595 men free from MI at baseline and with increased cholesterol levels, in which cholesterol lowering was achieved through an HMG-CoA reductase inhibitor, a non-significant reduction of 11% in risk of fatal and non-fatal stroke was observed (Shepherd *et al.* 1995). In the 4S trial among 4444 subjects with previous CHD and increased cholesterol levels, lipid lowering with an HMG-CoA reductase inhibitor resulted in a significant 30% reduction in cerebrovascular events (fatal and non-fatal stroke, and transient ischaemic attacks) (Scandinavian Simvastatin Survival Study Group 1994). Recently the effect of the HMG-CoA reductase inhibitor pravastatin on stroke events was investigated in a prospectively defined pooled analysis of three large, placebo-controlled, randomized trials that included 19 768 patients with 102 559 person-years of follow-up (Byington *et al.* 2001). In all, 598 participants had a stroke during ~5 years of follow-up. Pravastatin was associated with a 23% reduction in non-haemorrhagic strokes (95% CI: 6–37). The Heart Protection Study among 20 500 patients provides important new information on the effects of treatment with the HMG-CoA reductase inhibitor simvastatin for the elderly (Collins *et al.* 2002; Heart Protection Study Collaborative Group 2002). Preliminary results show a 12% reduction in total mortality, a 17% reduction in vascular mortality, a 24% reduction in CHD events, a 27% reduction in all strokes, and a 16% reduction in non-coronary revascularizations across all patient groups regardless of age, gender, or baseline cholesterol value. The results of all these trials support the view that the relation of cholesterol with stroke is not as strong as with CHD. The beneficial effect of cholesterol lowering on stroke may be attributable to reduced progression (or regression) of atherosclerosis or to prevention of secondary effects of MI, that is, embolic stroke or transient ischaemic attacks. The effects of cholesterol lowering with HMG-CoA reductase inhibitors have also been ascribed to their non-lipid lowering effects, such as cell function and proliferation (Soma *et al.* 1992), platelet function (Schror 1990), and migration of smooth muscle cells (Hidaka *et al.* 1992). It has therefore been questioned whether the results of the trials that studied the effects of HMG-CoA reductase inhibitors can be used as evidence that serum cholesterol is causally related to the occurrence of cardiovascular diseases (Ravnskov 1995).

35.4.3 Blood pressure and the incidence of cardiovascular diseases in older people

Population-based cohort studies have clearly established an increased risk of cardiovascular diseases with increasing blood pressure. In the Framingham Study of subjects aged 64–74 years, blood pressure >160/95 mmHg increased the incidence of cardiovascular diseases approximately three-fold for men and four-fold for women compared to normotensive individuals (Kannel and Gordan 1978). Although elevations of both systolic and diastolic blood pressure remain important risk factors, with advancing age, systolic blood pressure is the predominant determinant of cardiovascular disease (Stamler *et al.* 1993). The risk of all manifestations of cardiovascular diseases (coronary events, stroke, peripheral arterial disease, and congestive heart failure) rises sharply with systolic pressure in elderly men, but not as sharply in elderly women. There are similar associations between diastolic blood pressure and cardiovascular diseases in elderly men. For older women, the curve relating the incidence of cardiovascular diseases with diastolic blood pressure is relatively flat. Low, as well as high, diastolic blood pressure has been associated with an increased risk of cardiovascular diseases; and excessive lowering of diastolic blood pressures in hypertensive patients with known or unsuspected coronary artery disease has been related to an increase in the incidence of MI and sudden death (Alderman et al. 1989; Cruickshank et al. 1987). This paradoxical effect is known as the J-curve and has been ascribed to stiffening of the large arteries (Witteman et al. 1994) and to compromised coronary blood flow at lower diastolic blood pressures (Cruickshank et al. 1987).

In an 18-year follow-up study of low-risk subjects, the probability of developing cardiovascular disease within an 8-year period at a given age increased steeply and progressively between systolic blood pressures of 105 and 195 mmHg (Kannel et al. 1981). Elderly persons with borderline isolated systolic hypertension (defined as systolic blood pressure of 140–59 mmHg and diastolic blood pressure <90 mmHg) had an increased risk of a cardiovascular event compared to those with a systolic blood pressure <140 mmHg, and an even greater risk as compared to those with optimal blood pressure (defined as systolic blood pressure <140 mmHg and diastolic blood pressure <80 mmHg) (Sagie et al. 1993). In addition, during 24 years of follow-up, individuals with isolated systolic hypertension had a two- to four-fold increase in the incidence of strokes compared to normotensives (Kannel et al. 1981). This suggests that attention should be directed not only to the risk imparted by combined systolic and diastolic hypertension, but also to the enhanced risk posed by isolated systolic hypertension. Although the definition of isolated systolic hypertension varies between studies, its prevalence clearly increases with age (Wilking et al. 1988). Screening data from the Systolic Hypertension in the Elderly Program (SHEP), in which isolated systolic hypertension has been defined as systolic blood pressure >160 mmHg and diastolic blood pressure <90 mmHg, demonstrate that its percentage prevalence triples when comparing the >80 group with the 60–9-year-old age group (SHEP 1991). Elevated pulse pressure (systolic blood pressure – diastolic blood pressure), which results from loss of arterial compliance, may be an even better predictor of increased cardiovascular risk than systolic blood pressure (or diastolic blood pressure) alone, particularly in older persons (Lee et al. 1999; Mazza et al. 2001). Pulse pressure has been shown to be a predictor of MI and congestive heart failure in the elderly (Chae et al. 1999).

35.4.4 Benefit from blood pressure lowering for older people

The value of antihypertensive treatment in the elderly has been documented in several large prospective trials specifically designed to include older patients (Gong et al. 1996; MacMahon and Rodgers 1993; Staessen et al. 1997). The results of these trials show that treatment of isolated systolic hypertension or combined diastolic and systolic hypertension decreases cardiovascular morbidity (Gueyffier et al. 1999) and mortality in elderly patients (Cushman 2001; Wang and Staessen 2001). The SHEP is a landmark study that documented the benefits of treating isolated systolic hypertension in patients >60 years of age (SHEP 1991). The initial therapy was either diuretic chlorthalidone or placebo, and atenolol was added if needed. The study demonstrated reductions in total stroke incidence (36%), CHD (25%), and cardiovascular disease (32%) for active treatment compared with placebo. These reductions translate into a 5-year absolute benefit of 30 stroke events and 55 major cardiovascular events per 1000 participants. MacMahon's meta-analysis of five blood pressure trials in patients >60 years of age showed that active treatment resulted in reductions of 34% in strokes and 19% in CHD (MacMahon and Rodgers 1993). Although the proportional reduction was similar to that seen in younger individuals (stroke 43% and CHD 14%), the absolute reduction in elderly hypertensive patients was about twice that in younger hypertensive individuals (5.1 vs. 2.6/1000 for stroke and 2.5 vs. 1.0/1000 for CHD). Similarly, Mulrow *et al.* (1994) concluded that treating healthy, older hypertensive patients is efficacious, and that short-term morbidity and mortality benefits of therapy are greater for older than for younger individuals. Thus, the efficacy of treating hypertension in the elderly has been well documented. Blood pressure lowering also reduced the risk of major cardiovascular events among non-hypertensive individuals with a history of stroke or transient ischaemic attack (PROGRESS 2001). Current, ongoing trials have been designed to evaluate differences among antihypertensive agents with respect to their ability to reduce morbidity and mortality.

Although definite benefits are achieved for hypertensive patients <75 years of age, results from trials completed to date provide conflicting information on the benefits of treating hypertension in patients >80 years of age. A recent subgroup analysis of participants >80 years of age in randomized, controlled antihypertensive drug trials showed significant benefits for non-fatal events, such as stroke (Fig. 35.5) and congestive heart failure, but inconclusive findings for mortality (Gueyffier *et al.* 1999). To resolve this uncertainty, the Hypertension in the Very Elderly Trial (HYVET) is currently examining the relative benefits of the diuretic bendroflumethiazide and the ACE inhibitor lisinopril on stroke and other cardiovascular end points in patients >80 years of age (Bulpitt *et al.* 1994).

Comparative clinical trials have clearly established that treating elderly patients with hypertension is effective. However, the actual estimates of benefits and risks derived from trials with highly selective entry criteria for subjects may not be easily generalized to clinical practice. Age-related physiological and metabolic alterations, increased prevalence of risk factors and comorbidities, heterogeneity among the elderly, and physician attitudes are some factors that complicate the treatment of hypertension and must be considered in order to achieve effective blood pressure control in this population. Despite evidence of the usefulness of treating hypertension in the elderly, normotension is often not achieved. NHANES III showed that only 23–46% of individuals >70 years of age treated for hypertension have adequate blood pressure control (Burt *et al.* 1995).

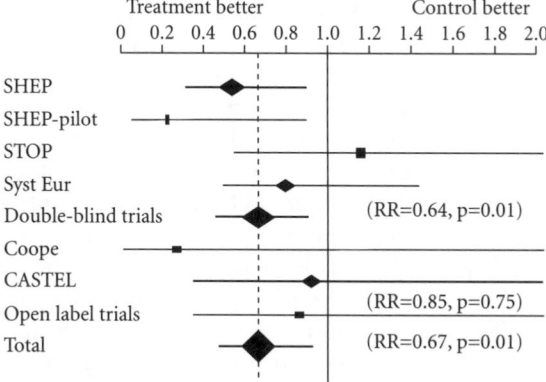

Fig. 35.5 Subgroup meta-analysis of randomized controlled trials assessing effects of treatment with antihypertensive drugs on the risk of stroke in patients over 80 years old. Treatment effect on relative risk (RR) of stroke. The areas of the symbols are proportional to the amount of information provided; error bars = 95% CIs. (Reproduced with permission from Gueyffier *et al.* 1999.)

35.4.5 **Smoking and cardiovascular disease risk in older people**

Smoking is an established risk factor for the development of new cardiovascular disease in the elderly (Aronow and Ahn 1996; Benfante *et al.* 1991; Hermanson *et al.* 1988; Houterman *et al.* 2002; Jajich *et al.* 1984; Kannel 1981; LaCroix *et al.* 1991; Siegel *et al.* 1987; Wolf *et al.* 1988). The relative contribution of smoking to the occurrence of cardiovascular diseases, however, decreases with increasing age. This is partly explained by the increasing prevalence of other risk factors with increasing age, and partly by the increased mortality among young smokers. At 6 year follow-up of older men and women in the Coronary Artery Surgery Study Registry (Hermanson *et al.* 1988), the relative risk of new MI or death was 2.9 for those 70 years of age and older who continued smoking, compared to persons who quit during the year before study enrolment. At 40-months follow-up of 664 men (mean age 80 years) and at 48 months follow-up of 1488 women (mean age 82 years), current cigarette smoking increased the risk of MI or sudden cardiac death by 2.2 times in men and 2.0 times in women (Aronow and Ahn 1996). It has been shown that after a cardiac event about 50% of patients continue their smoking habits (van Berkel *et al.* 1999). On the basis of available data, older men and women who smoke should be encouraged to undergo treatment for smoking cessation to decrease cardiovascular mortality and all-cause mortality.

35.4.6 **Diabetes mellitus type 2 and cardiovascular diseases in older people**

Type 2 diabetes mellitus (Casiglia *et al.* 2002) has been found to increase the risk for MI or sudden cardiac death by 1.9 times in elderly men (mean age 80 years) and by 1.8 times in elderly women (mean age 82 years) (Aronow and Ahn 1996; Psaty *et al.* 1999). Poor glycaemic control is associated with an increased incidence of cardiovascular events in older men and women (Kuusisto *et al.* 1994). In the United Kingdom Prospective Diabetes glucose reduction Study (UKPDS), the mean HbA1c, a measure for glycaemic control, over 10 years was 7.0% in the intensive treatment group versus 7.9% in the conventional treatment group. Despite the large number of subjects studied, the lengthy follow-up period and meticulous monitoring by the investigating team, no significant benefit was observed for reducing cardiovascular disease end points, stroke, or peripheral vascular disease (UKPDS 1998). In the same study, however, tight blood pressure control (target set at blood pressure <150/85 mmHg) considerably reduced both morbidity and mortality in hypertensive patients with type 2 diabetes mellitus, with largely the same benefit for beta-blockers as for ACE inhibitors (UKPDS 1998). For every 10 mmHg reduction in systolic blood pressure, a 12% risk reduction in diabetes-related end points was observed (risk reduction for strokes 44% (CI: 0.35–0.89), for heart failure 56% (0.20–0.94)). This suggests that the increased risk for cardiovascular diseases in patients with diabetes type 2 cannot be explained by poor glycaemic control, but that the effect of other cardiovascular disease risk factors such as hypertension may be enhanced by the presence of diabetes. Further support for this hypothesis comes from the findings of the Hypertension Optimal Treatment Trial (Hansson *et al.* 1998), which aimed to assess the optimal target diastolic blood pressure in the treatment of hypertension. Separate analysis of 1501 diabetic patients with hypertension in the study not only confirmed a lower risk of cardiovascular morbidity with diastolic blood pressure <90 mmHg (2.5-fold incidence compared to whole group), but also demonstrated additional benefit from blood pressure lowering, with a 51% risk reduction in major cardiovascular events in the group whose target blood pressure was <80 mmHg as compared to those whose target was <90 mmHg. The recently initiated ADVANCE trial will extend the findings by examining the benefits of glucose control versus blood pressure reduction in the normotensive range (ADVANCE 2001). Similarly, the effect of other cardiovascular disease risk factors may be modified by the presence of diabetes. Evidence on the effect of lipid lowering in older patients with type 2 diabetes is required.

35.5 Risk factors that are an expression of damage in the heart and arteries

35.5.1 ECG deviations

The ECG offers an inexpensive, non-invasive instrument to determine the presence of CHD, as well as other cardiac abnormalities such as ventricular hypertrophy and atrial fibrillation, known to be associated with the risk of future cardiovascular events. Especially in the elderly, in whom medical histories may be troubled by concomitant diseases, the ECG could be used as a useful diagnostic and prognostic instrument. Since the 1950s, large cohort studies among young and middle-aged men and women have provided important information on the prognostic value of ECG abnormalities. Relatively few studies have been performed in the elderly.

Myocardial infarction may occur with or without symptoms. Especially in the elderly, patients with MI often present themselves with atypical symptoms and signs; and the prevalence of silent MI increases with age (de Bruyne *et al.* 1997). The prognosis of silent MI with regard to the occurrence of new coronary events is similar to that of symptomatic MI (Aronow 1989*a*). A diagnosis of *left ventricular hypertrophy* by ECG has a poor sensitivity and predictive value in detecting echocardiographically determined left ventricular hypertrophy. *Repolarization disturbances* (ST-T wave changes), either isolated or in combination with other ischaemic or hypertrophic changes, have been associated with CHD and sudden cardiac death in the middle aged as well as in the elderly (Tervahauta *et al.* 1996). In the Framingham study in asymptomatic men and women non-specific ST-T abnormalities were associated with a two-fold risk for future cardiovascular events (Aronow 1989*b*). The risk associated with ST-T abnormalities is more pronounced in combination with other ECG abnormalities such as pathological Q-waves, left ventricular hypertrophy, or intraventricular conduction defects. Many studies have reported that chronic *atrial fibrillation* is associated with thrombo-embolic stroke (Boysen *et al.* 1988; Wolf *et al.* 1991). An association between atrial fibrillation and dementia was also reported (Ott *et al.* 1997). In addition, atrial fibrillation was a risk factor for all-cause mortality in the Coronary Drug Project (Coronary Drug Project 1972) and for cardiovascular mortality in the Framingham Heart Study (Kannel *et al.* 1982). ECG can also be used to study subclinical cardiac disease processes, such as disturbances in autonomic balance or repolarization, which may infer a poor prognosis even in the absence of symptoms. *Prolonged QTc interval* and *decreased heart rate variability* have been put forward as indicators of autonomic balance. With increasing age, sympathetic activity increases relative to vagal activity (Ziegler *et al.* 1976). Autonomic balance, in particular QTc interval and heart rate variability, is influenced by various physiological and pathophysiological conditions such as respiration, diabetic neuropathy, left ventricular function, and CHD. Both risk indicators have been associated with a poor prognosis of patients after a MI (Bigger *et al.* 1993; Cripps *et al.* 1991; Singh *et al.* 1996). Two new indicators of ventricular repolarization have been put forward as predictors of cardiac outcome in the elderly. First, interlead variability of the length of the QT interval in the standard ECG, defined as *QT dispersion*, was found to be a strong independent predictor of cardiac mortality in older men and women. Second, the *electrical T-axis* has been put forward as a general marker of repolarization abnormalitiy, indicative of subclinical myocardial damage. In the Rotterdam Study a four-fold risk for cardiac and sudden death was found in older men and women with an abnormal T-axis (Kors *et al.* 1998). In this study, T-axis was a stronger risk indicator than a history of MI or diabetes mellitus.

35.5.2 Left ventricular hypertrophy

Subjects with left ventricular hypertrophy are at increased risk of coronary events, atherothrombotic brain infarctions, congestive heart failure, peripheral artery disease, ventricular arrhythmias, and total mortality (Kahn *et al.* 1996). One of the most important causes of left ventricular hypertrophy is chronic hypertension. Prognosis of left ventricular hypertrophy in the elderly is reported to be similar to that of silent MI (Kannel *et al.* 1985). Treatment of left ventricular hypertrophy reduces the incidence of CHD (Cruickshank *et al.* 1992). Results from the Framingham Heart Study have shown that with an increasing awareness and treatment of severe hypertension, the frequency of left ventricular hypertrophy has markedly decreased over the last decades (Mosterd *et al.* 1999*b*).

35.5.3 Changes in the wall of the carotid artery

Angiography is the 'gold standard' technique for detecting atherosclerosis by visualization of vessel stenoses. However, due to the procedure's invasive nature, high cost, certain morbidity and mortality risks, and exposure to X-rays, its use as a CHD screening tool and for tracking the progression of disease is limited and alternative techniques have been sought. These include B-mode (two-dimensional) ultrasound, intravascular ultrasound (IVUS) and electron beam (computed) tomography (EB(C)T). The use of IVUS for large-scale intervention studies is constrained by the invasive nature of the procedure. EB(C)T is a non-invasive imaging technique that enables visualization and quantification of vascular calcification. Coronary calcium is a marker of atherosclerotic disease (O'Rourke *et al.* 2000) and is correlated with atherosclerosis in the carotid arteries, the abdominal aorta and the arteries of the lower extremities. It seems likely that EB(C)T or perhaps a substitute, multi-slice computed tomography (Achenbach *et al.* 2001; Nieman *et al.* 2001; Prokop 2000) will become a suitable technique for assessing changes in the rate of coronary atherosclerosis progression in the relatively near future, although few intervention studies using EBCT have been performed to date (O'Rourke *et al.* 2000).

B-mode ultrasound enables non-invasive, direct visualization of the arterial wall rather than estimation of atherosclerotic plaque from luminal stenosis. Several studies have examined the relationship between carotid intima media thickness (CIMT) and cardiovascular disease events. The relationship between the maximum CIMT of the common carotid artery and risk of incident MI in middle-aged men was assessed in the Kuopio Ischemic Heart Disease (KIHD) risk factor study (Salonen and Salonen 1993). Analysis of CIMT as a continuous variable revealed that for every 0.1 mm increment, risk of MI increased by 11%. Similar results were found for this age group in the Atherosclerosis Risk In Communities (ARIC) study (Chambless *et al.* 1997). The Cardiovascular Health Study (CHS) and the Rotterdam Study examined the association between CIMT of the common carotid artery and risk of MI and stroke in older male and female subjects. The association between CIMT and risk of coronary events was consistent with those of the KIHD and ARIC studies. In the CHS, for every 0.2 mm increase in CIMT, relative risk of MI or stroke increased by 47% and relative risk of MI increased by 46% (O'Leary *et al.* 1999). Subjects in the highest quintile for CIMT of the common carotid artery had an almost four-fold increase in risk compared with subjects in the lowest quintile (odds ratio 3.98 (CI: 2.88–5.51)), and consistent results were observed for CIMT of the internal carotid artery (odds ratio 4.22 (CI: 3.02–5.91)). Similarly, in the Rotterdam Study, the risk of MI increased by 43% for every 0.163 mm increase in CIMT of the common carotid artery (Bots *et al.* 1997). Following exclusion of subjects with a history of MI or stroke, a 0.163 mm increment in CIMT was associated with a 51% increase in the risk of MI. However, in contrast to the ARIC study, the strength of the association between CIMT and the incidence of coronary events was similar in men and women.

A significant relationship between CIMT and risk of coronary events was also demonstrated in patients with established CHD in a long-term follow-up of male CHD patients who had participated in the Cholesterol Lowering Atherosclerosis Study (CLAS) (Hodis *et al.* 1998). Furthermore, this study examined the association between the rate of progression of CIMT over the follow-up period and the risk of coronary events; the risk of MI or coronary death doubled (odds ratio 2.2 (CI: 1.4–3.6)) and that of MI, coronary death, or revascularization tripled (odds ratio 3.1 (CI: 2.1–4.5)) for every 0.03 mm/year increase in CIMT progression.

35.6 Conclusions

Atherosclerosis generally takes a lifetime to develop. Among the elderly a sizeable proportion of the population has developed some degree of atherosclerosis. In the presence of atherosclerosis 'trigger factors' and vulnerability of the myocardium to reduced coronary flow and ischaemia become important determinants of cardiovascular events. It is important to detect early atherosclerotic disease, because prevention of symptoms may be achieved by reduction of atherosclerosis through risk factor modification, but also by preventing triggers for sudden arterial occlusion and reduction of sensitivity for ischaemia of myocardial tissue that is already suffering from a compromised coronary circulation (left ventricular hypertrophy, heart failure). Several new methods for non-invasive assessment of presymptomatic atherosclerotic arterial disease have recently become available.

Decisions to apply a medical intervention are based on absolute benefits of interventions. Many of the older individuals are at higher absolute cardiovascular disease risk than any other section of the population and therefore are potentially more likely to benefit from risk reductions. It is important to note that risk factors can enhance each other and that the elevation of several risk factors has more impact than the sum of the individual parts. Additionally, the effects of drug therapies appear to decrease the risk for cardiovascular events independent of the baseline level of the risk factor (Yusuf 2002). Statins are as effective in reducing the risk among subjects with normal cholesterol levels as among those with increased cholesterol levels (Heart Protection Study Collaborative Group 2002; Scandinavian Simvastatin Survival Study Group 1995). Similarly, the cardiovascular benefit of ACE inhibitors is greater than that attributable to the decrease in blood pressure (Heart Outcomes Prevention Evaluation Study Investigators 2000). There is significant comorbidity among the elderly and clinical judgement is required about whether and, if so, how to decrease cardiovascular risk for the individual elderly patient. Additionally, evidence for some interventions, particularly in the very elderly is not available and judgement is again required on what action, if any, to take.

References

Achenbach, S., Giesler, T., Ropers, D., Ulzheimer, S., Derlien, H., Schulte, C. *et al.* (2001). Detection of coronary artery stenoses by contrast-enhanced, retrospectively electrocardiographically-gated, multislice spiral computed tomography, *Circulation*, **103** (21), 2535–8.

ADVANCE Study Group (2001). Study rationale and design of ADVANCE: action in diabetes and vascular disease–preterax and diamicron MR controlled evaluation, *Diabetologia*, **44** (9), 1118–20.

Alderman, M. H., Ooi, W. L., Madhavan, S., and Cohen, H. (1989). Treatment-induced blood pressure reduction and the risk of myocardial infarction. *Journal of the American Medical Association*, **262** (7), 920–4.

Aronow, W. S. (1989*a*). New coronary events at four-year follow-up in elderly patients with recognized or unrecognized myocardial infarction. *American Journal of Cardiology*, **63** (9), 621–2.

Aronow, W. S. (1989*b*). Correlation of ischemic ST-segment depression on the resting electrocardiogram with new cardiac events in 1,106 patients over 62 years of age. *American Journal of Cardiology*, **64** (3), 232–3.

Aronow, W. S. and Ahn, C. (1996). Risk factors for new coronary events in a large cohort of very elderly patients with and without coronary artery disease. *American Journal of Cardiology*, **77** (10), 864–6.

Benfante, R., Reed, D., and Frank, J. (1991). Does cigarette smoking have an independent effect on coronary heart disease incidence in the elderly? *American Journal of Public Health*, **81** (7), 897–9.

Benfante, R., Yano, K., Hwang, L. J., Curb, J. D., Kagan, A., and Ross, W. (1994). Elevated serum cholesterol is a risk factor for both coronary heart disease and thromboembolic stroke in Hawaiian Japanese men: implications of shared risk. *Stroke*, **25** (4), 814–20.

Bigger, J. T., Jr., Fleiss, J. L., Rolnitzky, L. M., and Steinman, R. C. (1993). Frequency domain measures of heart period variability to assess risk late after myocardial infarction. *Journal of American College of Cardiology*, **21** (3), 729–36.

Bots, M. L., Elwood, P. C., Nikitin, Y., Salonen, J. T., Freire, D. C., Inzitari, D. *et al.* (2002). Total and HDL cholesterol and risk of stroke. EUROSTROKE: a collaborative study among research centres in Europe. *Journal of Epidemiology and Community Health*, **56** (Suppl. 1), I19–I24.

Bots, M. L., Hoes, A. W., Koudstaal, P. J., Hofman, A., and Grobbee, D. E. (1997). Common carotid intima-media thickness and risk of stroke and myocardial infarction: the Rotterdam Study, *Circulation*, **96** (5), 1432–7.

Boysen, G., Nyboe, J., Appleyard, M., Sorensen, P. S., Boas, J., Somnier, F. *et al.* (1988). Stroke incidence and risk factors for stroke in Copenhagen, Denmark. *Stroke*, **19** (11), 1345–53.

Bulpitt, C. J., Fletcher, A. E., Amery, A., Coope, J., Evans, J. G., Lightowlers, S. *et al.* (1994). The Hypertension in the Very Elderly Trial (HYVET): rationale, methodology and comparison with previous trials. *Drugs Aging*, **5** (3), 171–83.

Burt, V. L., Whelton, P., Roccella, E. J., Brown, C., Cutler, J. A., Higgins, M. *et al.* (1995). Prevalence of hypertension in the US adult population: results from the Third National Health and Nutrition Examination Survey, 1988–1991. *Hypertension*, **25** (3), 305–13.

Byington, R. P., Davis, B. R., Plehn, J. F., White, H. D., Baker, J., Cobbe, S. M., and Shepherd, J. (2001). Reduction of stroke events with pravastatin: the Prospective Pravastatin Pooling (PPP) Project. *Circulation*, **103** (3), 387–92.

Casiglia, E., Mazza, A., Tikhonoff, V., Pavei, A., Privato, G., Schenal, N., and Pessina, A. C. (2002). Weak effect of hypertension and other classic risk factors in the elderly who have already paid their toll. *Journal of Human Hypertension*, **16** (1), 21–31.

Chae, C. U., Pfeffer, M. A., Glynn, R. J., Mitchell, G. F., Taylor, J. O., and Hennekens, C. H. (1999). Increased pulse pressure and risk of heart failure in the elderly. *Journal of the American Medical Association*, **281** (7), 634–9.

Chambless, L. E., Heiss, G., Folsom, A. R., Rosamond, W., Szklo, M., Sharrett, A. R., and Clegg, L. X. (1997). Association of coronary heart disease incidence with carotid arterial wall thickness and major risk factors: the Atherosclerosis Risk in Communities (ARIC) Study, 1987–1993. *American Journal of Epidemiology*, **146** (6), 483–94.

Collins, R., Peto, R., and Armitage, J. (2002). The MRC/BHF Heart Protection Study: preliminary results. *International Journal of Clinical Practice*, **56** (1), 53–6.

Comi, P., Chiaramonte, R., and Maier, J. A. (1995). Senescence-dependent regulation of type 1 plasminogen activator inhibitor in human vascular endothelial cells. *Experimental Cell Research*, **219** (1), 304–8.

Coronary Drug Project (1972). The prognostic importance of the electrocardiogram after myocardial infarction: experience in the Coronary Drug Project. *Annals of Internal Medicine*, **77** (5), 677–89.

Corti, M. C., Guralnik, J. M., Salive, M. E., Harris, T., Field, T. S., Wallace, R. B. *et al.* (1995). HDL cholesterol predicts coronary heart disease mortality in older persons. *Journal of the American Medical Association*, **274** (7), 539–44.

Corti, M. C., Guralnik, J. M., Salive, M. E., Harris, T., Ferrucci, L., Glynn, R. J., and Havlik, R. J. (1997). Clarifying the direct relation between total cholesterol levels and death from coronary heart disease in older persons. *Annals of Internal Medicine*, **126** (10), 753–60.

Cowie M. R., Mosterd, A., Wood, D., Deckers, J. W., Poole-Wilson P. A., Sutton G. C., and Grobbee D. E. (1997). The epidemiology of heart failure. *European Heart Journal*, **18** (2), 208–25.

Cripps, T. R., Malik, M., Farrell, T. G., and Camm, A. J. (1991). Prognostic value of reduced heart rate variability after myocardial infarction: clinical evaluation of a new analysis method. *British Heart Journal*, **65** (1), 14–19.

Cruickshank, J. M., Thorp, J. M., and Zacharias, F. J. (1987). Benefits and potential harm of lowering high blood pressure. *Lancet*, **1** (8533), 581–4.

Cruickshank, J. M., Lewis, J., Moore, V., and Dodd, C. (1992). Reversibility of left ventricular hypertrophy by differing types of antihypertensive therapy. *Journal of Human Hypertension*, **6** (2), 85–90.

Cushman, W. C. (2001). Clinical overview of hypertension and emerging treatment considerations. *American Journal of Hypertension*, **14** (7, Part 2), 226S–230S.

de Bruyne, M. C., Mosterd, A., Hoes, A. W., Kors, J. A., Kruijssen, D. A., van Bemmel, J. H. *et al.* (1997). Prevalence, determinants, and misclassification of myocardial infarction in the elderly. *Epidemiology*, **8** (5), 495–500.

Downs, J. R., Clearfield, M., Weis, S., Whitney, E., Shapiro, D. R., Beere, P. A. *et al.* (1998). Primary prevention of acute coronary events with lovastatin in men and women with average cholesterol levels: results of AFCAPS/TexCAPS. Air Force/Texas Coronary Atherosclerosis Prevention Study. *Journal of the American Medical Association*, **279** (20), 1615–22.

Egashira, K., Inou, T., Hirooka, Y., Kai, H., Sugimachi, M., Suzuki, S. *et al.* (1993). Effects of age on endothelium-dependent vasodilation of resistance coronary artery by acetylcholine in humans. *Circulation*, **88** (1), 77–81.

Enos W. F., Holmes R. H., and Beyer J. (1953). Coronary disease among United States soldiers killed in action in Korea: a preliminary report. *Journal of the American Medical Association*, **152**, 1090–3.

Esmon, C. T. (2000). Does inflammation contribute to thrombotic events? *Haemostasis*, **30** (Suppl. 2), 34–40.

Faergeman, O. (2002). Estimation and reduction of cardiovascular risk in old people. *European Heart Journal*, **23** (4), 261–3.

Fay, W. P., Murphy, J. G., and Owen, W. G. (1996). High concentrations of active plasminogen activator inhibitor-1 in porcine coronary artery thrombi. *Arteriosclerosis, Thrombosis, and Vascular Biology*, **16** (10), 1277–1284.

Fries J. F. (1980). Aging, natural death, and the compression of morbidity. *New England Journal of Medicine*, **303**, 130–5.

Gatchev, O., Rastam, L., Lindberg, G., Gullberg, B., Eklund, G. A., and Isacsson, S. O. (1993). Subarachnoid hemorrhage, cerebral hemorrhage, and serum cholesterol concentration in men and women, *Annals of Epidemiology*, **3** (4), 403–9.

Gong, L., Zhang, W., Zhu, Y., Zhu, J., Kong, D., Page, V. *et al* (1996). Shanghai trial of nifedipine in the elderly (STONE). *Journal of Hypertension*, **14** (10), 1237–45.

Gordon, T., Kannel, W. B., Castelli, W. P., and Dawber, T. R. (1981). Lipoproteins, cardiovascular disease, and death: The Framingham study. *Archives of Internal Medicine*, **141** (9), 1128–31.

Gueyffier, F., Bulpitt, C., Boissel, J. P., Schron, E., Ekbom, T., Fagard, R. *et al.* (1999). Antihypertensive drugs in very old people: a subgroup meta-analysis of randomised controlled trials. INDANA Group. *Lancet*, **353** (9155), 793–6.

Hager, K., Setzer, J., Vogl, T., Voit, J., and Platt, D. (1989). Blood coagulation factors in the elderly. *Archives of Gerontology and Geriatrics*, **9** (3), 277–82.

Haheim, L. L., Holme, I., Hjermann, I., and Leren, P. (1993). Risk factors of stroke incidence and mortality: a 12-year follow-up of the Oslo Study. *Stroke*, **24** (10), 1484–9.

Hansson, L., Zanchetti, A., Carruthers, S. G., Dahlof, B., Elmfeldt, D., Julius, S. *et al.* (1998). Effects of intensive blood-pressure lowering and low-dose aspirin in patients with hypertension: principal results of the Hypertension Optimal Treatment (HOT) randomised trial. HOT Study Group. *Lancet*, **351** (9118), 1755–62.

Harmsen, P., Rosengren, A., Tsipogianni, A., and Wilhelmsen, L. (1990). Risk factors for stroke in middle-aged men in Goteborg, Sweden. *Stroke*, **21** (2), 223–9.

Heart Outcomes Prevention Evaluation Study Investigators (2000). Effects of ramipril on cardiovascular and microvascular outcomes in people with diabetes mellitus: results of the HOPE study and MICRO-HOPE substudy. Heart Outcomes Prevention Evaluation Study Investigators. *Lancet*, **355** (9200), 253–9.

Heart Protection Study Collaborative Group (2002). MRC/BHF Heart Protection Study of cholesterol lowering with simvastatin in 20,536 high-risk individuals: a randomised placebo-controlled trial. *Lancet*, **360** (9326), 7–22.

Hebert, P. R., Gaziano, J. M., and Hennekens, C. H. (1995). An overview of trials of cholesterol lowering and risk of stroke. *Archives of Internal Medicine*, **155** (1), 50–5.

Hermanson, B., Omenn, G. S., Kronmal, R. A., and Gersh, B. J. (1988). Beneficial six-year outcome of smoking cessation in older men and women with coronary artery disease. Results from the CASS registry. *New England Journal of Medicine*, **319** (21), 1365–9.

Hidaka, Y., Eda, T., Yonemoto, M., and Kamei, T. (1992). Inhibition of cultured vascular smooth muscle cell migration by simvastatin (MK-733). *Atherosclerosis*, **95** (1), 87–94.

Hodis, H. N., Mack, W. J., LaBree, L., Selzer, R. H., Liu, C. R., Liu, C. H., and Azen, S. P. (1998). The role of carotid arterial intima-media thickness in predicting clinical coronary events. *Annals of Internal Medicine*, **128** (4), 262–9.

Houterman, S., Verschuren, W. M., Hofman, A., and Witteman, J. C. (1999). Serum cholesterol is a risk factor for myocardial infarction in elderly men and women: the Rotterdam Study. *Journal of Internal Medicine*, **246** (1), 25–33.

Houterman, S., Verschuren, W. M., Giampaoli, S., Nissinen, A., Feskens, E. J., Menotti, A., and Kromhout, D. (2000). Total but not high-density lipoprotein cholesterol is consistently associated with coronary heart disease mortality in elderly men in Finland, Italy, and The Netherlands. *Epidemiology*, **11** (3), 327–32.

Houterman, S., Boshuizen, H. C., Verschuren, W. M., Giampaoli, S., Nissinen, A., Menotti, A., and Kromhout, D. (2002). Predicting cardiovascular risk in the elderly in different European countries. *European Heart Journal*, **23** (4), 294–300.

Iribarren, C., Jacobs, D. R., Sadler, M., Claxton, A. J., and Sidney, S. (1996). Low total serum cholesterol and intracerebral hemorrhagic stroke: is the association confined to elderly men? The Kaiser Permanente Medical Care Program. *Stroke*, **27** (11), 1993–8.

Iso, H., Jacobs, D. R., Jr., Wentworth, D., Neaton, J. D., and Cohen, J. D. (1989). Serum cholesterol levels and six-year mortality from stroke in 350,977 men screened for the multiple risk factor intervention trial. *New England Journal of Medicine*, **320** (14), 904–10.

Jajich, C. L., Ostfeld, A. M., and Freeman, D. H., Jr. (1984). Smoking and coronary heart disease mortality in the elderly. *Journal of the American Medical Association*, **252** (20), 2831–4.

Kahn, S., Frishman, W. H., Weissman, S., Ooi, W. L., and Aronson, M. (1996). Left ventricular hypertrophy on electrocardiogram: prognostic implications from a 10-year cohort study of older subjects. A report from the Bronx Longitudinal Aging Study. *Journal of the American Geriatric Society*, **44** (5), 524–9.

Kalache, A. and Aboderin, I. (1995). Stroke: the global burden. *Health Policy Planning*, **10** (1), 1–21.

Kannel, W. B. (1981). Cigarettes, coronary occlusions, and myocardial infarction. *Journal of the American Medical Association*, **246** (8), 871–872.

Kannel, W. B. and Gordan, T. (1978). Evaluation of cardiovascular risk in the elderly: the Framingham study. *Bulletin of the New York Academy of Medicine*, **54** (6), 573–91.

Kannel, W. B., Wolf, P. A., McGee, D. L., Dawber, T. R., McNamara, P., and Castelli, W. P. (1981). Systolic blood pressure, arterial rigidity, and risk of stroke: The Framingham study. *Journal of the American Medical Association*, **245** (12), 1225–9.

Kannel, W. B., Abbott, R. D., Savage, D. D., and McNamara, P. M. (1982). Epidemiologic features of chronic atrial fibrillation: the Framingham study. *New England Journal of Medicine*, **306** (17), 1018–22.

Kannel, W. B., Dannenberg, A. L., and Abbott, R. D. (1985). Unrecognized myocardial infarction and hypertension: the Framingham Study. *American Heart Journal*, **109** (3, Part 1), 581–5.

Kors, J. A., de Bruyne, M. C., Hoes, A. W., van Herpen, G., Hofman, A., van Bemmel, J. H., and Grobbee, D. E. (1998). T axis as an indicator of risk of cardiac events in elderly people. *Lancet*, **352** (9128), 601–5.

Kronmal, R. A., Cain, K. C., Ye, Z., and Omenn, G. S. (1993). Total serum cholesterol levels and mortality risk as a function of age: a report based on the Framingham data. *Archives of Internal Medicine*, **153** (9), 1065–73.

Krumholz, H. M., Seeman, T. E., Merrill, S. S., Mendes de Leon, C. F., Vaccarino, V., Silverman, D. I. *et al.* (1994). Lack of association between cholesterol and coronary heart disease mortality and morbidity and all-cause mortality in persons older than 70 years. *Journal of the American Medical Association*, **272** (17), 1335–40.

Kuusisto, J., Mykkanen, L., Pyorala, K., and Laakso, M. (1994). NIDDM and its metabolic control predict coronary heart disease in elderly subjects. *Diabetes*, **43** (8), 960–7.

LaCroix, A. Z., Lang, J., Scherr, P., Wallace, R. B., Cornoni-Huntley, J., Berkman, L. *et al.* (1991). Smoking and mortality among older men and women in three communities. *New England Journal of Medicine*, **324** (23), 1619–25.

Lakatta, E. G. (2002). Age-associated cardiovascular changes in health: impact on cardiovascular disease in older persons. *Heart Failure Reviews*, **7** (1), 29–49.

Lee, M. L., Rosner, B. A., and Weiss, S. T. (1999). Relationship of blood pressure to cardiovascular death: the effects of pulse pressure in the elderly. *Annals of Epidemiology*, **9** (2), 101–7.

Lindenstrom, E., Boysen, G., and Nyboe, J. (1994). Influence of total cholesterol, high density lipoprotein cholesterol, and triglycerides on risk of cerebrovascular disease: the Copenhagen City Heart Study. *British Medical Journal*, **309** (6946), 11–15.

MacMahon, S. and Rodgers, A. (1993). The effects of blood pressure reduction in older patients: an overview of five randomized controlled trials in elderly hypertensives. *Clinical and Experimental Hypertension*, **15** (6), 967–78.

Mari, D., Mannucci, P. M., Coppola, R., Bottasso, B., Bauer, K. A., and Rosenberg, R. D. (1995). Hypercoagulability in centenarians: the paradox of successful aging. *Blood*, **85** (11), 3144–9.

Marinho, A., Soares, R., Ferro, J., Lacerda, M., and Schmitt, F. C. (1997). Angiogenesis in breast cancer is related to age but not to other prognostic parameters. *Pathology Research Practice*, **193** (4), 267–73.

Mazza, A., Pessina, A. C., Gianluca, P., Tikhonoff, V., Pavei, A., and Casiglia, E. (2001). Pulse pressure: an independent predictor of coronary and stroke mortality in elderly females from the general population. *Blood Pressure*, **10** (4), 205–11.

Miettinen, T. A., Pyorala, K., Olsson, A. G., Musliner, T. A., Cook, T. J., Faergeman, O. *et al.* (1997). Cholesterol-lowering therapy in women and elderly patients with myocardial infarction or angina pectoris: findings from the Scandinavian Simvastatin Survival Study (4S). *Circulation*, **96** (12), 4211–18.

Mosterd, A., Hoes, A. W., de Bruyne, M. C., Deckers, J. W., Linker, D. T., Hofman, A., and Grobbee, D. E. (1999*a*). Prevalence of heart failure and left ventricular dysfunction in the general population; The Rotterdam Study. *European Heart Journal*, **20** (6), 447–55.

Mosterd, A., D'Agostino, R. B., Silbershatz, H., Sytkowski, P. A., Kannel, W. B., Grobbee, D. E., and Levy, D. (1999*b*). Trends in the prevalence of hypertension, antihypertensive therapy, and left ventricular hypertrophy from 1950 to 1989. *New England Journal of Medicine*, **340** (16), 1221–7.

Mosterd, A., Cost, B., Hoes, A. W., de Bruijne, M. C., Deckers, J. W., Hofman, A., and Grobbee, D. E. (2001). The prognosis of heart failure in the general population: The Rotterdam Study. *European Heart Journal*, **22** (15), 1318–27.

Mulcahy, D., Purcell, H., and Fox, K. (1991). Should we get up in the morning? Observations on circadian variations in cardiac events. *British Heart Journal*, **65** (6), 299–301.

Mulrow, C. D., Cornell, J. A., Herrera, C. R., Kadri, A., Farnett, L., and Aguilar, C. (1994). Hypertension in the elderly: implications and generalizability of randomized trials. *Journal of the American Medical Association*, **272** (24), 1932–8.

Newman, W. P., III, Freedman, D. S., Voors, A. W., Gard, P. D., Srinivasan, S. R., Cresanta, J. L. *et al.* (1986). Relation of serum lipoprotein levels and systolic blood pressure to early atherosclerosis: The Bogalusa Heart Study. *New England Journal of Medicine*, **314** (3), 138–44.

Nieman, K., Oudkerk, M., Rensing, B. J., van Ooijen, P., Munne, A., van Geuns, R. J., and de Feyter, P. J. (2001). Coronary angiography with multi-slice computed tomography. *Lancet*, **357** (9256), 599–603.

O'Leary, D. H., Polak, J. F., Kronmal, R. A., Manolio, T. A., Burke, G. L., and Wolfson, S. K. (1999). Carotid-artery intima and media thickness as a risk factor for myocardial infarction and stroke in older adults: Cardiovascular Health Study Collaborative Research Group. *New England Journal of Medicine*, **340** (1), 14–22.

Oliver, M. F. (1986). Prevention of coronary heart disease: propaganda, promises, problems, and prospects. *Circulation*, **73** (1), 1–9.

O'Rourke, R. A., Brundage, B. H., Froelicher, V. F., Greenland, P., Grundy, S. M., Hachamovitch, R. *et al.* (2000). American College of Cardiology/American Heart Association Expert Consensus document on electron-beam computed tomography for the diagnosis and prognosis of coronary artery disease. *Circulation*, **102** (1), 126–40.

Ott, A., Breteler, M. M., de Bruyne, M. C., van Harskamp, F., Grobbee, D. E., and Hofman, A. (1997). Atrial fibrillation and dementia in a population-based study: The Rotterdam Study. *Stroke*, **28** (2), 316–21.

PDAY (Pathobiological Determinants of Atherosclerosis in Youth) Research Group (1990). Relationship of atherosclerosis in young men to serum lipoprotein cholesterol concentrations and smoking: a preliminary report from the Pathobiological Determinants of Atherosclerosis in Youth (PDAY) Research Group. *Journal of the American Medical Association*, **264** (23), 3018–24.

Pieper, C. F., Rao, K. M., Currie, M. S., Harris, T. B., and Chen, H. J. (2000). Age, functional status, and racial differences in plasma D-dimer levels in community-dwelling elderly persons. *The Journals of Gerontology: Series A, Biological Sciences and Medical Sciences*. **55** (11), M649–M657.

Pili, R., Guo, Y., Chang, J., Nakanishi, H., Martin, G. R., and Passaniti, A. (1994). Altered angiogenesis underlying age-dependent changes in tumor growth, *Journal of the National Cancer Institute*. **86** (17), 1303–14.

PROGRESS (2001). Randomised trial of a perindopril-based blood-pressure-lowering regimen among 6,105 individuals with previous stroke or transient ischaemic attack. *Lancet*, **358** (9287), 1033–41.

Prokop, M. (2000). Multislice CT angiography. *European Journal of Radiology*, **36** (2), 86–96.

Prospective Studies Collaboration (1995). Cholesterol, diastolic blood pressure, and stroke: 13,000 strokes in 450,000 people in 45 prospective cohorts. Prospective studies collaboration. *Lancet*, **346** (8991–2), 1647–53.

Psaty, B. M., Furberg, C. D., Kuller, L. H., Bild, D. E., Rautaharju, P. M., Polak, J. F. *et al.* (1999). Traditional risk factors and subclinical disease measures as predictors of first myocardial infarction in older adults: the Cardiovascular Health Study. *Archives of Internal Medicine*, **159** (12), 1339–47.

Ravnskov, U. (1995). Implications of 4S evidence on baseline lipid levels. *Lancet*, **346**, 181.

Reed, M. J., Corsa, A. C., Kudravi, S. A., McCormick, R. S., and Arthur, W. T. (2000). A deficit in collagenase activity contributes to impaired migration of aged microvascular endothelial cells. *Journal of Cell Biochemistry*, **77** (1), 116–26.

Ridker, P. M., Manson, J. E., Buring, J. E., Muller, J. E., and Hennekens, C. H. (1990). Circadian variation of acute myocardial infarction and the effect of low-dose aspirin in a randomized trial of physicians. *Circulation*, **82** (3), 897–902.

Robbie, L. and Libby, P. (2001). Inflammation and atherothrombosis. *Annals of the New York Academy of Sciences*, **947**, 167–79; discussion 179–80, 167–79.

Rubin, S. M., Sidney, S., Black, D. M., Browner, W. S., Hulley, S. B., and Cummings, S. R. (1990). High blood cholesterol in elderly men and the excess risk for coronary heart disease. *Annals of Internal Medicine*, **113** (12), 916–20.

Sagie, A., Larson, M. G., and Levy, D. (1993). The natural history of borderline isolated systolic hypertension. *New England Journal of Medicine*, **329** (26), 1912–17.

Salonen, J. T. and Salonen, R. (1993). Ultrasound B-mode imaging in observational studies of atherosclerotic progression. *Circulation*, **87** (3 Suppl.), II56–II65.

Salonen, J. T., Puska, P., Tuomilehto, J., and Homan, K. (1982). Relation of blood pressure, serum lipids, and smoking to the risk of cerebral stroke: a longitudinal study in Eastern Finland. *Stroke*, **13** (3), 327–33.

Sasayama, S. and Fujita, M. (1992). Recent insights into coronary collateral circulation. *Circulation*, **85** (3), 1197–204.

Scandinavian Simvastatin Survival Study Group (1994). Randomised trial of cholesterol lowering in 4444 patients with coronary heart disease: the Scandinavian Simvastatin Survival Study (4S). *Lancet*, **344** (8934), 1383–9.

Scandinavian Simvastatin Survival Study Group (1995). Baseline serum cholesterol and treatment effect in the Scandinavian Simvastatin Survival Study (4S). *Lancet*, **345** (8960), 1274–5.

Schror, K. (1990). Platelet reactivity and arachidonic acid metabolism in type II hyperlipoproteinaemia and its modification by cholesterol-lowering agents. *Eicosanoids*, **3** (2), 67–73.

SHEP (Systolic Hypertension in the Elderly Program) Cooperative Research Group (1991). Prevention of stroke by antihypertensive drug treatment in older persons with isolated systolic hypertension: final results of the Systolic Hypertension in the Elderly Program (SHEP). SHEP Cooperative Research Group. *Journal of American Medical Association*, **265** (24), 3255–64.

Shepherd, J., Cobbe, S. M., Ford, I., Isles, C. G., Lorimer, A. R., MacFarlane, P. W. *et al.* (1995). Prevention of coronary heart disease with pravastatin in men with hypercholesterolemia: West of Scotland Coronary Prevention Study Group. *New England Journal of Medicine*, **333** (20), 1301–7.

Siegel, D., Kuller, L., Lazarus, N. B., Black, D., Feigal, D., Hughes, G. *et al.* (1987). Predictors of cardiovascular events and mortality in the Systolic Hypertension in the Elderly Program pilot project. *American Journal of Epidemiology*, **126** (3), 385–99.

Simons, L. A., Friedlander, Y., McCallum, J., and Simons, J. (1995). Risk factors for coronary heart disease in the prospective Dubbo Study of Australian elderly. *Atherosclerosis*, **117** (1), 107–18.

Singh, N., Mironov, D., Armstrong, P. W., Ross, A. M., and Langer, A. (1996). Heart rate variability assessment early after acute myocardial infarction: pathophysiological and prognostic correlates. GUSTO ECG Substudy Investigators. Global Utilization of Streptokinase and TPA for Occluded Arteries. *Circulation*, **93** (7), 1388–95.

Soma, M. R., Corsini, A., and Paoletti, R. (1992). Cholesterol and mevalonic acid modulation in cell metabolism and multiplication. *Toxicology Letters*, **64–5**, Spec No: 1–15.

Staessen, J. A., Fagard, R., Thijs, L., Celis, H., Arabidze, G. G., Birkenhager, W. H. *et al.* (1997). Randomised double-blind comparison of placebo and active treatment for older patients with isolated systolic hypertension: The Systolic Hypertension in Europe (Syst-Eur). Trial Investigators. *Lancet*, **350** (9080), 757–64.

Stamler, J., Stamler, R., and Neaton, J. D. (1993). Blood pressure, systolic and diastolic, and cardiovascular risks: US population data. *Archives of Internal Medicine*, **153** (5), 598–615.

Strong, J. P. (1992). Atherosclerotic lesions: natural history, risk factors, and topography. *Archives of Pathological Laboratory Medicine*, **116** (12), 1268–75.

Taddei, S., Virdis, A., Mattei, P., Ghiadoni, L., Gennari, A., Fasolo, C. B. *et al.* (1995). Aging and endothelial function in normotensive subjects and patients with essential hypertension. *Circulation*, **91** (7), 1981–7.

Tanne, D., Yaari, S., and Goldbourt, U. (1997). High-density lipoprotein cholesterol and risk of ischemic stroke mortality: a 21-year follow-up of 8586 men from the Israeli Ischemic Heart Disease Study. *Stroke*, **28** (1), 83–7.

Tervahauta, M., Pekkanen, J., Punsar, S., and Nissinen, A. (1996). Resting electrocardiographic abnormalities as predictors of coronary events and total mortality among elderly men. *American Journal of Medicine*, **100** (6), 641–5.

Tunstall-Pedoe, H., Kuulasmaa, K., Mahonen, M., Tolonen, H., Ruokokoski, E., and Amouyel, P. (1999). Contribution of trends in survival and coronary-event rates to changes in coronary heart disease mortality: 10-year results from 37 WHO MONICA project populations. Monitoring trends and determinants in cardiovascular disease. *Lancet*, **353** (9164), 1547–57.

UKPDS (UK Prospective Diabetes Study) Group (1998a). Efficacy of atenolol and captopril in reducing risk of macrovascular and microvascular complications in type 2 diabetes: UKPDS 39. UK Prospective Diabetes Study Group. *British Medical Journal*, **317** (7160), 713–20.

UKPDS (UK Prospective Diabetes Study) Group (1998b). Intensive blood-glucose control with sulphonylureas or insulin compared with conventional treatment and risk of complications in patients with type 2 diabetes (UKPDS 33). UK Prospective Diabetes Study (UKPDS) Group. *Lancet*, **352** (9131), 837–53.

Van Berkel, T. F., Boersma, H., De Baquer, D., Deckers, J. W., and Wood, D. (1999). Registration and management of smoking behaviour in patients with coronary heart disease: The EUROASPIRE survey. *European Heart Journal*, **20** (22), 1630–7.

Van Der Bom, J. G., Bots, M. L., van Vliet, H. H., Pols, H. A., Hofman, A., and Grobbee, D. E. (1996). Antithrombin and atherosclerosis in the Rotterdam Study. *Arteriosclerosis, Thrombosis, and Vascular Biology*, **16** (7), 864–7.

Van Der Bom, J. G., Bots, M. L., Haverkate, F., Meyer, P., Hofman, A., Grobbee, D. E., and Kluft, C. (1999). Fibrinolytic activity in peripheral atherosclerosis in the elderly. *Thrombosis and Haemostasis*, **81** (2), 275–80.

Van Der Bom, J. G., Bots, M. L., Haverkate, F., Meijer, P., Hofman, A., Kluft, C., and Grobbee, D. E. (2001). Activation products of the haemostatic system in coronary, cerebrovascular and peripheral arterial disease. *Thrombosis and Haemostasis*, **85** (2), 234–9.

Vanhoutte, P. M. (2002). Ageing and endothelial dysfunction. *European Heart Journal Supplements*, **4** (Suppl. A), A8–A17.

Wang, J. G. and Staessen, J. A. (2001). The benefit of treating isolated systolic hypertension. *Current Hypertension Reports*, **3** (4), 333–9.

Weinsaft, J. W. and Edelberg, J. M. (2001). Aging-associated changes in vascular activity: a potential link to geriatric cardiovascular disease. *American Journal of Geriatric Cardiology*, **10** (6), 348–54.

Weverling-Rijnsburger, A. W., Blauw, G. J., Lagaay, A. M., Knook, D. L., Meinders, A. E., and Westendorp, R. G. (1997). Total cholesterol and risk of mortality in the oldest old. *Lancet*, **350** (9085), 1119–23.

Wilking, S. V., Belanger, A., Kannel, W. B., D'Agostino, R. B., and Steel, K. (1988). Determinants of isolated systolic hypertension. *Journal of the American Medical Association*, **260** (23), 3451–5.

Wiman, B., Andersson, T., Hallqvist, J., Reuterwall, C., Ahlbom, A., and deFaire, U. (2000). Plasma levels of tissue plasminogen activator/plasminogen activator inhibitor-1 complex and von Willebrand factor are significant risk markers for recurrent myocardial infarction in the Stockholm Heart Epidemiology Program (SHEEP) study. *Arteriosclerosis, Thrombosis, and Vascular Biology*, **20** (8), 2019–23.

Witte, D. R., Bots, M. L., Hoes, A. W., and Grobbee, D. E. (2000). Cardiovascular mortality in Dutch men during 1996 European football championship: longitudinal population study. *British Medical Journal*, **321** (7276), 1552–4.

Witteman, J. C., Grobbee, D. E., Valkenburg, H. A., van Hemert, A. M., Stijnen, T., Burger, H., and Hofman, A. (1994). J-shaped relation between change in diastolic blood pressure and progression of aortic atherosclerosis. *Lancet*, **343** (8896), 504–7.

Wolf, P. A., D'Agostino, R. B., Kannel, W. B., Bonita, R., and Belanger, A. J. (1988). Cigarette smoking as a risk factor for stroke: The Framingham Study. *Journal of the American Medical Association*, **259** (7), 1025–9.

Wolf, P. A., D'Agostino, R. B., Belanger, A. J., and Kannel, W. B. (1991). Probability of stroke: a risk profile from the Framingham Study. *Stroke*, **22** (3), 312–18.

Yusuf, S. (2002). Two decades of progress in preventing vascular disease. *Lancet*, **360** (9326), 2–3.

Ziegler, M. G., Lake, C. R., and Kopin, I. J. (1976). Plasma noradrenaline increases with age. *Nature*, **261** (5558), 333–5.

Zimetbaum, P., Frishman, W. H., Ooi, W. L., Derman, M. P., Aronson, M., Gidez, L. I., and Eder, H. A. (1992). Plasma lipids and lipoproteins and the incidence of cardiovascular disease in the very elderly: The Bronx Aging Study. *Arteriosclerosis and Thrombosis*, **12** (4), 416–23.

Section IV

Public health

Chapter 36

Strategies of prevention: the individual and the population

(reprinted from first edition)*

G. Rose

36.1 Aetiology: two different questions

The clinician asks: 'Why did this patient have a heart attack?' The public health doctor asks: 'Why do so many people have heart attacks?' These questions typify the two branches of aetiology: the causes of disease in individuals, and the determinants of its incidence rate in populations. Obviously each is relevant, but each calls for a different kind of research to provide the answers and those answers may not be the same.

Each approach to aetiology involves two further issues: susceptibility and exposure. In individuals, male sex identifies susceptibility, whereas smoking history and diet identify exposure to external causes. Both are called 'risk factors', but the distinction is important. Susceptibility cannot be changed. Its practical relevance is simply to indicate the individual's need for drug treatment or to attend to the modifiable external causes. Some risk factors, such as blood pressure and lipids, represent a complex outcome of both genetically determined susceptibility and modifiable behaviour, but in the main risk differences between individuals are due more to genetic than to modifiable factors (apart from smoking, and perhaps obesity). Thus a high level of blood cholesterol can be reduced by dietary change, but it will probably still fall in the upper part of the range for that population.

Results from migrant studies suggest that the reverse is true of risk differences between populations. Those of Asian extraction, it is true, seem to carry a high cardiovascular risk with them wherever they travel, but this is an exception, and migrants in general tend to acquire the disease rates of their adoptive countries. Incidence differences between countries, which are amazingly large, are due mainly to modifiable external factors rather than to differences in genetic susceptibility. The same must also, of course, apply to the rapid temporal changes in incidence which are occurring within so many countries: they must reflect changes in environment and behaviour.

Aetiologically there is thus a contrast: immutable genetic determinants of susceptibility play a much greater role in the risk differences between individuals within one population than in the incidence differences between populations. Conversely, the latter are much more the outcome of modifiable factors in the environment and behaviour. This creates a prior expectation of a greater potential for prevention at the population level.

36.2 **Prevention: two different strategies**

The two levels of aetiology have their counterparts in prevention. The individual or clinical approach seeks to identify and help those in whom an amalgam of genetic susceptibility and unhealthy lifestyle indicates unusual risk, but the public health approach seeks changes in those features of the population's behaviour or environment which are held responsible for the overall incidence rate. Thus the individual strategy is a rescue operation for individuals in need, whereas the population strategy is a radical attempt to deal with the underlying causes. The former is analogous to sending emergency aid for famine relief in the Third World: it is ethically compelling and it saves lives, but famines will continue to occur until there are changes in their underlying causes, which are economic, social, and agricultural. These radical changes are analogous to the population strategy of prevention.

36.2.1 **Sick individuals: the 'high risk strategy'**

Medicine's concern is with individuals. The main task of doctors will always be the care of sick patients, and many in fact see this as their only role, but preventive medicine is also essential because illness is unpleasant, care is expensive, and cure may be impossible. Nevertheless, even in preventive medicine doctors are naturally more attracted to a personal approach. High risk individuals are not really patients, but they are managed as though they were. Thus, for example, the care of hypertensives is really preventive medicine, but everyone speaks and thinks of it as treatment. For this to be possible, a label must first have been offered and accepted in order to justify the segregation of the high risk individuals from the 'healthy' population and their subsequent care alongside other patients.

Labelling, like diagnosis, implies a dichotomy. Medicine is heavily committed to dichotomous thinking. We speak of a risk factor as being present or absent. Screening involves recall of a high risk minority and reassurance of the rest. We say that a patient has or has not got coronary heart disease (CHD), even though pathologists tell us that it is all a matter of degree (nearly everyone has some of it). Coronary angiograms are reported as showing, for example, 'two-vessel disease' – as though coronary artery disease were either present or absent. It is nearly 40 years since Pickering produced clear evidence that hypertension is a man-made artefact, the result of an arbitrary split in a continuum. In nature, normality merges imperceptibly into abnormality, and most risk factors and diseases should be defined quantitatively and not qualitatively. He won the battle but he lost the war: medical thinking continues to espouse dichotomy.

The process of screening and high risk labelling thus necessarily involves a falsification. Nevertheless it may be quite appropriate to divide the population in this way if the purpose is to guide a decision on management which is itself necessarily dichotomous – such as giving or not giving some treatment or advice which is either not suitable or not available for everyone. But it should not be forgotten that this classification of the population is simply a matter of administrative convenience.

The large cohort studies have generally failed to identify any critical threshold level for the major risk factors (Martin *et al.* 1986; Rose and Shipley 1986): the lower the levels of blood pressure, cholesterol, and smoking, the lower is the long-term risk. If there are 'ideal' levels, then in Western populations they are rare, and a label of 'high risk' is affixed only to that proportion of the population to whom special help is to be offered. A management statement must not be confused with a prognostic statement. The public may readily misunderstand, and sometimes a screening examination with a 'normal' result can be a positive disincentive to preventive action (Kinlay and Heller 1990). This is not so much an argument against screening as a warning that the delivery of results needs to be accompanied by proper interpretation.

The point is further illustrated by our experience in the Whitehall Study of civil servants (Reid *et al.* 1976). For each participant we calculated a risk score based on smoking, blood pressure, and cholesterol, and the men were then classified into deciles of multivariate risk. Over the next 15 years the age-adjusted mortality from CHD was 10 times greater for men in the top decile relative to those in the lowest (Table 36.1 (previously unpublished)). For stroke, the difference was even larger. Men in the lowest-risk decile also had very favourable rates for cancers, especially of lung and stomach, and for respiratory disease. Their total mortality was about one-sixth of that for men in the top decile of coronary risk, which suggests that current advice on heart disease prevention should have favourable long-term effects on total mortality. It was, of course, to be expected that coronary mortality would be much reduced in the group with the lowest risk scores. The surprise was that, even in this group, CHD is still much the commonest single cause of death. Thus, although we can readily identify what we call a 'high risk' sector of the population, we cannot identify any such thing as a low risk group.

Potential benefits

It makes sense to focus preventive efforts on those who need them most, and so doctors and patients alike are better motivated. Thus, for example, the personal and service costs of achieving a change in eating habits are unrelated to the serum cholesterol level, but the potential rewards, which are substantial for high risk individuals, are statistically small (although still real) for the many with values around the average. An even stronger argument applies to the use of drugs, whether to control blood pressure or lipid levels, or to reduce the risk of thrombosis: the adverse effects are largely independent of cardiovascular risk, but it is only in high risk individuals that we can assert with sufficient confidence that the dangers are exceeded by the benefits. Therefore there can be no place for their mass use. Finally, in these days when 'Value for money!' is the cry, it has to be recognized that the cost per unit of benefit escalates rapidly as the clientele is enlarged. All these considerations argue potently for the advantages of focused preventive efforts.

Since it appears that disease is common even among those with low risk scores (see Table 36.1), it becomes important to know how the total case burden is distributed across different levels of risk. The more that cases are concentrated among an identifiable 'high risk' group, the better for a strategy based on screening: only a minority of people then need to take action. Conversely, this approach becomes less attractive if risk is more diffused and a higher proportion of people need to take action.

Table 36.1 Fifteen-year mortality (age-adjusted) among men in the Whitehall Study in whom values for smoking status, systolic blood pressure, and plasma cholesterol placed them in the top or bottom decile of multivariate risk

Cause of death	Percentage dead	
	Top decile	Bottom decile
All causes	36 (630)	7 (117)
CHD	17 (295)	2 (29)
Stroke	3 (53)	0.1 (2)
Cancer		
All sites	8 (141)	2 (45)
Lung	3 (57)	0.5 (9)
Stomach	1 (13)	0.2 (3)
Bronchitis/pneumonia	2 (37)	0.3 (6)

Widespread awareness of this issue originated with the World Health Organization (WHO) report (WHO 1982), where results of the Framingham Study were used to show that most of the excess cholesterol-associated risk of CHD did not occur among the clinically 'hypercholes-terolaemic' minority, but rather among the large numbers of men with values around or a little above the average. This illustrates an important general principle of preventive medicine: *many exposed to a small risk may generate more cases than a small number exposed to a conspicuous risk.* It also explains how a doctor can say: 'Most of my patients do not have risk factors.' It is all too easy to confuse statistical and biological normality. By definition, most people are within the statistical range of normal, but in Western populations most have (biologically speaking) high blood cholesterol levels and high blood pressure.

The efficiency of a screening strategy is further reduced by the error involved in characterizing individuals, particularly when this is based on a single examination. For example, within-subject variability for cholesterol is such that, it has been estimated, 28% of middle-aged men with a single value above 6.9 mmol/1 have a true (average) value below that level (Thompson and Pocock 1990). In order to avoid such frequent misclassifications, it is necessary to set the recall level for first screening examination well above the final action level and then to base the final decision on management on the mean of (say) three separate examinations. This is analogous to accepted good practice in blood pressure screening, but the costs and practical problems of implementing it are higher for a laboratory test.

The cardiovascular risks associated with raised blood pressure are rather more concentrated towards the high end of the distribution than those for raised cholesterol level, since the dose–response curve rises more sharply (particularly for stroke). Data from the Framingham Study for men and women aged 35–64 years indicate that nearly half of the excess strokes will occur among the 16% of the population with the highest pressures (diastolic blood pressure, >100 mmHg) (Royal College of Physicians 1989). This implies that, for a given recall and intervention rate, the potential for benefit is greater with screening for blood pressure than for cholesterol. (The actual benefit, of course, will also reflect the relative effectiveness of intervention.)

It has often been said that smoking is the chief preventable cause of heart disease, and the evidence for this view has (rather curiously) excited much less controversy than the case against dietary factors. It has perhaps not been sufficiently realized that the public health importance of a particular cause depends as much on the prevalence of exposure as on the risk to exposed individuals. In many countries smoking is now confined to a shrinking minority, and as its prevalence falls, so does its contribution to the total burden of illness. Advice to smokers is as important as ever it was for them as individuals, but its preventive potential for the community is falling rapidly (though it is still large).

Risk can be predicted better by a multivariate than a univariate score (Table 36.2). In the Whitehall Study 42% of the 15-year coronary deaths occurred among men in the top 20% of multivariate risk. (Interestingly, almost the same was true for total mortality.) This means that a screening strategy using a single examination of these three factors would require intervention in 20% of this population in order to offer help to 42% of the candidates for a heart attack. Intervention in only 10% would omit 75% of the candidates.

Realizable benefits

Achievement of these potential benefits is limited by factors of effectiveness, feasibility, and cost.

In the WHO European trial (WHO 1986) we estimated that the observed reduction in incidence of CHD was about two-thirds of what would have been expected if the observed

Table 36.2 Distribution of 15-year coronary and all-cause deaths according to quintile of a risk score based on smoking status, systolic blood pressure, and plasma cholesterol (Whitehall Study)

Quintile of risk	Percentage of deaths	
	CHD	All causes
1	7	10
2	11	13
3	17	17
4	24	24
5	42	36

changes in risk factors had led to an immediate and commensurate fall in risk. From this and other evidence it seems that a combined change in the major risk factors is likely to be reasonably and fairly rapidly effective.

The more serious problem is with feasibility. At present there is a disturbing lack of evidence on the long-term risk factor changes that can be achieved and sustained under ordinary practice conditions. A smoking cessation rate of 10–20% seems possible, but for cholesterol control the only evidence comes from relatively short follow-up in specialized clinics seeing selected referrals. This evidence is encouraging (Lewis and Rose 1991), but it may not be very relevant to the need to motivate and supervise ordinary people so that they will eat differently from their fellows for the rest of their lives.

Taking these problems together with the difficulties of screening those sections of the population that are most at risk, it seems unlikely that a high risk strategy could in practice achieve even half of its theoretical potential. If we accept the rather optimistic estimate from the European trial of about two-thirds effectiveness (relative to achieved risk factor reduction), taken with the earlier estimate that the 20% high risk segment of the population includes about 40% of future cases, we reach an overall (and probably overoptimistic) estimate of the maximum impact of a high risk preventive strategy in middle-aged men of $1/2 \times 2/3 \times 0.4 = 13\%$ reduction in total CHD in this group (probably less in older men and in women).

There are no realistic cost estimates for a national programme of screening and multifactorial prevention. Cost-effectiveness analyses of individual components (Lewis and Assmann 1989) suggest that general practitioners' advice against smoking is highly cost effective, and even cholesterol-lowering dietary advice calls for only half the cost of breast cancer screening per quality-adjusted life-year gained. The cost of a properly supported national programme would be high, but in relation to other accepted health service activities (not to mention governmental expenditure in other areas) it ought to be acceptable.

Outline principles for a risk factor screening programme

1 Screening without adequate advice and treatment has been shown to be a waste of time. Indeed, it can do positive harm by labelling people who previously thought that they were healthy. We are in danger of forgetting this lesson. There are strong pressures, backed by

lipidologists and some pharmaceutical companies, to institute mass screening for serum cholesterol, regardless of whether there are resources to deal adequately with the positive cases. But the first principle is: *no screening without adequate resources for long-term care.*

2 The second principle is that *selective screening and care are far more cost effective than mass screening*. It would cost 100 times as much to prevent one heart attack by cholesterol screening in 40-year-old women as in 60-year-old men (Khaw and Rose 1989).

3 The third principle is that *screening for a multifactorial disease should be multifactorial*. For cholesterol screening this means that the aim should not be to identify those with the highest cholesterol values, but those with the highest cholesterol-associated risk, for they are the ones who will receive most benefit from intervention. Thus in the population screened by the Multiple Risk Factor Intervention Trial (MRFIT) investigators (Martin *et al.* 1986), the 6-year follow-up found that the excess mortality associated with being in the top tertile of cholesterol was more than five times greater in a smoker whose blood pressure was in the top tertile than in a non-smoker with blood pressure in the lowest tertile. The importance of one risk factor or exposure depends on its context: isolated elevation of one factor may be relatively benign in individuals who are otherwise at low risk. Our aim should be to identify risk, not the individual risk factor. It makes little sense to define fixed action cut-points for cholesterol or blood pressure.

4 The fourth principle is a consequence of the third: *prevention of multifactorial disease must be multifactorial, not unifactorial.* Doctors treating hypertension are often satisfied if they can normalize the blood pressure. Lipid clinics concentrate on controlling blood lipid levels, and diabetic clinics on blood sugar. Yet in the Medical Research Council hypertension trial (MRC 1985) we found that the difference in the incidence of stroke between smokers and non-smokers was greater than the difference between treated and control patients. Risk factors interact. To control smoking in a hypertensive, or cholesterol in a diabetic, may be as important as to control the presenting problem. Management of multifactorial diseases should be multifactorial, but this is often not the case.

Conclusion

A high risk strategy for heart disease prevention is logical and scientifically well-founded, and it is attractive to doctors. Resources for adequate national implementation do not yet exist, and its long-term feasibility is unknown. It is unlikely that in any circumstances it could achieve a reduction of more than ~10–15% in the total incidence of CHD in middle-aged men. However, this does not condemn it, since *an intervention should be judged by what it achieves, not by what it fails to achieve*, but it does imply that we must look elsewhere for a more substantial answer to the problems of mass cardiovascular disease.

36.2.2 Sick populations: the public health approach

Pickering was the first to recognize that sick individuals may represent simply the extreme of a continuum, 'disease' being a quantitative rather than a qualitative phenomenon, but he did not generalize this revolutionary concept beyond blood pressure, nor did he recognize the idea of a sick population. That idea entered cardiovascular medicine with Keys' famous diagram demonstrating a near-complete separation of the Japanese and Finnish distributions of serum cholesterol. This told us that the root of the cholesterol problem lies in a characteristic of the population as a whole. To the extent that cholesterol differences determine incidence differences, this means that both

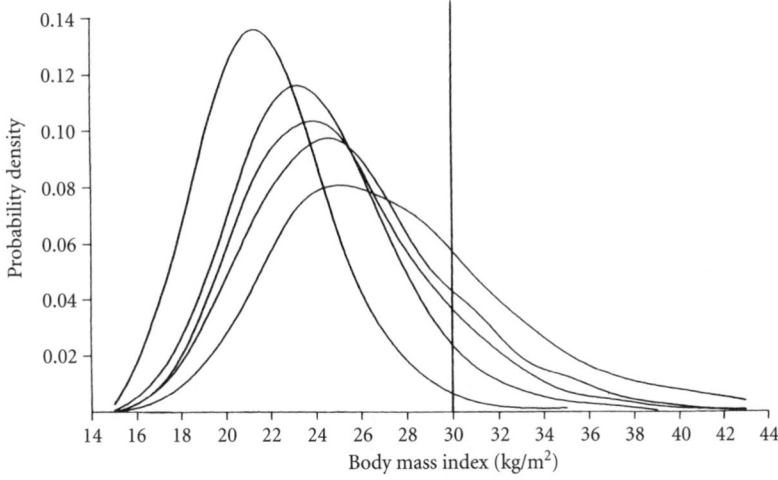

Fig. 36.1 Distributions of body mass index in five aggregated population groups of men and women aged 20–59 years, grouped according to increasing levels of the median.

research and prevention must be concerned with populations as a whole, not merely with deviant individuals, and this is the basis of the population or public health strategy of prevention.

We now know that what Keys demonstrated for one risk factor and one pair of populations is also true of many risk factors and population differences (Rose and Day 1990). Figure 36.1 illustrates the phenomenon for body mass index, using data from the INTERSALT study (INTERSALT Cooperative Research Group 1986). This study, which was undertaken for a different purpose, provided high quality standardized data on some cardiovascular risk factor distributions in 52 populations from 32 countries. For convenience of presentation in the figure, the 52 datasets have been aggregated into five groups, ranked according to their median values.

Several important points emerge, of which the chief is that the distributions shift up or down as a whole. Populations behave coherently: the range of difference between individuals is constrained, so that few move very far from their society's norm. Next, these whole-population shifts are large, with dramatic consequences for the prevalence of 'overweight'. In this particular instance an important part of the differences in prevalence results from variation in skewness, which is more pronounced for body weight than for other risk variables: the latter often show a striking consistency in the coefficient of variation.

Differences between populations in the incidence of cardiovascular disease are largely secondary to these whole-distribution shifts in major risk factors, and these in turn simply reflect mass differences in behaviour (principally eating, smoking, and exercise). Similar whole-distribution shifts probably also occur within populations over time, in company with secular changes in lifestyle, but unfortunately there are few datasets to test this supposition.

The aim of the population strategy of prevention is to seek means for promoting favourable shifts of these population distributions of risk factors – in other words, to tackle the underlying causes of a high incidence rate. The arguments for the desirability of such an approach are over-whelming. Unfortunately its realization is impeded by our scanty understanding of the determinants of population change.

Table 36.3 Reductions in population mean values associated with a halving of the prevalence of high values

Variable (definition of 'high')	Required reduction in mean
Systolic BP (≥140 mmHg)	8 mmHg
Diastolic BP (≥90 mmHg)	4 mmHg
Overweight (BMI ≥30 kg/m^2)	2.6 kg/m^2
Sodium intake (≥250 mmol/day)	39 mmol/d

BP: blood pressure; BMI: body mass index.

Potential benefits

The high risk strategy of prevention offers attractive rewards to individuals, but its probable impact on the total burden of disease is disappointingly small. The reverse is true of the population strategy (Table 36.3). Its potential for total benefit is large because a great many people are involved, each receiving a small reduction in risk, but the expectation of reward to individuals is small. Hence the 'prevention paradox': *a preventive measure which brings much benefit to the population offers little to each individual* (Rose 1981). This paradox applies to most public health measures (e.g. immunization, car seat belts, clean air legislation). It means that, if we are realistic, personal health rewards must be a weak motivator in health education.

Applied to blood pressure, a downwards shift of 2–3 mmHg in the whole distribution, if accompanied by corresponding reductions in risk, might save as many lives as all existing antihypertensive medication (Rose 1981). Applied to serum cholesterol, each 1% fall in the average level would lead (it has been estimated) to a 3% fall in the incidence of CHD. Applied to alcohol intake, a fall of 30% in average consumption might yield similar health benefits to the total elimination of all heavy drinking (Kreitman 1986).

Using data from the Whitehall Study we compared the relative size of predicted benefits from the population and high risk approaches to cholesterol reduction (Rose and Shipley 1990). A 10% reduction in the average level for the whole population (such as has probably already been achieved in some places) would be expected to reduce coronary mortality by more than twice as much as a reduction of 10% in the average for *all* members of the population with values in the top decile (which no one has yet been able to demonstrate as achievable by a screening programme).

Realizable benefits

The effectiveness of population-wide changes in coronary risk factors is amply demonstrated by the dramatic decline in coronary mortality for both men and women in a number of countries. What is not clear from such national experiences is which specific factors are responsible, nor how far they might have occurred in the absence of medical efforts.

The experience of the occupationally-based WHO European trial showed that advice aimed at the three major risk factors was effective to the extent that it was accepted (Rose 1987), but that acceptance was often disappointing in a low-cost health education effort and it was not sustained when the effort ceased. Medically led mass health education certainly seemed, after many years of sustained effort, to be effective against smoking, but in general it is ineffective if the timing is not right (the population must be in a receptive frame of mind) and it is probably much less powerful than economic and social forces. In developing countries the latter are exerting a seemingly irresistible adverse effect on coronary risk factors, but in Western countries they may have provided the prime mover behind declining coronary mortality. They have been a major force behind the impressive rise in the ratio of polyunsaturated to saturated fats in some national diets, and this has probably been a major factor in the declining incidence of heart disease. Thus an important decline in national consumption of saturated fats is clearly achievable, but so far a decline in total fat intake is not!

Estimates based on results from the INTERSALT study indicate that small but highly important falls in population levels of blood pressure might be expected to follow moderate changes in salt and alcohol intake and body weight (Stamler *et al.* 1989; Law *et al.* 1991). The first of these is now being realized in some countries, but unfortunately no one has yet much success to report in the control at population level of alcoholism or overweight.

Ethics and general principles

Doctors cannot decide how people are to live. As scientific experts we can say that a cholesterol-lowering dietary change will reduce the risk of heart disease, but the decision on whether the benefit justifies the costs is a matter for those whose lives are involved. This is difficult for doctors to accept, for their role in the care of acute illness leads them to expect a decision-taking role.

The concept of a need for mass change is also difficult for the community, for we are accustomed to believing that what most people do must be all right. They can readily accept the need for moderation – avoiding extremism and conforming with the average – but the suggestion that most people are living unhealthily is too threatening to be acceptable. Therefore the first need is for a changed perception of what is normal and socially desirable. The medical rewards for healthier living are remote in time and, for most individuals, small, but given a change in social norms of sensible behaviour the social rewards for a healthier lifestyle can be immediate and substantial.

The first necessity is a community will to change. For this to find practical expression calls for the support of educators and the mass media (so that people are properly informed about their choices) and of the suppliers of services and facilities for healthier eating and physical exercise (so that new demands can be met). There are different views on the role of government. Most seem to believe it to be legitimate for governments to seek to enforce virtue by heavy taxes on tobacco and alcohol, or even by legislation (car safety belts). This cannot be defended, either ethically or economically. Moreover, it is hypocritical if such governments are at the same time subsidizing and protecting the tobacco industry. The proper role of government in health promotion is (a) to protect the public from unbalanced or misleading information (the food and tobacco industries apply vast sums of money to encouraging people to eat unhealthy foods, to smoke, and to drink more alcohol); (b) to pursue economic policies which at least do not make it harder for people to pursue a healthier lifestyle (by, for example, subsidizing the production of saturated fats); and (c) to provide services which the public needs and wants in order to implement accepted health recommendations (such as intelligible food labelling and exercise facilities).

36.3 **Synthesis and conclusions**

High risk individuals need help, and this calls for screening and personal care to be provided by the medical services. But whatever it may offer to the individuals concerned, the high risk strategy is no more than an expensive rescue operation, offering disappointingly little towards solving the overall problem. This does not mean that it ought not to be pursued but only that it cannot be the main answer to the problems of a mass disease.

The two approaches (at individual and population levels) are interactive and mutually supportive, rather than rivals. Population-wide changes are essential if the attempts of individuals to change their lifestyles are not to turn them into social outcasts: people do not eat or live in isolation. Conversely, health education and advice given to individuals then diffuse outwards among their families, friends, and workmates, thus making the high risk strategy far more potent than if the targeted individuals were the only beneficiaries.

There are also deeper reasons why the two approaches must be seen as two components of a single preventive strategy. High risk individuals are quantitatively but not qualitatively different people: they are simply the tail of a continuous distribution, one part of their parent population. When different populations are compared (Fig. 36.1) it is seen that they behave as coherent entities, with their risk factor distributions shifting up or down as a whole. As a result of this coherence, population mean and the prevalence of deviance are necessarily highly correlated. Thus the prevalence of obesity, hypertension, or high intakes of fat or alcohol closely reflect the *average* weight, blood pressure, and dietary habits of the population as a whole; therefore the problems of deviance cannot be understood except in their societal context, and it is most unlikely that they can ever be successfully managed as isolated phenomena.

This means for research that in order to explain the prevalence of obesity, hypertension, hypercholesterolaemia, and alcoholism we need to understand the determinants of average weight, blood pressure, cholesterol, and drinking, and the dynamics of their changes. It means for preventive policy that it may be difficult or impossible to achieve any large fall in the prevalence of risk factors except as part of population-wide changes.

This population approach to prevention takes us beyond the responsibilities of medicine. The underlying causes for the rise and fall of major diseases, and for their national and regional differences, are related to the circumstances and manner of daily life. It is the responsibility of doctors to communicate their findings and expert opinions to the public and their governments, to exhort and support, and (if possible) to set a good personal example of healthy lifestyle, but society, not doctors, must decide how it wishes to live and what its priorities are. The prevention of heart disease is basically a matter of social, economic, and political policy.

Recent years have seen an astonishing growth in public concern about heart disease, health, and healthy living. Our task in the medical services is to work with this change. By more effective communication of medical knowledge (and its limitations) to the public, and by accepting that prevention is an integral part of all medical practice, we can hope to see greater improvements in health than could ever be achieved by therapeutic care alone. Treatment, preventive care for individuals, public health, and social policy are interlocking parts of a single strategy for better health.

References

INTERSALT Cooperative Research Group (1986). Intersalt study: an international co-operative study on the relation of blood pressure to electrolyte excretion in populations. 1. Design and methods. *Journal of Hypertension*, **4**, 781–7.

Khaw, K. T. and Rose, G. (1989). Cholesterol screening programmes: how much potential benefit? *British Medical Journal*, **299**, 606–7.

Kinlay, S. and Heller, R. F. (1990). Effectiveness and hazards of case finding for a high cholesterol concentration. *British Medical Journal*, **300**, 1545–7.

Kreitman, N. (1986). Alcohol consumption and the preventive paradox. *British Journal of Addiction*, **81**, 353–63.

Law, M. R., Frost, C. D., and Wald, N. J. (1991). Analysis of data from trials of salt reduction. *British Medical Journal*, **302**, 819–24.

Lewis, B. and Assmann, G. (eds) (1989). *The social and economic contexts of coronary prevention*. Current Medical Literature, London.

Lewis, B. and Rose, G. (1991). Prevention of coronary heart disease: putting theory into practice. *Journal of the Royal College of Physicians of London*, **25**, 21–6.

Martin, M. J., Hulley, S. B., Browner, W. S., Kuller, L. H., and Wentworth, D. (1986). Serum cholesterol, blood pressure, and mortality: implications from a cohort of 361 662 men. *Lancet*, **ii**, 933–6.

MRC (Medical Research Council) Working Party on Mild to Moderate Hypertension (1985). MRC trial of treatment of mild hypertension: principal results. *British Medical Journal*, **291**, 97–104.

Reid, D. D., Hamilton, P. J. S., McCartney, P., Rose, G., Jarrett, R. J., and Keen, H. (1976). Smoking and other risk factors for coronary heart-disease in British civil servants. *Lancet*, **ii**, 979–84.

Rose, G. (1981). The strategy of prevention: lessons from cardiovascular disease. *British Medical Journal*, **282**, 1847–51.

Rose, G. (1987). European collaborative trial of the multifactorial prevention of coronary heart disease. *Lancet*, **i**, 685.

Rose, G. and Day, S. (1990). The population mean predicts the number of deviant individuals. *British Medical Journal*, **301**, 1031–4.

Rose, G. and Shipley, M. (1986). Plasma cholesterol concentration and death from coronary heart disease: 10 year results of the Whitehall study. *British Medical Journal*, **293**, 306–7.

Rose, G. and Shipley, M. (1990). Effects of coronary risk reduction on the pattern of mortality. *Lancet*, **i**, 275–7.

Royal College of Physicians (1989). *Stroke: towards better management*. Royal College of Physicians, London, p. 9.

Stamler, J., Rose, G., Stamler, R., Elliott, P., Dyer, A., and Marmot, M. (1989). INTERSALT study findings: public health and medical care implications. *Hypertension*, **14**, 570–7.

Thompson, S. G. and Pocock, S. J. (1990). The variability of serum cholesterol measurements: implications for screening and monitoring. *Journal of Clinical Epidemiology*, **43**, 783–9.

WHO (World Health Organization) (1982). *Prevention of coronary heart disease: report of a WHO Expert Committee*. Technical Report Series 678. World Health Organization, Geneva.

WHO (World Health Organization) European Collaborative Group (1986). European collaborative trial of multifactorial prevention of coronary heart disease: final report on the 6-year results. *Lancet*, **i**, 869–72.

Chapter 37

Contributions to change: major risk factors and the potential for prevention

R. Beaglehole and A. Dobson

37.1 Introduction

The epidemics of coronary heart disease (CHD) apparently began in the early decades of the last century in many developed countries (Stallones 1980). However, it was not until the middle of the century that their importance for population health was appreciated. This recognition led to a major shift in the epidemiological paradigm from a sole focus on the causes of infectious diseases to consideration of the determinants of chronic diseases. During the last quarter of the twentieth century, as CHD in many developed countries declined, the disease was increasing elsewhere and in the last decade the growing global burden of cardiovascular disease has been recognized (WHO 2002).

The last 50 years has also seen a rapid development of the epidemiology of CHD and it is now established as a distinct discipline. The Framingham Study started in 1948 and examined the development of CHD in individuals followed over time (Kannel 2000). At about the same time, the Seven Countries study investigated characteristics which increased the risks of CHD at a population level (Keys 1980). Epidemiological and laboratory research has advanced our understanding of the causes of the CHD epidemics to the point where some commentators have suggested that the causes within populations are now essentially understood and the primary focus of public health should be to use this knowledge to strengthen prevention (Beaglehole and Magnus 2002; Magnus and Beaglehole 2001). Nevertheless, there is debate about the limitations of the 'risk factor' approach, applied to individuals, to understanding the underlying social causes of CHD epidemics (Marmot 2002; McKinlay and Marceau 1999). There is also debate about the value of searching for new biological risk factors (Beaglehole and Magnus 2002; Lefkowitz and Willerson 2001), although few would dispute the importance of a better understanding of the underlying mechanisms of CHD (Greenland *et al.* 2002).

A critical public health policy question is the extent to which the advances in epidemiological knowledge have contributed to the reductions in CHD mortality. Is the lack of application of this knowledge a factor in the failure to control the rising burden of CHD globally? The aim of this chapter is to assess the contribution of changes in the major CHD risk factors to changes in CHD event and mortality rates. The focus is on population trends using both theoretical and empirical approaches.

37.2 Burden of CHD and risk factors

It has been estimated that in 2002 there were 56 million deaths globally. The two leading causes of death, CHD (or ischaemic heart disease) and stroke (or cerebrovascular disease), were responsible for 7.0 million and 5.5 million deaths, respectively (WHO 2001). For demographic

Table 37.1 Ten leading causes of DALYs lost globally and in developed and developing countries, estimated for 2000

All countries	% total DALYs		Developed countries[a]	% total DALYs		Developing countries	% total DALYs
1 Lower respiratory infections	6.4	1	Unipolar depressive disorders	8.8	1	Lower respiratory infections	6.8
2 Perinatal conditions	6.2	2	Ischaemic heart disease	6.7	2	Perinatal conditions	6.7
3 HIV/AIDS	6.1	3	Alcohol use disorders	5.4	3	HIV/AIDS	6.6
4 Unipolar depressive disorders	4.4	4	Cerebrovascular disease	4.9	4	Meningitis	4.6
5 Diarrhoeal diseases	4.2	5	Alzheimer and other dementias	4.3	5	Diarrhoeal diseases	4.6
6 Ischaemic heart disease	3.8	6	Road traffic crashes	3.1	6	Unipolar depressive disorders	4.0
7 Cerebrovascular disease	3.1	7	Lung cancer	3.0	7	Ischaemic heart disease	3.5
8 Road traffic accidents	2.8	8	Osteoarthritis	2.7	8	Malaria	3.0
9 Malaria	2.7	9	COPD	2.5	9	Cerebrovascular disease	2.9
10 Tuberculosis	2.4	10	Hearing loss, adult onset	2.5	10	Road traffic crashes	2.8

Source: WHO 2001.

COPD: Chronic obstructive pulmonary disease.

[a] Developed countries include Established Market Economies (EMEs) and Former Socialist Economies (FSEs).

reasons, most of these deaths occur in the poorer regions of the world. Only in Africa are communicable diseases the leading cause of death (WHO 2001). In 2000 CHD and stroke together were estimated to be the leading cause of disability-adjusted life years lost (DALYs) (Table 37.1). The burden of specific cardiovascular disease varies by region (see Chapter 11), with stroke being much more common than CHD in east Asian populations.

The current burden of CHD reflects past and current risks. The future burden will be predicted in part by current population exposures to the major CHD risk factors. Fortunately, these risk factors are well known and are common to the other main categories of non-communicable diseases. Social and economic conditions are responsible for unhealthy diets, tobacco smoking, and physical inactivity (Yusuf *et al.* 2001*a*, *b*). Diets high in saturated fats and low in antioxidants lead to unfavourable lipid levels and hence to population-wide atherosclerosis. An atherogenic diet and lack of physical activity act together to produce excess weight and high levels of blood pressure.

The major risk factors for CHD (elevated levels of blood pressure, total cholesterol and body mass index, and tobacco smoking) have close and proximal relationships to CHD epidemics within populations. They are scientifically well established, with strong, dose-related, and biologically plausible associations with CHD shown observationally and experimentally in laboratory, clinical, and epidemiological studies conducted in many parts of the world (see Chapters 3 and 4).

37.3 **The public health potential of risk factor changes**

The evidence from cohort studies and randomized trials indicates that after adjusting for regression-dilution biases, a long-term change of 0.6 mmol/l in serum cholesterol concentration among middle-aged men corresponds to a coronary risk change of at least 25% (Law *et al.* 1994). Similarly, every 5 mmHg change in usual diastolic blood pressure corresponds to about a 20% change in coronary risk (MacMahon *et al.* 1990). Average population levels of 4 mmol/l or lower for cholesterol and 70 mmHg or lower for diastolic blood pressure are associated with very low rates of CHD (Law and Wald 2002; Stamler *et al.* 1999). On average, cigarette smoking increases the risk of CHD death by 70% compared with non-smoking (DHHS 1989). There is a lack of quantitative estimates of the CHD risk associated with physical inactivity; however, there is no doubt that changing activity patterns are contributing to the rapid development of obesity as a major public health problem in most countries (Paffenbarger *et al.* 2001; Prentice and Jebb 1995).

Although there is continuing research into new risk factors, the knowledge gained is unlikely to change rates of CHD (Beaglehole and Magnus 2002). In addition to evidence of causation, any new risk factor would have to have high prevalence in populations and to change rapidly within a population (for example, in response to social or environmental changes or to mass levels of treatment). Genetic research, for example, might improve our understanding of individual susceptibility to disease, but it cannot account for CHD epidemics which occurred within one generation; therefore it will contribute little to the control of CHD at the population level.

There are several strands of evidence that demonstrate the great potential of population-wide risk factor changes for reducing the burden of CHD. Firstly, and fundamentally, we know that the CHD epidemics are not inevitable. They are not a 'degenerative' consequence of ageing as described in the early formulations of the health transition theory (Omran 1971). The rapid changes in national rates of CHD mortality, both increases and decreases, indicate that these epidemics are modifiable within 5–10 years. Secondly, we know that in countries where population risk factor levels are low and do not increase with age, CHD is rare. Conversely, in populations undergoing rapid social and economic change, as with migration, risk factor levels change rapidly and in turn CHD emerges as an important cause of mortality and morbidity within a generation (Yusuf *et al.* 2001*a*, *b*). Thirdly, within Western populations the small proportion of young and middle-aged adults with optimal levels of risk factors do not experience CHD as a major cause of death (Stamler *et al.* 1999). The implication of these beneficial effects of low risk status is that there is a major preventive potential for increasing the proportion of the population with optimal levels of the major risk factors.

In terms of most efficiently maximizing the potential benefits of prevention, Rose has emphasized the need for small but population-wide changes in risk factor levels, rather than larger risk factor changes in the small proportion of the population at high risk of disease (Rose 1992). The goal of prevention policy and programmes is to shift the distribution to the 'left' (WHO 2001). Evidence is available in support of the policies required for the task of shifting risk distributions. The Asia Pacific Cohort Studies Collaboration indicates that a 2% reduction of mean blood pressure, achieved by a shift of the blood pressure distribution to the left, has the potential by the year 2020 to prevent annually 1.2 million stroke deaths (~15% of all stroke deaths) and 0.6 million coronary deaths (6% of all CHD deaths) (Rodgers *et al.* 2000). Reductions in blood pressure of this magnitude have been achieved in many countries and are achievable without expensive medical treatment, for example by reducing salt in manufactured food and salt used for cooking and food preservation (MacGregor and de Wardener 1998). Favourable shifts in the population distributions of abnormal blood lipid levels could be achieved by the wider adoption of healthy dietary patterns based on the traditional Mediterranean diet (Willett 1998). Much more attention should also be directed to modifying the environmental determinants of physical inactivity and obesity (Egger and Swinburn 1997).

The published data on the impact of risk factor changes and population event and mortality rates has been equivocal. Epidemiological studies from Finland (Vartiainen *et al.* 1999), Australia (Dobson *et al.* 1999), New Zealand (Beaglehole 1986; Capewell *et al.* 2000), Iceland (Sigfusson *et al.* 1991), the USA (Hunink *et al.* 1997), and Scotland (Capewell *et al.* 1999) have attempted to estimate the contribution of risk factor changes to changes, usually reductions, in CHD mortality rates. Several of these studies also estimated the contribution of improvements in the medical and surgical management of risk factors and coronary disease to the decline in CHD mortality rates. Many of these studies were conducted by collaborating centres in the WHO MONICA project (multinational **moni**toring of trends and determinants in **cardio**vascular disease), which is the 'definitive' study of this issue (Dobson *et al.* 1996; Kuulasmaa *et al.* 2000). All of the early results suggested a major contribution of population-wide risk factor changes to the reduction of mortality rates. It was claimed on the basis of the Finnish data that most of the decline in mortality rates in the province of North Karelia could be attributed to risk factor improvements, especially reductions in serum cholesterol levels. Similarly, estimates of the impact of demonstrated changes in risk factor levels in Australia and New Zealand suggested that more than half, and up to 100%, of the reduction in observed death rates could be explained by the improvements in population risk levels. A recent report from the UK has examined the contribution of changing prevalence of the major risk factors for CHD on time trends of CHD mortality and incidence (McPherson *et al.* 2002). A moderately optimistic summation of plausible improvements in the main risk factors predicts a change in incidence of CHD of ~30% in 10 years within the UK. By contrast, in the USA it was estimated that improvements in management of high risk and early disease were the most important determinants of the mortality improvements in the 1980s (Hunink *et al.* 1997). All of these studies attempted to examine a complex phenomenon indirectly and within a population. As a consequence, individually these studies had limited statistical power and were unlikely to provide definitive answers to an important public health question.

37.4 **Evidence from the WHO MONICA Project**

The WHO MONICA Project was established at the beginning of the 1980s to specifically examine the reasons for population changes in CHD mortality rates (see also Chapter 49). The main results have been published in the peer-reviewed literature (Kuulasmaa *et al.* 2000) and a detailed monograph describing the Project was recently published (Tunstall-Pedoe 2003). In brief, the Project used an ecological study design to examine trends in mortality and acute non-fatal events and associated risk factor changes over an approximately 10 year period in middle-aged people in 38 populations in 21 countries. Trends in mortality and disease rates were estimated through surveillance of all suspected CHD events in geographically defined populations, and trends in the major risk factor levels were assessed by repeated surveys on the same study populations. Considerable attention was given in the Project to achieving good quality data. Two main hypotheses were examined. The first studied the contribution of risk factor changes to the CHD event rate changes and the second examined the contribution of trends in case fatality to the CHD mortality trends.

The MONICA populations were mostly in Europe, but there were three in Asia, three in Australia and New Zealand, and two in North America. Table 37.2, derived from tables 2 and 3 of the paper by Kuulasmaa *et al.* (2000), shows that there was considerable variation among the study populations both in rates of CHD events and in risk factor levels. Notice firstly that the between-population variation in rates of CHD is considerably greater than the

Table 37.2 CHD event rates and risk factor levels near the end of the WHO MONICA Project

	Population statistics			
	Minimum	**Mean**	**Maximum**	**Standard deviation**
Men				
CHD event rate per 100 000	86	401	744	142
Daily smoking (%)	17	36	64	12
SBP (mmHg)	121	133	142	5
Cholesterol (mmol/l)	4.5	5.8	6.5	0.4
BMI (kg/m^2)	24.1	26.6	27.9	0.7
Risk score	6.6	7.1	7.5	0.2
Women				
CHD event rate per 100 000	33	98	269	46
Daily smoking (%)	4	21	45	9
SBP (mmHg)	117	129	139	6
Cholesterol (mmol/l)	4.5	5.8	6.2	0.3
BMI (kg/m^2)	24.5	26.5	29.3	1.2
Risk score	5.7	6.2	6.7	0.2

Data from tables 2 and 3 of the paper by Kuulasmaa *et al.* (2000).

BMI: body mass index; SBP: systolic blood pressure.

between-population variation in risk factor levels. (Similar 8–10-fold differences in rates of CHD have been noted in data from other countries) (Yusuf *et al.* 2001*a*). Secondly, the variation in mean levels of risk factors between the populations is less than the variation within populations; for example, the between-population standard deviation for systolic blood pressure was 5–6 mmHg whereas the within-population standard deviation is typically ~20 mmHg.

37.5 Modelling relationships between CHD event rates and risk factors

It has been noted by many people (for example, Law and Wald 2002) that within a population the logarithm of the CHD event rate increases linearly with level of each of the major risk factors. Thus proportional (or percentage) changes in event rates are linearly related to absolute changes in risk factor levels. The slope of the dose–response line for each risk factor has been found to be generally similar for men and women, in different age groups and in different populations using cohort studies and randomized trials (Dobson *et al.* 1998; Stamler *et al.* 1999). The magnitude of these effects is summarized in Table 37.3, which also shows the values used to calculate the composite risk scores used in the MONICA Project (Kuulasmaa *et al.* 2000).

The linear relationship is illustrated in Fig. 37.1 using data from tables 2 and 3 of the paper by Kuulasmaa *et al.* (2000) for the MONICA risk score, which combines effects of all four major risk factors. It suggests that the relationships found repeatedly within populations also apply between populations.

Table 37.3 Percentage changes in rate of CHD events predicted from absolute changes in risk factor levels

Risk factor	Change	Change in rates of CHD			
		Cohort studies[a]	Clinical trials[a]	NORA[b] (men)	NORA[b] (women)
DBP	5 mmHg	21	20		
SBP	10 mmHg			21	30
Total cholesterol	0.6 mmol/l	27	25	26	22.5
Smoking	100%	70		80.1	85.1
BMI	1 kg/m²	10		4.9	0.7

DBP: diastolic blood pressure.

[a] Calculated from NORA coefficients (Kuulasmaa et al. 2000).

[b] From Law and Wald 2002.

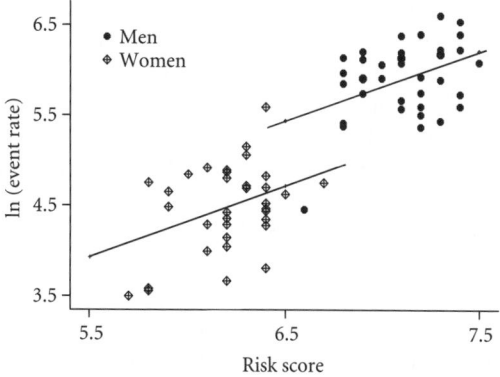

Fig. 37.1 Logarithm of event rates plotted against risk score. (Data from Kuulasmaa et al. 2000.)

The focus of the WHO MONICA Project was on the associations between **changes** in risk factor levels and **changes** in rates of CHD events. Less attention was paid to the associations between absolute levels of risk factor and event rates in the diverse study populations. It is this cross-sectional association towards the end of the study period that is depicted in Fig. 37.1. Data for men and women are displayed on the same graph, which increases the amount of heterogeneity between data points and hence makes the linear relationship more apparent than would be the case if data for each sex were presented separately. Clearly there are differences in levels of logarithm of event rate between men and women, but the dose–response lines are parallel.

The model to describe this relationship is given in eqn 37.1:

$$\ln y = b_0 + b_1 x_1 + b_2 x_2 + b_3 x_3 + e \tag{37.1}$$

where ln denotes the natural logarithm, y is the annual event rate per 100 000, x_1 denotes measured risk factors, x_2 denotes unmeasured risk factors (for example, level of physical inactivity), x_3 is an indicator variable for sex (with values 0 for men and 1 for women) and e denotes the error term. In eqn 37.1 the baseline hazard b_0, the effect b_2 of the unmeasured risk factors, and other sources of variation e, cannot be distinguished empirically, so in practice

Table 37.4 Results from fitting eqn 37.2 to the data in Fig. 37.1

	Estimate	Standard error	p-value
Intercept	0.305	1.546	0.840
Women	−0.7202	0.2194	0.002
Risk score	0.7896	0.2171	0.001

the following model is fitted:

$$\ln y = c + b_1 x_1 + b_3 x_3 + e^*. \tag{37.2}$$

In eqn 37.2 the intercept c includes the effects of unmodifiable risk factors such as age and unmeasured but potentially changing factors, and e^* is the term for the remaining random variation.

Table 37.4 shows the regression model (eqn 37.2) fitted to the data in Fig. 37.1. The model has an r-squared value of 77%. Both the effects of sex and risk score are strongly statistically significant while the intercept has a large standard error indicating considerable uncertainty.

This model allows prediction of event rates that might pertain under various conditions. For example, consider a population with plausibly low levels of risk factors, such as systolic blood pressure of 110 mmHg, total cholesterol of 3.5 mmol/l, body mass index of 22, and no smoking (Law and Wald 2002). In such a population the risk score would be 4.91 for men and 4.77 for women and so the predicted rates of CHD events would be 65.5 and 28.5 per 100 000, respectively (this event rate for women is similar to the rate in Beijing where smoking among women is rare).

This theoretical model of the relationship between CHD event rates and risk factor levels provides a framework for examining the effects of changes in risk factor levels at a population level.

37.6 Modelling relationships between changes in CHD event rates and changes in risk factor levels

Differentiation of eqn 37.1 with respect to time produces

$$\frac{\Delta y}{y} = b_1 \Delta x_1 + b_2 \Delta x_2 + e' \tag{37.3}$$

where Δ denotes the change over a specified time period and e' is an error term. This means that the percentage change in event rates should be linearly related to the absolute change in risk scores over a period of time. If the measured risk factors denoted by x_1 account for most of the changes in event rates, so that $b_2 \Delta x_2$ is approximately zero, then the line modelling the relationship between changes in event rates and changes in risk factor levels should go through the origin, the slope should be equal to the value b_1 estimated for eqn 37.2, and there should be no sex effect.

Figure 37.2 shows the MONICA data relating average annual changes in event rates (as percentage changes) plotted against the changes in risk scores (average annual absolute changes) with data for men and women on the same figure; this shows together the data in

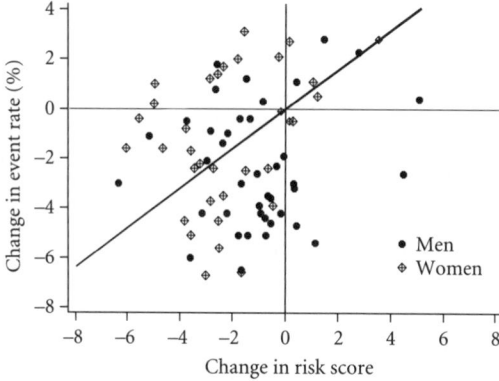

Fig. 37.2 Average annual percentage change in event rates plotted against average annual absolute change in risk score. (Data from Kuulasmaa *et al.* 2000.)

both parts of fig. 1 in the paper by Kuulasmaa *et al.* (2000). There is no clear sex-specific clustering of data for men and women, which is in accordance with eqn 37.3. However, there is considerable similarity in the sizes of the changes in both event rates and risk factor levels in most of the study populations. Therefore, it is difficult to test the adequacy of the model (given by eqn 37.3). Nevertheless, the regression line through the origin, corresponding to eqn 37.3 with no other time varying factors, gives an estimate of the slope b_1 of 0.523 (standard error = 0.124, *p*-value <0.001) which is consistent with the estimate in Table 37.4 (estimate of b_1 = 0.790, standard error = 0.217). Thus the data do not provide evidence against eqn 37.3.

This analysis shows that data from the MONICA project are consistent with a model, given by eqn 37.1, of how differences in CHD event rates between populations may be accounted for by the differences in average levels of risk factors in those populations.

There are several reasons why this view has not previously been apparent. Firstly, we started by looking at the bigger picture of whether the large differences in CHD event rates between populations can be explained by differences in risk factor levels. Using a proportional hazards model and MONICA data (combining data from men and women to get a broader range of CHD rates and risk levels) we have demonstrated that the hypothesized relationship describes the data quite well. Secondly, we have used this model to deduce the relationship that could be expected between changes in risk levels and changes in CHD rates at the population level. Figure 37.2 shows the straight line relating the two change measures going through the origin with the same slope as Fig. 37.1. The data are consistent with this model but the evidence is weak. The line is based on the strong assumption that the changes in event rates are related only to the risk factors considered in the calculation. Previous analysis of these data fitted both the level and the slope of the line separately for each sex, thus allowing for other factors that might affect event rates, but reducing the statistical power to detect effects (Kuulasmaa *et al.* 2000). The data for women are consistent with both these models, although the data for men are better described by a model that allows for other factors.

The model presented could be improved in various ways. For example, time lags between the changes in risk factors and changes in event rates were not considered. Evidence from randomized trials suggests that lag times for CHD are relatively short and Kuulasmaa *et al.* (2000) found that associations in MONICA data were improved when data were lagged by 4 years. The reliability of the estimates (summarized by standard errors) was not taken into account, although failure to do so attenuates the effects (Kuulasmaa *et al.* 2000).

37.7 **Discussion**

The theoretical model employed in this chapter, based on the assumption of proportional hazards and summarized by eqn 37.1, is well established within populations. The new aspects of our analysis are to extend the model to data from multiple populations, to deduce eqn 37.3 relating changes in disease rates to changes in risk factors and to test the model empirically using MONICA data. We have shown that the data are consistent with this model illustrating that the major risk factors of tobacco smoking and elevated blood pressure, total cholesterol, and body mass index can account for the wide range of CHD rates found among populations and that changes in these risk factors at a population level can account for observed trends in event rates.

Comparisons of the theoretical contribution of risk factor changes to event rates with the empirical evidence have until recently suggested discrepancies between these two approaches. The model we have presented provides a framework for combining them. Unfortunately the homogeneity of trends in the MONICA data means that the model could not be adequately tested.

Only observational epidemiological studies offer opportunities for examining secular trends within and among countries since formal experimental studies are out of the question. Some so-called 'natural experiments' provide interesting data, for example, the recent experience from Poland where a sharp decline in CHD mortality rates has been attributed to changes in the food supply at least in part as a consequence of major social and economic changes that took place in the early 1990s (Zatonski *et al.* 1998). Similarly, the recent increase in cardiovascular mortality in Russia is attributed to social factors (Leon *et al.* 1997). Many of the early epidemiological attempts to examine secular trends were limited by poor characterization of risk, lack of consideration of regression-dilution bias and time lags, lack of attention to the importance of low risk rather than 'normal risk', and a simple dichotomous approach to risk levels.

The MONICA Project, despite its many achievements, also had limited ability to examine the main hypotheses due to low statistical power. The Project was an ecological study design and was unable to involve a sufficient number of populations with enough variation in risk factor levels and trends; the project also included populations at different stages in the evolution of their CHD epidemics. Also, it was too short to examine time lags adequately. Nevertheless it does provide important insights into CHD from a population perspective.

37.8 **Conclusions**

Several important conclusions can be drawn from this chapter. The major risk factors can account for large differences on CHD event rates observed between populations. In turn this supports the argument that these major risk factors can account for most of the CHD epidemics seen in the second half of the twentieth century. It follows that the priority targets for prevention are to reduce levels of smoking, blood pressure, and total cholesterol in whole populations. In working towards this goal the two approaches enunciated by Rose (1992) have their place: firstly, to use all available means to help smokers to quit and to lower blood pressure and cholesterol in people at high absolute risk of a CHD event, if this is affordable for the population; and secondly, to use the full range of primary prevention measures to reduce smoking and to lower population blood pressure and lipid levels so that everyone in the population may benefit (with the added benefit of controlling other chronic diseases which share the same risk factors).

There remains a major gap between what we know about the causes of CHD and our willingness to act on this knowledge and prevent the most preventable of major epidemics (Beaglehole 2001). A striking deficiency has been in the development and application of appropriate prevention and control policies based on public health research evidence. The global public health context is increasingly complex and presents serious difficulties for public health practitioners more used to dealing with risk factors at the level of the individual and with traditional epidemiological study designs. However, this complexity must not become an excuse for inaction, especially since we have substantial evidence of the effectiveness of public health interventions; for example, the effect of coordinated and comprehensive tobacco control policies (see Chapter 45).

New research is required in certain areas, for example, concerning CHD prevention policy and programme effectiveness and on issues of importance for the spread of the epidemics to poor populations. There is also an urgent need for epidemiologists and other public health scientists to explore the applicability of new research methods to increasing understanding of the upstream determinants of CHD, for example, the adverse health effects of the globalization of the food, alcohol, and tobacco industry (Beaglehole and Yach 2003).

Policy-directed research will have the biggest public health payoff in the short term. The evidence is unequivocal: CHD epidemics can be prevented with no adverse population effects. The critical policy question now, especially for poor countries, is the appropriate balance between primary and secondary prevention and between the population and high risk approach to primary prevention. If the goal is to significantly increase the proportion of the population at low risk status, the only strategy with this potential is the population wide approach to primary prevention (Rose 1992). All other strategies will, at best, only restrain the epidemics and not prevent them. The challenge is to implement the population approach to primary prevention, that is, to shift the population risk factor distribution to the left. The ultimate public health goal is the reduction of population risk, and since 95% of the population, at least in developed countries, is not at the optimal risk level, it follows that substantial resources should be directed towards this goal (Ebrahim and Smith 2001).

References

Beaglehole, R. (1986). Medical management and the decline in coronary heart disease. *British Medical Journal*, **292**, 33–5.

Beaglehole, R. (2001). Global cardiovascular disease prevention: time to get serious. *Lancet*, **358**, 661–3.

Beaglehole, R. and Magnus, P. (2002). The search for new risk factors for coronary heart disease: occupational therapy for epidemiologists. *International Journal of Epidemiology*, **33**, 1117–22.

Beaglehole, R. and Yach, D. (2003). Globalisation and the prevention and control of noncommunicable diseases: the neglected chronic diseases of adults. *Lancet* **362**, 1763–4.

Capewell, S., Morrison, C. E., and McMurray, J. J. (1999). Contribution of medical care and risk factor changes to the decline in coronary heart disease mortality in Scotland, 1975–1994. *Heart*, **81**, 380–6.

Capewell, S., Beaglehole, R., Seddon, M., and McMurray, J. (2000). Explanation for the decline in coronary heart disease mortality rates in Auckland, New Zealand, between 1982 and 1993. *Circulation*, **102**, 1511–16.

DHHS (Department of Health and Human Services) (1989). Reducing the health consequences of smoking: 25 years of progress. A report of the Surgeon General. DHHS publication no. (CDC). 89–8411. Government Printing Office, Washington, DC.

Dobson, A., Filipiak, B., Kuulasmaa, K., Beaglehole, R., Stewart, A., Hobbs, M. *et al.* (1996). Relations of changes in coronary disease rates and changes in risk factor levels: methodological issues and a practical example. *American Journal of Epidemiology*, **143**, 1025–34.

Dobson, A. J., Evans, A., Ferrario, M., Kuulasmaa, K. A., Moltchanov, V. A., Sans, S. *et al.* for the WHO MONICA Project (1998). Changes in estimated coronary risk in the 1980s: data from the WHO MONICA Project. *Annals of Medicine*, **30**, 199–205.

Dobson, A. J., McElduff, P., Heller, R., Alexander, H., Colley, P., and D'Este, K. (1999). Changing patterns of coronary disease in the Hunter Region of New South Wales, Australia. *Journal of Clinical Epidemiology*, **52**, 761–1.

Ebrahim, E. and Smith, G. D. (2001). Exporting failure? Coronary heart disease and stroke in developing countries. *International Journal of Epidemiology*, **30**, 201–5.

Egger, G. and Swinburn, B. (1997). An 'ecological' approach to the obesity pandemic. *British Medical Journal*, **315**, 477–80.

Greenland, P., Gidding, S. S., and Tracy, R. P. (2002). Commentary: lifelong prevention of atherosclerosis: the critical importance of major risk factor exposures. *International Journal of Epidemiology*, **31**, 1129–34.

Hunink, M. G., Goldman, L., Tosteson, A. N., Mittleman, M. A., Goldman, P. A., Williams, L. W. *et al.* (1997). The recent decline in mortality from coronary heart disease, 1980–1990: the effects of secular trends in risk factors and treatment. *Journal of the American Medical Association*, **277**, 535–42.

Kannel, W. B. (2000). The Framingham Study: 50-year legacy and future promise. *Journal of Atherosclerosis and Thrombosis*, **6**, 60–6.

Keys, A. B. (1980). *Seven Countries: a multivariate analysis of death and coronary heart disease.* Harvard University Press, Cambridge, MA.

Kuulasmaa, K., Tunstall-Pedoe, H., Dobson, A., Fortmann, S., Sans, S., Tolonen, H. *et al.* for the WHO MONICA Project (2000). Estimating the contribution of changes in classical risk factors to trends in coronary-event rates across the WHO MONICA Project populations. *Lancet*, **355**, 675–87.

Law, M. R. and Wald, N. J. (2002). Risk factor thresholds: their existence under scrutiny. *British Medical Journal*, **324**, 1570–6.

Law, M. R., Wald, N. J., and Thompson, S. G. (1994). By how much and how quickly does reduction in serum cholesterol concentration lower risk of ischaemic heart disease? *British Medical Journal*, **308**, 367–73.

Lefkowitz, R. J. and Willerson, J. T. (2001). Prospects for cardiovascular research. *Journal of the American Medical Association*, **285**, 581–7.

Leon, D., Chenet, L., Shkolnikov, V. M., Zakharov, S., Shapiro, J., Rakhmanova, G. *et al.* (1997). Huge variation in Russian mortality rates 1984–94: artefact, alcohol or what? *Lancet*, **350**, 383–8.

MacGregor, G. A. and de Wardener, H. E. (1998). *Salt, diet and health: Neptune's poisoned chalice: the origins of high blood pressure.* Cambridge University Press.

MacMahon, S., Peto, R., Cutler, J., Collins, R., Sorlie, P., Neaton, J. *et al.* (1990). Blood pressure, stroke and coronary heart disease. Part 1. Prolonged differences in blood pressure: prospective observational studies corrected for the regression dilution bias. *Lancet*, **335**, 765–74.

Magnus, P. and Beaglehole, R. (2001). The real contribution of the major risk factors to the coronary epidemic: time to end the 50% myth. *Archives of Internal Medicine*, **161**, 2657–60.

Marmot, M. (2002). Commentary: occupational therapy or the major challenge? *International Journal of Epidemiology*, **31**, 1122–24.

McKinlay, J. B. and Marceau, L. D. (1999). A tale of 3 tails. *American Journal of Public Health*, **89**, 295–8.

McPherson, K., Britton, A., and Causer, L. (2002). *Coronary heart disease: estimating the impact of changes in risk factors.* National Heart Forum, London.

Omran, A. R. (1971). The epidemiologic transition: a theory of the epidemiology of population change. *Milbank Memorial Fund Quarterly*, **49**, 509–38.

Paffenbarger, R. S., Blair, S., and Lee, I-M. (2001). A history of physical activity and cardiovascular health and longevity: the scientific contributions of Jeremy Morris, DSc, DPH, FRCP. *International Journal of Epidemiology*, **30**, 1184–92.

Prentice, A. M. and Jebb, S. A. (1995). Obesity in Britain: gluttony or sloth? *British Medical Journal*, **311**, 437–9.

Rodgers, A., Lawes, C., and MacMahon, S. (2000). Reducing the global burden of blood pressure-related cardiovascular disease. *Journal of Hypertension Supplement*, **18**, S3–6.

Rose, G. (1992). *The strategy of preventive medicine*. Oxford University Press.

Sigfusson, N., Sigvaldason, H., Steingrimsdottir, L., Gudmundsdottir, II., Stefansdottir, I., Thorsteinsson, T., and Sigurdsson, G. (1991). Decline in ischaemic heart disease in Iceland and change in risk factor levels. *British Medical Journal*, **302**, 1371–5.

Stallones, R. A. (1980). The rise of ischemic heart disease. *Scientific American*, **243**, 53–9.

Stamler, J., Stamler, R., Neaton, J. D., Wentworth, D., Daviglus, M. L., Garside, D. *et al.* (1999). Low risk factor profile and long-term cardiovascular and non-cardiovascular mortality and life expectancy: findings from 5 large cohorts of young adult and middle-aged men and women. *Journal of the American Medical Association*, **282**, 2012–18.

Tunstall-Pedoe, H. (ed.). For the WHO MONICA Project (2003). *MONICA monograph and multimedia sourcebook*. World Health Organization, Geneva.

Vartiainen, E., Puska, P., Pekkanen, J. *et al.* (1999). Changes in risk factors explain changes in mortality from ischemic heart disease in Finland. *British Medical Journal*, **318**, 171–80.

Willett, W. (1998). *Nutritional epidemiology*, 2nd edn. Oxford University Press, New York.

WHO (World Health Organization) (2001). *World health report 2001*. World Health Organization, Geneva.

WHO (World Health Organization) (2002). *World health report 2002*. World Health Organization, Geneva.

Yusuf, S., Reddy, S., Ounpuu, S., and Anand, S. (2001*a*). Global burden of cardiovascular diseases. Part 1: general considerations, the epidemiologic transition, risk factors, and impact of urbanisation. *Circulation*, **104**, 2746–53.

Yusuf, S., Reddy, S., Ounpuu, S., and Anand, S. (2001*b*). Global burden of cardiovascular diseases. Part 2: Variations in cardiovascular disease by specific ethnic groups and geographic regions and prevention strategies. *Circulation*, **104**, 2855–64.

Zatonski, W. A., McMichael, A. J., and Powles, J. W. (1998). Ecological study of reasons for sharp decline in mortality from ischaemic heart disease in Poland since 1991. *British Medical Journal*, **316**, 1047–51.

Chapter 38

Prevention of coronary heart disease: findings from the Nurses' Health Study and Health Professionals' Follow-up Study

F. B. Hu and W. C. Willett

38.1 Introduction

In the last decade, our understanding of dietary and lifestyle factors most likely to promote cardiac health has improved substantially, owing in part to the data from several large and carefully conducted prospective cohort studies, including the Nurses' Health Study (NHS) and Health Professionals' Follow-up Study (HPFS). The contributions of these cohort studies to the nutritional epidemiology of coronary heart disease (CHD) are particularly noteworthy because these studies have used more detailed dietary assessment tools and multiple measurements to provide a wealth of information not only on major types of fat and different classes of fatty acids, but also other aspects of diet, including antioxidants, folate, fibre, dietary glycaemic load, and overall dietary patterns. Recent analyses from the NHS provide powerful evidence that CHD is largely preventable through diet and lifestyle modifications (Stampfer et al. 2000). Using 14-year follow-up data from the NHS, we estimated that 82% (95% confidence interval (CI): 58–93) of coronary events in the study cohort could be potentially prevented by improvements in behaviours, involving diet, exercise, body weight, and abstinence from smoking. In a subsequent analysis (Hu et al. 2000c) we estimated that the majority of decline in CHD incidence over time in the NHS was attributable to improvement in diet and decrease in smoking. In this chapter, we review major findings regarding dietary and lifestyle factors and CHD from the NHS and HPFS.

38.2 The NHS and HPFS

The NHS cohort was established in 1976 when 121 700 female registered nurses aged 30–55 years and residing in 11 large US states completed a mailed questionnaire on their medical history and lifestyle characteristics. Every 2 years, follow-up questionnaires have been sent to update information on potential cardiovascular risk factors. Starting in 1980, on a 2–4-year cycle, dietary information has been updated using validated food frequency questionnaires (FFQs). The HPFS began in 1986 when 51 529 US health professionals (dentists, optometrists, pharmacists, podiatrists, and veterinarians) aged 40–75 answered a detailed questionnaire that included a comprehensive diet survey, and items on lifestyle practice and medical history. Similar to the NHS, the cohort is followed through biennial mailed questionnaire. Dietary information is updated every 4 years. Biological specimens including blood samples, cheek cells, and toenails have been collected in both cohorts.

Substantial efforts have been devoted to the development and refinement of standardized dietary questionnaires that can be completed repeatedly by participants over a number of years. The dietary questionnaires have been shown to be reasonably reproducible and valid as compared with multiple week dietary records (considered as 'gold standards') in both cohorts (Feskanich *et al.* 1993; London *et al.* 1993; Michaud *et al.* 1998; Rimm *et al.* 1992; Salvini *et al.* 1989; Willett *et al.* 1985, 1988). In particular, nutrients calculated from the FFQ are correlated with their corresponding biochemical indicators: plasma vitamin E ($r = 0.41–0.53$) (Ascherio *et al.* 1992; Stryker *et al.* 1988), plasma folate ($r = 0.35–0.51$) (Jacques *et al.* 1993; Selhub *et al.* 1993), adipose linoleic acid ($0.35–0.37$) (Hunter *et al.* 1992; London *et al.* 1991), adipose trans fatty acids ($r = 0.51$) (London *et al.* 1991), and adipose n-3 fatty acids ($r = 0.48–0.49$) (Hunter *et al.* 1992; London *et al.* 1991). In addition, we have validated measures of alcohol consumption (Giovannucci *et al.* 1991), physical activity (Wolf *et al.* 1994), body weight (Willett *et al.* 1983), and waist and hip circumferences (Rimm *et al.* 1990).

38.3 **Major types of dietary fats**

Dietary fat intake is widely believed to be largely responsible for the development of CHD. This belief is primarily based on ecological studies relating dietary intakes of saturated fat and cholesterol to rates of CHD in different countries (Keys 1980). However, data from this kind of international comparison are seriously confounded by other aspects of diet, lifestyle, and economic development. Prospective cohort studies are more suitable for testing the diet–heart hypothesis because of the ability to measure and account for potential confounding factors. However, most previous cohort studies suffered from serious methodological limitations, including small study size, inadequate dietary assessment, incomplete adjustment for intake of total energy, failure to account for trans isomers of unsaturated fats, and lack of control for intakes of other types of fat (Willett 1998).

Using 14-year follow-up data from the Nurses' Health Study with repeated assessment of diet (Hu *et al.* 1997), we conducted detailed prospective analyses of dietary fat and CHD among 80 082 women aged 34–59. In multivariate analyses, 5% of energy from saturated fat, compared with equivalent energy from carbohydrates, was associated with a 17% greater risk of CHD (relative risk (RR) = 1.17, 95% CI: 0.97–1.41, $p = 0.10$). Compared with equivalent energy from carbohydrates, the RR for 2% of energy from trans fat was 1.93 (1.43–2.61, $p < 0.001$); for 5% of energy from monounsaturated fat, 0.81 (0.65–1.00, $p = 0.05$); and for 5% energy from polyunsaturated fat, 0.62 (0.46–0.85, $p = 0.002$). Total fat was not significantly related to risk (for 5% energy 1.02, 0.97–1.07, $p = 0.55$). It was estimated that replacement of 5% of energy from saturated fat by unsaturated fats would reduce risk by 42% (23–56, $p < 0.001$), and replacement of 2% of energy from trans fat by non-hydrogenated unsaturated fats would reduce risk by 53% (34–67, $p < 0.001$). These findings suggest that replacing saturated and trans fats with unhydrogenated mono- and polyunsaturated fats is more effective in preventing CHD than reducing overall fat intake. In support of these findings, several prospective cohort studies have found an inverse relation between nut consumption and CHD risk (Hu and Stampfer 1999). Nuts are high in fats, but most of the fats are unsaturated. In the NHS (Hu *et al.* 1998), compared to women who rarely ate nuts (never or less than once a month), those with frequent consumption (5+ times/week) had significantly lower risk of total CHD (RR = 0.65, 95% CI: 0.47–0.89, p for trend = 0.0009) after adjusting for a wide range of CHD risk factors. These results are consistent with findings from metabolic studies showing beneficial effects of a diet rich in nuts on blood lipids (Kris-Etherton *et al.* 2001). The beneficial effects of nut consumption observed in clinical and epidemiological studies underscore the importance of distinguishing different types of fat.

As with the NHS, we observed a weak positive association between saturated fat intake and risk of CHD in the HPFS (Ascherio *et al.* 1996), but in the HPFS, this association was largely attenuated after adjusting for dietary fibre. Overall, the observed relation in our cohorts for saturated fatty acids was much weaker than that predicted by international comparisons (Keys 1980), but is consistent with the possibility that the proportional increase in plasma high-density lipoprotein (HDL) concentration produced by saturated fatty acids (compared isocalorically to carbohydrate) tends to compensate for its adverse effect on low-density lipoprotein (LDL) level (Mensink and Katan 1992). In metabolic studies, different classes of saturated fatty acids have different effects on plasma lipid and lipoprotein levels (Kris-Etherton and Yu 1997). Specifically, myristic acid (14 carbons, mainly in dairy fat) is the most potent cholesterol-raising fatty acid, followed by palmitic acid (16 carbons, high in dairy and meat fats), and stearic acid (18 carbons, high in beef and chocolate), which does not elevate total serum cholesterol compared to carbohydrates. In an analysis of the NHS (Hu *et al.* 1999c), we found that all individual long-chain saturated fatty acids, including stearic acid, were associated with a small increase in risk of CHD.

We found a weak and non-significant positive association between dietary cholesterol and risk of CHD (RR for each increase of 200 mg/1000 kcal = 1.12, 95% CI: 0.91–1.40) (Hu *et al.* 1997). In a detailed analysis of egg consumption and incidence of CHD among 117 933 apparently healthy subjects in the NHS and HPFS (Hu *et al.* 1999e), we found no evidence of an overall positive association between moderate egg consumption and risk of CHD in either men or women. The RRs of CHD across categories of intake (<1/week, 1/wk, 2–4/week, 5–6/week, ≥1/day) were 1.0, 1.06, 1.12, 0.90, and 1.08 (*p* for trend = 0.75) in men and 1.0, 0.82, 0.99, 0.95, and 0.82 (*p* for trend = 0.95) in women.

38.4 **Trans fat**

The strong positive association between trans fat and risk of CHD observed in the NHS is noteworthy. Metabolic studies have consistently indicated adverse effects of trans fat intake on blood lipids and other cardiovascular risk factors (Ascherio *et al.* 1996). Trans fatty acids raise LDL cholesterol levels and lower HDL cholesterol relative to natural *cis* unsaturated fatty acids. As such, the increase in the ratio of total to HDL cholesterol for trans fat is approximately double that for the same amount of saturated fat (Ascherio *et al.* 1999). The NHS finding is broadly consistent with several prospective studies conducted in men, including the HPFS (Ascherio *et al.* 1996), the Alpha-Tocopherol Beta-Carotene Study (Pietinen *et al.* 1997), and the Zutphen Study (Oomen *et al.* 2001). These studies have provided a strong scientific basis for current dietary recommendations to minimize trans fat intake (USDA/USDHHS 2000).

38.5 **Omega-3 fatty acids**

Considerable interest exists in the role of fish and marine omega-3 fatty acids for the prevention of CHD (see Chapter 18). Several prospective cohort studies have found an inverse association between fish consumption and coronary mortality (Daviglus *et al.* 1997; Kromhout *et al.* 1985) and sudden cardiac death (Albert *et al.* 1998). In the HPFS, Ascherio *et al.* (1995)

found no appreciable association between dietary intake of n-3 fatty acids or fish intake and the overall risk of coronary disease, but there was a non-significant trend for a reduction in risk for fatal CHD with increasing fish consumption. Until recently, all studies had been limited to men. In a recent analysis of the NHS with 16 years of follow-up, we found strong evidence for beneficial effects of a higher consumption of fish and omega-3 fatty acids on risk of CHD, particularly CHD deaths, in women (Hu *et al.* 2002). Compared with women who rarely ate fish (less than once a month), the multivariate RRs (95% CI) adjusted for age, smoking, and other cardiovascular risk factors were 0.78 (0.63–0.97) for fish consumption 1–3 times per month, 0.71 (0.58–0.87) for once per week, 0.69 (0.54–0.87) for 2–4 times per week, and 0.66 (0.49–0.87) for five or more times per week (p for trend = 0.001). Similarly, women with a higher intake of omega-3 fatty acids (20:5 and 22:6) had a lower risk of CHD, with multivariate RRs of 1.0, 0.93, 0.78, 0.68, and 0.67 ($p < 0.001$) across quintiles of intake. The epidemiological findings are broadly consistent with results from two secondary prevention trials, the Diet and Reinfarction Trial (DART) (Burr *et al.* 1989) and the GISSI-Prevenzione trial (GISSI-Prevenzione Investigators 1999), which found that increasing fish consumption or fish oil supplementation significantly reduced coronary mortality among myocardial infarction (MI) patients.

We have also examined the association between intake of alpha-linolenic acid (ALA, an 18-carbon omega-3 fatty acid) and fatal CHD in the HPFS and NHS. In the HPFS (Ascherio *et al.* 1996), a 1% increase in linolenic intake expressed as percentage of energy was associated with a 40% lower risk of fatal CHD. In the NHS (Hu *et al.* 1999*d*), after adjusting for coronary risk factors, the RRs of fatal CHD from the lowest to highest quintiles of ALA intake were 1.0, 0.89, 0.90, 0.66, and 0.52 (95% CI: 0.30–0.90), p for trend = 0.01. Also, there was an ~50% lower fatal CHD risk among women who consumed oil and vinegar salad dressing (a major source of ALA in the cohort) frequently (5–6 times or more per week) compared to those who consumed this salad dressing less than once a month. These findings are consistent with the Lyon Diet Heart Trial (de Lorgeril *et al.* 1994, 1999), which demonstrated substantial reduction in cardiac deaths among MI patients assigned to a Mediterranean-type diet enriched with ALA.

38.6 Carbohydrates

Prevailing dietary guidelines recommend a low-fat, high-carbohydrate diet to lower blood cholesterol and prevent CHD (USDA/USDHHS 2000). However, low-fat, high-carbohydrate diets reduce HDL levels and raise fasting triglycerides (Mensink and Katan 1992), and the adverse metabolic effects are exacerbated in the presence of underlying insulin resistance (Jeppesen *et al.* 1997). Because low HDL and high triglyceride levels independently increase risk of CHD, the value of replacing overall fat with carbohydrates has been questioned (Katan *et al.* 1997). Indeed, in both the NHS (Hu *et al.* 1997) and HPFS (Ascherio *et al.* 1996), theoretical exchange of carbohydrates for total fat, according to the equations of Mensink and Katan (1992), was predicted to show no apparent benefit. More disturbingly, and as predicted by metabolic studies of blood lipids, theoretical exchange of carbohydrate for mono- or polyunsaturated fats was associated with significantly increased risk of CHD.

Traditionally, carbohydrates have been classified into simple or complex, based on chemical structures. Most dietary recommendations encouraged higher intake of complex carbohydrates or starches and avoidance of simple carbohydrates or sugars. This was based on the belief that simple sugars would be digested and absorbed more quickly, which would induce more rapid postprandial glucose response. Numerous metabolic studies have challenged this view and it is now recognized that many starchy foods such as baked potatoes and white bread produce even higher glycaemic responses than sucrose. That different carbohydrate-containing foods lead to different glycaemic responses has led to the development of the concept of glycaemic index (GI), a term first coined by Jenkins and coworkers (Jenkins *et al.* 1981). GI is a ranking of foods based on the extent that blood glucose rises (the area under the curve for blood glucose levels) after ingesting a test food as compared to a standard weight (50 g) of reference carbohydrate (glucose or white bread). The GI depends largely on the rate of digestion and rapidity of absorption of carbohydrate (Hallfrisch *et al.* 2000).

Until recently the influence of carbohydrate type and quality on risk of CHD has received little attention in epidemiological studies. To examine the influence of quality and quantity of carbohydrate, we examined the dietary glycaemic load (GL) in relation to incidence of type 2 diabetes in the HPFS (Salmeron *et al.* 1997*a*) and the NHS (Salmeron *et al.* 1997*b*). The glycaemic load was defined as the sum for all foods of the GI for each food multiplied by its total carbohydrate content, adjusted for total energy intake. In both studies, risk increased with higher GL, especially in combination with low intake of cereal fibre. In the NHS (Salmeron *et al.* 1997*b*), the RR of type 2 diabetes was 2.50 (95% CI: 1.14–5.51) for women with the combination of a high GL and a low cereal fibre intake compared with the opposite extreme. In a recent analysis (Liu *et al.* 2000), we found a strong positive association between GL and risk of CHD over 10 years of follow-up. The RR comparing women in the highest quintile vs. those in the lowest quintile of GL was 1.98 (95% CI: 1.41–2.77). The increased risk was more pronounced among overweight and obese women, suggesting that the adverse effects of a high GL diet are probably aggravated by underlying insulin resistance (Liu *et al.* 2001). Interestingly, neither total amount of carbohydrate nor simple sugars independently predicted risk of CHD. These results suggest that the GI and GL concepts are more useful than the traditional simple vs. complex classification of carbohydrate-containing foods in predicting risk of CHD.

38.7 Whole grains and fibre

Whole grain products such as coarsely ground whole wheat breads, brown rice, oats, and barley tend to produce slower glycaemic and insulinaemic responses than highly processed refined grains. Whole grains are also rich in fibre, antioxidant vitamins, magnesium, and phyto-chemicals, all of which can have cardioprotective effects. In the NHS (Liu *et al.* 1999), after adjustment for coronary risk factors, the RRs of CHD incidence across quintiles of whole grain consumption were 1.0, 0.92, 0.93, 0.83, and 0.75 (*p* for trend = 0.01). The inverse association was even stronger in the subgroup of never smokers (RR = 0.49 for extreme quintiles).

A number of prospective cohort studies, including NHS and HPFS, have examined the relationship between fibre intake and risk of CHD, and results from these studies are remarkably consistent. In the NHS (Wolk *et al.* 1999), for each 10 g/day increase in total fibre intake, the RR of CHD after adjustment for coronary risk factors was 0.81 (95% CI: 0.66–0.99). The inverse association appears to be stronger for cereal fibre than for fruit and vegetable fibre. The RRs of CHD for each 5 g/day increment were 0.63 (95% CI: 0.49–0.81) for cereal fibre, 1.06 (95% CI: 0.84–1.32) for vegetable fibre, and 0.93 (95% CI: 0.74–1.16) for fruit fibre. Similar results were observed in the HPFS (Rimm *et al.* 1996); the RRs of CHD comparing extreme quintiles were 0.71 (95% CI: 0.54–0.92) for cereal fibre, 0.81 (95% CI: 0.62–1.06) for fruit fibre, and 0.83 (0.64–1.08) for vegetable fibre. Despite a weak and non-significant association with fruit and vegetable fibres, our pooled analyses of NHS and HPFS indicate that a higher intake of fruits and vegetables was associated with a significant reduction in incidence of ischaemic stroke (Joshipura *et al.* 1999) and CHD (Joshipura *et al.* 2001). Each one serving per day increase in intake of fruits or vegetables was associated with a 4% lower risk for CHD and 6% lower risk for ischaemic stroke.

38.8 **Antioxidants and folate**

Among various antioxidants, vitamin E has attracted most attention as a potential agent for reducing CHD risk. A body of epidemiological evidence has linked intake of vitamin E and reduced risk of CHD. In both the NHS (Stampfer *et al.* 1993) and the HPFS (Rimm *et al.* 1993), we found a significantly lower risk for CHD in participants who had higher daily consumption of vitamin E, particularly in those subjects who took vitamin E supplements, after adjusting for coronary risk factors. The results from published clinical trials of vitamin E, all among patients with clinical CHD, however, have been inconsistent and largely disappointing (GISSI-Prevenzione Investigators 1999; HOPE Investigators 2000; Stephens *et al.* 1996; Virtamo *et al.* 1998) (see Chapter 15). Ongoing clinical trials among persons without CHD will hopefully provide more definitive data on the effects of vitamin E in primary prevention of CHD.

Growing evidence suggests that high folate intake is beneficial in preventing cardiovascular disease, possibly because folic acid and other B vitamins are the primary determinants of plasma homocysteine concentrations, a recognized independent cardiovascular risk factor (Boushey *et al.* 1995, and see Chapter 16). When we examined the association between folate intake and risk of CHD in the NHS (Rimm *et al.* 1998), the RR for CHD was 0.69 (95% CI: 0.55–0.87) for women in the highest quintile of folate intake (median 696 μg/day) compared to those in the lowest quintile of folate intake (median 158 μg/day). We also observed a reduction in risk for CHD with a higher intake of vitamin B_6 (RR comparing extreme quintiles = 0.67, 95% CI: 0.53–0.85). It is of interest that the inverse association between folic acid intake and CHD was strongest in women who had more than one alcoholic drink per day (RR = 0.27, 95% CI: 0.13–0.58). Several large, ongoing clinical trials of folate and MI and stroke may provide further data on the beneficial role of folic acid in reducing risk of CHD or stroke in both men and women, but results of supplementation could be unclear because of variations in dietary sources, including that due to fortification.

38.9 **Alcohol**

One of the most consistent findings from epidemiological studies of cardiovascular disease has been an inverse association between moderate alcohol consumption and risk of CHD (see Chapter 17). This was observed in both the NHS (Stampfer *et al.* 1988) and HPFS (Rimm *et al.* 1991). The apparent benefit was related to intake of alcohol per se, not specifically wine. Recently we examined the association between alcohol consumption and risk of CHD among patients with type 2 diabetes. In the NHS (Solomon *et al.* 2000) we found a 55% reduction in CHD incidence among diabetic women who consumed half a drink daily compared with non-drinkers. Similar results were observed in the HPFS (Tanasescu *et al.* 2001). Our results are consistent with two other published studies, the Wisconsin Epidemiologic Study of Diabetic Retinopathy (Valmadrid *et al.* 1999) and the Physicians' Health Study (Ajani *et al.* 2000). The inverse associations observed among diabetics appear to be stronger than those observed in the general population, suggesting that moderate alcohol consumption may have a particular cardiovascular benefit in this high-risk group.

38.10 **Dietary patterns**

Recently, dietary pattern analysis has emerged as an alternative and complementary approach to examining the relationship between diet and risk of chronic diseases (Hu 2002). Instead of looking at individual nutrients or foods, the pattern analysis examines the effects of overall diet. Using data from the HPFS (Hu *et al.* 1999*a*), we conducted a validation study to test the reproducibility and validity of dietary patterns assessed by an FFQ. Through factor analysis, we identified two major patterns. The first pattern (labelled the 'prudent pattern') was characterized by higher intake of vegetables, fruits, legumes, whole grains, fish, and poultry, while the second pattern (labelled the 'Western pattern') was characterized by higher intake of red meat, processed meat, refined grains, sweets/desserts, French fries, and high-fat dairy products. The reliability and validity coefficients were reasonably good for both patterns. The reliability correlations for the factor scores between the two FFQs were 0.70 for the prudent pattern and 0.67 for the Western pattern. The correlations (corrected for week-to-week variation in diet records) between the two FFQs and diet records ranged from 0.45 to 0.74 for the two patterns. In addition, we found significant positive correlations between the Western pattern and plasma insulin, C-peptide, leptin, and homocysteine concentrations, and an inverse correlation with plasma folate concentrations. The prudent pattern was positively correlated with plasma folate and inversely correlated with insulin and homocysteine concentrations (Fung *et al.* 2001*a*).

   In subsequent analyses, we found that the major dietary patterns significantly predicted incidence of CHD over 12 years of follow-up in the NHS (Fung *et al.* 2001*b*). After adjustment for age, smoking, body mass index, and other coronary risk factors, women at the top quintile of the 'prudent' diet score as compared with those in the bottom quintile had a RR of 0.76 (95% CI: 0.60–0.98, *p* for trend test = 0.03) for CHD, whereas women at the top quintile of the 'Western' diet score had a RR of 1.46 (95% CI: 1.07–1.99, *p* for trend test = 0.02). Similar associations were observed in the HPFS (Hu *et al.* 2000*a*). These findings are consistent with our previous finding that higher ratios of red meat (beef, pork, and lamb) to poultry/fish consumption and high-fat dairy to low-fat dairy consumption were associated with significantly increased risk of CHD in the NHS (Hu *et al.* 1999*c*). They are also consistent with ecological observations linking higher intakes of plant foods with a lower risk of CHD (Willett 1994), as well as with the prospective analyses of individual nutrients described above.

38.11 **Obesity and weight gain**

Although a detailed review of the relationship between adiposity and CHD risk is beyond the scope of this chapter (see Chapter 20), this is an important means by which diet influences risk of this disease. Excessive body weight, even at average levels for the US population, is associated with increased risk of both CHD incidence (Manson *et al.* 1990; Willett *et al.* 1995), and mortality (Manson *et al.* 1995) in the NHS. In particular, higher levels of body weight within the 'normal' range, as well as modest weight gains after 18 years of age, appear to increase risks of CHD in middle-aged women (Willett *et al.* 1995). Abdominal adiposity, reflected by a higher ratio of waist to hip circumferences, predicted risk of CHD among women in the NHS (Rexrode *et al.* 1998) and among men older than 65 years in the HPFS (Rimm *et al.* 1995). Given the high and increasing level of adiposity in our society, its contribution to population rates of CHD is large, and greater than any single component of the diet.

38.12 Cigarette smoking

Cigarette smoking is a well-established cause of CHD and the leading cause of death in the US. Smoking may confer even greater risk of CHD in women than in men. In the NHS (Willett *et al.* 1987), the number of cigarettes smoked per day was positively associated with the risk of fatal CHD (RR = 5.5 for ≥25 cigarettes/day) and non-fatal MI (RR = 5.8). Even smoking 1–4 or 5–14 cigarettes/day was associated with a two-fold to three-fold increase in the risk of fatal CHD or non-fatal infarction. Overall, cigarette smoking accounted for approximately half these events in the cohort.

Smoking cessation substantially reduces the risk of CHD. Using data from the NHS, we estimated that stopping smoking eliminates one-third of the excess risk of CHD within 2 years of cessation, and the risk returns to the level of those who never smoked after 10–14 years of cessation (Kawachi *et al.* 1994). Similar benefits were observed for total mortality. Therefore, people who stop smoking will experience an immediate benefit as well as a further longer-term decline in the excess risk of CHD and total mortality.

38.13 Physical activity

More than 40 epidemiological studies have addressed the relation between exercise and CHD and most of the studies have found an inverse association between increasing total and vigorous activity and risk of CHD (Pate *et al.* 1995). These studies indicate a 30–50% risk reduction in both men and women who engaged in regular physical activity, as compared with sedentary participants. In the NHS, we observed a strong inverse association between total physical activity and CHD risk in women, independent of body mass index and other coronary risk factors (Manson *et al.* 1999). Moreover, we found evidence to support that equivalent energy expenditure from moderate–intensity activity such as brisk walking and vigorous exercise confers similar cardiovascular benefits. In particular, we found a strong and graded inverse relation between energy expenditure in either walking or vigorous activity and the incidence of coronary disease. Among women who either walked briskly at least 3 h/week or exercised vigorously for 1.5 h/week, the risk was reduced by 30–40%. Similar benefits were observed for ischaemic stroke (Hu *et al.* 2000b) and type 2 diabetes (Hu *et al.* 1999b). These findings lend support to current federal guidelines that endorse moderate-intensity exercise, which is safe, achievable, and feasible for the majority of the population (Pate *et al.* 1995). Although vigorous exercise should not be discouraged for those who choose a higher intensity of activity, these results indicate that enormous public health benefits would accrue from the adoption of regular moderate-intensity exercise by those who are currently sedentary.

38.14 The combined effects of diet and lifestyle

The combination of dietary and lifestyle factors is more powerful than a single factor alone (Stampfer *et al.* 2000). In the NHS, women who did not smoke cigarettes, were not overweight, maintained a healthy diet (high in cereal fibre, fish, folate, and polyunsaturated fat and low in saturated and trans fat and glycaemic load), exercised moderately or vigorously for half an hour a day, and consumed alcohol moderately (half a drink per day) had an incidence of coronary events that was more than 80% lower than that in the rest of the population (Table 38.1). Thus, when combined with pharmacological treatment of hypertension and high

Table 38.1 Risk of coronary events in low-risk groups defined according to different constellations of modifiable risk factors for coronary disease in the NHS, 1980–94

Group	Women in group (%)	CHD events (n)	RR (95% CI)[a]	Population-attributable risk (95% CI) (%)[b]
Three low-risk factors[c] Diet score in upper two quintiles Non-smoking Moderate-to-vigorous exercise ≥30 min/day	12.7	62	0.43 (0.33–0.55)	54 (42–64)
Four low-risk factors[d] Diet score in upper two quintiles Non-smoking Moderate-to-vigorous exercise ≥30 min/day Body mass index <25	7.2	24	0.34 (0.23–0.52)	64 (46–76)
Five low-risk factors Diet score in upper two quintiles Non-smoking Moderate-to-vigorous exercise ≥30 min/day Body mass index <25 Alcohol ≥5g/day	3.1	5	0.17 (0.07–0.41)	82 (58–93)

Reproduced with permission from Stampfer *et al.* 2001.

[a] RR was estimated from a multiple logistic-regression model and adjusted for age (in 5-year categories), time periods (seven time periods). Presence or absence of a parental history of MI before the age of 60 years, menopausal status, and use or non-use of postmenopausal hormones, presence or absence of a history of hypertension, and presence or absence of a history of high cholesterol.

[b] The population-attributable risk is the percentage of coronary disease events in the population that are attributable to the non-adherence to the particular combination of lifestyle characteristics. Women with missing values were considered to be in the high-risk group.

[c] The model was also adjusted for body mass index and alcohol use.

[d] The model was also adjusted for alcohol use.

lipid levels (if necessary), diet and lifestyle modification could prevent the vast majority of CHD events.

In addition, we estimated that over 90% of type 2 diabetes cases could be prevented by adopting a healthy diet and lifestyle (Hu *et al.* 2001). However, only ~3% of the NHS cohort met the criteria for low risk defined by the guidelines, suggesting an even greater potential to prevent CHD in the general population by diet and lifestyle modification.

38.15 **Summary and conclusions**

Compelling evidence indicates that CHD is heavily influenced by dietary and lifestyle factors. While cigarette smoking, obesity, and physical inactivity have long been established as major causes of CHD, the role of specific dietary factors has not been clearly defined until more recently.

Further research will provide additional refinements about the relationship of diet to risk of CHD. In particular, future prospective studies including biochemical and genetic markers should be able to provide more evidence on biological mechanisms underlying diet–CHD associations and the effects of gene–diet interactions on CHD risk. However, evidence is now clear that replacing saturated and trans fats with unsaturated fats, including sources of n-3 fatty acids, substituting whole grain forms of carbohydrate for refined grains and potatoes, consuming an abundance of fruits and vegetables, and controlling body weight will dramatically reduce risk of CHD. The magnitude of benefit achievable through diet and lifestyle is large and substantially greater than that due to drug treatment of blood cholesterol or hypertension. Because these same dietary and lifestyle changes have many other health benefits, diet and lifestyle deserves far greater emphasis in the prevention of CHD.

References

Ajani, U. A., Gaziano, J. M., Lotufo, P. A., Liu, S., Hennekens, C. H., Buring, J. E., and Manson, J. E. (2000). Alcohol consumption, and risk of coronary heart disease by diabetes status [see comments], *Circulation*, **102**, 500–5.

Albert, C. M., Hennekens, C. H., O'Donnell, C. J., Ajani, U. A., Carey, V. J., Willett, W. C. *et al.* (1998). Fish consumption, and the risk of sudden cardiac death, *Journal of the American Medical Association*, **279**, 23–8.

Ascherio, A., Stampfer, M. J., Colditz, G. A., Rimm, E. B., Litin, L., and Willett, W. C. (1992). Correlations of vitamin A, and E intake with the plasma concentrations of carotenoids, and tocopherols among American men and women, *Journal of Nutrition*, **122**, 1792–801.

Ascherio, A., Rimm, E. B., Stampfer, M. J., Giovannucci, E. L., and Willett, W. C. (1995). Dietary intake of marine n-3 fatty acids, fish intake, and the risk of coronary heart disease among men, *New England Journal of Medicine*, **332**, 977–82.

Ascherio, A., Rimm, E. B., Giovannucci, E. L., Spiegelman, D., Stampfer, M. J., and Willett, W. C. (1996). Dietary fat and risk of coronary heart disease in men: cohort follow up study in the United States, *British Medical Journal*, **313**, 84–90.

Ascherio, A., Katan, M. B., Zock, P. L., Stampfer, M. J., and Willett, W. C. (1999). Trans fatty acids and coronary heart disease, *New England Journal of Medicine*, **340**, 1994–8.

Boushey, C. J., Beresford, S. A., Omenn, G. S., and Motulsky, A. G. (1995). A quantitative assessment of plasma homocysteine as a risk factor for vascular disease: probable benefits of increasing folic acid intakes, *Journal of the American Medical Association*, **274**, 1049–57.

Burr, M. L., Fehily, A. M., Gilbert, J. F., Rogers, S., Holliday, R. M., Sweetnam, P. M. *et al.* (1989). Effects of changes in fat, fish, and fibre intakes on death and myocardial reinfarction: diet and reinfarction trial (DART), *Lancet*, **2**, 757–61.

Daviglus, M. L., Stamler, J., Orencia, A. J., Dyer, A. R., Liu, K., Greenland, P. *et al.* (1997). Fish consumption and the 30-year risk of fatal myocardial infarction, *New England Journal of Medicine*, **336**, 1046–53.

de Lorgeril, M., Renaud, S., Mamelle, N., Salen, P., Martin, J. L., Monjaud, I. *et al.* (1994). Mediterranean alpha-linolenic acid-rich diet in secondary prevention of coronary heart disease, *Lancet*, **343**, 1454–9.

de Lorgeril, M., Salen, P., Martin, J. L., Monjaud, I., Delaye, J., and Mamelle, N. (1999). Mediterranean diet, traditional risk factors, and the rate of cardiovascular complications after myocardial infarction: final report of the Lyon Diet Heart Study [see comments], *Circulation*, **99**, 779–85.

Feskanich, D., Rimm, E. B., Giovannucci, E. L., Colditz, G. A., Stampfer, M. J., Litin, L. B., and Willett, W. C. (1993). Reproducibility and validity of food intake measurements from a semiquantitative food frequency questionnaire, *Journal of the American Dietetic Association*, **93**, 790–6.

Fung, T. T., Rimm, E. B., Spiegelman, D., Rifai, N., Tofler, G. H., Willett, W. C., and Hu, F. B. (2001*a*). Association between dietary patterns and plasma biomarkers of obesity and cardiovascular disease risk, *American Journal of Clinical Nutrition*, **73**, 61–7.

Fung, T. T., Willett, W. C., Stampfer, M. J., Manson, J. E., and Hu, F. B. (2001b). Dietary patterns and risk of coronary heart disease in women, *Archives of Internal Medicine*, **161**, 1857–62.

Giovannucci, E., Colditz, G., Stampfer, M. J., Rimm, E. B., Lihin, L., Sampson, L., and Willett, W. C. (1991). The assessment of alcohol consumption by a simple self-administered questionnaire, *American Journal of Epidemiology*, **133**, 810–17.

GISSI-Prevenzione Investigators (1999). Dietary supplementation with n-3 polyunsaturated fatty acids and vitamin E after myocardial infarction: results from the GISSI-Prevenzione trial, *Lancet*, **354**, 447–55.

Hallfrisch, J., Facn, and Behall, K. M. (2000). Mechanisms of the effects of grains on insulin and glucose responses [In Process Citation], *Journal of the American College of Nutrition*, **19**, 320S–325S.

HOPE Investigators (2000). Vitamin E supplementation and cardiovascular events in high-risk patients, *New England Journal of Medicine*, **342**, 154–60.

Hu, F. B. (2002). Dietary pattern analysis: a new direction in nutritional epidemiology, *Current Opinions in Lipidology*, **13**, 3–9.

Hu, F. B. and Stampfer, M. J. (1999). Nut consumption and risk of coronary heart disease: a review of epidemiologic evidence, *Current Atherosclerosis Reports*, **I**, 204–9.

Hu, F. B., Stampfer, M. J., Manson, J. E., Rimm, E., Colditz, G. A., Rosner, B. A. *et al.* (1997). Dietary fat intake and the risk of coronary heart disease in women [see comments], *New England Journal of Medicine*, **337**, 1491–9.

Hu, F. B., Stampfer, M. J., Manson, J. E., Rimm, E. B., Colditz, G. A., Rosner, B. A. *et al.* (1998). Frequent nut consumption and risk of coronary heart disease: prospective cohort study, *British Medical Journal*, **317**, 1341–5.

Hu, F. B., Rimm, E., Smith-Warner, S. A., Feskanich, D., Stampfer, M. J., Ascherio, A. *et al.* (1999a). Reproducibility and validity of dietary patterns assessed by a food frequency questionnaire, *American Journal of Clinical Nutrition*, **69**, 243–9.

Hu, F. B., Sigal, R. J., Rich-Edwards, J. W., Colditz, G. A., Solomon, C. G., Willett, W. C. *et al.* (1999b). Walking compared with vigorous physical activity and risk of type 2 diabetes in women: a prospective study, *Journal of the American Medical Association*, **282**, 1433–9.

Hu, F. B., Stampfer, M. J., Manson, J. E., Ascherio, A., Colditz, G. A., Speizer, F. E. *et al.* (1999c). Dietary saturated fat and their food sources in relation to the risk of coronary heart disease in women, *American Journal of Clinical Nutrition*, **70**, 1001–8.

Hu, F. B., Stampfer, M. J., Manson, J. E., Rimm, E. B., Wolk, A., Colditz, G. A. *et al.* (1999d). Dietary intake of alpha-linolenic acid and risk of ischemic heart disease among women, *American Journal of Clinical Nutrition*, **69**, 890–7.

Hu, F. B., Stampfer, M. J., Rimm, E. B., Manson, J. E., Ascherio, A., Colditz, G. A. *et al.* (1999e). A prospective study of egg consumption, and risk of cardiovascular disease in men and women, *Journal of the American Medical Association*, **281**, 1387–94.

Hu, F. B., Rimm, E. B., Stampfer, M. J., Ascherio, A., Spiegelman, D., and Willett, W. C. (2000a). Prospective study of major dietary patterns and risk of coronary heart disease in men, *American Journal of Clinical Nutrition*, **72**, 912–21.

Hu, F. B., Stampfer, M. J., Colditz, G. A., Ascherio, A., Rexrode, K. M., Willett, W. C., and Manson, J. E. (2000b). Physical activity and risk of stroke in women, *Journal of the American Medical Association*, **283**, 2961–7.

Hu, F. B., Stampfer, M. J., Manson, J. E., Grodstein, F., Colditz, G. A., Speizer, F. E., and Willett, W. C. (2000c). Trends in the incidence of coronary heart disease and changes in diet and lifestyle in women, *New England Journal of Medicine*, **343**, 530–7.

Hu, F. B., Manson, J. E., Stampfer, M. J., Colditz, G., Liu, S., Solomon, C. G., and Willett, W. C. (2001). Diet, lifestyle, and the risk of type 2 diabetes mellitus in women, *New England Journal of Medicine*, **345**, 790–7.

Hu, F. B., Bronner, L., Willett, W. C., Stampfer, M. J., Rexrode, K. M., Albert, C. M. *et al.* (2002). Fish and omega-3 fatty acid and risk of coronary heart disease in women, *Journal of the American Medical Association*, **287**, 1815–21.

Hunter, D. J., Rimm, E. B., Sacks, F. M., Stampfer, M. J., Colditz, G. A., Litin, L. B., and Willett, W. C. (1992). Comparison of measures of fatty acid intake by subcutaneous fat aspirate, food frequency questionnaire, and diet records in a free-living population of US men, *American Journal of Epidemiology*, **135**, 418–27.

Jacques, P. F., Sulsky, S. I., Sadowski, J. A., Phillips, J. C., Rush, D., and Willett, W. C. (1993). Comparison of micronutrient intake measured by a dietary questionnaire and biochemical indicators of micronutrient status, *American Journal of Clinical Nutrition*, **57**, 182–9.

Jenkins, D. J., Wolever, T. M., Taylor, R. H., Barker, H., Fielden, H., Baldwin, J. M. *et al.* (1981). Glycemic index of foods: a physiological basis for carbohydrate exchange, *American Journal of Clinical Nutrition*, **34**, 362–6.

Jeppesen, J., Schaaf, P., Jones, C., Zhou, M. Y., Chen, Y. D., and Reaven, G. M. (1997). Effects of low-fat, high-carbohydrate diets on risk factors for ischemic heart disease in postmenopausal women [published erratum appears in *Am. J. Clin. Nutr.* 1997 **66** (2), 437] [see comments], *American Journal of Clinical Nutrition*, **65**, 1027–33.

Joshipura, K. J., Ascherio, A., Manson, J. E., Stampfer, M. J., Rimm, E. B., Spiezer, F. E. *et al.* (1999). Fruit and vegetable intake in relation to risk of ischemic stroke, *Journal of the American Medical Association*, **282** (13), 1233–9.

Joshipura, K. J., Hu, F. B., Manson, J. E., Stampfer, M. J., Rimm, E. B., Spiezer, F. E. *et al.* (2001). The effect of fruit and vegetable intake on risk for coronary heart disease, *Annals of Internal Medicine*, **134**, 1106–14.

Katan, M. B., Grundy, S. M., and Willett, W. C. (1997). Should a low-fat, high-carbohydrate diet be recommended for everyone? Beyond low-fat diets [see comments], *New England Journal of Medicine*, **337**, 563–6; discussion 566–7.

Kawachi, I., Colditz, G. A., Stampfer, M. J., Willett, W. C., Manson, J. E., Rosner, B. *et al.* (1994). Smoking cessation and time course of decreased risks of coronary heart disease in middle-aged women, *Archives of Internal Medicine*, **154**, 169–75.

Keys, A. (1980). *Seven Countries: a multivariate analysis of death and coronary heart disease*, Harvard University Press, Cambridge, MA.

Kris-Etherton, P. and Yu, S. (1997). Individual fatty acids on plasma lipids and lipoproteins: human studies, *American Journal of Clinical Nutrition*, **65**(Suppl.), 1628S–1644S.

Kris-Etherton, P. M., Zhao, G., Binkoski, A. E., Coval, S. M., and Etherton, T. D. (2001). The effects of nuts on coronary heart disease risk, *Nutrition Reviews*, **59**, 103–11.

Kromhout, D., Bosschieter, E. B., and Coulander, C. (1985). The inverse relation between fish consumption and 20-year mortality from coronary heart disease, *New England Journal of Medicine*, **312**, 1205–9.

Liu, S., Stampfer, M. J., Hu, F. B., Giovannucci, E., Rimm, E., Manson, J. E. *et al.* (1999). Whole-grain consumption and risk of coronary heart disease: results from the Nurses' Health Study [see comments], *American Journal of Clinical Nutrition*, **70**, 412–19.

Liu, S., Willett, W. C., Stampfer, M. J., Hu, F. B., Franz, M., Sampson, L. *et al.* (2000). A prospective study of dietary glycemic load and risk of myocardial infarction in women, *American Journal of Clinical Nutrition*, **71**, 1455–61.

Liu, S., Manson, J. E., Stampfer, M. J., Holmes, M. D., Hu, F. B., Hankinson, S. E., and Willett, W. C. (2001). Dietary glycemic load assessed by food frequency questionnaire in relation to plasma high-density lipoprotein cholesterol and fasting triglycerides in postmenopausal women, *American Journal of Clinical Nutrition*, **73**, 560–6.

London, S. J., Sacks, F. M., Caesar, J., Stampfer, M. J., Siguel, E., and Willett, W. C. (1991). Fatty acid composition of subcutaneous adipose tissue and diet in post-menopausal US women, *American Journal of Clinical Nutrition*, **54**, 340–5.

London, S. J., Sacks, F. M., Stampfer, M. J., Henderson, I. C., Maclure, M., Tomita, A. *et al.* (1993). Fatty acid composition of the subcutaneous adipose tissue and risk of proliferative benign breast disease and breast cancer, *Journal of the National Cancer Institute*, **85**, 785–93.

Manson, J. E., Colditz, G. A., Stampfer, M. J., Willett, W. C., Rosner, B., Monson, R. R. *et al.* (1990). A prospective study of obesity and risk of coronary heart disease in women, *New England Journal of Medicine*, **322**, 882–9.

Manson, J. E., Willett, W. C., Stampfer, M. J., Colditz, G. A., Hunter, D. J., Hankinson, S. E. *et al.* (1995). Body weight and mortality among women, *New England Journal of Medicine*, **333**, 677–85.

Manson, J. E., Hu, F. B., Rich-Edwards, J. W., Colditz, G. A., Stampfer, M. J., Willett, W. C. *et al.* (1999). A prospective study of walking as compared with vigorous exercise in the prevention of coronary heart disease in women, *New England Journal of Medicine*, **341**, 650–8.

Mensink, R. P. and Katan, M. B. (1992). Effect of dietary fatty acids on serum lipids and lipoproteins: a meta-analysis of 27 trials, *Arteriosclerosis and Thrombosis*, **12**, 911–19.

Michaud, D. S., Giovannucci, E. L., Ascherio, A., Rimm, E. B., Forman, M. R., Sampson, L., and Willett, W. C. (1998). Associations of plasma carotenoid concentrations and dietary intake of specific carotenoids in samples of two prospective cohort studies using a new carotenoid database, *Cancer Epidemiology, Biomarkers & Prevention*, **7**, 283–90.

Oomen, C., Ocke, M. C., Feskens, J. M., van Erp-Barrt, M-J. J., Kok, F. J., and Kromhout, D. (2001). Association between trans fatty acid intake and 10-year risk of coronary heart disease in the Zutphen Elderly Study: a prospective population-based study, *Lancet*, **357**, 746–51.

Pate, R. R., Pratt, M., Blair, S. N., Haskell, W. L., Macera, C. A., Bouchard, C. *et al.* (1995). Physical activity and public health: a recommendation from the Centers for Disease Control and Prevention and the American College of Sports Medicine, *Journal of the American Medical Association*, **273**, 402–7.

Pietinen, P., Ascherio, A., Korhonen, P., Hartman, A. M., Willett, W. C., Albones, D., and Virtamo, J. (1997). Intake of fatty acids and risk of coronary heart disease in a cohort of Finnish men: The Alpha-Tocopherol, Beta-Carotene Cancer Prevention Study, *American Journal of Epidemiology*, **145**, 876–87.

Rexrode, K. M., Carey, V. J., Hennekens, C. H., Walters, F. E., Colditz, G. A., Stampfer, M. J. *et al.* (1998). Abdominal adiposity and coronary heart disease in women, *Journal of the American Medical Association*, **280**, 1843–8.

Rimm, E. B., Stampfer, M. J., Colditz, G. A., Chute, C. G., Litin, L. B., and Willett, W. C. (1990). Validity of self-reported waist and hip circumferences in men and women, *Epidemiology*, **1**, 466–73.

Rimm, E. B., Giovannucci, E. L., Willett, W. C., Colditz, G. A., Ascherio, A., Rosner, B., and Stampfer, M. J. (1991). A prospective study of alcohol consumption and the risk of coronary disease in men, *Lancet*, **338**, 464–8.

Rimm, E. B., Giovannucci, E. L., Stampfer, M. J., Colditz, G. A., Litin, L. B., and Willett, W. C. (1992). Reproducibility and validity of a expanded self-administered semiquantitative food frequency questionnaire among male health professionals, *American Journal of Epidemiology*, **135**, 1114–26.

Rimm, E. B., Stampfer, M. J., Ascherio, A., Giovannucci, E., Colditz, G. A., and Willett, W. C. (1993). Vitamin E consumption and the risk of coronary heart disease in men, *New England Journal of Medicine*, **328**, 1450–60.

Rimm, E. B., Stampfer, M. J., Giovannucci, E., Ascherio, A., Spiegelman, D., Colditz, G. A., and Willett, W. C. (1995). Body size and fat distribution as predictors of coronary heart disease among middle-aged and older US men, *American Journal of Epidemiology*, **141**, 1–11.

Rimm, E. B., Ascherio, A., Giovannucci, E., Spiegelman, D., Stampfer, M. J., and Willett, W. C. (1996). Vegetable, fruit, and cereal fiber intake, and risk of coronary heart disease among men, *Journal of the American Medical Association*, **275**, 447–51.

Rimm, E. B., Willett, W. C., Hu, F. B., Sampson, L., Colditz, G. A., Manson, J. E. *et al.* (1998). Folate and vitamin B6 from diet and supplements in relation to risk of coronary heart disease among women, *Journal of the American Medical Association*, 279, 359–64.

Salmeron, J., Ascherio, A., Rimm, E. B., Colditz, G. A., Spiegelman, D., Jenkins, D. J. *et al.* (1997*a*). Dietary fiber, glycemic load, and risk of NIDDM in men, *Diabetes Care*, 20, 545–50.

Salmeron, J., Manson, J. E., Stampfer, M. J., Colditz, G. A., Wing, A. L., and Willett, W. C. (1997*b*). Dietary fiber, glycemic load, and risk of non-insulin-dependent diabetes mellitus in women, *Journal of the American Medical Association*, 277, 472–7.

Salvini, S., Hunter, D. J., Sampson, L., Stampfer, M. J., Colditz, G. A., Rosner, B., and Willett, W. C. (1989). Food-based validation of a dietary questionnaire: the effects of week-to-week variation in food consumption, *International Journal of Epidemiology*, 18, 858–67.

Selhub, J., Jacques, P. F., Wilson, P. W. F., Rush, D., and Rosenberg, I. H. (1993). Vitamin status and intake as primary determinants of homocysteinemia in an elderly population, *Journal of the American Medical Association*, 270, 2693–8.

Solomon, C. G., Hu, F. B., Stampfer, M. J., Colditz, G. A., Spiezer, F. E., Rimm, E. B. *et al.* (2000). Moderate alcohol consumption and risk of coronary heart disease among women with type 2 diabetes mellitus [see comments], *Circulation*, 102, 494–9.

Stampfer, M. J., Colditz, G. A., Willett, W. C., Speizer, F. E., and Hennekens, C. H. (1988). A prospective study of moderate alcohol consumption and the risk of coronary disease and stroke in women, *New England Journal of Medicine*, 319, 267–73.

Stampfer, M. J., Hennekens, C. H., Manson, J. E., Colditz, G. A., Rosner, B., and Willett, W. C. (1993). Vitamin E consumption and the risk of coronary disease in women, *New England Journal of Medicine*, 328, 1444–9.

Stampfer, M. J., Hu, F. B., Manson, J. E., Rimm, E. B., and Willett, W. C. (2000). Primary prevention of coronary heart disease in women through diet and lifestyle, *New England Journal of Medicine*, 343, 16–22.

Stephens, N. G., Parsons, A., Schofield, P. M., Kelly, F., Cheeseman, K., and Mitchinson, M. J. (1996). Randomised controlled trial of vitamin E in patients with coronary disease: Cambridge Heart Antioxidant Study (CHAOS), *Lancet*, 347, 781–6.

Stryker, W. S., Kaplan, L. A., Stein, E. A., Stampfer, M. J., Sober, A., and Willett, W. C. (1988). The relation of diet, cigarette smoking, and alcohol consumption to plasma beta-carotene and alpha-tocopherol levels, *American Journal of Epidemiology*, 127, 283–96.

Tanasescu, M., Hu, F. B., Willett, W. C., Stampfer, M. J., and Rimm, E. B. (2001). Alcohol consumption and risk of coronary heart disease among men with type 2 diabetes mellitus, *Journal of the American College of Cardiology*, 38, 1836–42.

USDA/USDHHS (US Department of Agriculture/US Department of Health and Human Services) (2000). *Nutrition and your health: dietary guidelines for Americans*, Homes and Garden Bulletin No. 232, US Printing Office, Washington, DC.

Valmadrid, C. T., Klein, R., Moss, S. E., Klein, B. E., and Cruickshanks, K. J. (1999). Alcohol intake and the risk of coronary heart disease mortality in persons with older-onset diabetes mellitus, *Journal of the American Medical Association*, 282, 239–46.

Virtamo, J., Rapola, J. M., Ripatti, S., Heinonen, O. P., Taylor, P. R., Albones, D., and Huttunen, J. K. (1998). Effect of vitamin E and beta carotene on the incidence of primary nonfatal myocardial infarction and fatal coronary heart disease, *Archives of Internal Medicine*, 158, 668–75.

Willett, W. C. (1994). Diet and health: what should we eat?, *Science*, 264, 532–7.

Willett, W. C. (1998). *Nutritional epidemiology*, 2nd edn, Oxford University Press, New York.

Willett, W., Stampfer, M. J., Bain, C. *et al.* (1983). Cigarette smoking, relative weight, and menopause, *American Journal of Epidemiology*, 117, 651–8.

Willett, W. C., Sampson, L., Stampfer, M. J., Rosner, B., Bain, C., Witschi, J. *et al.* (1985). Reproducibility and validity of a semiquantitative food frequency questionnaire, *American Journal of Epidemiology*, **122**, 51–65.

Willett, W. C., Green, A., Stampfer, M. J., Speizer, F. E., Colditz, G. A., Rosner, B. *et al.* (1987). Relative and absolute excess risks of coronary heart disease among women who smoke cigarettes, *New England Journal of Medicine*, **317**, 1303–9.

Willett, W. C., Sampson, L., Browne, M. L., Stampfer, M. J., Rosner, B., Hennekens, C. H., and Speizer, F. E. (1988). The use of a self-administered questionnaire to assess diet four years in the past, *American Journal of Epidemiology*, **127**, 188–199.

Willett, W. C., Manson, J. E., Stampfer, M. J., Colditz, G. A., Rosner, B., Speizer, F. E., and Hennekens, C. H. (1995). Weight, weight change, and coronary heart disease in women: risk within the 'normal' weight range, *Journal of the American Medical Association*, **273**, 461–5.

Wolf, A., Hunter, D., Colditz, G. A., Manson, J. E., Stampfer, M. J., Corsano, K. A. *et al.* (1994). Reproducibility and validity of a self-administered physical activity questionnaire, *International Journal of Epidemiology*, **23**, 991–9.

Wolk, A. M., Manson, J. E., Stampfer, M. J., Colditz, G. A., Hu, F. B., Speizer, F. E. *et al.* (1999). Long-term intake of dietary fiber and decreased risk of coronary heart disease among women, *Journal of the American Medical Association*, **281**, 1998–2004.

Chapter 39

Risk scores for management and prevention of cardiovascular disease

D. A. Wood and K. Kotseva

39.1 **Introduction**

A physician intuitively assesses a patient's cardiovascular risk. This judgement is based on age, tobacco use, visible obesity, blood pressure, and other simple measurements. However, clinical judgement is often imprecise. So objective risk assessment using cardiovascular disease (CVD) risk charts, calculators, or computer programs is recommended. Such risk estimation methods do not exclude the need for clinical judgement as these tools do not incorporate all risk factors for atherosclerotic disease. The objective calculation of risk needs to be adjusted by the physician who takes account of other clinical factors. For example, clinical evidence of end organ damage, such as hypertensive retinopathy, or a family history of premature coronary heart disease (CHD) both increase cardiovascular risk, but may not be part of formal risk calculation. So the physician has to look at the complete clinical picture when judging an individual's absolute risk of developing CVD over time.

In defining objectives for CVD prevention in clinical practice it is implicit that priority is given to those patients who are at highest risk of developing it, rather than attempting to reach every adult in the population. Therefore, risk stratification is required. In the context of a comprehensive population strategy – to reduce tobacco smoking, encourage healthy food choices, and increase physical activity for the whole population – the medical priority is to focus on those with established atherosclerotic disease, and those apparently healthy individuals who are at high risk of developing atherosclerotic disease because of a combination of these risk factors.

So the priorities for preventive cardiology are:

1 Patients with established CVD.

2 Healthy individuals who are at high risk of developing CVD because of a combination of risk factors – including smoking, raised blood pressure, lipids (raised total cholesterol and low-density lipoprotein cholesterol (LDL-C), low high-density lipoprotein cholesterol (HDL-C) and raised triglycerides), raised blood glucose, family history of premature CHD – or those who have severe hypercholesterolaemia or other forms of dyslipidaemia, hypertension, or diabetes.

3 Close relatives of patients with early onset CVD and of healthy individuals at particularly high risk.

The overall objective of CVD prevention, both in patients with clinically established atherosclerotic disease and apparently healthy individuals at high risk of developing this disease, is the same: to reduce the risk of major atherosclerotic vascular events, and thereby reduce cardiovascular morbidity and mortality and prolong survival.

39.2 **Concept of cardiovascular risk**

The term risk factor describes those characteristics found in healthy individuals to be independently related to the subsequent occurrence of CVD and, where modifiable, to be reversible. This includes modifiable aspects of lifestyle and physiological and biochemical characteristics, as well as non-modifiable personal characteristics, such as age, sex, and family history of early onset atherosclerotic disease. When a person develops symptomatic atherosclerotic disease, the modifiable risk factors continue to contribute to disease progression and prognosis.

The determinants of atherosclerotic disease reflect a continuum of risk in the population. At one end of this risk spectrum are young individuals without atherosclerotic disease who are progressively exposed to lifestyle and environmental factors responsible for this disease and its complications. Then, as these individuals age, they develop asymptomatic atherosclerosis because of their increasing exposure to smoking, an unhealthy diet, and sedentary lifestyle resulting in obesity, elevated blood pressure, dyslipidaemia, hyperglycaemia, and other risk factors for atherosclerosis. At the far end of this risk spectrum symptomatic atherosclerosis manifests itself – as angina, myocardial infarction (MI), stroke, and peripheral arterial disease – and the patients' subsequent risk of recurrent disease and death is partly driven by those risk factors responsible for the disease's expression in the first place. Given this continuum of risk and atherosclerosis (both asymptomatic and symptomatic disease) in the population, the division of prevention into tertiary, secondary, and primary is artificial. While patients with symptomatic atherosclerotic disease are at high absolute risk of a further (or new) event compared to the healthy population, some apparently healthy individuals, for example, with diabetes mellitus, but without clinical atherosclerosis, may be at greater risk because of multiple predisposing factors. Therefore, it is appropriate to address lifestyle and other risk factors in the same way for both patients with symptomatic atherosclerosis and individuals at high absolute risk of developing symptomatic atherosclerosis. Risk stratification of asymptomatic individuals in the general population identifies those who are at highest risk who should be targeted first. The absolute risk of developing atherosclerotic disease is now widely recommended as the principal determinant of whether or not to introduce antihypertensive or lipid lowering drug therapy in apparently healthy individuals.

39.3 **CVD prevention strategies and absolute multifactorial risk**

The report of the World Health Organization Expert Committee on Prevention of Coronary Heart Disease (WHO 1992) considered that a comprehensive action for CHD prevention has to include three components:

1. A *population strategy* for altering, in the entire population, those lifestyle and environmental factors, and their social and economic determinants, that are the underlying causes of the mass occurrence of CHD.

2. A *high risk strategy* for identification of high risk individuals, and action to reduce their risk factor levels.

3. *Secondary prevention*: prevention of recurrent CHD events and progression of the disease in patients with clinically established CHD.

Patients with clinically established CVD have, at any level of a single risk factor or at any combination of risk factors, a much higher overall level of risk of recurrent disease than asymptomatic persons. Because modifiable risk factors continue to be important to the subsequent risk of atherosclerotic events in patients with clinically established CVD, comprehensive action aimed at reducing risk factors is of great importance in the proper care of such patients.

As CVD is multifactorial in its origins, it is important, in estimating the risk of apparently healthy individuals developing CVD, to consider all risk factors simultaneously. Traditionally, risk factor guidelines have been concerned with unifactorial assessment – in the management of hypertension or hyperlipidaemia – and this has resulted in undue emphasis being placed on individually high risk factors rather than the overall level of risk based on all factors taken together. In practice, clustering of risk factors will have a multiplicative effect and an individual with a number of modest risk factors may be at greater risk than someone with one very high risk factor.

The multifactorial aetiology of CVD and the contribution of all risk factors to the risk of developing a future CVD event are of great importance. For a proper assessment of CVD in an individual, the presence or absence and degree of severity of each individual risk factor has to be considered. In addition, the potential impact of modifying existing risk factors has to be assessed against the background set by the non-modifiable risk characteristics of each individual.

Risk factors have a multiplicative effect. In an asymptomatic man aged 50 years with a moderate elevation of plasma cholesterol, but without other risk factors, the absolute 10 year risk of CHD is relatively small (~10%), whereas in a man of the same age but with other risk factors, such as smoking and elevated blood pressure, the absolute risk is much higher (more than twofold). The absolute risk of an asymptomatic woman is, in both instances, lower than that of a man with a corresponding risk factor pattern. Because age has a major influence on the absolute risk of CVD events, the short-term impact of any risk factor, or any combination of risk factors, increases with age. Absolute risk of CVD helps the physician to focus preventive measures on those at highest risk and who are most likely to benefit. Relative risk is useful to patients to compare their absolute risk relative to the absolute risk of their peers.

The priority given to patients with symptomatic atherosclerosis is pragmatic. Such patients present to medical services by declaring themselves through symptoms to have the disease and to be at high risk of recurrent non-fatal disease or death. It is not necessary to risk stratify these patients for lifestyle and risk factor intervention. They all require intensive lifestyle intervention in relation to smoking, diet, and physical activity together with appropriate management of weight, blood pressure, lipids, and glycaemia. In addition, there are prophylactic drugs – aspirin or other platelet modifying agents, beta-blockers, angiotensin-converting enzyme inhibitors and AII receptor blockers, lipid modification therapies, and anticoagulants – which can reduce the risk of recurrent disease and improve survival. In contrast to patients with disease, apparently healthy asymptomatic high risk individuals in the population have to be identified through screening, whether opportunistic or systematic, in order to target risk factor interventions appropriately, and in particular drug therapies. For these individuals attendance at general practice or hospitals should be seen as an opportunity to assess the absolute risk of developing CVD – that is, the probability of developing CVD over a defined time period given a particular combination of risk factors – and to intervene appropriately depending on the degree to which they are at risk. Taking account of all major cardiovascular risk factors avoids undue emphasis on an individual risk factor at the expense of overall or absolute risk. This challenges the traditional approach to risk factor assessment and management where guidelines have focused on single risk factors, particularly for the management of hypertension or dyslipidaemia.

Because of the increased absolute risk of CVD events with increasing age (see Chapter 35), older people are more likely than younger ones to qualify for intervention on the basis of absolute risk. Therefore, there is a need to consider the benefits of intervention in the context of life expectancy. Younger individuals who are currently at lower absolute CVD risk stand to accumulate more benefit from preventive actions over their lifetime. To take account of lifetime exposure to risk factors it is appropriate both to estimate absolute CVD risk today, and to project that risk to, say, age 60 years, assuming no change in risk factor levels. In this way, the cumulative exposure to risk factors over a lifetime can be estimated, and individuals who are tracking towards a high risk category in later life can be identified at an earlier stage and appropriately managed.

39.4 Advantages and disadvantages of absolute risk prediction

The advantages of a multifactorial approach to treatment in primary prevention of CVD are that:

+ The concept of continuous risk replaces the dichotomous classification of risk factors.
+ The level of absolute (multifactorial) risk for which treatment is given is not fixed.
+ Treatment is targeted at those with the highest absolute CVD risk.
+ Benefit is potentially greatest in those at high multifactorial risk.
+ It avoids treatment of single risk factors in those at low multifactorial risk.

The disadvantage of a multifactorial approach to treatment in primary prevention of CVD is that treatment is concentrated in the older population unless the effect of lifetime exposure is taken into account.

39.5 Calculation of CVD risk

Cardiovascular risk calculation is now incorporated into international and national guidelines for the prevention of CVD. Practical methods – tables, charts, and computer programs – have been developed for the assessment of an individual's absolute risk of developing CVD on the basis of risk functions derived from prospective epidemiological studies. The majority of these methods are based on the risk function derived from the Framingham Study (Anderson *et al.* 1991*a, b*). This function has been widely used to predict CHD and CVD risk because it is the classical epidemiological study of risk and CVD and the data are in the public domain. Simplified forms of the Framingham risk function have been used in the New Zealand (Jackson 2000; Jackson *et al.* 1993; National Heart Foundation 1996), European (Pyörälä *et al.* 1994; Wood *et al.* 1998*a, b*), and UK (Haq *et al.* 1995; Joint British Recommendations on prevention of coronary heart disease in clinical practice 2000; Wallis *et al.* 2000; Wood *et al.* 1998*c*) guidelines for prevention of CHD, to target treatment at those at highest absolute risk. Framingham risk scoring has also been used in the National Cholesterol Education Program Adult Treatment Panel III (NCEP-ATP III) risk assessment for developing CHD (Executive Summary of the Third Report of the NCEP ATP III Panel 2001).

Using the context of absolute cardiovascular risk for managing individual risk factors was first proposed for the management of hypertension in New Zealand in 1993 (Jackson *et al.* 1993). The Joint European Societies' – European Society of Cardiology, European Society of Hypertension, and European Atherosclerosis Society – Task Force then proposed in 1994 that absolute risk should be the basis for prevention of CHD in the healthy population for the treatment of blood pressure, lipids, and diabetes. The Joint European Societies Task Force produced a coronary risk chart based on age, smoking, systolic blood pressure (SBP), and total cholesterol (Pyörälä et al. 1994). A separate coronary risk chart was produced for patients with diabetes mellitus. This was followed by the New Zealand cardiovascular risk chart based on a combination of systolic and diastolic blood pressure (DBP) values, the ratio of total cholesterol to HDL-C, and a 5 year rather than 10 year risk model (Jackson 2000).

The Sheffield Risk and Treatment Table differed from these initial risk assessment charts in that its first use was to determine whether total cholesterol and HDL-C needed to be measured. Then, if so, whether the lipid ratio conferred an absolute 10 year CHD risk of 30% or more in the context of other risk factors (Haq et al. 1995). Subsequently a Sheffield Table was published to identify individuals at ≥15% CHD risk (Wallis et al. 2000). The Joint British Societies produced a coronary risk prediction chart and an associated computer program 'Cardiac Risk Assessor', which estimated both 10 year CHD risk and cardiovascular risk (including stroke) over the same period (Joint British Recommendations on prevention of CHD in clinical practice 2000; Wood et al. 1998c).

The NCEP has produced three reports. The first, ATP I, outlined a strategy for primary prevention of CHD in persons with high levels of LDL-C (≥160 mg/dl) or those with border-line cholesterol (130–59 mg/dl) and multiple risk factors (NCEP 1988). In ATP II the intensive management of LDL-C in persons with established CHD was added (NCEP 1994). In ATP III Framingham projections of 10 year absolute CHD risk were used for the first time to identify certain patients with multiple (2+) risk factors for more intensive treatment (Executive Summary of the Third Report of the NCEP ATP III Panel 2001).

Using the Joint European Societies' Coronary Risk Charts (Fig. 39.1a, b), an individual's absolute risk of developing a CHD event (angina, non-fatal MI, or coronary death) over the coming years is found by locating the appropriate box in the charts in relation to patient's age, gender, smoking status, blood pressure, and cholesterol levels (Wood et al. 1998a, b). Systolic blood pressure is recorded vertically, and total cholesterol level is recorded horizontally. Total cholesterol concentrations (4–8 mmol/l) are used rather than total cholesterol to HDL-C ratios. Although this ratio improves CHD risk prediction, particularly in women, HDL-C is not routinely measured across Europe, whereas a measurement of total cholesterol is readily available in every European country. Therefore, the decision to use total cholesterol only was primarily made to ensure the widest possible application of the charts across Europe. It is assumed that the patient has an average HDL-C concentration of 1.0 mmol/l for men and 1.1 mmol/l per women. A further consideration was that a chart based on the ratio would have to assume an average European cholesterol value. Whilst this might be reasonable in a single country, it was not felt to be appropriate for Europe in view of the large differences in average cholesterol levels between countries. Compared to the 1994 Coronary Risk Chart, the range of total cholesterol in the 1998 Coronary Risk Chart was extended at the lower end by including 4.0 mmol/l. This is because a cholesterol goal of <5.0 mmol/l for CHD prevention was recommended and, therefore, the cholesterol range had to be extended below this level in the new chart. Age and cholesterol levels are rounded off to whole digits and SBP to 10 mmHg. The 10 year CHD risk is presented in five levels: low (<5%); mild (5–10%); moderate (10–20%); high (20–40%), and very high (>40%). An absolute risk of 20% or more was defined as the threshold for intensive risk factor intervention. An absolute CHD risk which exceeds 20% over the next 10 years, or will exceed 20% if projected to age 60, and which is sustained despite professional lifestyle intervention, is sufficiently high to justify the selective

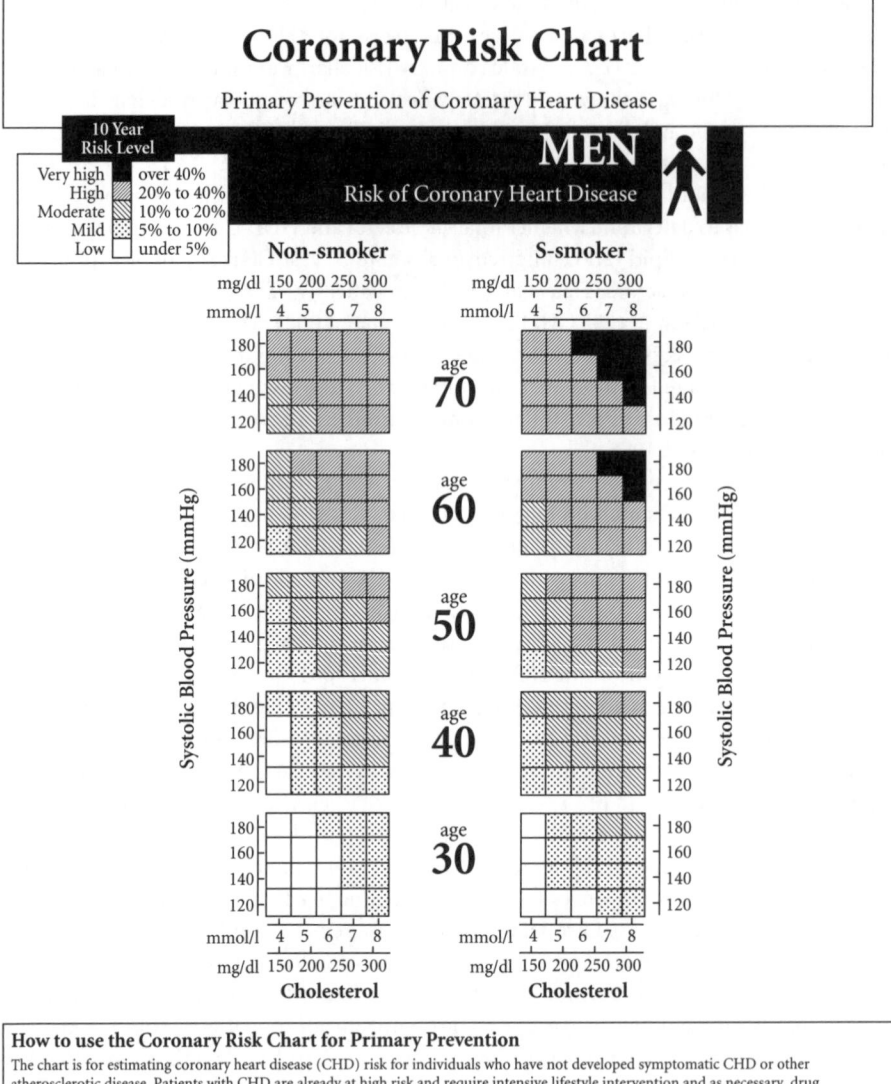

Fig. 39.1 (a) Coronary risk chart for primary CHD prevention in men. (b) Coronary risk chart for primary CHD prevention in women. (Reproduced from Wood 1998a.)

use of proven drug therapies. It should be stressed that certain individuals will be at higher risk than is evident from the coronary risk chart. The chart is not intended for patients with clinically manifest CHD or other atherosclerotic disease, who are already at high risk, over 20% and often over 40% over the next 10 years. Risk is also higher than indicated in the charts for

Coronary Risk Chart

Primary Prevention of Coronary Heart Disease

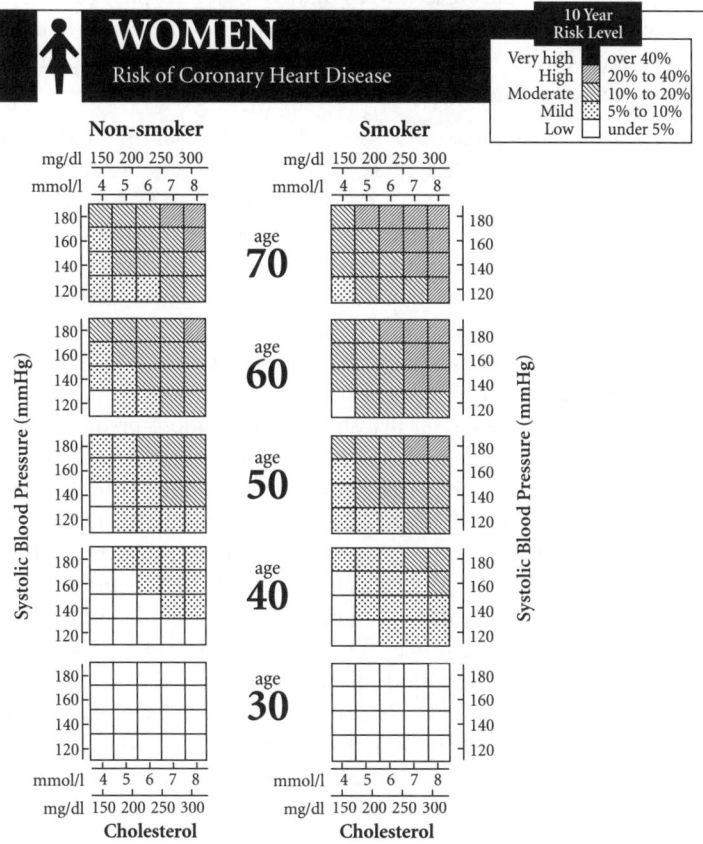

WOMEN
Risk of Coronary Heart Disease

10 Year Risk Level		
Very high		over 40%
High		20% to 40%
Moderate		10% to 20%
Mild		5% to 10%
Low		under 5%

- CHD risk is higher than indicated in the chart for those with:-
- Familial hyperlipidaemia
- Diabetes: risk is approximately doubled in men and more than doubled in women
- Those with a family history of premature cariovascular disease
- Those with low HDL cholesterol. Those tables assume HDL cholesterol to be 1.0 mmol/1 (39 mg/dl) in men and 1.1 (43) in women
- Those with raised triglyceride levels >2.0 mmol/1 (> 180 mg/dl)
- As the person approaches the next age category.

- To find a person's relative risk, compare their risk category with that for other people of the same age. The absolute risk shown here may not apply to all populations, especially those with a low CHD incidence. Relative risk is likely to be apply to most populations.
- The effect of changing cholesterol, smoking status or blood pressure can be read from the chart.

(continued)

patients with familial hyperlipidaemia, family history of premature CVD, and those with low HDL-C or raised triglycerides levels. With these caveats, the charts perform several functions:

- An individual's absolute risk of developing a CHD event in the next decade can be read from the chart without any calculations.

- Relative risk can be estimated by comparing the risk in one cell with any other in the same age group.

- ◆ The chart can be used to predict the effect of changing from one risk category to another. Thus, one can readily show a patient the reduction in risk associated with stopping smoking, or reducing blood pressure or total cholesterol.

- ◆ Although young people are at lower risk than older people, risk will rise steadily with increasing age. The chart can be used by following the boxes upwards to illustrate the effect of lifetime risk by observing the increased risk with increasing age if risk factors remain constant, or indeed if they increase further as age increases.

The New Zealand tables consist of a matrix of cells with four rows and five columns. The risk factors included in the tables are age, sex, smoking, blood pressure, diabetes, and total cholesterol to HDL-C ratio. Each row relates to a different band of SBP, which differs by 20 mmHg (120–80 mmHg), and each column relates to a different total to HDL-C ratio (4–8). The colour of the cell corresponds to a different 6 year cardiovascular risk level (<2.5%, 2.5–5%, 5–10%, 10–15%, 15–20%, and >20%) (National Heart Foundation 1996). A projected 5 year CVD risk of 20% is believed to be equivalent to a 10 year CHD risk of 30%. The updated New Zealand tables further stratify subjects with projected 5 year risk of CVD by including risk bands of 20–5%, 25–30%, and >30% (Jackson 2000).

The risk factors used in the Joint British recommendations prediction charts include age, sex, smoking, SBP, diabetes mellitus, and total cholesterol to HDL-C ratio. The projected 10 year CHD risk is represented graphically as a function of SBP (110–220 mmHg) on the vertical axis, and cholesterol to HDL ratio (3–12) on the horizontal axis. CHD risk is classified in three zones (<15%, 15–30%, and >30%; Wood et al. 1998c) (Fig. 39.2). High risk individuals are defined as those whose 10 year risk of CHD exceeds 15% (equivalent to a cardiovascular risk of 20% over the same period). As a minimum, those at highest risk (≥30%) should be targeted and treated, and as resources allow, others with a risk of >15% should be progressively targeted. The charts have recently been modified such that patients' age groups are classified as 35–44, 45–54, 55–64, or 65–74 years (Joint British Recommendations on prevention of CHD in clinical practice 2000). The British chart risk stratifies healthy individuals into three categories: those at highest CHD risk (30% or higher, red band); those at the next level of CHD risk (15% or higher, orange band); and finally those whose CHD risk is less than 15% (green band).

The original Sheffield tables have 12 vertical columns of cholesterol concentrations, each column applying to a different permutation of the four categorical risk factors: diabetes, smoking, left ventricular hypertrophy, and hypertension (defined as a SBP of >160 mmHg). There are separate tables for men and women. Each row in the table applies to a different age, with rows differing by intervals of 2 years. No account is taken of the HDL-C concentration, but the assumption is made that its average value is 1.15 mmol/l for men and 1.4 mmol/l for women (Haq et al. 1995). The modified Sheffield tables use the same design, but display total to HDL-C concentrations, and show the ratios that correspond to projected annual CHD risks of both ≥3.0% and ≥1.5%. Hypertension is defined as SBP >140 mmHg (Wallis et al. 2000).

The NCEP ATP III also focuses on a multiple risk factor approach (Executive Summary of the Third Report of the NCEP ATP III Panel 2001). ATP III identifies three categories of risk for different LDL-C goals and different intensities of LDL-lowering therapy: (a) CHD and CHD risk equivalents (other forms of clinical atherosclerotic disease); (b) Multiple (2+) risk factors (smoking, hypertension, low HDL-C, family history of premature CHD, age (male ≥45

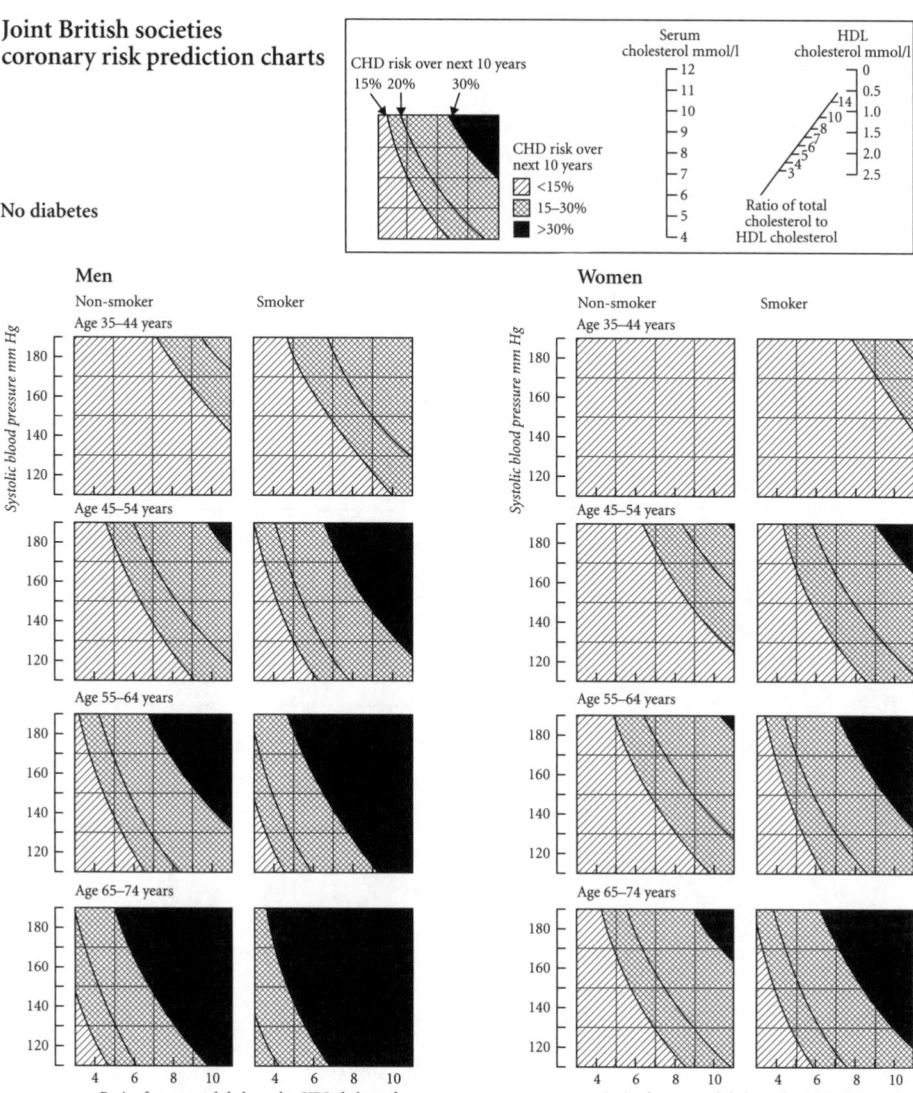

Fig. 39.2 Joint British Societies coronary risk prediction charts. (Reproduced from Joint British Recommendations on prevention of coronary heart disease in clinical practice 2000.)

years and female ≥55 years), and diabetes); 0–1 risk factor. One of the new features of ATP III is the focus on multiple risk factors using Framingham projections of 10 year absolute CHD risk to identify patients with multiple (2+) risk factors for more intensive treatment. The highest risk consists of CHD and CHD equivalents, which carry a risk for major coronary events of >20% per 10 years. The persons from this risk category have the lowest LDL-C goal (<100 mg/dl). The second category, which consists of persons with multiple (2+) risk factors and 10 year risk for CHD <20%, have a LDL-C goal of <130 mg/dl. The third category of persons, those with 0–1 risk factor, have a 10 year risk of <10% and their LDL-C goal is <160 mg/dl. Risk status in persons without clinically manifest CHD or other forms of atherosclerotic disease is determined by a two-step procedure. First, the number of risk factors is counted. Second, for persons with multiple (2+) risk factors, 10 year risk assessment is carried out with Framingham scoring to identify individuals whose risk warrants more intensive treatment. When 0–1 risk factors is present, Framingham scoring is not necessary because 10 year risk rarely reaches levels for intensive treatment. Risk factors used in

Age	Points
20-34	-9
35-39	-4
40-44	0
45-49	3
50-54	6
55-59	8
60-64	10
65-69	11
70-74	12
75-79	13

Total Cholesterol	Points				
	Age 20-39	Age 40-49	Age 50-59	Age 60-69	Age 70-79
<160	0	0	0	0	0
160-199	4	3	2	1	0
200-239	7	5	3	1	0
240-279	9	6	4	2	1
≥280	11	8	5	3	1

	Points				
	Age 20-39	Age 40-49	Age 50-59	Age 60-69	Age 70-79
Nonsmoker	0	0	0	0	0
Smoker	8	5	3	1	1

HDL (mg/dL)	Points
≥60	-1
50-59	0
40-49	1
<40	2

Systolic BP (mmHg)	If Untreated	If Treated
<120	0	0
120-129	0	1
130-139	1	2
140-159	1	2
≥160	2	3

Point Total	10-Year Risk %
<0	< 1
0	1
1	1
2	1
3	1
4	1
5	2
6	2
7	3
8	4
9	5
10	6
11	8
12	10
13	12
14	16
15	20
16	25
≥17	≥ 30

Fig. 39.3 (a) Estimate of 10 year risk for men (Framingham Point Scores). (b) Estimate of 10 year risk for women (Framingham Point Scores). (Reproduced from NCEP 2001.)

Age	Points
20-34	-7
35-39	-3
40-44	0
45-49	3
50-54	6
55-59	8
60-64	10
65-69	12
70-74	14
75-79	16

Total Cholesterol	Points				
	Age 20-39	Age 40-49	Age 50-59	Age 60-69	Age 70-79
<160	0	0	0	0	0
160-199	4	3	2	1	1
200-239	8	6	4	2	1
240-279	11	8	5	3	2
≥280	13	10	7	4	2

	Points				
	Age 20-39	Age 40-49	Age 50-59	Age 60-69	Age 70-79
Nonsmoker	0	0	0	0	0
Smoker	9	7	4	2	1

HDL (mg/dL)	Points
≥60	-1
50-59	0
40-49	1
<40	2

Systolic BP (mmHg)	If Untreated	If Treated
<120	0	0
120-129	1	3
130-139	2	4
140-159	3	5
≥160	4	6

Point Total	10-Year Risk %
<9	< 1
9	1
10	1
11	1
12	1
13	2
14	2
15	3
16	4
17	5
18	6
19	8
20	11
21	14
22	17
23	22
24	27
≥25	≥ 30

(continued)

Framingham scoring include age, total cholesterol, HDL-C, blood pressure, and cigarette smoking. The first step is to calculate the number of points for each risk factor and the total risk score sums. The 10 year risk for MI and coronary death is estimated from total points, and the person is categorized according to absolute 10 year risk (Fig. 39.3a, b). Framingham scoring divides persons with multiple risk factors into those with 10 year risk for CHD of >20%, 10–20%, and <10%. ATP III recommends a multifaceted lifestyle and drug therapy approach for CHD prevention.

39.6 **Comparison of risk prediction methods**

A comparison of the European, New Zealand, British, Sheffield, and NCEP-ATP III charts shows similarities and differences in these different approaches to prediction of risk of coronary and cardiovascular disease:

- The European, New Zealand (which was an adaptation of the European chart), British, Sheffield, and NCEP-ATP charts are all based on the Framingham function. The European risk function is based on angina, non-fatal MI, and coronary death over 10 years. The New Zealand chart uses all cardiovascular events (new angina, MI, coronary death, claudication, heart failure, and stroke or transient ischaemic attack) over 5 years, and the British version uses non-fatal MI and coronary death over 10 years.

- Cardiovascular risk is used only by the New Zealand tables and projected over a 5 year interval. All other tables and charts, with the exception of the Sheffield and modified Sheffield tables, use coronary risk projected over a 10 year interval. Both the original and modified Sheffield tables use CHD risk predicted for a 5 year interval, which was doubled to give a projected 10 year risk (Sheffield tables) or divided by five to give an annual risk (modified Sheffield tables).

- The Sheffield risk assessment uses tables for men and women. The European and New Zealand charts use coloured boxes. The British version directly plots the Framingham function for given levels of absolute CHD risk. Of these approaches the British one is more accurate, as the tables and boxes only give an approximation of risk.

- The estimation of absolute CHD (or cardiovascular) risk is less certain at both ends of the risk distribution, particularly for young people (especially <40 years) at lower levels of risk. This is because there are fewer clinical events and virtually none for the youngest. Therefore, both the European and New Zealand charts claim an accuracy which cannot be justified from the Framingham data. The European chart has five risk categories (<5% to >40% 10 year CHD risk) and the New Zealand charts (the original and updated) have six and eight risk categories, respectively (<2.5% to >30% 5 year cardiovascular risk), and both include ages 30–70 years. The British version has only three risk categories (<15%, 15–29%, and ≥ 30% CHD risk over 10 years) and excludes those <40 years of age. This simpler classification of CHD risk into three categories presents the Framingham data more appropriately than the other charts, particularly for those at both very high and very low risk. Those <40 years of age are completely excluded from the British chart. These three risk bands also represent the levels of risk targeted in the British recommendations: namely to target and treat those with an absolute CHD risk ≥30% (the red band), then move on to those with a CHD risk ≥15% (orange band), and to give lifestyle advice to those with a CHD risk <15% (green band). This simple traffic light system provides a powerful visual reinforcement of the order of priorities in primary CHD prevention. The NCEP-ATP III risk assessment has three risk categories: 10 year risk for CHD of <10%, 10–20%, and >20%.

- The New Zealand charts advise that the risk of CHD (or CVD) should be increased by one or two categories for patients with premature CHD. The European and British charts are for primary prevention only. Patients with established CHD or other atherosclerotic disease are managed as high risk and have specified lifestyle and risk factor targets. Using the chart solely for primary CHD prevention is better because it avoids classifying a patient with disease as anything other than high risk.

- The European and British charts use SBP (an alternative British Chart is available for diastolic pressure), but the New Zealand chart requires an interpolation of systolic and diastolic pressures (120/75, 140/85, 160/95, 180/105). The instruction on the New Zealand chart is to find the cell nearest to the person's blood pressure. Systolic blood pressure is a better predictor of CHD risk than diastolic pressure and therefore is the preferred variable for estimating coronary risk. The only other difference on blood pressure between the charts is the range: European and New Zealand have the same systolic ranges, 120–80 mmHg; the British chart goes from 110 to 210 mmHg; and diastolic pressure ranges from 75 to 105 mmHg in the New Zealand chart, and 70 to 120 mmHg in the British chart, but is not used in the European chart. Sheffield and NCEP-ATP III tables use hypertension as a categorical risk factor.

- The European chart uses total cholesterol only, but the New Zealand, British and NCEP-ATP III charts use the ratio of total to HDL-C. The range for this ratio in the New Zealand chart is 4–8 and in the British chart it is 3–12. The original Sheffield table uses total cholesterol and the modified Sheffield table uses total to HDL-C ratio.

- The European, New Zealand, and British charts are reproduced separately for patients with diabetes and both illustrate the higher coronary risk associated with diabetes. This is particularly so for women, whose risk is approximately that of non-diabetic men. Diabetes is used as a categorical risk factor in the Sheffield tables.

39.7 Application of absolute risk to management of blood pressure and lipids

In the management of blood pressure and lipids, assessing the absolute CHD or CVD risk is logical and the Joint European Societies produced algorithms based on this principle.

A decision to treat blood pressure with drugs depends on the absolute CHD risk as well as systolic and DBP levels, and target organ damage. As shown on the coronary risk chart, people with a mild elevation of blood pressure may have differences in their risks of coronary events depending on the number and severity of coexisting risk factors. A decision about the introduction of antihypertensive drug therapy should be based on the absolute risk of developing or having recurrent disease, not just the level of blood pressure. For subjects with a sustained SBP ≥180 mmHg and/or a DBP ≥100 mmHg, despite lifestyle interventions, the risk of CHD, stroke, or heart failure is so high that drug treatment is essential. Subjects with a SBP of 160–79 mmHg and/or a DBP of 95–9 mmHg often require drug treatment if these high blood pressure values are sustained. Those with a SBP of 140–59 mmHg and/or a DBP of 90–4 mmHg may also require drug treatment, but this will depend on the presence of other risk factors (an absolute CHD risk ≥20% over 10 years, or ≥20% if projected to age 60) and whether or not there is target organ damage. In contrast, at the same blood pressure levels antihypertensive therapy will not usually be needed in someone who is at lower absolute CHD risk.

A decision to treat blood lipids with drugs also depends on the absolute CHD risk as well as lipid levels, lipoprotein profile, and family history of premature CHD or other atherosclerotic disease. Patients with familial hypercholesterolaemia are at such high CHD risk of premature CHD that lipid-lowering therapy is always necessary. People at high CHD risk because of a combination of risk factors (an absolute CHD risk ≥20% over 10 years, or ≥20% if projected to age 60) and whose cholesterol levels are not lowered by diet, also require drug treatment.

39.8 Limitations of the Framingham risk function

The Framingham risk equation is based on measurements made at baseline on a single occasion and therefore it is appropriate to estimate risk in clinical practice in the same way. However, the slope of the relation between the true mean risk factor level and risk of developing disease is steeper than that shown between a single measurement and CVD risk because of regression-dilution bias. The slope of the regression line relating CVD risk to risk factor measurements based on a series of recordings is steeper because the effects of biological variation are reduced. Therefore CVD risk will be somewhat higher than the estimate based on the first blood pressure or cholesterol measurement made at an initial screening visit. Absolute risk will also be underestimated by using values of blood pressure on treatment, or cholesterol recorded after dietary intervention, because the true risk is likely to be closer to the lifelong habitual levels of these risk factors. By the same token, it would be inappropriate to classify a cigarette smoker, who has recently stopped, as a non-smoker because risk will reflect lifetime exposure to tobacco.

Although it is appropriate to estimate absolute CVD risk on the basis of single risk factor measurements, a decision to treat requires a series of recordings of, say, blood pressure or cholesterol over a period of time. So it is important to distinguish risk assessment from the final decision to introduce antihypertensive or lipid lowering therapy. The latter is dependent on both the context provided by absolute CVD risk and the long-term levels of individual risk factors observed over time. Lifestyle intervention will also impact on these levels.

Furthermore, the application of one coronary risk chart, based on a high risk middle-aged North American population, to European populations at different levels of CVD risk poses several problems. Since the inception of the Framingham study the incidence of CVD has fallen in many countries resulting in a decrease in absolute risk. Although the Framingham function still predicts absolute risk reasonably well in high risk populations, it over-predicts absolute risk in low risk European populations. It is known that the Framingham risk functions overestimate coronary risk when applied to a southern European population (Haq et al. 1999; Pyörälä 2000). Menotti et al. (2000) performed a systematic re-analysis of 10 year CHD incidence data from the northern and southern European cohorts of the Seven Countries study. The risk factors examined in this analysis were age, SBP, total serum cholesterol, and smoking habits. Risk functions were produced separately for northern European cohorts, the southern European cohorts, and all European cohorts pooled. Risk charts were created for northern and southern Europe showing the probability of CHD events over 10 years. They were based on three ages (40, 50, and 60 years), smoking habit (yes/no), four levels of SBP (120, 140, 160, and 180 mmHg), and five levels of total serum cholesterol (4, 5, 6, 7, and 8 mmol/l). The 10 year incidence rates of CHD events in northern European cohorts are much higher than in the southern European cohorts. The number of observed events is overestimated when the northern models are applied to the southern European cohorts (ratio of ~0.5). The risk charts show that, for the same levels of risk factors, the incidence of CHD in southern Europe is systematically lower than in northern Europe. The larger effect of age in the northern compared to the southern European cohorts might reflect a longer exposure to higher risk factor levels. Therefore, a single European risk chart is inappropriate because of the different CVD incidence rates and distributions of risk factors in different countries.

The other limitations of the original European Coronary Risk chart are:

♦ The modest size of the Framingham cohort: the risk function was based on 5573 individuals.

♦ The definition of non-fatal end points includes new onset angina, which differs from definitions used in other cohort studies, and also from end points used in treatment trials, making the function difficult to validate with data from other cohort studies.

♦ The small number of risk factors included in the risk chart, and in particular the omission of HDL-C.

The Joint European Task Forces were aware of the limitations of the Framingham-based coronary risk chart and emphasized these limitations in their recommendations. A special research project called SCORE (Systematic COronary Risk Evaluation), funded by the European Union Biomed 2 programme, was set up to develop European risk functions. The SCORE project is based on 12 European cohort studies, representing a wide range of CVD rates (De Backer *et al.* 2003). In round numbers, the SCORE risk prediction system is based on data for over 200 000 people, 3 million person years of observation, and over 7000 fatal cardiovascular events.

The main features of the SCORE risk prediction system are that:

1 The prediction is based on total cardiovascular deaths rather than the combination of non-fatal and fatal coronary events. Non-CHD cardiovascular mortality is especially important because it represents a greater proportion of all cardiovascular risk in European regions with low rates of CHD. An absolute fatal CVD risk ≥5% from SCORE is equivalent to a CHD event risk ≥20% based on the Framingham function.

2 A SCORE risk function has been calculated for high and low risk European regions. The cohorts from Denmark, Finland, and Norway were used to develop the high risk European region model, and the cohorts from Belgium, Italy, and Spain were used to develop the low risk European region model.

3 The risk in middle-aged subjects, in whom risk changes more rapidly, is provided in more detail.

4 The risk is displayed in each cell as a percentage (probability of fatal CVD over a 10 year period) rather than a broad risk category.

5 The cardiovascular risk is calculated in two ways: one based on total cholesterol and the other on the total cholesterol/HDL-C ratio.

There are several advantages of the European SCORE function. First, the function is based on a very large and representative European dataset with hard, reproducible, fatal cardiovascular end points. Second, fatal CHD and stroke risk can be derived separately. Third, the development of European high and low risk region charts improves the applicability of this scoring system across Europe (Fig. 39.4). Importantly, the risk SCORE function can be customized to any European country based on national mortality data. Therefore, it is possible to produce a risk score chart for each country.

The SCORE charts have several functions:

♦ An individual's risk of dying from CVD over the next 10 years can be read from the chart without any calculations.

♦ The chart illustrates the effect of lifetime risk by showing increasing risk as age increases.

♦ Relative risk can be estimated by comparing the risk in one cell with any other cell in the same age and sex group.

♦ The chart gives some indication of the effect of changing from one risk category to another.

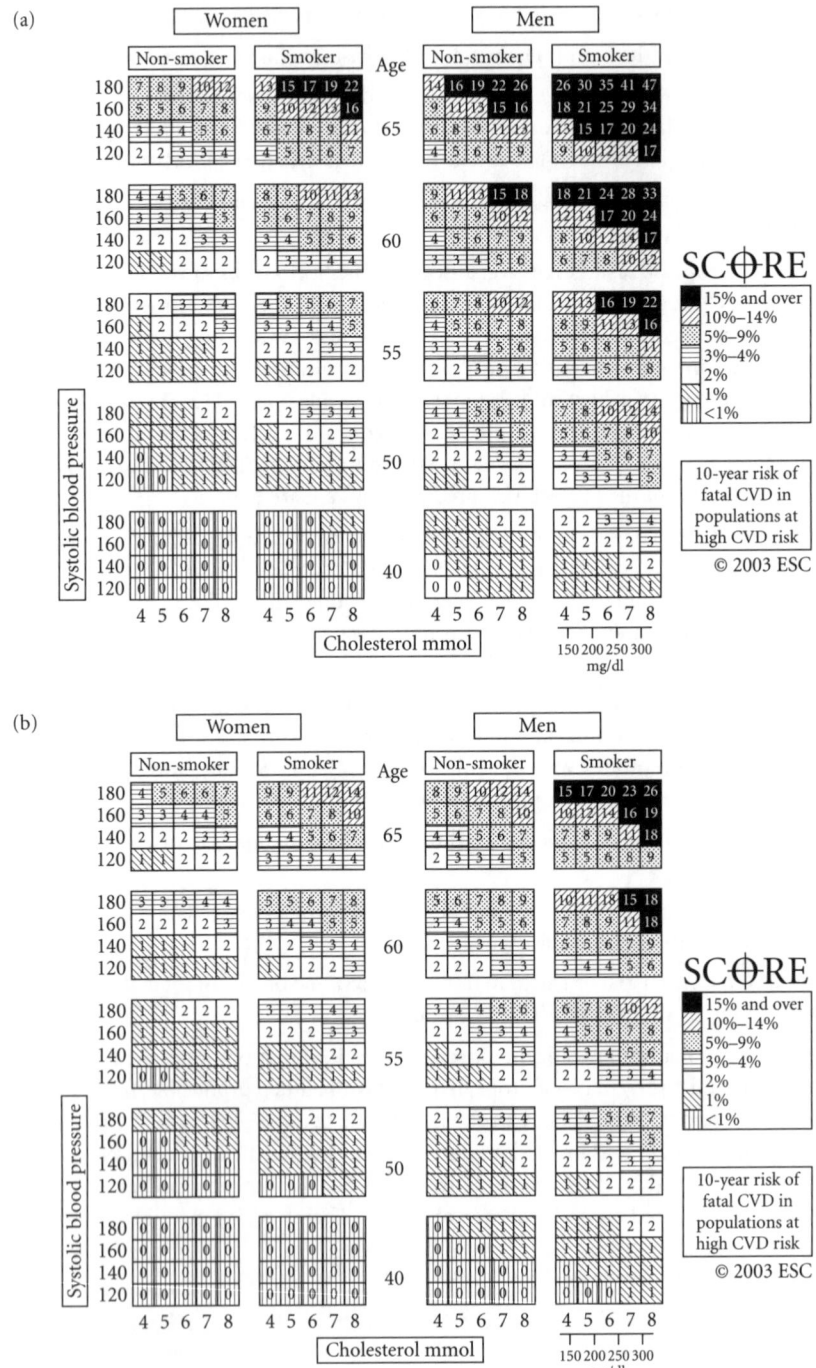

Fig. 39.4 Ten year risk of fatal CVD in (a) high risk and (b) low risk regions of Europe by gender, age, SBP, total cholesterol, and smoking status. (Reproduced from De Backer *et al.* 2003.)

A fatal CVD risk ≥5% based on SCORE is considered to be sufficiently high to justify intensive lifestyle intervention and, where appropriate, the use of drug therapies.

As in the original European charts, some CVD factors such as family history of CHD, triglycerides, fibrinogen, and homocysteine are not included in the SCORE risk prediction system. Future risk prediction systems may incorporate at least some of these risk factors. Patients with diabetes are included in the cohorts, but separate charts for diabetes mellitus cannot be produced because of the variation in the diagnostic criteria for diabetes between cohorts.

The development of a computerized electronic and interactive risk assessment model will allow more risk factor information to be included than can be incorporated in the simple paper charts. The new HeartScore program is a comprehensive computer-based CVD risk estimation and management program for prevention of CVD (Thomsen et al. 2001). The program gives a graphical and numerical presentation of absolute cardiovascular risk, the potential benefits of intervention, the relative impact of modifiable risk factors, and numbers needed to treat. The program provides individually tailored health messages in print for the patient. It can easily be adjusted for different national risk scores, other end points, and languages and will facilitate the practice of preventive cardiology.

39.9 Summary

A physician needs formally to be able to assess cardiovascular risk. This is the only way of distinguishing amongst apparently healthy people those who are at high multifactorial risk of developing CVD (see Chapter 40). This objective assessment using cardiovascular risk charts or computer programs is not a substitute for clinical judgement. The risk charts do not incorporate all risk factors for atherosclerotic disease and physicians need subjectively to adjust risk estimates for these other factors. For example, clinical evidence of end organ damage will increase the risk, as will a family history of premature CHD. With all this information an individual's absolute risk of developing CVD over 10 years can be estimated. A decision about antihypertensive or lipid lowering medication needs to be made in the context of absolute CVD risk and other clinical information, and a physician's judgement about individual management is always required.

To identify individuals at high multifactorial risk requires screening (see Chapter 41), which for the most part is undertaken in the primary care setting, either as new patient checks or opportunistically at other consultations. Other contacts with medical services through occupational health screening or specialized hospital clinics can afford the same opportunity. Risk estimation is based on an interview and some physical measurements including blood tests.

To estimate CHD or cardiovascular risk as accurately as possible the statistical models should be derived from prospective epidemiological data from the population to which the model is to be applied. The model should include all the important risk factors which are easily and routinely measured in clinical practice. The following variables are considered important: smoking, blood pressure, total cholesterol, HDL-C, diabetes, and family history of premature CHD. The Framingham model is widely used in the European, New Zealand, Sheffield, Joint British Societies', and NCEP-ATP III charts and related computer programs. However, the SCORE risk function is now more appropriate for CVD risk estimation in European countries. The HeartScore program provides a computer-based risk assessment and management tool for CVD prevention.

References

Anderson, K. M., Odell, P. M., Wilson, P. W., and Kannel, W. B. (1991a). Cardiovascular disease risk profiles. *American Heart Journal* **121** (1 Pt 2), 293–8.

Anderson, K. M., Wilson, P. W., Odell, P. M., and Kannel, W. B. (1991b). An updated coronary risk profile: a statement for health professionals. *Circulation* **83** (1), 356–62.

De Backer, G., Ambrosioni, E., Borch-Johnsen, K. *et al.* (2003). European guidelines on cardiovascular disease prevention in clinical practice. Executive Summary. Third Joint Task Force of European and other Societies on Cardiovascular Disease Prevention in Clinical Practice (constituted by representatives of eight societies and by invited experts). *European Journal of Cardiovascular Prevention and Rehabilitation* **10**(Suppl. 1), S2–S78.

Expert Panel on Detection, Evaluation, and Treatment of High Blood Cholesterol in Adults. Executive summary of the Third Report of the National Cholesterol Education Program (NCEP) (2001). Expert Panel on Detection, Evaluation, and Treatment of High Blood Cholesterol in Adults (Adult Treatment Panel III) final report. *Journal of the American Medical Association* **285**, 2486–97.

Haq, I. U., Jackson, P. R., Yeo, W. W., and Ramsay, L. E. (1995). Sheffield risk and treatment table for cholesterol lowering for primary prevention of coronary heart disease. *Lancet* **346**, 1467–71.

Haq, I. U., Ramsay, L. E., Yeo, W. W., Jackson, P. R., and Wallis, E. J. (1999). Is the Framingham risk function valid for northern European populations? A comparison of methods for estimating absolute coronary risk in high risk men. *Heart* **81**, 40–6.

Jackson, R. (2000). Updated New Zealand cardiovascular disease risk-benefit prediction guide. *British Medical Journal* **320** (7236), 709–10.

Jackson, R., Barham, P., Bills, J. *et al.* (1993). Management of raised blood pressure in New Zealand: a discussion document. *British Medical Journal* **307**, 107–10.

Joint British Recommendations on prevention of coronary heart disease in clinical practice: summary (2000). British Cardiac Society, British Hyperlipidaemia Association, British Hypertension Society, British Diabetic Association. *British Medical Journal* **320**, 705–8.

Menotti, A., Lanti, M., Puddu, P. E., and Kromhout, D. (2000). Coronary heart disease incidence in northern and southern European populations: a reanalysis of the Seven Countries study for a European coronary risk chart. *Heart* **84**, 238–44.

NCEP (National Cholesterol Education Program) (1988). Report of the NCEP Expert Panel on Detection, Evaluation, and Treatment of High Blood Cholesterol in Adults. *Archives of Internal Medicine* **148**, 36–9.

NCEP (National Cholesterol Education Program) (1994). Second Report of the Expert Panel on Detection, Evaluation, and Treatment of High Blood Cholesterol in Adults (Adult Treatment Panel II). *Circulation* **89**, 1333–445.

NCEP (National Cholesterol Education Program) (2002). *Expert Panel on Detection, Evaluation, and Treatment of High Blood Cholesterol in Adults (Adult Treatment Panel III.) Third Report of the National Cholesterol Education Program (NCEP).* Expert Panel on Detection, Evaluation, and Treatment of High Blood Cholesterol in Adults (Adult Treatment Panel III) final report. *Circulation* **106**, 3143–421.

National Heart Foundation (1996). Clinical Guidelines for the assessment and management of dyslipidaemia. *New Zealand Medical Journal* **109**, 224–32.

WHO (World Health Organization) (1992). *Prevention of coronary heart disease.* Report of a WHO Expert Committee. WHO technical Report Series 678. World Health Organization, Geneva.

Pyörälä, K. (2000). Assessment of coronary heart disease risk in populations with different levels of risk. *European Heart Journal* **21** (5), 348–50.

Pyörälä, K., De Backer, G., Graham, I., Poole-Wilson, P. A., and Wood, D. (1994). Prevention of coronary heart disease in clinical practice: recommendations of the Task Force of the European Society of Cardiology, European Atherosclerotic Society and European Society of Hypertension. *European Heart Journal* **15**, 1300–31.

Thomsen, T. F., Davidsen, M., Jorgensen, H. I. T., Jensen, G., and Borch-Johnsen, K. (2001). A new method for CHD prediction and prevention based on regional risk scores and randomized clinical trials: PRECARD and the Copenhagen Risk Score. *Journal of Cardiovascular Risk* **8** (5), 291–7.

Wallis, E. J., Ramsay, L. E., Haq, I. U. *et al.* (2000). Coronary and cardiovascular risk estimation for primary prevention: validation of a new Sheffield table in the 1995 Scottish health survey population. *British Medical Journal* **320**, 671–6.

Wood, D., De Backer, G., Faergeman, O., Graham, I., Mancia, G., and Pyörälä, K. (1998*a*). Prevention of coronary heart disease in clinical practice: recommendations of the Second Joint Task Force of European and other Societies on coronary prevention. *European Heart Journal* **19**, 1434–503.

Wood, D., De Backer, G., Faergeman, O., Graham, I., Mancia, G., and Pyörälä, K. (1998*b*). Prevention of coronary heart disease in clinical practice: recommendations of the Second Joint Task Force of European and other Societies on Coronary Prevention. *Atherosclerosis* **140** (2), 199–270.

Wood, D., Durrington, P., Poulter, N., McInnes, G., Rees, A., and Wray, R. on behalf of the British Cardiac Society, British Hyperlipidaemia Association, British Hypertension Society and British Diabetic Association (1998*c*). Joint British recommendations on prevention of coronary heart disease in clinical practice. *Heart* **80**(Suppl. 2), S1–S29.

Chapter 40

Non-invasive measures of preclinical coronary heart disease

P. Greenland

40.1 Introduction

Clinical characteristics such as sex, age, cigarette smoking, diabetes, blood lipids, and blood pressure are determinants of atherosclerosis and predictors of future coronary events (Grundy *et al.* 1999) as discussed in Chapters 10, 12, 21, 22, 35, and 43. Clinical practice guidelines for prevention of coronary heart disease (CHD) in Europe (Wood *et al.* 1998), the United States (NCEP 2002), and Canada (Stone *et al.* 2001) recommend measurement of these major cardiovascular disease (CVD) risk factors and estimation of global CHD risk, the primary goal being to aid the clinician in aligning intensity of risk reduction treatment with severity of overall cardiovascular risk (Califf *et al.* 1996). This alignment should maximize benefit/risk and efficacy/cost ratios. Although global risk assessment substantially improves CHD risk prediction over chance alone (Grover *et al.* 1998; Wilson *et al.* 1998), its predictive capacity is imperfect (Grundy *et al.* 1999; Smith *et al.* 2000). Therefore, a number of additional tests have been considered as alternatives or adjuncts to assess risk by detecting undiagnosed vascular disease at a preclinical stage (Smith *et al.* 2000).

In this chapter, we review four non-invasive tests for detection of preclinical CHD, and more importantly, for prediction of future coronary events in asymptomatic people: (a) coronary artery calcium detection by ultrafast computed tomography; (b) ankle-brachial blood pressure index; (c) B-mode ultrasound of the carotid artery for measurement of intima–media thickness; and (d) exercise stress testing. Each of these modalities has been studied in large samples of asymptomatic people in whom considerable follow-up and multivariable adjustment are available to determine incremental predictive value beyond standard risk factor measures.

40.2 Background: pretest and post-test probabilities

While early detection and early treatment of disease are appealing goals, the reality of most screening efforts is that they can create problems while trying to solve others (see Chapter 41). Since virtually all screening tests are imperfect, that is, they are not both 100% sensitive for the disease of interest (leading to false negatives and false reassurance), and 100% specific (leading to false positives and inappropriate labelling, further diagnostic work-up, and anxiety), any screening test must be targeted to the patient population that can benefit most, given the characteristics of the test. Efficacy of screening tests can be defined by the *predictive value* of the test, defined as the probability that the test result is a true reflection of the *presence* (predictive value of a positive test) or *absence* (predictive value of a negative test) of the disease. Thus, if sensitivity is below 100% (as is the case with nearly all tests), the predictive value of a negative test is always less than 100%, and many times, considerably below 100%. In addition, predictive value of a test also depends on prevalence of the disease in the population being studied. Prevalence is also frequently described as the *pretest probability* of disease, that is, the likelihood that disease is present *before* additional testing is employed.

An example of how the same test can be useful in one 'population' or patient sample, but not particularly useful in other 'populations', can be readily appreciated from a consideration of the use of exercise stress testing for screening of asymptomatic people versus testing of persons with symptoms suggestive of possible CHD. In the unselected screening situation, the pretest probability of CHD is estimated to be 10% among men, ages 50–59, with no cardiac symptoms (Diamond and Forrester 1979). From a meta-analysis of diagnostic utility of the standard exercise test (Gibbons *et al.* 1997), average sensitivity is 68% and specificity 77%. As shown in the 'Screening of 1000 low-risk people' section of Table 40.1, applying these estimates of test characteristics and pretest probability, predictive value of a positive exercise test is 25% (an increase from pretest probability of 10%). While the positive test result increased the probability of CHD, the likelihood of CHD is still relatively low; more likely that disease is absent than present. It is, therefore, unlikely that clinical decision-making will change based on positive test results in this type of patient population. Based on these considerations, screening for asymptomatic CHD in unselected populations is widely considered inappropriate (Gibbons *et al.* 1997; Screening for asymptomatic coronary artery disease 1996).

On the other hand, as shown in the lower part of Table 40.1, when pretest probability is intermediate, for example, in a 50–59-year-old man with atypical chest pain symptoms where pretest probability is estimated at ~59% (Diamond and Forrester 1979), a positive exercise test result yields a positive predictive value of 81%. This increase from pretest to post-test probability is very likely to lead to clinical action in this type of patient since the diagnosis of CHD is now fairly high (about 4 out of 5, versus only about 1 in 2 pretest). Consideration of test characteristics and pretest probabilities is well-established in the exercise testing literature (Diamond and Forrester 1979; Gibbons *et al.* 1997; Screening for asymptomatic coronary artery disease 1996). These principles have only recently been applied to CHD screening using other tests (Bielak *et al.* 2000; Callister and Raggi 2001; Greenland *et al.* 2001). In this chapter these principles will be considered in regard to each test in order to aid the clinician in deciding whether general screening, or more selected test use, is likely to be most appropriate.

Table 40.1 Estimates of test characteristics and pretest probability

		Disease		Totals
		−	+	
Screening of 1000 low-risk people[a]				
Test	−	693 TN	32 FN	725
	+	207 FP	68 TP	275
Pretest probability = 0.10		900	100	1000
Diagnosis of 1000 intermediate-risk people[b]				
Test	−	316 TN	189 FN	505
	+	94 FP	401 TP	495
Pretest probability = 0.59		410	590	1000

Sensitivity = 0.68; specificity = 0.77.

TN: true negative; FN: false negative; TP: true positive; FP: false positive.

[a] Predictive value positive = 68/275 = 0.25.

[b] Predictive value positive = 401/495 = 0.81.

40.3 **Thresholds for clinical action in an asymptomatic person**

In assessing an asymptomatic person, the clinician or researcher must decide the value of more firmly establishing the probability of CHD or other atherosclerotic disease. As discussed in the previous chapter, it has become standard practice to apply intensive risk reducing therapies in the clinical setting when global CHD risk is judged to be 'high'. In the United States, the threshold for intensive preventive action has been defined as 2% per year or higher for risk of a CHD event (NCEP 2002; Smith *et al.* 2000). Similar thresholds have been recommended by the Joint European Societies (Wood *et al.* 1998). In countries with more limited medical and financial resources, the threshold for intensive preventive action might be set higher than a risk of 2% per year (Wood *et al.* 1998). For purposes of discussion here, a threshold of 2% per year (or, 20% in 10 years) will be applied.

40.4 **Coronary calcium scores by computed tomography**

The presence of calcification within the coronary arterial wall is a highly specific marker of atherosclerosis; calcification is absent in the normal vessel wall (O'Rourke *et al.* 2000). Thus, the presence of coronary arterial calcification can be considered conclusive evidence of some degree of coronary atherosclerosis, and the test is 100% specific according to this definition. Coronary artery calcium can occur in early atherosclerotic lesions, but the amount of CC is greatest in advanced lesions in both men and women over the ages of 50–60 years (Raggi *et al.* 2000). Coronary calcium can be detected by various means, including cardiac fluoroscopy (Taylor *et al.* 2001) or conventional chest radiography, but CC detection is most commonly performed today using computed tomography (CT). In a direct comparison of electron-beam tomography (EBT) with digital subtraction cardiac fluoroscopy in 1309 subjects, the two measures were highly correlated for quantitation of CC (Taylor *et al.* 2001). In follow-up, both measures of CC predicted CVD events, but EBT calcium scores were slightly better predictors (Taylor *et al.* 2001). Cardiac fluoroscopy is also much less sensitive than CT for small degrees of calcium (Taylor *et al.* 2001), and fluoroscopy is more subjective and less quantitative than CT imaging. In addition, the preponderance of data on prognostic significance of CC is currently available from studies that used CT (mostly EBT). For these reasons, the remainder of this discussion will focus on CT imaging as the primary modality for detecting CC.

Two main approaches for CT detection of CC are in current use: spiral CT and electron beam CT. In either method, the amount of CC is typically quantitated using a scoring system developed by Agatston *et al.* (1990) in which the area of the calcified plaque is multiplied by an estimated coefficient based on the peak density of the calcified lesion. Scores range from 0 (no calcium) to 1000 − or even higher in severe cases. Mean and median values increase with age, and men generally have higher scores than women of same age (Raggi *et al.* 2000).

EBT uses an electron sweep of stationary tungsten target rings to generate X-ray images that can detect even small amounts of calcium. The rapid scan time allows for images that essentially 'freeze' the heart without motion artifact. Spiral CT imaging, which uses more standard CT hardware with recently developed software, has advanced rapidly and renewed interest in considering this technique for evaluation of coronary calcium (CC). Direct comparisons of the two techniques are uncommon, and most such studies are quite small due to the necessity to expose patients to radiation from both modalities. In one comparison study of 33 asymptomatic subjects who underwent both spiral CT and EBT within 4 weeks of one another (Budoff *et al.* 2001), quantitative CC scores were correlated ($R^2 = 0.68$), but EBT was more sensitive than spiral CT in detecting CC at the lowest end of the CC spectrum. In one direct comparison study (Budoff *et al.* 2001), high calcium scores (which have been found most predictive of future CVD events in various reports) were better correlated between the two modalities than were lower CC scores. Thus, it is possible that for detection of the most clinically important, that is, high amounts of CC, both types of scans may be acceptable. No studies have been conducted to compare the two types of CT for prediction of future CVD events. Whether it is critically important to detect very low calcium scores is unclear at the present time. However, more extensive data on CHD risk prediction are available using EBT. It is generally acknowledged that neither technique is reproducible enough to use serial scans to monitor patients with relatively low amounts of CC at first examination (O'Rourke *et al.* 2000).

EBT calcium scores correlate with extent of anatomical atherosclerosis and with risk of subsequent CHD events (Arad *et al.* 2000; Detrano *et al.* 1999; O'Malley *et al.* 2000; O'Rourke *et al.* 2000; Wong *et al.* 2000). Calcium scores can add incrementally to prediction of coronary angiographic findings beyond associations with conventional risk factors in *symptomatic* patients (O'Rourke *et al.* 2000). Several studies have also linked CC scores with risk of subsequent CHD events in *asymptomatic* persons (O'Malley *et al.* 2000). In published full reports, relative risks for coronary events in multivariate-adjusted models ranged from as high as 22 for extreme calcium score (Arad *et al.* 2000) to as low as 2.3 (Detrano *et al.* 1999). A meta-analysis (O'Malley *et al.* 2000) of five prospective studies (three full reports and two published abstracts) derived a summary relative risk for high calcium score of 4.2 (95% CI: 1.6–11.3) for hard events (myocardial infarction (MI) or sudden death). Summary data from the meta-analysis are shown in Table 40.2.

In a report published after the meta-analysis appeared, Wong *et al.* (2000) reported on a self-referred sample of 926 asymptomatic persons (735 men and 191 women, mean age 54 years) who were followed by questionnaire for a mean of 3.3 years after scanning; outcomes were

Table 40.2 Follow-up data from five studies of electron-beam computed tomography coronary calcium scores and coronary events in asymptomatic samples

Author, year	Number of people	Mean age (years)	Follow-up duration (months)	No. of hard events	RR for MI or death if high CC score
Arad, 1998	1173	53	43	2 deaths; 14 non-fatal MI	22.1, >160
Agatston, 1996	367	52	36–72	0 deaths; 10 non-fatal MI	16.9, >50
Sullivan, 1998	980	50	51	1 death; 7 non-fatal MI	1.0, >median for age
Raggi, 1999	632	52	37	8 deaths; 19 non-fatal MI	7.2, >median for age/sex
Detrano, 1999	1196	66	41	17 deaths; 33 non-fatal MI	2.3, >44
Overall (per O'Malley 2000)	4348	57	~42	28 deaths; 83 non-fatal MI	~4.2 (95% CI: 1.6–11.3)

After O'Malley *et al.* 2000.

CI: confidence interval; MI: myocardial infarction; RR: relative risk.

confirmed by medical record review. A graded relation was demonstrated between the extent of CC score and incidence of future CVD events. A score at or above the median in these relatively young people (CC score of 5 or greater) had a relative risk (RR) for new CVD events of 4.5 ($p < 0.01$) while a score at or above the mean (CC score of 143 or greater) had a RR of 4.6 ($p < 0.01$) for new CVD events. A score in the highest quartile (271 or greater) had a RR of 8.8 in proportional hazards models that adjusted for age, gender, high blood pressure, high cholesterol, past or current smoking, or diabetes. These results are generally consistent with the meta-analysis findings (O'Malley *et al.* 2000).

In another study published subsequent to the meta-analysis, Wayhs *et al.* (2002) reported on the prognostic significance of very high CC score (≥ 1000) in a case series of 98 asymptomatic people, ages 62 ± 10 years, who were followed for an average of 17 ± 11 months after undergoing EBT scan on self-referral. None of the patients had invasive or further non-invasive testing based on the abnormal EBT result. During follow-up, 35 patients (36%) experienced a coronary death or MI. Patients with coronary events had higher initial CC scores than patients not suffering an event (1561 ± 270 vs. 1199 ± 200, $p < 0.001$). The annualized event rate in subjects with a CC score ≥ 1000 was significantly greater than that of historical controls with severe abnormalities on myocardial perfusion imaging (25 vs. 7.4%, respectively; $p < 0.0001$). The authors suggested that an extreme CC score (≥ 1000) on a screening EBT in an asymptomatic person portends a very high risk of a CVD event in the short term. In general, these case series data are consistent with findings in other studies (Arad *et al.* 2000; O'Rourke *et al.* 2000; Wong *et al.* 2000) showing that patients with higher CC scores have a worse prognosis than patients with lower calcium scores.

Recommendations concerning appropriate clinical responses to high or low CC scores have been inconsistent (Hecht 2000; O'Rourke *et al.* 2000). For example, in reports in which the RR for high CC score is very high, authors have advocated relatively extensive use of EBT for screening asymptomatic people (Arad *et al.* 2000). Conversely, in studies in which the incremental values of EBT calcium scores are more modest (Detrano *et al.* 1999; Wong *et al.* 2000), as well as in the meta-analysis by O'Malley *et al.* (2000), a more cautious and targeted approach to the interpretation and use of CC scores has been advised. A technology assessment by the American Heart Association and the American College of Cardiology concluded that there is insufficient support to recommend EBT for general population screening (O'Rourke *et al.* 2000). However, given that the test appears to provide incremental risk information averaging in the range of RR = 4–5, EBT calcium scores are about as equally predictive as abnormal results from a number of other non-invasive modalities (to be discussed below). Thus, a strategy of applying this test indiscriminately (i.e., screening) does not appear justified, but selected use of the test in patients determined to be at intermediate pretest risk of CVD events seems appropriate (Greenland *et al.* 2001; O'Rourke *et al.* 2000; Smith *et al.* 2000). For example, if absolute pretest risk is judged to be only 5% in 10 years, a high CC score would be expected to yield a post-test risk estimate 4–5 times higher (20–5% in 10 years). Thus, CC testing should be worth consideration in such patients since it would cause the patient to cross the threshold for more intensive preventive action (Greenland *et al.* 2001).

40.5 Ankle–brachial blood pressure index

Peripheral arterial disease (PAD) typically refers to atherosclerosis of the arterial supply to the lower extremities and can be readily estimated non-invasively using the ankle–brachial index (ABI). To perform the ABI, the examiner measures systolic blood pressure in the brachial artery in both arms using a blood pressure cuff and Doppler detector in the antecubital fossa. The blood pressure cuff is then applied to the ankle, and the Doppler probe used to determine systolic blood pressure at the left and right posterior tibial and dorsalis pedis arteries. The ABI for each leg equals the ratio of the higher of the two systolic pressures (posterior tibial or dorsalis pedis) in the leg and the average of the right and left brachial artery pressures, unless there is a discrepancy ≥ 10 mmHg in blood pressure values between the two arms. In such a case, the higher reading is used for the ABI. Pressures in each leg should also be measured and ABI calculated separately for each leg. An ABI < 0.90 in either leg is considered evidence of PAD, and progressively lower ABI values indicate more severe obstruction.

When PAD is defined by ABI < 0.90, in general medical practice or in community studies, 15–20% of adults over age 55 have PAD, most of which is asymptomatic or produces atypical symptoms (McDermott et al. 2001; Weitz et al. 1996). Prevalence is markedly influenced by age such that few individuals under age 55 have abnormal ABI, but ABI < 0.90 is relatively common over age 70.

Asymptomatic PAD, or PAD that is clinically atypical, is at least 2–3 times as common as PAD with intermittent claudication (the best known symptom of PAD, described as pain, discomfort, or fatigue that occurs in a muscle or muscle group after repetitive use, and which subsides promptly with rest) (McDermott et al. 2001). Most patients with PAD will experience a benign course with regard to preservation of the affected extremity, but prognosis is most strongly influenced by occurrence of clinical CHD or stroke (Criqui et al. 1992; Weitz et al. 1996). Since atherosclerosis is a systemic disease, and many of the risk factors are identical in PAD and CAD, it is not surprising that patients with disease in one vascular bed experience increased risk of atherosclerosis in other vascular beds. Concurrence of PAD and CHD or stroke forms the rationale for considering PAD detection by ABI as a means of detecting asymptomatic patients who may be at heightened risk for CHD.

The ABI is a simple, non-invasive test that requires only inexpensive equipment. The procedure reliably identifies lower-extremity PAD. In experienced hands, test–retest reliability is excellent, and validity of the test for stenosis $\geq 50\%$ in leg arteries is considered to be high (sensitivity 90% and specificity 98%) (Ouriel et al. 1982). The ABI can be measured in a vascular laboratory or physician's office, and its more widespread use in general medical practice among asymptomatic people has been advocated by some clinical practice guidelines (Greenland et al. 2000).

ABI-detectable PAD correlates with clinical disease in the coronary and cerebral vascular beds. In population studies, persons with low ABI (<0.90) had higher prevalence of prior MI, coronary artery bypass graft, stroke, or stroke surgery, angina or congestive heart failure (Criqui et al. 1997). Prevalent CVD has been found in association with abnormal ABI in persons without symptoms of CVD in several studies (Criqui et al. 1991; Newman et al. 1993a; Ogren et al. 1993). A range of studies has also reported utility of ABI to predict future coronary, total CVD, and all-cause mortality (Criqui et al. 1992; Kuller et al. 1995; Leng et al. 1996; McKenna et al. 1991; Newman et al. 1993b, c, 1997; Vogt et al. 1993). For example, Criqui et al. (1992) found that ABI-detected PAD in men and women, average age 66 years, predicted a markedly increased risk of total CVD mortality (RR: 6.6; 95% CI: 2.9–14.9), CHD mortality (RR: 5.9; 95% CI: 3.0–11.4), and all-cause mortality (RR: 3.1; 95% CI: 1.9–4.9). These high RRs were obtained after excluding persons with known CVD at baseline and following adjustment for traditional CVD risk factors. Several other studies, in different asymptomatic populations, found similar results (Kuller et al. 1995; Leng et al. 1996; McKenna et al. 1991; Newman et al. 1993b, c, 1997; Vogt et al. 1993). Since, as noted, abnormal ABI is generally, but not exclusively, found in men and women >55 years of age (Criqui 2001; McDermott 1991;

Weitz *et al.* 1996), clinical use of the ABI for detection of PAD or risk assessment for CHD is applicable primarily in persons >55 years of age, or in smokers, or in persons with diabetes (Greenland *et al.* 2000). Individuals in these clinical categories with an ABI < 0.90 are typically at 2–5 times the risk of a CHD event compared to similar patients with normal ABI. Given that this age group, in the presence of CHD risk factors such as diabetes or smoking, is at least at intermediate pretest risk of CHD, an abnormal ABI can have the capability of influencing post-test treatment intensity.

40.6 B-mode ultrasound of the carotid artery for intima–media thickness

B-mode ultrasound is a safe, non-invasive procedure that can visualize the lumen and walls of selected arteries, including the carotid, aortic, and femoral. B-mode ultrasound has been validated for measuring intima–media thickness (IMT) in various research laboratories worldwide, and its reliability has been established in single- and multi-center studies (Chambless *et al.* 1996). Current ultrasound instrumentation with 8 MHz transducers is capable of identifying the two arterial interfaces (lumen–intima and media–adventitia) necessary for measuring IMT.

The carotid IMT measure is one of the best studied non-invasive markers of subclinical atherosclerosis (Barth 2002). The screening examination is performed bilaterally on the extracranial carotid artery segments. These segments are the distal straight 1 cm of the common carotid arteries and carotid bifurcations, and the proximal 1 cm of the internal carotid arteries. Circumferential longitudinal scans can identify IMTs that are >1.3 mm on the near and far walls of each segment (total of six walls per side). A template can be used to identify these IMT values. If the IMT value is >1.3 mm, the actual thickness of each lesion is measured with ultrasound instrument calipers.

IMT measures a single characteristic of atherosclerosis based on pathological studies documenting that both the intima and media are involved in atherogenesis and the anatomical progression of lesions. Increases in intimal thickness (fibromuscular hyperplasia) are associated with ageing, and medial thickness (smooth muscle hypertrophy) is associated with hypertension, even in the absence of atherosclerotic plaque. Associations between common carotid artery IMT and cardiovascular risk factors have been demonstrated in several cross-sectional studies (Mannami *et al.* 1997; O'Leary *et al.* 1992; Poli *et al.* 1988). Similarly, common carotid IMT has been associated with prevalent atherosclerotic CVDs in a number of cross-sectional studies (Bots *et al.* 1992; Burke *et al.* 1995; Mannami *et al.* 1997; O'Leary *et al.* 1992). Importantly, carotid IMT measurement is also a predictor of clinical coronary events (Bots *et al.* 1997; Chambless *et al.* 1997; Hodis *et al.* 1998; O'Leary *et al.* 1999; Salonen and Salonen 1991) as well as a harbinger of stroke (Chambless *et al.* 2000).

Among the strongest prospective data relating IMT measurement to incident cardiovascular events derive from the Atherosclerosis Risk in Communities (ARIC) Study (Chambless *et al.* 2000). In this study, the relation of carotid IMT to CHD events was studied over 4–7 years of follow-up in four US communities from samples of 7289 women and 5552 men aged 45–64 years who were free of clinical CHD at baseline. The hazard rate ratio comparing extreme mean IMT (1 mm) to not extreme IMT (<1 mm) was 5.07 for women (95% CI: 3.08–8.36) and 1.85 for men (95% CI: 1.28–2.69). The relation was graded (monotonic), and although the strength of the association was reduced by adjusting for major CHD risk factors, CHD risk remained elevated in the presence of higher IMT.

In the Cardiovascular Health Study (O'Leary *et al.* 1999), associations between the thickness of the carotid-artery intima and media and the incidence of new MI or stroke in persons without clinical CVD were studied in 5858 subjects ≥65 years of age. The RR of MI or stroke increased linearly with IMT. The RR of MI or stroke (adjusted for age and sex) for the quintile with the highest thickness compared with the lowest was 3.87 (95% CI: 2.72–5.51). The association between cardiovascular events and IMT remained significant after adjustment for traditional risk factors, showing increasing risk for each quintile of combined IMT, from the second quintile (RR: 1.54; 95% CI: 1.04–2.28), to the third (RR: 1.84; 95% CI: 1.26–2.67), fourth (RR: 2.01; 95% CI: 1.38–2.91), and fifth (RR: 3.15; 95% CI: 2.19–4.52).

A large number of clinical intervention or prevention trials have employed carotid B-mode ultrasound imaging to monitor changes in IMT over time (Blankenhorn *et al.* 1993; Furberg *et al.* 1994; Hodis *et al.* 1996; Lakka *et al.* 1999, 2001; Salonen *et al.* 1997). These studies have documented that the average annual IMT progression rates are 0.03 mm in the absence of intervention. In serial monitoring studies, careful quality control both of sonographers who perform the examinations and of readers who make the measurements is of critical importance. Although serial measurements can be standardized in well-controlled research settings, protocols for sonographers to monitor IMT over time in a valid and reliable manner may be difficult to implement in clinical practice environments. Thus, concern over lack of quality control represents a barrier to routine use of IMT for serial assessment of plaque progression/regression in medical practice. Provided that technical issues of this type can be resolved by using standardized protocols for scanning and monitoring of IMT, this method may be useful in follow-up of patients treated for plaque regression.

B-mode ultrasound may also be capable of providing information about susceptibility of individual plaques to rupture, with subsequent thrombosis and/or embolization. Several reports (Arnold *et al.* 2001; Lal *et al.* 2002; Matsagas *et al.* 2000) have indicated that B-mode densitometric evaluation grayscale intensity of plaques is feasible and valid when compared with the anatomical pathology of lesions. Although such information may not be specific for chemical components or metabolic by-products within the arterial wall, grayscale intensity tissue characteristics are known within reasonable limits. Highly echogenic structures include fibrous connective tissue such as collagen, minerals, and cholesterol monohydrate crystals. Hypoechoic tissue includes necrotic regions of the plaque, recent haemorrhage into lesions, and lipid-filled cores (Arnold *et al.* 2001; Lal *et al.* 2002; Lee *et al.* 1998; Matsagas *et al.* 2000). Hypoechoic plaques, particularly those with thin fibromuscular caps, in combination with carotid IMT measurements, may have the potential to identify unstable plaques prone to rupture. Further research is needed to establish this role for B-mode ultrasound (Fayad and Fuster 2001).

As discussed, measures of carotid IMT are independent predictors of transient cerebral ischaemia, stroke, and coronary events such as MI. Carotid IMT measurements are also incremental in risk prediction beyond risk factor scores alone. Based on this capacity, it can be concluded that carefully performed carotid ultrasound examination with IMT measurement can be considered for further clarification of CHD risk assessment. Relative incremental risk is in the range of 2–4, thus the use of this test should only be considered in highly selected patients in whom this level of incremental risk would lead to a change in clinical management (e.g., crossing a clinical threshold for action).

40.7 **Exercise electrocardiographic stress testing**

Exercise electrocardiographic testing is widely available and accessible, including in physicians' offices, and has been extensively studied in a large number of clinical and epidemiological settings. Several exercise protocols have been used in asymptomatic people, and various exercise-related and electrocardiographic parameters have been adopted to determine test outcome (Gibbons *et al.* 1997). The exercise electrocardiogram (ECG) is commonly used to assist in diagnosis of myocardial ischaemia in symptomatic patients, and guidelines have been developed and widely disseminated to define appropriate use of exercise testing in both symptomatic and asymptomatic patients (Gibbons *et al.* 1997).

In the most common approach to assessing the outcome of an exercise test, the examination relies on changes in the ST-segment to uncover evidence of ischaemia. Thus, exercise testing relies on the use of a physiological stressor (exercise) to provoke evidence of insufficient myocardial perfusion to meet the demands associated with this stress. In the asymptomatic person, the absence of ischaemic symptoms presumably derives from the individual's capacity to meet physiological demands of usual daily activity even in the presence of significant coronary arterial obstruction. However, with exertion and the attendant increase in myocardial oxygen demand, flow-limiting obstructive coronary atherosclerotic lesions commonly express themselves in exercise electrocardiographic findings (classically, a downsloping ST-segment characteristic of ischaemia) or by physiological abnormalities such as reduced exercise capacity, dyspnea, angina, or syncope. Since the findings associated with an abnormal exercise ECG test generally require substantial (flow-limiting) arterial blockages, more mild coronary arterial abnormalities usually result in normal exercise test results, leading to a so-called 'false-negative' test (Gibbons *et al.* 1997). Consequently, exercise testing for the purpose of identifying obstructive coronary lesions in asymptomatic people has been criticized because of a high rate of false-negative test outcomes (Gibbons *et al.* 1997; Screening for asymptomatic coronary artery disease 1996). In addition, many of the abnormal test results, especially in low-risk population or patient samples, are false positives. Predictive value of a positive test for significant angiographic stenosis in an unselected population has been reported to range from 25 to 72% (Gibbons *et al.* 1997). Some newer technologies, such as perfusion scintigraphy and stress echocardiography, may improve diagnostic and/or predictive capability compared to the exercise ECG alone (Blumenthal *et al.* 1996; O'Rourke *et al.* 2000). However, these newer tests are more costly, less widely available, and not as well-studied for risk prediction in asymptomatic populations as the traditional exercise ECG test. Therefore, this discussion focuses on the exercise ECG as the prototypical coronary perfusion stress test.

Despite general agreement that exercise testing should not be used in unselected people, a considerable number of studies have shown that an ischaemic finding in apparently healthy populations identifies heightened risk of future MI and sudden death. At least eight large studies have been conducted in asymptomatic people using exercise testing, multivariable adjustment, and long-term follow-up (Ekelund *et al.* 1989; Giagnoni *et al.* 1983; Gibbons *et al.* 2000; Gordon *et al.* 1986; Josephson *et al.* 1990; Laukkanen *et al.* 2001; Okin *et al.* 1991; Rautaharju *et al.* 1986). These studies are summarized in Table 40.3, and they permit an assessment of the incremental value of exercise testing in CHD risk prediction beyond standard risk factors.

Relative risks range from 2.8 to 10 for a positive test, with typical values in the 4–6 range. For example, Ekelund *et al.* (1989) studied 3806 asymptomatic hypercholesterolemic men in the Lipid Research Clinics Coronary Primary Prevention Trial. Each apparently healthy participant, aged 35–59 years, would have been judged to be at intermediate-to-high pretest CHD risk due to the presence of LDL-cholesterol $\geq$175 mg/dl as an entry criterion for the trial. All subjects underwent a submaximal treadmill exercise test at baseline before they

Table 40.3 Incremental prognostic value of exercise test in asymptomatic persons (studies using matching or multivariate analysis)

Author, year	n	Women?	Follow-up (years)	Type of multivariate adjustment	Relative risk for hard CHD event
Giagnoni, 1983	510	Yes	6.0 median	Matched w/controls on CHD risk factors	5.6
Gordon, 1986	3178	No	8.1 mean	MVA	4.2
Rautaharju, 1986	6205	No	6–8	MVA	3.5
Josephson, 1990	726	Yes	7.4 mean	MVA	2.8
Okin, 1991	3168	Yes	4.3 mean	MVA	4.7–6.2[a]
Ekelund, 1989	3806	No	7.4 mean	MVA	4.9–5.7
Gibbons, 2000	25 927	No	8.4 mean	Matched on number of CHD risk factors	8–10
Laukkanen, 2001	2682	No	10.2 mean	MVA	3.5–4.7

MVA: multivariable analysis.

[a] Positive test defined by non-standard ECG criteria.

were assigned to lipid-lowering drug (cholestyramine) or placebo groups. A positive exercise test was defined by ST-segment changes (ST-segment displacement ≥ 1 mm by visual examination, or ≥ 10 μV-s change in the ST-integral by computer code, or both). Prevalence of positive tests was 8.3%. During a follow-up period of 7–10 years (mean 7.4), mortality rate from CHD differed markedly based on exercise test results. In men with a positive test, CHD mortality was 6.7% versus only 1.3% in those with a negative test (placebo and cholestyramine groups combined). Age-adjusted RR for a positive test, compared to a negative test, was 6.7 in the placebo group and 4.8 in the cholestyramine group. In Cox proportional hazards models, risk of CHD death was 5.7 (95% CI: 2.7–12.2) for a positive test in the placebo group (4.9 (95% CI: 2.2–10.8) in cholestyramine group) after adjustment for age, smoking, systolic blood pressure, high-density lipoprotein cholesterol, and low-density lipoprotein cholesterol.

These results (Ekelund *et al.* 1989) are striking in several respects. First, they demonstrate that men with CHD risk factors can be stratified into low- and high-risk categories for future CHD events using non-invasive testing. Multivariable analysis conclusively demonstrated that exercise test results provided incremental risk prediction beyond standard risk factors. In addition, this study illustrates that high-risk individuals can benefit greatly from risk-factor modifying treatment. The investigators reported age-adjusted CHD and all-cause mortality rates per 1000 person years by treatment group and exercise test outcome. Comparing treatment effect in subjects with a positive exercise test, risk ratios for total and CHD mortality rates in cholestyramine versus placebo groups were 0.79 for all-cause and 0.55 for CHD mortality, respectively. Absolute risk reduction for CHD mortality was 5.8/1000 person years in the high-risk cholestyramine group. In contrast, the risk ratio in subjects with negative exercise tests in cholestyramine versus placebo groups was similar (0.79 for CHD mortality), but absolute risk reduction was only 0.4/1000 person years. There was almost no difference in age-adjusted total mortality rates between treatment groups in exercise-test negative subjects. These data are

Table 40.4 Potential role of exercise stress testing in asymptomatic men with CHD risk factors

Study, year	CHD mortality rates per 1000 person years		Absolute risk differences by exercise test outcome
	Exercise test −	Exercise test +	
LRC-CPPT, 1989	P: 1.9	P: 13.0	NEG: 0.4/1000 PY
	C: 1.5	C: 7.2	POS: 5.8/1000 PY
MRFIT, 1985	UC: 11.3	UC: 46.5	NEG: −1.0/1000 PY
	SI: 12.3	SI: 19.7	POS: 26.8/1000 PY

Refer to Rautaharju *et al.* 1986 and Ekelund *et al.* 1989.

C: cholestyramine group of LRC-CPPT; LRC-CCPT: Lipid Research Clinics–Coronary Primary Prevention Trial; MRFIT: Multiple Risk Factor Intervention Trial; NEG: negative exercise test; P: placebo group of LRC-CPPT; POS: positive exercise test; SI: Special Intervention group of MRFIT; UC: Usual Care group of MRFIT.

summarized in Table 40.4, along with similar data from the Multiple Risk Factor Intervention Trial (MRFIT). Using exercise testing to stratify risk in MRFIT, special risk intervention (SI) was associated with a marked risk reduction in exercise-test positive individuals while no effect of the special intervention was seen in exercise-test negative subjects. Data from these two trials suggest that exercise testing could be used to stratify apparently healthy intermediate-risk individuals into low- and high-risk groups and also identify patients most likely to benefit from risk-factor reducing therapies.

40.8 Summary and recommendations for using non-invasive tests for detection of subclinical CHD and prediction of CHD risk

Intensive reduction of CHD risk factors, including smoking, dyslipidaemia, and hypertension, has become the standard approach to CHD prevention in clinical medicine (NCEP 2002; Smith *et al.* 2000; Wood *et al.* 1998). Guidelines in various countries recommend that high-risk patients be identified by global risk assessment in the medical office setting (Califf *et al.* 1996; NCEP 2002; Wood *et al.* 1998). If patients can be shown to have coronary risk exceeding an agreed-upon threshold for intensive medical treatment (e.g., 20% CHD risk in 10 years) (NCEP 2002; Wood *et al.* 1998), the clinical management is straightforward. Based on evidence gleaned from the US National Health and Nutrition Examinations Survey (NHANES) III, ~25% of US adults fall into this high-risk stratum (Greenland *et al.* 2001). It has been suggested, based on Bayesian principles and standard clinical guidelines, that this quarter of the population, if asymptomatic, needs no further non-invasive testing to establish their high CHD risk (Greenland *et al.* 2001; NCEP 2002; Smith *et al.* 2000) and define appropriately intensive treatment.

Should non-invasive testing be considered in the remaining 75% of the US adult population? Based on NHANES III estimates (Greenland *et al.* 2001), ~35% of US adults are 'low-risk' for CHD, that is, <5–6% CHD risk in 10 years. These people have low global risk scores and no major CHD risk factor in the clinically important range (Greenland *et al.* 2001; NCEP 2002). Since all of the non-invasive tests described here have RR for a positive test in the 3–6 range (average ~4), it can be estimated that a pretest risk of <5% in 10 years would not quite achieve a post-test risk of 20% in 10 years in the presence of a positive ABI, exercise test, EBT, or carotid IMT study. Thus, such 'low-risk' persons are not good prospects for further risk stratification by non-invasive tests as the clinically important threshold of 20% in 10 years remains unbroken.

A large group of ~40% of US adults falls between the two extremes described above. This group has a global CHD risk estimate of 6–20% in 10 years, at least one major CHD risk factor above clinically important cut points, or a strong family history of CHD (Greenland *et al.* 2001). In these patients, a positive result with any of the non-invasive tests described here would yield a post-test probability of CHD events >20% in 10 years (assuming average RR of ~4.0). In addition, a negative test would sufficiently lower estimated risk and provide *additional* evidence against the need for intensive risk factor measures (especially drugs) (Greenland *et al.* 2001). Selective use of non-invasive tests, as summarized here, has been advocated (Greenland *et al.* 2001; Smith *et al.* 2000), and this approach is summarized in Table 40.5.

Finally, Table 40.6 provides an overview of the advantages, disadvantages, and proposed target populations for the four tests discussed here.

Table 40.5 Suggested approach to CHD risk assessment in asymptomatic patients

Risk level	Risk description	% of US population[a]	Recommendations
Low risk	Low global risk score and no major CHD risk factors	35	◆ Provide reassurance ◆ Encourage to adhere to healthy habits ◆ No further risk assessment for ~5 years
Intermediate risk	◆ One major risk factor outside desirable range or ◆ Positive family history ◆ Global risk assessment is 0.6–2%/year	40	◆ Consider further risk stratification by non-invasive procedures to test for myocardial ischemia and/or atherosclerotic burden
High risk	◆ Established CHD ◆ Other form of atherosclerotic diseases (stroke, abdominal aneurysm, peripheral artery disease) ◆ Middle-aged or older individuals with diabetes or multiple CHD risk factors ◆ CHD risk score >20% in 10 years	25	◆ Intensive risk factor intervention through a combination of life habit improvement and medical therapy ◆ Non-invasive testing not required to determine treatment goals

[a] Estimated from National Health and Nutrition Examination Survey (NHANES) III and adapted from Greenland *et al.* 2001.

Table 40.6 Non-invasive tests for CHD risk assessment in asymptomatic individuals

Test	Cut-off	Advantages	Disadvantages	Targeted population
Ankle–brachial index	<0.90	◆ Inexpensive ◆ Good reproducibility	◆ Not widely available outside vascular laboratories	Older than 55 years and smokers and/or diabetic
Carotid B-mode ultrasound	≥1.0 mm	◆ Safe ◆ Well-studied in research settings	◆ Not routinely performed ◆ Best validated predictive values of carotid IMT derived from highly controlled research labs (most clinical labs do not do this precise measurement); it is not clear if similar results can be derived in majority of clinical ultrasound laboratories	Older than 45 years of with ≥1 risk factor
Electron-beam tomography	Calcium score elevated (e.g., >75% tile for age and sex)	◆ 20 times faster than helical CT scan ◆ No contrast required ◆ Can play a role in accurately determining the coronary plaque burden	◆ Small dose of radiation	Intermediate-risk middle-aged adults with ≥1 risk factor
Exercise stress test	ST changes >1 mm	◆ Wide availability ◆ Low initial cost	◆ No data in elderly	Men older than 40 years with ≥1 risk factor; women with intermediate risk

References

Agatston, A. S., Janowitz, W. R., Hildner, F. J., Zusmer, N. R., Viamonte, M. Jr., Detrano, R. (1990). Quantification of coronary artery calcium using ultrafast computed tomography, *Journal of the American College of Cardiology*, **15**, 827–32.

Arad, Y., Spadaro, L. A., Goodman, K., Newstein, D., Guerci, A. D. (2000). Prediction of coronary events with electron beam computed tomography, *Journal of the American College of Cardiology*, **36**, 1253–60.

Arnold, A., Taylor, P., Poston, R., Modaresi, K., Padayachee, S. (2001). An objective method for grading ultrasound images of carotid artery plaques, *Ultrasound in Medicine and Biology*, **27** (8), 1041–7.

Barth, J. D. (2002). An update on carotid ultrasound measurement of intima-media thickness, *American Journal of Cardiology*, **89** (4A), 32B–38B; discussion 38B–39B. [Review.]

Bielak, L. F., Rumberger, J. A., Sheedy, P. F. 2nd, Schwartz, R. S., Peyser, P. A. (2000). Probabilistic model for prediction of angiographically defined obstructive coronary artery disease using electron beam computed tomography calcium score strata, *Circulation*, **102**, 380–5.

Blankenhorn, D. H., Selzer, R. H., Crawford, D. W., Barth, J. D., Liu, C. R., Liu, C. H. *et al.* (1993). Beneficial effects of colestipol-niacin therapy on the common carotid artery: two- and four-year reduction of intima-media thickness measured by ultrasound, *Circulation*, **88** (1), 20–8.

Blumenthal, R. S., Becker, D. M., Moy, T. F., Coresh, J., Wilder, L. B., Becker, L. C. (1996). Exercise thallium tomography predicts future clinically manifest coronary heart disease in a high-risk asymptomatic population, *Circulation*, **93** (5), 915–23.

Bots, M. L., Breslau, P. J., Briet, E., de Bruyn, A. M., van Vliet, H. H., van den Ouweland, F. A. *et al.* (1992). Cardiovascular determinants of carotid artery disease: the Rotterdam Elderly Study, *Hypertension*, **19** (6 Pt 2), 717–20.

Bots, M. L., Hoes, A. W., Koudstaal, P. J., Hofman, A., Grobbee, D. E. (1997). Common carotid intima-media thickness and risk of stroke and myocardial infarction: the Rotterdam Study, *Circulation*, **96** (5), 1432–7.

Budoff, M. J., Mao, S., Zalace, C. P., Bakhsheshi, H., Oudiz, R. J. (2001). Comparison of spiral and electron beam tomography in the evaluation of coronary calcification in asymptomatic persons, *International Journal of Cardiology*, **77**, 181–8.

Burke, G. L., Evans, G. W., Riley, W. A., Sharrett, A. R., Howard, G., Barnes, R. W. *et al.* (1995). Arterial wall thickness is associated with prevalent cardiovascular disease in middle-aged adults: the Atherosclerosis Risk in Communities (ARIC) Study, *Stroke*, **26** (3), 386–91.

Califf, R. M., Armstrong, P. W., Carver, J. R., D'Agostino, R. B., Strauss, W. E. (1996). 27th Bethesda Conference: matching the intensity of risk factor management with the hazard for coronary disease events. Task Force 5. Stratification of patients into high, medium and low risk subgroups for purposes of risk factor management, *Journal of the American College of Cardiology*, **27**, 1007–19.

Callister, T., Raggi, P. (2001). Electron-beam computed tomography: a Bayesian approach to risk assessment, *American Journal of Cardiology*, **88** (2-A), 39E–41E.

Chambless, L. E., Zhong, M. M., Arnett, D., Folsom, A. R., Riley, W. A., Heiss, G. (1996). Variability in B-mode ultrasound measurements in the atherosclerosis risk in communities (ARIC) study, *Ultrasound in Medicine & Biology*, **22** (5), 545–54.

Chambless, L. E., Heiss, G., Folsom, A. R., Rosamond, W., Szklo, M., Sharrett, A. R., Clegg, L. X. (1997). Association of coronary heart disease incidence with carotid arterial wall thickness and major risk factors: the Atherosclerosis Risk in Communities (ARIC) Study, 1987–1993, *American Journal of Epidemiology*, **146** (6), 483–94.

Chambless, L. E., Folsom, A. R., Clegg, L. X., Sharrett, A. R., Shahar, E., Nieto, F. J. *et al.* (2000). Carotid wall thickness is predictive of incident clinical stroke: the Atherosclerosis Risk in Communities (ARIC) study, *American Journal of Epidemiology*, **151** (5), 478–87.

Criqui, M. H. (2001). Peripheral arterial disease: epidemiological aspects, *Vascular Medicine*, **6** (3 Suppl.), 3–7. [Review.]

Criqui, M. H., Langer, R. D., Fronek, A., Feigelson, H. S. (1991). Coronary disease and stroke in patients with large-vessel peripheral arterial disease, *Drugs*, **42**(Suppl. 5), 16–21.

Criqui, M. H., Langer, R. D., Fronek, A. *et al.* (1992). Mortality over a period of 10 years in patients with peripheral arterial disease, *New England Journal of Medicine*, **326**, 381–6.

Criqui, M. H., Denenberg, J. O., Langer, R. D., Fronek, A. (1997). The epidemiology of peripheral arterial disease: importance of identifying the population at risk, *Vascular Medicine*, **2**, 221–6.

Detrano, R. C., Wong, N. D., Doherty, T. M., Shavelle, R. M., Tang, W., Ginzton, L. E. *et al.* (1999). Coronary calcium does not accurately predict near-term future coronary events in high-risk adults, *Circulation*, **99**, 2633–8.

Diamond, G. A., Forrester, J. S. (1979). Analysis of probability as an aid in the clinical diagnosis of coronary-artery disease, *New England Journal of Medicine*, **300**, 1350–8.

Ekelund, L. G., Suchindran, C. M., McMahon, R. P., Heiss, G., Leon, A. S., Romhilt D. W. *et al.* (1989). Coronary heart disease morbidity and mortality in hypercholesterolemic men predicted from an exercise test: the Lipid Research Clinics Coronary Primary Prevention Trial, *Journal of the American College of Cardiology*, **14** (3), 556–63.

NCEP (National Cholesterol Education Program) (2002). Executive Summary of The Third Report of The National Cholesterol Education Program (NCEP) Expert Panel on Detection, Evaluation, and Treatment of High Blood Cholesterol in Adults (Adult Treatment Panel III), *Journal of the American Medical Association*, **285** (19), 2486–97.

Fayad, Z. A., Fuster, V. (2001). Clinical imaging of the high-risk or vulnerable atherosclerotic plaque, *Circulation Research*, **89** (4), 305–16. [Review.]

Furberg, C. D., Adams, H. P. Jr., Applegate, W. B., Byington, R. P., Espeland, M. A., Hartwell, T. *et al.* (1994). Effect of lovastatin on early carotid atherosclerosis and cardiovascular events: Asymptomatic Carotid Artery Progression Study (ACAPS) Research Group, *Circulation*, **90** (4), 1679–87.

Giagnoni, E., Secchi, M. B., Wu, S. C., Morabito, A., Oltrona, L., Mancarella, S. *et al.* (1983). Prognostic value of exercise EKG testing in asymptomatic normotensive subjects: a prospective matched study, *New England Journal of Medicine*, **309** (18), 1085–9.

Gibbons, L. W., Mitchell, T. L., Wei, M., Blair, S. N., Cooper, K. H. (2000). Maximal exercise test as a predictor of risk for mortality from coronary heart disease in asymptomatic men, *American Journal of Cardiology*, **86** (1), 53–8.

Gibbons, R. J., Balady, G. J., Beasley, J. W., Bricker, J. T., Duvernoy, W. F., Froelicher, V. F. *et al.* (1997). ACC/AHA guidelines for exercise testing: executive summary. A report of the American College of Cardiology/American Heart Association Task Force on Practice Guidelines (Committee on Exercise Testing), *Circulation*, **96**, 345–54.

Gordon, D. J., Ekelund, L. G., Karon, J. M., Probstfield, J. L., Rubenstein, C., Sheffield, L. T., Weissfeld, L. (1986). Predictive value of the exercise tolerance test for mortality in North American men: the Lipid Research Clinics Mortality Follow-up Study, *Circulation*, **74** (2), 252–61.

Greenland, P., Abrams, J., Aurigemma, G. P. *et al.* (2000). Prevention Conference V: Beyond secondary prevention. Identifying the high-risk patient for primary prevention: noninvasive tests of atherosclerotic burden: Writing Group III, *Circulation*, **101**, E16–E22.

Greenland, P., Smith, S. C. Jr., Grundy, S. M. (2001). Improving coronary heart disease risk assessment in asymptomatic people: role of traditional risk factors and noninvasive cardiovascular tests, *Circulation*, **104**, 1863–7.

Grundy, S. M., Pasternak, R., Greenland, P., Smith, S. Jr., Fuster, V. (1999). Assessment of cardiovascular risk by use of multiple-risk-factor assessment equations: a statement for healthcare professionals from the American Heart Association and the American College of Cardiology, *Circulation*, **100**, 1481–92. Also available at <http://circ.ahajournals.org/cgi/content/full/100/13/1481>.

Grover, S. A., Coupal, L., Hu, X. P. (1998). Identifying adults at increased risk of coronary disease: how well do the current cholesterol guidelines work? *Journal of the American Medical Association*, **274**, 801–6.

Hecht H. S. (2000). Practice guidelines for electron beam tomography: a report of the Society of Atherosclerosis Imaging, *American Journal of Cardiology*, **86**, 705–6, A9.

Hodis, H. N., Mack, W. J., LaBree, L., Selzer, R. H., Liu, C., Liu, C. *et al.* (1996). Reduction in carotid arterial wall thickness using lovastatin and dietary therapy: a randomized controlled clinical trial, *Annals of Internal Medicine*, **124** (6), 548–56.

Hodis, H. N., Mack, W. J., LaBree, L., Selzer, R. H., Liu, C. R., Liu, C. H., Azen, S. P. (1998). The role of carotid arterial intima-media thickness in predicting clinical coronary events, *Annals of Internal Medicine*, **128** (4), 262–9.

Josephson, R. A., Shefrin, E., Lakatta, E. G., Brant, L. J., Fleg, J. L. (1990). Can serial exercise testing improve the prediction of coronary events in asymptomatic individuals? *Circulation*, **81** (1), 20–4.

Kuller, L. H., Shemanski, L., Psaty, B. M., Borhani, N. O., Gardin, J., Haan, M. N. *et al.* (1995). Subclinical disease as an independent risk factor for cardiovascular disease, *Circulation*, **92** (4), 720–6.

Lakka, T. A., Salonen, R., Kaplan, G. A., Salonen, J. T. (1999). Blood pressure and the progression of carotid atherosclerosis in middle-aged men, *Hypertension*, **34** (1), 51–6.

Lakka, T. A., Laukkanen, J. A., Rauramaa, R., Salonen, R., Lakka, H. M., Kaplan, G. A., Salonen, J. T. (2001). Cardiorespiratory fitness and the progression of carotid atherosclerosis in middle-aged men, *Annals of Internal Medicine*, **134** (1), 12–20.

Lal, B. K., Hobson, R. W. 2nd, Pappas, P. J., Kubicka, R., Hameed, M., Chakhtura, E. Y. *et al.* (2002). Pixel distribution analysis of B-mode ultrasound scan images predicts histologic features of atherosclerotic carotid plaques, *Journal of Vascular Surgery*, **35** (6), 1210–17.

Laukkanen, J. A., Kurl, S., Lakka, T. A., Tuomainen, T. P., Rauramaa, R., Salonen, R. *et al.* (2001). Exercise-induced silent myocardial ischemia and coronary morbidity and mortality in middle-aged men, *Journal of the American College of Cardiology*, **38** (1), 72–9.

Lee, D. J., Sigel, B., Swami, V. K., Justin, J. R., Gahtan, V., O'Brien, S. P. *et al.* (1998). Determination of carotid plaque risk by ultrasonic tissue characterization, *Ultrasound in Medicine & Biology*, **24** (9), 1291–9.

Leng, G. C., Fowkes, F. G., Lee, A. J., Dunbar, J., Housley, E., Ruckley, C. V. (1996). Use of ankle brachial pressure index to predict cardiovascular events and death: cohort study, *British Medical Journal*, **313** (7070), 1440–4.

Mannami, T., Konishi, M., Baba, S., Nishi, N., Terao, A. (1997). Prevalence of asymptomatic carotid atherosclerotic lesions detected by high-resolution ultrasonography and its relation to cardiovascular risk factors in the general population of a Japanese city: the Suita study, *Stroke*, **28** (3), 518–25.

Matsagas, M. I., Vasdekis, S. N., Gugulakis, A. G., Lazaris, A., Foteinou, M., Sechas, M. N. (2000). Computer-assisted ultrasonographic analysis of carotid plaques in relation to cerebrovascular symptoms, cerebral infarction, and histology, *Annals of Vascular Surgery*, **14** (2), 130–7.

McDermott, M. M. (1991). Ankle brachial index as a predictor of outcomes in peripheral arterial disease, *Journal of Laboratory and Clinical Medicine*, **133** (1), 33–40. [Review.]

McDermott, M. M., Greenland, P., Liu, K., Guralnik, J. M., Criqui, M. H., Dolan, N. C. *et al.* (2001). Leg symptoms in peripheral arterial disease: associated clinical characteristics and functional impairment, *Journal of the American Medical Association*, **286**, 1599–606.

McKenna, M., Wolfson, S., Kuller, L. (1991). The ratio of ankle and arm arterial pressure as an independent predictor of mortality, *Atherosclerosis*, **87** (2–3), 119–28.

Newman, A. B., Siscovick, D. S., Manolio, T. A., Polak, J., Fried, L. P., Borhani, N. O., Wolfson, S. K. (1993a). Ankle-arm index as a marker of atherosclerosis in the Cardiovascular Health Study: Cardiovascular Heart Study (CHS) Collaborative Research Group, *Circulation*, **88** (3), 837–45.

Newman, A. B., Sutton-Tyrrell, K., Vogt, M. T., Kuller, L. H. (1993*b*). Morbidity and mortality in hypertensive adults with a low ankle/arm blood pressure index, *Journal of the American Medical Association*, **270** (4), 487–9.

Newman, A. B., Sutton-Tyrrell, K., Kuller, L. H. (1993*c*). Lower-extremity arterial disease in older hypertensive adults, *Arteriosclerosis and Thrombosis*, **13** (4), 555–62.

Newman, A. B., Tyrrell, K. S., Kuller, L. H. (1997). Mortality over four years in SHEP participants with a low ankle-arm index, *Journal of the American Geriatric Society*, **45** (12), 1472–8.

Ogren, M., Hedblad, B., Jungquist, G., Isacsson, S. O., Lindell, S. E., Janzon, L. (1993). Low ankle-brachial pressure index in 68-year-old men: prevalence, risk factors and prognosis. Results from prospective population study 'Men born in 1914', Malmo, Sweden, *European Journal of Vascular Surgery*, **7** (5), 500–6.

Okin, P. M., Anderson, K. M., Levy, D., Kligfield, P. (1991). Heart rate adjustment of exercise-induced ST segment depression: improved risk stratification in the Framingham Offspring Study, *Circulation*, **83** (3), 866–74.

O'Leary, D. H., Polak, J. F., Kronmal, R. A., Kittner, S. J., Bond, M. G., Wolfson, S. K. Jr. *et al.* (1992). Distribution and correlates of sonographically detected carotid artery disease in the Cardiovascular Health Study: The CHS Collaborative Research Group, *Stroke*, **23** (12), 1752–60.

O'Leary, D. H., Polak, J. F., Kronmal, R. A., Manolio, T. A., Burke, G. L., Wolfson, S. K. Jr. (1999). Carotid-artery intima and media thickness as a risk factor for myocardial infarction and stroke in older adults: Cardiovascular Health Study Collaborative Research Group, *New England Journal of Medicine*, **340** (1), 14–22.

O'Malley, P. G., Taylor, A. J., Jackson, J. L., Doherty, T. M., Detrano, R. C. (2000). Prognostic value of coronary electron-beam computed tomography for coronary heart disease events in asymptomatic populations, *American Journal of Cardiology*, **85**, 945–8.

O'Rourke, R. A., Brundage, B. H., Froelicher, V. F. *et al.* (2000). American College of Cardiology/American Heart Association Expert Consensus document on electron-beam computed tomography for the diagnosis and prognosis of coronary artery disease, *Circulation*, **102**, 126–40.

Ouriel, K., McDonnell, A. E., Metz, C. E., Zarins, C. K. (1982). Critical evaluation of stress testing in the diagnosis of peripheral vascular disease, *Surgery*, **91** (6), 686–93.

Poli, A., Tremoli, E., Colombo, A., Sirtori, M., Pignoli, P., Paoletti, R. (1988). Ultrasonographic measurement of the common carotid artery wall thickness in hypercholesterolemic patients: a new model for the quantitation and follow-up of preclinical atherosclerosis in living human subjects, *Atherosclerosis*, **70** (3), 253–61.

Raggi, P., Callister, T. Q., Cooil, B., He, Z. X., Lippolis, N. J., Russo, D. J. *et al.* (2000). Identification of patients at increased risk of first unheralded acute myocardial infarction by electron-beam computed tomography, *Circulation*, **101**, 850–5.

Rautaharju, P. M., Prineas, R. J., Eifler, W. J., Furberg, C. D., Neaton, J. D., Crow, R. S. *et al.* (1986). Prognostic value of exercise electrocardiogram in men at high risk of future coronary heart disease: Multiple Risk Factor Intervention Trial experience, *Journal of the American College of Cardiology*, **8** (1), 1–10.

Salonen, J. T., Salonen, R. (1991). Ultrasonographically assessed carotid morphology and the risk of coronary heart disease, *Arteriosclerosis and Thrombosis*, **11** (5), 1245–9.

Salonen, J. T., Nyyssonen, K., Salonen, R., Porkkala-Sarataho, E., Tuomainen, T. P., Diczfalusy, U., Bjorkhem, I. (1997). Lipoprotein oxidation and progression of carotid atherosclerosis, *Circulation*, **95** (4), 840–5.

Smith, S. C. Jr., Greenland, P., Grundy, S. M. (2000) AHA Conference Proceedings. Prevention conference V: Beyond secondary prevention: Identifying the high-risk patient for primary prevention: executive summary. American Heart Association, *Circulation*, **101**, 111–16.

Stone, J. A., Cyr, C., Friesen, M., Kennedy-Symonds, H., Stene, R., Smilovitch, M. (2001). Canadian guidelines for cardiac rehabilitation and atherosclerotic heart disease prevention: a summary, *Canadian Journal of Cardiology*, **17**(Suppl. B), 3B–30B.

Taylor, A. J., O'Malley, P. G., Detrano, R. C. (2001). Comparison of coronary artery computed tomography versus fluoroscopy for the assessment of coronary artery disease prognosis, *American Journal of Cardiology*, **88**, 675–7.

US Preventive Services Task Force (1996). Screening for asymptomatic coronary artery disease. In *Guide to clinical preventive services*. 2nd edn, pp. 3–14. Williams & Wilkins, Baltimore.

Vogt, M. T., Cauley, J. A., Newman, A. B., Kuller, L. H., Hulley, S. B. (1993). Decreased ankle/arm blood pressure index and mortality in elderly women, *Journal of the American Medical Association*, **270** (4), 465–9.

Wayhs, R., Zelinger, A., Raggi, P. (2002). High coronary artery calcium scores pose an extremely elevated risk for hard events, *Journal of the American College of Cardiology*, **39**, 225–30.

Weitz, J. I., Byrne, J., Clagett, G. P. *et al.* (1996). Diagnosis and treatment of chronic arterial insufficiency of the lower extremities: a critical review, *Circulation*, **94**, 3026–49.

Wilson, P. W., D'Agostino, R. B., Levy, D., Belanger, A. M., Silbershatz, H., Kannel, W. B. (1998). Prediction of coronary heart disease using risk factor categories, *Circulation*, **97**, 1837–47.

Wong, N. D., Hsu, J. C., Detrano, R. C., Diamond, G., Eisenberg, H., Gardin, J. M. (2000). Coronary artery calcium evaluation by electron beam computed tomography and its relation to new cardiovascular events, *American Journal of Cardiology*, **86**, 495–8.

Wood, D., De Backer, G., Faergeman, O., Graham, I., Mancia, G., Pyorala, K. (1998). Prevention of coronary heart disease in clinical practice: recommendations of the Second Joint Task Force of European and other Societies on Coronary Prevention, *Atherosclerosis*, **140**, 199–270. Also available at <http://www.escardio.org/scinfo/slides/presentation.htm>.

Chapter 41

Screening for future coronary heart disease

N. J. Wald and M. R. Law

41.1 Introduction

Measuring risk factors such as blood pressure and serum cholesterol as a means of screening to identify people who will develop coronary heart disease (as well as stroke and other vascular diseases), has entered medical practice largely because of the aetiological importance of these factors. It has been assumed that an aetiologically important risk factor must also be a good screening test. In this chapter we examine risk factors considered as screening tests in general, and then examine how effective coronary heart disease (CHD) risk factors are in distinguishing individuals who will develop clinical CHD from individuals who will not.

41.2 Risk factors as screening tests

The *aetiological* strength of an association between a risk factor and a disorder is usually quantified by the dose–response relationship between the incidence of the disorder and increasing values of the risk factor. When risk (or incidence) is plotted on a logarithmic scale, a straight line relationship with increasing levels of the risk factor is commonly seen, indicating a constant proportional change in the risk of disease for a given change in the level of the risk factor from any pre-treatment level (see Fig. 41.1). The slope of the line indicates the magnitude of the proportional change. A convenient way of expressing this is to compare the risk in unaffected individuals in the highest fifth of the distribution of the risk factor with the risk in individuals in the lowest fifth of the distribution. In Fig. 41.1 the two risks are 50/1000/year and 10/1000/year. One divided by the other is the relative risk, which is 5. There are mathematical advantages in using the relative odds or odds ratio (i.e. $(50:950)/(10:990)$); the relative risk and the relative

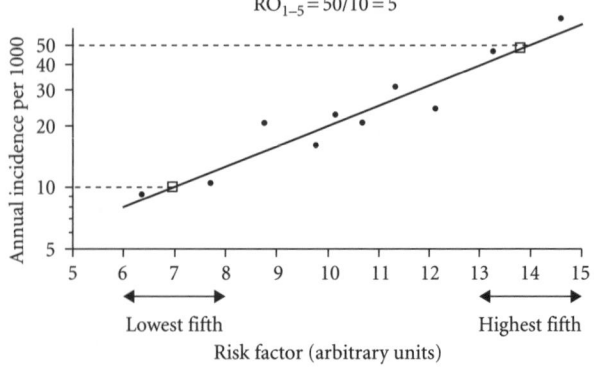

Fig. 41.1 Dose–response relation between incidence of a disorder and levels of a risk factor where the relative odds for people in the highest fifth of the risk factor distribution compared with people in the lowest fifth (RO_{1-5}) is ~5 $((50:950)(10:990))$. (Adapted from Wald *et al.* 1999.)

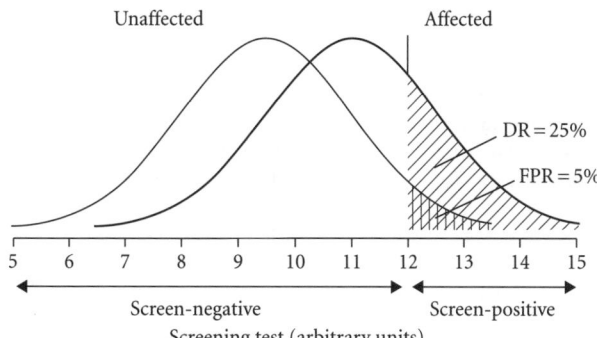

Fig. 41.2 Overlapping relative frequency distributions in affected and unaffected individuals where the detection rate for a 5% false-positive rate (DR_5) is 25%. The implicit vertical axis describes the percentage of affected and unaffected individuals according to the screening variable. (From Wald *et al*. 1999.)

odds are usually almost the same. The relative odds in the highest to the lowest fifth of the risk factor distribution can be abbreviated as the RO_{1-5}.

To assess the value of a risk factor as a *screening test*, on the other hand, the relationship between a risk factor and a disorder is best presented as two overlapping relative frequency distributions of the risk factor in two groups of people – those who will and those who will not develop the disorder in question. This is illustrated in Fig. 41.2. Individuals with positive results have values of the risk factor that are above some specified cut-off level. The detection rate (or sensitivity) of the risk factor used as a screening test is then defined as the proportion of all *affected* individuals (or those who become affected during a period of time) who have positive results. The false-positive rate (1-specificity) is defined similarly as the proportion of all *unaffected* individuals who have positive results. The performance of a screening test is often described in terms of the detection rate achieved for a 5% false-positive rate, which can be abbreviated as DR_5. In the example shown in Fig. 41.2, the DR_5 is 25%.

Provided, as is usually the case, the risk factor or screening test can be fitted to a Gaussian distribution, there is an algebraic relationship between the strength of the risk factor as measured by, say, the RO_{1-5} and the performance of the screening test as measured by, say, the DR_5 (Wald *et al*. 1999) This equivalence is independent of the prevalence of the disease.

Table 41.1 shows the quantitative relationship between a screening test and a risk factor in terms of the RO_{1-5} corresponding to a DR_5, assuming that the standard deviation in affected and unaffected individuals is the same, which is often the case, or approximately so. Serum cholesterol and blood pressure, both aetiologically important risk factors for coronary disease, have RO_{1-5} values of between 3 and 5 (i.e. the risk in people in the highest fifth of the distribution is 3–5 times higher than that in the lowest). Accordingly, from Table 41.2 they are very poor screening tests with detection rates of $\sim$15% for a 5% false-positive rate (DR_5 of 15%).

A screening test that is relatively poor, with a 30% detection rate for a 5% false-positive rate (DR_5 of 30%), is equivalent to a risk factor with an RO_{1-5} as high as 20, which is higher than most aetiological factors achieve. To achieve a DR_5 of 70% the RO_{1-5} would have to be $\sim$800.

It is not generally appreciated how strong a risk factor has to be before it can be considered a useful screening test. None of the cardiovascular 'causal' risk factors are anywhere near strong

Table 41.1 Quantitative comparison between a screening test and a risk factor

Variable considered as a screening test (Detection rate for a 5% (DR$_5$))	Variable considered as a risk factor (Risk in the highest fifth of the distribution of the risk factor relative to that in the lowest fifth (RO$_{1-5}$)
5%	1
10%	3
15%	5
20%	10
30%	20
40%	60
50%	100
60%	300
70%	80
80%	2000
90%	10 000
100%	∞

Adapted from Wald *et al.* 1999.

enough. There is therefore an apparent paradox. Causally important risk factors (which may account for most of the disease in a community) tend to be poor screening tests; they cannot discriminate within a population between those who will and those who will not develop clinical manifestation of that disease. The explanation is that, while many people are exposed to causes of a disease, not all succumb – there is sufficient variation within a population for many people to escape the hazards of exposure. Even if everyone smoked cigarettes throughout their lives, most people would not die of lung cancer, but smoking is still the major cause of lung cancer in the community.

The following may help to explain the paradox. In examining the aetiological potential of a risk factor, it is sensible to determine the relative risk of disease across the upper and lower tails of the distribution of the risk factor to maximize the chance of finding a difference comparing, for example, people in the top and bottom fifths of the distribution. In screening, however, the discriminatory potential is determined by examining the risk in the tail of the distribution (the screen-positives) with the risk in the whole population, including those who are screen-positive: that is, everyone in the population had they not been tested at all. This is appropriate because, by testing everyone, screening seeks to identify a small subgroup of the population that has a much higher risk than unscreened individuals. If the risk (or incidence) in an entire population is defined as 1 per 1000 and in the top fifth it is 3 per 1000 and in the bottom fifth 1/3 per 1000, the relative risk is 9 (3 divided by 1/3, since the 1000s cancel out), but the discriminatory potential (or likelihood ratio) is 3 divided by 1, or 3, much smaller than the relative risk of 9.

Table 41.2 Screening for CHD: detection rate (%) for a 5% and 10% false-positive rate according to combination of screening variables and number of measurements on different occasions. Men aged 35–64 years at entry to the study without a clinical history of CHD

Screening variables	No. of measurements (%)		
	1	2	3
For a 5% false-positive rate			
Total cholesterol alone	12	12	13
SBP alone	17	18	19
apoB	17	18	19
apoB, apoAI	18	19	19
apoB, apoAI, apo(a)	19	20	21
apoB, SBP	22	23	23
apoB, apoAI, apo(a), SBP	24	25	25
apoB, apoAI, apo(a), SBP, smoking	27	28	29
apoB, apoAI, apo(a), SBP, smoking, family history	28	29	29
For a 10% false-positive rate			
Total cholesterol alone	20	21	22
SBP alone	26	27	28
apoB	28	29	30
apoB, apoAI	29	30	31
apoB, apoAI, apo(a)	30	32	33
apoB, SBP	34	35	35
apoB, apoAI, apo(a), SBP	36	37	38
apoB, apoAI, apo(a), SBP, smoking	40	41	42
apoB, apoAI, apo(a), SBP, smoking, family history	41	42	43

Adapted from Wald *et al.* 1994, permission sought.

apoB ≡ LDL cholesterol; apoA1 ≡ HDL cholesterol; apo(a) ≡ Lipoprotein (a); SBP: systolic blood pressure.

In general, worthwhile screening tests measure some *consequence* of a disease, not a cause of it. For example, maternal serum alpha-fetoprotein, used in antenatal screening for open neural tube defects, is raised as a consequence of leakage of cerebral spinal fluid from the neural tube defect of the fetus into the amniotic fluid and thence into the maternal circulation. If alpha-fetoprotein were considered as a conventional risk factor, the risk of neural tube defect is ~2000 times greater in women in the top fifth of the distribution of maternal serum alpha-fetoprotein than in the bottom fifth (RO_{1-5} of 2000). This corresponds to a detection rate for a 5% false-positive rate of ~80% (DR_5 of 80%) (see Table 41.1). With modern antenatal screening tests for Down's syndrome the RO_{1-5} is ~5000, and the DR_5 ~85%.

In summary therefore: (a) to be a worthwhile screening test a risk factor has to be very strongly associated with a disorder; (b) causal risk factors are, in general, too weakly associated with the diseases they cause within a population to be useful as screening tests; and (c) useful screening tests are usually based on a measurement of a consequence of the disease process rather than a cause of it.

41.3 **CHD risk factors as screening tests**

Figure 41.3 shows the overlapping distributions of serum cholesterol and diastolic blood pressure in individuals who develop CHD. The detection rates for a 5% false-positive rate are only 15% and 13% respectively, even though, together with smoking, they account for the majority of cardiovascular disease in the western world.

It is often thought that combining information on several coronary risk factors would overcome the problem that individually they are poor screening tests, but this is not the case. Because the screening performance of each risk factor is low, the improvement in screening perform-ance from combining several of these risk factors is relatively small.

This was shown in an analysis from the BUPA cohort study, based on 229 men who had died from CHD by the end of 1987 (Wald *et al.* 1994). The serum concentration of apolipoproteins was measured on stored serum samples, including apoB (apolipoprotein B, the protein compon-ent of low-density lipoprotein (LDL) cholesterol, used as a measure of serum LDL cholesterol concentration), apoAI and apoAII (the protein components of high-density lipoprotein cholesterol), and apo(a) (the protein component of lipoprotein (a)). Data on smoking and family history had been collected and were used. The results are summarized in Table 41.2.

Using either systolic blood pressure or apoB in isolation, the detection rate was 17% (single measurement) for a 5% false-positive rate (i.e. the cut-off value that defines the 5% of men who did *not* die of CHD identifies only 17% of those who did). Using systolic blood pressure and apoB in combination, the detection rate increased to 22%. Additional risk factors added little to screening performance, and with six risk factors in combination the detection rate was only 28% for a 5% false-positive rate. The same conclusion is reached with a 10% false-positive rate. Multiple measurements of the same risk factor also add little to screening performance.

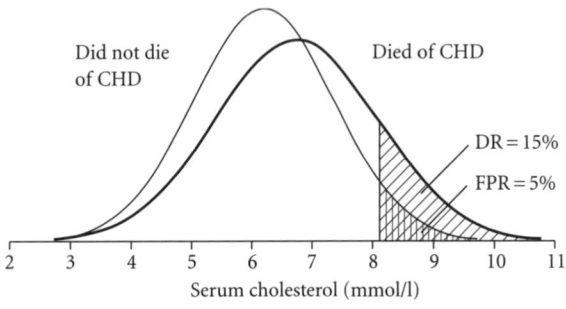

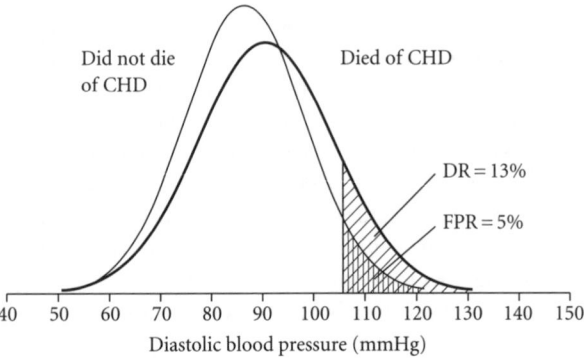

Fig. 41.3 Relative frequency distributions of serum cholesterol, blood pressure, and serum homocysteine in men who subsequently died of CHD and men who did not. (BUPA study data from Wald and Law 2003.)

The cardiovascular risk factors, even in combination, cannot be used to identify the majority of persons who will develop cardiovascular disease without also identifying a large proportion of those who will not.

The following illustrates why combining the cardiovascular risk factors does little to improve screening performance. Both systolic blood pressure alone and apoB alone detected 17% of those who died of heart disease at a 5% false-positive rate. If both were used together and a person were designated screen-positive (if either or both were positive), the detection rate would be a little less than twice as great (31%, calculated as follows: 17% of 100 cases detected by systolic blood pressure would leave 83, of which 17% would be detected by apoB, leaving 69, so 31% (100–31) would be prevented), but the false-positive rate would also be about twice as great – 10% (actually 9.75%). The critical question is whether this detection rate of 31% is substantially higher than those from using either blood pressure or apoB alone at a 10% false-positive rate. It is not: the detection rate is 26% for systolic blood pressure alone and 28% for apoB alone (Table 41.2) if the false-positive rate is set at 10% in each case. So the 'gain' in using both together rather than either one alone is an increase of only ~3–5% in the detection rate. Adding the second risk factor adds relatively little to the first one, and adding a third to two adds even less.

41.4 Existing cardiovascular disease as a screening test

In people who have had and survived a first myocardial infarction, the death rate from cardiovascular disease in the absence of any preventive treatment is ~5% per year for at least 15 years and probably for the rest of their life, regardless of their age (Law *et al.* 2002). The risk of a recurrent fatal or non-fatal coronary event is ~10% per year. This is an extremely high risk group. Identifying people in a population with existing cardiovascular disease should itself be regarded as a screening test, prompting medical intervention to reduce all known reversible risk factors. Adults with diabetes mellitus similarly have an increased risk of CHD and this itself should prompt preventive medical intervention.

41.5 Age as a screening test

In people without known cardiovascular disease age is the best predictor of CHD. From about the age of 25 the risk doubles every 8 years. Age itself can be regarded as a screening test. In respect of CHD and stroke, an age cut-off of 55 could be used as this would identify 96% of future fatal events which, with appropriate treatment, could be prevented or substantially delayed. Figure 41.4, taken from the Prospective Studies Collaboration (2002), illustrates several points of importance in relation to blood pressure as a risk factor for CHD; the same points apply to blood pressure and stroke. These are summarized in Box 41.1.

41.6 Is there any role for screening in the prevention of CHD?

The main reason for medical screening is to limit an intervention when the cost of intervening on everyone in a population is too great (either in terms of financial cost or in terms of the harm arising from the intervention). If a preventive intervention is inexpensive and either harmless or acceptably safe in light of the benefit achieved, there is no point in screening. In effect, screening is a barrier to entry, and it is probably not justified if there is no good reason for establishing such a barrier.

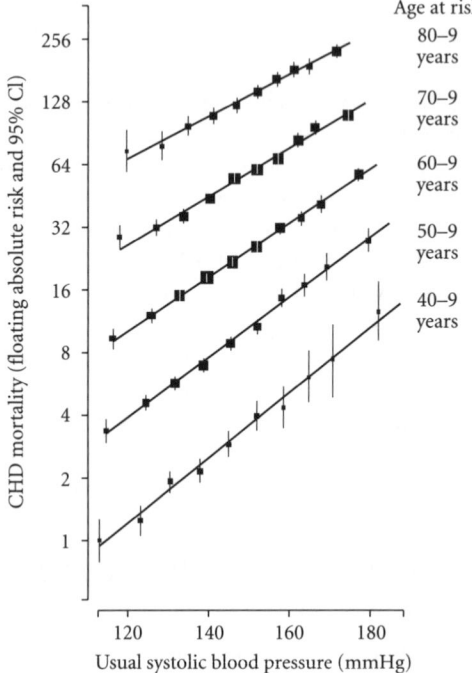

Fig. 41.4 CHD mortality rate in each decade of age versus usual blood pressure at the start of that decade. (Adapted from Prospective Studies Collaboration 2002, permission sought.)

Box 41.1 Coronary heart disease (CHD) risk associated with blood pressure (see Fig. 41.4)

1 At every age there is a straight-line relationship between disease risk and blood pressure with risk on a proportional (logarithmic) scale.

2 There is no threshold so a lower blood pressure is associated with a lower risk regardless of the starting level.

3 There is an approximate tripling of risk for every decade of life.

4 Risk approximately doubles from the 25th to the 75th centile of blood pressure.

5 The absolute risk of a disease event (vertical axis) is the same in a person with 'high' blood pressure as in a person 5–10 years older with 'normal' blood pressure or 10–15 years older with 'low' blood pressure.

6 It is illogical to treat a person aged 55 with 'high' blood pressure but not a person aged 65 with 'normal' blood pressure. Their risk is about the same so both will benefit to the same extent (both in relative and absolute terms).

7 Screening using blood pressure measurement simply identifies a small proportion of people for treatment a few years before the majority would achieve the same risk, and denies treatment to that majority even though they would benefit as much.

8 Age, not blood pressure, should be the main determinant for initiating treatment.

With CHD, prevention can be achieved through improvements in diet and lifestyle, and through the use of medicines to lower the reversible causal risk factors. In the first case, there is no disadvantage or cost (other than perhaps that healthy foods may be more expensive or less convenient). Here screening has no role to play.

Multiple risk factor modification achieved through taking a daily pill or pills – simultaneously lowering serum LDL cholesterol, blood pressure, serum homocysteine, and platelet 'stickiness' would prevent over 80% of first CHD events in an otherwise untreated population (Wald and Law 2003). The cost and side effects of such treatment would not justify its general use in younger adults, but for people who have a past medical history of cardiovascular disease or diabetes, and for those above an age of, say, 55, the benefits substantially outweigh the harm. Hence screening does have a role, but the screening is simple, involving only asking simple questions about a person's age and medical history.

References

Law, M. R., Watt, H. C., and Wald, N. J. (2002). The underlying risk of death after myocardial infarction in the absence of treatment. *Archives of Internal Medicine* **162**, 2405–10.

Prospective Studies Collaboration (2002). Age-specific relevance of usual blood pressure to vascular mortality: a meta-analysis of individual data for one million adults in 61 prospective studies. *Lancet* **360**, 1903–13.

Wald, N. J. and Law, M. R. (2003). A strategy to reduce cardiovascular disease by more than 80%. *British Medical Journal* **326**, 1419–23.

Wald, N. J., Law, M., Watt, H., Wu, T., Bailey, A., Johnson, M. *et al.* (1994). Apolipoproteins and ischaemic heart disease: implications for screening. *Lancet* **343**, 75–9.

Wald, N. J., Hackshaw, A. K., and Frost, C. D. (1999). When can a risk factor be used as a worthwhile screening test? *British Medical Journal* **319**, 1562–5.

Chapter 42

Screening for type 2 diabetes

D. G. Johnston, K. G. M. M. Alberti, I. F. Godsland,
M. Pierce, and S. Shepperd

42.1 Introduction

Macrovascular disease is the major cause of premature death in diabetes (Howard *et al.* 2002). The age-adjusted mortality from coronary heart disease (CHD) is 2–4 times higher than in the non-diabetic population. The risk is particularly high in the South Asian population in general (Balarajan 1991), and CHD and diabetes are recorded together on death certificates three times more frequently among those of South Asian origin compared with Europeans (Chaturvedi and Fuller 1996). There is a four-fold increase in cerebrovascular disease in African Caribbeans with diabetes relative to Europeans (Chaturvedi and Fuller 1996). Diabetes is the leading cause of renal failure, and of blindness in those of working age, in the UK (with type 2 diabetes predominant) and it accounts for one-quarter of those entering renal replacement programmes. Diabetes and its complications consume 5–15% of total healthcare budgets in the Western world, with the more recent estimates being at the upper end of this range (Laing and Williams 1989; ADA 1993a; Alberti 1997).

The major role of screening for diabetes is to diagnose it early in order to prevent or delay the complications. Macrovascular complications are often present when patients are diagnosed in the conventional way. At clinical presentation, 40–50% of people with type 2 diabetes are hypertensive (UKPDS Hypertension 1993), 14% have evidence of peripheral vascular disease, and >20% have evidence of CHD. The dyslipidaemia (elevated triglyceride; decreased high-density lipoprotein cholesterol (HDL-C)) of the pre-diabetic phase, particularly with impaired glucose tolerance (IGT), persists once diabetes has developed. The lipid disturbances are most marked in those with the most severe macrovascular disease (Panzram 1987) and it is believed the relationship is causative.

The arguments for and against screening for diabetes and how this should be done are presented in this chapter.

42.2 Definition of screening

We have adopted the World Health Organization definition of screening (WHO 2001):

> Screening is the process of identifying those individuals who are at sufficiently high risk of a specific disorder to warrant further investigation or direct action. It is systematically offered to a population of people who have not sought medical attention on account of symptoms of the disease for which screening is being offered and is normally initiated by medical authorities and not by patient's request for help on account of a specific complaint. The purpose of screening is to benefit the individuals being screened.

Table 42.1 Values for diagnosis of diabetes mellitus and other categories of hyperglycaemia

	Glucose concentration (mmol/l)		Plasma Venous
	Whole blood		
	Venous	Capillary	
Diabetes mellitus			
Fasting *or*	≥6.1	≥6.1	≥7.0
2 h post glucose load	≥10.0	≥11.1	≥11.1
IGT			
Fasting (if measured) *and*	<6.1 and	<6.1 and	<7.0 and
2 h post glucose load	≥6.7	≥7.8	≥7.8
IFG			
Fasting	≥5.6 and	≥5.6 and	≥6.1 and
and (if measured)	<6.1	≥6.1	<7.0
2 h post glucose load	<6.7	<7.8	<7.8

The term 'diagnosis' refers to confirmation of diabetes in people who have symptoms, or who have had a positive screening test (see also WHO 2003).

42.2.1 The definition of diabetes and other categories of impaired glucose regulation

Diabetes is diagnosed by WHO criteria (WHO 1999, Table 42.1) (in an asymptomatic patient, two of the following, or one test performed twice):

♦ Fasting plasma glucose (FPG) ≥7.0 mmol/l, and/or

♦ Casual plasma glucose ≥11.1 mmol/l, and/or

♦ 2 h plasma glucose in a 75 g oral glucose tolerance test (OGTT) ≥11.1 mmol/l.

Recent emphasis, at least in the USA, has been on the FPG criterion (≥7.0 mmol/l) (accepting that diabetes cannot be ruled out by a normal FPG alone).

An intermediate stage, impaired fasting glycaemia (IFG), is recognized where the FPG is ≥ 6.1 < 7.0 mmol/l. A 2 h OGTT value <7.8 mmol/l is normal, ≥11.1 mmol/l is diabetic, and intermediate values are impaired glucose tolerance (IGT) (when the FPG is <7.0 mmol/l).

42.3 Diabetes in the population

42.3.1 Plasma glucose in the population

The distribution of FPG, and the 2 h OGTT level, is bimodal in those populations where type 2 diabetes is highly prevalent, for example Pima Indians (Knowler *et al.* 1981). In other populations, the distribution curve is continuous without an obvious statistical cut-off. The WHO criteria have their basis partly in the bimodality of the plasma glucose distribution. They are also based on the fact that above the cut-offs the risk of developing retinopathy increases.

42.3.2 **Prevalence of diabetes**

Type 2 diabetes is the major form of diabetes in the population (90–5% worldwide). In UK adults >20 years, the prevalence is 3–5% and in those over 65 years it is >10% (Simmons *et al.* 1991). In some ethnic groups the prevalence is higher (e.g. for those of Indian origin in the UK, 11–13% if aged >20 years and 20–30% if 40–75 years, with similar figures for African-Caribbeans and intermediate figures for other ethnic groups such as the Chinese (Chaturvedi *et al.* 1994; Cruickshank 1997; Unwin *et al.* 1998; Pomerleau *et al.* 1999)). A high prevalence has also been observed in non-Europeans elsewhere (e.g. in the US, in the age range 45–74 years, the figures are 24% for Mexican Americans, 26% for Puerto Ricans, and 16% for Cubans (Flegal *et al.* 1991)). The prevalence of type 2 diabetes is rising (it has doubled in Australia in the last 20 years and tripled in the USA in the last 30 years). It has been predicted that the number worldwide will reach 210 million by 2010, from 110 million in 1994 (Alberti 1996; Dunstan *et al.* 2002).

The sexes are affected equally (King and Zimmet 1988). Both prevalence and incidence increase with age. In Europeans, the prevalence increases slowly until the mid-50s and rises more steeply thereafter. In some ethnic subgroups the prevalence rises linearly from an already high level in young adults (Zimmet 1989; Unwin *et al.* 1998).

In some population studies, there have been as many people with unknown as known diabetes (Keen 1966; Harris *et al.* 1987; Harris 1993; King and Rewers 1993; Jaber *et al.* 2003). In The Third National Health and Nutrition Examination Survey – NHANES-III, 5.3% of the population ≥20 years had known and 2.8% had undiagnosed diabetes (Harris *et al.* 1997, 1998). In developing countries, the percentage of people with previously unknown diabetes may be much higher (McLarty *et al.* 1989). The high prevalence of undiagnosed diabetes reflects the fact that 60% of patients diagnosed at screening do not volunteer symptoms (Keen 1966).

42.3.3 **The influence on population prevalence of recent modifications to diagnostic criteria**

Most prevalence studies are based on a single OGTT 2 h glucose (WHO 1985). It was calculated (based on NHANES) that FPG-defined diabetes prevalence would be lower (6.4% vs. 4.4%) (Harris *et al.* 1997). In the study of Unwin *et al.* (1998), the FPG criterion had the reverse effect, increasing the prevalence in three ethnic groups in the UK (Europeans aged 25–74 years, 7.1 vs. 4.8%; South Indians aged 25–74 years, 21.4 vs. 20.1%; Chinese aged 25–64 years, 6.2 vs. 4.7%). In a re-analysis of 16 European surveys totalling 26 190 people, the prevalence of diabetes was 4.1% with the FPG criteria and 3.6% with the 2 h OGTT (DECODE Study Group 1998). For individual surveys, the change in prevalence varied from –4% to +13%. Despite some extreme differences (Dinneen *et al.* 1998), overall no consistent difference has been observed. The individuals identified have, however, been different. In the DECODE study (1998), of 1517 people with diabetes by either criterion, only 28% met both criteria, 40% met only the FPG criterion, and 31% met only the 2 h criterion. In NHANES-III (Harris *et al.* 1998), 44% met both, 14% only the FPG criterion, and 41% only the 2 h criterion. The FPG criterion may select a greater proportion of middle-aged, obese subjects.

The new criteria have generally led to a lower prevalence of IFG in comparison with IGT (Harris *et al.* 1997; Mannucci *et al.* 1998; Larsson *et al.* 1998), although higher rates have been reported (Unwin *et al.* 1998). In eight populations, of those who had either, 16% had both, 23% had IFG alone, and 60% had IGT alone (Unwin *et al.* 2002). IFG could have a different metabolic basis from IGT (Tripathy *et al.* 2000; Hanefeld *et al.* 2003). IFG is 3–5 times more common in men than in women, whereas IGT is slightly more common in women (DECODE Study Group 1998, 2003; Unwin *et al.* 2002). IGT increases with increasing age whereas IFG plateaus in middle age.

42.4 **Selective screening for diabetes**

42.4.1 **Introduction**

There are several approaches:

- The whole population may be screened.
- Screening may be selective, targeted to high-risk subjects.
- Screening may be opportunistic, at a time of medical care or other screening.

The choice of approach is influenced by the characteristics of the screening test (sensitivity and specificity), and is critically affected by the disease prevalence. This can be illustrated as follows. If the whole population were screened, with FPG as the screening test, then a cut-off of 6.1 mmol/l might be selected, as this is the WHO lower value for IFG. If the population prevalence were 2%, this would have a sensitivity of 80% and specificity of 96% in comparison with the 2 h OGTT value (Hanson *et al.* 1993). For every 40 true positives, there would be 100 false positives and 10 false negatives. The predictive value positive (PVP) would be 29%. If the prevalence of diabetes in the population were 10%, then for every 40 true positives, there would be 18 false positives and 10 false negatives. The sensitivity would remain at 80%, the specificity would be 99%, and the PVP 69%.

Screening the entire population would be less efficient than screening subgroups with high prevalence, that is, selective or opportunistic screening.

42.4.2 **Selection of subgroups for screening**

Most of those discovered to have diabetes on screening have one or more predisposing factors (Cowie *et al.* 1994; Welborn *et al.* 1997) (Box 42.1).

Box 42.1 **Risk factors for type 2 diabetes**

1 Ethnicity

2 Age

3 IGT/IFT

4 Obesity

5 Physical inactivity

6 Hypertension

7 Previous gestational diabetes

8 Family history

9 Polycystic ovary syndrome

10 Dyslipidaemia

11 Established vascular disease

12 Others

Non-European subjects

In addition to ethnic influences on diabetes prevalence, there are ethnic influences on the frequency with which the diabetes is undiagnosed. In Coventry, UK, the proportion of the total with diabetes in whom it was previously undiagnosed was 0.65 in Europeans and 0.40 in Indian Asians (Simmons *et al.* 1991). In the northeast of England, the figures were 0.52 and 0.36, respectively (Unwin *et al.* 1998). The lower proportions in the Indian Asian populations may reflect a greater awareness of diabetes. In the USA, diabetes in adults was undiagnosed in 3.3% of whites, 4.1% of blacks, 4.2% of Mexican Americans, and 8.4% of American Indians (Flegal *et al.* 1991).

The middle aged and elderly

The prevalence of diabetes increases with age in all ethnic groups (Section 42.3.2). In those of European origin, the prevalence in the population >40 years is typically 5–8%. In those >65 years it is >10%. In Indian Asians, the figures have been typically >20% in the population >40 years. Diabetes also occurs at an younger age in ethnic groups where diabetes is most prevalent (Yue *et al.* 1996).

Known IGT and IFG

The prevalence of IGT in the USA is 6.4% at ages 22–44 years and 22% at 65–74 years (Harris *et al.* 1987; Harris 1989). Reported prevalence rates in the UK (Table 42.2) have ranged from 4.1% to 21.1% in those >40 years (Forrest *et al.* 1986; Williams *et al.* 1995; Unwin *et al.* 1998). Progression from IGT to diabetes occurs in 2–14.3% per year, depending on ethnic origin (Agner *et al.* 1982; Yudkin *et al.* 1990a; Motala *et al.* 1993; Heine *et al.* 1996; Alberti 1996).

Body mass index (BMI), FPG, plasma glucose levels after oral glucose, fasting insulin, fasting and 2 h proinsulin, insulin response to oral glucose, age, plasma triglyceride, and family history of diabetes influence the progression from IGT to diabetes (Box 42.2).

IGT is itself predicted, often by several years, by risk factors for CHD. Hypertension and hypertriglyceridaemia were predictive of both IGT and diabetes in the Rancho Barnardo study (McPhillips *et al.* 1990), while increased total and low-density lipoprotein cholesterol (LDL-C),

Table 42.2 Prevalence of IGT and IFG in the UK population

Population group	Age (years)	Prevalence (%)	Reference
Mainly white, IGT (London)	>40	4.1	Forrest *et al.* 1986
White with IGT (East Anglia)	40–65	16.7	Williams *et al.* 1995
African–Caribbean with IGT (London)	40–64	15.7	Chaturvedi *et al.* 1994
White with IGT (Newcastle)	25–74	12.5	Unwin *et al.* 1998
White with IFG (Newcastle)	25–74	18.9	Unwin *et al.* 1998
Chinese with IGT (Newcastle)	25–64	12	Unwin *et al.* 1998
Chinese with IFG (Newcastle)	25–64	14.5	Unwin *et al.* 1998
S. Asian with IGT (Newcastle)	25–74	18.7	Unwin *et al.* 1998
S. Asian with IFG (Newcastle)	25–74	19.0	Unwin *et al.* 1998

IGT was diagnosed in these studies using the WHO (1985) criteria, and IFG on the basis of WHO (1999) criteria.

Box 42.2 **Predictors of progression from IGT to diabetes**

1 *BMI.* The risk of diabetes increases when the BMI is >27 kg/m^2 (Knowler *et al.* 1981).

2 *Fasting plasma glucose >5.7 mmol/l.* This has been reported in South African Asians and Japanese (Motala *et al.* 1993; Kadowaki *et al.* 1984).

3 *High 2 h plasma glucose level following oral glucose.* Levels of >9.4 mmol/l and >10.6 mmol/l have been reported to be associated with an increased progression rate.

4 *Increased fasting insulin level.* Insulin has been predictive in the Paris Prospective Study, in the Nauruans, and in the Pimas (Charles *et al.* 1991; Sicree *et al.* 1987; Saad *et al.* 1988).

5 *Fasting and 2 h proinsulin.* This has been reported in the Dutch and Japanese (Heine *et al.* 1996; Inoue *et al.* 1996).

6 *Diminished insulin response to oral glucose.* This has been demonstrated to be predictive in Japanese, French, Nauruans, Italians, and Pimas (Kadowaki *et al.* 1984; Charles *et al.* 1991; Sicree *et al.* 1987; Riccardi *et al.* 1985; Saad *et al.* 1988).

7 *Others.* Other factors include age, plasma triglyceride, and a family history of diabetes (Harris 1989).

---

triglyceride and blood pressure (BP), and reduced HDL-C, were predictive in San Antonio (Haffner *et al.* 1990). Obesity, central fat, and physical inactivity have also been factors (Vaccaro *et al.* 1984; Fujimoto *et al.* 1994; Yamada *et al.* 1994).

IGT is a risk factor also for CHD, independently of diabetes. In the Paris Prospective Study, IGT increased CHD mortality two-fold at 2 years (Eschwege *et al.* 1985).

Since the introduction of the category of IFG, attempts have been made to determine its predictive value for diabetes. In Mauritius (Shaw *et al.* 1999), the sensitivity, specificity, and PVP were (respectively) 26, 94, and 29% for IFG, and 50, 84, and 24% for IGT. In most populations studied, the sensitivity of IFG as a predictor of later diabetes has been lower than that of IGT. The higher specificity of IFG warrants corroboration in other populations. In spite of its lower PVP, IGT identifies a larger number of subjects in the population who will develop diabetes, compared with IFG, in view of its higher prevalence (Section 42.2.3).

Attempts have been made to determine the FPG threshold for the prediction of diabetes (Shaw *et al.* 2000; ADA 2003). In Mauritius, 5.4 mmol/l was the value closest to the ideal 100% sensitivity and 100% specificity. In Holland, it was 5.7 mmol/l, for a Pima Indian population it was 5.4 mmol/l, and in San Antonio it was 5.2 mmol/l. For this reason, the American Diabetes Association (ADA 2003) is recommending reducing the normal FPG threshold (to 5.6 mmol/l). This would also render the prevalence of IFG and IGT more equivalent.

Indices of insulin resistance derived from the OGTT have been developed for diabetes prediction, such as the insulin sensitivity index based on glucose and insulin concentrations at 0 and 120 min (Hanley *et al.* 2003).

Obese individuals

In most studies, the risk of diabetes has increased progressively with increasing BMI (Westlund and Nicolaysen 1972; West 1978; Knowler *et al.* 1981). In Norwegian men aged 40–9 years, the incidence over 10 years was <1% if the BMI was 22–6, 4% if BMI 30–32.5, and 12% if BMI > 35. In the USA, the diabetes risk increased rapidly when the BMI was >24. The risk was 40-fold greater at BMI > 35 than at BMI < 23. A high BMI at age 21 years, and the weight gained in adult life, were also important risk factors (Chan *et al.* 1994). In Israel, although IGT increased progressively with BMI, diabetes was associated with a BMI > 31 (Modan *et al.* 1986). Obesity is a risk factor for diabetes in all ethnic groups (Daniel *et al.* 1999). Abdominal adipose tissue is especially important such that, even when BMI is taken into account, the waist-to-hip circumference ratio is significantly associated with diabetes risk (Ohlson *et al.* 1985).

The physically inactive

Physical training increases insulin sensitivity, muscle blood flow, and GLUT4 concentrations in muscle membranes (Koivisto *et al.* 1986). In retrospective studies, type 2 diabetes was three times more common in later life in former college students who had not been athletic at college in comparison with athletic students (Frisch *et al.* 1986). In prospective population studies, exercise protected against type 2 diabetes, the risk decreasing by 6% for each 500 kcal expended per week (Helmrich *et al.* 1991). The risk of diabetes over 13 years in UK subjects who took moderate physical activity was 0.4 (0.2–0.7) relative to physically inactive men (Perry *et al.* 1995). Differences in exercise may partly explain the ethnic variations in diabetes prevalence. In the UK Prospective Diabetes Study (UKPDS 1994), only 18% of South Asian women compared with 41% of European women were classified as physically active when they presented first with type 2 diabetes.

Hypertensive individuals

Most studies have investigated the prevalence of hypertension in established type 2 diabetes (typically a 1.5- to 2-fold increase compared with the population without diabetes (Drury 1988; Colhoun *et al.* 1999)). When the primary diagnosis was hypertension, the prevalence of both IGT and diabetes has been increased (Morales *et al.* 1993). In both untreated (Cederholm and Wibell 1985) and treated (Nilsson *et al.* 1990) hypertension, the prevalence of abnormal glucose tolerance (both type 2 diabetes and IGT) was 20–30%. In the Health Survey for England (1994), clinical diabetes was 2–3 times more common in older hypertensive individuals than in the age-matched normotensive population (Colhoun and Poulter, personal communication). In 12 550 US adults with hypertension aged 45–64 years, the prevalence of diabetes was increased 2.5-fold (Gress *et al.* 2000). The prevalence of diabetes was 28% greater in those who took a beta-blocker than in those on no medication. The evidence suggests that hypertension is associated with diabetes and that there might be an additional adverse influence of beta-blockers.

Women with previous gestational diabetes mellitus (GDM)

Type 2 diabetes is common following GDM (O'Sullivan 1984, 1988, 1991). This has been consistent in all ethnic groups. Predictive factors are:

◆ High initial FPG in pregnancy. In a European population (Damm *et al.* 1992), the odds ratio (OR) for the highest versus lowest quintile for FPG was 3.4 (confidence interval (CI): 1.8–6.1). In Californian women with previous GDM (Schaefer-Graf *et al.* 2002), the OR was 21-fold (95% CI: 5–96) greater in the highest quartile of FPG during pregnancy (FPG > 6.7 mmol/l; diabetes mellitus rate 37%) compared with the lowest quartile (FPG < 5.3 mmol/l; diabetes mellitus rate 0.5%).

♦ Abnormal post-partum OGTT. Although the majority of patients with an abnormal OGTT post-partum have a normal OGTT at 12 months (Damm 1998), the post-partum OGTT glucose area predicts a decline in glucose tolerance (OR upper versus lower quintile 4.9 (2.1–11.2)).

♦ Other predictors include the 2 h OGTT glucose, OGTT glucose area during pregnancy, the need for insulin therapy in pregnancy, low insulin levels in the pregnancy OGTT, pre-pregnancy weight, obesity in pregnancy, weight gain following pregnancy, previous GDM, and the occurrence of additional pregnancies (O'Sullivan 1979; Metzger et al. 1985, 1993; Kjos et al. 1995; Peters et al. 1996; Schaefer-Graf et al. 2002). Type 2 diabetes develops most frequently and most rapidly following GDM in those populations where type 2 diabetes is most prevalent (Yue et al. 1996).

Individuals with a family history of diabetes

Allowing for its late age of onset, Köbberling and Tillil (1982) calculated that 38% of siblings of patients with type 2 diabetes would develop diabetes by age 80 years. Similar results were reported for siblings by O'Rahilly et al. (1987), with a slightly lower risk for offspring of affected parents (Beaty and Fajans 1982). If both parents are diabetic, the risk for the offspring is greater than if only one is (Knowler et al. 1990). The familial tendency is increased when the diabetes develops early. It is increased also in some ethnic groups, for example Pima Indians and possibly in South Indians (McCarthy et al. 1992; Harrison et al. 2003). Features of the metabolic syndrome (Chapter 21) may be observed in relatives even when their glucose regulation is normal (Stewart et al. 1995).

Women with polycystic ovary syndrome (PCOS)

There is an increase in central body fat in PCOS even when women are matched for BMI (Robinson et al. 1992; Dunaif 1995; Franks 1995). PCOS is also associated with increased triglyceride and low HDL-C. The lifetime risk of diabetes has been estimated to be increased 6–7-fold (Dahlgren et al. 1992). In 254 women with PCOS aged 14–44 years, IGT or diabetes were increased 2.8-fold in comparison with 80 ethnically matched controls (Legro et al. 1999). A small retrospective survey has shown a 3- to 4-fold excess of deaths from diabetes in later life (Pierpoint et al. 1998). These women may also be at risk of CHD, as assessed by coronary calcification (Christian et al. 2003), although small prospective studies have not confirmed this (Pierpoint et al. 1998).

People with dyslipidaemia

When UK subjects in the upper quintile for serum triglyceride were compared with those in the lower quintile, the relative risk of developing diabetes over 13 years was 2.8 (1.4–5.8) (Perry et al. 1995). Low HDL-C was also predictive, but the significance was lost when triglyceride was taken into account.

Established macrovascular disease

In one UK series, undiagnosed diabetes was present in 4.3% of patients with myocardial infarction (Oswald and Yudkin 1987). Much higher rates have been reported. In a Swedish cohort of 181 patients, 40% had IGT and 25% had previously unrecognized diabetes at 3 months following discharge (Norhammar et al. 2002). The relative risk of developing diabetes on prolonged follow-up of a UK population of men with evidence of coronary artery disease was 1.53 (1.13–2.07) (Perry et al. 1995). A raised HbA1c on admission is also associated with a poorer prognosis (Yudkin et al. 1988).

Patients with peripheral vascular disease have a higher prevalence of diabetes (Gill *et al.* 1996; Treweek *et al.* 1998), as do patients with acute stroke (36% in one series, in the majority of whom the diabetes was undiagnosed (Gray *et al.* 1987)).

Others

Weight at birth is a determinant of later glucose tolerance. In early studies of 64-year-old men in Hertfordshire, UK (Hales *et al.* 1991), those <2.5 kg at birth were seven times more likely to have IGT or diabetes than those >4.4 kg at birth. Similar trends were found with infant weights at 1 year. With both birthweight and weight at 1 year, adult obesity compounded the risk. This relationship between birthweight and hyperglycaemia has been confirmed in other populations (Petry and Hales 1999). The relationship may be stronger for thinness at birth than for birthweight. In high-risk populations, for example Native or Mexican Americans, the relationship between glucose intolerance and size at birth is less clear and may be U-shaped.

Although an accepted factor in the pathogenesis of hyperglycaemia, the proportion of people with diabetes accounted for by smallness at birth may be small (McCance *et al.* 1994).

Spouses of patients with type 2 diabetes may be at increased risk. In a UK study (Khan *et al.* 2003), the relative risk of diabetes was 2.11 (95% CI: 1.74–5.10) and for any degree of glucose dysregulation, it was 2.32 (1.87–3.98).

Uric acid has been a risk factor in several studies (Herman *et al.* 1976; Perry *et al.* 1995).

42.4.3 The selection of individuals at risk of diabetes

Introduction

Prior selection can increase the yield of positive tests, that is, increase the PVP.

The ADA Expert Committee (1997, 2003) recommended the following criteria for screening:

1 Individuals >45 years.

2 Younger individuals if they fulfilled one of the following criteria;
   - BMI $\geq$ 27 kg/m^2.
   - Family history (first degree).
   - High-risk ethnic group.
   - Previous GDM or macrosomic baby (>4.1 kg).
   - Hypertension ($\geq$140/90).
   - HDL-C <0.9 mmol/l and/or triglyceride $\geq$2.8 mmol/l.
   - Previous known IGT or IFG.

The US Preventive Services Task Force (USPTF 2003) concluded that the evidence was insufficient to recommend routinely screening adults, unless they had hypertension or hyperlipidaemia.

Diabetes UK issued a Position Statement in November 2002 recommending screening for those at increased risk as follows:

- White people >40 years and people from black, Asian, and minority ethnic groups >25, with:
  - a first degree family history of diabetes and/or
  - who are overweight or obese (BMI 25–30 kg/m^2 and above), and who have a sedentary lifestyle and/or
  - who have CHD, cerebrovascular disease, peripheral vascular disease, or hypertension and/or

- women with previous GDM;
- obese women with PCOS;
- known IGT or IFG.

Other organizations have produced guidelines which vary in detail (Colagiuri *et al.* 2002*b*).

Selection using questionnaires

Self-reported questionnaires which focused on the symptoms of diabetes have been disappointing. For example, using an ADA questionnaire, 30–40% of a UK population reported feeling extremely tired and having urinary frequency, with 17% reporting excessive thirst (ADA 1993*b*; Burden and Burden 1994). The sensitivity was only 46% at specificity 59%.

Questionnaires based on risk factors for diabetes have performed better. One which used age, sex, obesity, sedentary lifestyle, family history, and a previous macrosomic baby, had a sensitivity of 79%, specificity 65%, PVP 10% (Herman *et al.* 1995). For a Caucasian Dutch population, a questionnaire contained items which were independently and significantly ($p < 0.05$) associated with undiagnosed diabetes (Ruige *et al.* 1997). These were: intermittent claudication; dyspnoea; thirst; age; sex; obesity; family history; use of antihypertensive drugs, and reluctance to exercise. In a comparison with this, the ADA questionnaire (1993*b*) and that of Herman *et al.* (1995), the sensitivities were 72, 59, and 72%, respectively; the specificities were 56, 57, and 55%; the PVPs were 6.5, 5.6, and 6.4%.

It is unlikely that a single questionnaire would be suitable for all ethnic groups.

Selection using existing primary care databases

A predictive model to identify undiagnosed diabetes, using only data routinely available in the individuals' primary care records (model 1), was compared with predictive models requiring other information (model 2), or requiring also a physical examination (model 3; Baan *et al.* 1999). For model 1, the routinely available data were as follows: age, sex, obesity, antihypertensive medication, lipid lowering medication, previous GDM, and known cardiovascular disease. For model 2, the questions covered BMI, family history, smoking, symptoms of cardiovascular disease, and an assessment of physical activity (only cycling – the study was based in Holland!). For model 3, the physical examination recorded BP and the waist:hip circumference ratio. The sensitivity and specificity of model 1 were 55% and 78%, respectively, with a PVP of 8%. Receiver operating characteristic (ROC) curves were constructed for the three models; physical examination added nothing of significance and, although the second model performed better than the first, the 95% confidence intervals for the areas under the ROC curves overlapped. This study suggested that even simple information on primary care databases may be valuable in selection. In other countries, even the basic information required for model 1 may not available. A risk score for use with some of the more comprehensive primary care databases in the UK has been described (Griffin *et al.* 2000; Park *et al.* 2002). This included age, height, weight, waist and hip circumferences, BP, medication, and family history of diabetes. For a specificity of 78%, it predicted an $HbA_{1c} \geq 7.0\%$ with a sensitivity of 51% in subjects aged 39–78 years and the area under the ROC curve was 74%. This Cambridge risk score has been applied to a Dutch population where 73% of those who turned out to have diabetes on an OGTT would have been detected by the risk score (Spijkerman *et al.* 2002). There was a high false positive rate (1037 of 2297) in this population, which would limit the usefulness of the risk score as an initial screen for diabetes. The false positives had increased mortality, however, suggesting that, even without diabetes, they constituted a subgroup for lifestyle or other intervention.

The likely efficiency of selective screening

In the National Health Interview Survey (NHIS) in the USA (Cowie *et al.* 1994), risk factors (age ≥ 40 years, black or Hispanic origin, parental history of diabetes, and body weight $\geq 120\%$ of desirable) were sought by questionnaire in 19 680 adults ≥ 18 years. Of those not known to have diabetes, 77% had one or more risk factors, age ≥ 40 years and obesity being the most frequent. Accepting that a high proportion of the adult population are eligible, the efficiency with which such subjects are in reality identified and screened has received minimal attention. In the NHIS survey, 39% of those with three or more risk factors had been screened in the previous 12 months (Cowie *et al.* 1994). In those with four or more risk factors, 57% had been screened.

42.4.4 **The site where screening should be implemented**

The most practical site for selective screening is primary care. Voluntary screening has had limited success when structured in other ways. For example, following an organized campaign in New Zealand, only 34% of those at risk were actually screened (Lawrenson *et al.* 1993). Higher proportions have presented for testing in other organized campaigns.

42.4.5 **Opportunistic screening**

Systematic opportunistic screening can be effective in call and recall, as demonstrated for cervical cytology (Pierce *et al.* 1989). There are no data for diabetes.

42.5 **The case for screening: potential benefits**

42.5.1 **Potential short-term benefit: acute symptoms**

Public awareness of the symptoms of diabetes is low (Jackson *et al.* 1991; Singh *et al.* 1994). When questioned directly, the majority of patients at clinical presentation have specific symptoms and in 40% these have been present for >12 months (Singh *et al.* 1992).

42.5.2 **Potential long-term benefit for complications**

Introduction

At clinical presentation, 40% of patients have microvascular complications (retinopathy, nephropathy, neuropathy; UKPDS 1991). These require a minimum of 5 years to develop and it has been estimated that the diabetes has been undetected for 9–12 years (Harris *et al.* 1992). There are suggestions that early diagnosis is associated with a decreased prevalence of microvascular disease. In 109 people diagnosed following screening, only 8% initially had retinopathy in comparison with 22% in those who presented clinically in the UKPDS (Davies *et al.* 1996). In the UKPDS, participants who at entry had the lowest FPG levels (<7.8 mmol/l), and may therefore have been detected at an early stage in their disease, had the lowest rates of retinopathy, abnormal biothesiometer measurements, and erectile dysfunction during follow-up (Colagiuri *et al.* 2002*a*). Although there are suggestive data from Germany that early diagnosis permitting early intervention may improve outcomes (Schneider *et al.* 1993, 1996), controlled trial data are lacking.

There is no evidence currently that those who are diagnosed early with diabetes, as a result of screening, show a decreased prevalence of macrovascular disease. In the small study of Davies *et al.* (1996), hypertension was present in those diagnosed following screening with the same or greater frequency as in patients who presented clinically; for example 48% had a systolic

BP >160 mmHg and 68% had a diastolic BP >90 mmHg. Both figures were slightly greater than in the conventionally diagnosed diabetic population.

Potential long-term benefit: CHD

In the UKPDS, intensive blood glucose control was associated with a statistically insignificant reduction in cardiovascular events (14.7 vs. 17.4 per 1000 patient years). Congestive cardiac failure, angina, and all-cause mortality were unaffected.

Effective BP control reduces cardiovascular events by 50% (Hansson *et al.* 1998; UKPDS 1998*b*). Therapy of isolated systolic hypertension in older patients with diabetes has led to a 34–69% reduction in events (Curb *et al.* 1996; Tuomilehto *et al.* 1999). Therapy with an angiotensin-converting enzyme (ACE) inhibitor, ramipril, in patients with type 2 diabetes and one additional risk factor led to a 22% reduction in events and 16% reduction in all-cause mortality, irrespective of the BP at the outset (Yusuf *et al.* 2000). Treatment of dyslipidaemia induces the same relative reduction in CHD events in diabetes as in the non-diabetic population (relative risk decreased by 19–42%) in secondary prevention studies (Pyorala *et al.* 1997; Elkeles *et al.* 1998; LIPID Study Group 1998; Haffner *et al.* 1999; Rubins *et al.* 1999; MRC/BHF Study 2002). In primary prevention studies, there have been insufficient patients with type 2 diabetes for conclusive evidence, although in the Heart Protection Study, vascular events were reduced by 20 to 25% over 5 years in diabetic patients receiving simvastatin (MRC/BHF 2002). Aspirin reduces CHD events by 30% in the diabetic and non-diabetic populations (Colwell 1997; ADA 2000; Hayden *et al.* 2002).

People with diabetes identified following screening would include many whose condition would never have become apparent clinically because they would have died, mainly from cardiovascular disease, with their diabetes undiagnosed (Goyder and Irwig 1999). Early diagnosis would provide an opportunity to initiate BP-lowering therapy and lipid modifying medication, and aspirin, before macrovascular complications developed. The management of type 2 diabetes in future will involve intervention to correct multiple risk factors, and there is preliminary evidence that this is beneficial (Gaede *et al.* 1999). If the UKPDS results, and the results from other intervention studies, can be extrapolated to diabetes diagnosed following screening, interventions could decrease the frequency and/or severity of complications in the first few years. It has not, however, been established that such early intervention is beneficial.

Potential long-term benefit: amputations

The cumulative incidence of amputation is 3–11% over 20–5 years (Humphrey *et al.* 1994; Resnick *et al.* 1999). In UKPDS, 1–2% of patients required amputation over 10 years follow-up. In Wisconsin, 7% of patients required amputation within 14 years (Moss *et al.* 1999).

In UKPDS (1998*a, b*), effective blood glucose and BP control did not reduce amputations significantly.

Intensive programmes may reduce the frequency of foot ulceration and amputations by 60% (Malone *et al.* 1989; Litzelman *et al.* 1993), although in a recent systematic review the effectiveness of such programmes overall was inconclusive (Mason *et al.* 1999*a, b*). There is no evidence that early intervention would have a better outcome.

Potential long-term benefit: retinopathy

In patients with diabetes of 20–5 years' duration, 5–15% will become blind over 10 years and 35–45% will develop significant visual deterioration (Moss *et al.* 1988, 1994). In prospective studies, intensive glucose control decreases retinopathy by 29–40% (Ohkubo *et al.* 1995;

UKPDS 1998*a*). In the UKPDS (1998*c*), intensive BP control in hypertensive patients reduced photocoagulation by 4.1% and prevented a decline in visual acuity by 9.2%, over 7.5 years. The incidence of blindness, however, was similar irrespective of BP control (3.3 and 2.4%, intensive and conventional treatment, respectively).

Although retinopathy may be present at clinical diagnosis, retinopathy requiring laser treatment is unusual at this stage. The patients at highest risk are those with an early age of onset (Eastman *et al.* 1997*a, b*). Laser treatment improves visual acuity in severe retinopathy or macular oedema, but most patients detected by screening will not need this treatment, at least for several years. The benefits for vision of glucose and BP control with early diagnosis are unclear (Harris *et al.* 2003; USPSTF 2003).

Potential long-term benefit: nephropathy

In patients without macroalbuminuria at clinical diagnosis, the incidence of chronic renal failure is 0.5% at 15 years, 10% at 30 years. When patients have macroalbuminuria at the outset, the incidence of chronic renal failure is 12% at 15 years. In the two large studies in which blood glucose and BP control were investigated, both diminished albuminuria. Neither reduced the incidence of chronic renal failure. Treatment with an ACE inhibitor or with an angiotensin receptor blocker in type 2 diabetes has reduced the frequency and progression of both albuminuria and chronic renal failure. Angiotensin receptor blockage diminished the progression to chronic renal failure in diabetic people with macroalbuminuria (Brenner *et al.* 2001; Lewis *et al.* 2001). At diagnosis, either conventionally or following screening, only 3–8% of patients have macroalbuminuria. Less than 1% of those detected at screening will progress to chronic renal failure within 15 years. Screening for diabetes to diminish the burden of chronic renal failure is, therefore, probably unjustified (USPSTF 2003). The economic costs of renal replacement therapy are, however, so large that the potential economic benefits could be considerable (Section 42.9).

42.6 Biochemical screening tests for diabetes

42.6.1 Introduction

Screening tests for diabetes have been validated mainly against the 2 h OGTT glucose (50, 75, or 100 g) (Table 42.3). The OGTT itself is imperfect, especially in view of its variability. For the 2 h value, coefficients of variation (CV) have ranged from 15–35% (Freeman *et al.* 1942; McDonald *et al.* 1965; O'Sullivan and Mahan 1966; Harding *et al.* 1973; Toeller and Knussmann 1973; Olefsky and Reaven 1974; Ganda *et al.* 1978; Riccardi *et al.* 1985; Forrest *et al.* 1988). Variation has been lower for FPG. In one study where repeated 75 g OGTTs were performed over 2–6 weeks in normal subjects, the CV was 6.4% for FPG and 17% for the 2 h level (Mooy *et al.* 1996). The definitive diagnostic procedure remains, however, the OGTT.

42.6.2 Circulating glucose estimations on fasting samples

A fasting test requires that the patient adheres to instructions for the overnight fast. Limited data suggest that compliance is not good. In the Health Survey for England, with nurses taking blood in individuals' homes, valid fasting samples were obtained in 50–64% of men and 38–64% of women (vs. 75–84% of men and 60–82% of women for non-fasting samples). A related disadvantage is that tests need to be performed in the morning. In NHANES, where subjects without known diabetes were studied fasting in the morning and compared with fasting in the afternoon (Troisi *et al.* 2000), the morning FPG (mean + standard deviation (SD)) was

Table 42.3 Selected screening tests for type 2 diabetes

	Cut-off	Sensitivity	Specificity	PVP	Reference
Urine glucose					
Fasting	≥Tr	16	98		Forrest *et al.* 1987a
Fasting	≥Tr	35	100		West and Kalbfleisch 1971
2–4 h post-prandial	≥Tr	39	98		West and Kalbfleisch 1971
1 h post-prandial	≥Tr	43	98		Davies *et al.* 1991, 1993
1–2 h post-prandial	≥Tr	21	99	47	Friderichsen and Maunsbach 1997
2 h post-OGTT	≥Tr	48	94		West and Kalbfleisch 1971
Random	≥Tr	18	99		Andersson *et al.* 1993
Random	≥Tr	64	99		Hanson *et al.* 1993
Venous plasma (mM)					
Fasting	≥6.7	44	98		West and Kalbfleisch 1971
Fasting	≥7.8	52	99		Simon *et al.* 1985
Fasting (US)	≥6.1	65	93	37	Modan and Harris 1994
Fasting (Israel)	≥6.1	81	84	27	Modan and Harris 1994
Fasting (US)	≥7.2	42	99	91	Modan and Harris 1994
Fasting (Israel)	≥7.2	49	99	87	Modan and Harris 1994
Fasting	≥6.5	74	93		Robertson *et al.* 1992
Fasting	≥6.1	80	96		Hanson *et al.* 1993
Fasting	≥6.1	95	90		Haffner *et al.* 1984
Fasting	≥6.0	68	93	48	Chang *et al.* 1998
Fasting	≥7.0	40	99	79	Chang *et al.* 1998
Fasting	≥7.0	58	97	94	Pauvilai *et al.* 1999
Random	≥6.7	50	98		West and Kalbfleisch 1971
Capillary blood (mM)					
Random	≥8.0	69	95		Andersson *et al.* 1993
Random	≥6.2	63	92		Qiao *et al.* 1995
2 h post-OGTT	≥11.1	69	98	16	Forrest *et al.* 1988
2 h post-OGTT	≥8.6	90	93	18	Hanson *et al.* 1993
1 h post-prandial	≥6.4 (30 yr)	82	78		Engelgau *et al.* 1995b
1 h post-prandial	≥7.8 (75 yr)	81	80		Engelgau *et al.* 1995b
HbA$_{1c}$ (%)	≥5.6	35	100		Robertson *et al.* 1992
	≥8.3	48	100		Santiago *et al.* 1978
	≥6.0	60	91		Simon *et al.* 1985
	≥6.03	85	91		Sekikawa *et al.* 1990
	≥7.5	98	79		Hanson *et al.* 1993
	+2 SDs	66	98	63	Peters *et al.* 1996
	+3 SDs	48	100	90	Meta-analysis with
	+4 SDs	36	100	97	Population prevalence 6%
	+1 SD	83	84		Rohlfing *et al.* 2000
	+2 SDs	63	97		Whole population
	+2 SDs	59	98		Whole population
	+2 SDs	76	93		Non-Hispanic white
	+2 SDs	84	98		Non-Hispanic black Mexican American
	≥5.9	76	86		Tanaka *et al.* 2001
	≥6.5	49	98		Japanese

Extended and modified from Engelgau *et al.* 1995a.

Sensitivity, specificity, and PVP data calculated with 2 h 75 g OGTT value as reference.

5.41 ± 0.01 mmol/l and the afternoon value was 5.12 ± 0.02 mmol/l ($p < 0.001$). Such a difference could reduce the prevalence of diabetes diagnosis by 50%.

Venous glucose estimations for screening have generally been performed on plasma, capillary analyses on whole blood. Using venous plasma, with a cut-off ≥6.1 mmol/l, specificity has usually been >90% (Table 42.3). Sensitivity has ranged from 44–65%, except in populations where known diabetic individuals were included (95% sensitivity has been reported).

With FPG, the screening test is the same as one diagnostic test. Two tests are required for diagnosis and if the second is a further FPG, the efficiency of screening becomes dependent on the test–retest differences for FPG. Contributors to test–retest differences include the assay CV (~3–4%) and the individual's preceding diet (inadequate intake worsens glucose tolerance, although the effects are greater on the 2 h OGTT value than on the FPG). The overall test–retest difference is 5% in the experimental situation (Godsland 1985), but may be somewhat higher in routine practice. As FPG provides one-half of the information required for diagnosis, it has an advantage over other measurements, such as glycosylated haemoglobin, where two additional diagnostic tests would be required. Other circulating glucose estimations, such as random or post-prandial values, could contribute to the diagnostic procedure (if ≥11.1 mmol/l), but their variability is greater.

If the screening procedure adopted the diagnostic cut-off (7.0 mmol/l), this would lead to misclassification due to the test–retest difference. The SD of these differences is ~0.5 mmol/l in the FPG range 6–8 mmol/l (i.e. 95% of people on retesting will have a second value within 1 mmol/l of the original). With such data, a cut-off for screening may be selected to achieve a desired sensitivity and specificity. For example, a cut-off at 6 mmol/l would ensure that <2.5% of those positive on both tests would have neither IFG nor diabetes following the second measurement.

Capillary glucose estimations on whole blood require only pin-prick samples and measurements are often made on the spot. In skilled hands portable methods, using for example reflectance meters, provide accurate capillary glucose estimations (Worth *et al.* 1981; Forrest *et al.* 1987*a*). In routine conditions, accuracy is inadequate for diagnosis (Campbell *et al.* 1992; Nichols *et al.* 1995). Fasting capillary glucose in routine hands has not been evaluated for screening (capillary studies have generally been non-fasting). The performance of some new point-of-care glucose meters, such as HemoCue (Dronfield, Derbyshire S18 2LX) (Torjman *et al.* 2001; Nichols 2002; Chen *et al.* 2003) requires study in field conditions.

42.6.3 Circulating glucose estimations on non-fasting samples

Casual (random) venous plasma or capillary whole blood glucose measurements require minimal preparation and may be checked at any time of day. The sensitivity is lower if a higher cut-off is selected for reasonable specificity (Engelgau *et al.* 1995). With a 6.7 mmol/l cut-off, venous plasma glucose 2–4 h post-prandially provided 50% sensitivity at 98% specificity (West and Kalbfleisch 1971). The cut-off for capillary glucose should be higher than for venous whole blood, in view of the higher glucose concentrations in non-fasting capillary blood. Using random capillary blood, with trained field workers and careful quality control, high sensitivities (60–70%) have been obtained at specificities >90% (Table 42.3). A major factor with random samples has been, as anticipated, the time since the last meal (Simmons and Williams 1994). Variation in sensitivity based on ethnic origin and age has been reported for random capillary samples (Simmons and Williams 1994).

42.6.4 Urine glucose analysis

Urine tests are easy and cheap (Bullimore and Keyworth 1997). Strips may be sent by post for self-testing (Davies *et al.* 1991, 1993). Response rates of >80% have been reported in Caucasian subjects in a semi-rural setting. The response has been less satisfactory in certain subgroups, such as older Asians in urban situations (Davies *et al.* 1999).

Fasting, random, post-prandial, and post-OGTT urine glucose samples have been employed (Table 42.3). Fasting tests have been less discriminatory than post-prandial (Forrest *et al.* 1987*b*). The main problem is that although specificity is high (>90%), sensitivity is low (16–64%).

42.6.5 Glycosylated haemoglobin (glycated haemoglobin, glycohaemoglobin)

Haemoglobin glycosylation gives an indication of the average blood glucose over preceding weeks (Ko *et al.* 1998*b*, *c*). It is not influenced acutely by meals.

Three glycosylated species are measured:

1. HbA_{1c}. This results from glucose attaching to the N-terminal valine of the haemoglobin β chain. It comprises 60–80% of the total.

2. HbA_1. This comprises HbA_{1c}, together with HbA_{1a1}, HbA_{1a2}, and HbA_{1b}, which result from the attachment of other carbohydrate moieties to the β chain N-terminal valine.

3. Total glycosylated haemoglobin. This comprises HbA_{1c} and glucose moieties attached to the ε amino group of lysine.

Measurement methods include ion exchange high-performance liquid chromatography (HPLC), gel electrophoresis, isoelectric focusing, low pressure chromatography, colorimetric methods, affinity chromatography, and immunoassays. HPLC has been the most widely employed. A bench-top device gives results within minutes.

HbA_{1c} is the measure for which data are available on the risks of complications in established diabetes. With differing methodologies, the normal ranges for HbA_{1c} have varied from 4.4–8.2% (Gillery *et al.* 1998). In 1996 the National Glycohemoglobin Standardization Program was established in the USA to certify that all HbA_{1c} methods gave results comparable to the Diabetes Control and Complications Trial (DCCT 1995). DCCT alignment was employed by the UKPDS. HbA_{1c} assays should now be DCCT-aligned or aligned to an alternative internationally recognized standard (Marshall and Barth 2000).

In a normal population, assay variability accounted for only 9% of the total variance of HbA_{1c} (Kilpatrick *et al.* 1998). The intra-individual variance (the real variance within a subject tested at different times, independent of assay variability) was 6%. There was wide inter-individual variance (85%). The implication is that some individuals with a naturally low HbA_{1c} will need to increase greatly (>12 SDs from their usual) before a diagnosis of diabetes can be made, while other subjects will need to increase only slightly (2 SDs). Furthermore, much of the inter-individual variability within the normal range is not due to glucose – the glucose contribution has ranged from 2–30% (Modan *et al.* 1988; Yudkin *et al.* 1990*b*).

At specificities >90%, HbA_{1c} has had moderate sensitivity (35–60%), when people with known diabetes were excluded (Table 42.3). HbA_{1c} has performed best in populations with a very high diabetes prevalence, where sensitivity has been reported at 85% with specificity 91%, using a cut-off >2 SDs above the mean (Little *et al.* 1988). In lower prevalence populations the results have been less impressive, with one study, for example, showing an elevated HbA_{1c} in only 23% of the population with diabetes (Gerken and van Lente 1990). A meta-analysis of 18 studies (Peters *et al.* 1996), comparing HbA_{1c} and the OGTT, provided specificity and sensitivity data based on results lying within 2, 3, or 4 SDs from the normal for each assay (Table 42.3). By selecting a cut-off >2 SDs, a sensitivity of 66% was observed at specificity 98%.

Most individual studies have concluded that low sensitivity at high specificity limits the value of HbA_{1c} in screening. The role of DCCT-aligned HbA_{1c} (or equivalent) warrants further investigation, in comparison with FPG as the gold standard in a multi-ethnic population. A sensitivity of 83% was obtained at a specificity of 84%, using as a cut-off >1 SD above the mean in a multi-ethnic US population, using FPG ≥7.0 mmol/l as the gold standard (Rohlfing *et al.* 2000). With a cut-off >2 SDs, the sensitivity was 63.2% and specificity 97.4%. The sensitivity was lowest in the white subpopulation and highest in the Mexican Americans (Table 42.3).

42.6.6 Other measurements and measurement combinations

Serum proteins (mainly albumin) become glycosylated. Fructosamine measurement is inexpensive and easily automated (Croxson *et al.* 1991; Kasezawa *et al.* 1993). It must be adjusted for albumin. Using two different assays in an elderly population, sensitivities of 75 and 81%, specificities of 83 and 87%, and PVP of 35 and 43%, were reported (Cefalu *et al.* 1993). Lower sensitivities have been reported (Sekikawa *et al.* 1990) and it has compared unfavourably with HbA_{1c} for screening (Tsuji *et al.* 1991).

Serum 1,5-anhydroglucitol is a naturally occurring glucose analogue. Most circulating 1,5-anhydroglucitol derives from food. Glucose competitively inhibits its renal tubular reabsorption and circulating levels are low in people with diabetes (Buse *et al.* 2003). Plasma concentrations show an inverse curvilinear relationship with urinary glucose. It reflects circulating glucose levels over the previous 24h. Good sensitivity (93%) and specificity (84%) at a cut-off <14 μg/ml have been reported (Yamanouchi *et al.* 1991) and 1,5-anhydroglucitol has compared favourably with HbA_{1c} and fructosamine. In another comparison in Japan, although the areas under the ROC curve were greatest for HbA_{1c} and fructosamine (Shirasaya *et al.* 1999), 1,5-anhydroglucitol was the most cost-effective. Neither fructosamine nor 1,5-anhydroglucitol assays have been internationally standardized.

Combinations of tests have been employed to identify individuals with FPG <7.0 mmol/l and 2 h OGTT values >11.1 mmol/l. Combining FPG and HbA_{1c} increased the area under the ROC curve ($p = 0.0008$) compared with FPG alone in a high prevalence population (Wang *et al.* 2002). In Poland, combining fructosamine and FPG produced larger ROC areas than HbA_{1c} + FPG (Herdzik *et al.* 2002). Two-step procedures, such as FPG followed by HbA_{1c} or fructosamine, have also been proposed (Ko *et al.* 1998a, b; Davidson *et al.* 1999).

42.6.7 Compliance with the diagnostic procedure following a positive screening test

Where studied, attendance for confirmatory testing has been >90% following detection in an organized campaign (Davies and Day 1994).

42.6.8 **Recommended practice**

The data are inadequate to recommend a biochemical screening test. It is likely that FPG will be the screening test most employed, with a cut-off of ∼5.6 mmol/l.

42.7 **The frequency of screening**

The data are inadequate to decide the optimal screening frequency in a multi-ethnic population. A recent Position Statement (2002) from Diabetes UK recommended screening every 3 years for those at increased risk. The ADA Expert Committee (1997) recommended screening those >45 years 3-yearly, with no distinction on the basis of risk factors. The 3 year interval was selected on the basis of a negligible likelihood of developing complications within this timescale. Other organizations, including the WHO and the Canadian Task Force on the Periodic Health Screen, did not specify a frequency. In one small study in the UK there were similar rates of diabetes, and similar response rates, when screening for glycosuria was repeated after 30 months, suggesting that a new cohort had been identified after this period, but other intervals were not examined (Davies and Day 1994).

The incidence of diabetes has been rarely studied (West 1978). In a US population aged 25–64 years, the 7–8 years incidence (both diagnosed and undiagnosed) was 9.4% in non-Hispanic whites and 15.7% in Mexican Americans (Burke *et al.* 1999). This had tripled between 1987 and 1996. Increases have been demonstrated in other subpopulations in the USA (Harris *et al.* 1998). The incidence of physician-diagnosed diabetes over 14.8 years in 5550 men aged 40–59 years from 18 British towns was 3% (Perry *et al.* 1999). Even allowing for half of those with diabetes to be undiagnosed, and for the majority of the UK population being white European, this is a lower incidence rate than in the USA. The best estimate is 0.4–2% per year. With screening every 5 years, the number of new cases in this interval would range from 2 to 10 per hundred, depending on ethnicity.

The more frequently a screening test is repeated, the higher will be the false positive rate (Park *et al.* 2000). Diminishing the frequency of testing will diminish the number of false positives, but increases the population exposure to undiagnosed diabetes.

42.8 **The case against screening**

42.8.1 **Introduction**

There are arguments against screening, some generic and some specific to diabetes.

42.8.2 **Early diagnosis may have no impact on disease progression: lead-time bias**

It is unknown if earlier diagnosis will increase total, or complication-free, survival. An increase in survival, or freedom from complications, may appear to have occurred merely as a consequence of the earlier diagnosis. As an example, if screening led to diagnosis being made 5 years earlier, the patients may appear to benefit from an extra 5 years of life, or an extra 5 years free of complications, when in reality the natural history of the disease had been unaltered ('lead-time bias').

42.8.3 The implications of the UKPDS results and other intervention trials

Intensive control of glycaemia, BP, and dyslipidaemia is now standard management for established type 2 diabetes. This will reduce complications and could reduce the benefits from screening, by permitting little additional improvement (Goyder and Irwig 1998).

42.8.4 Length-time bias

There is considerable inter-individual variability in the rate of progression of complications. The population diagnosed following screening could contain a high proportion of those with only slowly progressive complications and the group identified by screening might be those least in need of intervention ('length-time bias').

42.8.5 The initial intervention is likely to be lifestyle advice which should be given anyway

Initial management is likely to be lifestyle modification in the majority of people diagnosed following screening. As this is similar to 'healthy living' advice, which many people receive anyway, and to which they do not adhere, it could be argued that screening is unlikely to be effective. In other circumstances, however, knowledge of a personal medical condition has induced lifestyle changes (e.g. in hypercholesterolaemia, knowledge of the cholesterol level has resulted in improved cholesterol control (Elton *et al.* 1994)). In addition, modern management will often involve early drug therapy.

42.8.6 Potential harm from screening

Some people will have a false positive test and wrongly labelling people with diabetes could be a source of anxiety. The label of hypertension has been associated with increased work absenteeism, marital problems, and reduced income, and increased depression and perception of ill health (Bloom and Monterossa 1981). Psychological problems may be a lesser issue than for some disorders (e.g. breast cancer screening), in that it is possible to confirm or refute the screening result quickly and simply. Early results in diabetes screening have been encouraging (Kerbel *et al.* 1997). In a preliminary UK report, screening first-degree relatives had no adverse effect on those who were emotionally stable before screening (Farmer *et al.* 1998, 1999). It possibly increased anxiety in those who were anxious initially. In North Carolina, the health-related quality of life of people diagnosed following screening was similar to that in those with a negative screening test over 12 months (Edelman *et al.* 2002).

42.8.7 Lost opportunity costs

Even if cost-effective, it is uncertain if screening for diabetes is the best use of finite resources (UKPDS 1998c; Gray *et al.* 2000). UKPDS targets for BP, glucose, and lipids are not achieved in most instances. It could be argued that it would be better to use resources to treat properly those who are already diagnosed. Diagnosing more people earlier might exacerbate the problem.

42.9 **Cost–benefit analyses**

The CDC Diabetes Cost-Effectiveness Study Group (1998) used a Monte Carlo computer simulation model. The model consisted of:

◆ A screening module using an FPG cut-off of 6.1 mmol/l.

◆ A disease progression module which modelled the natural history and costs of treatment. Microvascular complications were modelled based on the studies of Eastman *et al.* (1997*a, b*) and the glycaemic changes observed with time in UKPDS. The progression was modelled as a function of blood glucose control using the benefits reported for type 1 diabetes in the DCCT (1995). The model did not attribute any benefit for macrovascular disease (it was performed before the UKPDS reported). It was assumed that screening would lead to the diagnosis 5 years earlier. Screening resulted in a reduction in lifetime cumulative incidence of end stage renal disease, blindness, and amputation by 26, 35, and 22% respectively. The years of life without major complications were increased and there were gains in both life years and quality-adjusted life years (QALYs). The incremental cost of screening per additional life year was estimated at \$236 449 and the cost per QALY was \$56 649. Although more expensive, the cost effectiveness was regarded as acceptable by the authors, in comparison with screening for breast cancer, cervical cancer, and hypertension. The cost effectiveness was greatest in black Americans where both the prevalence of diabetes and the frequency of complications were greatest. Although the cost per case was higher among younger subjects, the reduced costs from lifetime complications meant that the screening programme was most cost effective in those <30 years.

There is a need for a cost–benefit analysis for diabetes screening, taking account of the UKPDS results. Economics of screening and treatment of diabetes have been recently reviewed (Raikou and McGuire 2003).

42.10 **IFG and IGT**

IGT and IFG will be observed in up to 30% of adult individuals, depending on age and ethnicity. There is good evidence that intervention for the primary prevention of type 2 diabetes is effective. Initial evidence is derived from a prospective trial of lifestyle intervention (diet, exercise, diet plus exercise, or control) in Chinese individuals with IGT living in Da Qing (Pan *et al.* 1997). At 6 years, 68% of the control group had developed diabetes. The adjusted reductions in progression to diabetes for the diet, exercise, and diet plus exercise groups were 31% ($p < 0.03$), 46% ($p < 0.0005$), and 42% ($p < 0.005$) respectively. Other randomized controlled trials have confirmed that lifestyle or drug (metformin, acarbose, or troglitazone) interventions in people with impaired glucose regulation, or in women with previous GDM, have decreased the progression to diabetes by 42–58% over 3–6 years (Diabetes Prevention Program 1999; Eriksson *et al.* 1999; Tuomilehto *et al.* 2001; Wenying *et al.* 2001; Chiasson *et al.* 2002; Knowler *et al.* 2002).

Although it is possible to delay or prevent the progression from IGT or IFG to diabetes in trials, it is uncertain whether routine screening to permit earlier intervention would have a major impact on health. This is especially the case as any impact on diabetic complications would not be apparent for many years. The identification of individuals with impaired glucose regulation could permit intervention for control of other risk factors for vascular disease, for which treatment is effective. For patients with IGT, systolic BP, HDL-C, BMI, and insulin concentrations predicted CHD in the Whitehall Study (Fuller *et al.* 1980) and these risk factors are capable of being modified. Lipid and lipoprotein abnormalities have predicted CHD in other IGT populations (Pan *et al.* 1986; Fontbonne *et al.* 1989), suggesting that intervention could have particular benefit in this group. There is evidence that those with IFG have a less adverse cardiovascular disease risk factor profile than those with IGT (Tripathy *et al.* 2000; Hanefeld *et al.* 2003) and the bulk of the evidence suggests that IFG predicts cardiovascular disease and death less effectively than IGT (Barzilay *et al.* 1999; DECODE Study Group 1999).

Attempts have been made to identify, without blood tests, individuals with IFG or IGT, or those otherwise at risk of developing diabetes. A questionnaire-based risk score has been developed from a Finnish population followed over 10 years. Information was obtained on age, BMI, waist circumference, use of BP- and blood glucose-lowering medication, physical activity, and consumption of fruits, berries, and vegetables. The score had a sensitivity of 81%, a specificity of 76%, and a PVP of 5% in identifying individuals who progressed to develop type 2 diabetes (Lindstrom and Tuomilehto 2003).

The cost-effectiveness of intervention, combining screening for glycaemia with screening for other CHD risk factors, requires study. Preliminary modelling of the cost effectiveness of preventing diabetes has not been published at the time of writing and there is no consensus.

42.11 Conclusions

The UK National Screening Committee (1998) has outlined prerequisites for any screening programme. It is useful to conclude by examining these for diabetes (see also Wareham and Griffin 2001).

- *Diabetes as a health problem.* It has a high prevalence (3–5% of the adult population), highest of all in ethnic minorities, and the prevalence is increasing. The personal and economic consequences, particularly of complications, render it of major importance.

- *Epidemiology and natural history.* The epidemiology has been carefully studied. Groups within the population at high risk are identifiable. Symptoms are not prominent in the early stages, but IGT and IFG are measurable antecedents.

- *Preventive intervention.* The main purpose of screening for diabetes would be to prevent the long-term complications of diabetes. Primary prevention of diabetes in high risk individuals may be a future goal.

- *The screening test.* FPG provides diagnostic information in addition to screening. This is the case also with random plasma glucose estimations, but the sensitivity is lower. Urine glucose estimation has low sensitivity. DCCT-aligned HbA$_{1c}$ holds promise and does not require an overnight fast. The optimal screening procedure has not been established for the multi-ethnic UK population. The extent of screening (whole adult population over a certain age, selective or targeted) and the optimal frequency of screening, have not been established.

- *Population distribution of test values.* Plasma glucose distribution has been carefully studied and ethnic variations defined. Diagnostic criteria have been published (WHO 1999). Optimal cut-offs for positive results on screening have not yet been defined.

- *Test acceptability.* Blood and urine tests have proven acceptable in epidemiological studies. Ethnic differences in acceptability are unknown; for example blood versus urine, fasting versus random.

- *Policy in those who screen positive.* Diagnostic procedures are available (WHO 1999).

- *The effectiveness of therapy.* Treatment to reduce blood glucose, BP, and other risk factors delays complications in those with established diabetes. It is unknown if early diagnosis of diabetes following screening, to permit earlier intervention, would improve outcomes. Individuals with IFG or IGT could be offered lifestyle advice and management of the associated disorders (e.g. hypertension and dyslipidaemia).

- *Evidence base for therapy.* Strong evidence-based policies have been devised for the treatment of patients with established type 2 diabetes.

- *Optimization of existing healthcare for diabetes.* Guidelines for care have been published by many organizations in developed countries and attempts made to ensure their implementation.

- *Randomized controlled trials (RCTs).* There are no RCTs showing that screening for diabetes reduces complications. RCTs have shown that intervention in IGT/IFG delays the onset of diabetes.

- *Clinical, social, and ethical acceptability of the screening programme.* The screening tests, diagnostic procedures, and management protocols are established and ethical. Screening has been performed in pilot studies without evidence of serious problems. There is little information on acceptability of different screening procedures in population subgroups.

- *Benefits versus harm.* The psychological and other problems of false positive screens should be minimized by rapidly proceeding to the diagnostic procedure. The psychological aspects have not been extensively studied, but limited data do not suggest substantial harm.

- *Cost–benefit analysis.* Screening for diabetes has been regarded as cost effective in the USA. Further studies are required on screening to prevent diabetes in those at risk.

- *Monitoring and quality control.* National or international quality control mechanisms exist for most laboratory measurements. Quality control will need development for other aspects.

- *Staff and facilities.* A screening programme would probably be implemented in primary care. Adequate facilities, staff, and training would be mandatory in order to organize and perform the screening, and to deal effectively with those who screened positive.

Acknowledgements

Dr I. Godsland is supported by the Heart Disease and Diabetes Research Trust. The chapter is based on a Discussion Document written by the authors for Diabetes UK in 1999.

References

Agner, E., Thorsteinsson, B. and Eriksen, M. (1982). Impaired glucose tolerance and diabetes mellitus in elderly subjects. *Diabetes Care* 5, 600–4.

Alberti, K. G. M. M. (1996). The clinical implications of impaired glucose tolerance. *Diabetic Medicine* 13, 927–37.

Alberti, K. G. M. M. (1997). The costs of non insulin dependent diabetes mellitus. *Diabetic Medicine* 14, 7–9.

ADA (American Diabetes Association) (1993a). Direct and indirect costs of diabetes in the USA in 1992. American Diabetes Association, Alexandra, VA.

ADA (American Diabetes Association) (1993b). American diabetes alert. *Diabetes Forecast* **46**, 54.

ADA (American Diabetes Association) (1997). Report of the Expert Committee on the Diagnosis and Classification of Diabetes Mellitus. *Diabetes Care* **20**, 1183–97.

ADA (American Diabetes Association) (2000). Aspirin therapy in diabetes. *Diabetes Care* **23**, S61–S62.

ADA (American Diabetes Association) (2003). Follow-up report on the diagnosis and classification of diabetes mellitus. *Diabetes Care* **26**, 3160–7.

Andersson, D. K., Lundblad, E. and Svardsudd, K. (1993). A model of early diagnosis in type 2 diabetes mellitus in primary health care. *Diabetic Medicine* **10**, 167–73.

Baan, C. A., Ruige, J. B., Stolk, R. P., Witteman, J. C. M., Dekker, J. M., Heine, R. J. and Feskens, E. J. M. (1999). Performance of a predictive model to identify undiagnosed diabetes in a health care setting. *Diabetes Care* **22**, 213–19.

Balarajan, R. E. (1991). Ethnic differences in mortality from ischaemic heart disease and cerebrovascular disease in England and Wales. *British Medical Journal* **302**, 560–4.

Barzilay, J. I., Spiekerman, C. F., Wahl, P. W., Kuller, L. H., Cushman, M., Firberg, C. D. *et al.* (1999). Cardiovascular disease in older adults with glucose disorders: comparison of American Diabetes Association criteria for diabetes mellitus with WHO criteria. *Lancet* **354**, 622–5.

Beaty, T. H. and Fajans, S. S. (1982). Estimating genetic and non-genetic components of variance for fasting glucose levels in pedigrees ascertained through non-insulin dependent diabetes. *Annals of Human Genetics* **46**, 355–62.

Bloom, J. R. and Monterossa, S. (1981). Hypertension labeling and sense of well-being. *American Journal of Public Health* **71**, 1228–32.

Brenner, B. M., Cooper, M. E., de Zeeuw, D., Keane, W. F., Mitch, W. E., Parving, H. H. *et al.* (2001). Effects of losartan on renal and cardiovascular outcomes in patients with type 2 diabetes and nephropathy. *New England Journal of Medicine* **345**, 861–9.

Bullimore, S. P. and Keyworth, C. (1997). Finding diabetics: a method of screening in general practice. *British Journal of General Practice* **47**, 371–4.

Burden, M. L. and Burden A. C. (1994). The American Diabetes Association screening questionnaire for diabetes: is it worthwhile in the UK? [Letter.] *Diabetes Care* **17**, 97.

Burke, J. P., Williams, K., Gaskill, S. P., Hazuda, H. P., Haffner, S. M. and Stern, M. P. (1999). Rapid rise in the incidence of Type 2 diabetes from 1987 to 1996: results from the San Antonio Heart Study. *Archives of Internal Medicine* **159**, 1450–6.

Buse, J. B., Freeman, J. L., Edelman, S. V., Jovanovic, L. and McGill, J. B. (2003). Serum 1,5-anhydroglucitol (GlycoMark): a short-term glycemic marker. *Diabetes Technology and Therapeutics* **5**, 355–63.

Campbell, E. M., Redman, S., Dunkley, P. R. and Moffitt, P. S. (1992). The use of portable blood glucose monitors by trained lay operators. *Medical Journal of Australia* **157**, 446–8.

CDC Diabetes Cost-Effectiveness Study Group (1998). The cost-effectiveness of screening for Type 2 diabetes. *Journal of the American Medical Association* **280**, 1757–63.

Cederholm, J. and Wibell, L. (1985). Glucose intolerance in middle-aged males: a cause of hypertension? *Acta Medica Scandinavica* **217**, 363–71.

Cefalu, W. T., Ettinger, W. H., Bell-Farrow, A. D. and Rushing, J. T. (1993). Serum fructosamine as a screening test for diabetes in the elderly: a pilot study. *Journal of the American Geriatric Society* **41**, 1090–4.

Chan, J. M., Stampfer, M. J., Rimm, E. B., Willett, W. C. and Colditz, G. A. (1994). Obesity, fat distribution and weight gain as risk factors for clinical diabetes in man. *Diabetes Care* **17**, 961–9.

Chang, C. J., Wu, J. S., Lu, F. H., Lee, H. L., Yang, Y. C. and Wen, M. J. (1998). Fasting plasma glucose in screening for diabetes in the Taiwanese population. *Diabetes Care* **21**, 1856–60.

Charles, M. A., Fontbonne, A., Thibult, N., Warnet, J. M., Rosselin, G. E. and Eschwege, E. (1991). Risk factors for NIDDM in white population: Paris prospective study. *Diabetes* **40**, 796–9.

Chaturvedi, N. and Fuller, J. H. (1996). Ethnic differences in mortality from cardiovascular disease in the UK: do they persist in people with diabetes? *Journal of Epidemiology and Community Health* **50**, 137–9.

Chaturvedi, N., McKeigue, P. M. and Marmot, M. G. (1994). Relationship of glucose intolerance to coronary risk in Afro-Caribbeans compared with Europeans. *Diabetologia* **37**, 765–72.

Chen, E. T., Nichols, J. H., Duh, S. H. and Hortin, G. (2003). Performance evaluation of blood glucose monitoring devices. *Diabetes Technology and Therapeutics* **5**, 749–68.

Chiasson, J. L., Josse, R. G., Gomis, R., Hanefeld, M., Karasik, A. and Laakso, M. (2002). Acarbose for prevention of type 2 diabetes mellitus: the STOP-NIDDM randomized trial. *Lancet* **359**, 2072–7.

Christian, R. C., Dumesic, D. A., Behrenbeck, T., Oberg, A. L., Sheedy, P. F. 2nd, and Fitzpatrick, L. A. (2003). Prevalence and predictors of coronary artery calcification in women with polycystic ovary syndrome. *Journal of Clinical Endocrinology and Metabolism* **88**, 2562–8.

Colagiuri, S., Cull, C. A., Holman, R. R. and UKPDS Group (2002*a*). Are lower fasting plasma glucose levels at diagnosis of type 2 diabetes associated with improved outcomes? U.K. prospective diabetes study 61. *Diabetes Care* **25**, 1410–17.

Colagiuri, S., Zimmet, P., Hepburn, A., and Colagiuri, R. (2002*b*). *Evidence based guidelines for type 2 diabetes: primary prevention, case detection and diagnosis. Canberra, Australia.* Diabetes Australia and National Health and Medical Research Council (available at www.nhmrc.gov.au).

Colhoun, H. M., Dong, W., Barakat, M. T., Mather, H. M. and Poulter, N. R. (1999). The scope for cardiovascular disease risk factor intervention among people with diabetes mellitus in England: a population-based analysis from the Health Surveys for England 1991–94. *Diabetic Medicine* **16**, 35–40.

Colwell, J. A. (1997). Aspirin therapy in diabetes. *Diabetes Care* **20**, 1767–71.

Cowie, C. C., Harris, M. I. and Eberhardt, M. S. (1994). Frequency and determinants of screening for diabetes in the U. S. *Diabetes Care* **17**, 1158–63.

Croxson, S. C., Absalom, S. and Burden, A. C. (1991). Fructosamine in diabetes screening of the elderly. *Annals of Clinical Biochemistry* **28**, 279–82.

Cruickshank, K. (1997). Non-insulin-dependent diabetes. In *Textbook of diabetes*, 2nd edn (ed. J. C. Pickup and G. Williams), pp. 3.17–3.28. Blackwell Science, Oxford.

Curb, J. D., Pressel, S. L., Cutler, J. A., Savage, P. J., Applegate, W. B., Black, H. *et al.* (1996). Effect of diuretic-based antihypertensive treatment on cardiovascular disease risk in older diabetic patients with isolated systolic hypertension: Systolic Hypertension in the Elderly Program Cooperative Research Group. *Journal of the American Medical Association* **276**, 1886–92.

Dahlgren, E., Janson, P. O., Johansson, S., Lapidus, L. and Oden, A. (1992). Polycystic ovary syndrome and risk for myocardial infarction: evaluated from a risk factor model based on a prospective population study of women. *Acta Obstreticia et Gynecologica Scandinavica* **71**, 599–604.

Damm, P. (1998). Gestational diabetes mellitus and subsequent development of overt diabetes mellitus. *Danish Medical Bulletin* **45**, 495–509.

Damm, P., Kühl, C., Bertelsen, A. and Mølsted-Pedersen, L. (1992). Predictive factors for the development of diabetes in women with previous gestational diabetes mellitus. *American Journal of Obstetrics and Gynecology* **167**, 607–16.

Daniel, M., Rowley, K. G., McDermot, R., Mylvaganam, A. and O'Dea, K. (1999). Diabetes incidence in an Australian Aboriginal population. *Diabetes Care* **22**, 1993–6.

Davidson, M. B., Schriger, D. L., Peters, A. L. and Lorber, B. (1999). Relationship between fasting plasma glucose and glycosylated hemoglobin: potential for false-positive diagnosis of type 2 diabetes using new diagnostic criteria. *Journal of the American Medical Association* **281**, 1203–10.

Davies, M. and Day, J. (1994). Screening for non-insulin-dependent diabetes mellitus (NIDDM): how often should it be performed? *Journal of Medical Screening* **1**, 78–81.

Davies, M., Alban-Davies, H., Cook, C. and Day, J. (1991). Self testing for diabetes mellitus. *British Medical Journal* **303**, 696–8.

Davies, M. J., Williams, D. R. R., Metcalfe, J. and Day, J. L. (1993). Community screening for non-insulin-dependent diabetes mellitus: self-testing for post-prandial glycosuria. *Quarterly Journal of Medicine* **86**, 677–84.

Davies, M. J., Grenfell, A. and Day, J. L. (1996). Clinical characteristics and follow-up of subjects with non-insulin-dependent diabetes mellitus diagnosed by screening. *Practical Diabetes International* **13**, 75–8.

Davies, M. J., Ammari, F., Sherriff, C., Burden, M. L., Gujral, J. and Burden, A. C. (1999). Screening for Type 2 diabetes mellitus in the UK Indo-Asian population. *Diabetic Medicine* **16**, 131–7.

DECODE Study Group, on behalf of the European Diabetes Epidemiology Study Group (1998). Will new diagnostic criteria for diabetes mellitus change phenotype of patients with diabetes? Reanalysis of European epidemiological data. *British Medical Journal* **317**, 371–5.

DECODE Study Group, on behalf of the European Diabetes Epidemiology Study Group (1999). Glucose tolerance and mortality: comparison of WHO and American Diabetes Association diagnostic criteria. *Lancet* **354**, 617–21.

DECODE Study Group on behalf of the European Diabetes Epidemiology Study Group (2003). Age- and sex-specific prevalences of diabetes and impaired glucose regulation in 13 European cohorts. *Diabetes Care* **26**, 61–9.

DCCT (Diabetes Control and Complications Trial) Research Group (1995). Resource utilization and costs of care in the Diabetes Control and Complications Trial. *Diabetes Care* **18**, 1468–78.

Diabetes Prevention Program Research Group (1999). The Diabetes Prevention Program: design and methods for a clinical trial in the prevention of type 2 diabetes. *Diabetes Care* **22**, 623–34.

Dinneen, S. F., Maldonado, D. 3rd, Leibson, C. L., Klee, G. G., Li, H., Melton, L. J. 3rd, and Rizza, R. A. (1998). Effects of changing diagnostic criteria on the risk of developing diabetes. *Diabetes Care* **21**, 1408–13.

Dornhorst, A., Bailey, P. C., Anyaoku, V., Elkeles, R. S., Johnston, D. G. and Beard, R. W. (1990). Abnormalities of glucose tolerance following gestational diabetes. *Quarterly Journal of Medicine* **77**, 1219–28.

Drury, D. L. (1988). Hypertension. *Clinical Endocrinology and Metabolism* **2**, 375–9.

Dunaif, A. (1995). Hyperandrogenic anovulation (PCOS): a unique disorder of insulin action associated with an increased risk of non-insulin-dependent diabetes mellitus. *American Journal of Medicine* **98**, 33S–39S.

Dunstan, D. W., Zimmet, P. Z., Welborn, T. A., De Courten, M. P., Cameron, A. J., Sicree, R. A. *et al.* (2002). The rising prevalence of diabetes and impaired glucose tolerance: the Australian Diabetes, Obesity and Lifestyle Study. *Diabetes Care* **25**, 829–34.

Eastman, R. C., Javitt, J. C., Herman, W. H., Dasbach, E. J., Zbrozek, A. S., Dong, F., *et al.* (1997a). Model of complications of NIDDM. I: model construction and assumptions. *Diabetes Care* **20**, 725–34.

Eastman, R. C., Javitt, J. C., Herman, W. H., Dasbach, E. J., Copley-Merriman, C., Maier, W. *et al.* (1997b). Model of complications of NIDDM. II: analysis of the health benefits and cost-effectiveness of treating NIDDM with the goal of normoglycemia. *Diabetes Care* **20**, 735–44.

Edelman, D., Olsen, M. K., Dudley, T. K., Harris, A. C. and Oddone, E. Z. (2002). Impact of diabetes screening on quality of life. *Diabetes Care* **25**, 1022–6.

Efendic, S., Hanson, U., Wajnot, A. and Luft, R. (1987). Glucose tolerance, insulin release and insulin sensitivity in normal-weight women with previous gestational diabetes. *Diabetes* **36**, 413–19.

Elkeles, R. S., Diamond, J. R., Poulter, C., Dhanjil, S., Nicolaides, A. N., Mahmood, S. *et al.* (1998). Cardiovascular outcomes in Type 2 diabetes. A double-blind placebo-controlled study of bezafibrate: the St. Mary's, Ealing, Northwick Park Diabetes Cardiovascular Disease Prevention (SENDCAP) Study. *Diabetes Care* **21**, 641–8.

Elton, P. J., Ryman, A., Hammer, M. and Page, F. (1994). Randomised controlled trial in northern England of the effect of a person knowing their own serum cholesterol concentration. *Journal of Epidemiology and Community Health* **48**, 22–5.

Engelgau, M. M., Thompson, T. J., Smith, P. J., Herman, W. H., Aubert, R. E., Gunter, E. W. *et al.* (1995). Screening for diabetes mellitus in adults: the utility of random capillary blood glucose measurements. *Diabetes Care* **18**, 463–6.

Eriksson, J., Lindstrom, J., Valle, T., Aunola, S., Hamalainen, H., Hanne-Parikka, P. *et al.* (1999). Prevention of Type 2 diabetes in subjects with impaired glucose tolerance: the Diabetes Prevention Study (DPS) in Finland. Study design and 1-year interim report on the feasibility of the lifestyle intervention programme. *Diabetologia* **42**, 793–801.

Eschwege, E., Richard, J. L., Thibult, N., Ducimetiere, P., Warnet, J. M., Claude, J. R. and Rosselin, G. E. (1985). Coronary heart disease mortality in relation with diabetes, blood glucose and plasma insulin levels: the Paris Prospective Study, ten years later. *Hormone and Metabolic Research Supplement* **15**, 41–6.

Farmer, A. J., Levy, J. C. and Turner, R. C. (1998). Anxiety in first degree relatives screened for Type 2 diabetes. *Diabetes* **47**(Suppl. 1), 1262.

Farmer, A. J., Levy, J. C. and Turner, R. C. (1999). Knowledge of risk of developing diabetes mellitus among siblings of Type 2 diabetic patients. *Diabetic Medicine* **16**, 233–7.

Flegal, K. M., Ezzati, T. M., Harris, M. I., Haynes, S. G., Juarez, R. Z., Knowler, W. C. *et al.* (1991). Prevalence of diabetes in Mexican Americans, Cubans, and Puerto Ricans from the Hispanic Health and Nutrition Examination Survey, 1982–1984. *Diabetes Care* **14**(Suppl. 3), 628–38.

Fontbonne, A., Eschwege, E., Cambien, F., Richard, J. L., Ducimetiere, P., Thibult, N. *et al.* (1989). Hypertriglyceridaemia as a risk factor of coronary heart disease mortality in subjects with impaired glucose tolerance or diabetes: results from the 11-year follow-up of the Paris Prospective Study. *Diabetologia* **32**, 300–4.

Forrest, R. D., Jackson, C. A. and Yudkin, J. S. (1986). Glucose intolerance and hypertension in North London: The Islington Diabetes Survey. *Diabetic Medicine* **3**, 338–42.

Forrest, R. D., Jackson, C. A. and Yudkin, J. S. (1987*a*). Screening for diabetes mellitus in general practice using a reflectance meter system: the Islington Diabetes Survey. *Diabetes Research* **6**, 119–22.

Forrest, R. D., Jackson, C. A. and Yudkin, J. S. (1987*b*). The glycohaemoglobin assay as a screening test for diabetes mellitus: the Islington Diabetes Survey. *Diabetic Medicine* **4**, 254–9.

Forrest, R. D., Jackson, C. A. and Yudkin, J. S. (1988). The abbreviated glucose tolerance test in screening for diabetes: the Islington Diabetes Survey. *Diabetic Medicine* **5**, 557–61.

Franks, S. (1995). Polycystic ovary syndrome. *New England Journal of Medicine* **333**, 853–61.

Freeman, H., Looney, J. M. and Hoskins, R. G. (1942). 'Spontaneous' variability of oral glucose tolerance. *Journal of Clinical Endocrinology and Metabolism* **2**, 431–4.

Friderichsen, B. and Maunsbach, M. (1997). Glycosuric tests should not be employed in population screenings for NIDDM. *Journal of Public Health Medicine* **19**, 55–60.

Frisch, R. E., Wyshak, G., Albright, T. E., Albright, N. L. and Schiff, I. (1986). Lower prevalence of diabetes in female former college athletes compared with nonathletes. *Diabetes* **35**, 1101–5.

Fujimoto, W. Y., Bergstrom, R. W., Leonetti, D. L., Newell-Morris, L. L., Shuman, W. P. and Wahl, P. W. (1994). Metabolic and adipose risk factors for NIDDM and coronary disease in third-generation Japanese-American men and women with impaired glucose tolerance. *Diabetologia* **37**, 524–32.

Fuller, J. H., Shipley, M. J., Rose, G., Jarrett, R. J. and Keen, H. (1980). Coronary-heart-disease risk and impaired glucose tolerance: the Whitehall study. *Lancet* **1**, 1373–6.

Gaede, P., Vedel, P., Parving, H. H. and Pedersen, O. (1999). Intensified multifactorial intervention in patients with type 2 diabetes mellitus and microalbuminuria: the Steno type 2 randomised study. *Lancet* **353**, 617–22.

Ganda, O. P., Day, J. L., Soeldner, J. S., Connon, J. J. and Gleason, R. E. (1978). Reproducibility and comparative analysis of repeated intravenous and oral glucose tolerance tests. *Diabetes* **27**, 715–25.

Gerken, K. L. and Van Lente, F. (1990). Effectiveness of screening for diabetes. *Archives of Pathology and Laboratory Medicine* **114**, 201–3.

Gill, G. V., Lishman, M., Kaczmarczyk, E. and Tesfaye, S. (1996). Targeted screening for diabetes in community chiropody clinics. *Quarterly Journal of Medicine* **89**, 229–32.

Gillery, P., Dumont, G. and Vassault, A. (1998). Evaluation of GHb assays in France by national quality control surveys. *Diabetes Care* **21**, 265–70.

Godsland, I. F. (1985). Intra-individual variation: significant changes in parameters of lipid and carbohydrate metabolism in the individual and intra-individual variation in different test populations. *Annals of Clinical Biochemistry* **22**, 618–24.

Goyder, E. and Irwig, L. (1998). Screening for diabetes: what are we really doing? *British Medical Journal* **317**, 1644–6.

Goyder, E. and Irwig, L. (1999). Screening for Type 2 diabetes. *Journal of the American Medical Association* **281**, 1986–7.

Gray, C. S., Taylor, R., French, J. M., Alberti, K. G., Venables, G. S., James, O. F. *et al.* (1987). The prognostic value of stress hyperglycaemia and previously unrecognised diabetes in acute stroke. *Diabetic Medicine* **4**, 237–40.

Gray, A., Raikou, M., McGuire, A., Fenn, P., Stevens, R., Cull, C. *et al.* (2000). Cost effectiveness of an intensive blood glucose control policy in patients with type 2 diabetes: economic analysis alongside randomised controlled trial (UKPDS). *British Medical Journal* **320**, 1373–8.

Gress, T. W., Nieto, J., Shahar, E., Wofford, M. R., Brancati, F. L., for the Atherosclerosis in Communities Study (2000). Hypertension and antihypertensive therapy as risk factors for Type 2 diabetes. *New England Journal of Medicine* **342**, 905–12.

Griffin, S. J., Little, P. S., Hales, C. N., Kinmouth, A. L., and Wareham, N. J. (2000). Diabetes risk score: towards earlier detection of Type 2 diabetes in general practice. *Diabetes/Metabolism Research and Reviews* **16**, 164–71.

Haffner, S. M., Rosenthal, M., Hazuda, H. P., Stern, M. P. and Franco, L. J. (1984). Evaluation of three potential screening tests for diabetes in a biethnic population. *Diabetes Care* **7**, 347–53.

Haffner, S. M., Mitchell, B. D., Stern, M. P., Hazuda, H. P. and Patterson, J. K. (1990). Decreased prevalence of hypertension in Mexican-Americans. *Hypertension* **16**, 225–32.

Haffner, S. M., Alexander, C. M., Cook, T. J., Boccuzzi, S. J., Musliner, T. A., Pedersen, T. R. *et al.* (1999). Reduced coronary events in simvastatin-treated patients with coronary heart disease and diabetes or impaired fasting glucose levels: subgroup analyses in the Scandinavian Simvastatin Survival Study. *Archives of Internal Medicine* **159**, 2661–7.

Hales, C. N., Barker, D. J., Clark, P. M., Cox, L. J., Fall, C., Osmond, C. and Winter, P. D. (1991). Fetal and infant growth and impaired glucose tolerance at age 64. *British Medical Journal* **303**, 1019–22.

Hanefeld, M., Koehler, C., Fuecker, K., Henkel, E., Schaper, F. and Temelkova-Kurktschiev, T. (2003). Insulin secretion and insulin sensitivity pattern is different in isolated impaired glucose tolerance and impaired fasting glucose: the Risk Factor in Impaired Glucose Tolerance for Atherosclerosis and Diabetes Study. *Diabetes Care* **26**, 868–874.

Hanley, A. J., Williams, K., Gonzalez, C., D'Agostino, R. B. Jr, Wagenknecht, L. E., Stern, M. P., Haffner, S. M.; San Antonio Heart Study; Mexico City Diabetes Study; Insulin Resistance Atherosclerosis Study. (2003). Prediction of type 2 diabetes using simple measures of insulin resistance: combined results from the San Antonio Heart Study, the Mexico City Diabetes Study, and the Insulin Resistance Atherosclerosis Study. *Diabetes* 52, 463–9.

Hanson, R. L., Nelson, R. G., McCance, D. R., Beart, J. A., Charles, M. A., Pettitt, D. J. and Knowler, W. C. (1993). Comparison of screening tests for non-insulin-dependent diabetes mellitus. *Archives of Internal Medicine* 153, 2133–40.

Hansson, L., Zanchetti, A., Carruthers, S. G., Dahlof, B., Elmfeldt, D., Julius, S. *et al.* (1998). Effects of intensive blood-pressure lowering and low-dose aspirin in patients with hypertension: principal results of the Hypertension Optimal Treatment (HOT) randomised trial. HOT Study Group. *Lancet* 351, 1755–62.

Harding, P. E., Oakley, N. W. and Wynn, V. (1973). Reproducibility of oral glucose tolerance data in normal and mildly diabetic subjects. *Clinical Endocrinology* 2, 387–95.

Harris, M. I. (1989). Impaired glucose tolerance in the U. S. population. *Diabetes Care* 12, 464–74.

Harris, M. I. (1993). Undiagnosed NIDDM: clinical and public health issues. *Diabetes Care* 16, 642–52.

Harris, M. I., Hadden, W. C., Knowler, W. C. and Bennett, P. H. (1987). Prevalence of diabetes and impaired glucose tolerance and plasma glucose levels in U. S. population aged 20–74 yr. *Diabetes* 36, 523–34.

Harris, M. I., Klein, R., Welbourn, T. A. and Knuiman, M. W. (1992). Onset of NIDDM occurs at least 4–7 yr before clinical diagnosis. *Diabetes Care* 15, 815–19.

Harris, M. I., Eastman, R. C., Cowie, C. C., Flegal, K. M. and Eberhardt, M. S. (1997). Comparison of diabetes diagnostic categories in the US population according to 1997 American Diabetes Association and 1980–1985 World Health Organisation diagnostic criteria. *Diabetes Care* 20, 1859–62.

Harris, M. I., Flegal, K. M., Cowie, C. C., Eberhardt, M. S., Goldstein, D. E., Little, R. R. *et al.* (1998). Prevalence of diabetes, impaired fasting glucose, and impaired glucose tolerance in U. S. adults: the Third National Health and Nutrition Examination Survey, 1988–1994. *Diabetes Care* 21, 518–24.

Harris, R., Donahue, K., Rathore, S., Frame, P., Woolf, S. H. and Lohr, K. N. (2003). Screening adults for type 2 diabetes: a review of the evidence for the US Preventive Services Task Force. *Annals of Internal Medicine* 138, 215–29.

Harrison, T. A., Hindorff, L. A., Kim, H., Wines, R. C. M., Bowen, D. J., McGrath, B. B. and Edwards, K. L. (2003). Family history of diabetes as a potential public health tool. *American Journal of Preventive Medicine* 24, 152–159.

Hayden, M., Pignone, M., Phillips, C. and Mulrow, C. (2002). Aspirin for the primary prevention of cardiovascular events: a summary of the evidence for the US Preventive Services Task Force. *Annals of Internal Medicine* 136, 161–172.

Heine, R. J. and Mooy, J. M. (1996). Impaired glucose tolerance and unidentified diabetes. *Postgraduate Medical Journal* 72, 67–71.

Heine, R. J., Nijpels, G. and Mooy, J. M. (1996). New data on the rate of progression of impaired glucose tolerance to NIDDM and predicting factors. *Diabetic Medicine* 13, S12–14.

Helmrich, S. P., Ragland, D. R., Leung, R. W. and Paffenbarger, R. F. Jr. (1991). Physical activity and reduced occurrence of non-insulin-dependent-diabetes. *New England Journal of Medicine* 325, 147–52.

Herdzik, E., Safranow, K. and Ciechanowski, K. (2002). Diagnostic value of fasting capillary glucose, fructosamine and glycosylated haemoglobin in detecting diabetes and other glucose tolerance abnormalities compared to oral glucose tolerance test. *Acta Diabetologica* 39, 15–22.

Herman, J. B., Medalie, J. H. and Goldbourt, U. (1976). Diabetes, prediabetes and uricaemia. *Diabetologia* 12, 47–52.

Herman, W. H., Smith, P. J., Thompson, T. J., Engelgau, M. M. and Aubert, R. E. (1995). A new questionnaire to identify people at increased risk for undiagnosed diabetes. *Diabetes Care* 18, 382–7.

Howard, B. V., Rodriguez, B. L., Bennett, P. H., Harris, M. I., Hamman, R., Kuller, L. H. *et al.* (2002). Prevention Conference VI: Diabetes and Cardiovascular disease. Writing Group I: epidemiology. *Circulation* 105, e132–7.

Humphrey, L. L., Palumbo, P. J., Butters, M. A., Hallett, J. W. Jr, Chu, C. P., O'Fallon, W. M. and Ballard, D. J. (1994). The contribution of non-insulin-dependent diabetes to lower-extremity amputation in the community. *Archives of Internal Medicine* **154**, 885–92.

Inoue, I., Takahashi, K., Katayama, S., Harada, Y., Negishi, K., Ishii, J. *et al.* (1996). A higher proinsulin response to glucose loading predicts deteriorating fasting plasma glucose and worsening to diabetes in subjects with impaired glucose tolerance. *Diabetic Medicine* **13**, 330–6.

Jaber, L. A., Brown, M. B., Hammad, A., Nowak, S. N., Zhu, Q., Ghafoor, A. and Herman, W. H. (2003). Epidemiology of diabetes among Arab Americans. *Diabetes Care* **26**, 308–13.

Jackson, D. M., Wills, R., Davies, J., Meadows, K., Singh, B. M. and Wise, P. H. (1991). Public awareness of the symptoms of diabetes mellitus. *Diabetic Medicine* **8**, 971–2.

Kadowaki, T., Miyake, Y., Hagura, R., Akanuma, Y., Kajinuma, H., Kuzuya, N. *et al.* (1984). Risk factors for worsening to diabetes in subjects with impaired glucose tolerance. *Diabetologia* **26**, 44–9.

Kasezawa, N., Kiyose, H., Ito, K., Iwatsuka, T., Kawai, H., Goto, Y. *et al.* (1993). Criteria for screening diabetes mellitus using serum fructosamine level and fasting plasma glucose level: The Japanese Society of Multiphasic Health Testing and Services (JMHT), Fructosamine Working Party. *Methods of Information in Medicine* **32**, 237–40.

Keen, H. (1966). The presymptomatic diagnosis of diabetes. *Proceedings of the Royal Society of Medicine* **59**, 1169–74.

Kerbel, D., Glazier, R., Holzapfel, S., Yeung, M. and Lofsky, S. (1997). Adverse effects of screening for gestational diabetes: a prospective cohort study in Toronto, Canada. *Journal of Medical Screening* **4**, 128–32.

Khan, A., Lasker, S. S. and Chowdhury, T. A. (2003). Are spouses of patients with type 2 diabetes at increased risk of developing diabetes? *Diabetes Care* **26**, 710–12.

Kilpatrick, E. S., Maylor, P. W. and Keevil, B. G. (1998). Biological variation of glycated hemoglobin: implications for diabetes screening and monitoring. *Diabetes Care* **21**, 261–4.

King, H. and Rewers, M. (1993). Global estimates for prevalence of diabetes mellitus and impaired glucose tolerance in adults: WHO Ad Hoc Diabetes Reporting Group. *Diabetes Care* **16**, 157–77.

King, H. and Zimmet, P. (1988). Trends in the prevalence and incidence of diabetes: non-insulin-dependent diabetes mellitus. *World Health Statistics Quarterly* **41**, 190–6.

Kjos, S. L., Peters, R. K., Xiang, A., Henry, O. A., Montoro, M. and Buchanan, T. A. (1995). Predicting future diabetes in Latino women with gestational diabetes: utility of early postpartum glucose tolerance testing. *Diabetes* **44**, 586–91.

Knowler, W. C., Pettitt, D. J., Savage, P. J. and Bennett, P. H. (1981). Diabetes incidence in Pima indians: contributions of obesity and parental diabetes. *American Journal of Epidemiology* **113**, 144–56.

Knowler, W. C., Pettitt, D. J., Saad, M. F. and Bennett, P. H. (1990). Diabetes mellitus in the Pima Indians: incidence, risk factors and pathogenesis. *Diabetes Metabolism Reviews* **6**, 1–27.

Knowler, W. C., Barrett-Connor, E., Fowler, S. E., Hamman, R. F., Lachin, J. M., Walker, E. A., Nathan, D. M.; Diabetes Prevention Program Research Group (2002). Reduction in the incidence of type 2 diabetes with lifestyle intervention or metformin. *New England Journal of Medicine* **346**, 393–403.

Ko, G. T., Chan, J. C., Yeung, V. T., Chow, C. C., Tsang, L. W., Li, J. K. *et al.* (1998*a*). Combined use of a fasting plasma glucose concentration and HbA1c or fructosamine predicts the likelihood of having diabetes in high-risk subjects. *Diabetes Care* **21**, 1221–5.

Ko, G. T. C., Chan, J. C. N., Woo, J., Lau, E., Yeung, V. T. F., Chow, C-C. and Cockram, C. S. (1998*b*). The reproducibility and usefulness of the oral glucose tolerance test in screening for diabetes and other cardiovascular risk factors. *Annals of Clinical Biochemistry* **35**, 62–7.

Ko, G. T. C., Chan, J. C. N., Woo, J., Lau, E., Yeung, V. T. F., Chow, C-C. *et al.* (1998*c*). Glycated haemoglobin and cardiovascular risk factors in Chinese subjects with normal glucose tolerance. *Diabetic Medicine* **15**, 573–8.

Köbberling, J. and Tillil, H. (1982). Empirical risk figures for first degree relatives of non-insulin dependent diabetics. In *The genetics of diabetes mellitus* (ed. J. Kobberling and R. Tattersall), pp. 201–9. Academic Press, London.

Koivisto, V. A., Yki-Järvinen, H. and De Fronzo, R. (1986). Physical training and insulin sensitivity. *Diabetes Metabolism Reviews* **1**, 445–81.

Laing, W. and Williams, R. (1989). *Diabetes: a model for health care management.* No. 92 in a series of papers on current health problems. Office of Health Economics, London.

Larsson, H., Berglund, G., Lindegarde, F. and Ahren, B. (1998). Comparison of ADA and WHO criteria for diagnosis of diabetes and glucose intolerance. *Diabetologia* **41**, 1124–5.

Lawrenson, R. A., Dunn, P. J., Jury, D. and Sceats, J. (1993). Discover diabetes: screening for diabetes mellitus in the Waikato. *New Zealand Medical Journal* **106**, 522–4.

Legro, R. S., Kunselman, A. R., Dodson, W. C. and Dunaif, A. (1999). Prevalence and predictors of risk for type 2 diabetes mellitus and impaired glucose tolerance in polycystic ovary syndrome: a prospective, controlled study in 254 affected women. *Journal of Clinical Endocrinology and Metabolism* **84**, 165–9.

Lewis, E. J., Hunsicker, L. G., Clarke, W. R., Berl, T., Pohl, M. A., Lewis, J. B. *et al.* (2001). Renoprotective effect of the angiotensin-receptor antagonist irbesartan in patients with nephropathy due to type 2 diabetes. *New England Journal of Medicine* **345**, 851–60.

Lindstrom, J. and Tuomilehto, J. (2003). The diabetes risk score: a practical tool to predict type 2 diabetes risk. *Diabetes Care* **26**, 725–31.

LIPID Study Group (1998). Prevention of cardiovascular events and death with pravastatin in patients with coronary heart disease and a broad range of initial cholesterol levels: the Long-Term Intervention with Pravastatin in Ischaemic Disease (LIPID) Study Group. *New England Journal of Medicine* **339**, 1349–57.

Little, R. R., England, J. D., Wiedmeyer, H. M., McKenzie, E. M., Pettitt, D. J., Knowler, W. C. and Goldstein, D. E. (1988). Relationship of glycosylated hemoglobin to oral glucose tolerance: implications for diabetes screening. *Diabetes* **37**, 60–4.

Litzelman, D. K., Slemenda, C. W., Langefeld, C. D., Hays, L. M., Welch, M. A., Bild, D. E. *et al.* (1993). Reduction of lower extremity clinical abnormalities in patients with non-insulin-dependent diabetes mellitus: a randomized, controlled trial. *Annals of Internal Medicine* **119**, 36–41.

McCance, D. R., Pettit, D., Hanson, R. L., Jacobsson, L. T. H., Knowler, W. C. and Bennett, P. H. (1994). Birth weight and non-insulin dependent diabetes: thrifty genotype, thrifty phenotype, or surviving small baby genotype? *British Medical Journal* **308**, 942–5.

McCarthy, M. I., Hitman, G. A., Mohan, V., Ramachandran, A., Snehalatha, C. and Viswanathan, M. (1992). The islet amyloid polypeptide gene and non-insulin-dependent diabetes mellitus in south Indians. *Diabetes Research and Clinical Practice* **18**, 31–4.

McDonald, G. W., Fisher, G. F. and Burnham, C. (1965). Reproducibility of the oral glucose tolerance test. *Diabetes* **14**, 473–80.

McLarty, D. G., Swai, A. B., Kitange, H. M., Masuki, G., Mtinangi, B. L., Kilim, P. M. *et al.* (1989). Prevalence of diabetes and impaired glucose tolerance in rural Tanzania. *Lancet* **2**, 871–5.

McPhillips, J. B., Barrett-Connor, E. and Wingard, D. L. (1990). Cardiovascular disease risk factors prior to the diagnosis of impaired glucose tolerance and non-insulin-dependent diabetes mellitus in a community of older adults. *American Journal of Epidemiology* **131**, 443–53.

Malone, J. M., Snyder, M., Anderson, G., Bernhard, V. M., Holloway, G. A. Jr. and Bunt, T. J. (1989). Prevention of amputation by diabetic education. *American Journal of Surgery* **158**, 520–3; discussion 523–4.

Mannucci, E., Bardini, G., Ognibene, A. and Rotella, C. M. (1998). Screening for diabetes in obese patients using the new diagnostic criteria. [Correspondence.] *Diabetes Care* **21**, 468–9.

Marshall, S. M. and Barth, J. H. (2000). Standardization of HbA1c measurements: a consensus statement. *Diabetic Medicine* **17**, 5–6.

Mason, J., O'Keeffe, C., Hutchinson, A., McIntosh, A., Young, R. and Booth, A. (1999*a*). A systematic review of foot ulcer in patients with Type 2 diabetes mellitus. II: treatment. *Diabetic Medicine* **16**, 889–909.

Mason, J., O'Keeffe, C., McIntosh, A., Hutchinson, A., Booth, A. and Young, R. J. (1999*b*). A systematic review of foot ulcer in patients with Type 2 diabetes mellitus. I: prevention. *Diabetic Medicine* **16**, 801–12.

Metzger, B. E., Bybee, D. E., Frienkel, N., Phelps, R. L., Radvany, R. M. and Vaisrub, N. (1985). Gestational diabetes mellitus: correlations between the phenotypic and genotypic characteristics of the mother and abnormal glucose tolerance during the first year postpartum. *Diabetes* **34**(Suppl. 2), 111–15.

Metzger, B. E., Cho, N. H., Roston, S. M. and Radvany, R. (1993). Prepregnancy weight and antepartum insulin secretion predict glucose tolerance five years after gestational diabetes mellitus. *Diabetes Care* **16**, 1598–605.

Modan, M., Karasik, A., Halkin, H., Fuchs, Z., Lusky, A., Shitrit, A. and Modan, B. (1986). Effect of past and concurrent body mass index on prevalence of glucose intolerance and type 2 (non-insulin-dependent) diabetes and on insulin response: the Israel study of glucose intolerance, obesity and hypertension. *Diabetologia* **29**, 82–9.

Modan, M., Meytes, D., Rozeman, P., Yosef, S. B., Sehayek, E., Yosef, N. B. *et al.* (1988). Significance of high HbA1 levels in normal glucose tolerance. *Diabetes Care* **11**, 422–8.

Modan, M. and Harris, M. I. (1994). Fasting plasma glucose in screening for NIDDM in the U. S. and Israel. *Diabetes Care* **17**, 436–9.

Mooy, J. M., Grootenhuis, P. A., de Vries, H., Kostense, P. J., Popp-Snijders, C., Bouter, L. M. and Heine, R. J. (1996). Intra-individual variation of glucose, specific insulin and proinsulin concentrations measured by two oral glucose tolerance tests in a general Caucasian population: the Hoorn Study. *Diabetologia* **39**, 298–305.

Morales, P. A., Mitchell, B. D., Valdez, R. A., Hazuda, H. P., Stern, M. P. and Haffner, S. M. (1993). Incidence of NIDDM and impaired glucose tolerance in hypertensive subjects: the San Antonio Heart Study. *Diabetes* **42**, 154–61.

Moss, S. E., Klein, R. and Klein, B. E. (1988). The incidence of vision loss in a diabetic population. *Ophthalmology* **95**, 1340–8.

Moss, S. E., Klein, R. and Klein, B. E. (1994). Ten-year incidence of visual loss in a diabetic population. *Ophthalmology* **101**, 1061–70.

Moss, S. E., Klein, R. and Klein, B. E. (1999). The 14-year incidence of lower-extremity amputations in a diabetic population: the Wisconsin Epidemiologic Study of Diabetic Retinopathy. *Diabetes Care* **22**, 951–9.

Motala, A. A., Omar, M. A. and Gouws, E. (1993). High risk of progression to NIDDM in South-African Indians with impaired glucose tolerance. *Diabetes* **42**, 556–63.

MRC/BHF (2002). Heart protection study of cholesterol with simvastatin in 20,536 high-risk individuals: a randomised placebo-controlled trial. *Lancet* **360**, 7–22.

Nichols, J. H. (2002). Interpreting method evaluations. *Diabetes Technology and Therapeutics* **4**, 623–5.

Nichols, J. H., Howard, C., Loman, K., Miller, C., Nyberg, D. and Chan, D. W. (1995). Laboratory and bedside evaluation of portable glucose meters. *American Journal of Clinical Pathology* **103**, 244–51.

Nilsson, P., Lindholm, L. and Schersten, B. (1990). Hyperinsulinaemia and other metabolic disturbances in well-controlled hypertensive men and women: an epidemiological study of the Dally population. *Journal of Hypertension* **8**, 953–9.

Norhammar, A., Tenerz, A., Nilsson, G., Hamsten, A., Efendic, S., Ryden, L. and Malmberg, K. (2002). Glucose metabolism in patients with acute myocardial infarction and no previous diagnosis of diabetes mellitus: a prospective study. *Lancet* **359**, 2140–4.

Ohkubo, Y., Kishikawa, H., Araki, E., Miyata, T., Isami, S., Motoyoshi, S. *et al.* (1995). Intensive insulin therapy prevents the progression of diabetic microvascular complications in Japanese patients with non-insulin-dependent diabetes mellitus: a randomized prospective 6-year study. *Diabetes Research and Clinical Practice* **28**, 103–17.

Ohlson, L. O., Larsson, B., Svardsudd, K., Welin, L., Eriksson, H., Wilhelmsen, L. *et al.* (1985). The influence of body fat distribution on the incidence of diabetes mellitus: 13.5 years of follow-up of the participants in the study of men born in 1913. *Diabetes* **34**, 1055–8.

Olefsky, J. M. and Reaven, G. M. (1974). Insulin and glucose responses to identical oral glucose tolerance tests performed forty-eight hours apart. *Diabetes* **23**, 449–53.

O'Rahilly, S., Spivey, R. S., Holman, R. R., Nugent, Z., Clark, A. and Turner, R. C. (1987). Type II diabetes of early onset: a distinct clinical and genetic syndrome? *British Medical Journal (Clinical Research Edition)* **294**, 923–8.

O'Sullivan, J. B. (1979). Prevalence and course of diabetes modified by fasting blood glucose levels: implications for diagnostic criteria. *Diabetes Care* **2**, 85–90.

O'Sullivan, J. B. (1984). Subsequent morbidity among gestational diabetic women. In *Carbohydrate metabolism in pregnancy and the newborn* (ed. H. W. Sutherland and J. M. Stowers), pp. 174–80. Churchill Livingstone, Edinburgh.

O'Sullivan, J. B. (1988). The interaction between pregnancy, diabetes and long term maternal outcome. In *Diabetes mellitus in pregnancy: principles and Practice* (ed. E. A. Reece and D. R. Coustan), pp. 575–85. Churchill Livingstone, New York.

O'Sullivan, J. B. (1991). Diabetes mellitus after GDM. *Diabetes* **40**(Suppl. 2), 131–5.

O'Sullivan, J. B. and Mahan, C. M. (1966). Glucose tolerance test: variability in pregnant and non-pregnant women. *American Journal of Clinical Nutrition* **19**, 345–51.

Oswald, G. A. and Yudkin, J. S. (1987). Hyperglycaemia following acute myocardial infarction: the contribution of undiagnosed diabetes. *Diabetic Medicine* **4**, 68–70.

Pan, W. H., Cedres, L. B., Liu, K., Dyer, A., Schoenberger, J. A., Shekelle, R. B. *et al.* (1986). Relationship of clinical diabetes and asymptomatic hyperglycemia to risk of coronary heart disease mortality in men and women. *American Journal of Epidemiology* **123**, 504–16.

Pan, X. R., Li, G. W., Hu, Y. H., Wang, J. X., Yang, W. Y., An, Z. X. *et al.* (1997). Effects of diet and exercise in preventing NIDDM in people with impaired glucose tolerance: the Da Qing IGT and Diabetes Study. *Diabetes Care* **20**, 537–44.

Panzram, G. (1987). Mortality and survival in type 2 (non-insulin-dependent) diabetes mellitus. *Diabetologia* **30**, 123–31.

Park, P. J., Griffin, S. J., Duffy, S. W. and Wareham, N. J. (2000). The effect of varying the screening interval on false positives and duration of undiagnosed disease in a screening programme for type 2 diabetes. *Journal of Medical Screening* **7**, 91–6.

Park, P. J., Griffin, S. J., Sargeant, L. and Wareham, N. J. (2002). The performance of a risk score in predicting undiagnosed hyperglycemia. *Diabetes Care* **25**, 984–8.

Pauvilai, G., Chanprasertyotin, S. and Sriphraprdaeng, A. (1999). Diagnostic criteria for diabetes mellitus and other categories of glucose intolerance: 1997 criteria by the Expert Committee on the diagnosis and classification of diabetes mellitus (ADA), 1998 WHO criteria, and the 1985 WHO criteria. World Health Organization. *Diabetes Research and Clinical Practice* **44**, 21–6.

Perry, I. J., Wannamethee, S. G., Walker, M. K., Thomson, A. G., Whincup, P. H. and Shaper, A. G. (1995). Prospective study of risk factors for development of non-insulin dependent diabetes in middle aged British men. *British Medical Journal* **310**, 560–4.

Perry, I. J., Wannamethee, S. G., Shaper, A. G. and Alberti, K. G. (1999). Serum true insulin concentration and the risk of clinical non-insulin dependent diabetes during long-term follow-up. *International Journal of Epidemiology* **28**, 735–41.

Peters, A. L., Davidson, M. B., Schriger, D. L. and Hasselblad, V. (1996). A clinical approach for the diagnosis of diabetes mellitus: an analysis using glycosylated hemoglobin levels. Meta-analysis Research Group on the Diagnosis of Diabetes Using Glycated Hemoglobin Levels. *Journal of the American Medical Association* **276**, 1246–52.

Petry, C. J. and Hales, C. N. (1999). Intrauterine development and its relationship to Type 2 diabetes. In *Type 2 diabetes: prediction and prevention* (ed. G. A. Hitman), pp. 153–68. Wiley and Sons, Chichester.

Pierce, M., Lundy, S., Palanisamy, A., Winning, S. and King, J. (1989). Prospective randomised controlled trial of methods of call and recall for cervical cytology screening. *British Medical Journal* **299**, 160–2.

Pierpoint, T., McKeigue, P. M., Isaacs, A. J., Wild, S. H. and Jacobs, H. S. (1998). Mortality of women with polycystic ovary syndrome at long-term follow-up. *Journal of Clinical Epidemiology* **51**, 581–6.

Pomerleau, J., McKeigue, P. M. and Chaturvedi, N. (1999). Relationships of fasting and postload glucose levels to sex and alcohol consumption: are American Diabetes Association criteria biased against detection in women. *Diabetes Care* **22**, 430–3.

Pyorala, K., Pedersen, T. R., Kjekshus, J., Faergeman, O., Olsson, A. G. and Thorgeirsson, G. (1997). Cholesterol lowering with simvastatin improves prognosis of diabetic patients with coronary heart disease: a subgroup analysis of the Scandinavian Simvastatin Survival Study (4S). *Diabetes Care* **20**, 614–20.

Qiao, Q., Keinanen-Kiukaanniemi, S., Rajala, U., Uusimaki, A. and Kivela, S. L. (1995). Random capillary whole blood glucose test as a screening test for diabetes mellitus in a middle-aged population. *Scandinavian Journal of Clinical Laboratory Investigation* **55**, 3–8.

Raikou, M. and McGuire, A. (2003). The economics of screening and treatment of type 2 diabetes mellitus. *Pharmacoeconomics* **21**, 543–64.

Resnick, H. E., Valsania, P. and Phillips, C. L. (1999). Diabetes mellitus and nontraumatic lower extremity amputation in black and white Americans: The National Health and Nutrition Examination Survey Epidemiologic followup Study, 1971–1992. *Archives of Internal Medicine* **159**, 2470–5.

Riccardi, G., Vaccaro, O., Rivellese, A., Pignalosa, S., Tutino, L. and Mancini, M. (1985). Reproducibility of the new diagnostic criteria for impaired glucose tolerance. *American Journal of Epidemiology* **121**, 422–9.

Robertson, D. A., Alberti, K. G. M. M., Cowse, G. K., Zimmet, P., Toumilehto, J. and Gareeboo, H. (1992). Is serum anhydroglucitol an alternative to the oral glucose tolerance test for diabetes screening? *Diabetic Medicine* **10**, 56–60.

Robinson, S., Chan, S. P., Spacey, S., Anyaoku, V., Johnston, D. G. and Franks, S. (1992). Postprandial thermogenesis is reduced in polycystic ovary syndrome and is associated with increased insulin resistance. *Clinical Endocrinology* (Oxf) **36**, 537–43.

Rohlfing, C. L., Little, R. R., Wiedmeyer, H-M., England, J. D., Madsen, R., Harris, M. I. *et al.* (2000). Use of GHb (HbA1c) in screening for undiagnosed diabetes in the U. S. population. *Diabetes Care* **23**, 187–91.

Rubins, H. B., Robins, S. J., Collins, D., Fye, C. L., Anderson, J. W., Elam, M. B. *et al.* (1999). Gemfibrozil for the secondary prevention of coronary heart disease in men with low levels of high-density lipoprotein cholesterol. Veterans Affairs High-Density Lipoprotein Cholesterol Intervention Trial Study Group. *New England Journal of Medicine* **341**, 410–18.

Ruige, J. B., De Neeling, J. N., Kostense, P. J., Bouter, L. M. and Heine, R. J. (1997). Performance of a NIDDM screening questionnaire based on symptoms and risk factors. *Diabetes Care* **20**, 491–6.

Saad, M. F., Knowler, W. C., Pettitt, D. J., Nelson, R. G., Mott, D. M. and Bennett, P. H. (1988). The natural history of impaired glucose tolerance in the Pima Indians. *New England Journal of Medicine* **319**, 1500–6.

Santiago, J. V., Davis, J. E. and Fisher, F. (1978). Hemoglobin A1c levels in a diabetes detection program. *Journal of Clinical Endocrinology and Metabolism* 47, 578–80.

Schaefer-Graf, U. M., Buchanan, T. A., Xiang, A. H., Peters, R. K. and Kjos, S. L. (2002). Clinical predictors for a high risk for the development of diabetes mellitus in the early puerperium in women with recent gestational diabetes mellitus. *American Journal of Obstetrics and Gynecology* 186, 751–6.

Schneider, H., Lischinski, M. and Jutzi, E. (1993). Survival time after onset of diabetes: 29-year follow-up mortality study in a diabetes cohort from a rural district. *Diabete et Metabolisme* 19, 152–8.

Schneider, H., Ehrlich, M., Lischinski, M. and Schneider, F. (1996). Bewirkte das flächendeckende glukosurie-screening der 60er und 70er jahre im Osten Deutschlands tatsächlich den erhofften prognosevorteil für die frühzeitig entdeckten diabetiker? *Diabetes Stoffwechsel* 5, 33–8.

Sekikawa, A., Tominaga, M., Takahashi, K., Watanabe, H., Miyazawa, K. and Sasaki, H. (1990). Is examination of fructosamine levels valuable as a diagnostic test for diabetes mellitus? *Diabetes Research and Clinical Practice* 8, 187–92.

Shaw, J. E., Zimmet, P. Z., de Courten, M., Dowse, G. K., Chitson, P., Gareeboo, H. *et al.* (1999). Impaired fasting glucose or impaired glucose tolerance: what best predicts future diabetes in Mauritius? *Diabetes Care* 22, 399–402.

Shaw, J. E., Zimmet, P. Z., Hodge, A. M., de Courten, M., Dowse, G. K., Chitson, P. *et al.* (2000). Impaired fasting glucose: how low should it go? *Diabetes Care* 23, 34–9.

Shirasaya, K., Miyakawa, M., Yoshida, K., Takahashi, E., Shimada, N. and Kondo, T. (1999). Economic evaluation of alternative indicators of screening for diabetes mellitus. *Preventive Medicine* 29, 79–86.

Sicree, R. A., Zimmet, P. Z., King, H. O. and Coventry, J. S. (1987). Plasma insulin response among Nauruans: prediction of deterioration in glucose tolerance over 6 yr. *Diabetes* 36, 179–86.

Simmons, D. and Williams, D. R. (1994). Random blood glucose as a screening test for diabetes in a biethnic population. *Diabetic Medicine* 11, 830–5.

Simmons, D., Williams, D. R. R. and Powell, M. J. (1991). The Coventry Diabetes Study: prevalence of diabetes and impaired glucose tolerance in Europids and Asians. *Quarterly Journal of Medicine* 81, 1021–30.

Simon, D., Coignet, M. C., Thibilt, N., Senan, C. and Eschwege, E. (1985). Comparison of glycosylated hemoglobin and fasting plasma glucose with two-hour post-load plasma glucose in the detection of diabetes mellitus. *American Journal of Epidemiology* 122, 589–93.

Singh, B. M., Jackson, D. M., Wills, R., Davies, J. and Wise, P. H. (1992). Delayed diagnosis in non-insulin dependent diabetes mellitus. *British Medical Journal* 304, 1154–5.

Singh, B. M., Prescott, J. J., Guy, R., Walford, S., Murphy, M. and Wise, P. H. (1994). Effect of advertising on awareness of symptoms of diabetes among the general public: the British Diabetic Association Study. *British Medical Journal* 308, 632–6.

Spijkerman, A., Griffin, S., Dekker, J., Nijpels, G. and Wareham, N. J. (2002). What is the risk of mortality for people who are screen positive in a diabetes screening programme but who do not have diabetes on biochemical testing? Diabetes screening programmes from a public health perspective. *Journal of Medical Screening* 9, 187–90.

Stewart, M. W., Humphriss, D. B., Berrish, T. S., Barriocanal, L. A., Trajano, L. R., Alberti, K. G. and Walker, M. (1995). Features of syndrome X in first-degree relatives of NIDDM. *Diabetes Care* 18, 1020–2.

Tanaka, Y., Atsumi, Y., Matsuoka, K., Mokubo, A., Asahina, T., Hosokawa, K. *et al.* (2001). Usefulness of stable HbA(1c) for supportive marker to diagnose diabetes mellitus in Japanese subjects. *Diabetes Research and Clinical Practice* 53, 41–5.

Toeller, M. and Knussmann, R. (1973). Reproducibility of oral glucose tolerance tests with three different loads. *Diabetologia* 9, 102–7.

Torjman, M. C., Jahn, L., Joseph, J. I. and Crothall, K. (2001). Accuracy of the hemocue portable glucose analyser in a large nonhomogeneous population. *Diabetes Technology and Therapeutics* **3**, 591–600.

Treweek, S. P., Condie, M. E. and Gilmour, D. G. (1998). Screening for diabetes in lower limb amputees: a pilot study. *Journal of the Royal College of Surgeons of Edinburgh* **43**, 93–4.

Tripathy, D., Carlsson, M., Almgren, P., Isomaa, B., Taskinen, M-R., Tuomi, T. and Groop, L. C. (2000). Insulin secretion and insulin sensitivity in relation to glucose tolerance: lessons from the Botnia Study. *Diabetes* **49**, 975–80.

Troisi, R. J., Cowie, C. C. and Harris, M. I. (2000). Diurnal variation in fasting plasma glucose: implications for diagnosis of diabetes in patients examined in the afternoon. *Journal of the American Medical Association* **284**, 3157–9.

Tsuji, I., Nakamoto, K., Hasegawa, T., Hisashige, A., Inawashiro, H., Fukao, A. and Hisamichi, S. (1991). Receiver operating characteristic analysis on fasting plasma glucose, HbA1c, and fructosamine on diabetes screening. *Diabetes Care* **14**, 1075–7.

Tuomilehto, J., Rastenyte, D., Birkenhager, W. H., Thijs, L., Antikainen, R., Bulpitt, C. J. *et al.* (1999). Effects of calcium-channel blockade in older patients with diabetes and systolic hypertension. Systolic Hypertension in Europe Trial Investigators. *New England Journal of Medicine* **340**, 677–84.

Tuomilehto, J., Lindström, J., Eriksson, J. G., Valle, T. T., Hämäläinen, H., Ilanne-Parikka, P. *et al.* (2001). Prevention of type 2 diabetes mellitus by changes in lifestyle among subjects with impaired glucose tolerance. *New England Journal of Medicine* **344**, 1343–50.

UK National Screening Committee (1998). *First report of the National Screening Committee: the NSC handbook of population screening programmes*, Chapter 6. Health Departments of the United Kingdom.

UKPDS (UK Prospective Diabetes Study) Group (1991). UK Prospective Diabetes Study (UKPDS). VIII. Study design, progress and performance. *Diabetologia* **34**, 877–90.

UKPDS (UK Prospective Diabetes Study) Group (1994). UK Prospective Diabetes Study XII: differences between Asian, Afro-Caribbean and White Caucasian type 2 diabetic patients at diagnosis of diabetes. *Diabetic Medicine* **11**, 670–7.

UKPDS (UK Prospective Diabetes Study) Group (1998*a*). Intensive blood-glucose control with sulphonylureas or insulin compared with conventional treatment and risk of complications in patients with type 2 diabetes (UKPDS 33). *Lancet* **352**, 837–53.

UKPDS (UK Prospective Diabetes Study) Group (1998*b*). Tight blood pressure control and risk of macrovascular and microvascular complications in type 2 diabetes (UKPDS 38). *British Medical Journal* **317**, 703–13.

UKPDS (UK Prospective Diabetes Study) Group (1998*c*). Cost effectiveness analysis of improved blood pressure control in hypertensive patients with type 2 diabetes (UKPDS 40). *British Medical Journal* **317**, 720–6.

UKPDS (Hypertension) (1993). Hypertension in diabetes study (HDS): I. Prevalence of hypertension in newly presenting type 2 diabetic patients and the association with risk factors for cardiovascular and diabetic complications. *Journal of Hypertension* **11**, 309–17.

Unwin, N., Alberti, K. G. M. M., Bhopal, R., Harland, J., Watson, W. and White, M. (1998). Comparison of the current WHO and new ADA criteria for the diagnosis of diabetes mellitus in three ethnic groups in the UK. *Diabetic Medicine* **15**, 554–7.

Unwin, N., Shaw, J., Zimmet, P., and Alberti, K. G. M. M. for International Diabetes Federation IGT/IFG Consensus Statement (2002). Report of an Expert Consensus Workshop 1–4 August 2001, Stoke Poges, UK. Impaired glucose tolerance and impaired fasting glycaemia: the current status on definition and intervention. *Diabetic Medicine* **19**, 708–23.

USPSTF (US Preventive Services Task Force) (2003). Screening for Type 2 diabetes mellitus in adults: recommendations and rationale. February 2003. *Annals of Internal Medicine* **138**, 212–14.

Vaccaro, O., Rivellese, A., Riccardi, G., Capaldo, B., Tutino, L., Annuzzi, G. and Mancini, M. (1984). Impaired glucose tolerance and risk factors for atherosclerosis. *Arteriosclerosis* 4, 592–7.

Wang, W., Lee, E. T., Fabsitz, R., Welty, T. K. and Howard, B. V. (2002). Using HbA(1c) to improve efficacy of the American Diabetes Association fasting plasma glucose criterion in screening for new type 2 diabetes in American Indians: the strong heart study. *Diabetes Care* 25, 1365–70.

Wareham, N. J. and Griffin, S. J. (2001). Should we screen for type 2 diabetes? Evaluation against National Screening Committee criteria. *British Medical Journal* 322, 986–8.

Welborn, T. A., Reid, C. M. and Marriott, G. (1997). Australian Diabetes Screening Study: impaired glucose tolerance and non-insulin-dependent diabetes mellitus. *Metabolism* 46, 35–9.

Wenying, Y., Lixiang, L., Jimevu, Q., Zhiqing, Y., Haicheng, P., Guofeng, H. *et al.* (2001). The preventative effect of acarbose and metformin on the progression to diabetes mellitus in the IGT population: a 3 year multicenter prospective study. *Journal of Clinical Endocrinology and Metabolism* 17, 131–5.

West, K. M. (1978). Diabetes in American Indians. *Advances in Metabolic Disorders* 9, 29–48.

West, K. M. and Kalbfleisch, J. M. (1971). Sensitivity and specificity of five screening tests for diabetes in ten countries. *Diabetes* 20, 289–96.

Westlund, K. and Nicolaysen, R. (1972). Ten year mortality and morbidity related to serum cholesterol. *Scandinavian Journal of Clinical and Laboratory Investigation* 30(Suppl. 127), 1–24.

Williams, D. R., Wareham, N. J., Brown, D. C., Byrne, C. D., Clark, P. M., Cox, B. D. *et al.* (1995). Undiagnosed glucose intolerance in the community: the Isle of Ely Diabetes Project. *Diabetic Medicine* 12, 30–5.

WHO (World Health Organization) (1985). WHO Study Group on Diabetes Mellitus. Technical Report Series 727. World Health Organization, Geneva.

WHO (World Health Organization) (1999). *Definition, diagnosis and classification of diabetes mellitus and its complications*. Report of a WHO Consultation: World Health Organization, Geneva.

WHO (World Health Organization) (2001). Principles of Screening (draft). World Health Organization, Geneva.

WHO (World Health Organization) (2003). *Screening for type 2 diabetes*. Report of a World Health Organization and International Diabetes Federation meeting. World Health Organization, Geneva.

Worth, R. C., Harrison, K., Anderson, J., Johnston, D. G. and Alberti, K. G. M. M. (1981). A comparison of blood glucose test strips. *Diabetes Care* 4, 407–11.

Yamada, N., Yoshinaga, H., Gotoda, T., Harada, K., Shimada, M., Ohsuga, J. *et al.* (1994). Plasma lipid abnormalities and risk factors for coronary artery disease in Japanese subjects with diabetes mellitus and glucose intolerance. *Diabetes Research and Clinical Practice* 24(Suppl.), S215–220.

Yamanouchi, T., Akanuma, Y., Toyota, T., Kuzuya, T., Kawai, T., Kawazu, S. *et al.* (1991). Comparison of 1,5-anhydroglucitol, HbA1c, and fructosamine for detection of diabetes mellitus. *Diabetes* 40, 52–7.

Yudkin, J. S., Oswald, G. A., McKeigue, P. M., Forrest, R. D. and Jackson, C. A. (1988). The relationship of hospital admission and fatality from myocardial infarction to glycohaemoglobin levels. *Diabetologia* 31, 201–5.

Yudkin, J. S., Alberti, K. G. M. M., McLarty, D. G. and Swai, A. B. M. (1990*a*). Impaired glucose tolerance: is it a risk factor for diabetes or a diagnostic ragbag? *British Medical Journal* 301, 397–402.

Yudkin, J. S., Forrest, R. D., Jackson, C. A., Ryle, A. J., Davie, S. and Gould, B. J. (1990*b*). Unexplained variability of glycated haemoglobin in non-diabetic subjects not related to glycaemia. *Diabetologia* 33, 208–15.

Yue, D. K., Molyneaux, L. M., Ross, G. P., Constantino, M. I., Child, A. G. and Turtle, J. R. (1996). Why does ethnicity affect prevalence of gestational diabetes? The underwater volcano theory. *Diabetic Medicine* 13, 748–52.

Yusuf, S., Sleight, P., Pogue, J., Bosch, J., Davies, R. and Dagenais, G. (2000). Effects of an angiotensin-converting-enzyme inhibitor, ramipril, on cardiovascular events in high-risk patients. The Heart Outcomes Prevention Evaluation Study Investigators. *New England Journal of Medicine* **342**, 145–53.

Zimmet, P. (1989). Non-insulin-dependent (type 2) diabetes mellitus: does it really exist? *Diabetic Medicine* **6**, 728–35.

Chapter 43

Primary prevention of high blood pressure

P. Elliott and J. Stamler

43.1 Introduction

Raised blood pressure (BP) is a major risk factor for coronary heart disease (CHD) and the major risk factor for stroke (see Chapter 3). It is one of the most important underlying risk factors for cardiovascular and all-cause mortality in the world today, ranking above tobacco in estimates of the worldwide attributable burden of mortality (Ezzati and Lopez 2002). Demographic changes in the poorer countries (the so-called 'epidemiological transition'), together with adoption of Western lifestyle, mean that the poorer countries are set to experience an epidemic of cardiovascular diseases, as has been the case in the last century in the developed countries (Pearson *et al.* 1993). The rise of BP with age, leading to the development of unfavourable BP patterns in populations, along with smoking and unfavourable blood lipid profiles (related to diet), diabetes, and overweight–obesity are the key factors underlying this worldwide epidemic.

In this chapter, we review the risks of premature mortality and increased morbidity associated with raised BP, and the risk factors that lead to raised BP in individuals and populations. We then briefly address how this knowledge can inform preventive strategies to reduce the population burden of BP-related diseases.

43.1.1 Risks associated with raised BP in populations

As shown repeatedly by prospective population studies, the relationship between BP and disease risks is continuous, graded, strong, and independent of other risk factors. This relationship with BP is found for sudden cardiac death, CHD, stroke, abdominal aortic aneurysm, peripheral vascular disease, end-stage renal disease, and all-cause mortality. It prevails for women and men, young adult, middle-, and older-aged (Prospective Studies Collaboration 2002). It prevails for all ethnic and socio-economic strata (SES), even more severely for those of lower SES. It prevails internationally for populations from both industrialized and economically developing countries. It prevails for non-smokers and smokers, for non-diabetic and diabetic individuals, for persons at all levels of serum cholesterol, and for those without and with a history of heart attack (National High Blood Pressure Education Program Working Group 1993; Stamler *et al.* 1993a, b, 1996c; Klag *et al.* 1996; Lowe *et al.* 1998; Cooper *et al.* 2000; Miura *et al.* 2001; Rodin *et al.* 2003).

Excess risk is manifest for every systolic/diastolic BP (SBP/DBP) stratum above normal, that is, SBP above 120 mmHg and/or DBP above 80 mmHg (Chobanian *et al.* 2003). Population average BP higher by as little as 2–3 mmHg is associated with significant increases in risks of

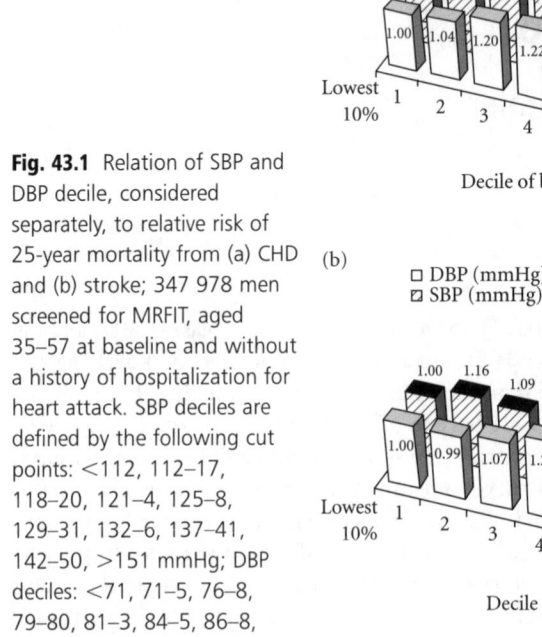
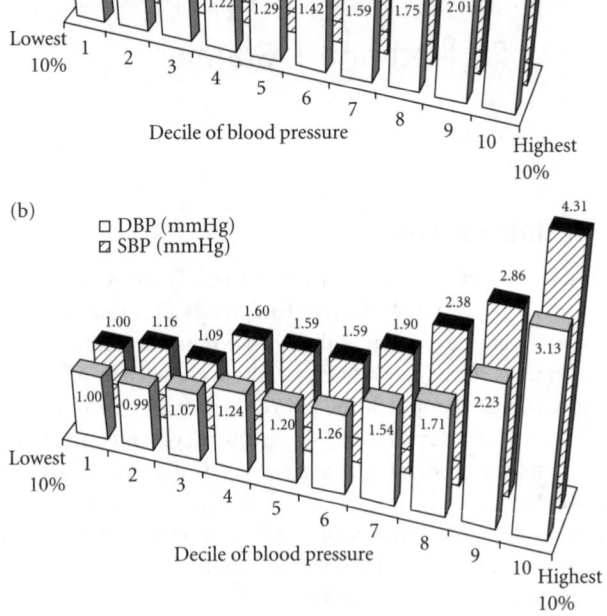

Fig. 43.1 Relation of SBP and DBP decile, considered separately, to relative risk of 25-year mortality from (a) CHD and (b) stroke; 347 978 men screened for MRFIT, aged 35–57 at baseline and without a history of hospitalization for heart attack. SBP deciles are defined by the following cut points: <112, 112–17, 118–20, 121–4, 125–8, 129–31, 132–6, 137–41, 142–50, >151 mmHg; DBP deciles: <71, 71–5, 76–8, 79–80, 81–3, 84–5, 86–8, 89–91, 92–7, >98 mmHg.

major diseases and death (Rose 1981; Stamler *et al.* 1993a, b; Klag *et al.* 1996; Miura *et al.* 2001). That is, *the BP problem goes beyond high BP as defined clinically* (SBP ≥ 140 mmHg and/or DBP ≥ 90 mmHg); risks are also higher for adults with BP levels in the pre-hypertension range as defined by the Joint National Committee on Prevention, Detection, Evaluation, and Treatment of High Blood Pressure (JNC) 7 Report, that is, SBP 120–39 mmHg and/or DBP 80–9 mmHg (Chobanian *et al.* 2003) (see Chapter 4).

This relationship of SBP/DBP to long-term risks is especially well demonstrated in the Multiple Risk Factor Intervention Trial (MRFIT) cohort of almost 350 000 men aged 35–57 screened in 18 US cities in 1973–75 (Fig. 43.1). Given large sample size and large numbers of deaths with 25-year follow-up, estimated mortality rates for each BP stratum are highly precise. The MRFIT cohort was the largest study contributing to a meta-analysis of 61 prospective studies, giving data on risks for women as well as men (Prospective Studies Collaboration 2002).

Only 18% of the MRFIT cohort had normal BP (SBP/DBP < 120/< 80 mmHg) (Neaton *et al.* 1994). Thus, adverse BP levels were the rule, not the exception, involving most (82%) of this sample of US men, young adult and early middle-aged, weighted toward higher SES levels. Some 47% had BP in the pre-hypertension range, about another quarter (26%) had Stage 1 hypertension (SBP 140–59 and/or DBP 90–9), and 9% Stage 2 hypertension (SBP ≥ 160 and/or DBP ≥ 100). Based on age-adjusted relative risk data, the estimate is that 50% of the 23 382 CHD deaths were excess deaths attributable to adverse SBP. While the highest *relative* risk was found for men with the highest BPs (Fig. 43.1), in terms of *attributable* risk 43% of these excess deaths

Table 43.1 Mean SBP and DBP, US Population, NHANES III, Phase I (1988–91), by age, ethnic group, and gender

Age (years)	Mean SBP (mmHg)				Mean DBP (mmHg)			
	Black men	Black women	White men	White women	Black men	Black women	White men	White women
18–29	119	108	117	106	72	65	70	65
30–9	122	115	119	110	78	73	77	70
40–9	128	123	122	114	82	76	79	72
50–9	136	132	127	123	84	76	79	74
60–74	140	142	134	132	79	73	75	70

Source: Data from Burt *et al.* 1995.

NHANES: National Health and Nutrition Examination Survey.

occurred among men in the pre-hypertension stratum, and a further 36% (2243 deaths) among men with Stage 1 hypertension at baseline. This is because nearly half the population had BPs in the pre-hypertension range. As Geoffrey Rose emphasized, many exposed to a 'small' excess relative risk may generate more cases than a small number exposed to a much higher risk (see Chapter 36).

In terms of disease prevention, pharmacological treatment of high BP is currently recommended for sustained systolic BP $\geq$ 140 mmHg (Chobanian *et al.* 2003). Even if a campaign to lower BPs in the community through pharmacological means were completely successful (implying a never-ending programme of screening and drug treatment, and assuming that anti-hypertensive drugs were 100% effective in achieving normal BP and preventing disease due to high BP, and without side effects), based on the above data around 43% of the BP-related mortality (and associated morbidity) would still not be prevented. To address (at the least) this part of the population BP problem requires a non-pharmacological approach alongside lifestyle plus drug treatment, to reduce the population burden of BP-related disease.

43.1.2 Low BP populations and the rise in BP with age

The rise in mean BP with age, and the potential for prevention if that rise could be stemmed, is demonstrated by data from the US National Health and Nutrition Examination Survey (Table 43.1). In each ethnic group and gender, the lowest average BPs are seen at ages 18–29, ranging from 106 mmHg (white women) to 119 mmHg (black men) for SBP and 65 mmHg (black and white women) to 72 mmHg (black men) for DBP, that is, average BPs within the normal BP range. Average BPs rise progressively with age thereafter, reaching at higher ages pre-hypertensive or (for black men and women aged 60–74 years) frank hypertensive levels. In terms of prevention of the CHD–cardiovascular disease (CVD) epidemic, the favourable BP patterns found in young adulthood need to be maintained throughout adult life; in addition the social and dietary factors underlying the higher mean BPs in black compared with white individuals, both men and women, apparent even at the youngest ages, need to be addressed (see later in this chapter).

Similarly, the data in Fig. 43.1 and Table 43.1 indicate that a substantial majority of the population develop adverse BP levels by middle age, and a substantial minority develop clinical

Fig. 43.2 BP distribution in London civil servants and Kenyan nomads. (Reproduced by permission of Oxford University Press from Rose, G (1985). Sick individuals and sick populations. *International Journal of Epidemiology* **14**, 32–8.)

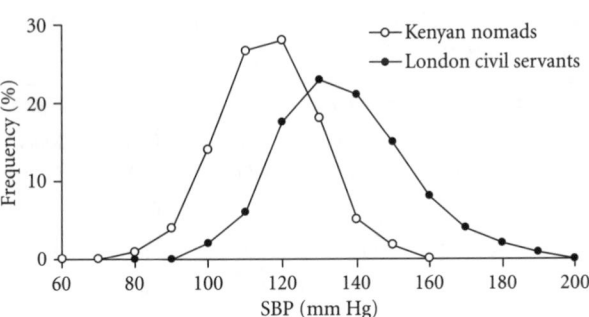

high BP; and given the rise of BP with age, this becomes even more so at older ages. For example, data from the Health Survey for England indicate that around 30% of both men and women have Stage 1 hypertension by ages of 55–64 years (Erens and Primatesta 1999).

A rise of BP with age is, however, not a universal finding in all societies. There are populations around the world where BP remains low throughout the lifespan, and hypertension is rare or absent. Figure 43.2 compares the BP distribution of Kenyan nomads with London civil servants (Rose 1985). While in both populations the BP distribution follows a familiar normal or log-normal curve, there is a striking shift to the right – toward higher BP levels – of the entire BP distribution for the London civil servants. The Kenyan population has much lower BP levels, and the prevalence of hypertension, even at older ages, is low.

Several other populations around the world have been studied where BPs are low and there is no or only minimal rise in BP with age (Shaper 1972; Carvalho *et al.* 1989). When people from low BP populations migrate, however, their BPs tend to rise. For example, among the Luo in Kenya, BPs were measured in the rural villages and then in an urban setting as men from the villages migrated to Nairobi (Poulter *et al.* 1990). SBPs were higher for the migrants compared with rural controls; the differences in BP between the two groups correlated with a number of variables, including higher urinary sodium:potassium (Na: K) ratio and higher bodyweight among the migrants.

43.2 **Implications for prevention**

Studies of low BP populations and the rise in BP when they migrate indicate that the reasons for the large differences in the position of the BP distribution between populations (Fig. 43.2) are due largely to environmental (not population genetic) factors. The key to prevention of the worldwide epidemic of BP-related morbidity and mortality is to identify and address those environmental factors (mainly dietary) that underlie the rise in BP with age, and result in the high prevalence of adverse BP levels and frank hypertension at older ages. For example, in the INTERSALT study, difference in average SBP for a 30-year period from average age 25 to average age 55 was around 16 mmHg (INTERSALT 1989) – around 11 mmHg greater average SBP difference for that period was associated with Na intake across population samples higher by 100 mmol/day (Elliott *et al.* 1996).

- ◆ Since risks of major diseases and death are importantly influenced by all levels of SBP/DBP above normal, and such raised BP levels prevail for the great majority of the adult population, the main and primary goal is to achieve a progressive downward shift in population average

SBP/DBP – so that the percentage of people with normal BP levels increases steadily over time, to become the norm (rather than the exception) at all adult ages.

♦ Effective population-wide strategies are required to reduce and eliminate the usual increases in SBP/DBP from youth into middle and older age.

♦ People with pre-hypertensive BP levels need to be identified early so that effective sustained improvements in lifestyles can be brought to bear – beyond general population-wide public health efforts – to restore BPs to normal levels (<120/80 mmHg).

♦ Simply relying on a high-risk strategy (Chapter 36) to identify and treat hypertensive individuals will not address risk among the important group with pre-hypertensive BP levels. Such a strategy is late, defensive, reactive (not proactive) and incomplete, ignoring adverse SBP/DBP levels among millions, and failing to achieve optimal BP levels for most patients. By definition it cannot put an end to the epidemic of adverse BP levels. Only primary prevention of this major risk factor can accomplish that task, and at the same time bring about a progressive large reduction in the burden of prevalent and incident cases of clinical high BP.

43.3 Established dietary and lifestyle risk factors for high BP

Four dietary and related factors are established risk factors for high BP: high NaCl (salt) intake, low K intake, calorie imbalance and overweight–obesity, and excessive alcohol drinking (Whelton *et al.* 2002*b*). In addition, the DASH (Dietary Approaches to Stop Hypertension) diet is beneficial with regard to BP reduction (Appel *et al.* 1997; Moore *et al.* 2001; Sacks *et al.* 2001; Svetkey *et al.* 1999) (see below). The evidence for these four factors – and the DASH diet – is now briefly reviewed.

43.3.1 Sodium chloride (salt)

Evidence of an adverse effect of Na intake on BP comes from animal experimental studies, anthropology, clinical observation, controlled clinical trials, and epidemiological studies both within and across populations.

Animal studies

There are various animal models of Na-induced hypertension, including dog and chicken, although the most commonly used experimental animal model is the rat. Several strains of rat develop hypertension and stroke when fed high doses of salt, while salt restriction attenuates the development of severe hypertension in spontaneously hypertensive rats. Increased K intake offsets to some extent the adverse effects of a high salt diet (National Research Council 1989). Denton and colleagues (1995) added up to 15 g/day salt to the diets of an experimental group of chimpanzees over a 20 month period; compared with a control group, SBP/DBP rose 33/10 mmHg, with rapid reversal to baseline values once the added salt was removed.

Evidence from anthropology

Several data sets on remote populations indicate the importance of salt intake in determining BP patterns, including the data cited above on the low salt intake of isolated populations with low normal BP at all ages and little or no rise in BP with age. By way of further examples, among six Solomon Islands population samples, only one, the Lau, had prevalent high BPs (Page *et al.* 1974). In contrast with the other five population samples that consumed low salt diets, the Lau cooked their food in brackish water from a Pacific inlet, hence had higher salt intake. The Qash'qai nomads of Iran had high salt intakes, with no rise of bodyweight with age, but a significant rise in SBP and DBP with age and prevalences of Stage 1 (or higher) hypertension at age 30 years or over of 12% in men and 18% in women (Page *et al.* 1981).

Consumption of Na in the UK, USA, and other Western countries averages around 140–50 mmol/day (8–9 g/day salt) (INTERSALT 1988). The addition of salt to the human diet is a relatively recent phenomenon, dating back only some 6–8000 years to when agriculture and animal husbandry were invented. Humans evolved on a low salt diet of no more than 20–40 mmol Na/day, and became (and remain) adapted to the physiological conservation of the limited salt naturally present in foods, not for excretion of a Na load some 10–20+ times the physiological need (8–10 mmol/day) (National Research Council 1989).

Clinical observations and controlled clinical trials

While Na reduction was advocated in the treatment of hypertension early in the last century, it was not until the 1940s that it gained favour when Kempner's low-Na rice diet proved to be an effective treatment of malignant hypertension. The introduction of diuretic therapy – which promotes both Na and water loss – revolutionized the management of hypertension. Subsequently, a number of controlled trials showed that lowered Na intake can reduce – or even obviate – the need for anti-hypertensive medication among people who have been treated for high BP (Elliott 1989).

Controlled clinical trials of Na reduction and BP have been the subject of various meta-analyses published in recent years (Midgley *et al.* 1996; Cutler *et al.* 1997; Graudal *et al.* 1998; He and MacGregor 2002). Despite different inclusion criteria, each of the meta-analyses reported a significant reduction in BP with lower Na intake. For example, Graudal *et al.* (1998) reported a mean decrease in SBP/DBP of 4.5/2.3 mmHg, and 1.6/0.4 mmHg, for mean Na reductions of 129 mmol/day and 165 mmol/day, among hypertensive and normotensive persons, respectively. Interpretation of the meta-analyses is not straightforward, however (Stamler 1997). Issues include the varying quality among the many trials, varying adherence of participants to counselling for salt intake reduction (leading to underestimation of true effects on BP), heterogeneity among trials, and, in two of the meta-analyses (Midgley *et al.* 1996; Graudal *et al.* 1998) inclusion of large numbers of short-duration trials with large fluctuations in Na intakes. Well-conducted trials of longer duration (4 weeks or more) tend to show larger effects (He and MacGregor 2002; Sacks *et al.* 2001).

Two high-quality trials have investigated effects of three different levels of Na intake on BP. The first used a double-blind randomized crossover design and either placebo or salt tablets to provide three Na intake levels among participants who had restricted Na intake to around 50 mmol/day. Comparison of the lowest Na group (49 mmol/day) with the highest (190 mmol/day) showed SBP/DBP reduction by 16/9 mmHg (MacGregor *et al.* 1989). The second study, the DASH-Na trial, was a feeding trial with all food supplied to participants to achieve high adherence; again its design provided for three levels of Na (Sacks *et al.* 2001) (Fig. 43.3). Results of the DASH and DASH-Na trials are considered further below.

From the perspective of primary prevention, results of a unique trial of lower Na intake in newborns are pertinent. The trial was carried out in the Netherlands in the early 1980s before no-added-salt baby feeds were widely available. With Na intake lower by about two-thirds, SBP at 6 months was significantly lower than in the 'usual' (high) Na group, by 2.1 mmHg (Hofman *et al.* 1983). At follow-up 15 years later, the reduced Na group continued to have lower BP than the 'usual' Na group, despite no further intervention since infancy (Geleijnse *et al.* 1997).

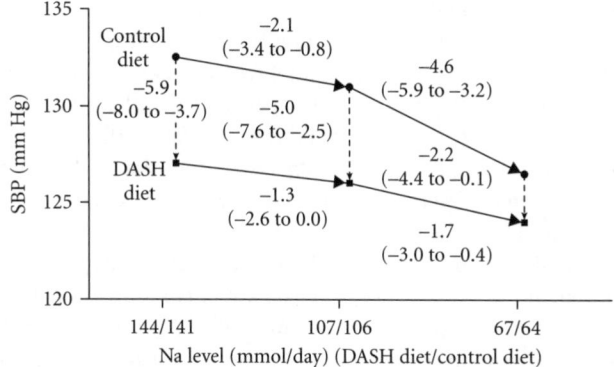

Fig. 43.3 DASH-Na Trial: effect of DASH diet and three different levels of Na intake on SBP. The figure gives reduction in SBP (95% CI) between control and DASH diets (Na (DASH/control) 144/141 mmol/day: −5.9 mmHg; 107/106 mmol/day: −5.0 mmHg; 67/64 mmol/day: −2.2 mmHg) and at different levels of Na control: 141 to 106 mmol/day: −2.1 mmHg; 106 to 64 mmol/day: −4.6 mmHg. DASH: 144 to 107 mmol/day: −1.3 mmHg; 107 to 67 mmol/day: −1.7 mmHg). (Adapted with permission from Sacks *et al.* (2001). Effects on blood pressure of reduced sodium and the Dietary Approaches to Stop Hypertension (DASH) diet. *New England Journal of Medicine* **344**, 3–10. Copyright © 2001 Massachusetts Medical Society. All rights reserved.)

Epidemiological studies

Epidemiological evidence for a positive association between Na and BP comes from both cross- and within-population studies. A positive cross-population association of salt and hypertension was first described by Dahl in 1960, and subsequently by other authors, though based on published data from different studies and subject to varying degrees of possible bias and confounding (Elliott 1991). By contrast, up until the 1980s, the within-population (individual) level studies were largely considered to be negative; because of methodological problems – especially large day-to-day variation in Na intake – estimates of association were biased toward the null ('regression dilution') and many were too small to find any effect (Elliott 1991). However, in an overview of 14 studies (16 populations) that reported BP and 24 h urinary Na excretion data (excluding INTERSALT – see below), a highly significant positive association of Na with both SBP and DBP was found, larger among women than men (Elliott 1991).

The INTERSALT study is the most extensive epidemiological investigation yet reported on the relation of Na to BP. It included over 10 000 men and women aged 20–59 years from 52 population samples in 32 countries (INTERSALT 1988). Sodium and K intakes were assessed by 24 h urinary excretion. A random 8% of participants provided two 24 h urine collections to estimate reliability (Dyer *et al.* 1994*a*, *b*) because known large day-to-day variability in Na intakes mean that estimates based on a single day's measure (e.g., a 24-h urinary collection) are imprecise measures of *usual* intake; this leads to attenuation of associations between Na and other variables such as BP (Liu 1988), so-called *regression-dilution bias*.

The study examined associations both across the 52 population samples and among the 10 000+ individuals who took part. In the cross-population analyses, a highly significant relationship of Na with upward slope of BP with age was found across the 52 population samples, such that SBP/DBP rise with age over a 30 year period (e.g., 25–55 years) was estimated to be 10/6 mmHg less for Na lower by 100 mmol/day. This finding was robust to different methods of estimating the upward slope with age in the 52 populations (Elliott *et al.* 1996). In addition, adjusted median SBP/DBP was lower by 4.5/2.3 mmHg for Na lower by 100 mmol/day (INTERSALT 1988) and Stage 1 (or greater) hypertension prevalence lower by 4.8 percentage points (Stamler 1997).

Results for the within-population analyses, both uncorrected and corrected for reliability (the regression-dilution problem) are shown in Table 43.2. The coefficients in the table are pooled from sample-specific multiple regression analyses, weighting each individual coefficient by the inverse of its variance. Data are shown both sample–age–sex adjusted and multiple adjusted, with and without BMI in the model. This is because inclusion of BMI may represent over-adjustment: Na and BMI are positively correlated and at least some of the BMI–BP relationship may be operating through association with Na. Also *usual* Na is estimated with limited reliability (because of the regression-dilution problem) while BMI is very precisely estimated and therefore tends to dominate in the regression models (Liu 1988; Dyer *et al.* 1994*a, b*). Table 43.2 shows that in the sample–age–sex adjusted models, and in the multiple adjusted models excluding BMI, Na is significantly associated positively with both SBP and DBP.

Table 43.2 INTERSALT study, pooled within-population regression estimates (SE) of BP difference per 100 mmol/day higher Na excretion, without and with correction for reliability, men and women combined (*n* = 10 074)

Reliability corrected[a]	Estimated difference in SBP (mmHg)			Estimated difference in DBP (mmHg)		
	Age–sex adjusted	Multiple adjustment[b]		Age–sex adjusted	Multiple adjustment[b]	
		With BMI	Without BMI		With BMI	Without BMI
No	1.6 (0.2)	1.0 (0.3)	2.1 (0.3)	0.7 (0.2)	0.04 (0.2)	0.9 (0.2)
Yes	4.3 (0.8)	3.1 (0.9)	6.0 (1.1)	1.8 (0.5)	0.1 (0.6)	2.5 (0.7)

BMI: body mass index.

[a] Multivariate correction for reliability (regression-dilution bias); standard error estimated approximately by bootstrap sampling.

[b] Adjusted for sample, age, sex, 24 h urinary K excretion, alcohol intake.

Table 43.3 INTERSALT Study: estimated differences in SBP and DBP for given differences in 24 h Na and K excretion, BMI, and alcohol intake

	SBP (mmHg)		DBP (mmHg)	
Na (100 mmol lower)	−3.1		−0.1	
without BMI		−6.0		−2.5
K (50 mmol higher)	−3.4		−1.8	
BMI (2 units lower)	−1.6		−1.2	
Alcohol (nil vs. ≥300 ml/week)[a]	−0.5		−0.3	
Total	−8.6	−11.5	−3.4	−5.9

10 074 men and women, 52 population samples. From individual-level regression models adjusted for sample, age, sex, and the other variables, except Na adjusted with/without BMI. Na, K corrected for reliability estimated from repeated measures on 8%.

[a] Regression estimates for alcohol intake are multiplied by 0.15 as overall 15% of the population sample had alcohol intake of ≥300 ml/week.

With BMI in the model, Na remains significantly associated with SBP. Associations of Na with BP tended to be larger in women than in men, and also at older compared with younger ages (not shown). Overall, in men and women combined with correction for reliability, 100 mmol lower Na intake was associated with SBP/DBP lower by 3–6/0–3 mmHg.

Few studies have investigated the association of Na intake and subsequent mortality; most were flawed methodologically (Chobanian and Hill 2000). Recently a Finnish group has reported up to 14 years mortality follow-up of over 1400 men and women from whom 24 h urinary Na excretion was obtained in the 1980s. There was a significant positive association between urinary Na excretion (based on a single 24 h urine collection) and subsequent CHD, CVD, and all-cause mortality. Multiple adjusted hazard ratios (men and women combined) were 1.56 (95% confidence interval (CI): 1.15–2.12), 1.36 (1.05–1.76), and 1.22 (1.02–1.47) per 100 mmol Na, respectively (Tuomilehto et al. 2001).

43.3.2 Calorie imbalance and overweight–obesity

Overweight and obesity reflect an imbalance (over time) between energy intake and energy expenditure. Extensive epidemiological data indicate that there is a strong, independent, direct association between bodyweight or BMI and BP (Stamler 1991; National High Blood Pressure Education Program Working Group 1993). For example, in the INTERSALT study, a 10 kg difference in bodyweight was associated with a 3 mmHg difference in SBP, and a difference in DBP that ranged from 2 to 3 mmHg (Dyer et al. 1990).

Larger effects of bodyweight on BP have been noted in clinical trials. An overview of 25 randomized controlled trials of weight reduction and BP published between 1966 and 2002, involving a total of 4874 participants, reported SBP lower by 4.4 mmHg and DBP by 3.6 mmHg for a net weight reduction of around 5 kg; per kilogram of weight loss, BP reductions were 1.1 mmHg systolic and 0.9 mmHg diastolic (Neter et al. 2003).

Weight loss has also been shown to reduce the incidence of hypertension. In phase I of the Trials of Hypertension Prevention study (TOHP-1), weight loss intervention produced a 34% reduction in risk of hypertension over a 12–18-month period among men with initial DBP 80–9 mmHg (TOHP 1992). Subsequently TOHP-1 participants from the Johns Hopkins clinical centre were followed up for 7 years; incidence of hypertension was ~19% in the weight loss group and 40% in its control group (He et al. 2000). In phase II of the TOHP, during up to 48 months of follow-up, there was a 21% reduction in hypertension incidence among participants assigned to weight loss intervention compared with those assigned to usual care (TOHP 1997).

Increased physical activity

Physical activity is an important component in maintaining optimal bodyweight. By the early 1990s, research reports from both observational studies and intervention trials indicated that regular, frequent, moderate isotonic exercise was associated with lower BP (National High Blood Pressure Education Program Working Group 1993). In a recent meta-analysis of 54 randomized controlled trials involving 2419 participants, aerobic exercise was associated with falls in SBP of 3.8 mmHg and DBP of 2.6 mmHg compared with control groups. Average overall weight change was small (–0.4 kg) and average BP reduction was not significantly associated with average change in bodyweight, suggesting that aerobic exercise may have an additional beneficial effect on BP independent of changes in bodyweight (Whelton et al. 2002a).

43.3.3 **Potassium**

The INTERSALT study found an independent, inverse association of urinary K excretion with both SBP and DBP (Table 43.3) and a positive association with the Na : K ratio (INTERSALT 1988). In China, in particular, K intakes are low, and in the face of high Na intake, Na : K ratios are high (Stamler *et al.* 1993*c*; Zhao *et al.* 2004). In a meta-analysis of the results of 32 randomized controlled trials involving 2561 participants, K supplementation (median: 75 mmol/day) resulted in SBP lower by ~3 mmHg and DBP by 2 mmHg. Potassium supplementation appeared to have a greater effect in those with higher levels of sodium intake (Whelton *et al.* 1997).

43.3.4 **Alcohol consumption**

Observational studies have documented a direct association of alcohol intake with BP (Dyer *et al.* 1977; Klatsky *et al.* 1977; Beilin *et al.* 1996). In the INTERSALT study, men who drank 300–499 ml alcohol per week had SBP/DBP on average higher by 2.7/1.6 mmHg than non-drinkers, and men who drank ≥500 ml alcohol per week had pressures 4.6/3.0 mmHg higher. For women, drinkers of ≥300 ml alcohol per week had SBP/DBP higher by 3.9/3.1 mmHg than non-drinkers (Marmot *et al.* 1994). In a meta-analysis of 15 randomized controlled trials, involving 2234 participants, reduction in alcohol intake was associated with reduction in SBP of ~3.3 mmHg and in DBP of 2.0 mmHg (Xin *et al.* 2001).

43.3.5 **Combined effects of the established risk factors for high BP**

The results of the INTERSALT study give an indication of the potential for BP reduction at the population level for realizable changes in each of the four established risk factors for high BP. Table 43.3 gives estimated differences in BP from multiple regression models for given differences in the four factors. For Na, the regression model was run with and without BMI. Note also that the estimate for alcohol has been adjusted for the fact that only ~15% of participants were consuming ≥300 ml/week absolute alcohol. Potentially these independent effects can be summed up to give an overall estimate of the potential population-wide BP lowering benefit that could be achieved by favourable changes in the combination of these risk factors. Depending on which of the Na models is selected (i.e., with or without BMI), the potential benefit is on average between 8 and 12 mmHg for SBP and 3 to 6 mmHg for DBP.

Data on the combined effect of dietary risk factors for high BP are also available from the INTERMAP cooperative study of macro- and micro-nutrient intakes and other factors in relation to BP, involving 4680 individuals from four countries (Japan, China, UK, USA) (Stamler *et al.* 2003). To assess diet, BP, and other variables, participants were seen at four visits, four 24 h in-depth dietary recalls were done, and two timed 24 h urine specimens collected (Stamler *et al.* 2003). Large BP differences were observed between samples in northern and southern China; average SBP/DBPs were 7.4/6.9 mmHg higher for northern than southern participants. North–south BP differences became much smaller (SBP/DBP –1.1/1.0 mmHg) with inclusion in multiple regression models of Na, K, and BMI, as well as magnesium or phosphorus, suggesting that these variables accounted importantly for the observed BP differences (Zhao *et al.* 2004).

Both the INTERSALT and INTERMAP studies indicate a significant association between higher SES and lower BP, which is largely explained by the tendency for lower SES groups to have more adverse patterns of the established dietary risk factors for high BP (Stamler *et al.* 1992; Stamler *et al.* 2003).

43.3.6 **DASH diet**

The DASH and DASH-Na trials both included adult men and women – African-American and non-Hispanic white – with pre-hypertensive and high BPs (Stage 1) (Appel *et al.* 1997; Svetkey *et al.* 1999; Moore *et al.* 2001; Sacks *et al.* 2001). Eligible participants were consumers of little or no alcohol and were on average overweight. Based on recent epidemiological findings indicating that multiple dietary factors influence BP, both trials assessed effects on BP of a 'combination diet' compared to a usual American diet. The combination diet was increased in fruits, vegetables, and fat-free and low-fat dairy products; it included whole grains, poultry, fish, and nuts; and it was reduced in fats, red meats, sweets, and sugar-containing beverages (Appel *et al.* 1997). Thus, it differed from the usual American diet in regard to many macro-and micronutrients – higher in total and vegetable protein, complex carbohydrates, fibre, K, magnesium, phosphorus, calcium, antioxidant and other vitamins, and lower in total fat, saturated fat, cholesterol, and sugars. In both DASH and DASH-Na, high-level adherence to the randomly assigned diet was achieved mainly by making all foods available to participants throughout the trials. That is, they were nutritional intervention trials of the feeding – not the counselling – type. Both were isocaloric by design, that is, energy content of supplied foods was serially adjusted to minimize loss or gain of weight. In the first trial, NaCl intake was deliberately maintained constant across groups at ~7.5 g/day (slightly below population average), so as not to be a trial confounder (Appel *et al.* 1997). In the second trial (Sacks *et al.* 2001), participants randomized to both groups (usual US diet and combination diet) were also randomly fed three levels of salt, designed to supply Na at 150, 100, and 50 mmol/day – 8.7, 5.8, and 2.9 g/day NaCl; that is, usual US intake, moderate reduction, more marked reduction.

Effects of the combination diet on SBP/DBP were similar in the two trials: reductions overall of ~6/3 mmHg (with NaCl at or near usual US average level) (Appel *et al.* 1997; Sacks *et al.* 2001). It was effective in all subgroups, defined by gender, age, income, education, ethnicity, body mass, and physical activity (Svetkey *et al.* 1999). Significant reductions in SBP and DBP occurred in response to the combination diet for both pre-hypertensive and hypertensive participants: ~4–5/2–3 mmHg and 12/5 mmHg, respectively (Appel *et al.* 1997; Sacks *et al.* 2001), including a net fall in SBP of 11 mmHg for a subgroup with isolated systolic hypertension (Moore *et al.* 2001).

For participants on both usual US and DASH combination diets, lower compared to higher salt intake substantially reduced SBP/DBP, for example by ~7/4 mmHg overall for those on usual American fare (Fig. 43.3); SBP was decreased by ~5 mmHg for pre-hypertensive and 9 mmHg for hypertensive participants (Sacks *et al.* 2001). Influence on BP was greater with reduction of NaCl from intermediate to lower level than from higher to intermediate level. The overall reduction of ~7/4 mmHg with Na lower by ~90 mmol/day in the DASH-Na trial is quantitatively concordant with the INTERSALT estimated effect of 6.0/2.5 mmHg with 100 mmol/day lower Na intake by individuals (Table 43.3) (Elliott *et al.* 1996).

Effects of the combination diet and of salt reduction were additive (partially, not completely). Thus, for the group on combination diet plus lower salt intake, SBP/DBP net reduction overall (compared to the group on usual US fare with higher salt intake) was ~9/6 mmHg; SBP was lowered 7 mmHg for pre-hypertensive participants and 12 mmHg for hypertensive participants (Sacks *et al.* 2001).

A further trial, PREMIER, compared an 'established' behavioural intervention (weight reduction, lower alcohol, lower Na, and increased exercise) with and without the DASH combination diet, versus an 'advice only' group. Both the 'established' and 'established plus DASH' groups recorded significant falls in both SBP and DBP, and hypertension incidence, compared with the 'advice only' group, though there were no significant differences in BP lowering or reduced incidence of hypertension between the two intervention groups (PREMIER 2003).

43.4 Other factors associated with BP

In addition to the established risk factors for high BP noted above, several other dietary factors have been implicated as influencing BP.

43.4.1 Macronutrients

In a second round of analyses, INTERSALT found an independent inverse relation to SBP/DBP of dietary total protein intake (measured by 24 h urinary total nitrogen or urea nitrogen) (Stamler *et al.* 1996*a*). Similar results were reported for 11 000+ middle-aged men randomized into the MRFIT study, based on analyses of average dietary data from 4 to 5 annual 24 h recalls done for each man and average annual SBP and DBP during the six trial years (Stamler *et al.* 1996*b*, 1997). The analyses for men in the MRFIT cohort also showed a direct relation of dietary cholesterol or Keys 3-factor dietary lipid score to BP, independent of age, ethnicity, education, BMI, reported Na, K, protein, and alcohol intake (Stamler *et al.* 1996*b*, 1997).

Other observational studies also report an inverse relation of dietary protein to BP. While in most studies this relates to markers of total protein and BP (Elliott 2003), cross-sectional data from the INTERMAP Study showed a significant inverse relation between vegetable protein and BP, but not animal or total protein and BP (Elliott 2001).

The Chicago Western Electric Study reported prospective data on diet and BP, for a cohort of over 1700 men who underwent two in-depth nutrition surveys in 1957–58 and 1958–59, and were followed annually for 9 years (Stamler *et al.* 2002). Data were not available on Na and K intake by these men. In multivariate analyses, dietary vegetable protein – but not total or animal protein – was inversely related to 9 year BP trend; dietary cholesterol or Keys score, heavy alcohol intake, and 9 year weight gain were directly related to 9 year BP change.

The observational epidemiological data on dietary vegetable protein and BP from the Western Electric and INTERMAP studies are concordant with findings from short-term intervention trials indicating that increase in vegetable protein intake from soy protein produces significant BP reduction (Elliott 2003).

43.4.2 Micronutrients, fibre, and foods

In the prospective analyses of the Western Electric Study, there was a significant independent inverse relation to average annual BP change of a combined antioxidant score based on beta-carotene and vitamin C intake (Stamler *et al.* 2002). Also, in analyses on food group–BP relations, intakes of vegetables and fruits were inversely related to SBP change, that is, average annual rise; intakes of beef–veal–lamb and of poultry related directly to SBP change (Miura *et al.* 2004). Data are also available indicating an inverse relation of dietary fibre to BP (Appel and Elliott 2003), small inverse associations with calcium (Allender *et al.* 1996) and magnesium (Mizushima *et al.* 1998), and an inverse association with phosphorus (Stamler *et al.* 2003; Zhao *et al.* 2004).

43.5 Strategies for the prevention of adverse BP levels

The *general strategy* is to implement – at national scale first and foremost – public policy to encourage improvements in population-wide eating patterns. This encompasses the DASH combination diet with lower salt intake, plus prevention and control of overweight–obesity, and of heavy alcohol consumption, alongside population-wide improvement in leisure-time physical activity – together with continued progress in achieving prevention and cessation of smoking. Such a strategy would be expected to lower average SBP/DBP, stem the rise in BP with age, and hence reduce the prevalence of pre-hypertension and hypertension at older ages, as well as increase the numbers of people with normal BP – with consequent reduction in BP-related disease.

43.5.1 **Specific strategies**

Conception and pregnancy

Low birthweight is associated with higher adult SBP/DBP, indicating a possible role for intrauterine nutrition in determining BP levels in later life (Barker 1998). There is need to extend and enhance prenatal care from conception on, to maximize favourable nutritional patterns and lifestyles for all pregnant women.

Infancy and childhood

Dietary composition and weight gain pattern in early childhood are especially important since they set the pattern for later life; it is easier to establish favourable lifestyle habits from the beginning than to decondition unfavourable habits later on. Commercial targeting of high salt, high sugar foods at children runs counter to this principle (see Chapter 46).

For teenagers and young adults

It is well established that adverse levels of SBP/DBP and other major risk factors in teenagers and young adults are already predictive of increased risk of CHD–CVD and shortened life expectancy. For the sizeable proportion of teenagers and especially young adults who already have SBP/DBP above normal, special targeted measures are needed at the individual level – that is, beyond general population-wide public health measures – to improve lifestyles and restore SBP/DBP to optimal levels.

For middle-aged and older adults

For most people BP becomes progressively higher at these stages of the lifespan, so that by early middle age only a minority have normal SBP/DBP. Since CHD–CVD are epidemic during these years, major strategic emphasis is needed on the primary prevention of the SBP/DBP rises of these years. These need to include detection and care of less severe adverse SBP/DBP levels in middle-aged and older adults as an ongoing clinical effort; that is, 'early' detection and care not only of people with high BP, but also those with pre-hypertensive BP levels. Care for all such people needs to include as a major ongoing component effective improvement of eating, drinking, exercise, and smoking habits, as well as antihypertensive drug therapy when indicated.

For persons from lower SES

As already noted, lower SES of the population have even more adverse SBP/DBP levels than others, associated with greater risks of CHD–CVD and shortened life expectancy (Davey Smith *et al.* 1996*a, b*). There are special challenges in terms of lifestyle improvement and access to healthcare, so particular efforts are needed to develop sustained effective approaches for application of the general and specific strategies throughout the lifespan for this group.

While seemingly a tall order, the foregoing set of strategic challenges is entirely realistic and achievable. Witness the substantial progress during the last four decades in improving diet composition to lower population-wide serum cholesterol levels; the progressive reduction in prevalence of smoking; and the evidence suggesting that SBP/DBP levels have begun to decline, independent of antihypertensive drug treatment (Burt *et al.* 1995). The efforts needed are substantial, at the levels of public health, medical care, and beyond. They include tackling special commercial interests opposed to the whole undertaking, and require the positive engagement of the food and communications industries, essential to accomplish population-wide improvements in eating patterns. For example, reduction of Na intakes to more favourable levels will require major cooperation from the food industry since ~75% of salt in the diet is added in food manufacture (James *et al.* 1987). Recent experience in the UK, where the Food Standards Agency has taken a lead in establishing a productive dialogue with the food manufacturers concerning reductions in Na content of foods, is encouraging. Further and continued efforts are required, but the rewards – ending the BP-related CHD–CVD epidemic – are high.

References

Allender PS, Cutler JA, Follman D, Cappuccio FP, Pryer J, Elliott P (1996). Dietary calcium and blood pressure: a meta-analysis of randomized clinical trials. *Annals of Internal Medicine* **124**, 825–31.

Appel LJ, Elliott P (2003). Macronutrients, fiber, cholesterol, and dietary patterns. In *Lifestyle modification for the prevention and treatment of hypertension* (ed. PK Whelton, J He, GT Louis), pp. 243–73. Marcel Dekker, New York.

Appel LJ, Moore TJ, Obarzanek E, Vollmer WM, Svetkey LP, Sacks FM *et al.* for the DASH Collaborative Research Group (1997). A clinical trial of the effects of dietary patterns on blood pressure. *New England Journal of Medicine* **336**, 1117–24.

Barker DJP (1998). *Mothers, babies, and health in later life.* Churchill Livingstone, Edinburgh.

Beilin LJ, Puddey IB, Burke V (1996). Alcohol and hypertension: kill or cure? *Journal of Human Hypertension* **10**(Suppl. 2), S1–S5.

Burt VL, Whelton P, Roccella EJ, Brown C, Cutler JA, Higgins M *et al.* (1995). Prevalence of hypertension in the U. S. adult population: results from the Third National Health and Nutrition Examination Survey, 1988–1991. *Hypertension* **25**, 305–13.

Carvalho JJM, Baruzzi RG, Howard P, Poulter N, Alpers MP, Franco LJ *et al.* (1989). Blood pressure in four remote populations in the INTERSALT study. *Hypertension* **14**, 238–46.

Chobanian AV, Bakris GL, Black HR, Cushman WC, Green LA, Izzo JL Jr *et al.* (2003). The Seventh Report of the Joint National Committee on Prevention, Detection, Evaluation, and Treatment of High Blood Pressure: the JNC 7 Report. *Journal of the American Medical Association* **289**, 2560–71.

Chobanian AV, Hill M (2000). National Heart, Lung, and Blood Institute Workshop on sodium and blood pressure: a critical review of current scientific evidence. *Hypertension* **35**, 858–63.

Cooper R, Cutler J, Desvigne-Nickens P, Fortmann SP, Friedman L, Havlik R *et al.* (2000). Trends and disparities in coronary heart disease, stroke, and other cardiovascular diseases in the United States: findings of the National Conference on Cardiovascular Disease Prevention. *Circulation* **102**, 3137–47.

Cutler JA, Follmann D, Allender PS (1997). Randomized trials of sodium reduction: an overview. *American Journal of Clinical Nutrition* **65**(Suppl.), 643S–651S.

Davey Smith G, Neaton JD, Wentworth D, Stamler R, Stamler J (1996*a*). Socioeconomic differentials in mortality risk among men screened for the Multiple Risk Factor Intervention Trial: I. White men. *American Journal of Public Health* **86**, 486–96.

Davey Smith G, Neaton JD, Wentworth D, Stamler R, Stamler J (1996*b*). Socioeconomic differentials in mortality risk among men screened for the Multiple Risk Factor Intervention Trial: II. Black men. *American Journal of Public Health* **86**, 497–504.

Denton D, Weisinger R, Mundy NI, Wickings EJ, Dixson A, Moisson P *et al.* (1995). The effect of increased salt intake on blood pressure in chimpanzees. *Nature Medicine* **1**, 1009–16.

Dyer AR, Stamler J, Paul O, Berkson DM, Lepper MH, McKean H *et al.* (1977). Alcohol consumption, cardiovascular risk factors, and mortality in two Chicago epidemiologic studies. *Circulation* **56**, 1067–74.

Dyer A, Elliott P, Shipley MJ (1990). Body mass index versus height and weight in relation to blood pressure: findings for the 10,079 persons in The INTERSALT Study. *American Journal of Epidemiology* **131**, 589–96.

Dyer AR, Shipley M, Elliott P (1994*a*). Urinary electrolyte excretion in 24-hours and blood pressure in the INTERSALT Study. I. Estimates of reliability. *American Journal of Epidemiology* **139**, 927–39.

Dyer AR, Elliott P, Shipley M (1994*b*). Urinary electrolyte excretion in 24-hours and blood pressure in the INTERSALT Study. II. Estimates of electrolyte-blood pressure associations corrected for regression dilution bias. *American Journal of Epidemiology* **139**, 940–51.

Elliott P (1989). The INTERSALT Study: an addition to the evidence on salt and blood pressure, and some implications. *Journal of Human Hypertension* **3**, 289–98.

Elliott P (1991). Observational studies of salt and blood pressure. *Hypertension* **17**(Suppl. I), I-3–I-8.

Elliott P, for the INTERMAP Cooperative Research Group (2001). *Dietary protein and blood pressure: findings from the INTERMAP Study.* Presented at the Symposium on the INTERMAP Study, Fifth International Conference on Preventive Cardiology, Osaka, Japan, May 29.

Elliott P (2003). Protein intake and blood pressure in cardiovascular disease. *Proceedings of the Nutrition Society* **62**, 495–504.

Elliott P, Stamler J, Nichols R, Dyer AR, Stamler R, Kestloot H, Marmot M for the INTERSALT Co-operative Research Group (1996). INTERSALT revisited: further analyses of 24-hour sodium excretion and blood pressure within and across populations. *British Medical Journal* **312**, 1249–53.

Erens B, Primatesta P (eds) (1999). *Health survey for England: risk factors for cardiovascular disease 1998.* The Stationery Office, London.

Ezzati M, Lopez AD (2002). Selected major risk factors and global and regional burden of disease. *Lancet* **360**, 1347–60.

Geleijnse JM, Hofman A, Witteman JC, Hazebroek AA, Valkenburg HA, Grobbee DE (1997). Long-term effects of neonatal sodium restriction on blood pressure. *Hypertension* **29**, 913–17.

Graudal NA, Galloe AM, Garred P (1998). Effects of sodium restriction on blood pressure, renin, aldosterone, catecholamines, cholesterols, and triglyceride: a meta-analysis. *Journal of the American Medical Association* **279**, 1383–91.

He FJ, MacGregor GA (2002). Effect of modest salt reduction on blood pressure: a meta-analysis of randomised trials. Implications for public health. *Journal of Human Hypertension* **16**, 761–70.

He J, Whelton PK, Appel LJ, Charleston J, Klag MJ (2000). Long-term effects of weight loss and dietary sodium reduction on incidence of hypertension. *Hypertension* **35**, 544–9.

Hofman A, Hazebroek A, Valkenburg HA (1983). A randomized trial of sodium intake and blood pressure in newborn infants. *Journal of the American Medical Association* **250**, 370–3.

INTERSALT Special Issue (1989). (Elliott P, ed.). *Journal of Human Hypertension* **3: 5**, Appendix Tables A1, A2, pp. 332–5.

INTERSALT Cooperative Research Group (1988). INTERSALT: an international study of electrolyte excretion and blood pressure. Results for 24-hour urinary sodium and potassium excretion. *British Medical Journal* **297**, 319–28.

James WP, Ralph A, Sanchez-Castillo CP (1987). The dominance of salt in manufactured food in the sodium intake of affluent societies. *Lancet* **1** (8530), 426–9.

Klag MJ, Whelton PK, Randall BL, Neaton JD, Brancati FL, Ford CE, *et al.* (1996). Blood pressure and end-stage renal disease in men. *New England Journal of Medicine* **334**, 13–18.

Klatsky AL, Friedman GD, Siegelaub AB, Gerard MJ (1977). Alcohol consumption and blood pressure Kaiser-Permanente Multiphasic Health Examination data. *New England Journal of Medicine* **296**, 1194–200.

Liu K (1988). Measurement error and its impact on partial correlation and multiple linear regression analyses. *American Journal of Epidemiology* **127**, 864–74.

Lowe LP, Greenland P, Ruth KJ, Dyer AR, Stamler R, Stamler J (1998). Impact of major cardiovascular disease risk factors, particularly in combination, on 22-year mortality in women and men. *Archives of Internal Medicine* **158**, 2007–14.

MacGregor GA, Markandu ND, Sagnella GA, Singer D, Cappuccio FP (1989). Double-blind study of three sodium intakes and long-term effects of sodium restriction in essential hypertension. *Lancet* **2**, 1244–7.

Marmot MG, Elliott P, Dyer AR, Shipley MJ, Ueshima H, Beevers DG *et al.* (1994). Alcohol and blood pressure: The INTERSALT Study. *British Medical Journal* **308**, 1263–7.

Midgley JP, Matthew AG, Greenwood CMT, Logan AG (1996). Effect of reduced dietary sodium on blood pressure: a meta-analysis of randomised controlled trials. *Journal of the American Medical Association* **275**, 1590–7.

Miura K, Daviglus ML, Dyer AR, Liu K, Garside DB, Stamler J, Greenland P (2001). Relationship of blood pressure to 25-year mortality due to coronary heart disease, cardiovascular diseases, and all causes in young adult men: The Chicago Heart Association Detection Project in Industry. *Archives of Internal Medicine* **161**, 1501–8.

Miura K, Greenland P, Stamler J, Liu K, Daviglus ML, Nakagawa H (2004). Relation of vegetable, fruit, and meat intake to 7-year blood pressure change in middle-aged men: The Chicago Western Electric Study. *American Journal of Epidemiology* **159**, 572–80.

Mizushima S, Cappuccio FP, Nichols R, Elliott P (1998). Dietary magnesium intake and blood pressure: a qualitative overview of the observational studies. *Journal of Human Hypertension* **12**, 447–53.

Moore TJ, Conlin PR, Ard J, Svetkey LP, for the DASH Collaborative Research Group (2001). DASH (Dietary Approaches to Stop Hypertension) diet is effective treatment for stage 1 isolated systolic hypertension. *Hypertension* **38**, 155–8.

National High Blood Pressure Education Program Working Group (1993). National High Blood Pressure Education Program Working Group Report on Primary Prevention of Hypertension. *Archives of Internal Medicine* **153**, 186–208.

National Research Council, Committee on Diet and Health, Food and Nutrition Board, Commission on Life Sciences (1989). *Diet and health: implications for reducing chronic disease risk.*, National Academy Press, Washington, DC.

Neaton JD, Kuller L, Stamler J, Wentworth DN (1994). Impact of systolic and diastolic blood pressure on cardiovascular mortality. In *Hypertension: physiology, diagnosis, and management*, 2nd edn (ed. JH Laragh, BM Brenner), Chapter 9. Raven Press, New York.

Neter JE, Stam BE, Kok FJ, Grobbee DE, Geleijnse JM (2003). Influence of weight reduction on blood pressure: a meta-analysis of randomised controlled trials. *Hypertension* **42**, 878–84.

Page LB, Damon A, Moellering RC (1974). Antecedents of cardiovascular disease in six Solomon Islands societies. *Circulation* **49**, 1132–46.

Page LB, Vandevert DE, Nader K, Lubin NK, Page JR (1981). Blood pressure of Qash'qai pastoral nomads in Iran in relation to culture, diet, and body form. *American Journal of Clinical Nutrition* **34**, 527–38.

Pearson TA, Jamison DT, Trejo-Gutierrez J (1993). Cardiovascular disease. In *Disease control priorities in developing countries* (ed. DT Jamison, WH Mosley, AR Measham, JL Bobadilla), pp. 577–94. Oxford University Press.

Poulter NR, Khaw KT, Hopwood BEC, Mugambi M, Peart WS, Rose G, Sever PS (1990). The Kenyan Luo migration study: observations on the initiation of a rise in blood pressure. *British Medical Journal* **300**, 967–72.

PREMIER Collaborative Research Group (2003). Effects of comprehensive lifestyle modification on blood pressure control: main results of the PREMIER clinical trial. *Journal of the American Medical Association* **289**, 2083–93.

Prospective Studies Collaboration (2002). Age-specific relevance of usual blood pressure to vascular mortality: a meta-analysis of individual data for one million adults in 61 prospective studies. *Lancet* **360**, 1903–13.

Rodin MB, Daviglus ML, Wong GC, Liu K, Garside DB, Greenland P, Stamler J (2003). Middle age cardiovascular risk factors and abdominal aortic aneurysm in older age. *Hypertension* **42**, 61–8.

Rose G (1981). Strategy of prevention: lessons from cardiovascular disease. *British Medical Journal* **282**, 1847–51.

Rose G (1985). Sick individuals and sick populations. *International Journal of Epidemiology* **14**, 32–8.

Sacks FM, Svetkey LP, Vollmer WM, Appel LJ, Bray GA, Harsha D *et al.* for the DASH-Sodium Collaborative Research Group (2001). Effects on blood pressure of reduced sodium and the Dietary Approaches to Stop Hypertension (DASH) diet. *New England Journal of Medicine* **344**, 3–10.

Shaper AG (1972). Cardiovascular disease in the tropics: III, Blood pressure and hypertension. *British Medical Journal* **3**, 805–7.

Stamler J (1991). Epidemiologic findings on body mass and blood pressure in adults. *Annals of Epidemiology* **1**, 347–62.

Stamler J (1997). The INTERSALT Study: background, methods, findings, and implications. *American Journal of Clinical Nutrition* **65**(Suppl.), 626S–642S.

Stamler R, Shipley M, Elliott P, Dyer A, Sans S, Stamler J (1992). Higher blood pressure in adults with less education: some explanations from INTERSALT. *Hypertension* **19**, 237–41.

Stamler J, Stamler R, Neaton JD (1993*a*). Blood pressure, systolic and diastolic, and cardiovascular risks: U. S. population data. *Archives of Internal Medicine* **153**, 598–615.

Stamler J, Dyer AR, Shekelle RB, Neaton J, Stamler R (1993*b*). Relationship of baseline major risk factors to coronary and all-cause mortality, and to longevity: findings from long-term follow-up of Chicago cohorts. *Cardiology* **82**, 191–222.

Stamler R, Liu LS, Nichols R, Huang DX, Long ZP, Xie JX, Elliott P (1993*c*). Blood pressure and life style in the People's Republic of China: three samples in the INTERSALT Study. *Journal of Human Hypertension* **7**, 429–35.

Stamler J, Caggiula A, Grandits GA, Kjelsberg M, Cutler JA, for the MRFIT Research Group (1996*a*). Relationship to blood pressure of combinations of dietary macronutrients: findings of the Multiple Risk Factor Intervention Trial (MRFIT). *Circulation* **94**, 2417–23.

Stamler J, Elliott P, Kesteloot H, Nichols R, Claeys G, Dyer AR, Stamler R, for the INTERSALT Cooperative Research Group (1996*b*). Inverse relation of dietary protein markers with blood pressure: findings for 10,020 men and women in the INTERSALT Study. *Circulation* **94**, 1629–34.

Stamler J, Stamler R, Garside D, Greenlund K, Archer S, Neaton JD, Wentworth DN (1996*c*). Socioeconomic status, cardiovascular risk factors, and cardiovascular disease: findings on U. S. working populations. In: *Report of the Conference on Socioeconomic Status and Cardiovascular Health and Disease*, 6–7 November 1995, pp. 109–118. National Institutes of Health; National Heart, Lung, and Blood Institute, Bethesda, MD.

Stamler J, Caggiula AW, Grandits GA (1997). Relation of body mass and alcohol, nutrient, fiber, and caffeine intakes to blood pressure in the special intervention and usual care groups in the Multiple Risk Factor Intervention Trial. *American Journal of Clinical Nutrition* **65**(Suppl. 1), 338S–365S.

Stamler J, Liu K, Ruth KJ, Pryer J, Greenland P (2002). Eight-year blood pressure change in middle-aged men: relationship to multiple nutrients. *Hypertension* **39**, 1000–6.

Stamler J, Elliott P, Appel L, Chan Q, Buzzard M, Dennis B *et al.* (2003). Higher blood pressure in middle-aged American adults with less education: role of multiple dietary factors. The INTERMAP study. *Journal of Human Hypertension* **17**, 655–775.

Svetkey LP, Simons-Morton D, Vollmer WM, Appel LJ, Conlin PR, Ryan DH *et al.* (1999). Effects of dietary patterns on blood pressure: subgroup analysis of the Dietary Approaches to Stop Hypertension (DASH) randomised clinical trial. *Archives of Internal Medicine* **159**, 285–93.

TOHP (Trials of Hypertension Prevention) Collaborative Research Group (1992). The effects of nonpharmacologic interventions on blood pressure of persons with high normal levels: results of the Trials of Hypertension Prevention, Phase I. *Journal of the American Medical Association* **267**, 1213–20.

TOHP (Trials of Hypertension Prevention) Collaborative Research Group (1997). Effects of weight loss and sodium reduction intervention on blood pressure and hypertension incidence in overweight people with high-normal blood pressure: the Trials of Hypertension Prevention, Phase II. *Archives of Internal Medicine* **157**, 657–67.

Tuomilehto J, Jousilahti P, Rastenyte D, Moltchanov V, Tanskanen A, Pietinen P, Nissinen A (2001). Urinary sodium excretion and cardiovascular mortality in Finland: a prospective study. *Lancet* **357**, 848–51.

Whelton SP, Chin A, Xin X, He J (2002*a*). Effect of aerobic exercise on blood pressure: a meta-analysis of randomised, controlled trials. *Annals of Internal Medicine* **136**, 493–503.

Whelton PK, He J, Appel LJ, Cutler JA, Havas S, Kotchen TA *et al.* (2002*b*). Primary prevention of hypertension: Clinical and Public Health Advisory from the National High Blood Pressure Education Program. *Journal of the American Medical Association* **288**, 1882–8.

Whelton PK, He J, Cutler JA, Brancati FL, Appel LJ, Follmann D, Klag MJ (1997). Effects of oral potassium on blood pressure: meta-analysis of randomized controlled clinical trials. *Journal of the American Medical Association* **277**, 1624–32.

Xin X, He J, Frontini MG, Ogden LG, Motsamai OI, Whelton PK (2001). Effects of alcohol reduction on blood pressure: a meta-analysis of randomised controlled trials. *Hypertension* **38**, 1112–17.

Zhao L, Stamler J, Yan LJ, Zhou B, Wu Y, Liu K *et al.*, for the INTERMAP Research Group (2004). Blood pressure differences between northern and southern Chinese: role of dietary factors. *Hypertension* **43**, 1332–7.

Chapter 44

The secondary prevention of cardiovascular disease

S. S. Anand, E. Lonn, and S. Yusuf

44.1 Introduction

In the twenty-first century, the absolute number of people who will suffer from cardiovascular disease (CVD) will increase dramatically, as CVD in countries such as India and China reaches epidemic proportions (Yusuf *et al.* 2001*b*). We embrace the viewpoint of the late Geoffrey Rose that the true gains in reducing the burden of CVD in the population will come from changes in the population averages of most conventional risk factors such as blood pressure, bodyweight, cholesterol, and tobacco (Rose 1981) (see Chapter 3). However, once an individual has developed CVD, their risk of experiencing recurrent CVD must be minimized. A combination of the two approaches (population-based and high-risk individual-based) is likely to lead to the greatest benefits. Observational studies and clinical trials provide evidence that lower levels of risk factors in patients with established vascular disease can substantially reduce their risk of suffering recurrent vascular events. Efforts directed towards reducing further CV events in patients with established CVD are known as secondary prevention. In this chapter we review the epidemiological evidence for risk factor control, lifestyle changes, and medical strategies in the secondary prevention setting.

44.2 Risk stratification: who should be treated?

Standard risk prediction models which are based on information derived from studies such as Framingham (Wilson *et al.* 1987) can assist clinicians in determining which patients are at low or high risk of suffering from recurrent CV events. In many cases this distinction is important, as it informs clinicians on how widely to search for risk states over and above conventional risk factors (e.g. homocysteine), as well as how 'aggressive' they should be from a medical standpoint. While these prediction models are helpful, they are also limited in the following ways:

1 They focus on absolute risk as a static estimate, as opposed to considering how a person's risk changes over time.

2 They are not comprehensive, as some important risk states are not figured into the calculation of risk (e.g. abdominal obesity).

3 They do not consider the number of years that the individual may have been exposed to the abnormal risk factor.

4 They classify risk factors are being 'present' or 'absent', and often ignore the continuous relationship that most factors share with CVD.

Table 44.1 The risk of suffering a recurrent vascular event[a] in subgroups of patients with established vascular disease

	1 year risk	(%) 5 year risk (%)
65-year-old man with one risk factor[b]	1.3	6.5
65-year-old man with DM and one risk factor[c]	2.4	11.5
Prior MI[c]	4.5	20.3
Non-ST elevation MI or unstable angina[c,d]	17.4	36.6
ST elevation MI	5	22.1
TIA/stroke[c]	5.6	24.4
PAD[c]	4.8	21.3

Adapted from the HOPE trial.

DM: diabetes mellitus.

[a] CV death, MI, or stroke.

[b] Framingham Risk Equation (Wilson *et al.* 1987).

[c] HOPE (Yusuf *et al.* 2000).

[d] OASIS Registry (Piegas *et al.* 1999).

5 They do not take into account regression-dilution biases, so the potential impact of interventions may be underestimated (Law and Wald 2002).

44.2.1 High risk groups

Determining whether a patient has 'established' vascular disease is important in determining their future vascular risk. Table 44.1 outlines the 1 and 5 year incidence of CV death, myocardial infarction (MI), and stroke for individuals who have suffered a prior vascular event. When compared to individuals with no history of vascular disease, the incidence of CVD among patients with established disease and among patients with diabetes is substantial. Therefore, individuals with established vascular disease or with diabetes should be treated aggressively with effective therapies (outlined below) to reduce their risk of suffering future vascular events.

44.2.2 Vascular territory

The pathogenesis of acute MI, unstable angina, ischaemic stroke, and peripheral arterial disease (PAD) is attributed to atherosclerosis, and superimposed thrombosis in a critical artery. Further, the determinants of atherothrombosis are similar and include all of the conventional risk factors for atherosclerosis. Interestingly, patients with evidence of PAD are also at substantial risk of suffering cardiovascular death, MI, or stroke (Criqui and Denenberg 1998). Therefore, aggressive risk factor reduction should not be overlooked in this high risk subgroup of vascular patients. Furthermore, the increased risk of future CV events is present in patients irrespective of the vascular territory (i.e. cerebrovascular, peripheral, or coronary vasculature) in which the first clinical manifestation has occurred, and risk factor modification should be aggressive in all vascular patients.

44.3 Approach to risk factors

The major risk factors of CVD in all populations (e.g. young or old, male or female, white or black) are cholesterol, blood pressure, glucose (all three are significantly influenced by body fat

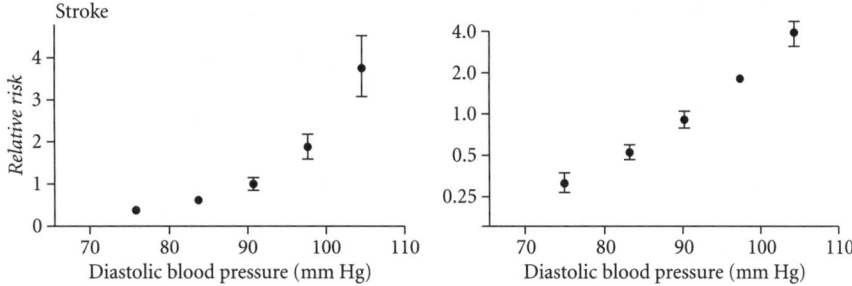

Fig. 44.1 The relationship between exposures and cerebrovascular disease.

and physical inactivity), and tobacco exposure. There is ample evidence that clinicians should not view risk factors as being 'present' or 'absent' because most risk factors share a continuous relationship with CVD (Law and Wald 2002). In this scenario, a given reduction in a risk factor, irrespective of its starting level, results in the same proportional CV event reduction (Fig. 44.1). Therefore, there is value in modifying risk factors in patients with established vascular disease no matter what the level of their risk factors. For example, blood pressure-lowering drugs should not be limited to people with high blood pressure, nor glucose-lowering drugs to people with diabetes. Below we review the evidence supporting the relationship between these factors and CVD, and highlight specific classes of medications, and lifestyle strategies that have been demonstrated in clinical trials to reduce risk factor levels and clinical events.

44.4 Secondary prevention

44.4.1 Cholesterol

Epidemiology

There is strong evidence that increasing serum cholesterol is an important cause of coronary heart disease (CHD), and that lowering serum cholesterol reduces the incidence of CHD (Law and Wald 1994; Law *et al.* 1994). The 'total' cholesterol measurement represents a summary measure of the lipid sub-fractions of low-density lipoprotein cholesterol (LDL-C), high-density lipoprotein cholesterol (HDL-C), triglycerides, and other lipoproteins. Data from 10 large cohort studies demonstrate that every 0.6 mmol/l decrease (~10%) in LDL-C is associated with a reduction in CHD of ~25% across all age ranges (Law *et al.* 1994). The proportional risk reduction is greater among younger individuals (i.e. at an age of 40 years the risk reduction is 54%), than for older individuals (i.e. at 80 years it is associated with a risk reduction of 19%). However, the absolute reduction in CHD is higher among older individuals because their baseline risk of suffering from a CHD event is greater. There does not appear to be a threshold (at least in Western populations) below which a decrease in serum cholesterol is not associated with a further decrease in the risk of ischaemic heart disease (Chen *et al.* 1991; Law 1998). An HDL concentration below 0.9 is also a risk factor for CV recurrence and elevated HDL is protective against CVD when values above 1.60 mmol/l are achieved (Boden 2000; Law *et al.* 1994). The risk that elevated blood triglycerides confer on vascular events in the presence of a normal HDL-C remains unclear (Jeppesen *et al.* 2000), although in the presence of an elevated LDL *or* low HDL, a triglyceride concentration of >2.30 mmol/l confers an additional risk of recurrent CV events, greater than does either abnormality alone (Pasternak *et al.* 2002).

Table 44.2 Changes in continuous risk factors and CHD events

	Change in factor	OES[+] (%)	RCTs[+] (%)
DBP + CHD	5 mm ↓	21	20 (16–23)
BMI + CHD	1 unit ↓	10	NA
Cholesterol + CHD	0.6 mmol/l ↓	27	25 (1–35)
DBP + CVA	5 mm ↓	34	33 (26–39%)
BMI + DM	1 unit BMI	10	NA

Adapted from Law and Wald 2002.

BMI: body mass index; CVA: cerebrovascular accidents; NA: not available; OES: observational epidemiological studies; RCT: randomized clinical trial.

[+] Corresponding reduction (%) in risk of disease.

Clinical trials

Observational epidemiology has informed the design and conduct of large clinical trials powered to detect significant reductions in hard outcomes such as total mortality, recurrent MI, and stroke. Clinical trials conducted among individuals with established vascular disease have demonstrated conclusively that lowering cholesterol substantially reduces the risk of cardiovascular mortality, and non-fatal MI and strokes (Table 44.2). These data show that while the proportional reduction in risk of lowering cholesterol is the same among people with and without established vascular disease, the absolute risk reduction is greater among individuals with established vascular disease because their baseline risks are higher. The class of medications called HMG CoA reductase inhibitors, or 'statins', decreases the synthesis of cholesterol by hepatocytes and results in up-regulation of LDL receptors, and lowering of serum cholesterol. Statins now constitute the single most effective type of treatment for reducing cholesterol and reducing cardiovascular risk. Use of a statin medication results on average in a 25% reduction in LDL, a 10–15% reduction in triglycerides, and an 8% increase in HDL-C (Opie and Gersh 2001).

Six large trials collectively demonstrate that among individuals with established vascular disease or high risk patients with elevated cholesterol who have not yet suffered a vascular event, statins reduce CHD mortality, cardiovascular mortality, and all-cause mortality compared with placebo over a mean of 5.4 years (CHD mortality: odds ratio (OR): 0.71 (95% confidence interval (CI): 0.63–0.80); CV mortality: OR: 0.73 (95% CI: 0.66–0.82); all-cause mortality: OR: 0.77 (95% CI: 0.70–0.85) (Downs *et al.* 1998; Heart Protection Study Collaborative Group 2002; LIPID Study Group 1998; Sacks *et al.* 1996; The Scandinavian Simvastatin Survival Study (4S) 1994; West of Scotland Coronary Prevention Study 1996). Recently the Heart Protection Study randomized 20 536 high risk patients (with coronary disease, other occlusive arterial disease, or diabetes) to receive simvastatin 40 mg/day versus placebo and included substantial representation of people older than 70 years, women, diabetics, patients with prior stroke, and PAD (HPS MRC/BHF Heart Protection Study 2002). Overall, simvastatin was associated with a significant reduction in CV events in the order of 24% (95% CI: 19–28%), a significant 18% reduction in coronary death ($p = 0.0005$), and a 13% relative risk reduction (RRR) in all-cause mortality ($p < 0.0003$), and these benefits were consistent among all subgroups. Overall, a 1 mmol reduction in LDL-C led to a 25% reduction in the relative risk of CHD and strokes irrespective of the starting cholesterol value.

While other treatments such as n-3 fatty acids, resins, hormones, and niacin, as well as surgery (ileal bypass) can also reduce cholesterol, statins are generally well-tolerated and highly effective, perhaps even more effective than predicted by their cholesterol-lowering effects. Recently, the hypothesis that statins may have more than one 'mechanism of action', including anti-inflammatory effects resulting in plaque stabilization, has been raised, and the evidence to support this hypothesis is accumulating (Albert *et al.* 2001).

Choosing a statin

Although most clinicians believe that HMG CoA reductase inhibitors are equivalent, their mechanism of action in the liver varies slightly, and this may lead to differences in their cholesterol-altering effects and safety profile. The majority of patients enrolled into the trials of cholesterol-lowering with a statin medication, received either pravastatin or simvastatin, and accordingly they should be the first line agents. Other statins have also been demonstrated to be effective in clinical trials; for example, atorvastatin (80 mg/day) was found to be superior to percutaneous coronary intervention among patients with chronic stable angina (Pitt *et al.* 1999), and among patients with unstable angina or non-Q wave MI (Schwartz *et al.* 2001).

Fibrates

Fibric acid derivatives work by stimulating fatty acid oxidation and reducing the rate of hepatic lipid generation. They reduce triglycerides by ~30% and raise HDL by 10–12%. Therefore, among vascular patients who have acceptable LDL concentrations but low HDL-C and/or elevated serum triglycerides, a fibrate may be chosen as the lipid-altering agent of choice. Six randomized trials have evaluated the effectiveness of fibrates versus placebo in people with known CHD (Pignone 2000). Specifically, among 2531 men with CHD, fibrates compared to placebo reduced the composite outcome of non-fatal MI plus death from CHD after a median of 5.1 years from 22% to 17% (RR 0.80, 95% CI: 0.68–0.94). Recently, the Veterans Affairs High-Density Lipoprotein Intervention Trial (VA-HIT) enrolled 2531 men with CHD who had an HDL concentration <1 mmol/l and a normal LDL (2.88 mmol/l) and found that gemfibrozil (1200 mg/day) reduced the composite outcome of non-fatal MI plus death from CHD after a median of 5.1 years compared to placebo (17% vs 22%; risk reduction of 20%, 95% CI: 6–32%) (Robins *et al.* 2001). CHD events were reduced by 11% with gemfibrozil for every 0.13 mmol/l increase in HDL-C. While fibrates are effective in raising HDL and lowering triglycerides, niacin is also effective and also lowers LDL-C. In the recently reported ADMIT trial, niacin (maximum tolerated dose) significantly increased HDL-C by 29%, and decreased triglycerides by 25% and LDL-C by 9% (Elam *et al.* 2000). However, niacin is more cumbersome to prescribe, as dose titration is required, and patients report more side effects with niacin than with statins or fibrates.

Side effects

A systematic review of long-term statin trials found no significant difference between statins and placebo in the incidence of non-cardiovascular mortality 0.93 (95% CI: 0.81–1.07), cancer incidence 0.99 (95% CI: 0.90–1.08), asymptomatic elevation of creatinine kinase (CK) (>10 times upper reference limit) 1.25 (95% CI: 0.83–1.89), or elevation of transaminases (>3 times upper reference limit) 1.13 (95% CI: 0.95–1.33) during a mean of 5.4 years of treatment (Pfeffer *et al.* 2002). In the Heart Protection Study 0.09% of patients who received simvastatin vs. 0.05% treated with placebo developed a CK elevation >10 times normal, and only 0.8% vs. 0.6% developed a transaminase elevation of three times normal (HPS MRC/BHF

Heart Protection Study 2002). Fibrates are also associated with a number of adverse effects, including liver enzyme elevations (6%) and gastrointestinal side effects; however, the incidence of life-threatening complications is low. Combination therapy of statin and fibrates may cause serious complications and should be avoided when possible. Recently cerivastatin was withdrawn from the public market as a result of 31 deaths from rhabdomyolysis in the United States attributable to cerivastatin. Close to half of these individuals were also taking a fibrate medication (Szarfman et al. 2002; Williams and Feely 2002).

44.4.2 Blood pressure lowering

Epidemiology

Observational epidemiology provides strong evidence that systolic blood pressure (SDP) and diastolic blood pressure (DBP) share a continuous relationship with CVD (MacMahon et al. 1990). The associations of DBP with stroke and with CHD were investigated in nine major prospective observational studies including 420 000 individuals, and prolonged differences in the DBP of 5, 7.5, and 10 mmHg were associated with at least 34%, 46%, and 56% less stroke and at least 21%, 29%, and 37% less CHD, respectively. Further, there was no evidence of any 'threshold' below which lower levels of DBP were not associated with lower risks of stroke and of CHD (MacMahon et al. 1990). Among a cohort of 12 031 middle-aged men observed over a 25 year period, the relative risk of death from CHD rose continuously with increasing levels of SDP and DBP (Van den Hoogen et al. 2000), and sustained differences of 10 mmHg in SBP and of 5 mmHg in DBP were each associated with a 28% difference in the risk of death from CHD. Therefore blood pressure, like cholesterol, should not be thought of as a categorical variable, but rather as a continuous exposure that warrants blood pressure-lowering interventions in high risk patients, regardless of whether they have hypertension by conventional standards or not (Rodgers and MacMahon 1999).

Clinical trials

As is the case for cholesterol, observational epidemiology has informed the design and conduct of large clinical trials of blood pressure-lowering which were powered to detect significant reductions in hard outcomes such as CHD and stroke. Placebo-controlled trials have confirmed that blood pressure-lowering reduces CHD and stroke. A recent meta-analysis of 18 trials including 48 220 patients followed for ~5 years (Psaty et al. 1992) demonstrated that (a) low dose diuretics reduced stroke and CHD, as well as CV and total mortality, and (b) beta-blockers prevent stroke and congestive heart failure (CHF) and are recommended as the first line agents in the treatment of hypertension. Another meta-analysis of four placebo-controlled trials of angiotensin converting enzyme (ACE) inhibitors including 12 124 patients, mostly with CHD, revealed reductions in stroke of 30% (95% CI: 15–43), CHD of 20% (11–28), and major cardiovascular events of 21% (14–27) (Neal and MacMahon 1999). The overview also included two placebo-controlled trials of calcium antagonists among 5520 patients, mostly with hypertension, and showed reductions in stroke of 39% (95% CI: 15–56) and major cardiovascular events of 28% (95% CI: 13–41). Given that blood pressure-lowering is effective, the question of which blood pressure-lowering agent to use is raised. The evidence from individual trials and meta-analysis indicates that blood pressure-lowering by any means does not result in similar reductions in CVD events, and suggests that the choice of blood pressure-lowering agents should be tailored to the individual patient and consider their risk factor profile and other comorbidities.

Choice of blood pressure agent

To help resolve the questions faced by clinicians as to how best to tailor blood pressure-lowering therapies, active controlled clinical trials have been conducted. A meta-analysis of nine randomized controlled trials of intermediate and long-acting calcium channels blockers compared to low dose diuretics, beta-blockers, and ACE inhibitors demonstrated that while the mean reduction in blood pressure achieved by calcium antagonists is similar, the calcium antagonists were associated with a 25% excess in CHF and (acute myocardial infarction) (AMI) (Pahor et al. 2000a). Another meta-analysis comparing ACE inhibitors to calcium antagonists in patients with diabetes suggested that ACE inhibitors reduce the risk of AMI and other vascular events despite achieving similar blood pressure reduction (Pahor et al. 2000b). More recently, the PROGRESS trial evaluated the ACE inhibitor perindopril (4 mg/day) in 6105 patients who had suffered prior stroke or transient ischaemic attack (TIA) (PROGRESS Collaborative Group 2001) 56% of patients also had indapamide added to increase blood pressure lowering when indicated. Over a 4 year period blood pressure was lowered by 9/4 mmHg with active therapy and stroke was reduced by 28%, $p < 0.0001$. Patents on combination therapy achieved reductions of 12/5 mmHg and stroke was reduced by 43%, compared to those who received perindopril alone whose reduction in blood pressure was 5/3 mm with no reduction in stroke observed (PROGRESS Collaborative Group 2001).

Given these data, low dose diuretics, beta-blockers, and ACE inhibitors are clearly effective in lowering blood pressure, and reducing clinical events and should be used as first line agents depending on a patient's risk factor profile. Although calcium antagonists lower blood pressure, they do not prevent CHF episodes or AMI events as effectively as other choices, especially among diabetics. Other emerging blood pressure-lowering therapies such as the angiotensin receptor blockers (ARBs) should also be considered in certain subgroups of patients (e.g. diabetics with contradiction to ACE inhibitors) or when patients require more than one or two agents to lower blood pressure (Dahlof et al. 2002).

Risks of therapy

The major risk of blood pressure-lowering therapy is lowering the blood pressure too much, to a point where patients experience dizziness and orthostatic hypotension. Certain categories of agents are associated with their own side effects, which need to be considered individually.

Lifestyle methods of lowering blood pressure

Weight reduction of 4.5 kg can lower blood pressure by 4/3 mmHg, sodium reduction of 80–100 mmol/day reduces blood pressure by 5/3 mmHg in hypertensives, and 2/1 mm in non-hypertensives (Sacks et al. 2001). There is some evidence that lifestyle changes may be additive in their effects on blood pressure lowering, although this has not been evaluated rigorously. There is also good evidence in support of the blood pressure-lowering effects of increased physical activity, moderation of alcohol consumption, and adequate potassium intake.

44.4.3 Glucose

Epidemiology

Patients with diabetes mellitus have a two- to four-fold increased risk of coronary, cerebrovascular, and peripheral vascular disease compared to non-diabetic people (Kannel and McGee 1979). There is increasing evidence that glucose shares a continuous relationship with atherosclerosis and CVD, and like total cholesterol or DBP, glucose appears to be a continuous risk factor for CVD. Observational data suggest that CV events rise by ~10–30% for every 1% increase in HbA1c (Coutinho *et al.* 1999; Gerstein and Yusuf 1996). In the UKPDS study, every 1% increase in HbA1c in subjects with type 2 diabetes increased the risk of death by 14%, MI by 14%, and stroke by 12% (Stratton *et al.* 2000). Taken together these studies suggest, but do not confirm, that lowering glucose levels into the normal range will prevent recurrent CV events (Coutinho *et al.* 1999).

Clinical trials

To date, several randomized controlled trials of intensive versus conventional glucose-lowering therapy have been conducted in people with type 2 diabetes mellitus. None of these trials was powered to determine whether or not glucose lowering reduced cardiovascular events. However, several trials did report a non-significant trend in favour of beneficial cardiovascular effects. Therefore, while randomized trials to date suggest that intensive glucose control reduces CV events, ongoing trials are needed to confirm these observations (Stratton *et al.* 2000). Until then, however, the totality of evidence suggests that tight glucose control among people with established CVD who have diabetes, impaired fasting glucose (fasting glucose 6.1–6.9 mmol/l), or impaired glucose tolerance (IGT) (fasting glucose <7.0 and 2 h post glucose load glucose of 7.8 to 11.1 mmol/l inclusive) is likely to be beneficial. While reduction in glucose concentration can be brought about by medication, weight reduction and regular exercise are effective methods of improving glucose control, can also decrease medication requirements among established diabetics, and decrease the development of type 2 diabetes among patients who are at risk of developing diabetes (e.g. patients with IGT) (Diabetes Prevention Program Research Group 2002; Tuomilehto *et al.* 2001).

44.4.4 **Tobacco cessation: epidemiology**

Tobacco exposure is a strong determinant of atherosclerosis and CVD (Kilaru *et al.* 2001). While there are no randomized trials which demonstrate the relative risk reduction associated with smoking cessation on CV events in people with CHD, observational epidemiology indicates that people with CHD who stop smoking attain the same risk of CVD as do non-smokers in 5 years (Peto *et al.* 2000). The risk decreases by 50% less than 2 years after quitting. Among patients with PAD for whom smoking is the primary determinant of their disease, smoking cessation leads to improved graft patency, improves walking distance, and decreases mortality (Anand and Creager 2002). Quit rates may be improved by the use of busproprion (Zyban) and/or nicotine patches which appear to be safe and effective for use among people with CHD who are motivated to quit smoking (Jorenby *et al.* 1999). Recently, the effectiveness of 'quit-lines', which are telephone services that offer smoking-cessation counselling was evaluated: 1309 controls received provision of smoking cessation materials only compared to 1973 smokers who received up to seven telephone counselling sessions. The smoking cessation rates at 1, 3, 6, and 12 months, according to an intention-to-treat analysis, were 23.7%, 17.9%, 12.8 %, and 9.1%, respectively, for those in the treatment group versus 16.5%, 12.1%, 8.6%, and 6.9 %, respectively, for those in the control group ($p < 0.001$). The 12-month abstinence rates for those who made at least one attempt to quit were 23.3% in the treatment group and 18.4% in the control group ($p < 0.001$) (Zhu *et al.* 2002). Therefore, among patients who have clinical evidence of vascular disease, smoking prevention and cessation should be vigorously promoted, and patients should be aided as much as possible by healthcare professionals providing advice and smoking cessation programs to increase the chances that patients will quit for a sustained period of time (Grover *et al.* 1994; Joseph *et al.* 1996) (Chapter 48).

44.4.5 **Physical exercise: epidemiology**

There is a large body of observational epidemiological data to support the hypothesis that regular physical exercise reduces the risk of future vascular events (see Chapter 19). Regular physical activity has a number of other beneficial effects on health such as improved glucose utilization, reduced blood pressure, and reduced chance of suffering a cardiovascular event (Pate *et al.* 1995; Ross *et al.* 2000). The 'optimal' type, intensity, duration, and frequency of physical exercise to 'prescribe' to individuals with established CVD depends in part on their specific manifestations of vascular disease (i.e. post-stroke patients vs. stable angina patients, vs. the claudicant). Supervised exercise has been proven to be effective for post-MI patients (Detry *et al.* 2001), post-coronary artery bypass graft patients (Hedback *et al.* 2001), and patients with intermittent claudication (Gardner and Poehlman 1995). One systematic review of 42 trials involving 7683 people with established vascular disease reported that cardiac rehabilitation including exercise reduces the risk of major cardiac events and mortality (Jolliffe *et al.* 2001). Comprehensive cardiac rehabilitation programs include medical evaluation, prescribed exercise, cardiac risk factor modification (directed towards smoking cessation, weight management, treatment of dyslipidemia, hypertension, and diabetes), education, and counselling. Such comprehensive cardiac rehabilitation programs were shown to reduce the risk of cardiovascular deaths by 20–5% and reduce cardiac morbidity (Richardson *et al.* 2000).

Despite the specific clinical manifestation of the vascular patient, however, in general a minimum of 120 min of moderate-intensity physical activity accumulated throughout the week will lead to improved CV health (US DHSS/NIH 1997). The type of exercise may be taken in the form of walking, which has been shown to be as effective as structured exercise for improving fitness in adults (Dunn *et al.* 1999). Even light-to-moderate activity (at least 1 h of walking per week predicted lower risk) is associated with lower CHD rates among women (Min *et al.* 2001). Simple messages from clinicians to patients about ways to increase physical activity (e.g. work in the garden, take short walks, take the stairs instead of the elevator) will likely lead to greater uptake and be sustained by patients over the long term.

44.4.6 **Antiplatelet therapy**

Clinical trials

There is strong evidence that antiplatelet therapies reduce the risk of serious vascular events in people at high risk of ischaemic cardiac events (Antithrombotic Trialists' Collaboration 2002). The Antithrombotic Trialists' Collaborative overview reported that a month or more of antiplatelet treatment significantly reduced the odds of a vascular event (non-fatal MI, non-fatal stroke, or vascular death) by 27% (95% CI: 24–30%) compared with control, among ~140 000 people with established vascular disease (Fig. 44.2). Along with subsequent randomized trials, prolonged use of aspirin at a dose of 75 mg/day appears to be as effective as higher doses of aspirin. There is no consistent evidence that any other antiplatelet regimen was superior to 75–325 mg of aspirin to prevent vascular events (Antithrombotic Trialists' Collaboration 2002). There is evidence that adenosine diphosphate receptor antagonists such as clopidogrel may be marginally more effective than aspirin in preventing recurrent vascular events in patients with established CVD. The APC overview demonstrated that compared to aspirin, thienopyridines such as ticlopidine and clopidogrel reduced the odds of a vascular event by 9% (OR: 0.91; 95% CI: 0.84–0.98; $p = 0.01$). This result is based primarily on the results of the CAPRIE trial, which was a large randomized trial of almost 20 000 patients in which a RRR of MI, stroke, and CV death of 8.7% ($p = 0.043$) with clopidogrel 75 mg/day compared to aspirin

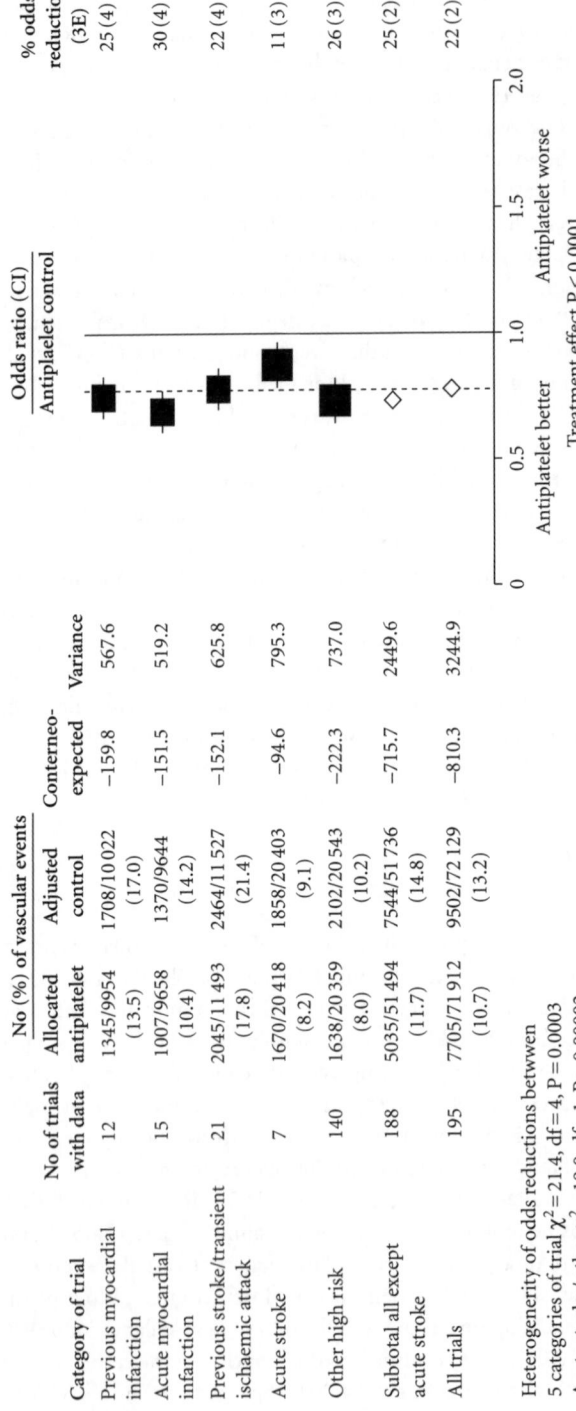

Category of trial	No of trials with data	No (%) of vascular events		Conterneo-expected	Variance	Odds ratio (CI) Antiplatelet control	% odds reduction (3E)
		Allocated antiplatelet	Adjusted control				
Previous myocardial infarction	12	1345/9954 (13.5)	1708/10022 (17.0)	−159.8	567.6		25 (4)
Acute myocardial infarction	15	1007/9658 (10.4)	1370/9644 (14.2)	−151.5	519.2		30 (4)
Previous stroke/transient ischaemic attack	21	2045/11493 (17.8)	2464/11527 (21.4)	−152.1	625.8		22 (4)
Acute stroke	7	1670/20418 (8.2)	1858/20403 (9.1)	−94.6	795.3		11 (3)
Other high risk	140	1638/20359 (8.0)	2102/20543 (10.2)	−222.3	737.0		26 (3)
Subtotal all except acute stroke	188	5035/51494 (11.7)	7544/51736 (14.8)	−715.7	2449.6		25 (2)
All trials	195	7705/71912 (10.7)	9502/72129 (13.2)	−810.3	3244.9		22 (2)

Heterogeneity of odds reductions betwwen
5 categories of trial $\chi^2 = 21.4$, df = 4, P = 0.0003
Acute stroke / other $\chi^2 = 18.0$, df = 1, P = 0.00002

Odds ratio (CI) Antiplatelet control

0   0.5   1.0   1.5   2.0
Antiplatelet better   Antiplatelet worse
Treatment effect P < 0.0001

Fig. 44.2 Proportional effects of antiplatelet therapy on vascular events (MI, stroke, or vascular death) in five main high risk categories. Meta-analysis of results for all trials (and 95% CI) is represented by an open diamond.

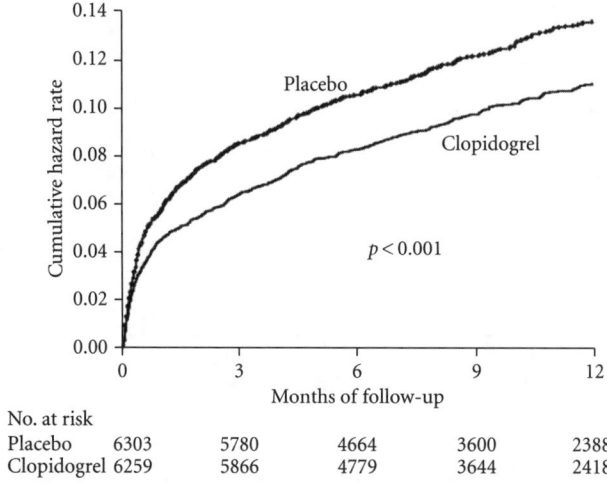

Fig. 44.3 CURE Study. Primary outcome: CV death, MI, or stroke. Placebo patients were taking aspirin; clopidogrel patients were taking clopidogrel and aspirin.

No. at risk

	0	3	6	9	12
Placebo	6303	5780	4664	3600	2388
Clopidogrel	6259	5866	4779	3644	2418

was observed (CAPRIE Steering Committee 1996). Furthermore, there is increasing evidence that combination antiplatelet therapy with a thienopyridine derivative and aspirin in high risk patients with vascular disease is more effective than aspirin alone (Yusuf *et al.* 2001*c*) (Fig. 44.3) and ongoing trials will help confirm this and inform clinicians if combination therapy can be extended to other subgroups of vascular patients.

Risks of prescribing long-term antiplatelet therapy

Bleeding is the most important adverse effect of antiplatelet treatment. The APTC overview reported that antiplatelet therapy is associated with an excess risk of intracranial bleeding in trials of long-term treatment. In addition, antiplatelet treatment is associated with a small but significant excess of non-fatal major extra cranial bleeds, but there is no clear excess of fatal extra cranial-bleeds. Higher dose antiplatelet therapy appears to be associated with more gastrointestinal bleeding than lower doses. The thienopyridines appear to be associated with significantly less gastrointestinal haemorrhage and upper gastrointestinal upset than aspirin (CAPRIE Steering Committee 1996). Clopidogrel is safer and more easily tolerated than ticlopidine. In the CURE trial of more than 12 000 patients with unstable angina or non-ST segment elevation MI, the combination of clopidogrel and aspirin is associated with a 38% increase in major bleeding, $p = 0.001$ (defined as intraocular, or requiring a transfusion of ≥ 2 units), but not life-threatening bleeds ($p = 0.13$) (defined as a haemoglobin drop of ≥ 5 g/dl, hypotension needing intravenous inotropes, surgery to stop bleeding, symptomatic intracranial haemorrhage, or transfusion or ≥ 4 units of blood) (Yusuf *et al.* 2001*c*).

44.4.7 **ACE inhibitors**

Clinical trials

Recently the ACE inhibitor ramipril (10 mg/day) was shown to reduce the composite primary outcome of cardiovascular death, stroke, or MI over an average of 4.7 years by 22% (95% CI: 14–30), $p < 0.00001$ compared to placebo (Yusuf *et al.* 2000*b*) (Fig. 44.4). Further, ramipril's effect appears to be greater than that accounted for by blood pressure lowering. Ramipril also prevented the progression of atherosclerosis (Lonn *et al.* 2001), and patients who were allocated to

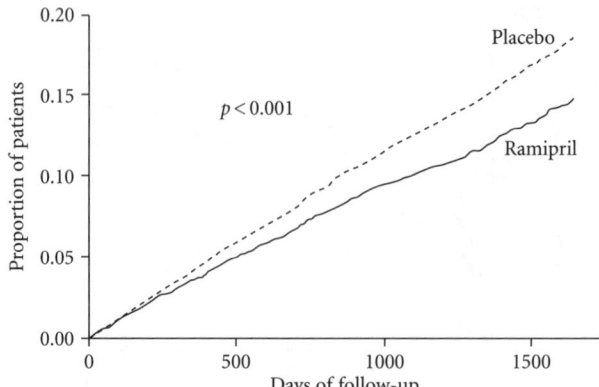

Fig. 44.4 HOPE Study. Incidence of primary outcome shown on *y* axis: CV death, MI, or stroke.

ramipril had a lower incidence of type 2 diabetes at the end of the trial (Yusuf *et al.* 2001*a*). Furthermore, the PROGRESS trial recently demonstrated that, among individuals who have suffered a prior TIA or stroke, treatment with the ACE inhibitor perindopril alone, or together with the diuretic indapamide, reduced the risk of recurrent stroke by 28% (20–38%) regardless of whether the patients were hypertensive or normotensive at entry (PROGRESS Collaborative Group 2001). Therefore, ACE inhibitors should be considered for use in all patients with established vascular disease, whether or not blood pressure lowering is required. Other blood pressure-lowering agents have also been demonstrated to effectively lower blood pressure, and may be needed when ACE inhibitors cannot be tolerated or when an additional blood pressure-lowering agent is required.

Risks of therapy

ACE inhibitors are generally well tolerated. The most common side effects include cough, occurring in 5–10% of patients. Dizziness, hypotension, renal dysfunction, and hyperkalaemia, are infrequent and can generally be avoided by careful drug titration and by avoiding the administration of ACE inhibitors in volume depleted patients. Angio-oedema is an uncommon but potentially life-threatening adverse event associated with ACE inhibitor therapy, which is due to potentiation of the vascular effects of bradykinin. In the HOPE trial among 4645 patients randomized to long-term ACE inhibitor use, the incidence of angio-oedema was 0.4% (Yusuf *et al.* 2000*b*).

44.4.8 Beta-blockers

Beta-blockers act by multiple mechanisms to improve outcomes following MI. These include blood pressure lowering, improved balance of oxygen demand and supply, and decreased ventricular irritability. Several randomized controlled trials have found benefits associated with the use of beta-blockers post-MI, and a large systematic overview of over 24 000 people reported that beta-blockers improved survival in patients with prior MI by 23%, reduced the risk of sudden death by 30%, and reduced the risk of non-fatal reinfarction by 25% (Yusuf *et al.* 1985). While some studies have suggested potential differences among beta-blockers, later studies and systematic overviews have not identified clear differences between beta-blockers with and without cardio-selectivity or membrane stabilizing properties, and between those with or without intrinsic sympathomimetic activity (Beta-Blocker Pooling Project Research

Group 1988; Yusuf *et al.* 1985). Subgroup analyses have demonstrated comparable benefits in men and women, and found that beta-blockers were particularly effective in subgroups with highest baseline risk, such as people over 50 years of age, and those with a history of previous MI, hypertension, or early heart failure symptoms. Therefore, beta-blockers are recommended in all post-MI patients who can tolerate them, and should be continued indefinitely post-MI. Patients with high baseline risk such as those with large infarcts, early heart failure symptoms, and hypertension are likely to derive the most benefit.

Risks of therapy

Adverse effects associated with beta-blocker use such as bronchospasm, bradycardia, hypotension, heart block, depression, nightmares, dizziness, and hallucinations have been reported. However, serious adverse effects are uncommon when patients are selected appropriately for treatment with beta-blockers.

44.4.9 Other therapies

Vitamin therapy: epidemiology

Large prospective epidemiological studies such as the US Nurses Health Study and the US male Health Professionals study have suggested that the use of vitamin E supplements (dose 200–400 IU) is associated with a 20–40% lower risk of CHD (Rimm *et al.* 1993; Stampfer *et al.* 1993). Other studies have identified vitamin E from food sources (but not supplements) as protective from CVD (Knekt *et al.* 1994). Further observational studies in which people who used beta-carotene were compared to people who did not have supported the notion that beta-carotene and foods which contain beta-carotene reduce the incidence of CVD among men, but not women (Hennekens *et al.* 1996).

Clinical trials

Large clinical trials conducted to date have failed to confirm the epidemiological findings. Six large randomized placebo-controlled trials of vitamin E supplementation with major CV morbidity and mortality end points have been completed (Alpha-Tocopherol, Beta Carotene Cancer Prevention Study Group 1994; de Gaetano 2001; Rapola *et al.* 1997; GISSI-Prevenzione Trial 1999; Stephens *et al.* 1996; Yusuf *et al.* 2000*a*). No convincing RRR with vitamin E in the primary or secondary prevention setting has been observed. Several large randomized trials with beta-carotene also failed to demonstrate a protective benefit of beta-carotene in the primary prevention setting (Heart Protection Study Collaborative Group 2002). More recently, 20 536 adults (aged 40–80) with coronary disease, other occlusive arterial disease, or diabetes in the UK were randomly allocated to receive a cocktail of antioxidant vitamins (600 mg vitamin E, 250 mg vitamin C, and 20 mg beta-carotene daily) or placebo. Allocation to this vitamin regimen approximately doubled the plasma concentration of alpha-tocopherol, increased that of vitamin C by one-third, and quadrupled that of beta-carotene (Heart Protection Study Collaborative Group 2002). However, there were no significant differences in all-cause mortality (14.1% vitamin-allocated vs. 13.5% placebo-allocated). Nor were there any significant differences in the numbers of participants having non-fatal MI or coronary death (10.4 vs. 10.2%), non-fatal or fatal stroke (5.0 vs. 5.0%), or coronary or non-coronary revascularization (10.3 vs. 10.6%). For the first occurrence of any of these 'major vascular events', there were no material differences either overall (22.5 vs. 22.5%) or in any of the various subcategories considered. Therefore, despite the predictions of benefit from observational studies, clinical trials to date do not support the efficacy of antioxidants in lowering clinical cardiovascular events among high risk patients (see Chapter 15).

Fish oils

Epidemiology The intake of n-3 polyunsaturated fatty acids (PUFA) that come mainly from marine sources is associated with a reduced incidence of CHD. Observational investigations raised the hypothesis that fish consumption was associated with a reduced incidence of CHD (Albert *et al.* 1998; Hu *et al.* 2002) (Chapter 18). Among almost 85 000 women initially free of heart disease followed for 16 years in the US Nurses Health Study, those who reported that they ate fish at least once a week were 30% less likely to have had a heart attack or have died of heart disease compared to those who ate fish less than once a month (Hu *et al.* 2002). In the US Physicians Health Study more than 22 000 healthy men were followed for 17 years, and the chance of dying suddenly was 80% lower among men with the highest blood levels of omega-3 fatty acids compared to those with the lowest levels (Albert *et al.* 1998).

Clinical trials In the GISSI-Prevenzione trial, more than 11 324 MI survivors were assigned to take capsules containing fish oil (1 g/day) or a placebo every day for 3.5 years (GISSI-Prevenzione Trial 1999). Treatment with n-3 PUFA significantly lowered the risk of death, non-fatal MI, and stroke (RRR: 10% (95% CI: 1–18)), and also resulted in a 50% reduction in sudden death (Marchioli *et al.* 2002). A meta-analysis of 11 randomized controlled trials, including almost 16 000 patients that compared dietary or non-dietary intake of n-3 PUFA with a control diet/placebo in patients with CHD, reported that the risk ratio of fatal MI in patients who were on n-3 PUFA-enriched diets compared with control diets or placebo was 0.7 (95% CI: 0.6–0.8) (Bucher *et al.* 2002). In five trials, sudden death was associated with a risk ratio of 0.7 (95% CI: 0.6–0.9), whereas the risk ratio of overall mortality was 0.8 (95% CI: 0.7–0.9) (Bucher *et al.* 2002).

Dietary modification

Dietary recommendations from the AHA/ACC Secondary Prevention Guidelines for patients with vascular disease (2001) include an emphasis by clinicians on promoting moderate sodium restriction, consumption of fruits, vegetables, and low fat dairy products, and increased consumption of omega-3 fatty acids (Smith *et al.* 2001). The results of the Lyon Diet Heart Study suggested that a Mediterranean-style diet, which emphasized consumption of more bread, root vegetables and green vegetables, fish, less beef, lamb and pork replaced with poultry, fruit, and butter and cream replaced with margarine high in linolenic acid, significantly lowered recurrent CV events among more than 400 survivors of a first MI (de Lorgeril *et al.* 1999). Subjects on the Mediterranean-style diet averaged 30% of calories from fat, 8% from saturated fat, 13% from monounsaturated fat, 5% from polyunsaturated fat, and 5.40 mmol/l of cholesterol. The trial was stopped early because subjects following the Mediterranean-style diet had a 50–70% lower risk of recurrent heart disease, including cardiac death and non-fatal heart attacks. Interestingly, the Mediterranean dietary pattern did not alter the independent association between major risk factors such as cholesterol and blood pressure with CV recurrence, suggesting that the protective effects of the Mediterranean diet are independent (and possibly additive) to CV prevention efforts attempted through medical therapy (de Lorgeril *et al.* 1997).

While dietary recommendations are based on randomized trials which have demonstrated that decreased consumption of certain foods and increased consumption of others lowers the risk of recurrent CHD (Chapter 14), clinicians deliver this advice poorly (or not at all), partly because they are unaware of the new information, have limited nutrition training (e.g. what are omega-3 fatty acids), or because they strongly embrace the medical model, believing that medical therapies are the only effective ways to reduce future cardiovascular risk. One way around this is for clinicians to refer patients to a professional dietitian for dietary counselling. However, it is incumbent upon the referring clinician to determine exactly what information the dietician is conveying to patients to ensure that their advice is based on up-to-date consensus recommendations (de Lorgeril *et al.* 1997). Poor dietary advice such as 'all fats are bad', and that 'patients should replace fat consumption with other nutrients such as carbohydrates' can have adverse effects on glycaemic control, triglycerides, and HDL-C (Knopp 2000).

Hormone replacement therapy (HRT)

Epidemiology More than 50 observational studies support the hypothesis that oestrogen use, alone or in combination with progesterone, significantly lowers the incidence of CHD and total mortality. The Nurses Health Study, involving over 59 337 women aged 30–55 years who were followed for 16 years, reported that the multivariate adjusted RR of CHD among HRT users was 0.39 (95% CI: 0.19–0.78) compared to non-users (Grodstein *et al.* 1997; Stampfer *et al.* 1991). Furthermore, studies of physiological parameters indicate that HRT has favourable effects on lipids, endothelial function, and arterial vasodilation (The PEPI Trial Writing Group 1995). All of these data led to the design and conduct of primary and secondary prevention clinical trials in which the role of HRT and vascular events was studied.

Clinical trials The largest secondary prevention trial testing the hypothesis that HRT reduced CV incidence was the HERS trial, in which 2763 women with prior CHD were randomized to receive HRT versus placebo; the trial was powered to detect at least a 24% RRR in the composite of CV death, MI, and stroke (Hulley *et al.* 1998). However, after a mean follow-up of 4.1 years no differences in cardiovascular outcomes were observed between the groups, and an excess of venous thromboembolic events occurred in patients allocated to HRT. This unexpected result was followed by the recent termination of one of the components of the primary prevention trial Women's Health Initiative (WHI), in which 16 608 women aged 50–79 years were randomized to receive conjugated equine oestrogen at a dose of 0.625 mg/day in combination with 2.5 mg of medroxy progesterone acetate versus placebo (Rossouw *et al.* 2002). After a mean of 5.2 years of follow-up, the trial was stopped because of an excess of breast cancer (hazard ratio (HR): 1.26, 95% CI: 1.00–1.59) and major cardiovascular events (CHD: HR of 1.29, 95% CI: 1.02–1.63; stroke: HR: 1.41, 95% CI: 1.07–1.85; pulmonary embolism: HR: 2.13, 95% CI: 1.39–3.25) (Fig. 44.5). Although there were fewer hip fractures (HR: 0.66, 95% CI: 0.45–0.98) and colorectal cancers (HR: 0.63, 95% CI: 0.43–0.92), a 'global index' that incorporated several prespecified outcomes (heart disease, breast cancers, hip fractures, colorectal cancers) was significantly adverse (HR: 1.15, 95% CI: 1.03–1.28). The excess of MI, strokes, and venous thromboembolism, suggests that a prothrombotic tendency occurs with HRT use and affects both the venous and arterial circulation. Taken together, the data from WHI and other smaller clinical trials are conclusive in that HRT increases the risk of vascular thrombosis.

The reasons why observational studies suggest a substantial reduction in CHD and total mortality are likely attributable to biases inherent in these types of studies (Grodstein *et al.* 2003). These include subjects who choose to take a given agent being very different from those who do not. For example, if women who choose to take HRT (as opposed to being randomized to it) are also of a higher socio-economic class, and engage in healthier lifestyle practices such as less smoking and more exercise, the apparent benefit attributed to HRT may in fact be due to other reasons. Randomized clinical trials avoid such biases because subjects are randomly

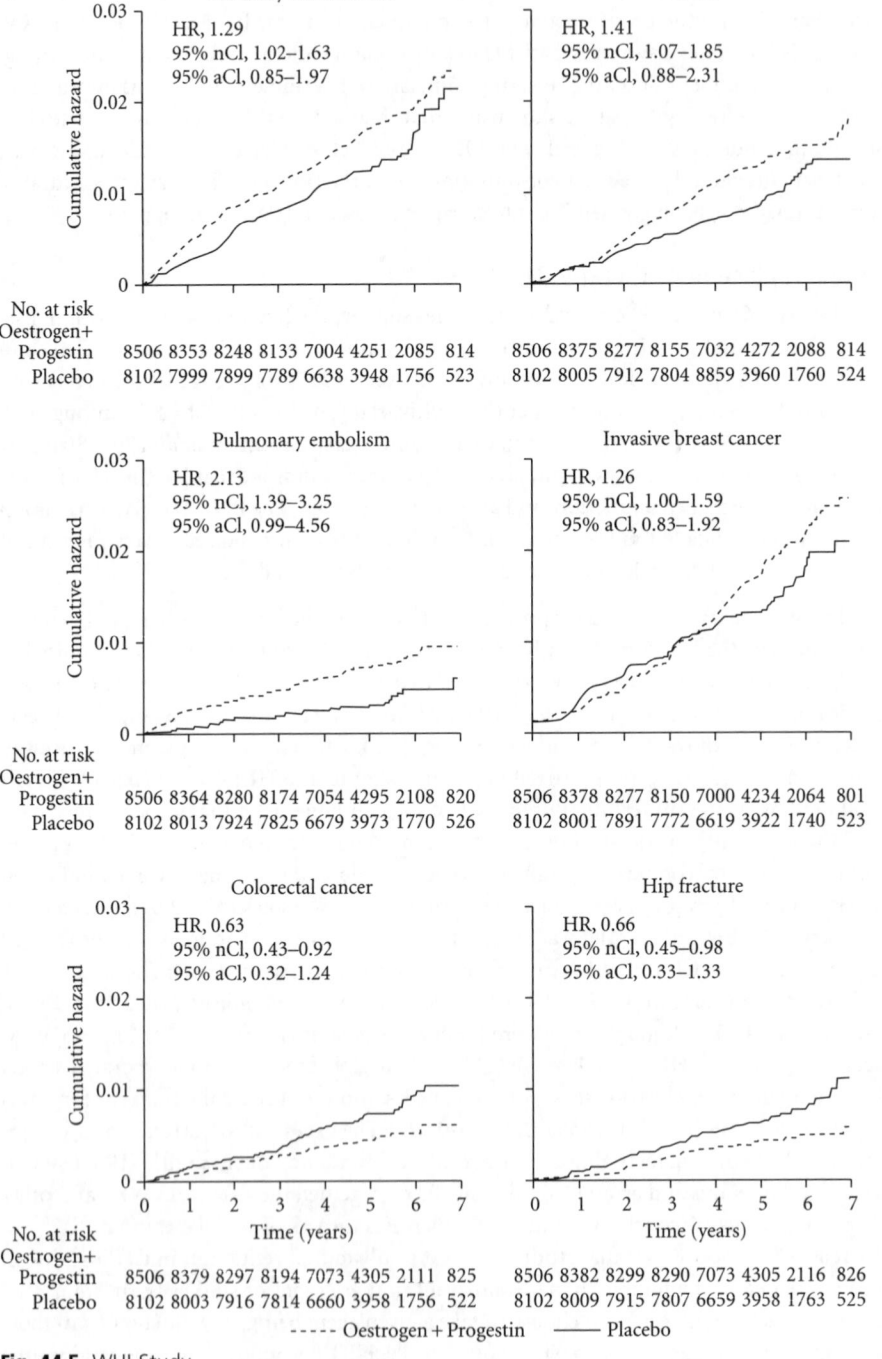

Fig. 44.5 WHI Study.

assigned to treatments, thereby minimizing possible differences between the groups in lifestyle or health-related factors. Other biases include the difficulty in cohort studies of ascertaining clinical events which occur early after therapy has begun, and compliance bias where confounding occurs because women who adhere to hormone therapy also tend to adhere to other protective types of behaviour (both measured and unmeasured) (Grodstein *et al.* 2003). Therefore, given current information from large randomized trials, HRT should not be given for the primary or secondary prevention of CVD.

44.5 Recommendations

44.5.1 Using risk

By definition 'secondary prevention' refers to preventing recurrent vascular events in patients who have vascular disease, and as such all major risk factors should be minimized and healthy lifestyles (e.g. smoking cessation, weight control, and physical exercise) should be promoted. Clinicians must avoid thinking of risk factors as being 'present' or 'absent', and think of them as being continuous exposures. For example, halving the CV risk of recurrence by lowering serum cholesterol is more important in a man who has an average serum cholesterol concentration but has suffered a prior MI, than in a man with high serum cholesterol who has no history of MI (Law and Wald 2002). Similar analogies hold true for blood pressure, glucose, and tobacco exposures. In Table 44.2 the proportional reductions in CHD incidence as predicted by observational epidemiological studies and clinical trials for a given change in selected exposures are provided.

44.5.2 Potential impact of proven medical therapies

Given the strong evidence from randomized trials that aspirin, beta-blockers, ACE inhibitors, and lipid-lowering therapies clearly reduce the risk of future vascular events by approximately a quarter each, and that their benefits appear to be largely independent, it is plausible to expect that, when used together, the cumulative RR of future vascular events approaches 75% (Yusuf 2002) (Table 44.3). Therefore, use of proven medical therapies and risk factor modification of lifestyle factors should be aggressively promoted among high risk patients.

Table 44.3 Cumulative benefits of multiple medical therapies

	RRR (%)	Two year event rate (%)[a]
No therapy	—	8
Aspirin	25	6
Beta-blocker	25	4.5
Lipid lowering ($\downarrow$ by 1.5 mmol/l)	30	3.0
ACE inhibitors	25	2.3

Adapted from Yusuf 2002.

Cumulative risk reduction if all four drugs are used is about 75%. To calculate the cumulative risk reduction, a multiplicative scale is used whereby two interventions each reducing the risk of an events by 30% would be expected to have a 50% RRR $(1 - (0.70 \times 0.70))$ (Yusuf 2002).

[a] CV death, MI, stroke.

44.6 **Conclusions**

Terms such as 'hypertension and hypercholesterolaemia' that focus medical attention on the tails of the distributions of physiological variables should be avoided (Law and Wald 2002). All reversible cardiovascular risk factors should be reduced in anyone who has established vascular disease. The best predictors of risk are factors that cannot be changed, such as previous disease (MI, stroke, or PAD), age, and sex. Interventions to change modifiable risk factors should therefore be determined by the individual's level of risk and not by the level of the risk factor. Attention to blood pressure lowering, glucose control, tobacco cessation, and optimizing an individual's cholesterol using proven medical therapies, together with sound dietary and physical activity programs, and regular use of antiplatelet agents, are the mainstay of secondary prevention.

References

Albert, C. M., Hennekens, C. H., O'Donnell, C. J., Ajani, U. A., Carey, V. J., Willett, W. C. *et al.* (1998). Fish consumption and risk of sudden cardiac death. *Journal of the American Medical Association*, **279** (1), 23–8.

Alpha-Tocopherol, Beta Carotene Cancer Prevention Study Group (1994). The effect of vitamin E and beta carotene on the incidence of lung cancer and other cancers in male smokers. *New England Journal of Medicine*, **330**, 1029–35.

Albert, M. A., Danielson, E., Rifai, N. and Ridker, P. M. (2001). Effect of statin therapy on C-reactive protein levels: the pravastatin inflammation/CRP evaluation (PRINCE). A randomized trial and cohort study. *Journal of the American Medical Association*, **286** (1), 64–70.

Anand, S. and Creager, M. (2002). Peripheral arterial disease. *Clinical Evidence*, **7**, 79–90.

Antithrombotic Trialists' Collaboration (2002). Collaborative meta-analysis of randomised trials of antiplatelet therapy for prevention of death, myocardial infarction, and stroke in high risk patients. *British Medical Journal*, **324** (7329), 71–86.

Beta-Blocker Pooling Project Research Group (1988). The beta-blocker pooling project (BBPP): subgroup findings from randomized trials in post infarction patients. *European Heart Journal*, **9**, 8–16.

Boden, W. E. (2000). High-density lipoprotein cholesterol as an independent risk factor in cardiovascular disease: assessing the data from Framingham to the Veterans Affairs High-Density Lipoprotein Intervention Trial. *American Journal of Cardiology*, **86** (12A), 19L–22L.

Bucher, H. C., Hengstler, P., Schindler, C. and Meier, G. (2002). N-3 polyunsaturated fatty acids in coronary heart disease: a meta-analysis of randomized controlled trials. *American Journal of Medicine*, **112** (4), 298–304.

CAPRIE Steering Committee (1996). A randomised, blinded, trial of clopidogrel versus aspirin in patients at risk of ischaemic events (CAPRIE). *Lancet*, **348**, 1329–39.

Chen, Z., Peto, R., Collins, R., MacMahon, S., Lu, J. and Li, W. (1991). Serum cholesterol concentration and coronary heart disease in population with low cholesterol concentrations. *British Medical Journal*, **303** (6797), 276–82.

Coutinho, M., Gerstein, H. C., Wang, Y. and Yusuf, S. (1999). The relationship between glucose and incident cardiovascular events: a metaregression analysis of published data from 20 studies of 95,783 individuals followed for 12.4 years. *Diabetes Care*, **22** (2), 233–40.

Criqui, M. H. and Denenberg, J. O. (1998). The generalized nature of atherosclerosis: how peripheral arterial disease may predict adverse events from coronary artery disease. *Vascular Medicine*, **3** (3), 241–5.

Dahlof, B., Devereux, R. B., Kjeldsen, S. E., Julius, S., Beevers, G., Faire, U. *et al.* (2002). Cardiovascular morbidity and mortality in the Losartan Intervention For Endpoint reduction in hypertension study (LIFE): a randomised trial against atenolol. *Lancet*, **359** (9311), 995–1003.

de Gaetano, G. (2001). Low-dose aspirin and vitamin E in people at cardiovascular risk: a randomized trial in general practice. Collaborative Group of the Primary Prevention Project. *Lancet*, **357** (9250), 89–95.

de Lorgeril, M., Salen, P., Monjaud, I. and Delaye, J. (1997). The 'diet heart' hypothesis in secondary prevention of coronary heart disease. *European Heart Journal*, **18** (1), 13–18.

de Lorgeril, M., Salen, P., Martin, J. L., Monjaud, I., Delaye, J. and Mamelle, N. (1999). Mediterranean diet, traditional risk factors, and the rate of cardiovascular complications after myocardial infarction: final report of the Lyon Diet Heart Study. *Circulation*, **99** (6), 779–85.

Detry, J. R., Vierendeel, I. A., Vanbutsele, R. J. and Robert, A. R. (2001). Early short-term intensive cardiac rehabilitation induces positive results as long as one year after the acute coronary event: a prospective one-year controlled study. *Journal of Cardiovascular Risk*, **6**, 355–61.

Diabetes Prevention Program Research Group (2002). Reduction in the incidence of type 2 diabetes with lifestyle intervention or metformin. *New England Journal of Medicine*, **346**, 393–403.

Downs, J. R., Clearfield, M., Weis, S., Whitney, E., Shapiro, D. R., Beere, P. A. *et al.* (1998). Primary prevention of acute coronary events with lovastatin in men and women with average cholesterol levels: results of AFCAPS/TexCAPS. Air Force/Texas Coronary Atherosclerosis Prevention Study. *Journal of the American Medical Association*, **279** (20), 1615–22.

Dunn, A., Marcus, B., Kampert, J., Garcia, M., Kohl, H. and Blair, S. (1999). Comparison of lifestyle and structured interventions to increase physical activity and cardiorespiratory fitness: a randomized trial. *Journal of the American Medical Association*, **281**, 327–34.

Elam, M. B., Hunninghake, D. B., Davis, K. B., Garg, R., Johnson, C., Egan, D. *et al.* (2000). Effect of niacin on lipid and lipoprotein levels and glycemic control in patients with diabetes and peripheral arterial disease: the ADMIT study. A randomized trial. Arterial Disease Multiple Intervention Trial. *Journal of the American Medical Association*, **284** (10), 1263–70.

Gardner, A. W. and Poehlman, E. T. (1995). Exercise rehabilitation programs for the treatment of claudication pain: a meta-analysis. *Journal of the American Medical Association*, **274** (12), 975–80.

Gerstein, H. C. and Yusuf, S. (1996). Dysglycaemia and risk of cardiovascular disease. *Lancet*, **347** (9006), 949–50.

Grodstein, F., Clarkson, T. B. and Manson, J. E. (2003). Understanding the divergent data on postmenopausal hormone therapy. *New England Journal of Medicine*, **348**, 645–50.

Grodstein, F., Stampfer, M. J., Colditz, G. A., Willett, W. C., Manson, J. E., Joffe, M. *et al.* (1997). Postmenopausal hormone therapy and mortality. *New England Journal of Medicine*, **336** (25), 1769–75.

Grover, S. A., Gray-Donald, K., Joseph, L., Abrahamowicz, M. and Coupal, L. (1994). Life expectancy following dietary modification or smoking cessation: estimating the benefits of a prudent lifestyle. *Archives of Internal Medicine*, **154** (15), 1697–704.

GISSI-Prevenzione Trial: Gruppo It Dietary supplementation aliano per lo Studio della Sopravvivenza nell'Infarto miocardico (1999). Dietary supplementation with n-3 polyunsaturated fatty acids and vitamin E after myocardial infarction: results of the GISSI-Prevenzione trial. *Lancet*, **354** (9177), 447–55.

Heart Protection Study Collaborative Group (2002). MRC/BHF Heart Protection Study of antioxidant vitamin supplementation in 20536 high-risk individuals: a randomised placebo-controlled trial. *Lancet*, **360** (9326), 23–33.

Hedback, B., Perk, J., Hornblad, M. and Ohlsson, U. (2001). Cardiac rehabilitation after coronary artery bypass surgery: 10-year results on mortality, morbidity and readmissions to hospital. *Journal of Cardiovascular Risk*, **8** (3), 153–8.

Hennekens, C. H., Buring, J. E., Manson, J. E., Stampfer, M., Rosner, B., Cook, N. R. *et al.* (1996). Lack of effect of long-term supplementation with beta carotene on the incidence of malignant neoplasms and cardiovascular disease. *New England Journal of Medicine*, **334** (18), 1145–9.

HPS Collaborative Group (2002). MRC/BHF Heart Protection Study of cholesterol lowering with simvastatin in 20,536 high-risk individuals: a randomised placebo-controlled trial. *Lancet*, **360** (9326), 7–22.

Hu, F. B., Bronner, L., Willett, W. C., Stampfer, M. J., Rexrode, K. M., Albert, C. M. *et al.* (2002). Fish and omega-3 fatty acid intake and risk of coronary heart disease in women. *Journal of the American Medical Association*, **287** (14), 1815–21.

Hulley, S., Grady, D., Bush, T., Furberg, C., Herrington, D., Riggs, B. and Vittinghoff, E. (1998). Randomized trial of estrogen plus progestin for secondary prevention of coronary heart disease in postmenopausal women: Heart and Estrogen/progestin Replacement Study (HERS) Research Group. *Journal of the American Medical Association*, **280** (7), 605–13.

Jeppesen, J., Hein, H. O., Suadicani, P. and Gyntelberg, F. (2000). High triglycerides and low HDL cholesterol and blood pressure and risk of ischemic heart disease. *Hypertension*, **36** (2), 226–32.

Jolliffe, J. A., Rees, K., Taylor, R. S., Thompson, D., Oldridge, N. and Ebrahim, S. (2001). Exercise-based rehabilitation for coronary heart disease. *Cochrane Database Systematic Reviews*, **1**, CD001800. John Wiley & Sons Ltd, Chichester.

Jorenby, D. E., Leischow, S. J., Nides, M. A., Rennard, S. I., Johnston, J. A., Hughes, A. R. *et al.* (1999). A controlled trial of sustained-release bupropion, a nicotine patch, or both for smoking cessation. *New England Journal of Medicine*, **340** (9), 685–91.

Joseph, A. M., Norman, S. M., Ferry, L. H., Prochazka, A. V., Westman, E. C., Steele, B. G. *et al.* (1996). The safety of transdermal nicotine as an aid to smoking cessation in patients with cardiac disease. *New England Journal of Medicine*, **335** (24), 1792–8.

Kannel, W. B. and McGee, D. L. (1979). Diabetes and cardiovascular disease: The Framingham study. *Journal of the American Medical Association*, **241** (19), 2035–8.

Kilaru, S., Frangos, S. G., Chen, A. H., Gortler, D., Dhadwal, A. K., Araim, O. and Sumpio, B. E. (2001). Nicotine: a review of its role in atherosclerosis. *Journal of the American College of Surgery*, **193** (5), 538–46.

Knekt, P., Reunanen, A., Jarvinen, R., Seppanen, R., Heliovaara, M. and Aromaa, A. (1994). Antioxidant vitamin intake and coronary mortality in a longitudinal population study. *American Journal of Epidemiology*, **139**, 1180–90.

Knopp, R. H. (2000). Introduction: low-saturated fat, high-carbohydrate diets. Effects on triglyceride and LDL synthesis, the LDL receptor, and cardiovascular disease risk. *Proceedings of the Society for Experimental Biology and Medicine*, **225** (3), 175–7.

Law, M. (1998). Lipids and cardiovascular disease. In *Evidence based cardiology* (ed. S. Yusuf, J. A. Cairns, A. J. Camm, E. L. Fallen, and B. J. Gersh), pp. 191–205. British Medical Journal Publishing Group, London.

Law, M. R. and Wald, N. J. (1994). An ecological study of serum cholesterol and ischaemic heart disease between 1950 and 1990. *European Journal of Clinical Nutrition*, **48** (5), 305–25.

Law, M. R. and Wald, N. J. (2002). Risk factor thresholds: their existence under scrutiny. *British Medical Journal*, **324** (7353), 1570–6.

Law, M. R. Wald, N. J. and Thompson, S. G. (1994). By how much and how quickly does reduction in serum cholesterol concentration lower risk of ischaemic heart disease? *British Medical Journal*, **308** (6925), 367–72.

LIPID (Long-term Intervention with Pravastatin in Ischaemic Disease) Study Group (1998). Prevention of cardiovascular events and death with pravastatin in patients with coronary heart disease and a broad range of initial cholesterol levels. *New England Journal of Medicine*, **339**, 1349–57.

Lonn, E., Yusuf, S., Dzavik, V., Doris, C., Yi, Q., Smith, S. *et al.* (2001). Effects of ramipril and vitamin E on atherosclerosis: the study to evaluate carotid ultrasound changes in patients treated with ramipril and vitamin E (SECURE). *Circulation*, **103** (7), 919–25.

MacMahon, S., Peto, R., Cutler, J., Collins, R., Sorlie, P., Neaton, J. *et al.* (1990). Blood pressure, stroke, and coronary heart disease. Part 1. Prolonged differences in blood pressure: prospective observational studies corrected for the regression dilution bias. *Lancet*, **335** (8692), 765–74.

Marchioli, R., Barzi, F., Bomba, E., Chieffo, C., Di Gregorio, D., Di Mascio, R. *et al.* (2002). Early protection against sudden death by n-3 polyunsaturated fatty acids after myocardial infarction: time-course analysis of the results of the Gruppo Italiano per lo Studio della Sopravvivenza nell'Infarto Miocardioco (GISSI)-Prevenzione. *Circulation*, **105** (16), 1897–903.

Min, L., Kathryn, M., Cook, N., Manson, J. and Buring, J. (2001). Physical activity and coronary heart disease in women. *Journal of the American Medical Association*, **285**, 1447–54.

Neal, B. and MacMahon, S. (1999). An overview of 37 randomised trials of blood pressure lowering agents among 270,000 individuals: World Health Organization–International Society of Hypertension Blood Pressure Lowering Treatment Trialists' Collaboration. *Clinical and Experimental Hypertension*, **21** (5–6), 517–29.

Opie, L. and Gersh, B. (2001). *Drugs for the heart*, 5th edn, Harcourt Health Sciences, W. B. Saunders, Philadelphia.

Pahor, M., Psaty, B. M., Alderman, M. H., Applegate, W. B., Williamson, J. D., Cavazzini, C. and Furberg, C. D. (2000*a*). Health outcomes associated with calcium antagonists compared with other first-line antihypertensive therapies: a meta-analysis of randomised controlled trials. *Lancet*, **356** (9246), 1949–54.

Pahor, M., Psaty, B. M., Alderman, M. H., Applegate, W. B., Williamson, J. D., Furberg, C. D. (2000*b*). Therapeutic benefits of ACE inhibitors and other antihypertensive drugs in patients with type 2 diabetes. *Diabetes Care*, **23** (7), 888–92.

Pasternak, R. C., Smith, S. C., Jr., Bairey-Merz, C. N., Grundy, S. M., Cleeman, J. I. and Lenfant, C. (2002). ACC/AHA/NHLBI Clinical Advisory on the Use and Safety of Statins. *Circulation*, **106** (8), 1024–8.

Pate, R. R., Pratt, M., Blair, S. N., Haskell, W. L., Macera, C. A., Bouchard, C. *et al.* (1995). Physical activity and public health: a recommendation from the Centers for Disease Control and Prevention and the American College of Sports Medicine. *Journal of the American Medical Association*, **273** (5), 402–7.

Peto, R., Darby, S., Deo, H., Silcocks, P., Whitley, E. and Doll, R. (2000). Smoking, smoking cessation, and lung cancer in the UK since 1950: combination of national statistics with two case-control studies. *British Medical Journal*, **321** (7257), 323–9.

Pfeffer, M. A., Keech, A., Sacks, F. M., Cobbe, S. M., Tonkin, A., Byington, R. P. *et al.* (2002). Safety and tolerability of pravastatin in long-term clinical trials: prospective Pravastatin Pooling (PPP) Project. *Circulation*, **105** (20), 2341–6.

PEPI (Postmenopausal Estrogen/Progestin Interventions) Trial Writing Group for the PEPI Trial (1995). Effects of estrogen or estrogen/progestin regimens on heart disease risk factors in postmenopausal women: the Postmenopausal Estrogen/Progestin Interventions (PEPI) Trial. *Journal of the American Medical Association*, **273** (3), 199–208.

Piegas, L. S., Flather, M., Pogue, J., Hunt, D., Varigos, J., Avezum, A. *et al.* (1999). The Organization to Assess Strategies for Ischemic Syndromes (OASIS) registry in patients with unstable angina. *American Journal of Cardiology*, **84** (5A), 7M–12M.

Pignone, M., Phillips, C., and Mulrow, C. (2000). Use of lipid lowering drugs for primary prevention of coronary heart disease: meta-analysis of randomised trials. *BMJ*, **321**, 983–6.

Pitt, B., Waters, D., Brown, W. V., van Boven, A. J., Schwartz, L., Title, L. M. *et al.* (1999). Aggressive lipid-lowering therapy compared with angioplasty in stable coronary artery disease: Atorvastatin versus Revascularization Treatment Investigators. *New England Journal of Medicine*, **341** (2), 70–6.

PROGRESS Collaborative Group (2001). Randomised trial of a perindopril-based blood-pressure-lowering regimen among 6,105 individuals with previous stroke or transient ischaemic attack. *Lancet*, **29**, 358 (9287), 1033–41.

Psaty, B. M., Furberg, C. D., Kuller, L. H., Borhani, N. O., Rautaharju, P. M., O'Leary, D. H. *et al.* (1992). Isolated systolic hypertension and subclinical cardiovascular disease in the elderly: initial findings from the Cardiovascular Health Study. *Journal of the American Medical Association*, **268** (10), 1287–91.

Rapola, J. M., Virtamo, J., Ripatti, S., Huttunen, J. K., Albanes, D., Taylor, P. R. *et al.* (1997). Randomised trial of alpha-tocopherol and beta-carotene supplements on incidence of major coronary events in men with previous myocardial infarction. *Lancet,* **349,** 1715–20.

Richardson, L. A., Buckenmeyer, P. J., Bauman, B. D., Rosneck, J. S., Newman, I. and Josephson, R. A. (2000). Contemporary cardiac rehabilitation: patient characteristics and temporal trends over the past decade. *Journal of Cardiopulmonary Rehabilitation,* **20** (1), 57–64.

Rimm, E. B., Stampfer, M. J., Ascherio, A., Giovannucci, E., Colditz, G. A. and Willett, W. C. (1993). Vitamin E consumption and the risk of coronary heart disease in men. *New England Journal of Medicine,* **328,** 1450–6.

Robins, S. J., Collins, D., Wittes, J. T., Papademetriou, V., Deedwania, P. C., Schaefer, E. J. *et al.* (2001). Relation of gemfibrozil treatment and lipid levels with major coronary events: VA-HIT: a randomized controlled trial. *Journal of the American Medical Association,* **285** (12), 1585–91.

Rodgers, A. and MacMahon, S. (1999). Blood pressure and the global burden of cardiovascular disease. *Clinical and Experimental Hypertension,* **21** (5–6), 543–52.

Rose, G. (1981). Strategy of prevention: lessons from cardiovascular disease. *British Medical Journal,* **282** (6279), 1847–51.

Ross, R., Dagnone, D., Jones, P. J., Smith, H., Paddags, A., Hudson, R., and Janssen, I. (2000). Reduction in obesity and related comorbid conditions after diet-induced weight loss or exercise-induced weight loss in men: a randomized, controlled trial. *Annals of Internal Medicine,* **133** (2), 92–103.

Rossouw, J. E., Anderson, G. L., Prentice, R. L., LaCroix, A. Z., Kooperberg, C., Stefanick, M. L. *et al.* (2002). Risks and benefits of estrogen plus progestin in healthy postmenopausal women: principal results from the Women's Health Initiative randomized controlled trial. *Journal of the American Medical Association,* **288** (3), 321–33.

Sacks, F. M., Pfeffer, M. A., Moye, L. A., Rouleau, J. L., Rutherford, J. D., Cole, T. G. *et al.* (1996). The effect of pravastatin on coronary events after myocardial infarction in patients with average cholesterol levels. Cholesterol and Recurrent Events Trial investigators. *New England Journal of Medicine,* **335** (14), 1001–9.

Sacks, F. M., Svetkey, L. P., Vollmer, W. M., Appel, L. J., Bray, G. A., Harsha, D. *et al.* (2001). Effects on blood pressure of reduced dietary sodium and the Dietary Approaches to Stop Hypertension (DASH) diet. DASH-Sodium Collaborative Research Group. *New England Journal of Medicine,* **344** (1), 3–10.

Scandinavian Simvastatin Survival Study (4S) (1994). Randomised trial of cholesterol lowering in 4444 patients with coronary heart disease. *Lancet,* **344** (8934), 1383–9.

Schwartz, G. G., Olsson, A. G., Ezekowitz, M. D., Ganz, P., Oliver, M. F., Waters, D. *et al.* (2001). Atorvastatin for acute coronary syndromes. *Journal of the American Medical Association,* **286** (5), 533–5.

Smith, S. C., Jr, Blair, S. N., Bonow, R. O., Brass, L. M., Cerqueira, M. D., Dracup, K. *et al.* (2001). AHA/ACC guidelines for preventing heart attack and death in patients with atherosclerotic cardiovascular disease: 2001 update. A statement for healthcare professionals from the American Heart Association and the American College of Cardiology. *Journal of the American College of Cardiology* **38,** 1581–3.

Stampfer, M. J., Colditz, G. A., Willett, W. C., Manson, J. E., Rosner, B., Speizer, F. E. and Hennekens, C. H. (1991). Postmenopausal estrogen therapy and cardiovascular disease: ten-year follow-up from the nurses' health study. *New England Journal of Medicine,* **325** (11), 756–62.

Stampfer, M. J., Hennekens, C. H., Manson, J. E., Colditz, G. A., Rosner, B. and Willett, W. C. (1993). Vitamin E consumption and the risk of coronary disease in women. *New England Journal of Medicine,* **328** (20), 1444–9.

Stephens, N. G., Parsons, A., Schofield, P. M., Kelly, F., Cheeseman, K. and Mitchinson, M. J. (1996). Randomised controlled trial of vitamin E in patients with coronary disease: Cambridge Heart Antioxidant Study (CHAOS). *Lancet,* **347** (9004), 781–6.

Stratton, I. M., Adler, A. I., Neil, H. A., Matthews, D. R., Manley, S. E., Cull, C. A. *et al.* (2000). Association of glycaemia with macrovascular and microvascular complications of type 2 diabetes (UKPDS 35): prospective observational study. *British Medical Journal,* **321** (7258), 405–12.

Szarfman, A., Machado, S. G. and O'Neill, R. T. (2002). Use of screening algorithms and computer systems to efficiently signal higher-than-expected combinations of drugs and events in the US FDA's spontaneous reports database. *Drug Safety,* **25** (6), 381–92.

Tuomilehto, J., Lindström, J., Eriksson, J. G., Valle, T. T., Hamalainen, H., Ilanne-Parikka, P. *et al.* (2001). Prevention of type 2 diabetes mellitus by changes in lifestyle among subjects with impaired glucose tolerance. *New England Journal of Medicine,* **344**, 1343–50.

US DHSS/NIH Physical Activity and Health (1997). A Report of the Surgeon General. Executive Summary US Department of Health and Human Services Centers for Disease Control and Prevention National Center for Chronic Disease Prevention and Health Promotion The President's Council on Physical Fitness and Sports: <http://www.fitness.gov/execsum.htm#majorconclu>.

Van den Hoogen, P. C., Feskens, E. J., Nagelkerke, N. J., Menotti, A., Nissinen, A. and Kromhout, D. (2000). The relation between blood pressure and mortality due to coronary heart disease among men in different parts of the world. *New England Journal of Medicine,* **342**, 1–8.

West of Scotland Coronary Prevention Study (1996). Identification of high-risk groups and comparison with other cardiovascular intervention trials. *Lancet,* **348** (9038), 1339–42.

Williams, D. and Feely, J. (2002). Pharmacokinetic-pharmacodynamic drug interactions with HMG-CoA reductase inhibitors. *Clinical Pharmacokinetics,* **41** (5), 343–70.

Wilson, P. W., Castelli, W. P. and Kannel, W. B. (1987). Coronary risk prediction in adults (the Framingham Heart Study). *American Journal of Cardiology,* **59** (14), 91G–94G.

Yusuf, S. (2002). Two decades of progress in preventing vascular disease. *Lancet,* **360** (9326), 2–3.

Yusuf, S., Peto, R., Lewis, J., Collins, R. and Sleight, P. (1985). Beta blockade during and after myocardial infarction: an overview of the randomized trials. *Progress in Cardiovascular Diseases,* **27** (5), 335–71.

Yusuf, S., Dagenais, G., Pogue, J., Bosch, J. and Sleight, P. (2000*a*). Vitamin E supplementation and cardiovascular events in high-risk patients. The Heart Outcomes Prevention Evaluation Study Investigators. *New England Journal of Medicine,* **342** (3), 154–60.

Yusuf, S., Sleight, P., Pogue, J., Bosch, J., Davies, R. and Dagenais, G. (2000*b*). Effects of an angiotensin-converting-enzyme inhibitor, ramipril, on cardiovascular events in high-risk patients. The Heart Outcomes Prevention Evaluation Study Investigators. *New England Journal of Medicine,* **342** (3), 145–53.

Yusuf, S., Gerstein, H., Hoogwerf, B., Pogue, J., Bosch, J., Wolffenbuttel, B. H. and Zinman, B. (2001*a*). Ramipril and the development of diabetes. *Journal of the American Medical Association,* **286** (15), 1882–5.

Yusuf, S., Reddy, S., Ounpuu, S. and Anand, S. (2001*b*). Global burden of cardiovascular diseases. Part I: general considerations, the epidemiologic transition, risk factors, and impact of urbanization. *Circulation,* **104** (22), 2746–53.

Yusuf, S., Zhao, F., Mehta, S. R., Chrolavicius, S., Tognoni, G. and Fox, K. K. (2001*c*). Effects of clopidogrel in addition to aspirin in patients with acute coronary syndromes without ST-segment elevation. *New England Journal of Medicine,* **16**, 345 (7), 494–502.

Zhu, S. H., Anderson, C. M., Tedeschi, G. J., Rosbrook, B., Johnson, C. E., Byrd, M. and Gutierrez-Terrell, E. (2002). Evidence of real-world effectiveness of a telephone quitline for smokers. *New England Journal of Medicine,* **347** (14), 1087–93.

Chapter 45

Smoke-free policies are an effective way to reduce heart disease rapidly

C. M. Fichtenberg and S. A. Glantz

45.1 Introduction

When people talk about smoking, the first disease that comes to mind is usually lung cancer; people rarely mention heart disease. In fact, heart disease accounts for more smoking-induced deaths than lung cancer (149 000 vs. 125 000 annual deaths in the US in 1995–99 (CDC 2002)) (see also Chapter 10) and smoking is the most important modifiable risk factor for heart disease. This situation is even more striking for passive smoking: heart disease kills over 10 times as many non-smokers as lung cancer (35 000 vs. 3000 (CDC 2002)). In addition, the risk of death from heart disease drops rapidly when an individual stops smoking, with half the risk gone in about a year and most gone in 3–5 years (Lightwood and Glantz 1997). This situation means that interventions that rapidly reduce cigarette consumption will rapidly reduce heart disease mortality and morbidity. The tobacco control experience in California demonstrates that this is true.

45.2 The California Tobacco Control Campaign

In 1989, California enacted a comprehensive tobacco control programme funded by a tax increase on cigarettes (Glantz and Balbach 2000). The programme combined the effect of the 25 cent tax increase (20% of which went to pay for the tobacco control programme) with an aggressive media campaign and with community-based interventions promoting clean indoor air policies. The programme was the largest such programme in history, averaging $74 million per year (about $2.40 per capita) for its first 7 years (Pierce et al. 1998).

The media campaign, instead of focusing on the health effects of smoking, broke new ground by attacking the tobacco industry and emphasizing non-smokers' rights to clean indoor air (Goldman and Glantz 1998) (Fig. 45.1). These messages reinforced the already-strong grass roots movement in California for local smoke-free legislation (Glantz and Balbach 2000). This grass roots movement was further strengthened by allocating substantial funds to local health departments to support the development of community-specific tobacco control interventions. One of the major activities carried out by the local groups was the promotion of local clean air ordinances. From 1990 to 1993 the proportion of local health departments involved in local policy interventions increased from 1% to 53% (Siegel 2002). Prior to the implementation of the programme, 213 communities had passed local clean air ordinances with the help of the California-based non-profit organization Americans for Nonsmokers' Rights (Glantz and Balbach 2000), but there were no 100% smoke-free restaurant ordinances (Siegel 2002). As a result of the combined effects of the media campaign and the community activities, between

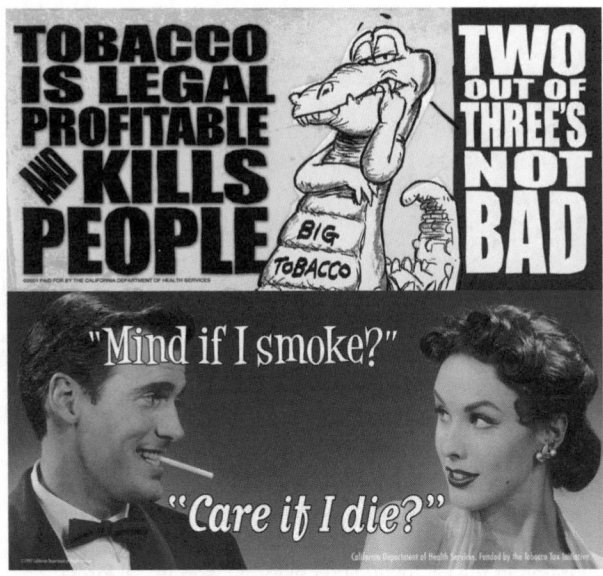

Fig. 45.1 Two billboards from the California Tobacco Control Program illustrate its central theme of educating people about the tobacco industry's behaviour and the dangers of second-hand smoke. The campaign also included paid television and radio advertising stressing these themes, as well as secondary components on cessation and youth. (Billboards courtesy of the California Department of Health Services.)

1989 and 2000, 139 new local laws were passed requiring that all workplaces be smoke-free (Siegel 2002). In the same time period, only 64 such laws were passed in the rest of the US (excluding Massachusetts, which had started a similar programme in 1993) (Siegel 2002). In 1994, after most of the state was already covered by local ordinances, California passed a state law that made all workplaces (including restaurants) smoke-free, starting in 1995, and extended the smoke-free policy to bars in 1998 (Glantz and Balbach 2000; Pierce *et al.* 1998).

The tobacco industry, working through political allies, including the California Medical Association, aggressively attacked both the content and funding of the programme, particularly the aggressive media campaign. In 1992, using claims that the media campaign was ineffective (claims that were contradicted by data that the Department of Health Services had collected), then-Governor Pete Wilson suspended the media campaign; it was restored only after the American Lung Association sued him (Glantz and Balbach 2000). Later, citing budgetary difficulties the state was facing, the Governor substantially cut the budget (Glantz and Balbach 2000). These cuts were only restored later, after a major political campaign by health advocates, led by the American Heart Association and Americans for Nonsmokers' Rights. These political difficulties served as a natural experiment to estimate the effects of the campaign independent of other underlying trends.

45.3 **Effects on smoking**

Cigarette consumption and smoking prevalence declined much faster in California after the programme launch than before, an improvement not seen during that same time period in the rest of the US. Tobacco industry sales data show that per capita cigarette consumption declined 26% faster during the 5 years following the implementation of the programme than in the period from 1983 to 1988 (Gilpin *et al.* 2001) (Fig. 45.2). This is almost twice as much of an acceleration as that seen in the rest of the US in the same time period, where cigarette consumption declined only 14% faster in 1989–93 than in 1983–88 (Gilpin *et al.* 2001).

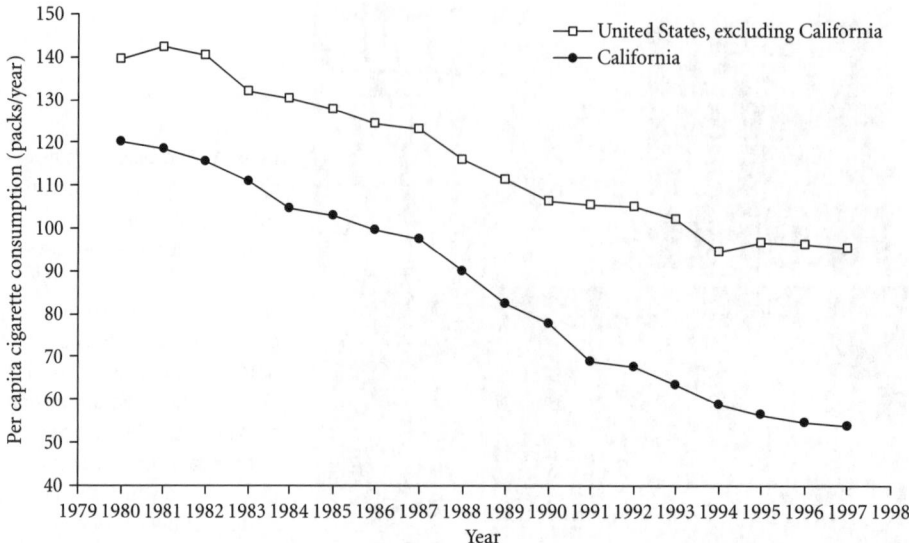

Fig. 45.2 Per capita cigarette consumption in the US (excluding California) and in California, 1980–97. Rates of per capita consumption were falling at roughly the same rate in both California and the rest of the US from 1980 to 1988. The rate of decline increased in California in 1989 when the California Tobacco Control Program was implemented. (Reproduced from Fichtenberg and Glantz 2000. Copyright 2000 Massachusetts Medical Society. All rights reserved.)

As with cigarette consumption, smoking prevalence in California decreased more rapidly during the early years of the tobacco control programme than it had before the existence of the programme, and those changes were not seen in the rest of the US. Between 1983 and 1989, adult smoking prevalence was dropping at roughly the same rate in California and the rest of the US (Gilpin *et al*. 2001). One analysis showed that the programme accelerated the rate of decline in the prevalence of smoking by one percentage point per year between 1989 and 1995, while there was no change in the rate of decline for that same time period for the rest of the US (Lightwood and Glantz 1997). Another analysis found that adult smoking prevalence rates were declining 20–30% faster in California than in the rest of the US from 1978 to 1990. From 1990 to 1994, however, the decline in California was almost eight times faster than in the rest of the country (Siegel *et al*. 2000).

The cutbacks and toning down of the programme beginning in 1992 were reflected in changes in smoking rates. Following the political and funding problems the programme faced starting in 1992, cigarette consumption declined more slowly than during the first 5 years of the programme (Fichtenberg and Glantz 2000, 2001; Gilpin *et al*. 2001). Likewise, smoking prevalence rates stagnated in California after 1994, while rates in the rest of the country continued to decrease slowly (Gilpin *et al*. 2001), although per capita consumption continued to decline (Fichtenberg and Glantz 2001). These results illustrate that the content of, and commitment to, the programme are essential for its success.

Despite the programme setbacks, the cumulative effects of the tobacco control programme on cigarette consumption in California are impressive. In the 10 years from 1989 to 1998, annual per capita consumption dropped a total of 57% in California, but only 27% in the rest of the US (Gilpin *et al*. 2001). Based on a comparison of trends in per capita consumption in

California and the rest of the US from 1980 to 1997, it is estimated that the programme was associated with 2.9 billion fewer packs of cigarettes sold between 1989 and 1997, costing the tobacco industry $4 billion in lost pretax sales (Fichtenberg and Glantz 2000, 2001). This drop in per capita consumption reflects declines in both the prevalence of smoking and the number of cigarettes smoked by continuing smokers.

The fact that cigarette consumption continued to drop after 1994 while prevalence remained at the same level indicates that while the number of smokers was unchanged after 1994, smokers were smoking less on average. In 1988, before the programme was implemented, per capita cigarette consumption was 23% lower in California than in the rest of the US while the prevalence of smoking was 12% lower. Eight years later, cigarette consumption in California was 56% lower than in the rest of the US and prevalence was 19% lower (Gilpin *et al.* 2001).

Thus there is a strong consensus that the California programme accelerated the rate of decline in cigarette smoking, both by reducing the prevalence of smoking and by reducing the number of cigarettes smoked per smoker.

45.4 The effect of tobacco control media campaigns

The California Tobacco Control Program's innovative media campaign was responsible for a significant portion of the programme's effect on smoking. As already discussed, the rate of decline in smoking seen in the early part of the programme slowed markedly when the anti-smoking media campaign was suspended in 1992 (Fichtenberg and Glantz 2000; Gilpin *et al.* 2001; Siegel *et al.* 2000). Likewise, the decline in smoking intensified again once the campaign was reinstated after the American Lung Association brought a successful lawsuit against the Governor. An econometric analysis of trends in cigarette consumption in California between 1980 and 1993 estimated that, after controlling for the 1989 tax increase, the media campaign accounted for 22% of the 1.1 billion pack decrease in cigarette sales which occurred between 1990 and 1992 (Hu *et al.* 1995). In addition to creating a political climate favourable to the passage of clean air ordinances, the media campaign directly influenced smokers to quit. A survey of California smokers who quit during the initial media campaign in 1990–91 found that 7% of those who successfully quit during that time period cited the media campaign as an important stimulus for quitting (Popham *et al.* 1993). A further 34% reported that the antismoking advertisements played some role in their decision to quit.

Media campaigns have proven themselves highly effective in other instances as well. In early 1998 the state of Florida initiated an anti-tobacco campaign (the 'truth' campaign) aimed at teenagers aged 12–17 years (Sly *et al.* 2001a). The campaign was similar to that in California in that it was centred on attacking the tobacco industry by portraying it as predatory and manipulative (Sly *et al.* 2001a). Several evaluations of the 'truth' campaign have demonstrated its success at changing teenagers' attitudes towards smoking and their smoking behaviour. A telephone survey of youths in Florida and in a national comparison group showed that attitudes towards tobacco industry tactics changed significantly in Florida compared to the rest of the US after the first year of the programme (Sly *et al.* 2001a). In addition, in the same time period, the prevalence of smoking among 12–17-year-olds decreased by 9% in Florida while it increased by 12% in the rest of the country (Sly *et al.* 2001a). Surveys in Florida middle and high schools in 1998 and 2000 showed that current cigarette use dropped by 40% among middle school students and by 18% among high school students over the first 2 years of the programme (Bauer and Johnson 2000). As further evidence that the media campaign was directly responsible for the changes in smoking, a longitudinal analysis of youth who were 12–17 years old during the first year of the programme linked exposure to the programme to smoking initiation in a dose dependent fashion. Youths who had a high awareness of the campaign were 2.4 times more likely to remain non-smokers than those who had no awareness of the campaign, while youths with a low awareness of the campaign were only 1.8 times more likely to remain smoke-free (Sly *et al.* 2001*b*).

A media campaign in Massachusetts is also credited with reductions in youth smoking rates. Youths who were 12–13 years old in 1993 and who recalled having seen an antismoking adver-tisement on television in 1993 were half as likely to have progressed to established smoking over the 4 year follow-up as those who did not remember seeing an advertisement (Siegel and Biener 2000).

Despite the success of these campaigns, not all tobacco media campaigns are effective. Focusing on tobacco industry practices, as was done in California and Florida, and now in a national 'truth' campaign launched by the American Legacy Foundation in 2000, is thought to be one of the most effective tactics to reduce smoking. A national sample of youth aged 12–17 years old was used to compare the effects of the Legacy's 'truth' campaign and Philip Morris' 'Think. Don't Smoke' campaign on youth attitudes, beliefs, and intentions towards smoking (Farrelly *et al.* 2002). Exposure to the 'truth' campaign was consistently associated with a higher likelihood of agreeing with anti-tobacco industry and antismoking beliefs as well as with a lower likelihood of intending to smoke in the following year. Exposure to the Philip Morris campaign had little effect on the likelihood of agreeing with anti-industry or antismoking beliefs and was associated with increased intention to smoke in the next year (Farrelly *et al.* 2002). An analysis of focus group reactions to different antismoking messages found that industry manipulation and second-hand smoke are the most effective messages for denormal-izing smoking behaviour and for reducing cigarette consumption (Goldman and Glantz 1998).

45.5 The effect of smoke-free workplaces

The California Tobacco Control Program's emphasis on clean indoor air legislation also had a significant impact on smoking rates. In California, the proportion of indoor workers covered by a smoke-free worksite policy (no smoking anywhere inside) increased from 35% in 1990 to more than 93% in 1999, and the proportion exposed to second-hand smoke at work decreased from 29% to 16% (Gilpin *et al.* 2002). This increase in smoke-free workplaces was associated with a decrease in smoking rates. A 1993 analysis found that the prevalence of smoking was statistically significantly lower in smoke-free workplaces than in those with no restrictions (13.7 vs. 20.6%) (Woodruff *et al.* 1993). Continuing smokers in smoke-free workplaces also smoked less than those in workplaces with no restrictions (296 vs. 341 packs/year).

The effects of smoke-free workplace policies were recently summarized in a meta-analysis (Fichtenberg and Glantz 2002*a*). A systematic review of the literature yielded 26 studies on the effects of smoke-free workplaces on cigarette consumption and smoking prevalence. In a random effects meta-analysis, totally smoke-free workplaces were associated with a 3.8% absolute reduction in prevalence and 3.1 cigarettes/day reduction per continuing smoker. Combining the effects of reduced prevalence and daily consumption per smoker yielded a mean reduction of 1.3 cigarettes/day/employee, which corresponded to a 29% reduction in employee consumption.

This effect is substantial; in order to achieve this large a reduction with the alternative policy option of price increases, one would need to raise the average tax in the US from \$0.76 to \$3.05 per pack and in the UK from £3.44 to £6.59 (Fichtenberg and Glantz 2002*a*). If all workplaces that were not smoke-free in 1999 were to prohibit smoking indoors, the authors estimated that consumption per capita in the entire population would drop by 4.5% in the US and 7.6% in the UK. Achieving this large a reduction with a tax increase would require the tax to increase to $1.11 in the US and to £4.26 in the UK. While the primary purpose of establishing smoke-free workplaces and public places is to protect people from the toxins in second-hand smoke, establishing smoke-free policies is probably the most cost-effective smoking reduction and cessation intervention.

45.6 The risk of heart disease drops rapidly when people stop smoking

In contrast to cancer and emphysema, excess smoking-related risk of heart disease and stroke decreases rapidly following cessation (USDHHS 1990). In the case of acute myocardial infarction, the relative risk of hospitalization declines exponentially immediately following cessation and, within 5 years of quitting, reaches an equilibrium level of 1.17 in males and 1.40 in females, compared to never smokers (Lightwood and Glantz 1997). Most importantly, the health benefits of quitting accrue immediately. Half of the 5 year decline in relative risk occurs within 1 year of cessation. The pattern of decline is the same in males and females.

45.7 Second-hand smoke and heart disease

Passive smoking is an important risk factor for heart disease, increasing the risk by about 30% (Glantz and Parmley 1991, 1995; Law et al. 1997; Office of Environmental Health Hazard Assessment 1997). While smaller than the risks of active smoking (which double to quadruple the risk of heart disease), this effect is substantial. This relatively large effect of second-hand smoke despite the low dose of toxins occurs because the cardiovascular system, particularly the vascular endothelium and platelets, is exquisitely sensitive to the toxins in smoke (Glantz and Parmley 2001; Otsuka et al. 2001). Just 30 min of second-hand smoke exposure at levels below that commonly seen in bars is enough to impact endothelial and platelet function to the same extent as being a pack-a-day smoker (Otsuka et al. 2001). Because more people are exposed to second-hand smoke than actually smoke, the impact on heart disease mortality among non-smokers is actually greater than among smokers (Ong et al. 2002).

An analysis of the health effects of providing smoke-free workplaces for the 31% of Americans who work indoors but whose workplaces are not yet smoke-free demonstrates this clearly (Ong et al. 2004). Among the non-smokers who would no longer be exposed to passive smoking, about 1500 acute myocardial infarctions (AMIs) and 350 strokes would be prevented in the first year alone. At steady state, 6250 AMIs and 1270 strokes would be prevented annually. Reduction in passive smoking accounts for about 60% of the effect, with the rest coming from increased cessation.

45.8 Effect of the California campaign on heart disease death rates

As could be expected, given how quickly smoking-related heart disease risk declines after cessation, the decreases in smoking due to the California Tobacco Control Program were closely followed by decreases in heart disease mortality. A comparison of age-adjusted heart disease mortality rates (including coronary heart disease (CHD), rheumatic fever and rheumatic heart disease, hypertensive heart disease, diseases of the endocardium, and all other forms of heart disease) in California and the rest of the US between 1980 and 1997 showed just that (Fichtenberg and Glantz 2000, 2001). In order to both model the changes in California over time and compare them to the changes that were happening in the country as a whole, California mortality rates were modelled as a function of rates in the rest of the country, allowing for changes in the slope when the programme was implemented and when programme funding was cut back in the early 1990s. Various possible break point years were investigated. Statistically 1988 and 1992 were the best break points for the analysis.

For 8 years preceding the programme, yearly mortality rates in California were approximately two-thirds of that in the rest of the country. While heart disease mortality was decreasing in the US as a whole, rates in California were decreasing a third less quickly. The implementation of the Tobacco Control Program was associated with a statistically significant increase in the yearly rate of decline of heart disease mortality by 2.9 deaths/100 000/year compared to the rest of the US, to the point that heart disease mortality was decreasing faster in California than in the rest of the country (Fig. 45.3). This acceleration in the decline of heart disease rates mimicked, with a 1 year lag, the acceleration in decline of cigarette consumption seen in California starting in 1988 (Fig. 45.2). Although the California death rate continued to decline after 1992, when the programme came under political assault and Governor Wilson cut it back and toned it down, the rate of decline was statistically significantly reduced by 1.7 deaths/100 000/year, bringing the rate in California in line with the rate in the rest of the US. This reduction in the effect of the programme on heart disease mortality again mirrors the reduction in the rate of decline of cigarette consumption seen in California in the early 1990s.

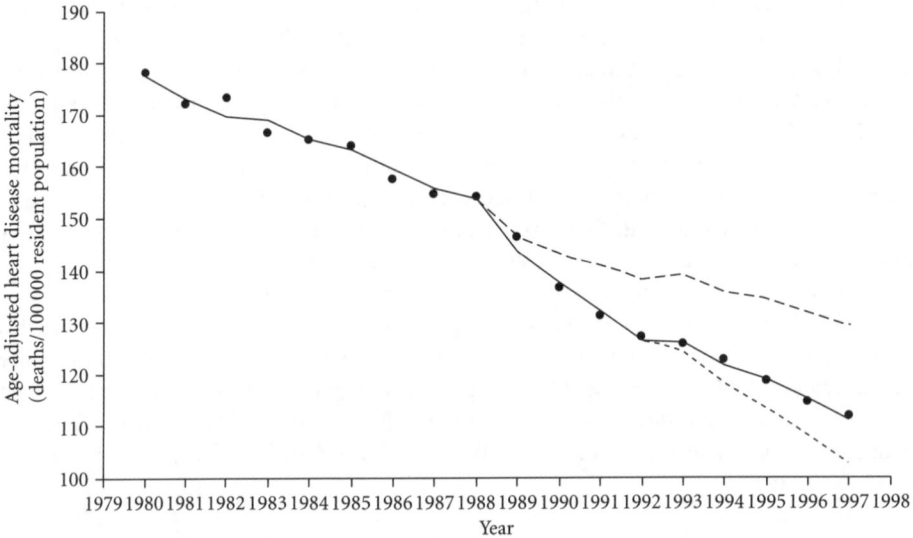

Fig. 45.3 Rate of age-adjusted mortality in California, 1980–97 (solid circles). The solid line represents the fit of the California rates to those in the rest of the country, allowing for changes in slope in 1988 and 1992. The dashed line represents what rates in California would have been if they had continued to be related to rates in the rest of the country as they had up to 1988. The dotted line represents what the rates would have been if they had continued to decrease as they had between 1989 and 1992. (Reproduced from Fichtenberg and Glantz 2000. Copyright 2000 Massachusetts Medical Society. All rights reserved.)

The trends in heart disease mortality in California are consistent with consumption trends not only in terms of timing but also in terms of magnitude. Estimates of the smoking-attributable risk of death from CHD vary between 40 and 55% (National Cancer Institute 1997). By 1997, the rate of per capita cigarette consumption in California was 21% lower than the predicted rate had the pre-1989 relation between rates in California and the rest of the US been maintained. If smoking is 21% lower than expected and 40–55% of CHD mortality is attributable to smoking, then we would expect CHD mortality to be 21% $\times$ 40–55% = 8–12% lower. In fact, the actual death rate in California in 1997 was 13% lower than the predicted rate had the pre-1989 trend been maintained.

By comparing the observed rates with those that would have happened if California rates had continued to follow US rates as they had before 1989, it was estimated that, between 1989 and 1997, the tobacco control programme was associated with 58 900 fewer deaths from heart disease, compared with the 611 500 deaths which actually occurred during this period (Fichtenberg and Glantz 2000, 2001) (Fig. 45.3). However, as a result of the programme cutbacks starting in 1992, it was estimated that 15 000 preventable deaths occurred in the 5 year period from 1993 to 1997 because the smoking rates were not decreasing as fast as they could have been.

This analysis presented the first evidence to date that an aggressive tobacco control programme can not only reduce smoking but also smoking-related mortality rates, and that these effects can occur within a year of the implementation of the programme. Equally significant, however, is the fact that failure to fully fund and politically support tobacco control programmes will lead to less effective programmes and therefore to unnecessary deaths.

45.9 **What about primary prevention and youth?**

There has been a strong emphasis among most tobacco control programmes on primary prevention and reduction of smoking initiation among youth. While it is always better not to smoke at all, the health benefits of smoking cessation, even late in life, are substantial enough to make smoking cessation among current smokers of all ages worthwhile. As we discussed previously, smoking-attributable risk of heart disease disappears almost entirely by 5 years after cessation (USDHHS 1990). In addition, smokers who quit even in middle age avoid most of the subsequent risk of lung cancer (Peto et al. 2000). As a result, smokers who quit at age 45 have a life expectancy that exceeds that of continuing smokers by 5.6–7.2 years for women and 5.6–7.1 years for men (Taylor et al. 2002). Even those who quit at age 65 can expect to live longer than those who continue to smoke: 2.7–3.7 years longer for women and 1.4–2.0 years for men. In contrast, a simulation of the effects of reducing youth initiation on overall smoking rates found that even if youth initiation were halted entirely, it would take 30 years before the number of smokers was even halved (Levy et al. 2000).

In addition to the fact that focusing on smoking prevention in children shifts limited resources to interventions which will not affect health-related end points for decades, the bulk of efforts aimed at children have not proven to be effective. The majority of youth-oriented interventions have focused on reducing availability of cigarettes to children on the grounds that this would reduce smoking initiation and, in the very long term, smoking-related disease and death. In the US there has been widespread support for the implementation of laws limiting the access of youth under the legal smoking age to commercial sources of cigarettes. Because of their broad political appeal, these 'youth access' laws have become a cornerstone of US federal tobacco control policy, as reflected in a 1992 law which requires states to enact and enforce a minimum age-of-sale law of 18 years in order to obtain funding for substance abuse programmes, as well as in the regulation of tobacco asserted by the Food and Drug Administration (but later struck down by the US Supreme Court). Both the US Centers for Disease Control and Prevention (Centers for Disease Control and Prevention 1999) and the Institute of Medicine (Institute of Medicine 2000) have recommended youth access laws as part of comprehensive tobacco control programmes. By August 2001, all 50 states and some 1139 local governments had passed youth access laws (Ling *et al.* 2002).

Unfortunately, while these laws can make it difficult for youths to purchase cigarettes, there is no evidence that they actually affect youth smoking (Fichtenberg and Glantz 2002*b*). A 2002 review of all published studies of the effects of youth access policies on youth smoking found no detectable correlation between the level of merchant compliance with the laws and prevalence of monthly or daily smoking among teens (Fichtenberg and Glantz 2002*b*) (Fig. 45.4a). No relationship was found either between increases in compliance and decreases in smoking (Fig. 45.4b). Several advocates of youth access laws have theorized that merchant compliance has to reach a critical threshold (90 or 95%) before access to cigarettes is sufficiently curbed to affect smoking rates. The study found no evidence of such a threshold. Smoking rates for communities with compliance above 90% varied between 19.4 and 32.5%, with a mean of 25.9%. In communities with compliance below 90%, smoking rates were between 15.6 and 37.7%, with a mean of 25.7%. One of the major reasons why youth access laws do not affect smoking, even though they may render commercial access more difficult, is that youth simply switch to other sources of cigarettes such as social sources (relatives, friends) (Castrucci *et al.* 2002;

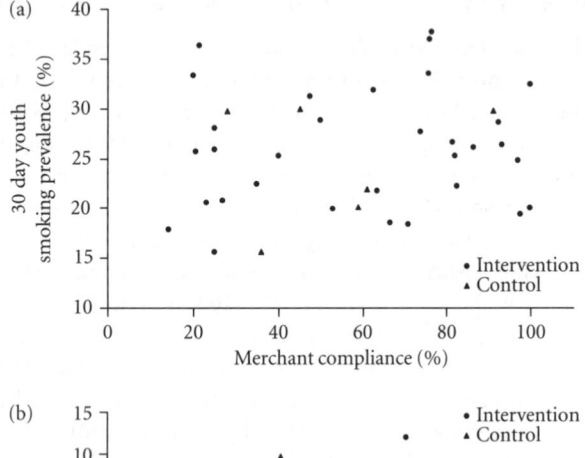

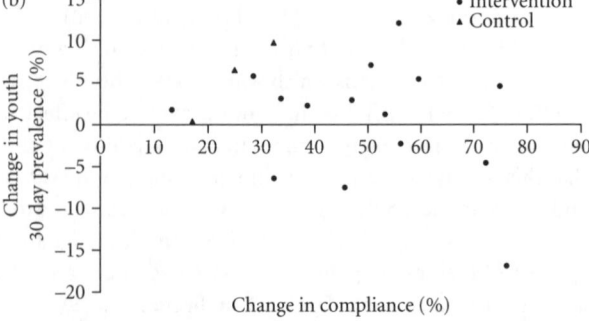

Fig. 45.4 (a) Thirty-day youth smoking prevalence as a function of merchant compliance with laws limiting sales of cigarettes to youth over 18 years of age in various communities in the US, UK, and Australia. (b) Changes in prevalence of 30-day youth smoking as a function of changes in merchant compliance with youth access laws over time (either as a result of an intervention to increase compliance or the secular changes in a control community). (Reproduced from Fichtenberg and Glantz 2002b by permission of *Pediatrics*.)

Cummings *et al.* 2003; DiFranza and Coleman 2001; Forster *et al.* 1998; Hinds 1992; Jones *et al.* 2002).

In addition to the fact that youth access laws do not reduce smoking rates, they actually help the tobacco industry in two ways. They create an opportunity for the industry to build coalitions with local merchants around youth access issues (Ling *et al.* 2002). These coalitions are then useful to the industry in fights against local laws which could hurt the industry. Further, youth access programmes reinforce the tobacco industry's central marketing message that kids should smoke because it will make them appear more 'adult' (Glantz 1996).

In contrast to youth access programmes, smoke-free workplaces and clean air legislation are effective at reducing youth smoking. In one study, teenagers who worked in totally smoke-free work sites were 32% less likely to ever smoke than teenagers who worked in less restricted worksites, after adjusting for demographics and parental smoking (Farkas *et al.* 2000). Several studies have also shown that teenagers living in locations with state and local clean air laws smoke less than teenagers living where there are no such laws (Chaloupka and Pacula 1999; Lewit *et al.* 1997; Wakefield *et al.* 2000; Wasserman *et al.* 1991). Voluntary action to make homes smoke-free is also associated with lower rates of smoking among US high school students. Teenagers living in smoke-free homes were 26% less likely to ever smoke than students living in homes with no restrictions, after adjusting for demographics and smoking status of other household members (Farkas *et al.* 2000).

Indeed, the California campaign, which has not concentrated on youth, has reduced adolescent smoking to 8%, one of the lowest rates in the US (Gilpin *et al.* 2001). During the mid-1990s, when Governor Wilson focused the California programme on youth, much as the tobacco industry does in its 'antismoking' campaigns, teen smoking actually increased. It dropped when the campaign returned to a broad adult-oriented message that was designed to engage teens.

45.10 **Conclusions**

Smoking reduction is probably the quickest, most effective prevention strategy for heart disease morbidity and mortality. The most effective components of tobacco control programmes are taxation of cigarettes, passage of clean air legislation, and media campaigns focusing on tobacco industry manipulation and second-hand smoke. Youth focused programmes such as legislation limiting commercial access to cigarettes or school education programmes are not as effective and, even if they are, will not have an impact on heart disease mortality for decades. In addition, since adults are the role models for teens, reducing adult smoking will contribute to preventing teen smoking.

The technology for rapidly reducing smoking and smoking-induced morbidity and mortality is now well established. The question is whether health professionals will muster the political resources to implement these programmes in the face of strong opposition from the tobacco industry, which loses billions of dollars in sales as these programmes succeed.

References

Bauer, U., and Johnson, T. (2000). 2000 Florida Youth Tobacco Survey Results. www.state.fl.us/tobacco. Florida Department of Health, Bureau of Epidemiology, Tallahassee, FL.

Castrucci, B., Gerlach, K., Kaufman, N., and Orleans, C. (2002). Adolescents' acquisition of cigarettes through non-commercial sources. *Journal of Adolescent Health*, **31**, 322–6.

CDC (2002). Annual smoking-attributable mortality, years of potential life lost, and economic costs: United States, 1995–1999. *MMWR Morbidity and Mortality Weekly Reports*, **51**, 300–3.

Centers for Disease Control and Prevention (1999). *Best practices for comprehensive tobacco control programs*. U.S. Department of Health and Human Services, Centers for Disease Control and Prevention, National Center for Chronic Disease Prevention and Health Promotion, Office on Smoking and Health, Atlanta, GA.

Chaloupka, F., and Pacula, R. (1999). Sex and race differences in young people's responsiveness to price and tobacco control policies. *Tobacco Control*, **8**, 373–7.

Cummings, K., Hyland, A., Perla, J., and Giovino, G. (2003). Is the prevalence of youth smoking affected by efforts to increase retailer compliance with a minors' access law? *Nicotine Tobacco Research* **5** (4), 465–71.

DiFranza, J. R., and Coleman, M. (2001). Sources of tobacco for youths in communities with strong enforcement of youth access laws. *Tobacco Control*, **10**, 323–8.

Farkas, A. J., Gilpin, E. A., White, M. M., and Pierce, J. P. (2000). Association between household and workplace smoking restrictions and adolescent smoking. *Journal of the American Medical Association*, **284**, 717–22.

Farrelly, M. C., Healton, C. G., Davis, K. C., Messeri, P., Hersey, J. C., and Haviland, M. L. (2002). Getting to the truth: evaluating national tobacco countermarketing campaigns. *American Journal of Public Health*, **92**, 901–7.

Fichtenberg, C. M., and Glantz, S. A. (2000). Association of the California Tobacco Control Program with declines in cigarette consumption and mortality from heart disease. *New England Journal of Medicine*, **343**, 1772–7.

Fichtenberg, C. M., and Glantz, S. A. (2001). Controlling tobacco use. *New England Journal of Medicine*, **344**, 1798–9.

Fichtenberg, C. M., and Glantz, S. A. (2002*a*). Effect of smoke-free workplaces on smoking behaviour: systematic review. *British Medical Journal*, **325**, 188–91.

Fichtenberg, C. M., and Glantz, S. A. (2002*b*). Youth access interventions do not affect youth smoking. *Pediatrics*, **109**, 1088–92.

Forster, J., Murray, D., Wolfson, M., Blaine, T., Wagenaar, A., and Hennrikus, D. (1998). The effects of community policies to reduce youth access to tobacco. *American Journal of Public Health*, **88**, 1193–8.

Gilpin, E., Emery, S., Farkas, A., Distefan, J., White, M., and Pierce, J. (2001). *The California Tobacco Control Program: a decade of progress. Results from the California Tobacco Surveys, 1990–1998*. University of California, San Diego, La Jolla.

Gilpin, E. A., Farkas, A. J., Emery, S. L., Ake, C. F., and Pierce, J. P. (2002). Clean indoor air: advances in California, 1990–1999. *American Journal of Public Health*, **92**, 785–91.

Glantz, S. A. (1996). Preventing tobacco use: the youth access trap [editorial] [see comments]. *American Journal of Public Health*, **86**, 156–8.

Glantz, S., and Balbach, E. (2000) *Tobacco war: inside the California battles*. University of California Press, Berkeley.

Glantz, S. A., and Parmley, W. W. (1991). Passive smoking and heart disease: epidemiology, physiology, and biochemistry. *Circulation*, **83**, 1–12.

Glantz, S., and Parmley, W. (1995). Passive smoking and heart disease: mechanisms and risk. *Journal of the American Medical Association*, **273**, 1047–53.

Glantz, S., and Parmley, W. (2001). Even a little secondhand smoke is dangerous. *Journal of the American Medical Association*, **286**, 462–3.

Goldman, L., and Glantz, S. (1998). Evaluation of antismoking advertising campaigns. *Journal of the American Medical Association*, **279**, 772–7.

Hinds, M. (1992). Impact of local ordinance banning tobacco sales to minors. *Public Health Reports*, **82**, 355–8.

Hu, T. W., Sung, H. Y., and Keeler, T. E. (1995). Reducing cigarette consumption in California: tobacco taxes vs an anti-smoking media campaign. *American Journal of Public Health*, **85**, 1218–22.

Institute of Medicine (2000). State programs can reduce tobacco use, pp. 1–9 <www.nap.edu>. National Cancer Policy Board, Institute of Medicine, National Research Council, Washington, DC.

Jones, S. E., Sharp, D. J., Husten, C. G., and Crossett, L. S. (2002). Cigarette acquisition and proof of age among U.S. high school students who smoke. *Tobacco Control*, 11, 20–5.

Law, M., Morris, J., and Wald, N. (1997). Environmental tobacco smoke exposure and ischaemic heart disease: an evaluation of the evidence. *British Medical Journal*, 315, 973–80.

Levy, D., Cummings, K., and Hyland, A. (2000). A simulation of the effects of youth initiation policies on overall cigarette use. *American Journal of Public Health*, 90, 1311–14.

Lewit, E., Hyland, A., Kerrebrock, N., and Cummings, K. (1997). Price, public policy and smoking in young people. *Tobacco Control*, 6, S17–S24.

Lightwood, J. M., and Glantz, S. A. (1997). Short-term economic and health benefits of smoking cessation: myocardial infarction and stroke. *Circulation*, 96, 1089–96.

Ling, P. M., Landman, A., and Glantz, S. A. (2002). It is time to abandon youth access tobacco programmes. *Tobacco Control*, 11, 3–6.

National Cancer Institute (1997). *Changes in cigarette-related disease risks and their implication for prevention and control.* National Cancer Institute, Bethesda, MD.

Office of Environmental Health Hazard Assessment (1997). *Health effects of exposure to environmental tobacco smoke.* California Environmental Protection Agency, Sacramento.

Ong, M., and Glantz, S. (2004). Cardiovascular health and economic impacts of smoke-free workplaces. *American Journal of Medicine,* 117, 32–8.

Otsuka, R., Watanabe, H., Hirata, K., Tokai, K., Muro, T., Yoshiyama, M. *et al.* (2001). Acute effects of passive smoking on the coronary circulation in healthy young adults. *Journal of the American Medical Association*, 286, 436–41.

Peto, R., Darby, S., Deo, H., Silcocks, P., Whitley, E., and Doll, R. (2000). Smoking, smoking cessation, and lung cancer in the UK since 1950: combination of national statistics with two case-control studies. *British Medical Journal*, 321, 323–9.

Pierce, J. P., Gilpin, E. A., Emery, S. L., White, M., Rosbrook, B., and Berry, C. (1998). Has the California Tobacco Control Program reduced smoking? *Journal of the American Medical Association*, 280, 893–9.

Popham, W. J., Potter, L. D., Bal, D. G., Johnson, M. D., Duerr, J. M., and Quinn, V. (1993). Do anti-smoking media campaigns help smokers quit? *Public Health Rep*, 108, 510–13.

Siegel, M. (2002). The effectiveness of state-level tobacco control interventions: a review of program implementation and behavioral outcomes. *Annual Reviews of Public Health*, 23, 45–71.

Siegel, M., and Biener, L. (2000). The impact of an antismoking media campaign on progression to established smoking: results of a longitudinal youth study. *American Journal of Public Health*, 90, 380–6.

Siegel, M., Mowery, P. D., Pechacek, T. P., Strauss, W. J., Schooley, M. W., Merritt, R. K. *et al.* (2000). Trends in adult cigarette smoking in California compared with the rest of the United States, 1978–1994. *American Journal of Public Health*, 90, 372–9.

Sly, D. F., Heald, G. R., and Ray, S. (2001a). The Florida 'truth' anti-tobacco media evaluation: design, first year results, and implications for planning future state media evaluations. *Tobacco Control*, 10, 9–15.

Sly, D. F., Hopkins, R. S., Trapido, E., and Ray, S. (2001b). Influence of a counteradvertising media campaign on initiation of smoking: the Florida 'truth' campaign. *American Journal of Public Health*, 91, 233–8.

Taylor, D. H., Jr., Hasselblad, V., Henley, S. J., Thun, M. J., and Sloan, F. A. (2002). Benefits of smoking cessation for longevity. *American Journal of Public Health*, 92, 990–6.

USDHHS (1990). *The health benefits of smoking cessation: a report of the Surgeon General.* DHHS Publication No. (CDC) 90-8416. U.S. Department of Health and Human Services, Public Health Service, Centers for Disease Control, Center for Chronic disease Prevention and Health Promotion, Office on Smoking and Health. Atlanta, GA.

Wakefield, M., Chaloupka, F., Kaufman, N., Orleans, C., Barker, D., and Ruel, E. (2000). Effect of restrictions at home, at school, and in public places on teenage smoking: cross sectional study. *British Medical Journal*, **321**, 333–7.

Wasserman, J., Manning, W., Newhouse, J., and Winkler, J. (1991). The effects of excise taxes and regulations on cigarette smoking. *Journal of Health Economics*, **10**, 43–64.

Woodruff, T., Rosbrook, B., Peirce, J., and Glantz, S. (1993). Lower levels of cigarette consumption found in smoke-free workplaces in California. *Archives of Internal Medicine*, **153**, 1485–93.

Chapter 46

Nutrition policy: national strategies for dietary change

W. P. T. James and N. J. Rigby

46.1 Introduction

After the Second World War self-sufficiency in food production was seen as essential to national security and, therefore, governmental approaches were dominated by agriculture pressures and perceptions. Indeed, the development of the original European Common Agricultural Policy was based both on the need to guarantee adequate food supplies and the social and political benefits in maintaining an economically active rural community. Health issues in relation to food supply seemed to have been solved by pre-war and wartime experience of the value of food rationing. This had been based on human experimental studies showing the importance of animal protein from milk and meat for ensuring children's growth and the importance of enough energy from butter, sugar, and other energy-rich sources to meet the needs of a very active population.

Only in the 1960s in Scandinavia, and later in the 1970s and 1980s for many parts of Europe, were national strategies for dietary change proposed, aimed at preventing cardiovascular and other adult chronic diseases such as cancer. These proposals were often in conflict with agricultural priorities, which even now dominate the thinking of finance ministries.

However, huge changes in the European and, indeed, global perspective of the food chain, were precipitated by the bovine spongiform encephalopathy (BSE) epidemic in cattle, first observed in the UK in 1986 and subsequently elsewhere in Europe. The realization that this was a global crisis arose in 1996 with the discovery of variant Creutzfeldt–Jakob disease (vCJD) in 10 surprisingly young adults who, it had to be assumed, had become infected from eating beef and its products, which the British and other governments had declared were entirely safe. This led to a collapse of public confidence in any governmental statement relating to the food chain, in its scientists, in industry and, of course, in farming, this distrust being amplified by outbreaks of *Escherichia coli* $_{0157}$ both in the UK and abroad. Attempts by ministries of agriculture to play down the importance of these developments only reinforced the crisis in confidence in government handling of public health issues. In turn this led to the establishment of Food Standards Agencies in the UK and several other countries. In Europe a new system of independent scientific evaluation was developed as the European Union (EU) Commission and its President were threatened with dismissal by the European Parliament in 1997, accused of incompetent handling of the BSE problem.

The public disquiet about governmental approaches to food was heightened by a new focus in the media on scientific debate about the safety of genetically modified foods. The media and the public then automatically tended to assume that any scientist receiving money from industry had been 'bought', and that even organizations such as the UK Royal Society were biased towards dramatic discoveries and interesting manipulations of plant genomic structures. The public's perception was that their wellbeing and the principles of public health as a societal priority seemed to have been forgotten in favour of industrial opportunities and exciting science.

46.2 The development of current perceptions of the need for dietary change

Although the American Heart Association had set out its advice for Americans in the late 1950s, Norway had started a national policy in 1962 (Norum *et al.* 1997), in Finland the North Karelia Project was underway from 1972 (Puska *et al.* 1995), it was not until the early 1980s that there was a change in international thinking on national diets. The US initiative had been amplified by the US Senate hearings, chaired by Senator George McGovern and published as 'Dietary Goals for the United States' in 1977, which had led to extreme disquiet in the food manufacturing sector (Walker and Cannon 1984). The Royal College of Physicians of London (1976) had also published an elegant and very specific set of dietary targets for the prevention of coronary heart disease (CHD) in 1976. Following the UK Government's failure to act on the London Royal College report, its contributors, including Geoffrey Rose, set up the Coronary Prevention Group to lobby for change in the UK. They organized the Canterbury Conference in 1983 to set out plans for action (Health Education Council 1984).

These national initiatives finally led the World Health Organization (WHO) to develop a series of reports concentrating on cardiovascular disease. These built on Rose and Blackburn's seminal WHO report (WHO 1982) on the prevention of CHD with its clear enunciation, as in the London Royal College 1976 report, of the concept of population attributable risks. This highlighted the need to shift the national distributions of serum cholesterol within the populations of the world to a lower level. Rose and Blackburn were careful to highlight the range of intakes implied by a population's mean intake: individuals with different genotypes within populations – and therefore with greater or smaller responses to a dietary change – would all be involved in the general shifts in saturated fat intakes to more beneficial levels. They illustrated these points by using data from the national cohorts on diet from the Seven Country Study (Keys 1980) and set out a perspective far broader than the then current American or European focus. Other countries were recognized as having very different intakes of fats, for example China and Japan, and had incidences and mortality rates of CHD – but not cerebrovascular disease – which were 10 or more times lower than those then found in Northern Europe and North America. They, therefore, contrived a range of 'moderate' total fat intakes of 15–30%, which implied that within this range there was a health equivalence.

Once this report was produced, there quickly followed the report on the primary prevention of hypertension (WHO 1983), which even then considered excess weight gain as the principal factor enhancing blood pressure and suggested that 25% of hypertensive cases could be prevented by avoiding excess weight gain in the young and maintaining bodyweight throughout adult life.

This was the background to a new effort by WHO, again chaired by Geoffrey Rose, to consider what to do about 'community prevention and control of cardiovascular diseases' (WHO 1986). This went considerably further than the 1982 report, which called for national action plans, but still emphasized the concept of education as the major route for change. Nevertheless, a major section was devoted to the role of government, albeit dealing with surveillance, coordination, health care, mass media responsibilities, and statistical analyses.

There was then one small paragraph specifying the notion that legislation and fiscal policies could contribute greatly to public health.

46.3 The WHO 797 report on diet and the prevention of chronic diseases

The next major development came in 1990 when WHO undertook its first ever global analysis of nutrition and diet in the prevention of chronic diseases (WHO 1990). This development followed the publication of the first European report on diet and health for the WHO Europe Regional Office (James *et al.* 1988) and a recognition by the then WHO Geneva Director of Chronic Diseases, Dr Vilius Grabauskas, that there was a need to consider the issue of diet on a global basis where hitherto the traditional concern was the prevention of childhood protein–energy malnutrition, and iodine, vitamin A, and iron deficiencies. An integrated approach to the analysis and prevention of cardiovascular diseases, cancers, diabetes, and dental caries was produced together with an assessment of the problem of vitamin and nutrient deficiencies. Nutrient goals were combined with a new dietary population goal of 400 g vegetables and fruit per day, based on our rapid estimation of the consumption in the classic Mediterranean diet, which Keys and his colleagues had found to be so associated with low rates of CHD in the Seven Country Study (Keys 1980). The range of food intakes internationally was also considered and this led to a series of lower and upper limits for the final recommendations. Total fat intakes were recognized to be only 14–15% in China and Japan, with minimal intakes of saturated fatty acids. A lower goal of 15% total fat was maintained, recognizing that a lower fat content could be so energy dilute that energy intake could be compromised and induce malnutrition in children in East Africa. Even then, however, the 30% upper population limit was termed an 'interim goal', which might need to be lower because of concerns about the impact of fat on cancer and obesity. For saturated fatty acid intakes the lower limit was set at 0%, since there is no biological necessity for these fatty acids and there was no discernible lower limit to their effects on serum cholesterol levels. No figure was defined for the lower limit for sodium and again a zero value was chosen for what were termed 'free sugars'. This was simply based on the recognition that added refined sugar had no intrinsic value except as a source of energy and that patients with genetic abnormalities of fructose metabolism were perfectly well-nourished with no intakes of sucrose and other refined sugars at all. There was also no lower limit to their impact on dental caries, although the impact of dental hygiene and fluoride complicated the analysis.

46.4 Industrial responses to public policy making

The reaction to the finalization of this report was astonishingly rapid. It appeared that some representatives of industry, classified as non-governmental organizations (NGOs), who attended the consultation, lost no time in alerting their relevant industrial contacts. Within days an organization representing the interests of the world sugar industry had contacted numerous countries at a very high level so that 40 ambassadors then wrote to WHO demanding the withdrawal of this WHO/Food and Agricultural Organization (FAO) report. The US State Department was also being lobbied intensely on the grounds that the sugar and dental caries analyses were scientifically flawed. At the Executive Board, which formally accepts any WHO Technical Report, questions were posed by the US and UK delegates regarding the validity of the report, despite assurances from the then Chief Medical Officer that he was totally behind the report's analysis and findings.

46.5 **The battle over nutritional policies in the 1990s** *

The WHO/FAO 1990 report proved to be a turning point and heralded a 10 year battle by the sugar, soft drink, and confectionery industries to question the validity and block the implementation of the report. This was led by a series of initiatives from FAO, following a change in senior personnel, which convened new consultations on fats (FAO/WHO 1994) and carbohydrates (FAO/WHO 1998). Some of their scientific experts seemed to have been chosen because their views reflected the interests of the food industry and were at odds with those expressed in the WHO/FAO 1990 report.

46.6 **The Eurodiet Project**

The industrial need to defend and maintain its interests then focused on Europe because, with the BSE crisis, it was becoming clear in the late 1990s that other aspects of diet could well be included in any new portfolio of responsibilities assigned to the European Commission. Nutritional concerns were not only potentially threatening to the sugar, confectionery, soft drink, and fast food industries, but there was also an opportunity to portray nutritional questions in a new light. 'Functional' foods were now the new opportunity for the food industry if special foods could be portrayed as having unusually valuable health promoting properties.

At this time the WHO Europe Regional Office proposal for its First Action Plan for Food and Nutrition Policy was unanimously accepted by 50 European ministers of health. This, for the first time, combined food safety, environmental aspects of food sustainability, and a drive to change the nutritional quality of the diet. This was important because, with Central and Eastern European countries attempting to join the EU, the WHO and ministers not only had to contend with very high levels of cardiovascular disease, but also the food safety demands of the EU. The renewed pressures to alter the EU's Common Agriculture Policy also put the whole range of food issues up the priority list of prime ministers and presidents.

The EU responded to these WHO initiatives by convening, with industrial support, a nutrition and health group to assess the need for any changes in nutrition policies within the EU. This rapidly proved to be controversial because several independent scientists (including one of the authors, WPTJ) appointed to the group objected to what they perceived as an attempt to manipulate the outcome to minimize the role of sugars, fats, and salt in precipitating the major diseases currently afflicting Europe. Additional independent scientists were eventually appointed and a final meeting had to compromise on these issues of diet in relation to public health (EURODIET 2001).

46.7 **A new 2003 WHO analysis of nutritional causes of chronic diseases**

In 2002 the WHO convened a new expert consultation to revise the original 1990 WHO report. This reached the same general conclusions regarding weight gain underlying the

* The FAO suspended collaboration with the International Life Sciences Institute (ILSI) following allegations of clandestine funding and influence by the sugar industry and ILSI over the FAO/WHO carbohydrate consultation in 1998 made in a BBC Panorama documentary, *The Trouble With Sugar*, broadcast October 10 2004. The FAO announced its intention to reconvene the carbohydrate consultation in 2005

Table 46.1 Summary of the level of evidence on factors that might promote or protect against weight gain and obesity

Evidence	Decreases risk	No relationship	Increases risk
Convincing	Regular physical activity High dietary NSP (fibre) intake		High intake of energy-dense, nutrient-poor foods Sedentary lifestyles
Probable	Home and school environments that support healthy food choices for children[a] Promoting linear growth		Heavy marketing of energy-dense foods[a] and fast-food outlets Adverse social and economic conditions (in developed countries, especially for women) Sugar-sweetened soft drinks and fruit juices
Possible	Low glycaemic index foods Breastfeeding	Protein content of the diet	Large portion sizes; high proportion of food prepared outside the home (Western countries) 'Rigid restraint / periodic disinhibition' eating patterns
Insufficient	Increasing eating frequency		Alcohol

Source: WHO 2003.

[a] Associated evidence and expert opinion.

major public health problems of cardiovascular disease and several cancers as well as diabetes (see Table 46.1).

The nutrient goals are unremarkable, but the inclusion of such environmental issues as the heavy promotion of high-density foods put the public health issues into a different context. The report rapidly gained a high profile after it was issued in draft form for formal consultations with both industry and the NGO community. As expected, there was again intense industrial lobbying claiming that there was no evidence that the consumption of refined sugars promoted weight gain. The launch of the report at the FAO headquarters in Rome in April 2003 was preceded by a frenzied episode when embarrassed US Federal Secretaries of State found themselves pressurized by an industry consortium fronted by the Sugar Association, which wanted to withdraw US funding from WHO (but not the FAO) if the report went ahead.

46.8 A global strategy for the prevention and control of non-communicable diseases

With the successful publication of the report, WHO embarked on the development of a new global strategy, which involved further extensive consultations and a series of negotiations with industry prior to its global strategy receiving approval by ministers at the World Health Assembly in 2004.

Given the clear perspective on dietary goals, the issue is: What can be done to establish proper nutritional policies? These clearly have to take account of the first ever analyses of risk factors contributing to global ill-health (Ezzati *et al.* 2002, 2003) and the dominance of cardiovascular deaths – and cancers – in the developing as well as in the developed world (WHO 2002) (see Chapters 10 and 11).

46.9 **The dilemma in prevention**

Most national diets and physical activity patterns are far from the optimum. Thus total fat and saturated fat intakes in most European countries are so far removed that only a very small proportion of the population would have intakes equivalent to current recommendations. Therefore, it is inappropriate to engage in health education – advocating consumption of more or less amounts of particular foods because there is no obvious section within most populations which can readily be identified by the public as enjoying a good diet. Furthermore, it has been clearly shown, for example, in the Minnesota cardiovascular prevention programmes, that general health education, or even personalized advice to adults aimed at improving their diet, is very ineffective in terms of blood cholesterol changes or weight management (Jeffery 1993, 1995). Personalized effective advice can work with some adults who know that they are at a high risk of developing serious disease. Thus dietary fat changes with weight reduction, sugar avoidance, and the consumption of vegetables and fruits can prevent the development of hypertension (Stamler *et al.* 1980) and type 2 diabetes (Pan *et al.* 1997; Tuomilehto *et al.* 2001; Diabetes Prevention Program 2002). If drastic changes in diet and exercise patterns can be made, then Ornish and colleagues (Ornish *et al.* 1990) have shown that it is possible to even reverse arterial atherosclerosis. Comprehensive lifestyle modification can produce individual benefits in blood pressure control, as demonstrated in the Premier Collaborative Research Group's evaluation of the DASH diet, with implications for population-wide adoption of healthier diets (Appel *et al.* 1997, 2003).

46.10 **The toxic environment**

Why should it be so difficult to get people to change their diets and physical activity patterns when the benefits are so obvious? Analyses have now made it clear that altering diet and physical activity is very difficult when most, if not all, the environmental circumstances promote an inappropriate diet and a sedentary lifestyle. This is first illustrated in terms of physical inactivity. The advent of the motor car has led to multi-billion dollar investments by governments, aided by the highly influential car and oil industries, in road systems which have resulted in the complete redesign of towns and cities. The construction of out-of-town shopping complexes, which necessitate the use of motor vehicles, and the steady concentration of public services into larger hospitals and schools, again demand motorized transport for ready access. These changes, together with the neglect of cycle path provision or safe streets for children's play outside their home means that there has been a complete societal emphasis on the car to the detriment of walking and cycling. Then there is increasing mechanization at work and in the home, widespread computer use, the provision of multiple television channels, and the explicit encouragement of all women, including mothers with small children, to work. These developments, together with long commutes to work, all contribute to increasingly sedentary behaviour.

The well-off can afford to join leisure centres to counteract the environmental pressures to lead a sedentary existence, but this choice is often too expensive for the majority of people. Furthermore, it is naïve to expect everyone from the age of 5 years to 85 years of age to circumvent these enormous societal constraints on physical activity. It is, therefore, only logical to engender change in our 'toxic' physical environment. For example, street design must be changed to produce places for children, women, and the elderly to move at their ease, that is, so that they alter their every-day behaviour and feel safe day or night. This requires very careful town planning with readily accessible play areas for children so they are automatically encouraged to move outside the house or apartment without inducing parental anxiety. Street lighting and other features of road design have a huge impact on the sense of space and safety for all age groups. Cycle path provision needs to be as routine as it is in Copenhagen or the Netherlands, and town centres need to be dominated by the needs of pedestrians.

All these issues are the province of governmental sectors other than health and so far health issues relating to transport have been confined to the avoidance of traffic accidents and drunken driving with no recognition of the importance of preventing chronic diseases such as cardiovascular disease and excess weight gain by encouraging general physical activity.

46.11 Toxic food environments

Some groups assign the blame for chronic diseases to poor education with a failure of the public to choose a 'balanced diet' and to engage in sports. Some food industrial groups also prominently promote sporting activities, which divert attention from their own involvement in the dietary transformation. Yet, for decades governments have been advocating dietary change in line with current recommendations with only modest effects. To sustain the educative 'balanced diet' approach to health promotion demands some evidence of effectiveness after so many decades of trying to reduce cardiovascular morbidity and mortality by this means. So we must ask why this approach does not work.

Firstly it is important to remember that it has been the accepted practice of many agricultural ministries worldwide to maintain the post-Second World War strategies of increasing meat and milk consumption as a means of providing cheaper foods from animal sources. This emphasis on animal-derived foods continues, with huge financial farming subsidies that exceed by far the total health budgets of the world. Farming groups, particularly with surpluses of meat and fats, then do everything in their power to dispose of these foods at a profit.

Many companies have discovered the benefits of targeting young children to establish brand preferences for foods and drinks as well as sportswear in just the same way that tobacco companies are targeting older children and adolescents. Food patterns in less affluent as well as wealthy nations are now, therefore, being driven by intensive marketing by manufacturers and producers to sell their cheap vegetable oils and soft drinks, their 'fast foods' high in fat, sugars, and salt, and confectionery because these provide far better profit margins than the traditional foods.

Large portion sizes are also now being promoted as 'bargains' and more profitable than standard portion sizes. This is a new marketing strategy. There has also been a major societal shift to eating outside the home as more women work and have less time to cook. Ready-made meals and largely processed food purchased outside the home are far more common, so that the average consumer has no idea of the composition of what they are eating and no real control over their diet. Even buying food in a supermarket presents difficulties from a nutritional perspective, since food labelling is based on analytical criteria developed for statutory disclosure, which are incomprehensible to most consumers.

46.12 Some unrecognized features of inappropriate food

In addition to the classic major agricultural distortions of the food supply with all their implications for food prices, there are previously unrecognized issues in the way in which crops have been selected and developed to serve the needs of the food industry to extend shelf life and reduce wastage. In the 1970s and 1980s there was a major drive to enhance the n-6 polyunsaturated fatty acid content of the oils so that food manufacturers could respond to the prevailing health advice that polyunsaturated fatty acids should be substituted for saturated fats. However, n-3 polyunsaturated fats were systematically minimized in crop researchers' plant breeding selection because these contribute markedly to the speed at which food becomes rancid. This decline in n-3 intake may well have been matched by a reduction in the folic acid content of plant foods since this vitamin has rarely, if ever, been monitored in plant selection programmes. Thus, two important contributors to cardiovascular (as well as reproductive) health have been neglected when considering the fundamental composition of our modern food supply.

46.13 Food labelling and standards

The current labelling system is incomprehensible. One example is the way that fat or saturated fat content is often displayed on a g/100 g basis. To make sense of what proportion of calories this signifies means this then has to be recalculated and related to the energy needs of individual adults and children. So current approaches are conceptually flawed. The original 1990 WHO proposals set out a new simplified and comprehensible system with banding of high, medium, and low levels of fats and sugars, salt, etc. This system would then automatically be suitable for everybody's individual need and should be re-explored.

46.14 The rural/urban transition

It has been shown over almost half a century that the transition from a rural to an urban environment precipitates weight gain, hypertension, disadvantageous changes in plasma lipids, and the progressive development of CHD. Poor city dwellers in Asia, Africa, and South America, who have migrated from the countryside to find work in the cities, are confronted by the need to find accommodation, often in poorly served slums with no running water or sanitation facilities. The traditional fruits and vegetables, available in their rural setting, have now to be transported, with poor preservation facilities, into cities where their costs are substantial compared with the locally made fast foods containing extra fat, sugars, and salt which keep better in hot environments.

Therefore, systematic policies are needed for urban planning, to improve facilities for the local production of foods, and for the transport, preservation, and storage of perishable foods, as well as for ensuring adequate water and sanitation provision.

46.15 Catering and restaurants

Catering establishments and restaurants have rarely been targeted for improvements and few countries seem to have followed the Finnish approach of routinely including the cost of vegetables or a salad bar within the price of the main dish in all catering facilities. This simple device trebled the national vegetable consumption in 20 years – the biggest nutritional gain from health promotional efforts probably ever achieved. This is of particular importance in many poor countries, for example, in Asia, given the endemic vitamin A deficiency and the newly recognized benefits of vegetable and fruit consumption in preventing chronic diseases, including cancers.

46.16 School children

National policies are needed for regulating the food environment in schools, as well as for nutrition education. Agreements by schools to install vending machines supplying sugary drinks and confectionery to raise funds for the school is now considered, even in the US, as a real hazard. Meals in most schools worldwide are poorly regulated and of low nutritional content. There is also a mistaken belief that young children are capable of making informed, healthy choices despite evidence to the contrary and an acceptance of the idea that school meals have an educational as well as nutritional purpose. Where school councils or committees, made up of teacher, parent, and school governor representatives, as well as the children themselves, have been introduced to consider issues relating to nutrition, physical activity and health, they have been found to be of considerable benefit (see Chapter 48).

46.17 **Marketing to pre-school children**

The diets of pre-school children are deteriorating dramatically in many societies in association with weight gain and increasing evidence of cardiovascular risk factors as well as the pre-diabetes condition of impaired glucose tolerance. In many developing countries pre-school children still have high stunting rates, but they are also showing clear evidence of overweight, incipient diabetes, and emerging hypertension associated with the so-called nutrition transition. Type 2 diabetes is already emerging rapidly in adolescents.

46.18 **Effective approaches to implementation**

The WHO, or indeed any ministry of health, needs to involve all its expert health groups concerned with important aspects of diet and physical activity, for example child nutrition, maternal and child care, food safety, and sustainable development. This will ensure that the ministries are not confronted by discordant, competitive proposals in the health sector. The need for a broad approach is illustrated in Fig. 46.1, which highlights the requirement of all ministries of health to interact collegially with other governmental ministries.

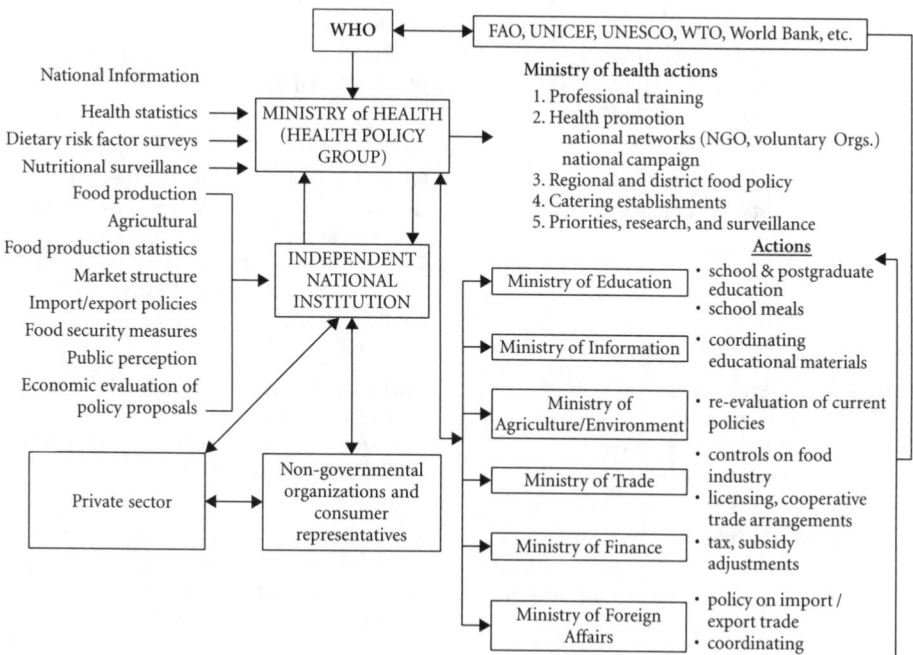

Fig. 46.1 Formulating a nutrition policy for the prevention of non-communicable diseases.

The challenge for ministries of health, therefore, is how best to move away from current approaches, which often evade the environmental and marketing issues and opt for 'health education'. They need instead to work out the principal forces and processes involved in the current 'toxic environment'. Then, where possible, they have to develop, with other ministries, new countermeasures to those factors promoting sedentaryism and inappropriate diets. Ministries of health are traditionally one of the weakest government departments because their portfolio is not seen to relate to economic benefits for society, but to costs. Now the health costs of chronic diseases are of concern to sophisticated treasuries, but the health impact assessments of different options for change have not been made available to them. Nor has the public, the media, or the politically active sector been nurtured by many ministries of health to gain the political backing needed for change. A powerful role for civil society focused in a major national institution of eminence with independence from the government seems to be crucial. This is also illustrated in Fig. 46.1.

In attempting to develop a logical approach, the ANGELO (Analysis Grid for Environments Linked to Obesity) model for assessing the environmental contributors to one non-communicable disease (obesity), developed by Egger and Swinburn (1997), has been transformed into a scheme appropriate for global application. Table 46.2 takes a similar format and considers the big issues in terms of the need to consider the physical facilities and

Table 46.2 Action points as determinants of a sustainable high quality diet and appropriate physical activity

	Focused settings	Broad sectoral influences
Physical	Easier access to fresh fruit and vegetable supplies Efficient/affordable public transport/safe path- and cycle ways, public spaces Access to appropriate self-monitoring systems, e.g. weight, blood pressure	Improve provision for: Public transport Pedestrian and cyclist movement Constraints on car use in urban environments Play/sports facilities in schools/public spaces Urban growing zones for food production
Economic	Rewards for meeting specific targets in primary care	Review food subsidy/taxation policies and impact on production/consumption to remove the 'health premium' Favour fruit and vegetable market expansion using public procurement powers Constrain oil/fat/sugar consumption with price penalties
Policy	Baby Friendly Hospitals Targeted dietary guidelines Fortification policies Effective policies on health claims, e.g. functional foods	Health impact assessment of the EU's Common Agricultural Policy Food labelling with appropriate, understandable, health-related information
Socio-cultural	Health education / promote positive initiatives to inhibit 'junk food culture' and promote healthier options as goals	Promote physical activity in the workplace with required breaks for sedentary staff Support breastfeeding with better workplace facilities

Source: developed from the ANGELO Framework (Egger and Swinburn 1997).

arrangements for food provision and physical activity and economic issues where the ministry itself or its associated ministries may be required to contribute public finance or specify charging schemes for public services. A separate category relates to policy development and the fourth category relates to socio-cultural issues. This last category is explicitly included because policy makers are often concerned that particular sectors of society have an inappropriate perception or a culturally based conviction that a particular approach to a problem is appropriate or wrong, and where health education, advocacy, and promotional campaigns can help.

46.19 Promoting change

Governments tend to assume that their own initiatives are the only basis for change whereas many analyses show that the most effective, marked, and rapid changes come when the community is also heavily involved and where the media and public can trust the process of transparent policy analysis with recommendations to parliament as well as ministers. There are several European examples, notably in Scandinavia (Chapter 51).

46.20 Focusing on dietary priorities

The WHO 2000 review focused on seven features of the diet once children have been weaned: total fat, the dietary fatty-acid composition with a special emphasis on the saturated and n-3 polyunsaturated fatty acids, refined sugars, sodium, vegetables, and fruit intakes. Although there are other important issues, for example, fibre and folate, these are likely to be encompassed by the programmes focusing on the seven components above.

Given the different settings for the importation, production, food processing, retailing, and catering systems, a plan can be developed which not only prioritizes the desirable changes, but also specifies the multiple levels at which action can be taken. The constraints on change, for example pricing policies and their determinants, will soon emerge. Nordic and developing country experience, such as in Thailand, show the importance of governmental, academic, political, and local authority participation in producing a socially and locally relevant series of operational goals.

46.21 Operational approaches

Ministries of health should lead the way and consider a variety of initiatives within their own area of responsibility, as illustrated in Table 46.3. These include the transformation of catering and physical activity services in healthcare facilities, and primary care guidelines for patient and community action on diet and physical activity. Regional centres of public health should be expected to develop partnerships at the community level, involving local government, large and small industries, sports councils, and transport planning groups so that recreational facilities and opportunities are targeted at the more disadvantaged sectors of society, with a particular focus on the young and the old.

Schemes are also needed for developing strategies so that ministries of health can engage the public. Thus modest support for NGOs can go a long way towards allowing them to function effectively as a community forum. Mechanisms need to be established involving the NGOs and public health groups, as well as government sources, in briefing and responding to the media. Relying on governmental sources alone has not proved to be an effective mechanism of gaining public trust in many societies.

Table 46.3 Potential avenues of action for ministries of health to improve diet, physical activity, and health. Sections are classified in relation to the life course and different health professional groups

Health professional groups	Diet and physical activity	
	Macro	**Micro**
(a) Health professionals dealing with preconception, pregnancy, infancy, e.g. obgyn midwives, paediatricians, PHC doctors, paediatric nurses	Audit policies, e.g. on anaemia, weight gain, optimum diet in pregnancy and breastfeeding. Lead initiatives of Baby Friendly Hospitals. Establish immediate breastfeeding (0–6 months inclusive) and appropriate complementary foods	Establish optimum techniques, e.g. limiting low birthweight, anaemia, pregnancy diabetes, neural tube defects; specify local breastfeeding strategies
(b) Health professionals dealing with pre-school and school-age children, e.g. paediatricians/school medical officers/paediatric and school nurses/health visitors	Establish policies to promote physical activity in pre-school and school. Work with Ministry of Education to develop policies for monitoring child weight/BMI. Training of nurses/school dietitians/canteen staff on healthy diet	Establish policies to monitor iodine levels of population. Promote the consumption of iodized salt with simultaneous education about the need to consume limited amounts of salt. Support or initiate policies to reduce the number of vending machines in schools
(c) Health professionals dealing with adults, e.g. PHC doctors, adult specialists	Education of health professionals about the particular dietary needs of adults	Establish policies so that health professionals speak to their patients about healthy diet, particularly low saturated fat and salt intake and high fruit and vegetable intake; monitor their patients' BMI
(d) Health professionals dealing with older people, e.g. geriatricians, nursing home personnel	Establish policies to promote physical activity (especially weight bearing) in older people via nursing home/caregiver/community centre	Establish policies so that health professionals regularly monitor bone density and micro/macronutrient deficiencies
(e) Public health professionals involved in hospital and community care, e.g. dietitians and nutritionists in hospitals, schools	Initiating and monitoring a range of public health initiatives involving both hospital and community policies	Major role in promoting specific initiatives, e.g. local community demonstration projects for physical activity and dietary change
(f) Public health professionals dealing with migrant populations	Establish policies to properly train volunteers and medical staff to particular needs of immigrants with obesity and particularly the metabolic syndrome	Support initiatives that monitor BMI of migrant populations, particularly children, and micronutrient deficiencies

BMI: body mass index, PHC: primary healthcare.

46.22 **Conclusions**

Although for decades there has been an emphasis on the need for appropriate diets to prevent cardiovascular disease, the practical changes to improve diets on a global basis have been very modest indeed. We have now entered a phase when global industrial interests are so powerful and focused on maintaining profits that governments are going to find it very difficult to promote radical dietary changes. The recent emphasis on individual responsibility and the importance of the free market further limits the likelihood of governments accepting the importance of major public health initiatives to alter the toxic environment affecting most societies in the world. Therefore, we face a greater challenge than ever before in putting across the need for priority-setting for the public good.

References

Appel, L. J., Moore, T. J., Obarzanek, E., Vollmer, W. M., Svetkey, L. P., Sacks, F. M. *et al.* (1997). A clinical trial of the effects of dietary patterns on blood pressure. DASH Collaborative Research Group. *New England Journal of Medicine,* **17**, 336 (16), 1117–24.

Appel, L. J., Champagne, C. M., Harsha, D. W., Cooper, L. S., Obarzanek, E., Elmer, P. J. *et al.* (2003). Effects of comprehensive lifestyle modification on blood pressure control: main results of the PREMIER clinical trial. *Journal of the American Medical Association,* **289** (16), 2083–93.

Health Education Council (1984). *Coronary heart disease prevention: plans for action* Pitman, London.

Diabetes Prevention Program Research Group (2002). Reduction in the incidence of Type 2 diabetes with lifestyle intervention or Metformin. *New England Journal of Medicine,* **346**, 393–403.

Egger, G. and Swinburn, B. (1997). An 'ecological' approach to the obesity pandemic. *British Medical Journal,* **315** (7106), 477–80.

EURODIET Reports and Proceedings (2001) (Also Volume 4(2B). April 2001: Nutrition and Diet for Healthy Lifestyles in Europe: the EURODIET evidence.) *Public Health Nutrition,* Volume 4(2A). April 2001.

Ezzati, M., Lopez, A. D., Rodgers, A., Vander Hoorn, S. and Murray, C. J.; Comparative Risk Assessment Collaborating Group (2002). Selected major risk factors and global and regional burden of disease. *Lancet,* **360** (9343), 1347–60.

Ezzati, M., Hoorn, S. V., Rodgers, A., Lopez, A. D., Mathers, C. D. and Murray, C. J. (2003). Comparative Risk Assessment Collaborating Group: estimates of global and regional potential health gains from reducing multiple major risk factors. *Lancet,* **362** (9380), 271–80.

FAO/WHO (Food and Agricultural Organization/World Health Organization) (1994). *Fats and oils in human nutrition: report of a joint expert consultation.* FAO Food and Nutrition Paper 57. Food and Agricultural Organization, Rome.

FAO/WHO (Food and Agricultural Organization/World Health Organization) (1998). *Carbohydrates in human health.* FAO Food and Nutrition Papers, No. 66. Food and Agriculture Organization, Rome.

James, W. P. T. in collaboration with Ferro-Luzzi, A., Isaksson, B. and Szostak, W. B. (eds) (1988). *Healthy nutrition: preventing nutrition-related diseases in Europe.* WHO Regional Publications, European Series, No. 24. WHO Europe, Copenhagen.

Jeffery, R. W. (1993). Minnesota studies on community-based approaches to weight loss and control. *Annals of Internal Medicine,* **119**, 7(2), 719–21.

Jeffery, R. W. (1995). Community programs for obesity prevention: The Minnesota Heart Health Program. *Obesity Research,* **3**, 283s–288s.

Keys, A. (ed.) (1980). *Seven countries: a multivariate analysis of death and coronary heart disease.* Harvard University Press, Cambridge, MA.

Norum, K. R., Johansson, L., Botten, G., Bjorneboe, G.-E. and Oshaug, A (1997). Nutrition and food policy in Norway: effects on reduction of coronary heart disease. *Nutrition Reviews*, 55 (11), S32–S39.

Ornish, D., Brown, S. E., Scherwitz, L. W., Billings, J. H., Armstrong, W. T., Ports, T. A. *et al.* (1990). Can lifestyle changes reverse coronary heart disease? The Lifestyle Heart Trial. *Lancet*, 336, 129–33.

Pan, Xiao-Ren, Li, Guang-wei, Hu, Ying-Hua *et al.* (1997). Effects of diet and exercise in preventing NIDDM in people with impaired glucose tolerance: the Da Qing IGT and Diabetes Study. *Diabetes Care*, 20, 537–44.

Puska, P., Tuomilehto, J., Nissinen, A. and Vartiainen, E. (1995). *The North Karelia Project: 20 year results and experiences*. National Public Health Institute, KTL Helsinki.

Royal College of Physicians of London and British Cardiac Society (1976). Prevention of coronary heart disease: Chairman A. G. Shaper. *Journal of the Royal College of Physicians of London*, Vol. 10.

Stamler, J., Farinaro, E., Mojonnier, L., Hall, Y., Moss, D. and Stamler, R. (1980). Prevention and control of hypertension by nutritional-hygienic means: long-term experience of the Chicago Coronary Prevention Evaluation Program. *Journal of the American Medical Association*, 243, 1819–23.

Tuomilehto, J., Lindstöm, J., Eriksson, J. G. *et al.* (2001). Prevention of type 2 diabetes mellitus by changes in lifestyle among subjects with impaired glucose tolerance. *New England Journal of Medicine*, 344, 1343–50.

Walker, C. and Cannon, G. (1984). *The food scandal*. Century Publishing, London.

WHO (World Health Organization) (1982). *Prevention of coronary heart disease*. Technical Report Series No. 678. World Health Organization, Geneva.

WHO (World Health Organization) (1983). *Primary prevention of essential hypertension*. Technical Report Series 686. World Health Organization, Geneva.

WHO (World Health Organization) (1986). *Community prevention and control of cardiovascular diseases*. Technical Report Series 732. World Health Organization, Geneva.

WHO (World Health Organization) (1990). *Diet, nutrition and the prevention of chronic diseases*. WHO Technical Report, Series 797. World Health Organization, Geneva.

WHO (World Health Organization) (2000). *Obesity: preventing and managing the global epidemic*. WHO Technical Report Series No. 894. World Health Organization, Geneva.

WHO (World Health Organization) (2002). *World health report*. World Health Organization, Geneva. Website: <http://www.who.int/whr/en/>.

WHO (World Health Organization) (2003). *Diet, nutrition and the prevention of chronic diseases*. Technical Report Series 916. World Health Organization, Geneva

Chapter 47

Lessening inequalities and effect on coronary heart disease

M. Whitehead and M. Marmot

47.1 Background

Rose's conceptual framework for prevention, presented at the beginning of this section of the book, has particular value when considering the enormity of the challenge of lessening some inequalities in coronary heart disease (CHD) and the possible strategies for doing so. Inequalities provide a perfect illustration of why the 'high risk', individualistic approach is inadequate and why a 'population' or ecological approach is imperative to make significant inroads into the problem.

This chapter starts by summarizing the evidence on the social patterning of CHD, before going on to outline some of the main pathways leading to this marked social gradient in disease. An understanding of these pathways and mechanisms is needed in order to devise plausible, and theoretically sound strategies to intervene along the pathways. The second half of the chapter applies an equity perspective in a discussion of the effectiveness of these strategies, with a particular focus on the potential to reduce differential exposure, vulnerability, and consequences of CHD.

47.2 The social patterning of CHD

When referring to disease prevalence and population risks, figures are frequently quoted for the population as a whole. But the burden of CHD and its risk factors is not spread evenly across society: there are systematic social, ethnic, and gender inequalities.

CHD death rates increase with decreasing social class, for example, resulting in unskilled manual workers in England and Wales having three times the mortality rate of professionals, with an even greater gap at ages 45–9, when there is a four-fold difference (Drever and Whitehead 1997). This social class gradient is also reflected in morbidity rates, with prevalence of angina, heart attack, and stroke all more common amongst those in manual social classes. Even in non-manual groups there is a social gradient in CHD prevalence, incidence, and mortality. The Whitehall studies of British civil servants, all employed in offices, showed a clear inverse gradient: the lower the employment grade the higher the risk (Marmot *et al.* 1984, 1991, 1997, 2001). Furthermore, while CHD mortality in the UK has declined overall over the last 20 years, the gap has widened between social classes, as death rates have declined rapidly for professionals and managers, while little or no improvement has been observed for unskilled manual workers (Drever and Whitehead 1997).

There are also ethnic differentials. In the UK, the death rate for CHD for people born in the Indian subcontinent is 38% higher for men and 43% higher for women than rates for the country as a whole. CHD mortality is higher for people living in the north of England and for geographic areas with high deprivation. Mortality in Manchester, which is one of the most deprived health authorities, is three times higher than in the more affluent Kingston and Richmond (Department of Health 2000).

There appear to be critical stages in the life course for the development of CHD, none more so than fetal and early life (discussed in Chapters 32–4). People who had low birthweight, or who were thin or stunted at birth, are at increased risk of cardiovascular disease (CVD) and the disorders related to it in later life (Barker 1998). Birthweight is determined by the weight and height of the mother, which in turn reflects her own growth in childhood. Low birthweight, however, is itself socially patterned – the babies of women in disadvantaged groups, for example, are more likely to have reduced growth *in utero*. Babies with fathers in semi- and unskilled manual jobs have a birthweight which is on average 100 g lower than that of babies with fathers in professional and managerial jobs (ONS 2001*a*). Babies of mothers born in the Indian subcontinent are on average 200 g lighter than those born to mothers in the UK (ONS 2001*a*).

47.3 **The pathways to inequalities in CHD**

The most critical element of a strategy to tackle these inequalities in CHD is to identify points for entry for action on root causes. In line with the weight of scientific evidence presented in the Acheson Report (Acheson *et al.* 1998), a socio-economic model of the determinants of health and its inequalities needs to be adopted. Figure 47.1 illustrates one such model, in which the main determinants of health *in general* are thought of as layers of influence (Dahlgren and Whitehead 1991). Individuals have age, sex, and constitutional characteristics that influence their health (largely fixed), but surrounding them are influences that are modifiable by policy. First, there are personal behavioural factors such as smoking habits and physical activity. Second, individuals interact with their peers and immediate community and come under social and community influences, factors represented in the next layer. The wider influences on a person's ability to maintain health (in the third layer) include their living and working conditions, food supplies, and access to essential goods and services. Finally, as an overarching mediator of population health, there are the economic, cultural, and environmental conditions prevailing in society as a whole. Figure 47.1 emphasizes interactions: individual lifestyles are embedded in social and community networks, and in living and working conditions, which in turn are related to the wider cultural and socio-economic environment.

Many of these determinants have a direct influence on CHD, but what causes such a marked social gradient in the disease to develop? What are the key pathways leading to inequalities in CHD? A prominent route is through *differential exposure* to health-damaging factors and conditions across the social spectrum (Diderichsen *et al.* 2001). There is a gradient in exposure to important health risks such as poverty, nutritional deficiencies, dangerous physical and psychosocial working conditions, health-damaging behaviours, and so on, depending on a person's social position (defined by their gender, occupational class, or ethnic origin, for example). The lower down the social scale, the greater the exposure to health-damaging factors. Furthermore, this exposure is cumulative over the life course, as has been shown when cohorts have been followed from childhood into adult and older ages (Holland *et al.* 2000). In addition, certain exposures may or may not lead to CHD, depending on whether other contributory risk factors are present. A certain combination of risk factors may interact to produce a *higher vulnerability* to the health-damaging effects of an exposure, and as the number of risk factors and comorbidity increases with decreasing social position, the chance of such an interaction

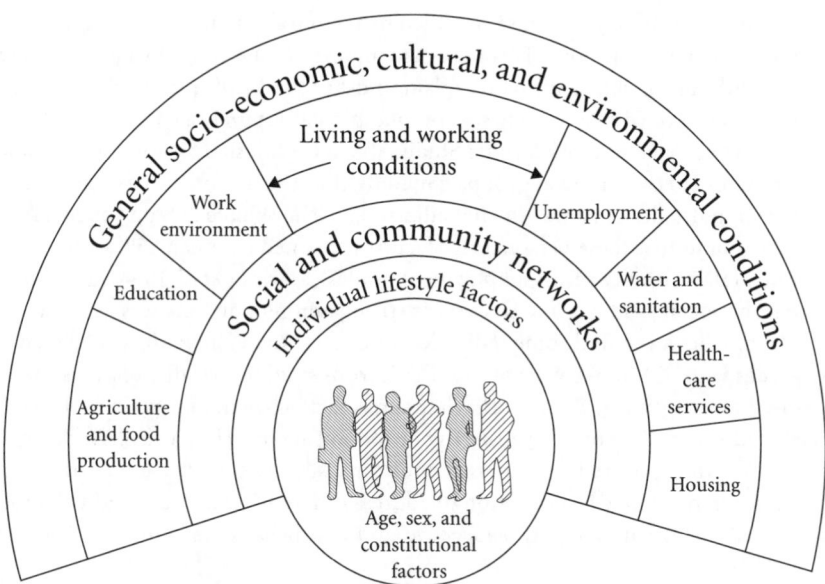

Fig. 47.1 The main determinants of health. (Reproduced from Dahlgren and Whitehead 1993.)

occurring increases (differential vulnerability; Hallqvist *et al.* 1998). This can be seen in the relation between early life conditions, adult conditions, and their interaction: in Barker's work, thinness at birth (low ponderal index) was related to CHD incidence only in the presence of low adult social class. Alternatively, low adult social class was related to CHD more strongly in men who had been thin at birth (Barker *et al.* 2001). It is also evident in relation to smoking and its interaction with other risk factors, which produces a magnified effect on CHD rates.

A further pathway may be through *differential social consequences* – the social and economic consequences of having CHD may vary for different groups. CHD itself may have social and economic consequences such as loss of job with increased exposure to poverty, social exclusion, and other health risks, which, if socially patterned, may lead to a vicious circle of more severe illness and disability for those in lower social groups.

The scope for intervening along these pathways is evident at a number of distinct policy entry points, to tackle differential exposure, vulnerability, and consequences. An important conclusion, however, drawn by the Acheson Inquiry into inequalities in health, is that a concerted effort is needed across a broad front, addressing many factors both 'upstream' and 'downstream', but also to do so with a multi-level approach. In the following sections, we select strategies on some key risk factors and risk conditions, to illustrate this multi-level approach with an equity perspective.

47.4 Reducing differential exposure and vulnerability to CHD risks

The major proximal risk factors for CHD for the population as a whole, as Chapters 3 and 4 detail, are inappropriate diet and physical activity (resulting in unfavourable lipid concentrations, high body mass index (BMI) and raised blood pressure) coupled with tobacco use. Together, these are said to explain at least 75% of new cases of CVD (Beaglehole 2001, and

Chapter 37 in this volume). All these so-called behavioural risk factors, however, exhibit a social gradient as detailed above. This raises the important question of whether differential exposure to these major risk factors also explains most of the *social gradient* observed in CVD. Is increasing incidence with decreasing socio-economic status purely a reflection of the similar gradient in these behavioural risk factors? Studies that have adjusted for variations in smoking and other factors between social groups conclude that this is not the case, as substantial differentials in mortality remain even after adjustment. The Whitehall Study of civil servants, for instance, found that these personal risk factors explained less than 25% of the observed gradient in CHD mortality across employment grades (Marmot *et al.* 1984). The study also found that the social gradient in CHD was as strong among non-smokers as it was among smokers. It did, however, find some indication of differential vulnerability. The men in the higher grades who did smoke were at lower risk from smoking-related diseases than were smokers in the lower grades. Clearly, behavioural risk factors are not the main explanation for the social gradient in CHD, but they make a contribution and may be particularly damaging in combination with exposure to other risk conditions, such as poverty, and poor living and working conditions. Public health action to address differential exposure and vulnerability, therefore, needs to take on an equity perspective, and view behaviours in their social context.

47.4.1 Tobacco control with an equity perspective

In many countries in Europe and North America there is a higher prevalence of cigarette smoking in lower socio-economic groups. In 2000, 29% of men and 25% of women in Britain smoked overall, but this ranged from 15% of professional men (13% for women) to 39% of unskilled manual men (34% of women) (ONS 2001*b*). Even among smokers, professionals smoked fewer cigarettes than those from unskilled manual occupations. The problem is compounded by the fact that nicotine dependence is higher in people experiencing disadvantage, with higher plasma cotinine levels even after adjusting for the number of cigarettes smoked. The increased dependency is one reason why lower socio-economic groups have lower cessation rates. Since 1973 rates of cessation have more than doubled in the most advantaged groups, from 25 to over 50%. In the least well-off groups, there has been a very limited increase in cessation rates, from 8 to 9% in 1973 to 10 to 13% in 1996 (Jarvis 1997).

Indeed, smoking is becoming a condition of poverty in some countries. Smoking maps on to areas of deprivation so closely in Britain that it has been suggested that smoking rates be used as an indicator of deprivation. The risk of smoking increases with each additional marker of disadvantage, reaching a prevalence of nearly 70% for lone parents with low incomes, no educational qualifications, and manual occupations, living in social housing (Marsh and McKay 1994). This illustrates vividly the interaction between behavioural and environmental factors, and the need to be sensitive to the social context in which the behaviours are being played out.

To make inroads into these inequalities in smoking, there are two main ways in which smoking could be reduced:

◆ by preventing uptake of smoking, particularly in the critical adolescent years and among more disadvantaged social groups;

◆ by helping current smokers quit or cut down.

While in the long term prevention is better, the benefits will not be seen for some time, and the more immediate gains in population health will come from smoking cessation, particularly if the disadvantaged smokers, who are at greatest risk, can be helped to quit. As Chapter 45 outlines, an effective tobacco control strategy for prevention and cessation needs to encompass policies at all levels – from global to local, and from legal and fiscal to community development and individual support. From an equity perspective, there are a number of additional factors to take into account in formulating an effective strategy. First, it is not sufficient to rely on the standard health education approaches, giving antismoking information to individuals, as this has been differentially effective – influencing advantaged social groups more than disadvantaged, and men more than women (Townsend *et al.* 1994). Educational programmes are unlikely to be effective with disadvantaged groups unless sensitive to the circumstances in which groups in hardship live, and backed up by wider policies to create supportive environments. This includes interventions that help lift some of the material and emotional pressures that work against smoking cessation for low-income women (Graham 1993).

Second, fiscal policy to regulate the price of cigarettes is an important arm of any comprehensive tobacco control policy, but sensitivity to some of the complexities of using this tool in relation to inequalities is needed. For the population as a whole, tobacco consumption falls when the real price of tobacco rises. This affects young people particularly strongly. Studies in the US and Canada indicate that young people's intention to start smoking and their uptake are highly price-sensitive. This is partly due to the fact that most young people are not yet nicotine-dependent. Price rises can therefore be an effective way of preventing the onset of regular smoking in adolescence.

However, the evidence in relation to people with disadvantaged socio-economic circumstances is mixed and requires careful interpretation. On the one hand, evidence from the UK suggests that unskilled manual workers reduce not only levels of consumption, but also total expenditure on cigarettes when there is a price rise (Townsend *et al.* 1994). On the other hand, a direct consequence of such price rises is a further reduction in the real incomes of people in hardship who continue to smoke – and as noted above, people in such circumstances are more likely to be nicotine-dependent and find it harder to quit. The solution to this dilemma is not to abandon pricing policy altogether, as it has positive benefits for the population as a whole, but to make concurrent attempts to reduce the financial and social hardship of those on low income, particularly women bringing up children on their own, and to have a complementary strategy to reduce nicotine dependence, through, for example, the provision of free nicotine replacement therapy (Townsend 1995; Acheson *et al.* 1998).

47.4.2 Improving nutrition and food policy

Low-income households tend to consume less fruit and vegetables, and less food that is rich in fibre. As a consequence, they have lower intakes of antioxidants, and other vitamins and some minerals, than high-income households (DEFRA 2000). Breastfeeding is also socially graded. High intake of sodium, across the board, but especially by disadvantaged groups, is a serious problem: people of lower education, worldwide, have higher levels of sodium excretion. This, together with higher rates of obesity and lower intakes of food rich in potassium, places those from lower socio-economic groups at higher risk of hypertension and its related risks (COMA 1994). Average blood pressure increases as social class decreases. Moreover, at any level of blood pressure, people from lower socio-economic groups appear to be more vulnerable to the associated diseases, including higher rates of heart disease and stroke.

A component part of the picture is obesity, which in women is more prevalent in lower social classes – the gradient ranges from 25% in social class V women to 14% of professional women. This is compounded by the pattern of physical activity in men. Among women, there is no social class gradient, but among men those in non-manual occupations have higher rates of leisure time activity. On the other hand, manual men take more work-related physical activity.

The reasons behind these patterns need to be examined to devise effective action. For a start, people on low incomes eat less healthily because of cost, rather than lack of concern or information. Lack of money is often cited as the reason why low-income families have not bought more fresh fruit and vegetables, even though they say they would like to provide their children with these foods. Parents report that they cut down on the food budget and miss meals for themselves when in financial difficulties (Kempson *et al.* 1994; Dowler and Calvert 1995). These reports are backed up by studies of the cost of a recommended healthy diet, which is unaffordable from the social security benefits on which many families with small children are living (Dallison and Lobstein 1995). It is certainly not through lack of awareness or inefficiency. In fact, low-income households tend to be much more efficient in buying nutrients than their higher-income counterparts, with the exception of vitamin C (Leather 1996). They make meagre resources stretch a long way to feed their families, but the problem is that, as calories from foods richer in fat and sugar are cheaper than those from other foods, they tend to buy fattier, less nutritious food products. The problem is compounded by poorer access to retail food outlets in deprived areas (necessitating additional expenditure on transport) and the higher price of food in small corner shops (Piachaud and Webb 1996). At the macro-economic level, the Acheson Report has also drawn attention to the role of the Common Agricultural Policy of the European Union, and its effect on food pricing, with its particularly strong impact on low-income families (Acheson *et al.* 1998).

In line with the recommendations of the Acheson Report, this calls for policies sensitive to these circumstances, and the creation of supportive environments for good nutrition, stretching from local to global, aimed at:

◆ increasing the availability and accessibility of food;

◆ adjusting national and European food and agriculture policies;

◆ working with food producers to reduce the sodium content of processed foods (without increasing the cost to the consumer);

◆ provision of adequate social security benefits for families with children to buy a nutritious diet;

◆ working with schools and the education sector, including the promotion of school food policies and the preservation of free school meals entitlement.

47.4.3 Improving living and working conditions

Many of the behavioural risk factors for CHD are embedded in more distal 'risk conditions' – health-damaging environmental conditions—including psychosocial stress in the living and working environment.

Employment, or lack of it, can have a major impact on economic circumstances and on health, and is socially patterned. The risk of being unemployed is much higher for young adults, people from minority ethnic groups, disabled people, and for people in less skilled occupations. For example, unemployment rates are four times higher among unskilled workers than among professional groups, and three times higher for groups with disability compared to those without. Unemployed people are found to have lower levels of psychological well-being, ranging from symptoms of depression and anxiety to self-harm and suicide. In relation to physical health, mortality from all major causes, including CHD, is consistently higher than average among unemployed men and women (Drever and Whitehead 1997).

A number of studies from the UK, Europe, and USA show that an imbalance between psychological demands and control, and a lack of control at work, are associated with increased risk of CHD (Hemingway and Marmot 1999). Workers at the lower end of the labour market are affected the most in terms of exposure to high demands and low control. As detailed in Chapter 26, the work factors resulting in the highest cardiovascular risk are those where people have little control over how they meet the job's demands and how they use their skills, coupled with little emotional support or feedback from superiors and fellow workers. These conditions are found to be more common among workers with low-status jobs, many of whom are rated as having psychological demands as heavy as those of executives, but who lack the freedom to make decisions about how to do their work.

As these psychosocial factors are related to the organization of work – together with related employment policies – there are opportunities for change. There are four main policy areas to address employment and health issues:

- Ameliorating the health damage among people experiencing unemployment, through ensuring adequate income levels for unemployed people and their families.

- Increasing training and education opportunities for population groups at greatest risk, to help prevent unemployment in the future.

- Removing barriers to employment through, for example, the provision of adequate child care, family-friendly employment policies, and employment generation.

- Improving employment conditions and health-enhancing quality of the work environment for people in employment.

In relation to reducing inequalities due to psychosocial conditions in the work environment, Karasek (1992) has suggested four main points for intervention: person-based approaches (offering counselling and education to enhance skill in coping with stress); improvements in communication patterns and human relations (e.g. providing more opportunities to exercise 'control', to make decisions, and for constructive feedback from colleagues); large-scale organizational changes (e.g. redesigning production processes); and making changes in external pressures, such as labour market conditions and rules for competition, that are largely outside an individual company's control. A review of international case studies found that it was possible to prevent or at least reduce stress in the work environment by tailoring changes to specific workplaces, especially with a multi-level approach to creating a supportive environment (International Labour Office 1992).

47.5 Tackling differential consequences of ill health

Once people become ill with CHD, further mechanisms may come into play to influence inequalities in the disease. First, inadequate access to effective treatment may directly cause a deterioration in the patient's health. Second, poor health may cause a slide in socio-economic circumstances, due to loss of employment and subsequent poverty, for instance, which in turn may damage health and wellbeing still further.

The evidence for poorer access to coronary care for poorer patients is mounting, and relates right through from screening and diagnosis to secondary care treatment.

Even though patients in more disadvantaged social groups are at greater risk of developing CHD and dying from it, they are less likely to be investigated once the disease develops

(Findlay *et al.* 1990; Keskimaki *et al.* 1997; Payne and Saul 1997; Manson-Siddle and Robinson 1998) and are less likely to be referred for cardiac surgery once diagnosed (Ben-Shlomo and Chaturvedi 1995; Payne and Saul 1997; MacLeod *et al.* 1999). In a study of referral from primary care for investigation and/or treatment for CHD, for example, practices with high deprivation scores had significantly lower rates of utilization of angiography and revascularization procedures. Their patients also waited longer for angiography, as did patients from practices far from a revascularization centre (Hippisley-Cox and Pringle 2000).

Furthermore, recent studies in Scotland have found that once socio-economically deprived patients reached secondary care, they were given lower priority on the waiting list for cardiac surgery, and were further disadvantaged by having to wait longer for surgery because of being classed as non-urgent (Pell *et al.* 2000). Age- and sex-related bias has also been found in the management of heart disease in a general hospital. In a study in a London hospital, for instance, patients aged under 75 were significantly more likely than older patients to be given thrombolysis after acute myocardial infarction, to be given secondary prevention with aspirin and beta-blockers, to undergo exercise testing and coronary angiography, and to receive an echocardiogram. Men were also more likely than women to have these investigations (Dudley *et al.* 2002). Part of the apparent sex bias may be due more to ageism – one study in the north of England found that much of the disparity in treatment between men and women was attributable to less intensive treatment of older people (Hanratty *et al.* 2000).

How can these inequalities in care and adverse social consequences of illness be prevented or at least ameliorated? There are several complementary strategies that need to be put in place to respond to these inequalities, outlined below.

47.5.1 Tackling the inverse care law in CHD services

The first response to tackling the inverse care law is to match resources for services more closely to increased need in disadvantaged populations. An essential task of the traditional resource allocation mechanisms in the NHS has been concerned with this goal, and other countries with national systems are also pursuing the quest to find a more equitable formula (Diderichsen *et al.* 1997). Although there is some evidence that these efforts have improved the regional distribution of resources (Carr-Hill *et al.* 1994; Smith *et al.* 1994), the pattern of fewer, less well-resourced services in more disadvantaged areas remains a stubborn problem. With more of the funding for services being devolved to primary care agencies, the quest to find an equitable formula for distributing resources to take full account of increased need will be more important than ever. There is no guarantee, of course, that resources allocated to tackling the inverse care law will be used for the intended purposes.

Part of the root cause of the observed inequalities in access to CHD services detailed above, however, may have nothing to do with inadequate resourcing. The gradient in access and uptake of services raises the question of whether somewhere along the pathways from first presentation to referral and treatment, discrimination in the selection of patients may be coming into play. Whether this bias is conscious or unconscious, there needs to be more awareness among professionals in the service of the possibility that this may occur and how to guard against it. This requires input in training, but also inclusion in the process of audit – both internal and external performance review.

47.5.2 Proactive initiatives with effective treatments

The central question needs to be asked: Which are the healthcare interventions for CHD known to be effective *and* for which there is a social gradient in access/utilization, with lower utilization in more disadvantaged groups? This process of identification would provide pointers to the scope for reducing under-utilization among less advantaged groups. Important interventions, across the spectrum of preventative care, curative care, and rehabilitation fields have already been identified in quality assurance initiatives such as the National Service Framework for CHD (Department of Health 2000). A further step of identifying differential access or uptake across the social scale now needs to be taken, and this needs to form the basis of supplementary resource allocations and efforts to reach under-served groups. There have been some successes in this respect, for example, with systematic case finding and audit within primary care (Tudor Hart *et al.* 1991). The National Service Framework now needs to be developed to take on board these equity of access and uptake issues much more thoroughly. Some of this work is hampered by failure of medical and health services research to assess whether CHD interventions have a differential impact for different social and ethnic groups. It is rare to find evaluations in which the possibility of differential impact has been systematically investigated; rather the reverse is true. Socio-economic status and ethnicity are variables that are controlled out of the study, rather than being the focus of investigation.

47.5.3 Rehabilitation and labour market policies

Although the National Service Framework for CHD specifies a standard for cardiac rehabilitation (Department of Health 2000, pp. 52–5), as yet there is very little acknowledgement within this initiative of the socio-economic consequences of suffering from CHD and the need to ameliorate adverse developments on this front. From an equity perspective, there are two further aspects of the situation that need to be recognized. First, there is evidence of differential employment consequences in Britain, with a steep gradient in employment rates for men with chronic illness by socio-economic group, ranging from 43% for unskilled manual workers in work to 79% for professionals. Crucially, Sweden, with much more proactive rehabilitation and labour market policies, has a much shallower social gradient in employment for men with chronic illness, ranging from 78% of unskilled workers to 89% of professionals (Burström *et al.* 2000). Second, there is a risk, when the resources for rehabilitation are scarce, that priority is given to those with highest earning potential, argued on the grounds that they have greater potential for future productivity and usefulness to the economy. This can only exacerbate the situation and leads to inequitable service provision.

Rehabilitation services, if sensitive to these equity issues, could make a particularly important contribution to helping people remain in work, thus preventing unemployment and poverty, in those recovering following treatment. Cardiac rehabilitation provided by health services needs to be coordinated with social security and labour market programmes to be optimally effective. Monitoring of the provision of services and their impact by socio-economic group is an essential component of performance assessment.

47.6 Conclusions

Any attempts to reduce inequalities in CHD need to be grounded in an understanding of how these inequalities are generated and maintained. As we learn more about the pathways and mechanisms behind the observed social patterning of the disease, it becomes clearer that the causes are many-layered, but the roots stretch back to wider determinants linked to socio-economic inequalities in society as a whole. This wider social context needs to be taken into account fully – a single risk factor cannot be considered in isolation. It also follows, from a deeper understanding of pathways, that the action required to lessen CHD inequalities cannot be limited solely to the health sector, but must encompass action at many different levels and across various sectors. Moreover, a population, rather than a high-risk, individualistic approach is the most appropriate. Health services cannot be let off the hook, however.

As outlined in this chapter, there is much to be done for the health sector to get its own house in order. Every aspect of promotion, prevention, treatment, and rehabilitation in relation to CHD can, and should, be made more equitable.

References

Acheson, D., Barker, D., Chambers, J., Graham, H., Marmot, M. and Whitehead, M. (1998). *Report of the Independent Inquiry into Inequalities in Health*. The Stationery Office, London.

Barker, D. (1998). *Mothers, babies and health in later life*. Churchill Livingstone, Edinburgh.

Barker, D., Forsen, T., Uutela, A., Osmond, C. and Eriksson, J. (2001). Size at birth and resilience to effects of poor living conditions in adult life: longitudinal study. *British Medical Journal*, **323**, 1273–6.

Beaglehole, R. (2001). Global cardiovascular prevention: time to get serious. *Lancet*, **358**, 661–3.

Ben-Shlomo, Y. and Chaturvedi, N. (1995). Assessing equity in access to health care provision in the UK: does where you live affect your chances of getting coronary artery bypass graft? *Journal of Epidemiology and Community Health*, **49**, 200–4.

Burström, B., Whitehead, M., Lindholm, C. and Diderichsen, F. (2000). Inequalities in the social consequences of illness: how do people with long-term illness fare in the British and Swedish labour markets? *International Journal of Health Services*, **30**, 435–51.

Carr-Hill, R., Sheldon, T., Smith, P., Martin, S., Peacock, S. and Hardman, G. (1994). Allocating resources to health authorities: development of methods for small area analysis and use of inpatient services. *British Medical Journal*, **309**, 1046–9.

COMA (1994). *Report on health and social subjects no. 46: nutritional aspects of cardiovascular disease*. Committee on Medical Aspects of Food Policy. HMSO, London.

Dahlgren, G. and Whitehead, M. (1993). *Tackling inequalities in health: what can we learn from what has been tried?* Background paper for Ditchley Park Seminar, September. King's Fund, London.

Dallison, J. and Lobstein, T. (1995). *Poor expectations: poverty and under-nourishment in pregnancy*. NCH Action for Children and the Maternity Alliance, London.

DEFRA (2000). *National food survey for 2000*. Department of Environment, Food and Rural Affairs. The Stationery Office, London.

Department of Health (2000). *National Service framework for coronary heart disease: modern standards and service models*. Department of Health, London.

Diderichsen, F., Varde, E. and Whitehead, M. (1997). Resource allocation to health authorities: the quest for an equitable formula in Britain and Sweden. *British Medical Journal*, **315**, 875–8.

Diderichsen, F., Evans, T. and Whitehead, M. (2001). The social basis of disparities in health. In *Challenging inequities in health: from ethics to action* (ed. T. Evans, M. Whitehead, F. Diderichsen, A. Bhuiya and M. Wirth), pp.13–23. Oxford University Press, New York.

Dowler, E. and Calvert, C. (1995). *Nutrition and diet in lone-parent families in London*. Family Studies Centre, London.

Drever, F. and Whitehead, M. (eds) (1997). *Health inequalities*, Decennial Supplement. Series DS No. 15. Office for National Statistics, The Stationery Office, London.

Dudley, N., Bowling, A., Bond, M., McKee, D., McClay Scott, M., Banning, A. *et al.* (2002). Age- and sex-related bias in the management of heart disease in a district general hospital. *Age and Ageing*, **31**, 37–42.

Findlay, I., Dargie, H., Dyke, T. and Archibald, M. (1990). Who gets coronary angiography in Scotland? *British Heart Journal*, **66**, 43–4.

Graham, H. (1993). *When life's a drag: women, smoking and disadvantage*. Department of Health. HMSO, London.

Hallqvist, J., Diderichsen, F., Theorell, T., Teuterwall, C. and Ahlbom A. (1998). Is the effect of job strain on myocardial infarction risk due to interaction between high psychological demand and low decision latitude? *Social Science and Medicine*, **46**, 1405–15.

Hanratty, B., Lawlor, D., Robinson, M., Sapsford, R., Greenwood, D. and Hall, A. (2000). Sex differences in risk factors, treatment and mortality after acute myocardial infarction: an observational study. *Journal of Epidemiology and Community Health*, **54**, 912–16.

Hemingway, H. and Marmot, M. (1999). Psychosocial factors in the aetiology and prognosis of coronary heart disease: systematic review of prospective cohort studies. *British Medical Journal*, **318**, 1460–7.

Hippisley-Cox, J. and Pringle, M. (2000). Inequalities in access to coronary angiography and revascularisation: the association of deprivation and location of primary care services. *British Journal of General Practice*, **50**, 449–54.

Holland, P., Berney, L., Blane, D., Davey Smith, G., Gunnell, S. and Montgomery, S. (2000). Life course accumulation of disadvantage: childhood health and hazard exposure during adulthood. *Social Science and Medicine*, **50**, 1285–95.

International Labour Office (ed.) (1992). Preventing stress at work: *Conditions of Work Digest*, 11 (2). International Labour Office, Geneva.

Jarvis, M. (1997). Patterns and predictors of smoking cessation in the general population. In *The tobacco epidemic. Progress in respiratory research*. (ed. C. Bolliger and K. Fagerström), pp. 151–64. Karger, Basel.

Karasek, R. (1992). Stress prevention through work reorganisation: a summary of 19 case studies. In: Preventing stress at work: *Conditions of Work Digest*, 11 (2) (ed. International Labour Office), pp. 23–40. International Labour Office, Geneva.

Kempson, E., Bryson, A. and Rowlingson, K. (1994). *Hard times? How poor families make ends meet*. Policy Studies Institute, London.

Keskimaki, I., Koskinen, S., Salinto, M. and Aro, S. (1997). Socio-economic and gender inequities in access to coronary artery bypass grafting in Finland. *European Journal of Public Health*, **7**, 392–7.

Leather, S. (1996). *The making of modern malnutrition: an overview of food poverty in the UK*. Caroline Walker Trust, London.

MacLeod, M., Finlayson, A., Pell, J. and Findlay, I. (1999). Geographical, demographic and socioeconomic variations in the investigation and management of coronary heart disease in Scotland. *Heart*, **81**, 252–6.

Manson-Siddle, C. and Robinson, M. (1998). Profile analysis of socio-economic variations in coronary investigation and revascularisation rates. *Journal of Epidemiology and Community Health*, **52**, 507–12.

Marmot, M., Shipley, M., Brunner, E. and Hemingway, H. (2001). Relative contribution of early life and adult socioeconomic factors to adult morbidity in the WII study. *Journal of Epidemiology and Community Health*, **55**, 301–7.

Marmot, M., Shipley, M. and Rose, G. (1984). Inequalities in death: specific explanations of a general pattern. *Lancet*, **323**, 1003–6.

Marmot, M. G., Bosma, H., Hemingway, H., Brunner, E. and Stansfeld, S. (1997). Contribution of job control and other risk factors to social variations in coronary heart disease. *Lancet*, **350**, 235–40.

Marmot, M. G., Davey Smith, G., Stansfeld, S. A., Patel, C., North, F., Head, J. *et al.* (1991). Health inequalities among British Civil Servants: the Whitehall II study. *Lancet*, **337**, 1387–93.

Marsh, A. and McKay, S. (1994). *Poor smokers*. Policy Studies Institute, London.

Piachaud, D. and Webb, J. (1996). *The price of food: missing out on mass consumption*. LSE Suntory and Toyota International Centre for Economics and Related Disciplines, London.

ONS (Office for National Statistics) (2001a). *Series DH3 mortality statistics: perinatal and infant: social and biological factors*. The Stationery Office, London.

ONS (2001*b*). *General household survey for 2000*. The Stationary Office, London

Payne, N. and Saul, C. (1997). Variations in use of cardiology services in a health authority: comparison of coronary artery revascularisation rates with prevalence of angina and coronary mortality. *British Medical Journal*, **314**, 257–61.

Pell, J., Pell, A., Norrie, J., Ford, I. and Cobbe, S. (2000). Effect of socio-economic deprivation on waiting time for cardiac surgery: retrospective cohort study. *British Medical Journal*, **320**, 15–19.

Smith, P., Sheldon, T., Carr-Hill, R., Martin, S., Peacock, S. and Hardman, G. (1994). Allocating resources to health authorities: results and policy implications of small area analysis of use of inpatient services. *British Medical Journal*, **309**, 1050–4.

Townsend, J. (1995). The burden of smoking. In *Tackling inequalities in health: an agenda for action* (ed. M. Benzeval, K. Judge and M. Whitehead), pp. 82–94. King's Fund, London.

Townsend, J., Roderick, P. and Cooper, J. (1994). Cigarette smoking by socio-economic group, sex, and age: effects of price, income and health publicity. *British Medical Journal*, **309**, 923–7.

Tudor Hart, J., Thomas, C., Gibbons, B., Edwards, C., Hart, M., Jones, J. *et al.* (1991). Twenty five years of case finding and audit in a socially deprived community. *British Medical Journal*, **302**, 1509–13.

Chapter 48

Behaviour change

L. J. Cooke, M. J. Jarvis, and J. Wardle

48.1 **Introduction**

Ten years after the publication of the first edition of this book, the need for health behaviour change is no less pressing if we are to reduce rates of coronary heart disease (CHD) in the UK. Trends in overweight and obesity, physical activity, diet, and smoking are either going in the wrong direction or remain at unacceptably high levels. Interventions aimed at high risk groups are unlikely to make enough impact to warrant the expense and difficulty of identifying potential participants. Instead, we need to improve population health behaviour with interventions from which every individual may not benefit, but in which all have to take part. Some of the most effective strategies for reducing disease at the population level have required no input from individuals, but instead involved modification of the environment – increasing taxation on cigarettes or fluoridation of water. Unfortunately, long-term health behaviour change frequently involves considerable individual effort. A major challenge of the twenty-first century will be to establish effective ways of supporting people to make healthy behavioural choices in the face of 'societal and industrial counterforces' (Orleans 2000) and a 'lay epidemiology' which observes frequent 'anomalous deaths' and 'unwarranted survivals' and remains sceptical of the real worth of health behaviour change (Hunt and Emslie 2001).

48.2 **Models of health behaviour**

It is well-documented that adopting health-enhancing behaviours (e.g. regular physical activity) and avoiding health-compromising behaviours (e.g. smoking) can enable individuals to reduce their cardiovascular disease risk; but there are wide variations in the extent to which people perform them. Behavioural science has been engaged both to explain these variations and to provide conceptual and empirical knowledge to inform interventions aimed at changing health behaviours. A number of theoretical models have been proposed which attempt to identify the factors most predictive of behaviour. Whilst extrinsic factors are acknowledged to play a part, most of these models focus on the intrinsic factors – typically cognitive and emotional – that have been identified as important, and potentially manipulable, determinants of behaviour.

The most influential social cognitive models (e.g. Theory of Planned Behaviour (Ajzen 1985); Health Belief Model (Janz and Becker 1984); Theory of Reasoned Action (Fishbein and Ajzen 1975); Social Cognitive Theory/Self-Efficacy Theory (Bandura 1986)) share many similarities at a conceptual level. The decision to act is considered to be the end result of a quasi-rational – although not necessarily deliberate – analysis of the relative costs and benefits associated with that action. Self-efficacy and outcome expectancies also appear in most models, although they may be labelled differently. These are assumed to be linked with intentions to act, which in turn translate to actions unless there are barriers. Barriers might include remembering to act (if the intention–behaviour interval is large), or a whole range of external events that make the act more difficult or less rewarding than had been anticipated.

Although social cognition models have provided a valuable framework for understanding the determinants of health behaviour and have guided interventions aimed at changing them, their explanatory value is limited. For example, in a recent meta-analytic review, the Theory of Planned Behaviour elements (Ajzen 1985) accounted for 39% and 27% of the variance in intention and behaviour, respectively (Armitage and Conner 2001). Possible reasons for this relatively poor predictive performance have been discussed in detail elsewhere (Conner and Norman 1995), but include unreliable measurement of variables, the omission of highly influential variables (e.g. past behaviour), and a failure to address the problem of translating intentions into actual behaviour.

A more recent development has been the Transtheoretical Model of Behaviour Change (TTM) (Prochaska and DiClemente 1983), otherwise known as the Stages of Change Model (SCM); this represents a more dynamic approach in which a temporal perspective is emphasized. Individuals are assumed to pass through a set sequence of stages of behaviour change from 'pre-contemplation' through 'contemplation' to 'initiation' and 'maintenance' of behaviour. The TTM proposes that different cognitions are influential for different transitions, and that interventions should therefore be tailored to the individual's stage. Like the continuum models (e.g. Weinstein's (1988) Precaution Adoption Process Model) it has been influential in the design of interventions which can be targeted at populations of resistant pre-contemplators as well as the usual well-motivated volunteers. Despite being devised for application to smoking cessation, the TTM has been applied to a variety of other health behaviours such as diet and physical activity, for which, some have suggested, it may be less appropriate (Marshall and Biddle 2001; Ni et al. 1998). Critics point to the somewhat arbitrary time periods specified for movement between stages and the lack of qualitative difference between stages as limiting the utility of these models (Sutton 1999). There is some evidence to suggest that interventions tailored to stage of change can be more effective than standardized interventions (Dijkstra et al. 1998), although other results have been less supportive (Aveyard et al. 2003).

It is beyond the scope of this chapter to provide a comprehensive review of studies of health behaviour change for CHD risk reduction. Instead the focus will be on recent reviews in the key areas of smoking, diet, and physical activity, including the emergence of interventions which utilize new technology to tailor messages to the specific concerns of individuals.

48.3 Smoking cessation

Cessation of cigarette smoking reduces the risk of cardiovascular disease towards that of never-smokers. Some studies have indicated that the effect is rapid, occurring within 2–3 years (Dobson et al. 1991; Rosenberg et al. 1985), while others have pointed to a slower decline in risk (Ben-Shlomo et al. 1994; Cook et al. 1986). The difficulty of achieving cessation is notorious. Most quit attempts are unaided, and the success rate from such attempts is estimated at no higher than 1 or 2 in 100 (Jarvis 1997). Cigarette smoking prevalence in the UK has declined by around 1 percentage point per year over the past 30 years, the main predictors of cessation being broader social influences rather than individual dependence (Jarvis 1997). Efforts to reduce smoking uptake among the young have met with little success (Lynch et al. 1994; Nutbeam et al. 1993). At the same time, there has been considerable success in developing effective treatments (Fiore et al. 2000). The challenge has been to find ways of delivering effective individual interventions sufficiently widely to impact significantly on population prevalence.

48.3.1 **Effective treatments for smoking cessation**

Both behavioural and pharmacological treatments are effective. Brief advice from a health professional increases the likelihood of a quit attempt and of successful cessation (Fiore *et al.* 2000; Raw *et al.* 1998). The increase in long-term cessation from brief advice is of the order of 2% (Silagy 2000). More intensive behavioural support and counselling are associated with better outcomes. Pharmacological adjuncts which mitigate the severity of nicotine withdrawal reliably increase the chances of successful quitting. Meta-analysis of over 100 randomized controlled trials indicates an increase in the odds of successful cessation of about 70% from the use of the various forms of nicotine replacement (Silagy *et al.* 2000). Similar efficacy is evident from the much smaller literature on bupropion. A recent meta-analysis conducted by the National Institute for Clinical Excellence found an odds ratio of 2.16 (95% CI: 1.51–3.10) for continuous abstinence compared to placebo (National Institute for Clinical Excellence 2002). A trial of bupropion in patients with established cardiovascular disease has shown clear efficacy with acceptable safety (Tonstad *et al.* 2003). The cardiovascular risk profile of nicotine replacement is good (Benowitz 1999; Benowitz and Gourlay 1997), and concerns over the use of nicotine replacement in patients with heart disease may have been overstated (Joseph *et al.* 1996).

48.3.2 **Smoking cessation as part of multiple risk factor interventions for preventing CHD**

Interventions against smoking have formed a part of a number of randomized controlled trials of primary prevention of CHD. These trials typically used counselling and educational approaches, and were carried out in general population samples, occupational settings, and high risk groups. In a meta-analysis of 14 trials, the net reduction in smoking prevalence in intervention subjects compared with controls was 4.2% (Ebrahim and Smith 1997). However, most studies showed no or only small effects, and the overall outcome was strongly influenced by the Multiple Risk Factor Intervention Trial (MRFIT 1982). An analysis of objective markers of smoke intake has shown that the smoking outcomes in this trial may have been very considerably overstated (Jarvis *et al.* 1984).

Ebrahim and Davey Smith concluded that this type of health promotion intervention may have limited use in the general population, and advocated wider use of fiscal and legislative measures as alternatives deserving higher priority (Ebrahim and Smith 1997). However, before dismissing the potential value of such interventions some limitations of the approaches used need to be considered. Most trials used a 'negotiated behaviour change' model in which participants could choose the risk behaviour they wished to prioritize (Imperial Cancer Research Fund OXCHECK study group 1995; Wood *et al.* 1994). This may have led to a lowered emphasis on difficult behaviours such as smoking and an uneven implementation of the smoking protocol. In addition, these trials were based on behavioural counselling methods and did not incorporate pharmacological adjuncts such as nicotine replacement. The value of a well-specified and vigorously implemented smoking intervention is demonstrated by the Lung Health Study, which achieved both a clear effect on smoking prevalence and a benefit in its respiratory end point (Anthonisen *et al.* 1994).

48.3.3 **Community-based health promotion for smoking cessation**

The challenge of achieving population-level change in common health behaviours such as cigarette smoking has led to the development of community-based interventions. In these the unit of randomization is the community, not the individual. The rationale for community-based health promotion is the notion that the individuals cannot be considered separately from their social milieu, and that programmes incorporating intervention beyond the individual level have the potential to be more successful in changing behaviour. For smoking, interventions have included activities such as information campaigns, 'Quit and Win' competitions, involvement of community associations, and local ordinances to restrict youth access to tobacco, in addition to increased availability of cessation services (Chapter 45). The largest such trial to date (the COMMIT study) found some evidence for an impact on light to moderate smokers, but did not change the smoking behaviour of heavy smokers, the primary target population (COMMIT Research Group 1995). Similarly modest effects have been observed in other trials (Carleton et al. 1995; Lando et al. 1995; Tudor-Smith et al. 1998). A review of community-based health promotion programmes has summarized the results and set out some of the possible reasons for the relatively poor outcomes (Merzel and D'Affliti 2003). Some problems stem from inherent methodological difficulties relating to study design, small anticipated effect sizes, and detecting these against the background of concurrent secular trends. Other issues relate to achieving sufficient programme penetration to influence behaviour at the individual level, and the timescale necessary for altering behaviours that are highly entrenched in the community.

48.3.4 **Wide-reach behavioural interventions based on the stages of change model**

The SCM (Prochaska et al. 1992) has been very popular with clinicians. In part this may be because it provides them with a road-map for assessing smokers' readiness to quit, but another attraction may be that it suggests the value of intermediate goals, such as a move from precontemplation to contemplation, in addition or as an alternative to complete cessation.

A further advantage could potentially come from greater population reach. In contrast to traditional cessation interventions, which appeal to highly motivated smokers and have low recruitment rates, stages of change interventions place less emphasis on readiness to quit at the time of recruitment, and so could have a wider appeal. Prochaska and colleagues reported that 80% of a community sample of smokers cold-called by telephone were successfully recruited to a trial in which they were randomized to either an Expert System condition involving a series of tailored stage-matched self-help manuals or to an assessment-only condition (Prochaska et al. 2001). An increasing advantage for the Expert System condition emerged over time: by 24 months 7-day point prevalence abstinence was 25% compared with 19% in controls. These outcomes were reported to be similar to those from more intensive clinic-based interventions. However, these figures were based on subjects successfully followed up rather than on an intention-to-treat analysis. Prochaska argued that the high recruitment rate coupled with the good cessation outcomes indicated that the programme had the capacity to impact significantly on population-wide cessation.

However, a recent attempt to replicate these results in a British sample has failed to confirm the findings (Aveyard et al. 2003). Only 9% of smokers participated, and retention in the study to generate individualized feedback was poor. There was no evidence for an advantage of the intervention, especially when an intention-to-treat analysis was employed. Similar difficulties with recruitment to a primary care intervention based on the SCM have been reported by others (Steptoe *et al.* 1999*a, b*). The SCM has also not performed well in other empirical tests. Analysis of the California Tobacco Survey showed that assessed stage membership at baseline did not predict smoking cessation at follow-up after allowing for cigarette consumption and quitting history (Farkas *et al.* 1996).

48.4 **Dietary interventions**

In attempting to review the effectiveness of different interventions aimed at improving dietary quality, a number of methodological issues arise. Although some studies target a single behaviour (e.g. fat intake) others are multi-factorial (targeting fat, and fruit and vegetable consumption, or combining dietary intervention with exercise promotion). Where a programme has been ineffective it may be the result of one goal being emphasized more than another, rather than a poorly designed programme per se. Alternatively, one outcome may be easier to achieve than another. Increasing fruit and vegetable consumption, for example, may be simpler than reducing fat intake since the latter demands extensive knowledge of the fat contents of foods whereas the former merely relies on the recognition of fruit and vegetables. A majority of studies rely on self-report to track outcomes, with the associated problems of social desirability and memory bias affecting the validity of findings (Bingham 1991; Tinker *et al.* 2001). Firm conclusions as to the characteristics of effective interventions are hard to draw for such reasons.

Many trials have examined the impact of intensive intervention on the behaviour of motivated individuals. The evidence is clear that some people can make and maintain substantial changes in dietary composition. In the Women's Health Trial, for example (White *et al.* 1992), fat intake was reduced by half. The challenge from the population perspective is to translate this so that smaller changes can be achieved across the whole population. Most of these studies have targeted communities at some level – most often schools and workplaces.

48.4.1 **Effectiveness of interventions with children**

Although improving eating habits in early childhood will have no immediate effect on rates of CHD, there is evidence to suggest that early intervention may reap health dividends in the longer term. A recent review of interventions with pre-school children (Tedstone *et al.* 1998) identified only 12 studies of high quality, of which 11 were based in the USA. Positive changes in nutrition knowledge were observed in many studies, although impact on eating behaviour was more variable. Findings were that pre-school and day-care were appropriate settings for interventions and that parental involvement tended to enhance effectiveness. Knowledge was increased with traditional, video-based, or computer-based teaching methods, but changes in actual eating behaviour were best achieved using behavioural modification techniques. Repeated exposure to the taste of initially novel foods was successful in increasing willingness to consume them, whereas rewards to encourage healthy food selection only worked as long as rewards were in place.

A review of interventions aimed at increasing fruit and vegetable consumption in children of 4 years and older (Ciliska *et al.* 2000) concluded that the most effective interventions included gave clear messages about fruit and vegetable consumption and reinforced these messages using multiple strategies. In addition, those that involved the family, were longer and more intensive, and based on a theoretical framework were more likely to achieve significant increases in intake. However, it is important to note that these guidelines are not fail-safe and one of the most intensive trials, the Child and Adolescent Trial for Cardiovascular Health (Perry *et al.* 1998) failed to achieve any impact at all on fruit and vegetable intake.

Since these reviews were published, further intervention studies have been carried out, mostly with 3rd, 4th and 5th graders, although some have targeted college students. Adolescents are still neglected, although promising signs of research taking place outside the USA (Friel *et al.* 1999; Sahota *et al.* 2001), or with longer follow-ups are evident (Nader *et al.* 1999). In the CATCH trial, which examined the effectiveness of a multi-component school- and home-based intervention, a 3 year follow-up found that although the difference between intervention and control groups had declined, the intervention group remained significantly lower in self-reported energy intake from fat. Results from school-based studies in Ireland (Friel *et al.* 1999) and the UK (Parker and Fox 2001; Sahota *et al.* 2001), however, suggest that achieving dietary change in school-aged children remains a significant problem. In the former, a 10 week, multi-component intervention achieved only a very small percentage increase in the number of children in the intervention group eating four or more servings of fruit and vegetables daily (from 1 to 2%). Parker and Fox (2001) found no significant changes in school-based eating at the end of 2 years of an intervention involving catering provision and curriculum activities aimed at increasing the availability and consumption of fruit, vegetables, and fibre-rich foods, and Sahota *et al.*'s (2001) extensive intervention achieved a modest increase in vegetable consumption in intervention children (0.3 portions/day), but no improvements in any other nutritional or anthropometric outcomes.

Overall, the results of interventions with children in school settings have been disappointing. The reason for the popularity of school settings for interventions is clearly the unique opportunity they provide to reach everyone, not just highly motivated volunteers, but the importance of the home environment and the family in influencing children's diets should not be underestimated. Where interventions have included parental involvement, findings have generally been more positive. Where they have not (as in the recent British studies cited above), a great deal of effort has resulted in very little positive change.

48.4.2 Effectiveness of interventions with adults

Dietary interventions with adults have met with some degree of success. A recent meta-analysis of 17 randomized controlled trials aimed at CHD risk factor reduction (Brunner *et al.* 1997) concluded that individual dietary interventions in primary prevention can result in some improvements in risk status that are maintained for 9–18 months. If sustained, the authors estimated that these changes could lead to a 14% reduction in the incidence of CHD. Longer duration and higher levels of contact appeared to be associated with larger effect sizes, although this finding is confounded by differences in the motivations of the study populations (greatest effects were seen in breast cancer prevention trials (Henderson *et al.* 1990).

A systematic review of the effectiveness of 76 healthy eating interventions in a wide variety of settings from worksites to supermarkets (Roe *et al.* 1997) highlighted a number of characteristics of successful interventions. A focus on diet alone, or diet in conjunction with physical activity, was associated with more successful outcomes than those that were multi-factorial. In common with the interventions directed at children, the provision of information alone was rarely effective. Those that incorporated behavioural change theories tended to be more effective, as were those that set clear goals for participants. Goal setting, together with small group interaction, also emerged as promising intervention components in one of the most extensive reviews recently undertaken (Ammerman *et al.* 2002). In contrast, a quantitative review of 32 diet and physical activity interventions (Wilcox *et al.* 2001) found that effect sizes were larger in dietary fat reduction studies where no explicit behaviour theory was used. It is possible, however, that systematic behavioural principles were incorporated, but not reported. Roe *et al.* (1997) found that other features of effective interventions were sustained personal contact, personalized feedback on changes made, and local environment changes that promoted healthy eating (e.g. in catering establishments or supermarkets). The magnitude of change achieved in many of the studies remains modest, for example a decrease in fat intake of between 1 and 4% of energy, or a reduction in blood cholesterol of 2–5%; but the latter would still be estimated to result in a 4–10% lower risk of heart disease on a population basis, which should result in substantial saving of lives.

Some recent studies have used information technology to better tailor interventions to the motivations and concerns of participants. Baker and Wardle (2002) evaluated a brief tailored psycho-educational intervention for increasing fruit and vegetable consumption in older adults attending a cancer-screening clinic. Messages were tailored to stage of change of participants and addressed their barriers and existing knowledge as assessed from questionnaires. An increase of almost 0.6 portions of fruit and 0.5 of vegetables in the intervention group compares favourably with the results of previous successful interventions, and are similar to those reported by Marcus and colleagues (Marcus *et al.* 2001) using a tailored intervention to callers to the Cancer Information Service. Likewise, a healthcare practice-based intervention delivered by interactive, computer-controlled telephone system (Delichatsios *et al.* 2001a) increased fruit intake by 1.1 servings/day and improved overall diet quality in intervention participants after 6 months. Even more impressive are the results of the PACE+ for adults program (Calfas *et al.* 2002). Here, participants completed a computerized assessment and were encouraged to target a specific nutrition behaviour. Where an increase in consumption of fruit and vegetables was the target, increases of over one and a half servings a day were achieved. Other recent personalized interventions have had similarly positive results (Delichatsios *et al.* 2001b; Kristal *et al.* 2000) and in a recent large-scale randomized controlled trial of a brief, interactive, computer-based intervention (Stevens *et al.* 2003) increases of almost one whole serving a day and significantly reduced fat intake was sustained at a 12-month follow-up. Compared with many intensive interventions detailed above, these interventions are both brief and cost-effective and have the potential to reach a large population.

There are still shortcomings to be addressed in research into the adoption and maintenance of dietary change. Adolescents, people on lower incomes, and ethnic minority populations are neglected, although some recent community-based interventions have begun to target the latter (Resnicow *et al.* 2002). Dietary change must be sustained to effect reductions in CHD morbidity and mortality, but there are still very few studies that undertake long-term follow-up of participants. Outcomes are often based on self-reported food intake despite the poor reliability and the likely bias when interventions increase the social desirability of healthy behavioural choices. Few studies include even proxy clinical end points and, therefore, the contribution of behaviour change to health outcomes can only be estimated. Study samples are frequently restricted to highly motivated volunteers and it remains to be seen how these findings can be generalized to less enthusiastic populations. Some of the reviews discussed here comment on the poor quality of many studies in terms of design, implementation, measurement, statistical analysis, and reporting of results. Nevertheless, it appears that in several areas we are moving in the right direction and new technology offers considerable promise in dietary interventions.

48.4.3 Ecological interventions for dietary change

The majority of research into dietary behaviour change has grown out of an individual-level perspective – albeit the participants might be recruited from community settings or through the internet, and the intervention might be delivered in the form of posters or group programmes. The aim is either to encourage all members of the study population to make healthier food choices or to help those whose intake is particularly at odds with healthy eating guidelines become aware of the need to change and acquire the appropriate skills. However, an analysis of dietary trends over time suggests that the causes of the unhealthy diets of today are more likely to lie with the food supply than with the consumers. There is no evidence that consumers are either less knowledgeable about diet and health or less concerned about being healthier than they used to be – in fact trends are probably in the opposite direction. The rise of commercial food production and distribution over the twentieth century has meant that the food supply has become progressively safer, more consistent, more convenient to consume, and cheaper, as well as offering a wider range of foods. This has remedied shortfalls in food availability, and limited seasonal variation, as well as reducing the risk of food-borne diseases. At the same time, however, developments in food processing have created a smorgasbord of new foods and drinks that are almost all high in sugar, salt, or fat; the very properties which are (not by coincidence) most well-liked by consumers (Nestle 2002). Laboratory studies of human eating behaviour show that supplying foods which are varied, cheap, highly flavoured (e.g. sweet or salty), high in energy density, and served in large portions, tends to promote higher food intake (Raynor and Epstein 2001; Rolls *et al.* 2004*a, b*; Stubbs *et al.* 2000). Changes in the food supply are, therefore, likely to have contributed substantially to the positive energy balance and the consequent rise in obesity that has been seen across the world (World Health Organization 1998).

Behaviour change approaches described earlier in this section have been directed largely towards shoring up people's resistance to the temptations of the food supply – encouraging them to resist sugary, salty, and fatty foods and seek out less palatable, but nutrient-rich foods such as vegetables. Helping consumers resist the damaging features of their environment is a worthy goal, but perhaps a more logical alternative – or supplement – to this Sisyphean task might be to change the environment. If the food supply could be modified so that 'healthy' foods were more widely promoted and accessible, and cheaper than the less healthy foods, consumers could change their diets without the need for any intensive individual effort.

Some community interventions, such as the North Karelia study (Puska *et al.* 1979), have incorporated strategies to change the food supply along with more conventional health promotion approaches. These are described in the chapter on community level interventions (Chapter 51). A series of smaller-scale studies have shown that pricing changes can influence both fruit and vegetable intake and fat intake (French *et al.* 1997*a, b*, 2001). However, there is an urgent need for a more systematic research effort into the environmental determinants of dietary behaviour (Jeffery and Utter 2003). Behavioural scientists should create new alliances with economists, policy makers, engineers, and food producers to identify acceptable and effective ways of creating food environments which support, rather than undermine, healthy food choices (see Chapter 46).

48.5 Physical activity interventions

There is a vast literature on physical activity interventions, a comprehensive review of which is beyond the scope of this chapter. A number of excellent reviews and meta-analyses are available (Dishman and Buckworth 1996; Hillsdon *et al.* 1995; Marcus *et al.* 2000; Wilcox *et al.* 2001) and an entire issue of the American *Journal of Preventive Medicine* (1998, Vol. 15, Part 4) is devoted to reviews of interventions segmented by type, setting, and target population. Many of the methodological problems associated with dietary interventions discussed earlier also apply to exercise promotion, not least that of lack of long-term follow-up and measurement issues. Maintenance of physical activity behaviour change represents a significant challenge, as dropout rates are notoriously high. Although no official definition exists, one that is widely accepted holds that successful maintenance is the continuation of regular physical activity for at least 6 months post-intervention (Marcus *et al.* 2000).

Establishing the characteristics of effective physical activity interventions is extremely difficult. The factors that determine adoption, maintenance, and relapse may differ and may also vary with age, culture, ethnicity, and socio-economic status. What appears certain is that the provision of information is not sufficient to effect behaviour change, as the results of a number of mass media campaigns have demonstrated. For example, a 3 year prospective longitudinal survey to assess the impact of a national awareness campaign on knowledge of recommendations and engagement in physical activity: ACTIVE for LIFE (Hillsdon *et al.* 2001) found no significant improvements in physical activity overall or in any subgroup. Mass media campaigns in Australia (Booth *et al.* 1992)) and Scotland (Wimbush *et al.* 1998) have had broadly similar results (see Marcus *et al.* 1998*b* for a review).

48.5.1 Effectiveness of interventions with children

The finding that a decline in physical activity begins in adolescence and that inactivity tends to track into adulthood (Malina 1996) (i.e. that the less active adolescents become the less active adults) has led to the suggestion that childhood is an important time for intervention. This, of course, assumes that getting an adolescent 'off-course' with an intervention can be sustained. Typically, youth intervention studies have been conducted in school settings for the obvious reasons of good reach and resources. A recent review of interventions in youth (Stone *et al.* 1998) found 14 completed school-based studies and 8 in progress. Of the 14 completed studies, 11 were carried out in the USA as were all those in progress. All employed a sound theoretical framework, usually Social Learning Theory or Social Cognitive Theory, although many used a multiple theoretical approach. Studies varied considerably in length, scope, and content, although most included a dietary component in addition to physical activity. The most common strategy was modification of existing physical education (PE) classes, although some offered out-of-school physical activity sessions. Most studies measured changes in knowledge, attitudes, and self-reported physical activity or measures of activity levels during PE lessons.

While improvements in knowledge and attitudes were often achieved, increases in physical activity were more elusive. Despite considerable investment of time and effort a number of studies reported no increases at all in out-of-school physical activity after as much as 2 years of intervention (McKenzie *et al.* 1997; Perry *et al.* 1987; Simons-Morton *et al.* 1991); indeed one study reported less out-of-school physical activity for the intervention group (Donnelly *et al.* 1996). A rare and recent study in the UK (Sahota *et al.* 2001) comprised a 1 year programme aimed at improving diet and increasing physical activity in 7–11-year-old children. Again, results were disappointing with no significant intervention effects on exercise. There have been some successes, however, most notably in the large-scale Child and Adolescent Trial for Cardiovascular Health (CATCH) (Luepker *et al.* 1996; Nader *et al.* 1999). Not only did intervention schools achieve higher rates of out-of-school physical activity and more moderate to vigorous activity during PE lessons post-intervention, but they also maintained differences between intervention and control schools at 3 year follow-up. It is possible that the involvement of the family contributed to better outcomes in this study. The Oslo Youth Study (Tell and Vellar 1987) included a 12 year follow-up, with the finding that early physical activity was predictive of behaviour in early adulthood.

It appears that school-based interventions can increase physical activity in the short, and occasionally in the long term. Unfortunately, the enormous variation in content of interventions and measurement of outcomes makes it difficult to draw conclusions as to the characteristics of effective interventions. Effects appear to vary with intensity, duration, and frequency of intervention and with the sex (Dale et al. 1998) and age of the children involved. Interventions are sometimes poorly described so that the effectiveness of individual components in multi-component programs cannot be assessed. Nevertheless, Stone et al (1998) conclude that the best results have been obtained using valid and reliable measures and more extensive interventions. Given the likely health benefits associated with establishing good exercise habits in childhood, the development of effective school-based physical activity interventions must be a priority for future research.

48.5.2 Effective interventions with adults

Interventions with adults have been carried out in a wide variety of settings, including primary care, workplaces, and fitness centres, and have taken a number of different approaches, among them home-based programmes, lifestyle activity programmes, structured activity, and environmental changes. In a quantitative synthesis of 127 studies involving in excess of 130 000 people, Dishman and Buckworth (1996) examined intervention effects and the moderating variables influencing these effects. They concluded that 'interventions for increasing physical activity have a moderately large effect' at least in the short term (only ~25% of studies reported follow-up measures). Effect sizes (weighted by sample size) were larger when the interventions used the principles of behaviour modification, used mediated delivery, targeted groups of mixed ages, sampled apparently healthy people, and encouraged active leisure. Similarly, a review of randomized controlled trials of physical activity (Hillsdon et al. 1995) concluded that sustained high levels of participation were associated with home-based programmes that were informal and unsupervised, but involved frequent professional contact (usually by telephone). Where moderate intensity exercise (e.g. brisk walking) was promoted, adherence was more likely. The success of lifestyle interventions probably lies in their flexibility. Personal, cultural, and social factors can be taken into account and everyday activities such as gardening, doing the shopping on foot, and climbing stairs rather than taking the lift can all contribute to the recommended 30 min/day physical activity.

The finding that the promotion of active leisure or lifestyle, rather than structured, exercise produces greater improvement has a good deal of support, particularly with regard to maintenance of physical activity (Dunn et al. 1998 for a review; Hillsdon et al. 1999; Koffman et al. 2001). However, a recent randomized controlled trial comparing lifestyle and structured interventions found no difference in any outcome after 24 months (Dunn et al. 1999). Both groups had significantly increased their physical activity from baseline and both had declined in the 18 month maintenance period, but it was evident that the decline was less pronounced in the lifestyle exercise group. Likewise, a home-based programme with older adults (King et al. 1995) resulted in significantly greater adherence after 1 year than a structured programme.

The reviews by Dishman and Buckworth (1996) and Hillsdon et al (1995) also highlighted the utility of mediated delivery approaches for long-term adherence.

A recent review by (Marcus *et al*. 1998*b*) also concluded that media-based approaches are effective and economical in a variety of settings, both to enhance face-to-face counselling and as the sole intervention technique. At present, however, the most effective type, frequency, and form of media remains unclear.

Physical activity promotion is an area in which the use of newer interactive technologies may have great potential since the scale of the problem makes face-to-face delivery impractical and prohibitively costly. The proliferation of home computers and their widespread use as a reliable source of health information suggest that the Internet represents an ideal medium for intervention delivery. Not only does it allow proactive recruitment from a vast audience, but also the ability to tailor and target feedback to the characteristics and needs of participants, at times convenient to them (Marcus *et al*. 1998*b*). To date few studies have been published on the use of the Internet to promote physical activity, but the results of a recent pilot study suggest that the situation is set to change rapidly. McKay *et al*. (2001) randomized sedentary diabetes patients to an Internet information-only condition or to an intervention which provided goal-setting and personalized feedback, strategies to overcome barriers, and an online 'personal coach'. There was an overall moderate improvement in levels of physical activity within both intervention and control groups, but patients in the intervention condition who used the site more regularly derived significantly greater benefits than less regular users and control participants. It remains to be seen whether these improvements would be seen in non-clinical populations, and long-term effects remain unknown, but it can be concluded that Internet-based interventions show promise and deserve further investigation.

As previously discussed, computer technology has facilitated the development and delivery of interventions tailored to the specific needs of individuals. Only recently has this approach been applied to physical activity. Bull *et al*. (1999) compared the effectiveness of advice from a family physician plus a standard pamphlet with advice plus a computer-generated tailored pamphlet addressed at stage of change. In contrast to findings in the areas of smoking cessation (Strecher *et al*. 1994) and nutrition (Delichatsios *et al*. 2001*b*), there were no additional benefits of the tailored over the standard intervention. More encouraging are the preliminary results of the PACE+ program for adults (Calfas *et al*. 2002), which was directed at both physical activity and nutrition behaviours. The utility of computer-guided, tailored 'action plans' targeting one exercise and one dietary behaviour was demonstrated by significant improvements in targeted behaviours. Likewise, (Marcus *et al*. 1998*a*) found that participants receiving motivation-matched materials together with individual tailoring via computer expert system took part in significantly more minutes of exercise per week and maintained this level through the 12 month follow-up compared to those receiving standard self-help materials.

The use of computer technology in physical activity promotion is still in its infancy, but its potential to reach large numbers of people is clear. Unfortunately, the very populations that we most need to reach are the least likely to have a computer at home or to even have sufficient experience to use one, although touch-screen technology and audio components may improve applicability to a broader audience.

In the meantime, socio-economically deprived populations remain a neglected focus for research into physical activity promotion, despite the fact that they are twice as likely to be sedentary as more affluent groups (Gordon *et al*. 1999). A review by Taylor *et al*. (1998) found only 4 studies with disabled participants and 10 with ethnic minority populations carried out between 1983 and 1997. Of the latter only two achieved positive improvements and both were weight control programmes for women. Effective interventions with these groups must acknowledge that additional barriers to participation such as language, racism, and cultural appropriateness (e.g. lack of single sex facilities) must be overcome.

48.5.3 Ecological interventions for activity change

An exclusive focus on changing the activity levels of individuals, as has been argued in relation to diet and smoking, is unlikely to result in the development of effective strategies for population-wide change. Environmental and policy interventions are also required to create the conditions in which individual behaviour change is facilitated and supported.

There has been a reduction in the amount of physical activity in daily life over the past few decades, but this does not appear to have been the result of lack of public interest in physical activity. On the contrary, many people now engage in leisure time physical activities, with gyms and jogging being increasingly popular along with home exercise equipment (Tracking the fitness movement 2003: http://www.sgma.com/reports/2003/report1062016991–24961.html). The one exception might be physical activity in the school curriculum, which does appear to have declined substantially. The most dramatic changes have been in the environment. The necessary activity of daily life has decreased as a result of the development of energy saving devices, the use of ergonomic interior designs, and high levels of car ownership, and over recent years the built environment has been increasingly designed for car drivers. Walking and cycling have reduced as a form of transport in many Western countries. The range of attractive and absorbing sedentary activities has increased, with multiple televisions, video, and DVD players in homes, and an increasing range of computer games.

The behaviour change studies described earlier in this section, like the dietary intervention studies, are based on encouraging people to resist the option to be sedentary: to take the stairs when there is the option of the escalator, to walk when transport is available, and to select active rather than passive leisure time activities. There may be additional leverage to be gained from 're-engineering' activity back into the environment. Area-level analyses suggest that people walk more when they live in areas with parks and with traditional street designs, and they take up more sports when sports facilities are available locally (Sallis *et al.* 1998). Of course part of this may be due to different people choosing to live in different environments, but these are questions which could be addressed in a new paradigm of behaviour change research, where behavioural scientists can work with planners, designers, transport experts, and architects to create environments which support, rather than curtail, physical activity.

48.6 Conclusions

In looking at three aspects of health behaviour vital to the reduction of CHD: smoking cessation, increased physical activity, and improved diet, it is clear that the successes achieved at the population level in reducing tobacco use are not yet evident for unhealthy eating and exercise practices. As Mercer *et al.* (2003) suggest, there is much to be learnt from the tobacco experience. Social, cultural, economic, and legislative changes have resulted in a reduction in smoking that has been hailed as 'one of America's 10 greatest public health achievements of the 20th Century' (Centers for Disease Control and Prevention 1999*a, b*) and other countries have seen similar declines. However, even for tobacco the role of specific individual treatments in achieving population level change is limited. In order to make healthy choices of food and physical activity the easy choices, similar structural change may be necessary to complement more micro-level dietary and exercise activity interventions.

Reflecting this, there has been a recent move away from a solely individual-level approach to behaviour change, and what have been termed social ecological models have been proposed (McKinlay 1995; McLeroy *et al.* 1988; Stokols 1992). Their general thesis is that behaviours are promoted and others discouraged by the immediate environment and that environmental and policy variables can add explanatory value above that provided by individual-level factors. McKinlay (1995) argues that achieving long-term behaviour change in the population as a whole requires a combination of 'downstream' (individually based), 'midstream' (organizational/ workplace), and 'upstream' (environmental and policy level) interventions. This multi-level approach is claimed to have greater potential to effect *maintenance* of behaviour change – an aspect sometimes ignored or more often merely assumed to be associated with the same factors as initiation (see Health Psychology 2000). Individual-level interventions may help people to change behaviour in the short term, but once treatment has ceased, powerful societal and industry counterforces may undermine attempts at maintenance, and strong public policy and environmental interventions may be required to overcome these (McKinlay 1995; McKinlay and Marceau 1999).

References

Ajzen, I. (1985). From intention to actions: a theory of planned behavior. In *Action control: from cognitions to behavior* (ed. J. Kuhl and J. Beckman), pp. 11–39. Springer-Verlag, New York.

Ammerman, A. S., Lindquist, C. H., Lohr, K. N., and Hersey, J. (2002). The efficacy of behavioural interventions to modify dietary fat and fruit and vegetable intake: a review of the evidence, *Preventive Medicine*, **35**, 25–41.

Anthonisen, N. R., Connett, J. E., Kiley, J. P., Altose, M. D., Bailey, W. C., Buist, A. S. *et al.* (1994). Effects of smoking intervention and the use of an inhaled anticholinergic bronchodilator on the rate of decline of FEV1: The lung health study, *Journal of the American Medical Association*, **272** (19), 1497–505.

Armitage, C. J. and Conner, M. (2001). Efficacy of the Theory of Planned Behaviour: a meta-analytic review, *British Journal of Social Psychology*, **40**, 471–99.

Aveyard, P., Griffin, C., Lawrence, T., and Cheng, K. (2003). A controlled trial of an expert system and self-help manual based on the stages of change versus standard self-help materials in smoking cessation, *Addiction*, **98**, 345–54.

Baker, A. H. and Wardle, J. (2002). Increasing fruit and vegetable intake among adults attending colorectal screening: the efficacy of a brief tailored intervention, *Cancer Epidemiology, Biomarkers and Prevention*, **11**, 203–6.

Bandura, A. (1986). *Social foundations of thought and action.* Prentice-Hall, Englewood Cliffs, NJ.

Ben-Shlomo, Y., Smith, G. D., Shipley, M. J., and Marmot, M. G. (1994). What determines mortality risk in male former cigarette smokers? *American Journal of Public Health*, **84** (8), 1235–42.

Benowitz, N. L. (1999). Treatment of nicotine dependence in clinical cardiology, *CVD Prevention*, **2**, 135–9.

Benowitz, N. L. and Gourlay, S. G. (1997). Cardiovascular toxicity of nicotine: implications for nicotine replacement therapy, *Journal of the American College of Cardiology*, **29**, 1422–31.

Bingham, S. A. (1991). Limitations of the various methods for collecting dietary intake data, *Annals of Nutrition and Metabolism*, **35** (3), 117–27.

Booth, M., Bauman, A., and Oldenburg, B. *et al.* (1992). Effects of a national mass media campaign on physical activity participation, *Health Promotion International*, **7**, 241–7.

Brunner, E., White, I., Thorogood, M., Bristow, A., Curle, D., and Marmot, M. (1997). Can dietary interventions change diet and cardiovascular risk factors? A meta-analysis of randomized controlled trials, *American Journal of Public Health*, **87**, 1415–22.

Bull, F. C., Jamrozik, K., and Blanksby, B. A. (1999). Tailored advice on exercise: does it make a difference? *American Journal of Preventive Medicine*, **16**, 230–9.

Calfas, K. J., Sallis, J. F., Zabinski, M. F., Wilfley, D. E., Rupp, J., Procaska, J. J. *et al.* (2002). Preliminary evaluation of a multicomponent program for nutrition and physical activity change in primary care: PACE+ for adults, *Preventive Medicine*, **34**, 153–61.

Carleton, R. A., Lasater, T. M., Assaf, A. R., Feldman, H. A., and McKinlay, S. (1995). The Pawtucket Heart Health Program: community changes in cardiovascular risk factors and projected disease risk, *American Journal of Public Health*, **85** (6), 777–85.

Centers for Disease Control and Prevention (1999a). *Achievements in public health, 1900–1999: tobacco use – United States 1900–1999*. Morbidity and Mortality Weekly Reports. Centers for Disease Control and Prevention. Atlanta, GA.

Centers for Disease Control and Prevention (1999b). *Ten greatest public health achievements: United States 1900–1999*. Morbidity and Mortality Weekly Reports. Centers for Disease Control and Prevention. Atlanta, GA.

Ciliska, D., Miles, E., O'Brien, M. A., Turl, C., Tomasik, H. H., Donovan, U., and Beyers, J. (2000). Effectiveness of community-based interventions to increase fruit and vegetable consumption, *Journal of Nutrition Education*, **32**, 341–52.

COMMIT Research Group (1995). Community Intervention Trial for Smoking Cessation (COMMIT), I: cohort results from a four-year community intervention, *American Journal of Public Health*, **85**, 183–92.

Conner, M. and Norman, P. (1995). *Predicting health behaviour: research and practice with social cognition models*. Open University Press, Buckingham.

Cook, D. G., Shaper, A. G., Pocock, S. J., and Kussick, S. J. (1986). Giving up smoking and the risk of heart attack, *Lancet*, **2**, 1376–9.

Dale, D., Corbin, C. B., and Cuddihy, T. F. (1998). Can conceptual physical education promote physically active lifestyles? *Pediatric Exercise Science*, **10**, 97–109.

Delichatsios, H. K., Friedman, R. H., Glanz, K., Tennstedt, S., Smigelski, C., Pinto, B. M. *et al.* (2001a). Randomized trial of a 'talking computer' to improve adults' eating habits, *American Journal of Health Promotion*, **15**, 215–24.

Delichatsios, H. K., Hunt, M. K., Lobb, R., Emmons, K., and Gillman, M. W. (2001b). EatSmart: efficacy of a multifaceted preventive nutrition intervention in clinical practice, *Preventive Medicine*, **33**, 91–8.

Dijkstra, A., De Vries, H., Roijackers, J., and van Breukelen, G. (1998). Tailoring information to enhance quitting in smokers with low motivation to quit: three basic efficacy questions, *Health Psychology*, **17** (6), 513–19.

Dishman, R. K. and Buckworth, J. (1996). Increasing physical activity: a quantitative synthesis, *Medicine and Science in Sports and Exercise*, **28**, 706–19.

Dobson, A. J., Alexander, H. M., Heller, R. F., and Lloyd, D. M. (1991). How soon after quitting smoking does risk of heart attack decline? *Journal of Clinical Epidemiology*, **44** (11), 1247–53.

Donnelly, J. E., Jacobsen, D. J., and Whately, J. E. *et al.* (1996). Nutrition and physical activity program to attenuate obesity and promote physical and metabolic fitness in elementary school children, *Obesity Research*, **4**, 229–43.

Dunn, A. L., Anderson, R. E., and Jakicic, J. M. (1998). Lifestyle physical activity interventions: History, short-and long-term effects, and recommendations, *American Journal of Preventive Medicine*, **15**, 398–412.

Dunn, A. L., Marcus, B. H., Kampert, J. B., Garcia, M. E., Kohl, H. W., and Blair, S. N. (1999). Comparison of lifestyle and structured interventions to increase physical activity and cardiorespiratory fitness: a randomised trial, *Journal of the American Medical Association*, **281**, 327–34.

Ebrahim, S. and Smith, G. D. (1997). Systematic review of randomised controlled trials of multiple risk factor interventions for preventing coronary heart disease, *British Medical Journal*, **314** (7095), 1666.

Farkas, A. J., Pierce, J. P., Zhu, S. H., Rosbrook, B., Gilpin, E. A., Berry, C., and Kaplan, R. M. (1996). Addiction versus stages of change models in predicting smoking cessation, *Addiction*, **91** (9), 1271–80.

Fiore, M., Bailey, W., Cohen, S. *et al.* (2000). *Treating tobacco use and dependence*. Clinical practice guideline. US Department of Health and Human Services, Public Health Service, Rockville, MD.

Fishbein, M. and Ajzen, I. (1975). *Belief, attitude, intention and behavior: an introduction to theory and research*. Addison-Wesley, Reading, MA.

French, S. A., Jeffery, R. W., Story, M., Hannan, P., and Snyder, M. P. (1997*a*). A pricing strategy to promote low-fat snack choices through vending machines, *American Journal of Public Health*, **87** (5), 849–51.

French, S. A., Story, M., Jeffery, R. W., Snyder, P., Eisenberg, M., Sidebottom, A., and Murray, D. (1997*b*). Pricing strategy to promote fruit and vegetable purchase in high school cafeterias, *Journal of the American Dietetic Association*, **97** (9), 1008–10.

French, S. A., Jeffery, R. W., Story, M., Breitlow, K. K., Baxter, J. S., Hannan, P., and Snyder, M. P. (2001). Pricing and promotion effects on low-fat vending snack purchases: the CHIPS Study, *American Journal of Public Health*, **91** (1), 112–17.

Friel, S., Kelleher, C., Campbell, P., and Nolan, G. (1999). Evaluation of the Nutrition Education at Primary School (NEAPS) programme, *Public Health Nutrition*, **2**, 549–55.

Gordon, D., Shaw, M., Dorling, D., and Smith, G. D. (1999). *Inequalities in health: the evidence presented to the independent enquiry into inequalities in health, chaired by Sir Donald Acheson*. Policy Press, Bristol.

Health Psychology (2000). Supplement re papers from a conference 'Maintenance of Behaviour Change in Cardiorespiratory Risk Reduction', **19** (1).

Henderson, M. M., Kushi, L. H., Thompson, D. J., Gorbach, S. L., Clifford, C. K., Insull, W., Jr *et al.* (1990). Feasibility of a randomized trial of a low-fat diet for the prevention of breast cancer: dietary compliance in the Women's Health Trial Vanguard Study, *Preventive Medicine*, **19** (2), 115–33.

Hillsdon, M., Thorogood, M., and Morris, J. (1995). Randomised controlled trials of physical activity promotion in free living populations: a review, *Journal of Epidemiology and Community Health*, **49**, 448–53.

Hillsdon, M., Thorogood, M., and Foster, C. (1999). A systematic review of strategies to promote physical activity. In *Benefits and hazards of exercise* (ed. D. MacAuley), pp. 25–46. British Medical Journal Publications, London.

Hillsdon, M., Cavill, N. A., Nanchahal, K., Diamond, A., and White, I. R. (2001). National level promotion of physical activity: results from England's ACTIVE for LIFE campaign, *Journal of Epidemiology and Community Health*, **55**, 755–61.

Hunt, K. and Emslie, C. (2001). Commentary: the prevention paradox in lay epidemiology, *International Journal of Epidemiology*, **30**, 442–6.

Imperial Cancer Research Fund OXCHECK study group (1995). Effectiveness of health checks conducted by nurses in primary care: final results of the OXCHECK study, *British Medical Journal*, **310**, 1099–104.

Janz, N. K. and Becker, M. H. (1984). The health belief model: a decade later, *Health Education Quarterly*, **11**, 1–47.

Jarvis, M. J. (1997). Patterns and predictors of unaided smoking cessation in the general population. In *The tobacco epidemic*, 28th edn (ed. C. T. Bolliger and K. O. Fagerstrom), pp. 151–64. Karger, Basel.

Jarvis, M., West, R., Tunstall Pedoe, H., and Vesey, C. (1984). An evaluation of the intervention against smoking in the multiple risk factor intervention trial, *Preventive Medicine*, **13** (5), 501–9.

Jeffery, R. W. and Utter, J. (2003). The changing environment and population obesity in the United States, *Obesity Research*, **11**(Suppl.), 12S–22S.

Joseph, A. M., Norman, S. M., Ferry, L. H., Prochazka, A. V., Westman, E. C., Steele, B. G. *et al.* (1996). The safety of transdermal nicotine as an aid to smoking cessation in patients with cardiac disease, *New England Journal of Medicine*, **335** (24), 1792–8.

King, A. C., Haskell, W. L., Young, D. R., Oka, R. K., and Stefanick, M. L. (1995). Long-term effects of varying intensities and formats of physical activity on participation rates, fitness and lipoproteins in men and women aged 50 to 65 years, *Circulation*, 9 (2596), 2604.

Koffman, D. M., Bazzarre, T., Mosca, L., Redberg, R., Schmid, T., and Wattigney, W. A. (2001). An evaluation of Choose to Move 1999: an American Heart Association physical activity program for women, *Archives of Internal Medicine*, 161, 2193–9.

Kristal, A. R., Curry, S. J., Shattuck, A. L., Feng, Z., and Li, S. (2000). A randomized trial of a tailored self-help dietary intervention: The Puget Sound Eating Patterns Study, *Preventive Medicine*, 31, 380–9.

Lando, H. A., Pechacek, T. F., Pirie, P. L., Murray, D. M., Mittelmark, M. B., Lichtenstein, E. *et al.* (1995). Changes in adult cigarette smoking in the Minnesota Heart Health Program, *American Journal of Public Health*, 85 (2), 201–8.

Luepker, R. V., Perry, C. L., McKinlay, S. M., Nader, P. R., Parcel, G. S., Stone, E. J. *et al.* (1996). Outcomes of a field trial to improve children's dietary patterns and physical activity, *Journal of the American Medical Association*, 275 (768), 776.

Lynch, B. S. and Bonnie, R. J. (eds) (1994). *Growing up tobacco free: preventing nicotine addiction in children and youths*. National Academy Press, Washington, DC.

Malina, R. M. (1996). Tracking of physical activity and physical fitness across the lifespan, *Research Quarterly in Exercise and Sport*, 57, 48–57.

Marcus, A. C., Heimendinger, J., Wolfe, P., Fairclough, D., Rimer, B. K., Morra, M. *et al.* (2001). A randomized trial of a brief intervention to increase fruit and vegetable intake: a replication study among callers to the CIS, *Preventive Medicine*, 33, 204–16.

Marcus, B. H., Bock, B. C., Pinto, B. M., Forsyth, L. H., Roberts, M. B., and Traficante, R. M. (1998*a*). Efficacy of an individualized, motivationally-tailored physical activity intervention, *Annals of Behavioural Medicine*, 20 (3), 174–80.

Marcus, B. H., Owen, N., Forsyth, L. H., Cavill, N. A., and Fridinger, F. (1998*b*). Physical activity interventions using mass media, print media, and information technology, *American Journal of Preventive Medicine*, 15 (4), 362–78.

Marcus, B. H., Dubbert, P. M., Forsyth, L. H., McKenzie, T. L., Stone, E. J., Dunn, A. L., and Blair, S. N. (2000). Physical activity behavior change: issues in adoption and maintenance, *Health Psychology*, 19 (1) (Suppl.), 32–41.

Marshall, S. J. and Biddle, S. J. (2001). The transtheoretical model of behavior change: a meta-analysis of applications to physical activity and exercise, *Annals of Behavioural Medicine*, 23 (4), 229–46.

McKay, H. G., King, D., Eakin, E. G., Seeley, J. R., and Glasgow, R. E. (2001). The diabetes network internet-based physical activity intervention: a randomised pilot study, *Diabetes Care*, 24, 1328–34.

McKenzie, T. L., Sallis, J. F., Kolody, B., and Faucett, F. N. (1997). Long-term effects of a physical education curriculum and staff development work: SPARK, *Research Quarterly in Exercise and Sport*, 68, 280–91.

McKinlay, J. B. (1995). The new public health approach to improving physical activity and autonomy in older populations. In *Preparation for aging* (ed. E. Heikkinen), pp. 87–103. Plenum Press, New York.

McKinlay, J. B. and Marceau, L. D. (1999). A tale of 3 tails. *American Journal of Public Health*, 89, 295–8.

McLeroy, K. R., Bibeau, D., Steckler, A., and Glanz, K. (1988). An ecological perspective on health promotion programs, *Health Education Quarterly*, 15, 351–77.

Mercer, S. L., Green, L. W., Rosenthal, A. C., Husten, C. G., Khan, L. K., and Dietz, W. H. (2003). Possible lessons from the tobacco experience for obesity control, *American Journal of Clinical Nutrition*, 77(Suppl.), 1073S–1082S.

Merzel, C. and D'Affliti, J. (2003). Reconsidering community-based health promotion: promise, performance and potential, *American Journal of Public Health*, 93, 557–74.

MRFIT (Multiple Risk Factor Intervention Trial) Research Group (1982). Multiple Risk Factor Intervention Trial: risk factor changes and mortality results, *Journal of the American Medical Association*, 248 (12), 1465–77.

Nader, P. R., Stone, E. J., Lytle, L. A., Perry, C. L., Osganian, S. K., Kelder, S. *et al.* (1999). Three-year maintenance of improved diet and physical activity: the CATCH cohort. Child and Adolescent Trial for Cardiovascular Health, *Archives of Pediatric and Adolescent Medicine*, **153**, 695–704.

National Institute for Clinical Excellence (2002). *Guidance on the use of nicotine replacement therapy (NRT) and bupropion for smoking cessation.* Technology appraisal guidance no. 39. National Institute for Clinical Excellence, London.

Nestle, M. (2002). *Food politics: how the food industry influences nutrition and health.* University of California Press, Berkeley.

Ni Mhurchu, C., Margetts, B. M., and Speller, V. (1998). Randomized clinical trial comparing the effectiveness of two dietary interventions for patients with hyperlipidaemia, *Clinical Science*, **95**, 479–87.

Nutbeam, D., Macaskill, P., Smith, C., Simpson, J. M., and Catford, J. (1993). Evaluation of two school smoking education programmes under normal classroom conditions, *British Medical Journal*, **306** (6870), 102–7.

Orleans, C. T. (2000). Promoting the maintenance of health behavior change: recommendations for the next generation of research and practice, *Health Psychology*, **19** (1) (Suppl.), 76–83.

Parker, L. and Fox, A. (2001). The Peterborough Schools Nutrition Project: a multiple intervention programme to improve school-based eating in secondary schools, *Public Health Nutrition*, **4**, 1221–8.

Perry, C. L., Bishop, D. B., Taylor, G., Murray, D. M., Mays, R. W., Dudovitz, B. S. *et al.* (1998). Changing fruit and vegetable consumption among children: the 5-a-Day Power Plus program in St. Paul, Minnesota, *American Journal of Public Health*, **88**, 603–9.

Perry, C. L., Klepp, K. I., and Halper, A. (1987). Promoting healthy eating and physical activity patterns among adolescents: a pilot study of 'Slice of Life', *Health Education Research*, **1**, 93–103.

Prochaska, J. O. and DiClemente, C. C. (1983). Stages and processes of self-change in smoking: toward an integrative model of change, *Journal of Consulting and Clinical Psychology*, **51**, 390–5.

Prochaska, J. O., DiClemente, C. C., and Norcross, J. C. (1992). In search of how people change. Applications to addictive behaviors, *American Psychologist*, **47** (9), 1102–14.

Prochaska, J. O., Velicer, W. F., Fava, J. L., Rossi, J. S., and Tsoh, J. Y. (2001). Evaluating a population-based recruitment approach and a stage-based expert system intervention for smoking cessation, *Addictive Behaviours*, **26** (4), 583–602.

Puska, P., Tuomilehto, J., Salonen, J., Neittaanmaki, L., Maki, J., Virtamo, J. *et al.* (1979). Changes in coronary risk factors during comprehensive five-year community programme to control cardiovascular diseases (North Karelia project), *British Medical Journal*, **2** (6199), 1173–8.

Raw, M., McNeill, A., and West, R. (1998). Smoking cessation guidelines for health professionals, *Thorax*, **53**, S1–S38.

Raynor, H. A. and Epstein, L. H. (2001). Dietary variety, energy regulation, and obesity, *Psychological Bulletin*, **127** (3), 325–41.

Resnicow, K., Jackson, A., Braithwaite, R., DiIorio, C., Blisset, D., Rahotep, S., and Periasamy, S. (2002). Healthy Body/Healthy Spirit: a church-based nutrition and physical activity intervention, *Health Education Research*, **17**, 562–73.

Roe, L., Hunt, P., Bradshaw, H., and Rayner, M. (1997). *Health promotion interventions to promote healthy eating in the general population: a review.* Health Education Authority, London.

Rolls, B. J., Roe, L. S., Kral, T. V., Meengs, J. S., and Wall, D. E. (2004*a*). Increasing the portion size of a packaged snack increases energy intake in men and women, *Appetite*, **42** (1), 63–9.

Rolls, B. J., Roe, L. S., Meengs, J. S., and Wall, D. E. (2004*b*). Increasing the portion size of a sandwich increases energy intake, *Journal of the American Dietetic Association*, **104** (3), 367–72.

Rosenberg, L., Kaufman, D. W., Helmrish, S. P., and Shapiro, S. (1985). The risk of myocardial infarction after quitting smoking in men under 55 years of age, *New England Journal of Medicine*, **313**, 1511–14.

Sahota, P., Rudolf, M. C. J., Dixey, R., Hill, A. J., Barth, J. H., and Cade, J. (2001). Randomised controlled trial of primary school based intervention to reduce risk factors for obesity, *British Medical Journal*, **323**, 1029–32.

Sallis, J. F., Bauman, A., and Pratt, M. (1998). Environmental and policy interventions to promote physical activity, *American Journal of Preventive Medicine*, **15**, 379–97.

Silagy, C. (2000). Physician advice for smoking cessation (Cochrane Review). In *The Cochrane Library*, Issue 3, 2000. Update Software, Oxford.

Silagy, C., Lancaster, T., Stead, L., Mant, D., and Fowler, G. (2000). Nicotine replacement therapy for smoking cessation (Cochrane Review). in *The Cochrane Library*, Issue 1, 2003 (ed. T. Lancaster, C. Silagy, and D. Fullerton). Update Software, Oxford.

Simons-Morton, B., Parcel, G. S., Baranowski, J., Forthofer, R., and O'Hara, N. M. (1991). Promoting physical activity and a healthful diet among children: results of a school-based intervention study, *American Journal of Public Health*, **81**, 986–91.

Steptoe, A., Doherty, S., Rink, E., Kerry, S., Kendrick, T., and Hilton, S. (1999a). Behavioural counselling in general practice for the promotion of healthy behaviour among adults at increased risk of coronary heart disease: randomised trial, *British Medical Journal*, **319**, 943–7.

Steptoe, A., Doherty, S., Rink, E., Kerry, S., Kendrick, T., Hilton, S., and Day, S. (1999b). Behavioural counselling in general practice for the promotion of healthy behaviour among adults at increased risk of coronary heart disease: randomised trial. Commentary: Treatment allocation by the method of minimisation, *British Medical Journal*, **319** (7215), 943–8.

Stevens, V. J., Glasgow, R. E., Toobert, D. J., Karanja, N., and Smith, K. S. (2003). One-year results from a brief, computer-assisted intervention to decrease consumption of fat and increase consumption of fruit and vegetables, *Preventive Medicine*, **36**, 594–600.

Stokols, D. (1992). Establishing and maintaining healthy environments: toward a social ecology of health promotion, *American Psychologist*, **47** (1), 6–22.

Stone, E. J., McKenzie, T. L., Welk, G. J., and Booth, M. L. (1998). Effects of physical activity interventions in youth, *American Journal of Preventive Medicine*, **15**, 298–315.

Strecher, V. J., Kreuter, M., Den Boer, D. J., Kobrin, S., Hospers, H., and Skinner, C. S. (1994). The effects of computer-tailored smoking cessation messages in family practice settings, *Journal of Family Practice*, **39**, 262–70.

Stubbs, J., Ferres, S., and Horgan, G. (2000). Energy density of foods: effects on energy intake, *Critical Reviews in Food Science and Nutrition*, **40** (6), 481–515.

Sutton, S. (1999). A critical review of the transtheoretical model applied to smoking cessation. In *Understanding and changing health behaviour: from health beliefs to self-regulation* (ed. P. Norman, C. Abraham, and M. Conner), pp. 207–25. Harwood Academic, New York.

Taylor, W. C., Baranowski, T., and Young, D. R. (1998). Physical activity interventions in low-income, ethnic minority, and populations with disability, *American Journal of Preventive Medicine*, **15**, 334–43.

Tedstone, A. E., Aviles, M., Shetty, P., and Daniels, L. A. (1998). *Effectiveness of interventions to promote healthy eating in pre-school children aged 1–5 years: a review*. Health Education Authority, London.

Tell, G. S. and Vellar, O. D. (1987). Noncommunicable disease risk factor intervention in Norwegian adolescents: The Oslo Youth Study. In *Cardiovascular risk factors in childhood: epidemiology and prevention* (ed. B. Hetzel and G. Berenson), pp. 123–49. Elsevier Science, Amsterdam.

Tinker, L. F., Patterson, R. E., Kristal, A. R., Bowen, D., Kuniyuki, A., Henry, H., and Shattuck, A. (2001). Measurement characteristics of 2 different self-monitoring tools used in a dietary intervention study, *Journal of the American Dietetic Association*, **101**, 1031–40.

Tonstad, S., Farsang, C., Klaene, G., Lewis, K., Manolis, A., Perruchoud, A. P. *et al.* (2003). Bupropion SR for smoking cessation in smokers with cardiovascular disease: a multicentre, randomised study, *European Heart Journal*, **24** (10), 946–55.

Tudor-Smith, C., Nutbeam, D., Moore, L., and Catford, J. (1998). Effects of the Heartbeat Wales programme over five years on behavioural risks for cardiovascular disease: quasi-experimental comparison of results from Wales and a matched reference area, *British Medical Journal*, **316** (7134), 818–22.

Weinstein, N. D. (1988). The precaution adoption process, *Health Psychology*, **7**, 355–86.

White, E., Shattuck, A. L., Kristal, A. R., Urban, N., Prentice, R. L., Henderson, M. M. *et al.* (1992). Maintenance of a low-fat diet: follow-up of the Women's Health Trial, *Cancer Epidemiology, Biomarkers & Prevention*, **1** (4), 315–23.

Wilcox, S., Parra-Medina, D., Thompson-Robinson, M., and Will, J. (2001). Nutrition and physical activity interventions to reduce cardiovascular disease risk in health care settings: a quantitative review with a focus on women, *Nutrition Reviews*, **59**, 197–215.

Wimbush, E., MacGregor, A., and Fraser, E. (1998). Impacts of a national mass media campaign on walking in Scotland, *Health Promotion International*, **13**, 45–53.

Wood, D. A., Kinmonth, A. L., Davies, G. A., Yarwood, J., Thompson, S. G., Pyke, S. D. M. *et al.* (1994). Randomised controlled trial evaluating cardiovascular screening and intervention in general practice: principal results of British family heart study, *British Medical Journal*, **308** (6924), 313–20.

World Health Organization (1998). *Obesity: preventing and managing the global epidemic.* WHO Technical Report 894. World Health Organization, Geneva.

Chapter 49

Contributions to change: treatment

H. Tunstall-Pedoe

49.1 **Does treatment work?**

At the beginning of the 1980s, while working on the protocol for the WHO MONICA Project (Tunstall-Pedoe 1988, 2003), I visited the World Health Organization Headquarters in Geneva. Among other things, I was there to speak to an expert on medical care about our need to define an index of coronary care that we could use in this study. We had hypothesized that, at the population level, trends in coronary risk factors determined the trends in coronary event rates (by coronary events we meant acute myocardial infarctions and coronary deaths). We also had hypothesized that trends in 28 day case fatality (percentage of events that were fatal at 28 days from the onset – the complement of survival rates) were determined by trends in the acute treatment of the attack, known as acute coronary care.

There was an extensive literature at that time on measurement of risk factors and on coronary risk-factor scoring systems. It was less obvious how we were to measure coronary care and therefore how to score it. For one thing, we knew that most coronary deaths occurred suddenly outside hospital. Although many victims had seen a doctor within the last month or so, these were for varied reasons. The bulk of sudden deaths outside hospital were medically unattended in that there was no direct contact with doctors or other medical workers between the onset of the acute episode and the sudden death that followed. Indeed previous work in Belfast (McNeilly and Pemberton 1968) and on the European Myocardial Infarction Community Registers had suggested that half of all coronary deaths occurred suddenly or within a very few minutes (World Health Organization Regional Office for Europe 1976). Two-thirds of coronary deaths occurred in the same place as the onset (Tunstall-Pedoe *et al.* 1975). Our hypothesis on coronary care at that time, therefore, seemed less credible than that on risk factors, but worth testing nonetheless, as a huge amount of medical effort was being put into coronary care.

The expert advice I was given by the World Health Organization's leading authority on medical care was essentially negative. The influence of doctors on disease was generally harmful, I was told. There was no good evidence that medical care affected the course of any of the chronic non-infectious diseases of middle and old age. MONICA was wasting its time. There was no such thing as good or bad coronary care. We would not be able to measure or score coronary care because it was ineffective. There was nothing relevant to measure. Fortunately we ignored this advice (see later).

49.2 **Public health, therapeutic nihilism, and the noble savage**

My adviser followed a distinguished tradition in the public health medicine of the early decades after the Second World War. Doctors who believed in treatment became physicians, surgeons, and general practitioners, where they could prescribe medicines and plan operations and other interventions without limit. Many of the then conventional drugs and interventions were of unproven benefit, and some, in retrospect, were definitely harmful. In the absence of real evidence, doctors deluded themselves and their patients with claims and anecdotes. Their critics in the profession, the sceptics and agnostics, were often recruited into public health medicine. This took an environmental or ecological attitude. Going back to the classic and later physicians such as Hippocrates and Thomas Sydenham, it was also strongly influenced by nineteenth century reformers, such as Rudolf Virchow, and by social and political theories. Disease was not so much an individual as a social problem, which could be prevented by drains and clean water, by good diet, good housing, benign employment which did not involve too much real work, and by social engineering to reduce inequality. In a healthy environment most diseases would disappear, or would get better by themselves without medical intervention. In the words of his Second World War prisoner-of-war camp Kommandant quoted by the late Archie Cochrane (after whom the Cochrane Collaboration is named), 'Doctors are superfluous' (Cochrane 1972).

In the 1970s a nihilistic or agnostic approach to existing therapies for many diseases, other than for relief of symptoms, was justified. For example, it was possible to superimpose the charts for incidence rates of cancer of the lung and the stomach, derived from cancer registers, on top of those for national mortality rates from the Registrar General. Incidence and death rates were virtually identical. Five-year survival rates after treatment were so low that if you came across a long-term survivor you wondered if the tumour had been atypical, or the diagnosis incorrect. While the protagonists of new treatments and 'breakthroughs' trumpeted their success and ability to save thousands of lives, concurrent epidemiological data of mortality rates often showed monotonous consistency: either no change, or even trends going in the wrong direction – upwards.

For much of the twentieth century, trends in mortality from different diseases seemed to be more influenced by whatever was causing them in the first place than by later interventions. Many diseases went through a progression of first attacking the wealthy, then the whole population indiscriminately, and then the poor, before declining. Peptic ulcers were an example. Of course, antibiotics had been a triumphant success, but only applicable to certain infections. 'Concentrate on causation or immunization' seemed the best precept for public health. This was shown by the legislation on atmospheric air pollution in the 1950s, and more recent campaigns to control cigarette smoking, which have led to a greater fall in deaths from chronic obstructive lung disease than was achieved by the millions of antibiotic prescriptions used for it over the years.

Some of the ideas of public health medicine at that time resonated with the myth of the noble savage. This is still prevalent both among some public health people and in the public fascination with alternative and traditional medicine. Somewhere, out of touch with modern civilization, like biblical man in a state of grace in the Garden of Eden before the Fall, were healthy, long-living noble savages. They had no need for modern medicine, only for simple folk and herbal remedies, because they had not been corrupted and ruined by industrialization and its morbid lifestyles. This attractive myth remains surprisingly prevalent, by implication even if not spoken out loud, despite much evidence that the life of primitive man was often brutish and short. Most twentieth century exemplars live on the edge of starvation, often stunted, anaemic, malarious, and riddled with other parasites such as worms. But in the mythical past, and the mythical future, whether Eden or Utopia, neither expensive doctors treating disease, nor multinational, profit-making drug companies, would be really necessary.

An innocent medication free state of nature was equated with health. This attractive myth (attractive because it implied that the expense of medical care was not necessary – all that was needed was merely a radical change in society) was subsequently overtaken by a revolutionary era in treatment of heart disease. This dated approximately from the end of the 1970s to 1995.

Before that happened, however, there were a number of false dawns that were greeted with fanfares of trumpets at the time, and tremendous enthusiasm. Subsequent disappointment that they had not fulfilled their promise at the time reinforced the polarization of convictions between enthusiasts that treatment did work, and sceptics that it did not. This further explains the reluctance of the latter to recognize the real dawn when it occurred. Two such examples were oral anticoagulation and acute coronary care. The history of these treatments illustrates the problems of obtaining evidence on the impact of treatment on cardiovascular disease, and the pitfalls arising from erroneous interpretation of data.

49.3 The first false dawn: oral anticoagulation for myocardial infarction

During the 1950s and early 1960s one false dawn was the use of oral anticoagulation for patients with myocardial infarction. It was initiated (correctly, despite a subsequent fashion for claiming the opposite) on the argument that myocardial infarction was a consequence of thrombosis in the coronary arteries and that long-term oral anticoagulation should reduce the tendency to further thrombosis. Cardiologists were passionately committed on whether or not to use anticoagulants on their patients. At the London Hospital in the late 1960s I was told of one eminent (then retired) cardiologist from that era who would not have his patients 'fed rat poison'. The junior medical staff were so convinced that he was wrong that all his patients had two drug charts, one without anticoagulants for his ward rounds, and another for daily use, the nursing staff being party to the conspiracy. (It might even have been true that later on he knew about it and connived at it to save public recantation.) In 1965, as a junior doctor at the Brompton Hospital managing the anticoagulant clinic, I was under instruction to wean coronary patients off long-term anticoagulation, despite the great Paul Wood having told them years earlier that their lives depended on it and they must take the tablets for life. He had died and was not able to revise his opinion.

The benefits claimed and looked for in the initial studies did not seem to be borne out by experience, probably because they were exaggerated. Clinical trials tended to be too small to demonstrate a size of effect that would be modest, but still useful in practice. Anticoagulants were greeted with enthusiasm, became standard therapy in many units for some years, and then went out of fashion. Various attempts at reviews and analyses have been made over the years (International Anticoagulant Review Group 1970; Anand and Yusuf 1999). The latest incorporate the newer trials. The conclusion is that long-term oral anticoagulation does work, but not as dramatically as was originally claimed. Further very large studies would be needed to establish this comprehensively. Oral anticoagulants are not entirely safe and there are now newer treatments that are more up to date. The fashion has passed.

49.4 The second false dawn: acute coronary care and mobile coronary care units

Next in the 1960s came claims of remarkable results for acute coronary care. Admission of all patients with suspected myocardial infarction into specialized hospital units was widely claimed to drop the mortality of myocardial infarction by half. In these units cardiac rhythm was monitored on oscilloscopes and harmful rhythms were to be controlled by suppressive drugs or reversed by electric defibrillation. The claims were sustained by eyewitness accounts of the results of cardiopulmonary resuscitation in which sufferers from myocardial infarction were apparently raised from the dead. A bandwagon began to roll faster and faster, apparently sweeping all before it. Acute coronary care could halve the burden of coronary deaths, given the resources it increasingly demanded (Day 1962; Caswell 1967).

However, closer examination showed that numbers did not add up. Numbers of lives known to be saved directly by resuscitation and intervention were disproportionate to the alleged numbers of deaths prevented. Successful cardiopulmonary resuscitation in the coronary care unit was comparatively uncommon, although it undeniably occurred. More cardiac arrests occurred in the accident and emergency department before the patient was formally admitted to hospital, and many more deaths than that occurred outside hospital. Hospital clinicians' claims to halve 'mortality' were seen to apply only to patients coming under their care, not the population as a whole. What they called 'mortality rates' were what epidemiologists called the 'case fatality', inherently different things. The hospital and whole population perspective are quite different (Chambless et al. 1997).

Most of the triumphant reporting of acute coronary care was based either on case series of successful resuscitations – numerators without denominators – or on before-and-after comparisons of what happened when coronary care units were opened in large hospitals where they had not previously existed. Such comparisons showed that, in general, case fatality fell dramatically, indeed it often halved.

Another indicator of success was that the workload for myocardial infarction increased considerably. There was now an imperative to recognize potential cases of myocardial infarction, whether in the community, the emergency department, or the general hospital wards, and to send the patients for coronary care. Clinicians were delighted to be making a real impact on a major killer and felt the sacrifice of their (or their junior staff's) time and leisure was worthwhile. It was obvious to them that a major increase in hospital resources for coronary care was needed to sustain and generalize this manifest improvement over the longer term (Joint Working Party 1975).

It was Geoffrey Rose, to whom this book is dedicated, who put these two observations on coronary care together in what should be a classic paper. It appeared in a specialist epidemiological journal that was not read by clinicians. One wonders whether it had been rejected previously elsewhere. The findings did not support the enthusiasm for coronary care (Rose 1975).

Rose compared hospital figures for admissions and deaths from myocardial infarction with those from national mortality statistics over the period in which coronary care was introduced in England and Wales. Hospital admissions for myocardial infarction had increased dramatically at the same time that hospital case fatality had fallen. Overall numbers of deaths from coronary disease in the population of England and Wales had not substantially changed, neither had the number or proportion of such deaths occurring in hospital. Hospital coronary care, therefore, had sucked a large number of previously undiagnosed or unreported cases of myocardial infarction into specialized hospital units and had diagnosed them. Other than that, it was difficult to demonstrate what coronary care had done at that time, despite the anecdotal evidence. Whatever it did or did not do for patients, it trained a generation of cardiologists to be concerned with coronary heart disease, a disease previously neglected, although it was killing more people than any other single cause in industrialized countries.

At about this time Archie Cochrane was proselytizing for a group that was trying to put the '50% mortality reduction' to the test by persuading coronary care physicians and general practitioners to collaborate in a regional study in which, where it was feasible, myocardial infarction cases recognized in the community were randomized to home care or to hospital coronary care unit management. At that time, many myocardial infarction patients were being diagnosed or suspected in general practice. Some patients insisted on staying at home. Others had to be sent to hospital for medical or social reasons. In-between was a group which, at that time, it was considered ethical (after argument) to randomize to home or hospital care. Setting the study up was a considerable undertaking, and the proportion of cases randomized was not great.

Part-way through the study one of the coordinators who was in the know claims that he wickedly showed a cardiologist that there was a non-significant trend developing in favour of hospital coronary care. He was told that home care was unethical. He then revealed that he had swapped the labels and it was actually home care that was winning. He then asked the cardiologist whether hospital care should be abandoned (Cochrane 1972). Final results showed no definite statistical advantage to either, but definitive publication was delayed for a long time while the authors of the paper wrangled over what the study really showed and what it really meant (Mather et al. 1971, 1976). The study was criticized for the low proportion of cases that were randomized. It was also suggested, to explain the result, which was in an era before mobile coronary care units or ambulances equipped with defibrillators were common, that it was the transport to hospital in an attack which did the damage, neutralizing the benefit of coronary care after arrival. Evidence for the harmful effects of ordinary transport by ambulance was not forthcoming and is still controversial.

Home care for myocardial infarction must now be exceptionally rare in economically advanced countries unless there is a misdiagnosis. Hospital care is now almost universal. It is now better justified by what can be done in hospital. However, the change in medical management that occurred from the 1960s through to the early 1980s – implying that everyone with myocardial infarction must have coronary care – preceded the real evidence that this was necessary. Propaganda for benefit ran well ahead of the evidence, making it risky in terms of the relationship between the general practitioner and his or her patients and their families to keep someone at home in a heart attack and run the risk of losing them unattended. Better to die in hospital surrounded by specialists and nurses and lots of equipment. Publicity for coronary care therefore led to universal hospitalization for myocardial infarction of those who were alive.

However, the majority of coronary deaths were known to occur outside hospital (McNeilly and Pemberton 1968) and this had led to the idea of mobile coronary ambulances, manned by doctors in the Belfast model (Pantridge and Geddes 1967), by ambulancemen in Brighton (Briggs et al. 1976), and by firemen and other paramedics in Seattle and other cities (Cobb et al. 1976). In the last 15 years it has become standard to equip emergency ambulances with defibrillators and with crews equipped to use them. Although able to achieve worthwhile saving of lives when well-organized in cities where the geography favours rapid communication and access, such savings are modest compared with the death toll from coronary heart disease, a large proportion of which occurs at home and unwitnessed (Cobb and Hallstrom 1982; Pell et al. 2001). Now electronic witnesses can provide the answer coupled to implantable cardioverter defibrillators, but these are expensive and can only be used in persons previously identified as at high risk (Brodsky et al. 2002).

During the decade in which hospital coronary care was first introduced, early 1960s to early 1970s, population mortality rates in some countries began to come down. In others they remained stable or even increased. The claimed mortality reduction in hospital coronary care units was not obviously impacting on the bottom line, population mortality rates. It is arguable that the natural history and prognosis of coronary heart disease was unaffected by coronary care at that time. There were some drugs being used that were shown subsequently to be beneficial. There were others in common use that were probably harmful, and others still which have never been properly investigated (for example, the widespread use of benzodiazepine tranquillizers in coronary care units).

49.5 Randomized controlled trials and the coronary care revolution

Beginning in the 1960s, but reaching its peak between the early 1980s and the end of the century, there occurred a revolution in coronary care based on the development of new treatments, their formal testing in really large, well-designed, randomized controlled trials (RCTs), and their widespread adoption into clinical practice, often by the clinicians and units who had participated in testing them. RCTs had been developed by British statisticians for agricultural experiments and first appeared in clinical medicine at the end of the 1940s in Medical Research Council trials of anti-tuberculous drugs (Daniels and Hill 1952), but were slow to catch on. Many clinicians in the 1960s and 1970s considered that elaborate testing protocols for treatments were not necessary and should not replace clinical judgement, and that randomization itself was unethical, a viewpoint shared by some journalists who labelled randomization 'an obscene lottery'. Introduced first into some English-speaking countries, the RCT was adopted in Scandinavia, but met resistance elsewhere in Europe where clinicians in the 1970s still preened themselves that: 'In my country, thank God, randomized controlled trials are still illegal and unethical.' In the middle 1970s a trainee physician from a middle-European country spent some weeks with us in Geoffrey Rose's Department of Epidemiology at St Mary's Hospital Medical School in London, where I was then senior lecturer. He returned home to his university medical school, where he was asked to address the postgraduate weekly meeting. 'In future' he told the assembly, 'doctors will only use those treatments that have been validated as beneficial and safe by properly conducted randomized controlled trials.' For this outrage he was immediately exiled to a provincial hospital, where, he wrote to tell us, patients waiting to see him in the outpatient clinic had a view of the local cemetery. It made them very thoughtful.

49.6 Can results of trials be generalized?

Although RCTs had appeared in the 1940s, many early trials were insufficiently powerful to detect anything other than major benefits or risks. As a consequence, results were often inconclusive or contradictory. Too much information and consequent time and effort were involved in each case. It took some decades for it to be accepted that very large trials were needed, owing much to the leadership of the Oxford ISIS group, involving the disciplined participation of clinicians in many different centres. Such studies could not be done without major funding by government agencies or interested drug companies. Entry criteria had to be very simple, as did the treatment protocol and information requested. These studies involved the sacrifice of individual judgement as most clinician participants were not contributing intellectually to the study, although they were contributing cases (Vanuzzo *et al.* 2000).

When treatments are being pioneered there may be restrictions and disqualifications that appear wise at the time and which are built into the definitions of eligibility for large trials. Trials may be restricted by age and sex, even ethnicity, and may exclude some common comorbidities or subtypes of the disease being investigated. The responsible clinicians may have the option not to randomize particular patients unless they wish to do so, and the list of exclusions gives an opportunity for such an excuse.

This means that some trials of treatment by drug D for disease X involve only a minority of patients seen with X. The result of the trial may be to show significant benefit to those patients with X who were treated. There may then be doubts as to whether the results can be generalized to all patients with X and whether mass use of D across whole populations would produce the same benefit as is seen in the trials. Doubters might argue that misuse or abuse of the drug may result in harm as well as good, leading to no net benefit, or even harm. Enthusiasts may argue that the high-risk exclusions from trials may be exactly those cases that would benefit most. Even, therefore, when major studies have demonstrated substantial benefit from use of drug D, its use in practice outside the original study group may be controversial, and its impact in population terms, after widespread introduction on disease X, unknown.

A drug whose impact appears to be miraculous in a specific trial can have no impact on the population burden of the disease if it is prohibitively expensive, if it is only used in specialist units, and if its use is inhibited by alarming restrictions – all of these would result in failure to use it across the spectrum of the disease. A drug cannot work if it is not used. For reasons given, where it is widely adopted, it is still not possible to state categorically what its impact is going to be, although estimates would be enhanced by knowing on whom, when, and where it is being used.

49.7 Acute coronary care versus secondary prevention

Successful intervention between the onset of an acute coronary event and its potential fatal outcome cannot be guaranteed. One half of coronary deaths occur instantaneously or within the first hour, whereas the majority of cases of myocardial infarction have not come under care within that time (McNeilly and Pemberton 1968; Tunstall-Pedoe *et al.* 1975). In the age groups in which coronary deaths occur, victims spend most of their time in their own homes where a good half of coronary deaths are not witnessed – any spouse or partner often being in a different room in the home. So-called 'acute coronary care', even in the best hands, was therefore always arguably sub-acute. It was available for those who had survived the initial impact of the coronary event. Those who came under care or reached hospital had weathered the initial storm.

It can be shown in the findings from population registration of coronary events in high incidence countries that approximately half of new events in those below age 65 occur in subjects with a previous history of myocardial infarction or diagnosed angina pectoris. Really sudden death in an attack is relatively more common in younger victims, particularly men, with no previous history of coronary heart disease. This means that some 30% of coronary deaths occur suddenly in those with no previous history of vascular disease (Tunstall-Pedoe *et al.* 1996). But there are 70% of deaths in which death is delayed or has some coronary disease precedent. Thus, while half of all coronary deaths are so sudden that they may not be suitable for coronary care *in the attack itself*, when previous history is taken into account the statistics are less depressing. The argument that I once used that two-thirds of coronary deaths are so sudden that intervention in the attack is problematic, approximating to Russian roulette, presupposes that it is acute coronary care (treatment in the attack itself) that matters and not what came before.

RCTs of medical interventions in coronary care have tended to show that drug treatments used acutely in myocardial infarction also have a continuing action during convalescence from the acute event. They may also be long-term prophylactics in terms of acute recurrence of a coronary event in survivors of myocardial infarction or first event in those with angina pectoris. Whereas 30 years ago drugs were considered to be specific for acute coronary care, beta-blockers, aspirin, and angiotensin-converting enzyme (ACE) inhibitor drugs are used both in acute management of myocardial infarction and in its long-term prophylaxis. These drugs are increasingly used in 'secondary prevention', that is, to prevent the progression of symptomatic vascular disease (Vanuzzo *et al*. 2000).

It is arguable that ensuring that a coronary patient has secondary prophylactic drugs on board before he or she has a potential acute event is more important and reliable than the inevitably delayed treatment they may or may not receive once such an event has started (Tunstall-Pedoe 2002). The most dramatic change in philosophy over the last 10–15 years has, therefore, been the swing in emphasis away from exclusive emphasis on management of an acute coronary event and towards ensuring that patients with evidence of vascular disease and/or angina receive adequate 'secondary prevention' with aspirin (or other platelet inhibitor drug), beta-blockers, and ACE inhibitors and lipid-lowering medication such as statins (Chapter 44).

The exceptions to the *treatment for acute is the same as chronic* story is thrombolysis in myocardial infarction, which usually reverses the acute coronary arterial thrombosis, and also coronary artery surgery. Given intravenously, thrombolytic therapy is fulfilling the old dream of anticoagulation, but it is not used long term. Coronary artery procedures have been shown to reduce the long-term risk of subsequent coronary events in patients with angina pectoris if the degree of arterial disease at surgery exceeds a certain degree of severity. Their benefit in acute myocardial infarction has been less obvious until recently, when there have been trials suggesting that percutaneous coronary artery angioplasty is beneficial in the acute stage. Making this procedure available to all potential sufferers from acute myocardial infarction would involve having teams of interventional cardiologists available within every community, able to respond immediately to any and every emergency admission (Vanuzzo *et al*. 2000).

49.8 **Primary prevention, lifestyle, and drugs**

At the opposite end of the scale is primary prevention, which was the main area of attention of cardiovascular epidemiologists in the 1970s and 1980s. Atheromatous coronary artery disease takes decades to develop in an individual. The priority here is that intervention should be effective and sustained, although this does not stop some protagonists of prevention promoting it as if it was an emergency measure for an imminent catastrophe. Two decades ago the focus of primary prevention was on lifestyle factors. Serum cholesterol levels were modulated by diet. Smokers should choose to quit. Those with mild hypertension in particular, but really almost everybody, could and should lose weight, cut the amount of salt and alcohol that they consumed, and take more exercise. In the carefully controlled conditions of a metabolic ward it is possible to derive formulae which show that the blood level of serum cholesterol responds to change in the diet. These results correlate well with classical studies on differences in diet and blood lipids in different populations. Dietary advice based on these formulae has not proved particularly effective in changing serum cholesterol in a clinical context. The formulae predicted cholesterol change in captive or unsophisticated populations, but not in urban sophisticates subjected to multiple media pressures and cynical about the veracity of what the experts tell them. Hence the clinical myth of 'diet-resistant hyperlipidaemia'. It is not the hyperlipidaemia that is resistant to a change in diet so much as the patient failing to make the recommended dietary change in the first instance.

Disappointingly for those early idealists (like Geoffrey Rose at one time) who considered that controlling disease was a matter of informed choice, individual human behaviour has proved remarkably resistant to change (Rose *et al.* 1983; Rose 1987). Mass behaviour does change, but slowly. It is possible to secure greater mean changes in serum cholesterol in a whole population, such as parts of Finland (Vartiainen *et al.* 1994), over 20 years than may be possible in one individual over the short term, when that individual is being asked to go against his or her previous experience and peer-group pressures. As discussed in the previous chapter, telling an individual to be healthy and be good may not achieve much in terms of sustained changes in lifestyle. What is true for serum cholesterol is also true for diet and obesity, for taking more exercise, and for lifestyle contributions to control of mild hypertension. The MONICA Project was observing the effect of slow changes in lifestyles in populations, good and bad, populations which were also simultaneously subjected to the systematic introduction of powerful and effective drugs and treatments.

49.9 The WHO MONICA Project, disease trends, risk factors, and the effects of treatment

As was stated at the beginning of this chapter, the WHO MONICA Project was established to monitor changes in coronary heart disease event rates and their case fatality, and also change in population risk factors and in what we then called acute coronary care, but which for reasons given above should now be called coronary care. The influence of risk factors on coronary event rates is discussed in Chapter 37. The first WHO MONICA Project paper on disease trends showed that the major contribution to falling mortality rates from coronary heart disease (Tunstall-Pedoe *et al.* 1999) was change in coronary event rates rather than case fatality, in a ratio of two-thirds to one-third (see Fig. 49.1). Employing the conceptual model that we had originally used, that risk factors drove event rates and treatment drove case fatality, some observers took this paper to mean that primary risk factors were what contributed most (Capewell 1999), but they had jumped to conclusions prematurely.

When the separate analyses of our two hypotheses were published in parallel a year later they showed a somewhat confusing and disappointing relationship of trends in event rates to trends in calculated risk factor scores (Kuulasmaa *et al.* 2000) (see Chapter 37). The findings from our second hypothesis on coronary care, rather put on the back-burner by MONICA investigators in the early 1980s for reasons already given, were overwhelmingly positive. A treatment score used to assess what proportion of myocardial infarction patients had four evidence-based treatments before the onset of the attack, and four during the attack (Tunstall-Pedoe *et al.* 2000; Tunstall-Pedoe 2003) had a very strong negative relationship with trends not only in community case fatality (see Fig. 49.2a), but also with coronary event rates, and most dramatically with population mortality rates from coronary heart disease (see Fig. 49.2b). The conclusion was inescapable that, at the population level, those populations in which new evidence-based treatments were being rapidly introduced for myocardial infarction and secondary prevention

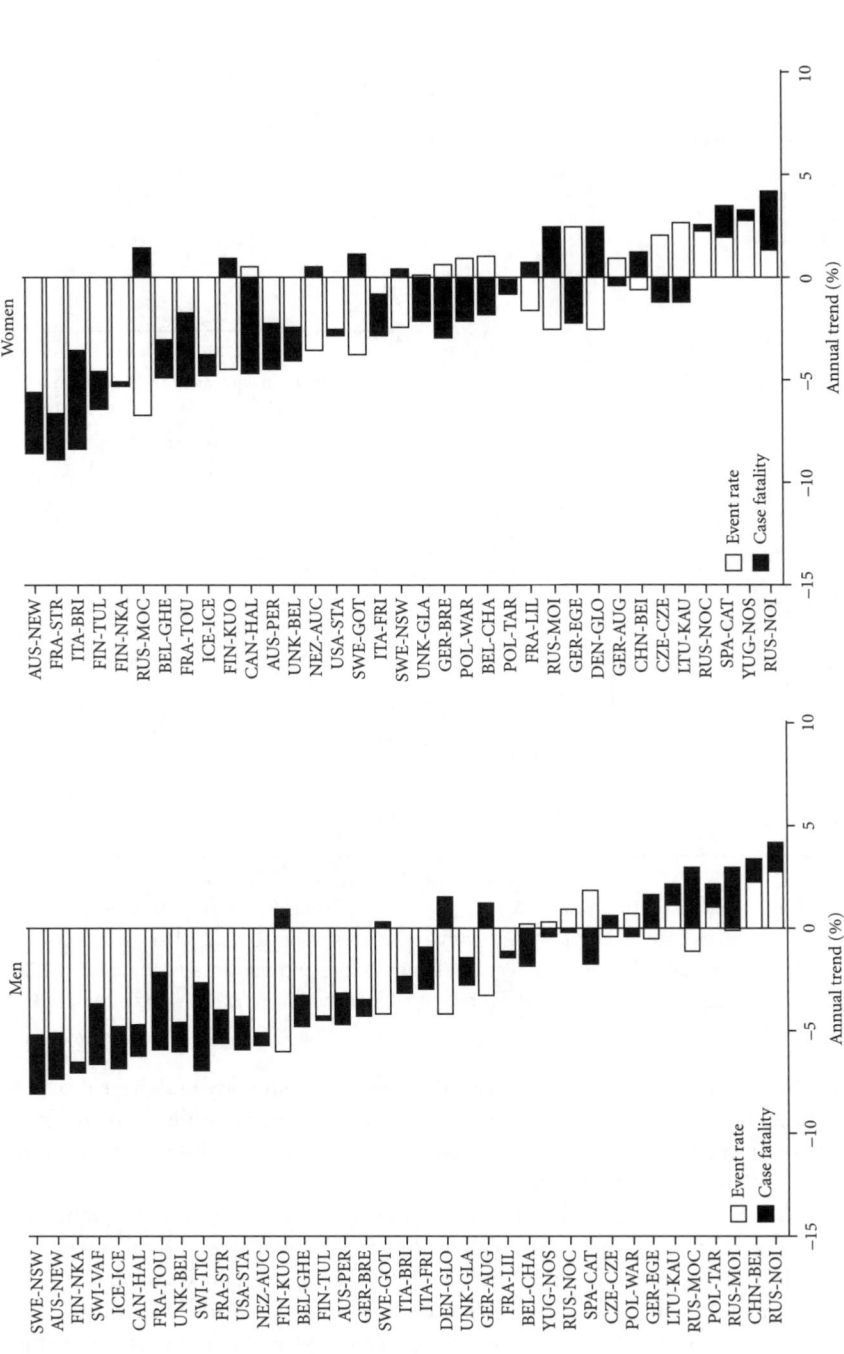

Fig. 49.1 Annual trends in coronary mortality rates apportioned between changes in event rates and case fatality. (Reproduced with permission. Previously published in Tunstall-Pedoe *et al.* 1999 and Tunstall-Pedoe 2003.)

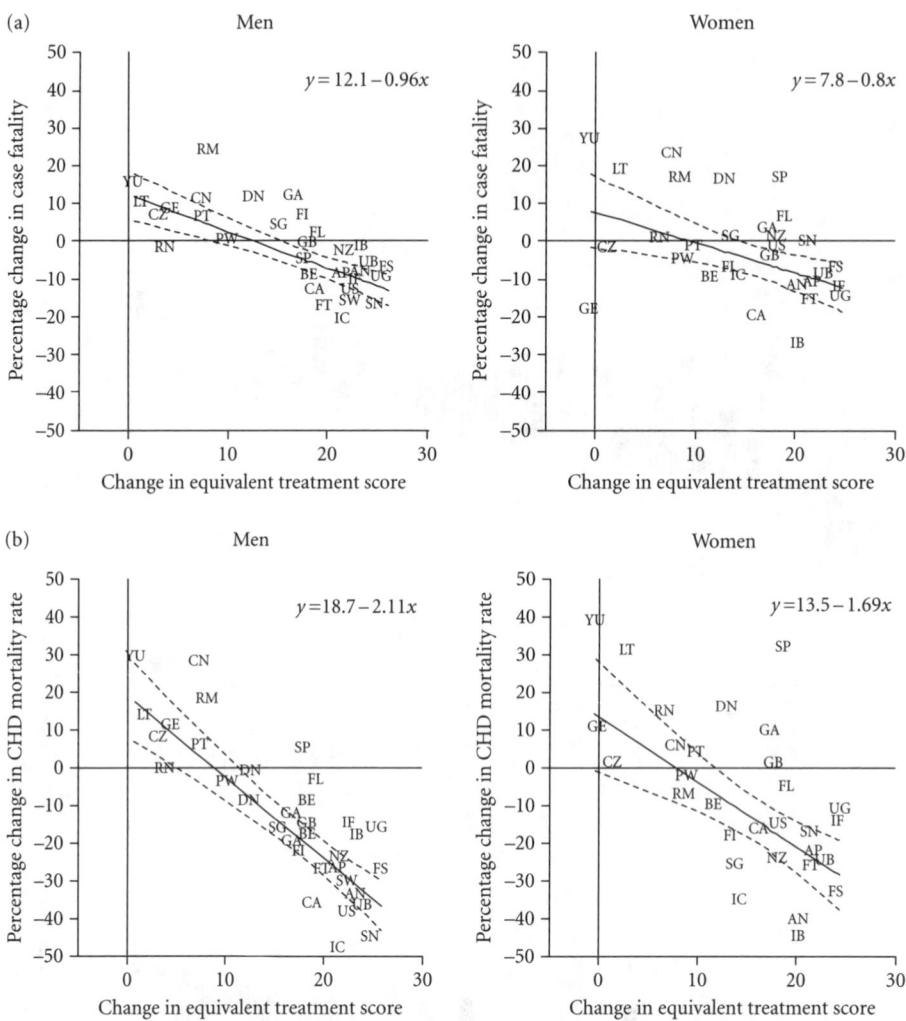

Fig. 49.2 (a) Correlation between equivalent treatment score and percentage change in coronary case fatality. (b) Correlation between equivalent treatment score and percentage change in CHD mortality rates. (Reproduced with permission. Previously published in Tunstall-Pedoe et al. 2000 and Tunstall-Pedoe 2003.)

of coronary heart disease were overwhelmingly those in which mortality rates were dropping at their fastest. The results were more powerful than would be possible from any other community study because MONICA recorded standard data in over 30 different populations across Europe and three other continents.

The WHO MONICA Project was best equipped to say what was happening at a population level, and to assess relationships across populations, but not to give an unequivocal answer as to why. Unlike RCTs where the only factor that should differ substantially between treatment groups is the treatment, this is not true of an ecological analysis (Morgenstern 1982). The simplest explanation for the MONICA result is that evidence-based treatments are having a major effect on the attack rate, case fatality, and mortality rate from coronary heart disease.

The most likely mechanism is through secondary prevention and acute coronary care, rather than by primary prevention acting through the classic risk factors, as this latter relationship would have then appeared stronger in the first hypothesis paper. Really widespread use of lipid-lowering statins is a recent phenomenon, whereas MONICA finished data collection in the early 1990s. Possibly the next decade will be that in which the pharmacological revolution has a real impact on the primary classic risk factors, of smoking, blood pressure, and blood cholesterol.

However, there are alternative explanations for the WHO MONICA Project results. Implementation of evidence-based treatments could be taken to be an indicator of an economically successful, dynamic society able to change behaviours in the light of evidence. Perhaps that extended to protection from coronary disease in other highly correlated ways such as diet, although not reflected through the classic primary risk factors. However, it is not possible to name what this overwhelming dietary or other factor might be. The least successful populations in implementing coronary care were those geographically clustered in the old Soviet sphere of influence, where things went badly wrong for cardiovascular mortality and indeed for many causes of death in the early 1990s (see Chapter 6). The MONICA results were weakened slightly by omitting Russian centres from analyses, and weakened more substantially by omitting all populations from the former Soviet sphere of influence (Tunstall-Pedoe et al. 2000). Whilst it is possible to make alternative suggestions, Occam's razor persuades us to go for the simplest explanation. If we have treatments that really work when formally tested, why should they not have an impact at the population level when rapidly introduced in a wholesale systematic manner?

The WHO MONICA Project results were at variance with those published shortly beforehand from the American multicentre ARIC (Atherosclerosis Risk In Communities) study (Rosamond et al. 1998), which suggested that over an 8 year period the major contributor to change in mortality had been from change in case fatality rather than in event rates, which were rather stable. The ARIC criteria for myocardial infarction were less demanding than those used by MONICA for definite myocardial infarction. Results were more similar if criteria were adjusted. It is possible that a contribution to the stability of American event rates was the introduction of increasingly sensitive serological tests, a cause of confusion now being exacerbated further with the redefinition of myocardial infarction to include troponin testing (Joint Committee 2000; Tunstall-Pedoe 2001), causing problems for epidemiological monitoring of coronary heart disease. Whatever the problems with increasing sensitivity in the diagnosis of non-fatal myocardial infarction, which would produce the appearance of declining case fatality, the MONICA relationship between declining mortality rates and increasingly effective coronary care would be unaffected.

Although MONICA was concerned with short-term (28 day) case fatality, several MONICA and other population-based coronary registers have reported declining mortality during follow-up beyond that time, most prominently in men. Given the results of RCTs, it would be wrong to deny both the potential and the actual contribution of systematic introduction of aspirin, beta-blockers, and other drugs, although lifestyle management through better rehabilitation must also contribute to better prognosis after myocardial infarction (Abrahamsson et al. 1998; Stewart et al. 1999; Peltonen et al. 2000; Bronnum-Hansen et al. 2001).

49.10 Conclusion

Despite excited claims to the contrary, for the first two decades of the last half century it is unlikely that treatment had much impact on coronary heart disease, which followed its own natural history. The development of powerful new pharmacological agents along with the discovery of new uses for old ones, coupled with really large RCTs, enabled effective treatments to be introduced, firstly in the acute phase, but probably more effectively for secondary prevention. The WHO MONICA Project results are very impressive in suggesting that treatment has an effect at the population level. Where old-style public health could largely ignore treatment as often random or idiosyncratic, and likely to be mixing some potential good and some potential harm with general futility, and could therefore concentrate on aetiology and prevention and the contribution of lifestyles, this is no longer true. It is no longer possible to study the natural history of coronary disease in terms of classic factors without considering treatments. Good public health now demands widespread use of effective treatments and an understanding of their impact on disease patterns and outcomes. This should be reflected in the emphasis given to treatment in any further editions of this book.

References

Abrahamsson, P., Dellborg, M., Rosengren, A., and Wilhelmsen, L. (1998). Improved long-term prognosis after myocardial infarction 1984–1991. *European Heart Journal*, **19**, 1512–17.

Anand, S. S. and Yusuf, S. (1999). Oral anticoagulant therapy in patients with coronary artery disease: a meta-analysis. *Journal of the American Medical Association*, **282**, 2058–67.

Briggs, R. S., Brown, P. M., Crabb, M. E., Cox, T. J., Ead, H. W., *et al.* (1976). The Brighton resuscitation ambulances: a continuing experiment in pre-hospital care by ambulance staff. *British Medical Journal*, **2**, 1161–5.

Brodsky, M. A., Mitchell, L. B., Halperin, B. D., Raitt, M. H., Hallstrom, A. P., *et al.* (2002). Prognostic value of baseline electrophysiological studies in patients with sustained ventricular tachyarrhythmia: the Antiarrhythmic Versus Implantable Defibrillators (AVID) trial. *American Heart Journal*, **144**, 478–84.

Bronnum-Hansen, H., Jorgensen, T., Davidsen, M., Madsen, M., Osler, M., *et al.* (2001). Survival and cause of death after myocardial infarction: the Danish MONICA study. *Journal of Clinical Epidemiology*, **54**, 1244–50.

Capewell, S. (1999). Survival trends, coronary event rates and the MONICA project. *Lancet*, **354**, 862–3.

Caswell, J. E. (1967). A brief history of coronary care units. *Public Health Reports*, **82**, 1105–7.

Chambless, L., Keil, U., Dobson, A., Mähönen, M., Kuulasmaa, K., *et al.* for the WHO MONICA Project (1997). Population versus clinical view of case fatality from acute coronary heart disease: results from the WHO MONICA Project 1985–1990. *Circulation*, **96**, 3849–59.

Cobb, L. A. and Hallstrom, A. P. (1982). Community-based cardiopulmonary resuscitation: what have we learned? *Annals of the New York Academy of Science*, **382**, 330–42.

Cobb, L. A., Alvarez, H. 3rd, and Kopass, M. K. (1976). A rapid response system for out-of-hospital cardiac emergencies. *Medical Clinics of North America*, **60**, 282–93.

Cochrane, A. L. (1972). *Effectiveness and efficiency: random reflections on health services*. Rock Carling Fellowship 1971/Nuffield Provincial Hospitals Trust, London.

Daniels, M. and Hill, A. B. (1952). Chemotherapy of pulmonary tuberculosis in young adults: an analysis of the combined results of three Medical Research Council trials. *British Medical Journal*, **1**, 1162–8.

Day, H. W. (1962) An intensive coronary care area. *Diseases of the Chest*, **44**, 423–27.

International Anticoagulant Review Group (1970). Collaborative analysis of long-term anticoagulant administration after acute myocardial infarction. *Lancet*, **I**, 203–9.

Joint Committee (2000). Myocardial infarction redefined: a consensus document of The Joint European Society of Cardiology/American College of Cardiology Committee for the redefinition of myocardial infarction. *European Heart Journal*, **21**, 1502–13.

Joint Working Party of the Royal College of Physicians of London and the British Cardiac Society (1975). The care of the patient with coronary heart disease. *Journal of the Royal College of Physicians of London*, **10**, 5–46.

Kuulasmaa, K., Tunstall-Pedoe, H., Dobson, A., Fortmann, S., Sans, S., *et al.* for the WHO MONICA Project (2000). Estimation of contribution of changes in classic risk factors to trends in coronary-event rates across the WHO MONICA Project populations. *Lancet*, **355**, 675–87.

Mather, H. G., Pearson, N. G., Read, K. L. Q., Shaw, D. B., Steed, G. R., *et al.* (1971). Acute myocardial infarction: home and hospital treatment. *British Medical Journal*, **3**, 334–8.

Mather, H. G., Morgan, D. C., Pearson, N. G., Read, K. L. Q., Shaw, D. B., *et al.* (1976). Myocardial infarction: a comparison between home and hospital care for patients. *British Medical Journal*, **1**, 925–9.

McNeilly, R. H. and Pemberton, J. (1968). Duration of last attack in 998 cases of coronary artery disease and its relation to possible cardiac resuscitation. *British Medical Journal*, **3**, 139–42.

Morgenstern, H. (1982). Uses of ecological analysis in epidemiological research. *American Journal of Public Health*, **72**, 1336–44.

Pantridge, J. F. and Geddes, J. S. (1967). A mobile intensive care unit in the management of myocardial infarction. *Lancet*, **ii**, 271–5.

Pell, J. P., Sirel, J. M., Marsden, A. K., Ford, I., and Cobbe, S. M. (2001). Effect of reducing ambulance response times on deaths from out of hospital cardiac arrest: cohort study. *BMJ*, **322**, 1385–8.

Peltonen, M., Lundberg, V., Huhtasaari, F., and Asplund, K. (2000). Marked improvement in survival after myocardial infarction in middle-aged men but not in women: The Northern Sweden MONICA study 1985–94. *Journal of Internal Medicine*, **247**, 579–87.

Rosamond, W. D., Chambless, L. E., Folsom, A., Cooper, L. S., Conwill, D. E., *et al.* (1998). Trends in the incidence of myocardial infarction and in mortality due to coronary heart disease 1987–94. *New England Journal of Medicine*, **339**, 861–7.

Rose, G. (1975). The contribution of intensive coronary care. *British Journal of Preventive and Social Medicine*, **29**, 147–50.

Rose, G. (1987). European collaborative trial of multifactorial prevention of coronary heart disease. *Lancet*, **1**, 685.

Rose, G., Tunstall-Pedoe, H., and Heller, R. F. (1983). UK heart disease prevention project: incidence and mortality results. *Lancet*, **1**, 1062–6.

Stewart, A. W., Beaglehole, R., Jackson, R., and Bingley, W. (1999). Trends in three-year survival following acute myocardial infarction, 1983–1992. *European Heart Journal*, **20**, 803–7.

Tunstall-Pedoe, H. for the WHO MONICA Project (1988). The World Health Organization MONICA Project (Monitoring Trends and Determinants in Cardiovascular Disease): a major international collaboration. *Journal of Clinical Epidemiology*, **41**, 105–14.

Tunstall-Pedoe, H. (2001). Comment on the ESC/ACC redefinition of myocardial infarction by a consensus dissenter. *European Heart Journal*, **22**, 613–16.

Tunstall-Pedoe, H. (2002). What was preventing coronary heart disease (CHD) prevention and why its time has now come. In *Effective secondary prevention and cardiac rehabilitation* (ed. D. Wood, A. McLeod, M. Davis and A. Miles), pp. 3–13. Key Advances Series. Aesculapius Press, London.

Tunstall-Pedoe, H. (ed.) for the WHO MONICA Project (2003). *MONICA monograph and multimedia sourcebook*. World Health Organization, Geneva.

Tunstall-Pedoe, H., Clayton, D., Morris, J. N., Brigden, W., and McDonald, L. (1975). Coronary heart attacks in East London. *Lancet*, **2**, 833–8.

Tunstall-Pedoe, H., Morrison, C., Woodward, M., Fitzpatrick, B., and Watt, G. (1996). Sex differences in myocardial infarction and coronary deaths in the Scottish MONICA population of Glasgow 1985–91: presentation, diagnosis, treatment and 28-day case fatality of 3991 events in men and 1551 events in women. *Circulation*, **93**, 1981–92.

Tunstall-Pedoe, H., Kuulasmaa, K., Mähönen, M., Tolonen, H., Ruokokoski, E., *et al.* for the WHO MONICA Project (1999). Contribution of trends in survival and coronary-event rates to changes in coronary heart disease mortality: 10-year results from 37 WHO MONICA Project populations. *Lancet*, **353**, 1547–57.

Tunstall-Pedoe, H., Vanuzzo, D., Hobbs, M., Mahonen, M., Cepaitis, Z., Kuulasmaa, K., *et al.* for the WHO MONICA Project (2000). Estimation of contribution of changes in coronary care to improving survival, event rates, and coronary heart disease mortality across the WHO MONICA Project populations. *Lancet*, **355**, 688–700.

Vanuzzo, D., Pilotto, L., Pilotto, L., Mahonen, M., and Hobbs, M. for the WHO MONICA Project (2000). Pharmacological treatment during AMI and in secondary prevention: the scientific evidence. Available from URL: <http://ktl.fi/publications/monica/carpfish/appenda/evidence.htm> and also on CD-ROM attached to Tunstall-Pedoe *et al.* (2003).

Vartiainen, E., Puska, P., Pekkanen, J., Tuomilehto, J., and Jousilahti, P. (1994). Changes in risk factors explain change in mortality from ischaemic heart disease in Finland. *BMJ*, **309**, 23–7.

World Health Organization Regional Office for Europe (1976). Myocardial infarction community registers. Public Health in Europe No 5. Copenhagen.

Chapter 50

Intervention in high risk groups: hypertension

P. S. Sever and N. R. Poulter

50.1 Introduction

Prospective epidemiological data have shown that an increased risk of cardiovascular disease is predicted by increments both in systolic and diastolic blood pressure (SDP/DBP) (MacMahon *et al.* 1990) (see Chapter 43). This increase in risk is continuous and graded with no evidence of a J-shaped relationship. It is estimated that in middle-aged men, a 20 mmHg higher SBP is associated with a 60% increase in cardiovascular mortality, and with a 50% higher all-cause mortality over a 10 year period.

50.2 The early trials

Prior to the introduction of drug therapy for severe hypertension, associated morbidity and mortality from stroke, coronary heart disease (CHD), congestive heart failure and renal failure were high. In the Mayo Clinic reports of 1939 (Keith *et al.* 1939), 80% of hypertensive patients who developed papilloedema died within a year, 90% were dead within 2 years, and few remained alive after 3 years. With the introduction of drug therapy, survival was dramatically improved; in an early study from the Hammersmith Hospital, 50% of treated patients survived 2 years (Harrison *et al.* 1970). The introduction of therapy changed not only the associated mortality rates, but also the relative importance of the causes of death, such that congestive heart failure and renal disease were virtually eliminated and stroke was no longer the main cause of death. The results of the Veterans Administration study laid to rest any doubts about the advantages of treating moderate (DBP 105–114 mmHg) and severe (DBP $\geq$115 mmHg) levels of blood pressure (Veterans Administrative Cooperative Study Group on Antihypertensive Agents 1967, 1970). Drug treatment reduced strokes, heart failure, other cardiovascular and renal end points, but not myocardial infarction.

From this and other early trials, a number of observations were made: a greater reduction in morbid events was seen among men compared with women and in the higher blood pressure groups at entry; the incidence of accelerated phase hypertension was greatly reduced by treatment; and older patients gained more absolute benefit than the young. On the whole, the limited number of participants in these early trials reduced their power to answer the question as to whether lowering blood pressure reduced coronary events.

The question then arose as to whether the benefits of treating hypertension could be extended to the larger population at risk from mild hypertension. In these patients, for whom the individual attributable risk is relatively small, it was particularly important to demonstrate that the advantages of blood pressure reduction were not counterbalanced by long-term adverse responses to the antihypertensive drugs.

In all the trials that have involved patients with mild hypertension, active treatment has conferred benefits when compared with placebo or, in the case of the Hypertension Detection and Follow-up Program (HDFP) (HDFP Cooperative Group 1979, 1982) and the Multiple Risk Factor Intervention trial (MRFIT) (MRFIT Research Group 1982), the outcome in the special care group was better than in those patients who continued with 'usual' medical care.

In the Australian trial (entry diastolic pressures 95–109 mmHg), active treatment reduced the incidence of stroke (Australian Therapeutic Trial in Mild Hypertension 1980). Although fewer cases of fatal CHD occurred in the active treatment group, the numbers were small and the difference just failed to achieve statistical significance.

In the Medical Research Council Trial of mild hypertension (diastolic pressure 90–109 mmHg) (MRC Working Party 1985), stroke rate was again reduced by active treatment, but there was no overall reduction in coronary events. The results of subgroup analysis from this trial require cautious interpretation. However, comparing the two active regimens, the diuretic was more effective than the beta-blocker, propranolol, in reducing stroke rate. Strokes were reduced in both smokers and non-smokers by the diuretic, but only in non-smokers by propranolol. With the exception of non-smoking males, in whom a modest reduction in coronary events was associated with a beta-blocker, there was no effect of either treatment on coronary morbidity. When overall morbidity was assessed, including silent infarcts diagnosed electrocardiographically, the beta-blocker group fared significantly better than the diuretic or placebo group. In the HDFP (HDFP 1979, 1982), which also included patients in the mild hypertension category, special treatment conferred additional benefits over usual care, both in respect of stroke prevention and coronary morbidity. However, because neither this study nor the MRFIT were placebo-controlled, no conclusive statement can be made about the definitive benefits of antihypertensive treatment. The International Prospective Primary Prevention Study in Hypertension (IPPPSH) (IPPPSH 1985) addressed the question of whether the incidence of cardiac and cerebrovascular events could be influenced by the inclusion in an antihypertensive regimen of a beta-blocker (oxprenolol), compared with treatment not containing a beta-blocker. No overall differences were found between treatment groups in total mortality, cardiac events, or strokes. However, as in the MRC trial, subgroup analysis suggested that beta-blockers may confer some benefit in terms of a reduction in cardiac events in non-smoking men.

Another trial, the Heart Attack Primary Prevention Trial in Hypertension (HAPPHY) (Wilhelmsen et al. 1987), also addressed the question of whether a beta-blocker-based regimen differed from the diuretic-based regimen with regard to the prevention of coronary artery disease in men with mild to moderate hypertension. The outcome of the trial was similar for the two groups and neither regimen preferentially reduced the incidence of hypertensive complications, including CHD events. Further analysis failed to confirm the observations (from the MRC and IPPPSH studies) that non-smokers benefited from beta-blockers compared with diuretics with respect to coronary morbidity.

Patients in the HAPPHY trial received one of two beta-blockers, atenolol or metoprolol. Those receiving metoprolol were followed for a slightly longer period and the data were analysed separately (Wikstrand et al. 1988). In the metoprolol-treated group overall mortality was lower than in the thiazide group because of fewer deaths from CHD and stroke. However, the number of end points was small in this subgroup analysis, so these data should be interpreted with caution.

The absolute benefits of active treatment of hypertension in reducing the incidence of cardiovascular events as observed in the trials may underestimate the real benefits. For example it was reported, based on the MRC trial data, that 850 mildly hypertensive patients must be treated for 1 year to prevent one stroke. This estimate may grossly underestimate the benefits of treatment to ordinary hypertensive individuals (Collins and Peto 1994) for the following reasons. First, the ranges of blood pressure entry criteria in the MRC and Australian trials were 90–109 and 95–109 mmHg, with mean entry levels of 98 and 100.4 mmHg, respectively. However, 'actual' mean blood pressures (those recorded a few weeks post-randomization and on placebo) were 91 and 93 mmHg, respectively. Presumably the benefits observed in the trials therefore relate to these lower actual blood pressure levels, and thus underestimate benefits which would accrue from lowering blood pressures which are genuinely maintained as high as 95–100 mmHg. Second, the mortality rates in the controls in the MRC and Australian trials were low, in part because of the study exclusion criteria and the healthy volunteer effect, as most of the volunteers were middle-class patients, who generally enjoy better cardiovascular health. Third, the intention to treat analyses makes no allowance for the effects of a significant proportion of the most at-risk controls who received active antihypertensive medication. Furthermore, because treatment is more likely to be initiated in those controls with highest blood pressures (and hence at greatest risk) and those who stop active treatment are likely to be at least risk by virtue of their blood pressure levels, 'on treatment' analyses do not solve all these problems. Fourth, because inflexible drug regimens often using high dosages are inevitably followed in trials, side effects are likely to be more prevalent and severe (with implications for compliance) than in everyday clinical practice.

Trial data have also shown that, if left untreated, a significant number of people with mild hypertension progress to more severe hypertension in a relatively short time, demonstrating the clear benefits of treatment in preventing the progression of hypertension. These comments have not usually been incorporated into the often quoted evaluation of benefits in the treatment of mild hypertension, but need to be borne in mind when considering the introduction of therapy for patients potentially at risk from hypertension-related cardiovascular disease.

When the results of these intervention trials with older drug regimens were pooled in 1994 (Collins and Peto 1994), treatment was found to have reduced the risk of stroke by 38% and that of non-fatal myocardial infarction and CHD death by 16% (Fig. 50.1). This represented an apparent shortfall in benefit from drug treatment on risk of coronary disease expected from prospective observational data (MacMahon et al. 1990). The important question arising from this meta-analysis was whether lowering blood pressure with new treatment strategies would reduce the shortfall in protection against CHD especially in the elderly.

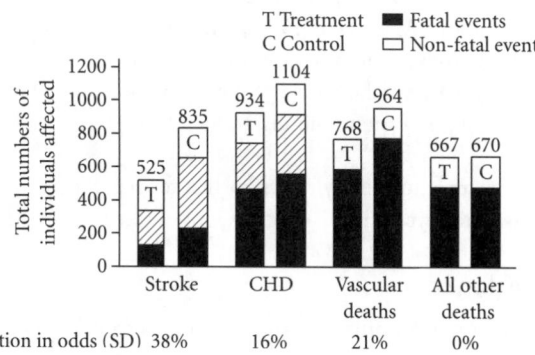

Fig. 50.1 Meta-analysis of blood pressure-lowering trials (17 trials, 47 653 patients; SBP difference: 10–12 mmHg, DBP difference: 5–6 mmHg. (Reproduced from Collins and Peto 1994).

50.3 **Unresolved issues in drug treatment**

As of the early 1990s, despite 17 major morbidity/mortality trials, several key unresolved issues in the treatment of hypertension remained. These included:

1 Whether treatment with more contemporary drugs such as calcium channel blockers (CCBs), angiotensin-converting enzyme (ACE) inhibitors, and angiotensin receptor blockers (ARBs), compared with diuretics or beta-blockers, would result in greater protection against CHD events.

2 Whether specific combinations of antihypertensive agents would confer benefits over other combinations.

3 At what level should blood pressure therapy be initiated (thresholds) and to what level should blood pressure be lowered (targets).

4 Whether other concomitant medications (e.g. lipid-lowering) would provide further benefits.

5 To what extent the answers to the above questions vary in specific subgroups of patients.

50.3.1 **Non-pharmacological measures**

There is increasing evidence that a population strategy could reduce the rise in blood pressure with age, decrease the prevalence of hypertension, the need for drug therapy and lower overall cardiovascular risk (Appel *et al.* 1997; Applegate *et al.* 1992; National High Blood Pressure Education Program Working Group 1993; Stamler 1998; Watt 1995; Whelton 1994). Such a strategy, outlined by Stamler (1998) includes a diet high in fruit and vegetables, high in legumes and whole grain, high in fat-free or low fat dairy products, poultry, fish, shellfish, and meat products, and high in essential nutrients; low in salt; reduced total and saturated fat and low cholesterol; alcohol restricted to 2–3 units/day; calorie-controlled to prevent obesity; and regular physical exercise.

In established hypertension, intervention trials have confirmed the benefits of changes in lifestyle both on blood pressure and on reducing overall cardiovascular risk (Appel *et al.* 1997; Applegate *et al.* 1992; Braith *et al.* 1994; Fotherby and Potter 1992, 1993; Geleijnse *et al.* 1994; Kokkinos *et al.* 1995; McCarron *et al.* 1997; Trials of Hypertension Prevention Collaborative Research Group 1997; Whelton *et al.* 1998).

Measures that lower blood pressure include: weight reduction (Appel *et al.* 1997; Applegate *et al.* 1992; Trials of Hypertension Prevention Collaborative Research Group 1997; Whelton *et al.* 1998), reduced salt intake (Law *et al.* 1991; Midgley *et al.* 1996; Whelton *et al.* 1998), limited alcohol consumption (Kaplan 1995), regular physical exercise (Applegate *et al.* 1992), increase in fruit and vegetable consumption (Appel *et al.* 1997), and reduction in total fat and saturated fat intake (Appel *et al.* 1997). These should be combined with measures to reduce overall cardiovascular risk (Sever *et al.* 1993), which include: stopping smoking, reducing total fat intake and replacing saturated fat with poly- and monounsaturated fats, and increasing oily fish consumption.

These non-pharmacological measures constitute lifestyle changes that form part of a treatment strategy irrespective of whether the hypertensive patient is on drugs or not (see Chapter 43).

50.3.2 **More recent trial evidence**

Given that in previous trials (based largely on diuretics and beta-blockers) the benefits of blood pressure-lowering on stroke prevention had been as large as prospective observational data had predicted, the newer agents (CCBs, ACE inhibitors, etc.) – hitherto untested – were only likely to prove superior to the older agents in relation to CHD prevention. Therefore, trials thereafter should have focused on, and been powered to, differentiate the effects of the drug classes on CHD events.

Unfortunately most studies comparing drug classes have used total cardiovascular events – including a large proportion of stroke for which differential effects were not predicted – as the primary end point. These trials were, therefore, largely underpowered to evaluate significant differences between drug classes.

The results of several large trials have been reported since the meta-analysis published in 1994 (Collins and Peto 1994). The key findings of these more recent trials are presented in relation to their potential impact on the unresolved issues.

50.4 Benefits of more contemporary drugs over standard therapy?

50.4.1 Systolic Hypertension in Europe Trial (SYST-EUR) (Staessen et al. 1997)

This was an important trial in two respects. It was designed to answer the question of whether drug treatment of isolated systolic hypertension (ISH) improves cardiovascular outcome. This trial was also the first prospective, randomized, placebo-controlled trial to evaluate, as first line active treatment, a drug class other than a diuretic or beta-blocker – in this case a dihydropyridine CCB. During the earlier stages of this trial of 4695 patients the results of a similar study in ISH – the SHEP trial (SHEP Co-operative Research Group 1991) – were reported, which clearly identified major cardiovascular benefits from the drug treatment of ISH, although in this case with a diuretic-based treatment regimen. The results of SHEP were conclusive, and in keeping with subgroup analyses of the MRC trial of the treatment of older patients (MRC Working Party 1992), which confirmed reductions in cardiovascular events with diuretic-based treatment of older patients with ISH. On the basis of SHEP, some physicians questioned whether it was appropriate to continue SYST-EUR – an ethical issue that was vigorously defended by the investigators. Using a Bayesian approach to analysis they justified the continuation of SYST-EUR, although in the construction of their 'prior hypothesis' it is likely that they did not include data from the MRC trial.

In the event, the continuation of SYST-EUR allowed the important question as to whether the diuretic-based benefits seen in SHEP could be attained using a CCB. SYST-EUR was stopped early by the Steering Committee because of unequivocal benefits from the CCB-based treatment – the magnitude of the benefit being at least as great as for other drug treatments in earlier trials.

50.4.2 The Captopril Primary Prevention Project (CAPPP) (Hansson et al. 1999b)

Although several trials incorporating ACE inhibitors as components of therapeutic regimens have demonstrated convincing benefits in the treatment of heart failure and left ventricular dysfunction (Konstam et al. 1992), and other studies suggest treatment benefits in subgroups of patients with renal disease and type I diabetes (Lewis et al. 1993), there have been no placebo-controlled trials of ACE inhibitors in hypertension. CAPPP was the first trial of 'old' versus new drug classes and attempted to compare cardiovascular morbidity and mortality in 10 985 hypertensive patients randomized to treatment with either a captopril-based regimen or 'usual' treatment (predominantly beta-blocker-based). The primary outcome measure of cardiovascular morbidity and mortality was not differentially influenced by the two treatment regimens, but a number of secondary end points were differentially affected, for example, stroke incidence was higher in the captopril group. Regrettably this study was seriously flawed in two respects. First, despite randomization, the two groups were markedly unbalanced at baseline, probably because the randomization process (by sealed letter) gave the investigator the potential to influence the choice of treatment patients received. Thus, for example, there were more diabetic patients in those randomized to captopril. Second, blood pressure levels were higher throughout the trial in those randomized to the ACE inhibitor. This reflects the fact that up to two-thirds of the patients in the captopril group were given the drug once daily, rather than three times daily – the ideal necessary to provide adequate blood pressure control over 24 h. This study, therefore, could not help in addressing the important question of whether drugs that block the renin–angiotensin system confer additional cardiovascular protection over conventional therapy.

50.4.3 The Swedish Trial in Older Patients with Hypertension-2 (STOP 2) (Hansson *et al*. 1999*a*)

STOP-2 was a further study designed to compare conventional drug treatment (thiazide ± beta-blocker) with newer treatments, which in this case was either CCB-based or ACE inhibitor-based. This study of older patients involved 6614 patients followed up for an average of 5 years. As with CAPPP, the design of this trial was based on a hypothesis that newer treatments would reduce cardiovascular mortality by 25% compared with older drugs, perhaps unrealistic given the former discussion and results of older trials. On all cardiovascular end points, including stroke, myocardial infarction, and cardiovascular mortality, there was no significant difference in outcome when comparing newer drugs with conventional drugs. One difficulty associated with interpreting these results, however, was the contamination across the three groups under investigation by the use of drugs from one of the competing limbs as add-on therapy. Furthermore, this trial was underpowered to address the key question of differential effects of treatment regimens on CHD events – the end point around which controversy over differential drug effects was centred.

50.4.4 International Nifedipine gastro-intestinal transport-system (GITS) Study: intervention as a Goal in Hypertension Treatment (INSIGHT) (Brown *et al*. 2000)

INSIGHT was designed to test the primary hypothesis that a dihydropyridine CCB (nifedipine GITS) would reduce the combined cardiovascular end points of cardiovascular death, myocardial infarction, heart failure, and stroke by 25% (once again an unlikely difference) compared with thiazide/amiloride-based treatment regimens. In both limbs of the study atenolol was the add-on therapy.

The study included 6321 hypertensive patients, with at least one additional cardiovascular risk factor, who were randomized and followed-up for a median period of ~3.5 years. There was no overall difference in the incidence of primary events in the two treatment groups. There were significantly fewer fatal myocardial infarcts and cases of heart failure in the diuretic limb of the trial, but the number of events was small. There were more withdrawals from treatment (mainly due to oedema) in the nifedipine group, but more serious adverse events were reported with the diuretic.

50.4.5 **Nordic Diltiazem Study (NORDIL) (Hansson et al. 2000)**

NORDIL was a further study comparing a CCB (in this case the non-dihydropyridine, diltiazem) with a reference regimen of either diuretic or beta-blocker. The study, involving 10 916 patients, was powered to detect a 20% relative risk reduction (RRR) in combined cardiovascular events, not dissimilar from INSIGHT. After an average follow-up period of 4.5 years, all cardiovascular events in the two limbs of the trial were almost identical. There were, interestingly, significantly fewer strokes in the diltiazem arm (RRR 20%) despite if anything smaller falls in pressure in the diltiazem group.

50.4.6 **The Antihypertensive and Lipid-Lowering treatment to prevent a Heart Attack Trial (ALLHAT) (Davis et al. 1996)**

This is, to date, the largest hypertension study conducted. It was unique in attempting to discover the optimal first-line agent for preventing CHD in hypertensive subjects. An outline of the design of ALLHAT is shown in Fig. 50.2. Initially over 40 000 patients were randomized, double-blind, to receive either the CCB amlodipine, the ACE inhibitor lisinopril, the alpha-blocker doxazosin, or a reference diuretic, chlorthalidone. Using a factorial design, the effects of the cholesterol-lowering drug, pravastatin, were compared with usual care in a subgroup (see Section 50.8.3). The study was planned for an average follow-up period of 6 years (Davis et al. 1996).

After a mean follow-up period of ~3 years, the alpha-blocker limb of the trial was terminated prematurely on the grounds that there was an apparent excess of cardiovascular events (mainly heart failure) in those allocated to the alpha-blocker, compared with the diuretic (ALLHAT Officers and Co-ordinators for the ALLHAT Collaborative Research Group 2000). No outcome differences were observed in the primary end point, fatal CHD and non-fatal myocardial infarction, nor in all-cause mortality despite less blood pressure reduction achieved in the alpha-blocker limb.

For the remainder of the trial, following an average intervention period of ~5 years, the primary outcome of combined fatal CHD or non-fatal myocardial infarction was not significantly different between the treatment arms of the study (ALLHAT Officers and Co-ordinators for the ALLHAT Collaborative Research Group 2002a). In the ALLHAT population, which consisted of 47% women and 32% African-Americans, the ACE inhibitor

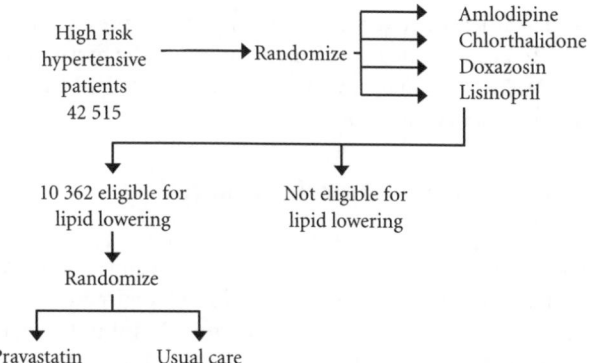

Fig. 50.2 Outline of ALLHAT. (Reproduced from Davis et al. 1996)

lisinopril was significantly less effective at lowering blood pressure than either the diuretic or the CCB. The differences in secondary end points, notably stroke incidence (higher on the ACE inhibitor) could be explained by the relative lack of efficacy on blood pressure reduction with the ACE inhibitor compared with the other drugs. The most striking and controversial finding in ALLHAT was an apparent excess of congestive heart failure seen both with the CCB (increased by 38% compared with a diuretic) and the ACE inhibitor (increased by 20% compared with a diuretic). However, the lack of any increased mortality associated with the increased heart failure raises the question, as it did in the case of the alpha-blocker limb, of whether this largely unvalidated end point was indeed heart failure in the strict sense of the definition. Recruitment into ALLHAT necessitated the withdrawal of previous therapies which would have included diuretics in many patients, the withdrawal of which could have (a) led to fluid retention, (b) unmasked previously treated or pre-empted heart failure, and (c) led to an apparent excess of heart failure in those patients not allocated chlorthalidone. The diagnosis of heart failure may have been further complicated or confused by the side effect of pedal oedema, which is frequently induced by the CCB and, to a lesser extent, doxazosin.

One clear piece of evidence from ALLHAT was that there was no excess of coronary events associated with the CCB and this important finding from a randomized controlled study highlights serious flaws in the interpretation of earlier uncontrolled observational studies, suggesting that CCBs were associated not only with increased coronary risk, but also with other non-cardiovascular events (Stanton 1998).

An advantage of ALLHAT is that, by virtue of its design and study size, meaningful analyses of subgroups of patients such as diabetics, African-Americans, and females were undertaken. Clearly blacks were disadvantaged by ACE inhibitor-based treatment compared with diuretics, presumably reflecting the lack of efficacy of the ACE inhibitor on blood pressure control in this ethnic group. ALLHAT did not confirm significant advantages of any of the treatment limbs, notably ACE inhibitors, compared with chlorthalidone in the subgroup of patients with diabetes.

The extrapolation of ALLHAT data to more contemporary treatment regimens is problematic in many respects. The diuretic chlorthalidone used in ALLHAT is rarely used outside North America and it is questionable as to whether the nature of the drug and the average doses used in ALLHAT are equivalent to 'low dose thiazides' such as bendrofluazide and hydrochlorthiazide. There are important pharmacological differences between chlorthalidone and thiazides, and the significant hypokalaemia observed and treated in many patients receiving chlorthalidone in ALLHAT raises the question of dose equivalence to more usual low dose thiazide treatment.

In addition, most patients needed at least two drugs to reach the blood pressure targets stipulated in the trial, and in order to avoid crossover treatments affecting the first-line drug comparisons, a number of largely obsolete add-on drugs were incorporated into the treatment strategies, including reserpine, clonidine, and hydralazine.

50.4.7 The second Australian National Blood Pressure Study (ANBP2) (Wing et al. 2003)

This trial of 6083 patients aged 65–84 was designed to compare the effects of an ACE inhibitor-based regimen (usually enalapril) with those of a thiazide-based regimen (usually hydrochlorothiazide). The results suggested that those allocated to ACE inhibition had a non-significant reduction in the primary end point of death or total cardiovascular events. These benefits were peculiar to men and interpretation was further complicated by the fact that compliance was only ~60% with a minority (38%) taking monotherapy. These data appear to conflict with the ALLHAT results and generally appear to be less reliable.

50.5 Overview and meta-analyses to date

Based on evidence from interventional trials and meta-analyses, the most recent of which was published in 2003, it appears that cardiovascular outcome is influenced to a greater extent by better pressure lowering than by choice of initial drug (Turnbull/BPLTTC 2003). Overall, there is no evidence that any one class of drug is more effective than another, but within the hypertensive population there are potentially important variations in blood pressure-lowering efficacy of individual drugs (Attwood et al. 1994). In many cases clinical practice is simply 'trial and error'. The heterogeneity of hypertensive patients accounts for varying and often unpredictable blood pressure responses to individual anti-hypertensive drugs (Sever 1999a) and, with one or two exceptions (Materson et al. 1993; Brown et al. 2003), no distinct patient phenotypes dictate the choice of individual drugs.

In general, in relation to blood pressure, older patients and those of African origin tend to respond better to diuretics and CCB drugs, in contrast with young or Caucasian patients whose response to beta-blockers and either ACE inhibitors or ARBs is greater than to diuretics or CCBs (Mallion and Goldberg 1996; Materson et al. 1993). It must be emphasized that these are broad generalizations and there are many exceptions to the rule.

For each major class of antihypertensive drug there are compelling indications and contraindications for their use in particular patient groups based on trial experience (Table 50.1) (ESH–ESC Guidelines Committee 2003; Williams et al. 2004). In other instances recommendations may be made based upon evidence that is less robust.

In the absence of special considerations, cost is an important issue, and the least expensive agent – which is a low dose diuretic in most countries – should be used, particularly since this class of agent is a good companion with most other drug classes.

Dose titration is recommended, where necessary, to achieve target blood pressures for all drugs except diuretics, but may be limited by the appearance of side effects. This may be avoided by either dose reduction and combination therapy or a switch to an alternative agent.

The obvious deficiency of many of these recently reported trials comparing 'new' and 'older' therapies was that they lacked the power to detect differences in CHD outcome which, based on earlier meta-analysis, was the source of a shortfall in benefit. A realistic hypothesis might be that newer drugs would confer greater protection against CHD, and several studies (not designed in hypertensive subjects) provide credence for this idea. In order to test this hypothesis, two courses of action have been followed. The first demanded studies with adequate numbers of patients randomized to detect a 20% RRR in CHD end points between treatment groups. Two studies were powered to address this critical question, ALLHAT (Davis et al. 1996) as detailed above, and the Anglo-Scandinavian Cardiac Outcomes Trial (ASCOT) (Sever et al. 2002), which is described later in this chapter.

The second course of action was to conduct further pooled analyses of available trial data. The Blood Pressure Lowering Treatment Trialists' Collaboration (BPLTTC) reported overviews of data from 22 trials comparing different treatment strategies in ~125 000 patients (Turnbull/BPLTTC 2003). It is important to emphasize that all eligible trials had to conform to pre-specified criteria and the collaborators agreed to a programme of prospectively designed overviews (WHO–ISH 1998).

The main conclusions from these important analyses (Fig. 50.3) is that, overall cardiovascular events are not differentially influenced by different treatment regimens based on older or newer

Table 50.1 Guidelines for management of hypertension. Compelling and possible indications, contraindications, and cautions for the major classes of antihypertensive drug

Class of drug	Compelling indications	Possible indications	Possible contraindications	Compelling contraindications
Alpha-blockers	Benign prostatic hypertrophy	–	Postural hypotension Heart failure	Urinary incontinence
ACE-inhibitors	Heart failure LV dysfunction post-myocardial infarction or established coronary heart disease Type 1 diabetic nephropathy Secondary stroke prevention[b]	Chronic renal disease[c] Type 2 diabetic nephropathy Proteinuric renal disease	Renal Impairment[c] PVD[d]	Pregnancy Renovascular disease[e]
AII receptor blockers	ACE inhibitor intolerance Type 2 diabetic nephropathy Hypertension with LV hypertrophy Heart failure in ACE intolerant patients, after myocardial infarction	LV dysfunction after myocardial infarction Intolerance of other antihypertensive drugs Proteinuric renal disease, chronic renal disease[e] Heart failure	Renal impairment[c] PVD[d]	Pregnancy Renovascular disease[e]
Beta-blockers	Myocardial infarction Angina	Heart failure[f]	Heart failure[f] PVD Diabetes (except with CHD)	Asthma/COPD Heart block
Calcium channel blockers (dihydropyridine)	Elderly patient ISH	– Angina	–	–
Calcium channel blockers (rate-limiting)	Angina	Elderly patient	Combination with beta-blockade	Heart block Heart failure
Thiazides or thiazide-like diuretics	Elderly patient ISH Heart failure Secondary stroke prevention	–	–	Gout[g]

Source: Williams *et al.* 2004.

COPD: chronic obstructive pulmonary disease; ISH: isolated systolic hypertension; LV: left ventricular; PVD: peripheral vascular disease.

[a] In heart failure when used as monotherapy; [b] In combination with a thiazide or thiazide-like diuretic; [c] ACE-inhibitors or AII receptor blockers may be beneficial in chronic renal failure but should only be used with caution, close supervision, and specialist advice when there is established and significant renal impairment; [d] Caution with ACE-inhibitors and AII receptor blockers in peripheral vascular disease because of association with renovascular disease; [e] ACE-inhibitors and AII receptor blockers are sometimes used in patients with renovascular disease under specialist supervision; [f] Beta-blockers are used increasingly to treat stable heart failure but may worsen heart failure; [g] Thiazides or thiazide-like diuretics may sometimes be necessary to control blood pressure in people with a history of gout, ideally used in combination with allopurinol.

drugs. This latest analysis has, however, shown certain trends of differences; for example, stroke events appeared somewhat lower and heart failure somewhat higher with CCB regimens than with older drugs. In the case of ACE inhibitors, compared with diuretic or beta-blocker-based regimens, there was a trend towards more stroke events with ACE inhibitors, but no differences in CHD.

In this most recent analysis, with over one million patient years follow-up during which over 25 000 strokes and CHD events occurred, compared with older treatment strategies, the earlier reports of advantages of ACE inhibitor-based treatments and disadvantages of CCB-based treatment on coronary events were not confirmed.

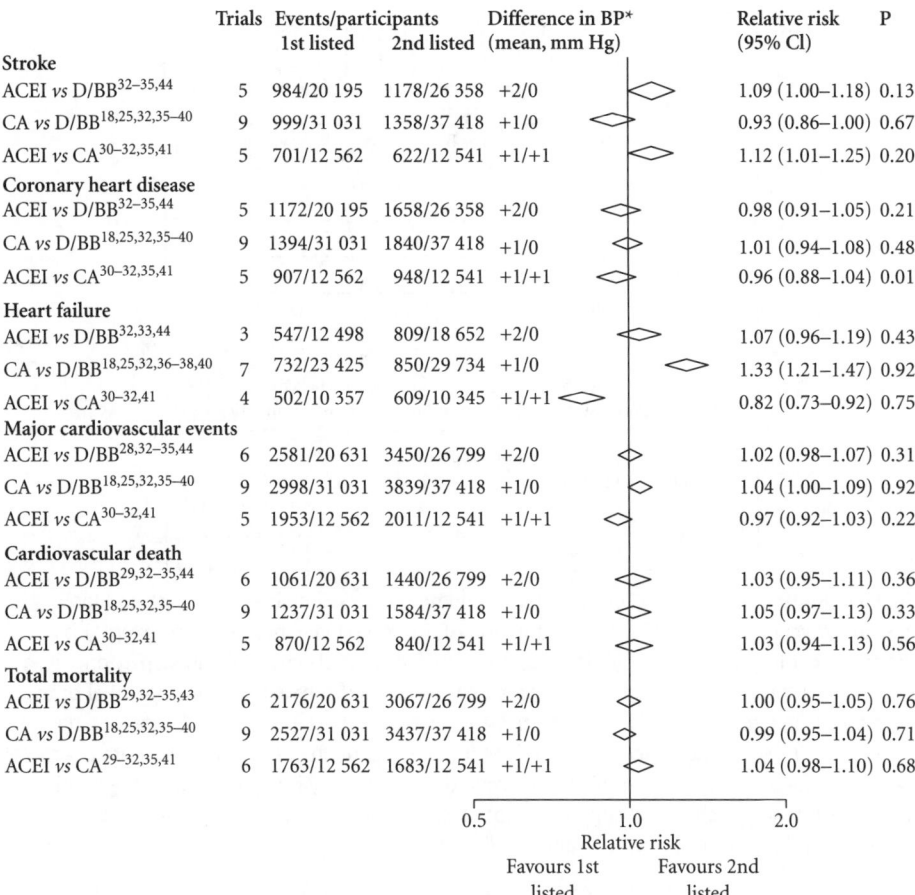

	Trials	Events/participants		Difference in BP*		Relative risk	P
		1st listed	2nd listed	(mean, mm Hg)		(95% CI)	
Stroke							
ACEI vs D/BB[32–35,44]	5	984/20 195	1178/26 358	+2/0		1.09 (1.00–1.18)	0.13
CA vs D/BB[18,25,32,35–40]	9	999/31 031	1358/37 418	+1/0		0.93 (0.86–1.00)	0.67
ACEI vs CA[30–32,35,41]	5	701/12 562	622/12 541	+1/+1		1.12 (1.01–1.25)	0.20
Coronary heart disease							
ACEI vs D/BB[32–35,44]	5	1172/20 195	1658/26 358	+2/0		0.98 (0.91–1.05)	0.21
CA vs D/BB[18,25,32,35–40]	9	1394/31 031	1840/37 418	+1/0		1.01 (0.94–1.08)	0.48
ACEI vs CA[30–32,35,41]	5	907/12 562	948/12 541	+1/+1		0.96 (0.88–1.04)	0.01
Heart failure							
ACEI vs D/BB[32,33,44]	3	547/12 498	809/18 652	+2/0		1.07 (0.96–1.19)	0.43
CA vs D/BB[18,25,32,36–38,40]	7	732/23 425	850/29 734	+1/0		1.33 (1.21–1.47)	0.92
ACEI vs CA[30–32,41]	4	502/10 357	609/10 345	+1/+1		0.82 (0.73–0.92)	0.75
Major cardiovascular events							
ACEI vs D/BB[28,32–35,44]	6	2581/20 631	3450/26 799	+2/0		1.02 (0.98–1.07)	0.31
CA vs D/BB[18,25,32,35–40]	9	2998/31 031	3839/37 418	+1/0		1.04 (1.00–1.09)	0.92
ACEI vs CA[30–32,41]	5	1953/12 562	2011/12 541	+1/+1		0.97 (0.92–1.03)	0.22
Cardiovascular death							
ACEI vs D/BB[29,32–35,44]	6	1061/20 631	1440/26 799	+2/0		1.03 (0.95–1.11)	0.36
CA vs D/BB[18,25,32,35–40]	9	1237/31 031	1584/37 418	+1/0		1.05 (0.97–1.13)	0.33
ACEI vs CA[30–32,41]	5	870/12 562	840/12 541	+1/+1		1.03 (0.94–1.13)	0.56
Total mortality							
ACEI vs D/BB[29,32–35,43]	6	2176/20 631	3067/26 799	+2/0		1.00 (0.95–1.05)	0.76
CA vs D/BB[18,25,32,35–40]	9	2527/31 031	3437/37 418	+1/0		0.99 (0.95–1.04)	0.71
ACEI vs CA[29–32,35,41]	6	1763/12 562	1683/12 541	+1/+1		1.04 (0.98–1.10)	0.68

0.5 1.0 2.0
Relative risk
Favours 1st listed   Favours 2nd listed

Fig. 50.3 Comparisons of blood-pressure-lowering regimens based on different drug classes. ACEI:ACE inhibitor; BP: blood pressure; CA: calcium antagonist; CI: confidence interval; D/BB: diuretic or beta-blocker. p values from χ^2 test for homogeneity. *Overall mean blood pressure difference (systolic/diastolic) during follow-up in the group assigned the 1st-listed treatment compared with the group assigned the 2nd-listed treatment, calculated by weighting the difference observed in each contributing trial by the number of individuals in the trial. Positive values indicate a higher mean follow-up blood pressure in the 1st-listed group (ACEI and CA) than in the 2nd-listed group (D/BB and CA). (Reproduced with permission from Turnbull/BPPLTTC 2003).

As the authors of this overview emphasize, substantial new information has been provided, but many questions remain unanswered. Future overviews from the BPLTTC will provide vital new evidence, particularly with respect to high-risk subgroups, such as those with diabetes, renal disease, and cerebrovascular disease.

50.6 Optimal combinations of antihypertensive therapies?

This question is particularly important since earlier studies (Hansson *et al.* 1998; UKPDS 38 1998) have shown that the majority of patients require at least two drugs to reach currently recommended targets. Combination therapies may enable target blood pressures to be achieved with lower doses of the individual drugs than would be required to achieve similar targets with

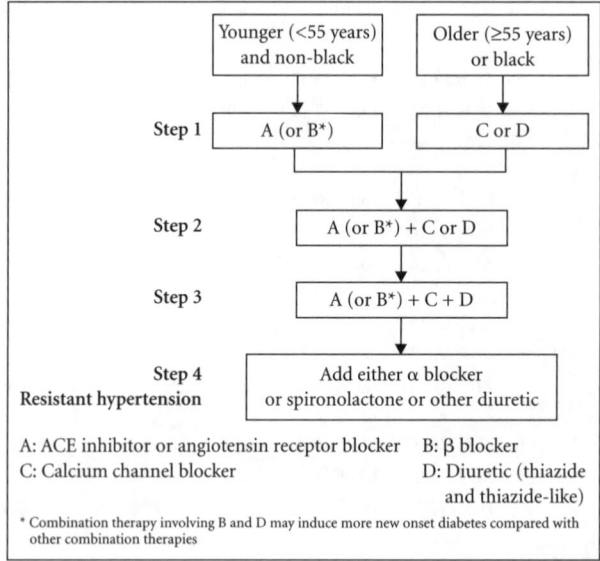

Fig. 50.4 British Hypertension Society Recommendations for a Simplified Approach to Blood Pressure Lowering Therapy. Modified Cambridge AB/CD Rule. Initial monotherapy (step 1) is selected according to age and ethnic group, as surrogates for plasma renin. In step 2, one drug from each of the AB and CD categories combined. Because of the diabetogenic potential of the older classes in older patients, B is shown in parenthesis at step 2, and is dropped altogether from step 3 (triple therapy). Recommendations for step 4 (quadruple therapy) are more anecdotal and may require secondary referral. Non-thiazide diuretic therapy is most appropriate in patients with normal renal function and suppression of plasma renin despite receiving the A + C + D combination. (Reproduced from Williams et al. 2004.)

monotherapy. Dose titration of many blood pressure-lowering drugs is associated with the emergence of unwanted side effects (e.g. lethargy, gout, oedema) which may be avoided by combinations of drugs using lower doses. In theory it is logical to combine agents that act on different pathophysiological mechanisms involved in blood pressure regulation or to add a second agent that counteracts neurohumoral responses to the first drug, which may limit blood pressure-lowering efficacy (Sever 1999a). In practice, we have as yet no trial evidence to guide the selection of optimal combinations in terms of the prevention of cardiovascular events.

Pending the availability of such data, a scheme for the selection of preferred combinations and subsequent add-on therapy is shown in Fig. 50.4.

50.6.1 **ASCOT (Sever et al. 2002)**

This was designed to compare two combinations of drugs in preventing coronary events among patients with hypertension. The design of ASCOT (Fig. 50.5), with its common third-line add on drug allows a direct comparison of the 2 drug combinations – the standard beta-blocker plus diuretic with the more contemporary regimen of CCB plus ACE inhibitor.

ASCOT also incorporated a lipid-lowering arm (see Section 44.8.3) and has the further advantage that meaningful subgroup analyses will be feasible on important subgroups such as diabetic patients, since over 4000 diabetic patients with hypertension have been randomized into this trial.

Clearly, further trials which allow comparisons of pairs of antihypertensive agents are required.

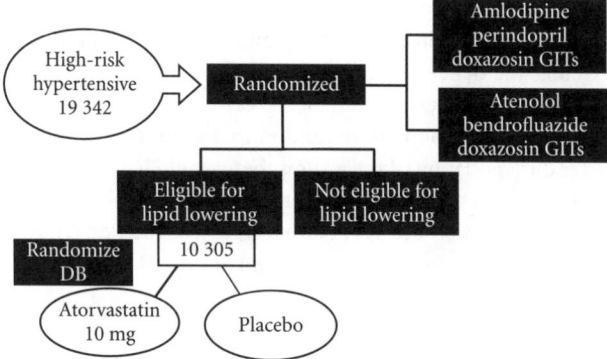

Fig. 50.5 Outline of ASCOT. (Reproduced from Sever *et al.* 2002.) DB: double-blind.

50.7 **Thresholds and targets for antihypertensive drug therapy**

50.7.1 **Thresholds**

Outcome data from interventional studies provide clear evidence of benefit from treating patients with blood pressures over 160 mmHg systolic and 100 mmHg diastolic, throughout most of the age range. Evidence of benefit over 84 years remains to be established (Sever *et al.* 1993).

No guidelines recommend across-the-board treatment for pressures less than 140 mmHg systolic and 90 mmHg diastolic, except in pre-specified high risk groups for example, diabetes, post-stroke, and other high cardiovascular risk patients. Different approaches have been taken to provide recommendations for treatment to patients in the borderline range for whom information from outcome trials is either lacking or inconsistent. Contemporary guidelines (Chobanian *et al.* 2003; ESH–ESC Guidelines Committee 2003; Williams *et al.* 2004) favour the concept of assessment of absolute cardiovascular or coronary risk in these patients, based either on the presence of target organ damage, or additional cardiovascular risk factors including older age, male sex, elevated serum lipids, smoking, diabetes, and family history. This is normally done using a modified Framingham risk score (Williams *et al.* 2004). A 10 year CHD risk ≥15% is deemed an indication for drug treatment. This is roughly equivalent to a 10 year cardiovascular event rate of ≥20%.

It should be noted that placebo-controlled trial evidence is as yet only available to confirm the benefits of blood pressure lowering among those with a SBP in the range 140–159 in certain subgroups of patients (see Section 50.9).

50.7.2 **Treatment targets**

Recent guidelines all recommend target SBPs and DBPs, although the evidence from intervention trials to support these recommendations is limited.

The Hypertension Optimal Treatment Trial (HOT) (Hansson *et al.* 1998)

This is, as yet, the only trial designed to evaluate how far blood pressure should be lowered and was a potentially important study in the light of concerns expressed about a possible J-shaped relationship between blood pressure lowering and cardiovascular risk. The trial design aimed for three target blood pressure groups of ≤90, ≤85, and ≤80 mmHg DBP in a randomized allocation of 18 790 patients with hypertension. In the event, the three random-ized groups differed by only ~4 mmHg DBP instead of the planned 10 mmHg and, with the lower than expected cardiovascular incidence rate observed, the trial was underpowered to answer the primary question. It would have been preferable, if feasible, once it was discerned that there was inadequate separation of the groups, to re-randomize the 'middle' group to ≤90 or ≤80 mmHg DBP. With greater differentiation of the groups there would have been a greater chance to test the original hypothesis. Regrettably the steering committee had to revert to 'on-treatment' analyses of the data, which are less robust because the benefits of the randomization process are foregone. Even so, the reported nadir of blood pressure

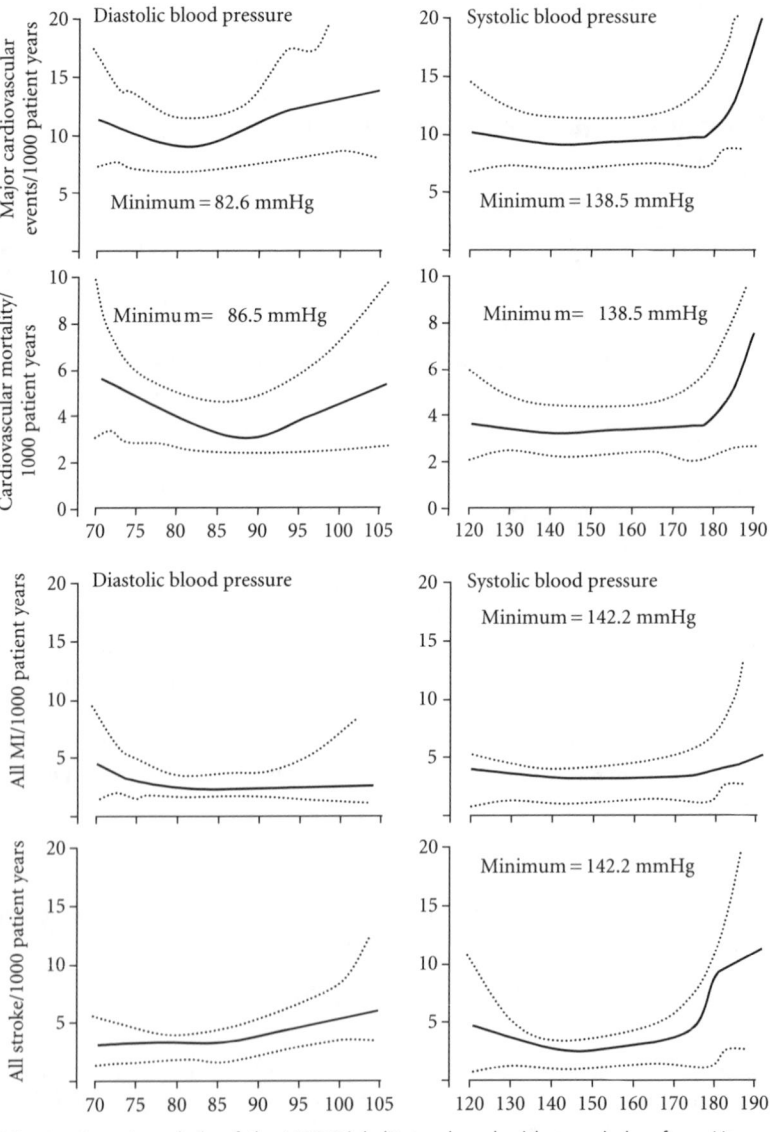

Fig. 50.6 On-treatment analysis of the HOT Trial. (Reproduced with permission from Hansson *et al.* 1998.)

(138.5/82.6 mmHg) associated with the fewest cardiovascular events was not convincingly apparent in the data provided (Fig 50.6). HOT also addressed the question of potential benefits from aspirin in treated hypertensives (see Section 50.8.1).

Despite a general consensus among guidelines for thresholds and targets, reference to clinical practice provides widespread disturbing evidence of major discrepancies between guidelines and practice with poor blood pressure control in the majority of cases (Andersson *et al.* 1998; Primatesta *et al.* 2001). Hence there is a major need to address this important issue, which remains responsible for a high residual (and potentially remedial) cardiovascular risk in the hypertensive population. Whilst many explanations have been proffered to account for the problem, observations in several European countries point to physicians failing to modify treatment (dose or drug) in the circumstance of poor blood pressure control. The complexity of guidelines is one potential contributor to suboptimal practice and in response to such criticisms one simplified guideline for primary care (Sever 1999*b*), which may be used to good effect in the developing world, was recommended: a simple goal of 150 mmHg SBP (ignoring DBP). The arguments supporting this recommendation were that SBP is a better predictor of risk for most hypertensive individuals, isolated diastolic hypertension is uncommon, and once decisions have been made, based on SBP measurements (both thresholds and goals) in the majority of patients the DBP is controlled if SBP is.

One important message arising from trials which include treatment algorithms targeted at pre-specified goals is that in nurse-led clinics where such pre-specified treatment algorithms are followed, substantially better control of blood pressure is achieved in a greater proportion of hypertensive patients.

50.8 Concomitant therapy

50.8.1 Aspirin

In both the HOT trial and among hypertensive patients in the Thrombosis Prevention Trial (1998) aspirin reduced cardiovascular events by 15% and 16%, respectively, and myocardial infarction by 36% and 20%, respectively. However, in both studies there was a narrow margin between risk of haemorrhage and benefit. For example, in the placebo-controlled arm of the HOT trial 15% fewer cardiovascular events occurred in the aspirin-treated group, but these events were outnumbered by an excess of major gastrointestinal bleeds, leading to the appropriate conclusion that the use of aspirin in hypertensive subjects should be restricted to those with controlled blood pressure and at least a 20%, 10 year risk of a future major cardiovascular event (Williams *et al.* 2004).

50.8.2 Antioxidants

The Heart Outcomes Prevention Evaluation (HOPE 2000) and the Heart Protection Study (HPS 2002) trials have emphasized the total lack of any cardiovascular benefits associated with the use of antioxidants (see Chapter 15). Pending further information, these agents should not be prescribed except for nutritional deficiencies.

50.8.3 Lipid-lowering agents

Subgroup analyses of the primary and secondary prevention trials of CHD have demonstrated similar benefits of treatment with statins in the hypertensive patients as in the total trial population. On average, ~30% reduction in major coronary events was observed, and stroke was also importantly reduced by between 15 and 30%.

In two hypertension trials – ALLHAT and ASCOT – the impact of lipid lowering in hypertensive patients was addressed by way of factorial design. In ALLHAT patients were randomized to pravastatin versus usual care (ALLHAT Officers and Coordinators for the ALLHAT Collaborative Research Group 2002b), and in ASCOT, to atorvastatin versus placebo (Sever et al. 2003). ALLHAT included some patients who had previously sustained a myocardial infarction, whereas in ASCOT prior myocardial infarction was an important exclusion criterion.

In ALLHAT, no significant difference in outcome for the primary end point, all-cause mortality, and a modest but non-significant reduction in CHD events (9%) and stroke (9%) is best explained by the extensive use of statins in the 'usual' care limb. This accounts for a much smaller difference in total cholesterol levels (9%) achieved between the two limbs of the trial.

In ASCOT, however, the lipid-lowering limb of the trial was terminated early owing to a highly significant (36%) reduction in the primary end point of CHD mortality and non-fatal myocardial infarction, together with a significant reduction in stroke incidence (27%). These benefits were associated with a 24% reduction in total cholesterol after $\sim$3 years of follow-up. The results of ASCOT have important implications for the management of hypertensive patients with regard to lipid-lowering since the RRRs in CHD outcome were independent of baseline cholesterol values and the overall CHD event rate of 9.4% over 10 years in the placebo group clearly falls below some recommended treatment thresholds in guidelines for cholesterol lowering in the primary prevention of CHD (NCEP 2001; Wood et al. 1998).

In light of increasing trial evidence, including ASCOT, thresholds for intervention with drug therapy have been reduced to 15% CHD risk, 20% cardiovascular disease risk over 10 years.

50.9 Patient subgroups

50.9.1 Diabetes

Cardiovascular morbidity and mortality rates are high in patients with hypertension and diabetes. Higher blood pressure levels are instrumental in the pathophysiology of macrovascular and microvascular disease and the potential benefits of therapeutic intervention are therefore large. Only one major trial of blood pressure-lowering in patients with non-insulin dependent diabetes (NIDDM) has been carried out to date: the United Kingdom Prospective Diabetes Study (UKPDS 38 1998). This long-awaited study included a blood pressure-lowering limb which evaluated macrovascular and microvascular end points as a function of different degrees of blood pressure lowering in 1148 hypertensive patients with NIDDM. There were unequivocal benefits associated with tight compared with less tight blood pressure control in terms of any diabetes-related end point (34%) and macrovascular outcomes (stroke reduction 44%, CHD reduction 31%). These benefits were significantly greater than those associated with greater or lesser improvements in HbA$_{1C}$, which did not impact significantly on macrovascular events.

Similar findings were supported from a subgroup analysis of the HOT study, and provide good support for the recommendations to lower target blood pressures in patients with NIDDM (Williams et al. 2004).

A critical issue about UKPDS concerns the investigators' attempts to compare outcome in the two blood pressure treatment groups – one ACE inhibitor-based and one beta-blocker-based (UKPDS 39 1998). Here, in a randomized comparison of 400 patients allocated to captopril and 358 patients allocated to atenolol (a surprising disparity), cardiovascular event rates were similar in the two groups. This is hardly surprising since this aspect of the study had negligible power to detect potentially important differences between the two groups. What is surprising is the uncritical way that the apparent 'equivalence' of treatment has been accepted both by diabetologists and indeed by the journals responsible for publishing the UKPDS results, where the obvious potential for a type 2 statistical error was not commented upon.

Three studies have shown that ARBs provide a renoprotective effect and reduce renal morbidity independent of blood pressure reduction in type 2 diabetics with nephropathy.

Study of the effects of irbesartan on microalbuminuria in hypertensive patients with type 2 diabetes (IRMA2) (Parving *et al*. 2001)

In this trial 590 hypertensive patients with type 2 diabetes and microalbuminuria were randomized to either irbesartan (150–300 mg/day) or placebo, added to usual antihypertensive therapy (excluding ACE inhibitors). The primary outcome, of progression to overt proteinuria and a 30% increase in urinary albumin excretion rate, was significantly reduced by 70% in the group treated with the higher dose of irbesartan and 30% in that treated with the lower dose.

Reduction of Endpoints in Non-Insulin Dependent Diabetes Mellitus with the Angiotensin 2 Antagonist Losartan (RENAAL) (Brenner *et al*. 2001)

RENAAL included 1513 patients with type 2 diabetes, proteinuria, and raised serum creatinine, who were randomized to either losartan (maximum dose 100 mg) or placebo in addition to other antihypertensive drugs. The primary outcome of a composite end point, including doubling of serum creatinine, end-stage renal failure, or death, was significantly reduced (by 16%) in the losartan group. The trial was stopped prematurely over ethical concerns about withholding inhibitors of the renin-system in diabetics with renal impairment.

Irbesartan type-2 Diabetic Nephropathy Trial (IDNT) (Lewis *et al*. 2001)

In this trial, 1715 patients were randomized to receive either irbesartan (maximum dose 300 mg), amlodipine (maximum dose 10 mg), or placebo (other antihypertensive drugs), and with a similar primary end point as RENAAL. For similar falls in blood pressure in the two pre-specified active treatment groups of 140/77 mmHg and 141/77 mmHg, respectively, there was a significant, 23% RRR with irbesartan compared with amlodipine, and a 20% reduction compared with placebo in the primary end point, due mainly to a reduction in the time to doubling of creatinine. However, further information is needed on secondary cardiovascular end points, which were marginally higher in the irbesartan group.

This raises the important issue, when interpreting trials in high risk patients, of demonstrating major cardiovascular benefits from a particular treatment strategy rather than surrogate end points, before recommendations can be made for the use of particular drug classes.

From trials restricted to patients with diabetes and from subgroup analyses of diabetic patients recruited into other hypertension trials, the benefits of blood pressure lowering to prevent cardiovascular events were observed to be substantial (Staessen *et al*. 1997; UKPDS 38 1998). On this basis, and in consideration of outcome data for diabetics in the HOT trial (Hansson *et al*. 1998), lower goal blood pressures on treatment are recommended (Williams *et al*. 2004).

In patients with type 1 diabetes, treatment regimens based on ACE inhibitors have been claimed to reduce the rate of decline in renal function (Lewis *et al*. 1993), although to what extent these benefits were independent of blood pressure reduction remains controversial (Perkins *et al.* 2003).

Among patients with type 2 diabetes, of whom 70% or more are hypertensive, trial evidence supports the need for at least two therapies to control blood pressure and thereby to reduce cardiovascular events (Hansson *et al.* 1998; Staessen *et al.* 1997). There is increasing evidence that, for equivalent reductions in blood pressure, preservation of renal function and reductions in the rate of decline of renal function are seen to a greater extent with drug regimens based upon either ARBs (Brenner *et al.* 2001; Lewis *et al.* 2001; Parving *et al.* 2001) or ACE inhibitors (Agodoa *et al.* 2001). However, further evidence is needed to ensure that this is achieved without any compromise in the protection against cardiovascular events in this population. Results from the diabetic subgroup in the LIFE (Losartan Intervention For Endpoint) reduction in hypertension trial (Lindholm *et al.* 2002) (see Section 50.9.4) provide strong evidence to support the use of ARBs in patients with hypertension and diabetes, especially when complicated by left ventricular hypertrophy (LVH).

50.9.2 Those at high risk of cardiovascular disease

The HOPE Trial (HOPE 2000) was not, in the strict sense, a trial in hypertensive patients, indeed blood pressure was not measured in any standardized way. It was designed to assess the role of an ACE inhibitor (ramipril) in patients at high risk for cardiovascular events. A total of 9297 high risk patients who had evidence of vascular disease or diabetes plus one other cardiovascular risk factor were randomly assigned to receive either ramipril or placebo for a 5 year follow-up period. Ramipril reduced the rates of death from cardiovascular disease by 26 % compared with placebo and a host of other cardiovascular end points were similarly reduced. The small differences in blood pressure initially reported between the two groups of ~3 mmHg systolic have resulted in discussion and debate about how much of the ACE inhibitor-induced benefit could be blood pressure related. From the early meta-analyses of prospective observational studies and intervention trials, this difference in blood pressure might account for one-third of the benefit observed in the HOPE trial.

A more recent report of a HOPE substudy (Svenson *et al.* 2001) further challenges the HOPE investigators' claims that the benefits observed in this trial are drug (or class) related, rather than due to blood pressure differences. In this, albeit very small, substudy blood pressure was more carefully evaluated by ambulatory blood pressure monitoring. Significant differences in 24 h blood pressures of 10/4 mmHg and night-time differences of 17/8 mmHg were observed with lower pressures in the ramipril group. Such differences are totally commensurate with the cardiovascular benefits observed in the trial overall.

50.9.3 Those with established cerebrovascular disease

In 1997 the INDANA (INdividual Data ANalysis of Antihypertensive intervention trials) project provided evidence that patients having already suffered from a stroke were likely to benefit from antihypertensive treatment (Gueyffier *et al.* 1997).

The Perindopril Protection Against Recurrent Stroke Study (PROGRESS) (MacMahon *et al.* 2001) trial was initiated in 1996, and designed to assess the effects of blood pressure lowering with a regimen including the ACE inhibitor perindopril, with or without the diuretic indapamide, in patients with a history of transient ischaemic attacks or minor strokes, when compared with placebo. In this study 6105 patients, who did not necessarily have raised blood pressure, were randomized and followed-up for an average of 4 years.

Active treatment reduced blood pressure by 9/4 mmHg and recurrent stroke incidence by 28%. These benefits were seen in patients irrespective of baseline blood pressure. The combination of perindopril and indapamide was more effective in both lowering blood pressure and reducing recurrent stroke incidence than monotherapy with either the ACE inhibitor or diuretic alone.

This important trial confirms the need to consider blood pressure-lowering treatment in patients suffering from transient ischaemic attacks or who have recovered from a stroke, irrespective of the blood pressure level. However, further issues remain unanswered, including the extent to which blood pressure should be lowered and how blood pressure should be managed in the context of acute stroke.

50.9.4 Those with LVH

Many small, usually inadequately designed, trials evaluating the effects of various drug classes on regression of LVH have been published. Meta-analyses of these studies (Dahlöf *et al.* 1992; Jennings and Wong 1998) suggest that ACE inhibitors and CCBs may be more effective at achieving LVH regression than other drug classes. However, the implications of these findings, if true, on major cardiovascular events, remains unclear. One trial has compared the impact of two blood pressure regimens on major cardiovascular events in patients with LVH, the LIFE reduction in hypertension study (Dahlöf *et al.* 2002).

This trial investigated the effects of the ARB losartan, compared with a beta-blocker, atenolol, in 9222 patients with essential hypertension and ECG-based LVH. Hydrochlorthiazide was used as a common second-line add-on therapy. Following an average follow-up period of 4 years, blood pressures were reduced to similar levels by both treatment strategies. The regression of LVH was significantly greater in the losartan than in the atenolol group. There was a clinically significant reduction of 13% in the combined primary end point of cardiovascular death, myocardial infarction, and stroke in the losartan compared with the atenolol limb of the trial. This difference was chiefly accounted for by reductions in stroke. In a separate analysis of diabetic subjects the benefits of losartan were confirmed, and if anything larger than in the non-diabetic group (Lindholm *et al.* 2002).

This was the first trial to show a convincing difference in the primary cardiovascular outcome among hypertensive patients treated with different drug classes, for an equivalent degree of blood pressure lowering, with the inference that treatment effects may be independent of blood pressure lowering. The question arises, therefore, as to whether the differential outcome was due to a particular benefit of the ARB or whether, as in the MRC Trial, a treatment regimen based on a beta-blocker is simply less effective in protecting against certain cardiovascular events. Would the same result have occurred in LIFE had the comparator not been atenolol?

50.9.5 Elderly patients

In most populations SBP rises with age, and DBP rises up to ~60–70 years and falls thereafter. Consequently the prevalence of hypertension including ISH is high in the elderly (Primatesta *et al.* 2001). The elderly are at higher absolute cardiovascular risk than the young for any given level of blood pressure, and are more likely to have concomitant conditions that may influence treatment choices.

Intervention trials failed to confirm historical dogma that treating the elderly would do more harm than good. On the contrary, treating the elderly with hypertension, including ISH up to the age of 80 years and possibly beyond, confers major benefits from reduction in cardiovascular risk, including heart failure (Amery *et al.* 1985; Collins and Peto 1994; Coope and Warrender Thomas 1986; Dahlöf *et al.* 1991; MRC Working Party 1992; SHEP Cooperative Research Group 1991; Staessen *et al.* 1997). The magnitude of the RRR is similar for younger and older patients, but because the absolute risk is higher in the elderly, the absolute risk reduction is substantially greater than in younger hypertensive people.

Concerns that tolerance of antihypertensive drugs was worse in the elderly have not been borne out in the trials (Hansson *et al.* 1998) and non-pharmacological treatment is at least as effective in the elderly. Treatment thresholds and goals of therapy are broadly similar to those recommended to younger patients, except that in patients with resistant elevated SBPs, despite multiple drug therapy, it may be necessary to accept somewhat less stringent blood pressure control.

The percentage reduction in the incidence of strokes in elderly hypertensive patients receiving drug treatment is similar to that seen in the young (Collins and Peto 1994). In at least two studies a significant reduction in cardiac mortality has also been observed and in two recent trials there has been a significant reduction in the incidence of coronary events. The cardiovascular benefits of therapy were also seen in the first treatment trial of ISH in the elderly (SHEP Cooperative Research Group 1991; Staessen *et al.* 1997). In these studies, and in the MRC trial of treatment of older patients (MRC Working Party 1992), the reduction in coronary events appeared to be linked to therapy with a diuretic-based regimen. Whether there are indeed benefits in terms of coronary event outcome from diuretics as opposed to beta-blocker regimens remains uncertain.

Trial data indicate that diuretics and CCBs are particularly effective in this population and are the recommended first line therapy (Materson *et al.* 1993). Furthermore, a subgroup analysis of SYST-EUR demonstrated substantial cardiovascular benefits associated with CCB treatment in patients with NIDDM (Tuomilehto *et al.* 1999). The results of the LIFE trial (Dahlöf *et al.* 2002) suggest that an ARB, if required for additional blood pressure reduction – particularly for those with LVH – would make a suitable additional drug for either the diuretic or the CCB. The ANBP2 (Wing *et al.* 2003) trial included patients between age 65 and 84 years and the Study on COgnition and Prognosis in the Elderly (SCOPE) trial (Hansson *et al.* 1999c) included over 1000 patients aged over 80 years. These trials provide the most data currently available in the very elderly. Although no true placebo-controlled limb was included in the SCOPE trial, side effect and withdrawal rates were low and additional good blood pressure lowering with an ARB was achieved in association with a modest reduction in cardiovascular events, including non-fatal stroke.

One trial, the Hypertension in the Very Elderly Trial (HYVET) is currently in progress. This trial (Bulpitt *et al.* 1994) is unique in evaluating benefits of blood pressure lowering exclusively in those aged over 80 years, a group for whom the benefits of treatment are not fully established, despite the SCOPE and ANBP2 trials. In addition, SCOPE formally evaluated benefits on cognitive function associated with blood pressure lowering which, in view of the reduced rates of dementia observed among those treated with nitrendipine in the SYST-EUR trial (Forette *et al.* 1998), is potentially an important and exciting focus for intervention. However, perhaps because of the limited blood pressure reduction achieved in this trial, and because of the insensitivity of the mini mental state examination (MMSE) score for the large number of patients with high baseline scores, no significant benefits in cognitive function were apparent.

50.9.6 **Different ethnic groups**

Hypertension poses particular problems in different ethnic groups. Hypertension in blacks (African, Afro-Caribbean, African-American) is common, often severe, and is frequently associated with increased rates of cerebrovascular (often small vessel) disease, renal impairment, LVH, and heart failure (Saunders and Hildreth 1991; see also Chapter 9).

Salt sensitivity and blood pressure responses to reductions in dietary sodium may be more apparent in black than white hypertensive patients, although this is relative rather than absolute. A volume dependent, low renin hypertension is more commonly seen in blacks and accounts for their relative lack of response to beta-blockers, ACE inhibitors, and ARBs, in contrast with diuretics and CCBs, which are the preferred first line agents (Materson *et al.* 1993).

Hypertensive subjects from the Indian subcontinent have a high prevalence of the metabolic syndrome and other abnormalities which make up the insulin resistance syndrome (McKeigue *et al.* 1991). No outcome trials have focused on this important subgroup of patients. In the absence of such trial data it seems prudent to avoid drug regimens that exacerbate or worsen these abnormalities (e.g. beta-blockers).

Optimal strategies for the treatment of each ethnic group throughout the developing world remain to be determined. This should be a major area for further research in hypertension (see Section 50.10). The high prevalence of hypertension in Japan and in some Chinese populations, the high cardiovascular risk in certain Polynesian/Micronesian populations, and the uncertainties around preferred drug choices in those of Arab origin present particular challenges for future trials. In the meantime, emphasis must be placed on achieving goal pressures as the primary objective and further studies and meta-analyses will hopefully shed light on this important international problem, which contributes substantially to the global burden of disease (see Chapter 11).

The ALLHAT trial (ALLHAT Officers and Coordinators for the ALLHAT Collaborative Research Group 2002*a*) included, by design, a large proportion of African-American patients and this trial suggested that diuretics may overall be preferred to ACE inhibitors for such patients. However, it may be that these apparent benefits merely relate to the better blood pressure reduction achieved in the diuretic group.

One recent trial has compared three drug classes in African-American patients, although the findings and interpretation are controversial. The African-American Study of Kidney Disease (AASK) (Agodoa *et al.* 2001) study compared the effects of three drugs: amlodipine, ramipril, and metoprolol, on the progression of renal disease in 1094 African-Americans with renal impairment. Following an interim analysis after an average of 3 years follow-up, amlodipine was discontinued following a comparison of the amlodipine and ramipril arms of the trial (a comparison which was not planned a priori), in a subset of patients (selected post hoc) with proteinuria greater than 300 mg/day, in whom ramipril had a 36% slower mean decline in glomerular filtration rate (GFR) and a 48% reduced risk of clinical end points compared with amlodipine, despite similar blood pressure-lowering effects.

The authors reported no overall differences in the primary outcome of GFR decline for the whole cohort, but after adjusting for baseline covariates the ramipril group had a 38% reduced risk of clinical end points and a 36% slower decline in GFR after 3 months. However, for the majority of randomized patients who had a urinary protein:creatinine ratio of <0.22 and a baseline GFR >40 ml/min there was a smaller loss of GFR over 3 years in the amlodipine group. The premature closure of this trial highlights the difficulty of stopping trials on the basis of results relating to subgroup, post-hoc secondary end points, which were not pre-specified among a subgroup, which was also not pre-specified.

50.10 **Other trials needed**

It is clear that, assuming adequate power, the blood pressure-lowering trials in progress will contribute individually and collectively towards answering many of the outstanding questions relating to hypertension management.

Current recommendations for treating SBP levels of ~140 mmHg (Williams *et al.* 2004; Chobanian *et al.* 2003) are not based on randomized trial evidence (except in high risk groups). Despite the limitations of the data (Sever 1999c), the results of the HOT trial (Hansson *et al.* 1998) were influential in determining the optimal target blood pressures recommended in the 2004 BHS management guidelines (Williams *et al.* 2004). However, whilst the HOT data are perhaps the best available they were, as discussed above, by no means definitive in determining the optimal diastolic target and even less robust for systolic targets. Given the prime importance of systolic rather than diastolic blood pressure for most hypertensive subjects, further trials to determine optimal systolic targets are required.

Hitherto two morbidity/mortality trials have been carried out in China (Gong *et al.* 1996; Liu *et al.* 1998) and some developing countries have contributed patients to other hypertension trials. However, with these exceptions, despite the increasing global problem of hypertension, most trial data hail from the developed Western world and no trials have been carried out purely in the developing world in, for example, black or south Asian hypertensive patients. Given ethnic differences in blood pressure responses for various antihypertensive agents (Materson *et al.* 1993), the results of such trials may have major implications for the majority of the world's hypertensive populations who hail from such countries. As the majority of the world is developing, hypertension and its adverse sequelae will increase in relative and absolute terms as a global source of cardiovascular burden. It is, therefore, critical that trials in such populations are carried out to determine country-specific effective ways of treating or, ideally, preventing raised blood pressure.

50.11 **Summary and conclusion**

Few, if any, areas of medicine have as many large randomized trials to help guide practice as hypertension. Despite this, by the year 1994 (MacMahon *et al.* 1990) objective decisions on several key management issues could not be made on the basis of randomized trial evidence. Progress since that time has been limited, despite the publication of several major new trials including tens of thousands of patients. However, prospects for the future are more exciting, with over 30 major trials in progress, and the potentially large advantages of a prospective collaboration among these triallists.

References

Agodoa, L. Y., Appel, L., Bakris, G. L., Beck, G. *et al.* (2001). Effect of ramipril vs amlodipine on renal outcomes in hypertensive nephrosclerosis: a randomised controlled trial. *Journal of the American Medical Association*, **285**, 2719–28.

ALLHAT Officers and Co-ordinators for the ALLHAT Collaborative Research Group (2000). Major cardiovascular events in hypertensive patients randomized to Doxazosin vs Chlorthalidone: the antihypertensive and lipid-lowering treatment to Prevent heart Attack Trial (ALLHAT). *Journal of the American Medical Association*, **283**, 1967–75.

ALLHAT Officers and Coordinators for the ALLHAT Collaborative Research Group (2002a). The Antihypertensive and Lipid-Lowering Treatment to Prevent Heart Attack Trial. Major outcomes in high-risk hypertensive patients randomized to angiotensin-converting enzyme inhibitor or calcium channel blocker vs diuretic: The Antihypertensive and Lipid-Lowering Treatment to Prevent Heart Attack Trial (ALLHAT). *Journal of the American Medical Association*, **23**, 2981–97.

ALLHAT Officers and Coordinators for the ALLHAT Collaborative Research Group (2002*b*). The Antihypertensive and Lipid-Lowering Treatment to Prevent Heart Attack Trial. Major outcomes in moderately hypercholesterolemic, hypertensive patients randomized to pravastatin vs usual care: The Antihypertensive and Lipid-Lowering Treatment to Prevent Heart Attack Trial (ALLHAT-LLT). *Journal of the American Medical Association*, **23**, 2998–3007.

Amery, A., Birkenhäger, W., Brixho, P. *et al.* (1985). Mortality and morbidity results from the European Working Party on High Blood Pressure in the Elderly trial. *Lancet*, **i**, 1349–54.

Andersson, O. K., Almgren, T., Persson, B., Samuelsson, O., Hedner, T. and Wilhelmsen, L. (1998). Survival in treated hypertension: follow up study after two decades. *British Medical Journal*, **317**, 167–71.

Appel, L. J., Moore, T. J., Obarzanek, E., Vollmer, W. M., Svetkey, L. P., Sacks, F. M. *et al.* for the DASH Collaborative Research Group (1997). A clinical trial of the effects of dietary patterns on blood pressure. *New England Journal of Medicine*, **336**, 1117–24.

Applegate, W. B. Miller, S. T., Elam, J. T., Cushman, W. C., el Derwi, D., Brewer, A., Graney, M. J. (1992). Nonpharmacologic intervention to reduce blood pressure in older patients with mild hypertension. *Archives of Internal Medicine*, **152**, 1162–66.

Attwood, S., Bird, R., Burch, K., Casadei, B., Coats, A., Conway, J. *et al.* (1994). Within-patient correlation between the antihypertensive effects of atenolol, lisinopril and nifedipine. *Journal of Hypertension*, **12**, 1053–60.

Australian Therapeutic Trial in Mild Hypertension (1980). Report by the Management Committee. *Lancet*, **1**, 1261–7.

Braith, R. W., Pollock, M. L., Lowenthal, D. T., Graves, J. E. and Limacher, M. C. (1994). Moderate- and high-intensity exercise lowers blood pressure in normotensive subjects 60–79 years of age. *American Journal of Cardiology*, **73**, 1124–8.

Brenner, B. M., Cooper, M. E., de Zeeuw, D. *et al.* for the RENAAL Study Investigators (2001). Effects of losartan on renal and cardiovascular outcomes in patients with type 2 diabetes and nephropathy. *New England Journal of Medicine*, **345**, 861–9.

Brown, M. J., Palmer, C. R., Castaigne, A., de Leeuw, P. W., Mancia, G., Rosenthal, T. and Ruilope, L. M. (2000). Morbidity and mortality in patients randomised to double-blind treatment with a long-acting-calcium channel blocker of diuretic in the International Nifedipine GITS study: Intervention as a Goal in Hypertension Treatment (INSIGHT). *Lancet*, **356**, 366–72.

Brown, M. J., Cruickshank, J. K., Dominiczak, A. F., MacGregor, G. A., Poulter, N. R., Russell, G. I. *et al.* (2003). Better blood pressure control: how to combine drugs. *Journal of Human Hypertension*, **17**, 81–6.

Bulpitt, C. J., Fletcher, A. E., Amery, A., Coope, J., Evans, J. G., Lightowlers, S. *et al.* (1994). The Hypertension in the Very Elderly Trial (HYVET): rationale, methodology and comparison with previous trials. *Drugs Ageing*, **5**, 171–83.

Chobanian, A. V., Bakris, G. L., Black, H. R., Cushman, W. C., Green, L. A. *et al.* and the National High Blood Pressure Education Programme Coordinating Committee (2003). The Seventh Report of the Joint National Committee on Prevention, Detection, Evaluation, and Treatment of High Blood Pressure: The JNC 7 Report. *Journal of the American Medical Association*, **289**, 2560–72.

Collins, R. and Peto, R. (1994). Antihypertensive drug therapy: effects on stroke and coronary heart disease. In *Textbook of Hypertension* (ed. J. D. Swales), pp. 1156–64. Blackwell Scientific, Oxford.

Coope, J. and Warrender Thomas, S. (1986). Randomised trial of treatment of hypertension in elderly patients in primary care. *British Medical Journal*, **293**, 1145–51.

Dahlöf, B., Devereux, R. B., Kjeldsen, S. E., Julius, S., Beevers, G., Faire, U. *et al.* (2002). Cardiovascular morbidity and mortality in the Losartan Intervention For Endpoint reduction in hypertension study (LIFE): a randomised trial against atenolol. *Lancet*, **359** (9311), 995–1003.

Dahlöf, B., Lindholm, L. H., Hansson, L., Schersten, B., Ekbom, T. and Wester, P. O. (1991). Morbidity and mortality in the Swedish Trial in Old Patients with Hypertension (STOP-Hypertension). *Lancet*, **338**, 1281–5.

Dahlöf, B., Pennert, K. and Hansson, L. (1992). Reversal of left ventricular hypertrophy in hypertensive patients: a meta-analysis of 109 treatment studies. *American Journal of Hypertension*, **5**, 95–110.

Davis, B. R., Cutler, J. A., Gordon, D. J., Furberg, C. D., Wright, J. T., Cushman, W. C. et al. (1996). Rationale and design for the antihypertensive and lipid lowering treatment to prevent heart attack trial (ALLHAT). *American Journal of Hypertension*, **9**, 342–60.

ESH–ESC (European Society of Hypertension–European Society of Cardiology) Guidelines Committee (2003). 2003 European Society of Hypertension-European Society of Cardiology guidelines for the management of arterial hypertension. *Journal of Hypertension*, **6**, 1011–53.

NCEP (National Cholesterol Education Programme) executive summary of the third report (2001). Expert Panel on detection, evaluation and treatment of high blood cholesterol in adults. *Journal of the American Medical Association*, **285**, 2487–97.

Forette, F., Seux, M. L., Staessen, J. A., Thijs, L., Birkenhager, W. H., Babarskiene, M. R.et al. (1998). Prevention of dementia in randomised double-blind placebo-controlled Systolic Hypertension in Europe (Syst-Eur) trial. *Lancet*, **352**, 1347–51.

Fotherby, M. D. and Potter, J. F. (1992). Potassium supplementation reduces clinic and ambulatory blood pressure in elderly hypertensive patients. *Journal of Hypertension*, **10**, 1403–8.

Fotherby, M. D. and Potter, J. F. (1993). Effects of moderate sodium restriction on clinic and twenty-four hour ambulatory blood pressure in elderly hypertensive subjects. *Journal of Hypertension*, **11**, 657–63.

Geleijnse, J. M., Witteman, J. C., Bak, A. A., den Breeijen, J. H. and Grobbee, D. E. (1994). Reduction in blood pressure with a low sodium, high potassium, high magnesium salt in older subjects with mild to moderate hypertension. *British Medical Journal*, **309**, 436–40.

Gong, L., Zhang, W., Zhu, Y., Zhu, J., Kong, D., Page, V.et al. (1996). Shanghai trial of nifedipine in the elderly (STONE). *Journal of Hypertension*, **14**, 1237–45.

Gueyffier, F., Boissel, J. P., Boutitie, F., Pocock, S., Coope, J., Cutler, J.et al. (1997). Effect of antihypertensive treatment in patients having already suffered from stroke: gathering the evidence. The INDANA (INdividual Data ANalysis of Antihypertensive intervention trials) Project Collaborators. *Stroke*, **12**, 2557–62.

Hansson, L., Zanchetti, S., Carruthers, S., Dahlof, B., Elmfeldt, D., Julius, S. et al. for the HOT Study Group (1998). Effects of intensive blood pressure lowering and low-dose aspirin in patients with hypertension: principal results of the Hypertension Optimal Treatment (HOT) randomised trial. *Lancet*, **351**, 1755–62.

Hansson, L., Lindholm, L. H., Ekborn, T., Dahlof, Lanke, J., Schersten, B.et al. for the STOP-2 Hypertension Study Group (1999a). Randomised trial of old and new antihypertensive drugs in elderly patients: cardiovascular mortality and morbidity. The Swedish Trial in Old Patients with Hypertension-2 study. *Lancet*, **354**, 1751–6.

Hansson, L., Lindholm, L. H., Niskanen, L., Lanke, J., Hedner, T., Niklason, A. et al, for the Captopril Prevention Project (CAPPP) study group (1999b). Effect of angiotensin-converting-enzyme inhibition compared with conventional therapy on cardiovascular morbidity and mortality in hypertension: the Captopril Prevention Project (CAPPP) randomised trial. *Lancet*, **353**, 611–16.

Hansson, L., Lithell, H., Skoog, I., Baro, F., Banki, C. M., Breteler, M. et al. (1999c). Study on COgnition and Prognosis in the Elderly (SCOPE). *Blood Pressure*, **8**, 177–83.

Hansson, L., Hedner, T., Lund-Johansen, P., Kjeldsen, S. E., Lindholm, L. H., Syvertsen, J. O.et al. (2000). Randomised trial of the effects of calcium antagonists compared with diuretics and β-blockers on cardiovascular morbidity and mortality in hypertension on the Nordic Diltiazem study NORDIL. *Lancet*, **356**, 359–65.

Harrison, M., Kincaid-Smith, P. and McMichael, J. (1970). Results of treatment in malignant hypertension. *Journal of the American Medical Association*, **213**, 1143–92.

HDFP (Hypertension Detection and Follow-up Program) Cooperative Group (1979). Five-year findings of the Hypertension Detection and Follow-Up program: reduction in mortality in persons with high blood pressure, including mild hypertension. *Journal of the American Medical Association*, **242**, 2562–71.

HDFP (Hypertension Detection and Follow-up Program) Cooperative Group (1982). The effect of treatment on mortality in 'mild' hypertension. *New England Journal of Medicine*, **307**, 976–80.

HOPE (Heart Outcomes Prevention Evaluation) Study Investigators (2000). Effect of ramipril on cardiovascular and microvascular outcomes in people with diabetes mellitus: results of the HOPE study and MICRO-HOPE substudy. *Lancet*, **355**, 253–9.

HPS (Heart Protection Study) Collaborative Group (2002). MRC/BHF Heart Protection Study of antioxidant vitamin supplementation in 20,536 high-risk individuals: a randomised placebo-controlled trial. *Lancet*, **360**, 23–33.

IPPPSH (International Prospective Primary Prevention Study in Hypertension) Collaborative Group (1985). Cardiovascular risk and risk factors in a randomised trial of treatment on the beta-blocker oxprenolol. *Journal of Hypertension*, **3**, 379–92.

Jennings, G. and Wong, J. (1998). Regression of left ventricular hypertrophy in hypertension: changing patterns with successive meta-analyses. *Journal of Hypertension Supplement*, **6**, S29–S34.

Kaplan, N. M. (1995). Alcohol and hypertension. *Lancet*, **345**, 1588–9.

Keith, N. M., Wagener, H. P. and Barker, N. W. (1939). Some different types of essential hypertension: their cause and prognosis. *American Journal of Medical Science*, **197**, 332–43.

Kokkinos, P. F., Narayan, P., Colleran, J. A., Pittaras, A., Notargiacomo, A., Reda, D. and Papademetriou, V. (1995). Effects of regular exercise on blood pressure and left ventricular hypertrophy in African-American men with severe hypertension. *New England Journal of Medicine*, **333**, 1462–7.

Konstam, M. A., Rousseau, M. F., Kronenberg, M. W., Udelson, J. E., Melin, J., Stewart, D., *et al.* (1992). Effects of the angiotension converting enzyme inhibitor enalapril on the long-term progression of left ventricular dysfunction in patients with heart failure. SOLVD Investigators. *Circulation*, **2**, 431–8.

Law, M. R., Frost, C. D. and Wald, N. J. (1991). III Analysis of data from trials of salt reduction. *British Medical Journal*, **302**, 819–24.

Lewis, E. J., Hunsicker, L. G., Bain, R. P., Rohde, R. D., for the Collaborative Study Group (1993). The effect of angiotensin converting-enzyme inhibition on diabetic nephropathy. *New England Journal of Medicine*, **329**, 1456–62.

Lewis, E. J., Hunsicker, L. G., Clarke, W. R. *et al.* for the Collaborative Study Group (2001). Renoprotective effects of the angiotensin-receptor antagonists irbesartan in patients with nephropathy due to type 2 diabetes. *New England Journal of Medicine*, **345**, 851–60.

Lindholm, L. H., Ibsen, H., Dahlof, B., Devereux, R. B., Beevers, G., de Faire, U.*et al.* (2002). Cardiovascular morbidity and mortality in patients with diabetes in the Losartan Intervention For Endpoint reduction in hypertension study (LIFE): a randomised trial against atenolol. *Lancet*, **359**, 1004–10.

Liu, L., Wang, J. G., Gong, L., Liu, G. and Staessen, J. A. (1998). Comparison of active treatment and placebo for older patients with isolated systolic hypertension. *Journal of Hypertension*, **16**, 1823–9.

MacMahon, S., Peto, R., Cutler, J., Collins, R., Sorlie, P., Neaton, J.*et al.* (1990). Blood pressure, stroke and coronary heart disease. Part 1, prolonged differences in blood pressure: prospective observational studies corrected for the regression dilution bias. *Lancet*, **335**, 765–74.

MacMahon, S., Neal, B., Tzouirio, C., *et al.* for the PROGRESS Collaborative Group (2001). Randomised trial of a perindopril-based blood-pressure-lowering regimen among 6105 individuals with previous stroke or transient ischaemic attack. *Lancet*, **358**, 1033–41.

Mallion, J. M. and Goldberg, A. I. (1996). Global efficacy and tolerability of losartan, an angiotensin II subtype 1-receptor antagonist, in the treatment of hypertension. *Blood Pressure Supplement*, **2**, 82–6.

Materson, B. J. Reda, D. J., Cushman, W. C., Massie, B. M., Freis, E. D., Kochar, M. S. *et al.*, for the Department of Veterans Affairs Cooperative Study Group on Antihypertensive Agents (1993). Single-drug therapy for hypertension in men: a comparison of six antihypertensive agents with placebo. *New England Journal of Medicine*, **328**, 914–21.

McCarron, D. A., Oparil, S., Chait, A., Haynes, R. B., Kris-Etherton, P., Stern, J. S. *et al.* (1997). Nutritional management of cardiovascular risk factors: a randomised clinical trial. *Archives of Internal Medicine*, **157**, 169–77.

McKeigue, P. M., Shah, B. and Marmot, M. G. (1991). Relation of central obesity and insulin resistance with diabetes prevalence and cardiovascular risk in south Asians. *Lancet*, **337**, 382–6.

MRC (Medical Research Council) Working Party (1985). MRC Trial of mild hypertension: principal results. *British Medical Journal*, **291**, 97–104.

MRC (Medical Research Council) Working Party (1992). Medical Research Council trial of treatment of hypertension in older adults: principal results. *British Medical Journal*, **304**, 405–12.

Midgley, J. P., Matthew, A. G., Greenwood, C. M. T. and Logan, A. G. (1996). Effect of reduced dietary sodium on blood pressure: a meta-analysis of randomized controlled trials. *Journal of the American Medical Association*, **275**, 1590–7.

MRFIT (Multiple Risk Factor Intervention Trial) Research Group (1982). Multiple Risk Factor Intervention Trial: risk changes and mortality results. *Journal of the American Medical Association*, **248**, 1465–77.

National High Blood Pressure Education Program Working Group (1993). National High Blood Pressure Education Program: Working Group report on primary prevention of hypertension. *Archives of Internal Medicine*, **153**, 186–208.

Parving, H. H., Lehnert, H., Brochner-Mortensen, J., Gomis, R., Andersen, S., and Arner, P. for the Irbesartan in Patients with Type 2 Diabetes and Microalbuminuria Study Group (2001). The effect of irbesartan on the development of diabetic nephropathy in patients with type 2 diabetes. *New England Journal of Medicine*, **345**, 870–8.

Perkins, B. A., Ficociello, L. H., Silva, K. H., Finkelstein, D. M., Warram, J. H. and Krolewski, A. S. (2003). Regression of microalbuminuria in Type 1 diabetes. *New England Journal of Medicine*, **348**, 2285–2293.

Primatesta, P., Brookes, M. and Poulter, N. R. (2001). Improved hypertension management and control: results from the Health Survey for England 1998. *Hypertension*, **38**, 827–32.

Saunders, E. and Hildreth, C. (1991). Hypertension in blacks: a clinical overview. In *Cardiovascular disease in blacks* (ed. E. F. A. Saunders), pp. 85–96. Davis, Philadelphia.

Sever, P. (1999*a*). The heterogeneity of hypertension. *European Society of Cardiology*, **1**, L11–L13.

Sever, P. (1999*b*). Simple blood pressure guidelines for primary health care. *Journal of Human Hypertension*, **131**, 725–7.

Sever, P. (1999*c*). Recent clinical trials: a critical appraisal. *Current Hypertension Reports*, **1**, 333–6.

Sever, P., Beevers, G., Bulpitt, C., Lever, A., Ramsay, L., Reid, J. and Swales, J. (1993). Management guidelines in essential hypertension: report of the second working party of the British Hypertension Society. *British Medical Journal*, **306**, 983–7.

Sever, P. S., Dahlof, B., Poulter, N. R., Wedel, H., Beevers, G., Caulfield, M. *et al.* (2002). Rationale, design, methods, and baseline demography of participants of the Anglo-Scandinavian Cardiac Outcomes Trial. *Journal of Hypertension*, **19**, 1139–47.

Sever, P. S., Dahlof, B., Poulter, N. R., Wedel, H., Beevers, G., Caulfield, M. *et al.*(2003). Prevention of coronary and stroke events with atorvastatin in hypertensive patients who have average or lower-than-average cholesterol concentrations, in the Anglo-Scandinavian Cardiac Outcomes Trial. *Lancet*, **361**, 1149–58.

SHEP (Systolic Hypertension in the Elderly Program) Co-operative Research Group (1991). Prevention of stroke by antihypertensive drug treatment in older persons with isolated systolic hypertension:

final results of the Systolic Hypertension in the Elderly Program (SHEP). *Journal of the American Medical Association*, **265**, 3255–64.

Staessen, J. A., Fagard, R., Thijs, L., Celis, H., Arabidze, G. *et al.*, for the Systolic Hypertension in Europe (Syst-Eur) Trial Investigators (1997). Randomised double-blind comparison of placebo and active treatment for older patients with isolated systolic hypertension. *Lancet*, **350**, 757–64.

Stamler, J. (1998). Setting the TONE for ending the hypertension epidemic. *Journal of the American Medical Association*, **279**, 878–9.

Stanton, A. V. (1998). Calcium channel blockers: the jury is still out on whether they cause heart attacks and suicide. *British Medical Journal*, **316**, 1471–3.

Svenson, P., de Faire, U., Sleight, P., Yusuf, S. and Ostergren, J. (2001). Comparative effects of ramipril on ambulatory and office blood pressures: a HOPE Substudy. *Hypertension*, **38**, e28.

Thrombosis Prevention Trial (1998). Randomised trial of low-intensity oral anticoagulation with warfarin and low-dose aspirin in the primary prevention of ischaemic heart disease in men at increased risk. The Medical Research Council's General Practice Research Framework. *Lancet*, **351**, 233–41.

Trials of Hypertension Prevention Collaborative Research Group (1997). Effects of weight loss and sodium reduction intervention on blood pressure and hypertension incidence in overweight people with high-normal blood pressure: the Trials of Hypertension Prevention, Phase II. *Archives of Internal Medicine*, **157**, 657–67.

Tuomilehto, J., Rastenyte, D., Birkenhager, W. H., Lutgarde, T., Antikainen, R., Bulpitt, C. J. *et al.* (1999). Effects of calcium channel blockade in older patients with diabetes and systolic hypertension. *New England Journal of Medicine*, **340**, 677–84.

Turnbull, F./BPLTTC (Blood Pressure Lowering Treatment Trialists' Collaboration) (2003). Effects of different blood-pressure-lowering regimens on major cardiovascular events: results of prospectively-designed overviews of randomised trials. *Lancet*, **362**, 1527–35.

UKPDS 38 (1998). Tight blood pressure control and risk of macrovascular and microvascular complications in type 2 diabetes. *British Medical Journal*, **317**, 703–13.

UKPDS 39 (1998). Efficacy of atenolol and captopril in reducing risk of macrovascular and microvascular complications in type 2 diabetes. *British Medical Journal*, **317**, 713–26.

Veterans Administrative Cooperative Study Group on Antihypertensive Agents (1967). Effects of treatment on morbidity in hypertension: results in patients with diastolic blood pressures averaging 115 through 129 mmHg. *Journal of the American Medical Association*, **202**, 116–22.

Veterans Administrative Cooperative Study Group on Antihypertensive Agents (1970). Effects of treatment on morbidity in hypertension: results in patients with diastolic blood pressures averaging 90 through 114 mmHg. *Journal of the American Medical Association*, **213**, 1143–52.

Watt, G. C. M. (1995). Prevention of high blood pressure and its complications: strategic issues in a local context. *Journal of Hypertension*, **13**, 377–83.

Whelton, P. K. (1994). Epidemiology of hypertension. *Lancet*, **344**, 101–6.

Whelton, P. K., Appel, L. J., Espeland, M. A., Applegate, W. B., Ettinger, W. H. Jr., Kostis, J. B. *et al.* for the TONE Collaborative Research Group (1998). Sodium reduction and weight loss in the treatment of hypertension in older persons: a randomized controlled trial of nonpharmacologic interventions in the elderly (TONE). *Journal of the American Medical Association*, **279**, 839–46.

Wikstrand, J., Warnold, I., Olsson, G. *et al.* (1988). Primary prevention with Metoprolol in patients with hypertension. *Journal of the American Medical Association*, **259**, 1976–82.

Wilhelmsen, L., Berglund, G., Elmfeldt, D. *et al.* (1987). Beta-blockers versus diuretics in hypertensive men: main results from the HAPPHY Trial. *Hypertension*, **5**, 561–74.

Williams, B., Poulter, N. R., Brown, M. J., Davis, M., McInnes, G. T., Potter, J. F., *et al.*; BHS Guidelines Working Party for the British Hypertension Society (2004). British Hypertension Society Guidelines for Hypertension Management 2004 (BHS-IV): Summary. *British Medical Journal*, **328**, 634–40.

Wing, L. M. H., Reid, C. M., Ryan, P., Beilin, L. J., Brown, M. A., Jennings, G. L. R. *et al.* (2003). A comparison of outcomes with angiotensin-converting-enzyme inhibitors and diuretics for hypertension in the elderly. *New England Journal of Medicine*, **348**, 583–92.

Wood, D., Durrington, P., Poulter, N., McInnes, G., Rees, A., Wray, R. for the British Cardiac Society, British Hyperlipideamia Association, British Hypertension Society, and British Diabetic Association (1998). Joint British recommendation on prevention of coronary heart disease in clinical practice. *Heart*, **80**, S1–29.

WHO–ISH (World Health Organization–International Society of Hypertension) Blood Pressure Lowering Treatment Trialists' Collaboration (1998). Protocol for prospective collaborative overviews of major randomized trials of blood-pressure-lowering treatments. *Journal of Hypertension*, **16**, 127.

Chapter 51

Community change and the role of public health

P. Puska

51.1 Summary

Strong medical evidence exists on the important role of some behavioural risk factors in the prevention of cardiovascular and many other chronic diseases. Community-based preventive programmes start from the fact that people's behaviours are strongly determined by their social and physical environment. Thus the intervention target is the community and not the individual. Successful programmes call for understanding the basic concepts of social change; while epidemiological knowledge guides the choice of target risk factors, behavioural and social frameworks help plan actual interventions.

This chapter discusses some relevant theories as well as the basic principles of planning, implementation, and evaluation of community programmes. Important aspects are leadership and community ownership. Community-based programmes are often carried out as pilot or demonstration programmes for wider, usually national applications.

Reviews of community-based heart health programmes have often shown smaller effects than initially anticipated. On the other hand, experiences like those from the North Karelia Project in Finland show the great public health potential of long-term sustained intervention on lifestyles.

51.2 Introduction

For several decades non-communicable diseases (NCDs), and especially cardiovascular diseases (CVDs), have been the main public health problem in industrialized countries. What is more recent is that the rates of these diseases have, during the last few years, rapidly increased in most of the developing countries. According to the latest WHO data in 1999, NCDs contributed ~60% of deaths in the world and 43% of the global burden of disease (WHO 2001). About half of these deaths were attributable to CVD. On the basis of current estimates, NCD deaths are expected to account in 2020 for 73% of deaths and 60% of the disease burden worldwide (WHO 2002). Already 79% of NCD deaths occur in developing countries, where most of the people affected are between 45 and 65 years of age. In China and India alone, the burden of CVD is greater than in the industrialized countries as a whole.

Much research has, during the last few decades, been carried out to study the causes and mechanisms of the major NCDs. Research has involved large epidemiological studies within and between populations, as well as basic biochemical and animal studies, intervention trials, and large-scale, community-based preventive studies. This research has clearly shown that NCDs have their roots in unhealthy lifestyles. Such factors as unhealthy nutrition, smoking, physical inactivity, excess use of alcohol, and psychosocial stress are among the major lifestyle issues.

These observations have provided a firm basis for modern public health work to prevent NCDs as outlined, for example, in the *WHO global strategy for NCD prevention and control* (WHO 2000). There is little doubt that strong evidence is available concerning the possibilities of preventing at least the premature occurrence of these diseases. NCDs are to a great extent preventable diseases and potential for public health gain is huge.

Although further research will undoubtedly improve our knowledge of the medical basis for prevention, the big challenge is how to apply the knowledge for disease prevention in real life. Knowledge of the causes is not enough for successful prevention. The key question is the *strategy for prevention.*

51.3 **Community in key position**

The identification of certain behaviours as key risk factors has often led to an emphasis on individual responsibility for prevention and to messages for individuals to change their behaviour (see Chapter 48). Obviously, individuals can do much for their health through adoption of healthy lifestyles; but there are great limitations. The basic notion is that an *individual's behaviour is strongly determined by their social and physical environment.* In other words, *lifestyles and behaviours are deeply rooted in the community.* People often tend to behave like others in the community due to the cultural, political, economical, and physical features of the community.

Thus in the 1970s, people in the province of North Karelia in Finland, for example, had a very unhealthy, high saturated fat diet, because it was a dairy farming area and butter and fatty milk were culturally very much appreciated. Food items high in dairy fat were most commonly available in groceries, school meals, restaurants, etc., and the local recipes were based on these food items. An obvious consequence of this was a high general blood cholesterol level and very high rates of coronary heart disease (CHD).

An opposite example was southern Italy where the diet was largely based on vegetables, olive oil, fish, pasta, and wine. This was not for health reasons, but because there was a strong culture and tradition, and these products were commonly available. This situation was, as is well-known, associated with low blood cholesterol and low rates of CHD.

These two examples show how the lifestyles (diets) of the respective populations were strongly determined by community features. These in turn were strongly associated with national features, including agricultural and fiscal policies. Thus, for example in Finland, the agricultural policy supported dairy production and taxation favoured butter instead of vegetable oil products. In a similar way, in Italy wine and olive production was favoured. These examples also help us to understand how changing dietary habits in these communities essentially calls for changes in the community structures and the determinants of dietary habits. In Finland this notion led to the start of the North Karelia Project with a 'community-based approach', that is the idea that the intervention target is the community and not the individual.

This thinking leads us back to the classical wisdom of public health teachings, such as the observation of R. Wirchow that public health is ultimately a matter of social policy. We can also usefully be reminded of the basic principles of public health, according to which disease is dependent on agent, host, and the environment. Although the agent (lifestyle) is important, the role of environment is often crucial.

51.4 **Community change**

The big challenge for public health, therefore, is to understand and be able to promote community change for health. Community change relates to the concept of social change. There are a number of, often overlapping, theories on social change that are relevant to understanding changes in behaviours and their determinants in the community.

Essentially, community change can take place through decisions made by an authority or by a process of social change. In democratic societies an interrelated mix often occurs; that is, administrative decisions reflect changes in people's opinions, intentions, and behaviour.

The classical theory of *innovations diffusion* is highly relevant to community change (Rogers 1983). New lifestyles can be seen as innovations that diffuse with time through the natural networks in the community to its members. This diffusion, which causes social change, occurs through communication over time. The innovation-diffusion theory argues that mass media are more effective in creating knowledge of innovations and are useful for 'agenda-setting' purposes, while interpersonal channels are more effective in actually changing attitudes and behaviours.

The innovation-diffusion theory classifies people on the basis of their innovativeness as either innovators, early adopters, early majority, late majority, or laggards. The social structure has several norms (system effects) that have a strong influence on the rate of diffusion. Early adoption and a greater diffusion rate are more likely to occur in modern rather than traditional community norms. The early adopters usually have the greatest social influence in the community and are thus in key positions to influence a wider adoption of the innovation.

An agent of change is a professional who attempts to influence this innovation–decision process. Typically, health projects can also be seen as agents of change trying to promote health-related innovations in the community.

Another general aspect that relates to community change is *communication*. Lifestyle changes are often related to communication: mass communication or interpersonal communication. The 'two steps flow' of communication is important. Mass communication can reach a great number of people, increase their knowledge, and shape the public agenda, but local opinion leaders, or 'gate keepers', are in a key position in interpreting the messages and in influencing attitudes and behaviours. Several classical theories provide well-documented frameworks for community change related to communication: Bandura's social learning theory (Bandura 1977), the communication persuasion model of McGuire (1969), and the belief–attitude–intention model of Ajzen and Fishbein (1975).

In the modern world communication relates closely to marketing and to journalism. *Marketing* uses all available methods of communication and often huge resources to influence behaviour and change lifestyles; commercial marketing usually relates to consumption of particular products, but sometimes it leads the way to deeper social change. *Journalism* through various media reflects and shapes lifestyles and social change, and is in many cases linked to commercial interests. On the other hand, journalism can also be used in health programmes – a special approach sometimes called behavioural journalism.

Community organization is another concept often linked to community change. Broad-ranging and permanent changes in the community usually have to relate to a whole range of community structures. Every community has a complex network of social organizations, both official and unofficial, that exercise great influence over people's behaviour and lifestyles. The concept of community organization involves both community self-development (when the community initially detects a problem and organizes itself to cope with it) and the outside influences promoting re-organization towards particular needs (such as health needs).

51.5 **Influencing community change**

When trying to influence community change, as in community-based health programmes, one has to pay attention to the aspects described above. No single theory can tell us what to do, but sound behavioural and social theories are most useful for the framework of programme planning and evaluation.

Community diagnosis or community analysis is a useful concept for the planning of community projects. The aim is to have a comprehensive understanding of the situation for planning purposes (Haglund 1983). To the greatest extent possible, the community diagnosis should provide a comprehensive understanding of the situation at the start of the programme. It should provide the basis for selecting priorities and particularly for decisions as to appropriate and effective methods of intervention. Existing data from previous studies, statistics, and expert opinions should be collected and reviewed. At a later stage, the results of a baseline survey can also be used to complement the picture. It is also important to interview key local people. Special focus groups involving local community representatives can be used to find out relevant information about the background on lifestyles and possible channels of influence.

Important information for the community analysis includes epidemiological data from the area, taking in mortality and morbidity rates of possible health problems among the total population and various subgroups, and prevalence rates of possible factors influencing these diseases in the target population. Geographical, demographic, and socio-economic features of the community should be reviewed. Information needs to be obtained concerning the various lifestyles related to the risk factors, about the various community features influencing these behaviour complexes, about the community leadership and social interaction/communication channels, and about other factors relevant to the adopted behavioural/social framework.

Because much of the success of such a programme depends on the support of the population, information is needed on how people and their representatives see the problems and how they feel about the possibilities of solving them. As the programme will depend on the cooperation of local decision-makers and health personnel, their opinions and attitudes should also be surveyed at the outset. The community resources and service structure, too, need to be considered before deciding on the actual forms of programme implementation.

In addition to good community diagnosis, there are other important aspects in planning a community-based health programme. The main *objectives of the programme* are usually set by the objective and/or perceived health needs of the community. They usually relate to the most common and serious NCDs. The intermediate objectives are designed on the basis of the available medical/epidemiological knowledge concerning how to influence the health problem(s) and on local prevalence rates of the risk factors.

The practical objectives and actual intervention measures should then be based on a careful analysis of the community and on an understanding of the strategic determinants of the intermediate objectives. This, of course, relates to the choice of theoretical behavioural/social frameworks previously discussed.

Figure 51.1 describes the hierarchy of objectives in a community programme. The general aim is improved health and wellbeing of the population. The main objectives concern reduction of CVDs or other specified NCDs. The choice is dependent on local mortality/incidence/prevalence rates and on public concerns.

After selection of the main objectives, the intermediate objectives are defined. This is based on the medical/epidemiological knowledge from the literature concerning well-established risk

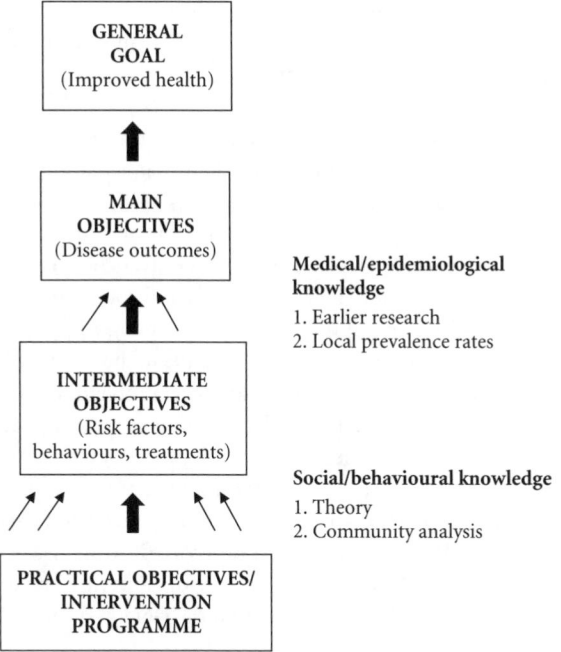

Fig. 51.1 Hierarchy of objectives in a community health programme.

factors of given diseases and on information on the local prevalence rates of these factors. Clear definitions of the main and intermediate objectives are needed in order to decide on the respective indicators and data sources for monitoring and evaluation.

Once the intermediate objectives have been defined, the immediate objectives or the contents of a practical programme are decided upon. Because the task primarily concerns influencing health behaviours and related lifestyles, behavioural and social theories are needed as well as the lessons from the community diagnosis. Advantage should be taken of practical opportunities available in the community.

A key feature of a community-based prevention programme is that it simultaneously applies medical and epidemiological knowledge to identify health problems and target risk factors in selecting the intervention objectives, and behavioural and social knowledge to design the actual programme's contents and activities. This implies an interdisciplinary approach, both in planning and implementation, and in the evaluative research.

Although good planning, definition of objectives, and theoretical frameworks are needed, it should be emphasized that the actual implementation of a community programme should be flexible and respond sensitively to the various possibilities that occur in the community. For this, the programme should be in daily contact with the community, be able to 'listen as much as speak', know the community structures well, and have a good feedback system.

As to the *implementation* of the programme, the goal is to systematically implement the programme according to its aims and principles and, as discussed, to be sufficiently flexible to adjust in response to opportunities that may arise in the community.

Integrating the programme into the community's social organization is important, because in so doing, the participation of the community and the availability of community resources can be strengthened. Thus the project usually sets the objectives and develops the general framework, while the activities are carried out mainly by the community. The programme catalyses this work by providing materials, training, necessary official support, mass media support, and follow-up.

To identify and mobilize community resources, the programme should work closely with community agencies and voluntary organizations. Thus participation in preventive activities should form part of the regular work of the health professional, and not be simply an extra job or hobby. In many instances a community programme can combine 'top-down' decisions with training and motivation of personnel. Close personal contacts between the project team and local health personnel are important to help motivation and compliance.

The use of local organizations and opinion leaders can encourage population participation. Many such organizations appreciate being able to contribute to the success of an important health project. Numerous personal contacts need to be made, local problems discussed, and possibilities for practical contributions reviewed. The population's interest and support generated by such activities can be harnessed by the mass media to establish further intervention activities.

Since the motivation and support of the general population forms a cornerstone of the project intervention, lay people and voluntary organizations often carry out much of the practical work. In some cultures, trained and motivated public health nurses can be an important professional group. The role of medical doctors is at its best very important, but in many programmes they act as medical experts within the general framework.

51.6 Community programme as a national demonstration project

In principle, a community-based project can vary from a relatively restricted academic study or local effort to a major programme with strong national involvement. The North Karelia Project and many of the demonstration projects in WHO networks on integrated NCD prevention fall definitely in the latter category (Puska 1993).

An advantage of an intervention programme in a small community would be that an intensive intervention reaching every inhabitant could be used. However, there are also major disadvantages. Many important environmental decisions can be made only at a higher level, that is, at a provincial or national level. This concerns both legislation and private action, such as by the food industry. Another disadvantage with a small community intervention would be the lower generalizability of such experience to the national level.

In the national demonstration projects, the aim is to take a rather large community (country, province, or other large geographically defined area) in which comprehensive intervention is implemented in a well-conceived way and with careful evaluation. In addition to innovative educational interventions, community organization and major environmental modifications are applied – measures that could possibly be implemented nationally.

Because it may often be difficult to implement many of the necessary, often innovative and somewhat contradictory measures directly at a national level, they are first tested in a demonstration area, which therefore acts as a 'pilot' area. Thus the national pilot area, with proper evaluation, gives good information on feasibility, effects, and other experiences of such action. When several measures are implemented in an integrated and comprehensive way in the same area, a national pilot area gives information on the overall experience of this kind of intervention package, where several activities implemented at the same time may support each other.

The term 'pilot' means implementation first in a restricted area and later on, if experience of the intervention is positive, nationally. The terms 'demonstration' or 'model' have the connotation that the preventive activities are done in a more planned and 'better' way in that area – to demonstrate an example of good implementation and to learn what the lessons are. Thus national activities and activities in the demonstration area may well take place at the same time and support each other, as is usually the case with many demonstration projects in industrialized countries. In fact, many current demonstration projects first started as a 'pilot' activity, but later on clearly became more a 'demonstration' for ongoing national activities (Puska 1988).

For a national demonstration project to be useful and effective, a few important rules should be observed. The project should obviously be professionally well planned, implemented, and evaluated. The available resources and input, that is, 'the dose of intervention', should be sufficient for meaningful results to be achieved. Also, an effective national demonstration project should have not only good support from the national health authorities, but also close operational links with them. Thus communication should continually operate in both directions. This ensures that relevant national aspects are well considered in the demonstration project and also that the decision-makers are familiar and well informed about the experiences of the demonstration project as a basis for national decisions.

51.7 **Leadership and ownership**

A key question in community programmes concerns their leadership and ownership. Success clearly calls for strong and visible leadership but also, at the same time, strong ownership by the community concerned. How can these two be achieved?

These questions also deal with the basic philosophy of the project: Is it a top-down or a bottom-up approach? The former refers to the situation where usually the experts define the problem (in epidemiological terms) and from this the required actions for planned change are determined. The latter refers to the situation where basically the people decide on the actions required and then take action for some good purpose.

Both approaches have their merits and are not mutually exclusive. For maximum effect, sound epidemiological and behavioural principles should be applied. On the other hand, without strong ownership by, and involvement of, the local population, it is impossible to consider that any major changes in community lifestyles would take place.

These considerations also refer to the question of leadership. Should the leader be a strong academic/professional person or a local representative? And should the focal point/coordinating centre of the project be an academic institution or a local office?

In the North Karelia Project in Finland, attempts were made to blend these different needs (Puska et al. 1995). Leadership was based on partnership. While on the one hand the project was sparked by people's petition to reduce heart disease and improve health in North Karelia, it was the project leaders and experts who acted collectively as the change agent, showing the community how to achieve the objectives that the people had themselves set. The project director and central project team formed a visible leadership that people could clearly identify with and support, and their support has come in many ways. The strength of the partnership model is also demonstrated by the numerous initiatives and activities that took place over the years.

This mixed model of leadership contrasts with community-based pressure groups on the one hand (there are numerous examples in the environmental field), and on the other with the majority of academic projects, which are carefully designed and directed from above using skilful behaviour-modification techniques.

A central underlying principle from the very start of the programme in North Karelia was that the project itself would not carry out the activities, but that the various bodies and sectors of the community would perform them. Thus local health services, for example, featured strongly in the activities. The local provincial medical officers were leading figures and effective activators, as were many of the head physicians of health centres. The public health nurses were frequently active participants and leaders in their own project-related activities.

Several major voluntary organizations were enthusiastic contributors to the project. The powerful housewives' organization (Martta) carried out major campaigns for a healthy diet in collaboration with the project. There were similar examples with sports organizations, heart associations, etc., as well as with local food manufacturers and storekeepers. Many enterprises picked up useful business ideas, and initiated development, production, and marketing activities for healthier foods in collaboration with the project.

In the field of agriculture, the local berry and vegetable farmers eagerly allied themselves with the project. These cooperative efforts took the form of projects for promoting the consumption of local berries and vegetables. The resultant success meant that dairy farmers, under pressure from the declining consumption of dairy fat, were able to switch to the more promising business of berry farming. Over the years the local media (newspapers and radio) publicized many initiatives that have grown into major collaborative efforts involving the project.

The principles of partnership and leadership were maintained throughout. The central project leadership carefully scrutinized the evaluation results and feedback, and was in daily contact with the community to guide overall development. Within this framework various community bodies themselves carried out activities, innovation was encouraged, and new ideas were often realized after consultation with the central project office.

51.8 Evaluation of community programmes

Numerous textbooks and articles have dealt with aspects of evaluating community-based health programmes. There are many different perspectives and certainly no one standard approach exists.

It is common to divide evaluation into *formative vs. summative* and *internal vs. external* evaluation. Internal evaluation is carried out during and within the programme to give rapid feedback to the programme workers and management. An overlapping concept is formative evaluation, which provides data during the programme about the experience with the various programme components and thus helps further to develop (formulate) the programme. The summative evaluation of the programme assesses over a given time the overall effects and other results, usually by an expert group in some way external to the daily community work.

The evaluation aims can, as was done in the North Karelia Project (Puska *et al.* 1995), be divided into assessment of various aspects of the programme:

1 Feasibility/performance.

2 Effects (behaviours and risk factors, disease rates).

3 Process.

4 Costs.

51.8.1 **Feasibility/performance**

The programme feasibility or performance evaluation assesses the extent to which it was possible to implement the planned activities, that is, what actually happened in the community. This concerns the amount of resources available to the project, how they were used in the community, and how well the activities reached the target populations.

A feasibility evaluation is especially important in a large and comprehensive programme, where the community itself carries out the activities in a large geographical area. Before the question of effect can be meaningfully addressed, the actual intervention must be defined. Results of the feasibility assessment can be based on a log of activities, on statistical data within the community, or on survey and other data (project statistics) collected during and after certain programme periods.

51.8.2 **Effect**

The effect evaluation is carried out to assess whether, and to what extent, objectives of the programme were achieved. Thus indicators of the different objectives need to be defined, and these need to be measured in the community at the outset and after the given programme period(s). The effect assessment should in particular answer the question: 'Did the programme cause changes in target behavioural and/or biological risk factors?' If the community size allows it, and follow-up time is long enough, the evaluation can also try to assess whether these changes were associated with changes in NCD rates (mortality/incidence). However, because significant changes in NCD rates call for quite large population size, relatively major changes in risk factors, and several years' duration, changes in NCD rates are often not a stated aim of the effect evaluation. This is also not needed, since the relationships between 'hard risk factors' and the main NCDs are convincingly demonstrated (see Chapters 3 and 4).

Because the target of the programme is usually the whole community, information is collected to represent the whole population (with certain appropriate age limits). For prevalence data (behaviours, risk factors), a representative population sample is usually surveyed at the outset and at the main summative evaluation points. Independent, cross-sectional population samples are preferred so that the baseline measurements or selective loss at follow-up will not influence the findings of subsequent follow-ups.

Relatively large sample sizes are used to detect changes in risk factor means that would be small for individuals but meaningful for the health of the population as a whole. Large sample sizes also enable interesting subgroup analyses to be carried out.

Comparison of results from baseline and follow-up surveys reveals the changes that take place in the target community during the programme period. However, changes over several years could well partly or completely be due to reasons other than the intervention programme. Thus a reference area is often used. The baseline and follow-up surveys should be carried out simultaneously in the programme and reference areas, and with strict adherence to identical methodology and sampling procedures.

The reference area should be as similar to the programme area as possible ('matched'), but without the input of the programme. This study design can be called 'quasi-experimental', whereby the study controls the experimental intervention and the choice of reference area, but not the allocation to experimental or reference area.

There are several problems concerning the use of a reference area. One is that a major national demonstration programme is likely also to have an impact in the reference area.

To eliminate the possibility of unexpected events in the reference area (that will harm the comparison) in many cases the whole country (the rest of the country) is used as reference/comparison.

51.8.3 Process

The process evaluation concerns both changes in the intervening variables and the change trends with time in different population subgroups during the programme. The main goal of process evaluation is to get a good picture of what happens between the input (i.e. the work of the project) and the output (i.e. changes in behaviours and risk factors). The process evaluation is related to the behavioural/social framework adopted and to definition of the intended intervening (independent) variables. Measurement of these factors shows how the change process in the community led, or did not lead, to the desired behavioural and risk factor changes.

Process variables include such factors as exposure to the various intervention measures, changes in health knowledge, attitudes and intentions, social support, environmental changes, etc. In process evaluation it is also of interest to learn how the changes take place over time (concerning different variables) and in the different subgroups of the population. Process evaluation is at its best really interdisciplinary work, which often emphasizes behavioural/social sciences.

51.8.4 Costs

The cost evaluation assesses the total project resources and how they were allocated. In addition, efforts can be made to assess the community costs. This can concern both total community costs, or specifically the extra costs involved for the community. In addition to direct community costs (i.e. mainly health service-related costs), attempts can be made to estimate indirect community costs and savings related to the programme.

51.9 Evidence of effectiveness of community-based interventions

Since the early 1980s, a number of publications have tried to summarize the results of major community-based preventive projects, particularly concerning CVD prevention. At the same time methodological aspects of the projects have been discussed from several perspectives (Flay and Best 1982; Puska 1985; Altman 1986; Sellers *et al.* 1997). One of the most thorough summaries of the preventive cardiovascular community projects was made by the Swedish Council on Technology Assessment in Health Care (SBU 1997).

The task of summarizing the experience of preventive heart health interventions is not an easy one. In these projects a set of different strategies has been used. The scientific literature describes 50–100 projects or studies that in one way or another have aimed at community-based prevention of CVDs. In most of them the evaluation is, however, not sufficient to draw valid conclusions on impact or effectiveness. The Swedish work determined that only eight of the community-based heart health projects met with the given criteria for study design and evaluation: North Karelia Project (Finland), Stanford Three Community Study (USA), Stanford Five City Project (USA), Minnesota Heart Health Program (USA), Pawtucket Heart Health Program (USA), Swiss National Research Program (Switzerland), German Cardiovascular Prevention Study (Germany), Kilkenny Health Project (Ireland).

51.10 **Should these studies be referenced?**

Both the Swedish (SBU 1997) and the US (Schooler *et al.* 1997) reviews agree that the most rigid evaluation of the projects usually shows only modest or no 'hard' effects on target risk factors or CVD rates. At the same time they discuss the difficulties in assessing the true overall impact. This is because of the comprehensive nature of the intervention, caused by diffusion to other areas and linkage with national trends. A recent British review dealt with both trials and community studies and arrived at rather similar conclusions (Ebrahim and Smith 1997). It stated that for pooled effects on mortality, a small but potentially significant ($\sim$10% reduction) effect may have been missed.

Work at the New England Research Institutes in USA by Sellers *et al.* (1997) also collected information on community interventions to reduce CVDs during the past 25 years. This study used meta-analysis, particularly to assess the variability in the effectiveness of community heart health programmes. These results suggested that some of the variation is attributable to different evaluation methods, but that characteristics of the intervention also play a role.

The US (Schooler *et al.* 1997) synthesis responds to criticism of 'meagre effects' by stating that expectations for community level interventions are often unrealistic, that is, based on overly high estimates of effect size and insufficient samples to detect smaller effects. Commercial advertising campaigns, which generally have substantially more resources than community prevention trials, are typically satisfied with quite modest increases in market share. Further, Mittelmark *et al.* (1993) call for 'realistic outcomes' in their review. The US summary further recognized that 'subgroup component studies demonstrate the efficacy of many risk reduction strategies'. Mittelmark *et al.* conclude that it has been demonstrated that a broad range of intervention strategies can favourably modify the health behaviours of specific groups in communities such as employees and school children.

A very important aspect is the dose of the intervention, because most of the projects in larger communities over a number of years have had only very limited resources – and thus the dose is small. The US synthesis (Schooler *et al.* 1997) found that the 'results support a dose-response relationship by evidence of stronger effects where adequate exposure to the intervention was achieved'.

The importance of dose is further strengthened by the observation that more restricted interventions have repeatedly demonstrated greater effects than large comprehensive community projects. A recent meta-analysis of dietary trials analysed the experience of 17 trials on dietary behaviour interventions. According to the analysis the mean net changes for dietary fat as per cent of energy was −2.5% and for serum cholesterol −0.22 mmol/l (Brunner *et al.* 1997). Such changes permanently established in the population would already have a major impact on CHD rates. Another case illustration is the recent cholesterol lowering village competition in North Karelia, Finland, where the 16 participating villages lowered their average serum cholesterol level by 9% and the winning village by 16%, although only for a short period (Puska *et al.* 1998a).

The US synthesis concludes finally that 'the community approach to CVD prevention has a high degree of generalizability, cost effectiveness due to the use of mass communication methods, ability to diffuse information successfully through use of community networks, and potential for influencing environmental, regulatory, and institutional policies that shape health' (Schooler *et al.* 1997).

These conclusions are supported by the fact that countries with major heart health demonstration projects have usually been in many ways active in heart health promotion and have also had major declines in CVD rates. Thus it is evident that major heart health promotion projects are linked with national progress in a complex way. This finding is illustrated by the principles used, for example, in the WHO CINDI programme: 'A major national demonstration programme can be a powerful tool for generating favourable nation-wide developments in chronic disease prevention and health promotion' (Puska *et al.* 1995).

Perhaps the best example to illustrate the long-term experience and potential of sustained community-based and national heart health work is the experience in Finland. The North Karelia Project was started in the early 1970s in the province of North Karelia, which acted as a pilot area. After the early success in the 1970s, and with significant net reductions in both risk factors and CHD mortality, intensive national work was started to which the project actively contributed. During this latter period the decline in risk factors and disease rates accelerated in parallel between North Karelia and the whole of Finland.

After 25 years a remarkable decline has taken place in smoking among men, major dietary changes have occurred, and serum cholesterol and blood pressure levels have markedly reduced. At the same time in North Karelia (among the male population of 35–64 years) CVD mortality has declined by 68%, CHD mortality by 73%, cancer mortality by 44%, lung cancer mortality by 71%, and all-cause mortality by 49% (Puska *et al.* 1998*b*). During the original project period, 1972–77, the reductions in target risk factors and in CHD mortality were significantly greater in North Karelia than in the reference area or nationally. At the end of 25 years, the respective changes in the whole of Finland have been nearly as great; for example, there has been a reduction in CHD mortality of 65%. Separate analyses have shown that most of this decline in CHD mortality is explained by population level changes in the main risk factors (Vartiainen *et al.* 1994). General dietary changes seem to have been the most important determinant.

51.11 **Discussion on evaluation**

The principles and methods of evaluation have been developed and discussed along with the community-based or population-based intervention studies which have been carried out, for the prevention of CVDs and also for the prevention of other related chronic diseases (Puska 1985).

In general, evaluation is concerned with outcome. Different levels of objectives have been used: mortality, incidence, risk factors, health behaviours, etc. At the same time it is very useful to understand how and why the programme has worked, so that a possible success can be replicated. This process evaluation is concerned with assessing changes in the intervening variables and calls for a theoretical framework for an intervention.

A key issue is evaluation of the study design. A truly experimental design would allocate a number of communities randomly into intervention and control communities. This is seldom possible and one might also ask how much this would comply with the basic idea of community intervention, that is, broad community participation and comprehensive community organization that benefit from a bottom-up approach. Instead, quasi-experimental designs have often been used with a reference community, or sometimes with national changes as comparison. In a number of studies no comparison community has been used, and in these cases process evaluation becomes crucial.

Other evaluation issues deal with the target population and time frame. Different age limits have been used. Older age groups are more relevant for disease rates in the near future; younger age groups are preferred when interest is focused on lifestyle changes and a long-term public health perspective. A short period of evaluation may not be sufficient to show the effects of an intervention whereas longer follow-up may dilute the actual effect. Furthermore, the ideal assessment period probably varies for different end points: mortality, incidence, risk factors, behaviours, etc.

As mentioned earlier, changes in risk factors should be preferred as outcome measures over mortality or morbidity (Lindholm and Rosen 2000). The arguments behind this are sound: the medical and epidemiological evidence of the benefits of reduction of, for example, smoking rates, low-density lipoprotein cholesterol levels and blood pressure levels is overwhelming (see Chapters 3 and 4). Thus, if we can convincingly show an effect on these indicators, we can be assured that useful prevention has been achieved. With a smaller community it is unrealistic to expect to detect statistically significant effects on disease rates despite effective intervention.

Discussion has also taken place as to whether cross-sectional, independent population samples or a cohort design should be used in assessment. Obviously, independent samples will assess the magnitude of changes in the whole population better than follow-up of a cohort, but the cohort approach can give more information on the type of changes that have actually taken place at individual level.

One of the most crucial questions that has persisted over the years is how actually to evaluate the intervention. Obviously, assessment of possible effects is meaningful only if we can be sure that a proper intervention has taken place. This relates both to choosing appropriate theoretical frameworks and to having enough intensity in the intervention. A common problem for most community programmes is the small dose of these interventions in relation to their stated ambitious aims.

The question of proper assessment of the input of programmes is extremely important for understanding the public health implications. Negative or meagre results from some community-based interventions are often interpreted as proof that population-based interventions are not effective, while the reason may be that actually very little happened in the community.

In addition to the intensity or dose of the intervention, even more difficult is to assess the quality or type of the intervention. A population-based community intervention typically uses a whole range of intervention modalities ranging from media campaigns and health service interventions to community organization and environmental and policy changes. Some work has been done to assess factors like exposure to media or to preventive services, but assessment of factors such as community organization or environmental changes that may be crucial is even more difficult. Despite efforts, there has been little progress concerning assessment of these aspects.

It is highly desirable that discussion and work concerning the concepts and evaluation of population-based community intervention programmes should continue and further development will occur (Puska 2000). Despite many critical comments, modern public health is very dependent on changes in the major, well-established risk factors in the community and in the national population. In addition to national policy decisions and actions, numerous local, regional, and national programmes will be implemented to change lifestyles and they need to be thoroughly evaluated. Development in both our concepts and measurement tools will be important so that we can better learn our lessons to serve public health.

In summary, it could be said that successful community-based programmes should aim to do the 'right' things and enough of them, that is, use sound theoretical frameworks and apply them with sufficient 'dose'. Usually, environmental and policy decisions are key, but such can often be achieved only in conjunction with health promotion activities that influence the public agenda and people's intentions. At the same time, the human factor is crucial: persistent and dedicated work is needed, combining enthusiastic and credible leadership with close involvement of, and ownership by, the population.

References

Altman, D. G. (1986). A framework for evaluating community-based heart disease prevention programs. *Social Science and Medicine*, **22** (4), 479–87.

Ajzen, J. and Fishbein, M. (1980) 1975 in text. *Understanding attitudes and predicting social behaviour.* Prentice Hall, Englewood Cliffs, NJ.

Bandura, A. (1977). *Social learning theory.* Prentice Hall, Englewood Cliffs, NJ.

Brunner, E., White, I., Thorogood, M., Bristow, A., Curle, D. and Marmot, M. (1997). Can dietary interventions change diet and cardiovascular risk factors? A meta-analysis of randomized controlled trials. *American Journal of Public Health*, **87**, 1415–22.

Ebrahim, S. and Smith, G. D. (1997). Systematic review of randomized controlled trials of multiple risk factor interventions for preventing coronary heart disease. *British Medical Journal*, **314**, 1666–74.

Flay, B. R. and Best, J. A. (1982). Overcoming design problems in evaluating health behavior change programs. *Evaluation for Health Professions*, **5**, 43–69.

Haglund, B. (1983). Community diagnosis: a theoretical model for prevention in primary health care. *Scandinavian Journal of Primary Health Care*, **1**, 12–19.

Lindholm, L. and Rosen, M. (2000). What is the 'golden standard' for assessing population-based interventions? Problems of dilution bias. *Journal of Epidemiology and Community Health*, **54**, 617–22.

McGuire, W. J. (1969). The nature of attitudes and attitude change. In *Handbook of social psychology*, Vol. III (ed. G. Lindsay and E. Aronson), pp. 136–311. Addison-Wesley, Reading, MA.

Mittelmark, M., Hunt, M., Heath, G. and Schmid, T. (1993). Realistic outcomes: lessons from community-based research and demonstration programs for prevention of cardiovascular diseases. *Journal of Public Health Policy*, **14** (4), 437–62.

Puska, P. (1985). Intervention and experimental studies. In *Oxford textbook of public health* (ed. W. Holland, R. Detels and G. Know), pp. 113–22. Oxford University Press, New York.

Puska, P. (ed.) (1988). *Comprehensive cardiovascular community control programmes in Europe.* WHO EURO Reports and Studies 106. World Health Organization, Copenhagen.

Puska, P. (1993). CINDI demonstration projects for national policy development. *Canadian Journal of Cardiology*, **9**, 43–4D.

Puska, P. (2000). Do we learn our lessons from the population-based interventions? *Journal of Epidemiology and Community Health*, **54**, 562–3.

Puska, P., Tuomilehto, J., Nissinen, A. and Vartiainen, E. (eds) (1995). *The North Karelia Project: 20 year results and experiences.* National Public Institute, Helsinki.

Puska, P., Isokaanta, M., Korpelainen, V. and Vartiainen, E. (1998a). Village competition as an innovative method for lowering population cholesterol. *European Heart Journal*, **5**, 561–72.

Puska, P., Vartiainen, E., Tuomilehto, J., Salomaa, V. and Nissinen, A. (1998b). Changes in premature deaths in Finland: successful long-term prevention of cardiovascular diseases. *Bulletin of the World Health Organization*, **76** (4), 419–25.

Rogers, E. (1983). *Diffusion of innovations.* Free Press, New York.

SBU (The Swedish Council on Technology Assessment in Health Care) (1997). Att forebygga sjukdom i hjarta och karl genom befolknings – inriktade program – en systematisk litteraturoverskit. SBU-rapport nr. 134. Stockholm.

Schooler, C., Farquhar, J. W., Fortmann, S. P. and Flora, J. A. (1997). Synthesis of findings and issues from community prevention trials. *Annals of Epidemiology*, **S7**, S54–S68.

Sellers, D. E., Crawford, S. L., Bullock, K. and McKinlay, J. B. (1997). Understanding the variability in the effectiveness of community heart health programs: a meta-analysis. *Social Science and Medicine,* **44** (9), 1325–39.

Vartiainen, E., Puska, P., Pekkanen, J., Tuomilehto, J. and Jousilahti, P. (1994). Changes in risk factors explain changes in mortality from ischaemic heart disease in Finland. *British Medical Journal,* **309**, 23–7.

WHO (World Health Organization) (2000). *WHO global strategy for NCD prevention and control.* Report by Director General. WHA/53. World Health Organization, Geneva.

WHO (World Health Organization) (2001). *Mental health: new understanding, new hope.* World Health Report 2001. World Health Organization, Geneva.

WHO (World Health Organization) (2002). *Diet, physical activity and health.* WHO/EB 109/14. World Health Organization, Geneva.

Index